YOUR GUIDE TO

Essentials of Psychiatric Mental Health Nursing

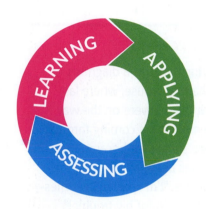

Everything you need to succeed...

in class, in clinical, on exams, and on the NCLEX®

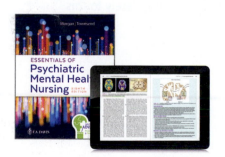

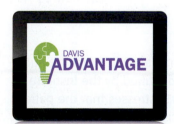

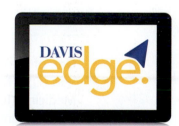

LEARNING   **APPLYING**   **ASSESSING**

Your journey to success
BEGINS HERE!

Your text works together with an interactive, personalized learning and quizzing experience that makes this often-intimidating, but must-know content easier to master.

Don't miss everything that's waiting online to make learning less stressful...and save you time. Follow the instructions on the inside front cover to use the access code to unlock your resources today.

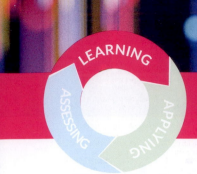
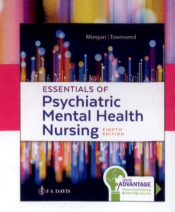

Morgan | Townsend

ESSENTIALS OF
**Psychiatric
Mental Health
Nursing** EIGHTH EDITION

F.A. DAVIS

DAVIS ADVANTAGE

STEP #1
Build a solid foundation.

Communication Exercises let you practice your communication skills with vignettes and questions that prepare you for clinical and practice.

Communication Exercises

1. Hal, a patient on the psychiatric unit, has a diagnosis of schizophrenia. He lives in a halfway house, where last evening he began yelling that "aliens were on the way to take over our bodies! The message is coming through loud and clear!" The residence supervisor became frightened and called 911. As Hal was being admitted to the psychiatric unit, he told the nurse, "I'm special! I get messages from a higher being! We are in for big trouble!" How would the nurse respond appropriately to this statement by Hal?

One of the Quality and Safety in Nursing Education (QSEN) criteria identified by the Institute of Medicine (IOM) (2003) stresses that the patient must be at the center of decisions about treatment (patient-centered care), and this type of assessment tool provides an opportunity to actively engage the patient in describing what medications have been effective or ineffective and identifying side effects that may impact willingness to adhere to a medication regimen.

Quality and Safety Education for Nurses (QSEN) activities and content, highlighted with a special icon, help you attain the knowledge, skills, and attitudes required to fulfill the initiative's quality and safety competencies.

Real People, Real Stories: Dr. Fred Frese

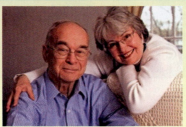

People with schizophrenia continue to be disenfranchised, misunderstood, and stigmatized. Even within healthcare, evidence has shown that some settings have been very hostile to people with severe mental illnesses. One way to begin combating stigmatization of people with mental illness is to get to know them personally. Dr. Fred Frese is a licensed psychologist and an internationally renowned speaker, writer, and advocate in the field of mental illness.

Karyn: Could you share a little bit about your history with the illness of schizophrenia?

Dr. Frese: I was 25 when I had my first episode. I was in the Marines and—I know I had seen the movie *The Manchurian Candidate* previously—and I began to think

me. During the last attempt to hospitalize me, I actually escaped and ran away, even though I was in pretty bad shape.

Karyn: So since you were knowledgeable about the laws, you could essentially be your own self-advocate and argue your case, so to speak?

Dr. Frese: Yes, and by that time, I was in grad school and had secured a job at what is now the Department of Mental Health and Addiction Services. I remember I was living in the hallway of some university housing, and one of the students, who saw me day after day just hanging around and not really doing anything, suggested that I might be eligible for a government job because of my military background. When I applied, the receptionist saw my history of mental health commitments and said I would never get the job, but I did. The last time I went to the hospital, I went voluntarily because I knew I needed more medication, but they thought I needed to be hospitalized and I didn't; so I ran away.

Karyn: Sounds like you were managing a lot of stuff—grad school, working—and, at the same time, episodically struggling with symptoms of illness. You were working in the field of mental health, too. Was the work environment supportive?

Dr. Frese: Not always. It seemed like even among my coworkers, when something strange happened, they thought it was something wrong with me.

Karyn: What do you mean by "something strange"?

Dr. Frese: Like one time when they perceived I was spending too much time interacting with patients, they assumed I was "going off again," and next thing I knew, they called a "blue alert" and wanted to hospitalize me. But that time, the medical director just told me to take some time off. I never did find out why they called that blue alert.

Karyn: So you haven't been hospitalized for a very long time, and you are internationally renowned for all of your work and advocacy in the field of mental health. What do you think has contributed most to your recovery?

Dr. Frese: No, I haven't been hospitalized since I got married. I think that has been central in my recovery: having a person who you trust to give you feedback and let me know when I need more medication.

Karyn: What role do medications play in recovery?

Dr. Frese: It's very individual. We need more research to identify who, among people with schizophrenia, will benefit most by continuous medication versus episodic, reduced doses, or no medication. Genetic research is hopeful, but we're not there yet. It's hard to advise any individual what to do without knowing their individual circumstances, and even knowing, it can be very hard.

TABLE 15–2 | CARE PLAN FOR THE PATIENT WITH SCHIZOPHRENIA–cont'd

NURSING DIAGNOSIS: DISTURBED THOUGHT PROCESSES

RELATED TO: Inability to trust, panic anxiety, possible hereditary or biochemical factors

EVIDENCED BY: Delusional thinking; inability to concentrate; impaired volition; inability to problem solve, abstract, or conceptualize; extreme suspiciousness of others

OUTCOME CRITERIA	NURSING INTERVENTIONS	RATIONALE
Short-Term Goal ■ By the end of 2 weeks, patient will recognize and verbalize that false ideas occur at times of increased anxiety. **Long-Term Goals** ■ By time of discharge from treatment, patient's verbalizations will reflect reality-based thinking with no evidence of delusional ideation. ■ By time of discharge from treatment, the patient will be able to differentiate between delusional thinking and reality.	1. Convey acceptance of patient's need for the false belief but indicate that you do not share the belief. 2. 💬 Do not argue or deny the belief. Use "reasonable doubt" as a therapeutic technique: "I understand that you believe this is true, but I personally find it hard to accept." 3. Reinforce and focus on reality. Discourage long ruminations about the irrational thinking. Talk about real events and real people. 4. If patient is highly suspicious, the following interventions may be helpful: a. Use same staff as much as possible; be honest and keep all promises.	1. Patient must understand that you do not view the idea as real. 2. Arguing with the patient or denying the belief serves no useful purpose, because delusional ideas are not eliminated by this approach, and the development of a trusting relationship may be impeded. 3. Discussions that focus on the false ideas are purposeless and useless and may even aggravate the psychosis. 4. To decrease patient's suspiciousness: a. Familiar staff and honesty promotes trust.

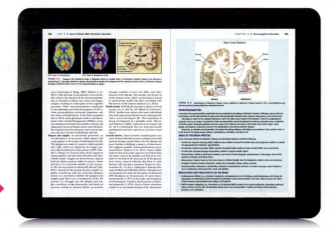

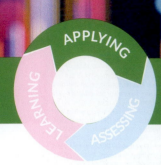

APPLYING

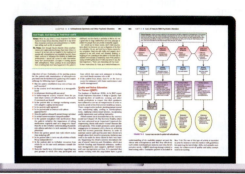

STEP #2
Apply your knowledge and make the connections.

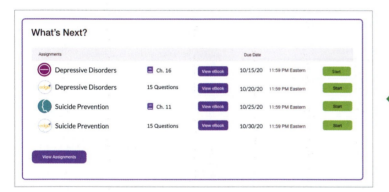

What's Next?

Assignments				Due Date		
⊖ Depressive Disorders	📖 Ch. 16	View eBook		10/15/20	11:59 PM Eastern	Start
Depressive Disorders	15 Questions	View eBook		10/20/20	11:59 PM Eastern	Start
Suicide Prevention	📖 Ch. 11	View eBook		10/25/20	11:59 PM Eastern	Start
Suicide Prevention	15 Questions	View eBook		10/30/20	11:59 PM Eastern	Start

View Assignments

Assignments in Davis Advantage correspond to key topics in your book. Begin by reading from your printed text or click the eBook button to be taken to the **FREE integrated eBook.**

Pre-Assessment for Psychotic Disorders

Question 2 of 5

Which of the following are common side effects of antipsychotic medications? Select all that apply.

○ Dry mouth and urinary retention
○ Sedation and orthostatic hypotension
○ Extrapyramidal symptoms
○ Tardive dyskinesia
○ Gynecomastia

Submit

Pre-Assessment for Psychotic Disorders

Results

 You answered 3 out of 5 correctly.

To receive full credit for this assignment, you must complete the remaining content. Click Start to begin.

View PLP   Start

Following your reading, take the **Pre-Assessment** quiz to evaluate your understanding of the content. You'll receive **immediate feedback** that identifies your strengths and weaknesses.

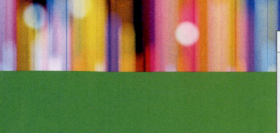

Psychosis

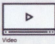
Video

Activity

Post-Assessment

Question 2 of 10

Make the connection. Drag and drop the symptom exemplified by the patient scenario.

The nurse asks his patient, Scott, "Did you shower this morning?" Scott states, "When did I shower? I love to take showers. I love to do a lot things, like cook breakfast. Speaking of breakfast, it was great! Oh yeah, I took a shower after breakfast this morning."

What positive symptom of schizophrenia is the patient experiencing?

hallucinations   delusions of persecution   delusions of reference

somatic delusions   circumstantiality   neologisms   word salad

Answer: Circumstantiality

CORRECT: There are many different types of speech disturbances that represent disorganized thinking. With circumstantiality, the patient is delayed in reaching the point of communication because of unnecessary and over-the-top details. The patient will eventually answer the question but with numerous interruptions by the nurse to keep the person on track.

Next

Animated mini-lecture videos make key concepts easier to understand, while **interactive learning activities** allow you to apply your knowledge and make the connections.

Post-Assessment for Psychotic Disorders

Question 2 of 5

Which of the following patients with schizophrenia is at highest risk for injury to self or others?

- ○ Has little to no family support
- ○ Has a family history of mood disorders
- ● Has command hallucinations
- ○ Has delusions of reference

Submit

After working through the video and activity, a **Post-Assessment** quiz tests your mastery. The results feed into your **Personalized Learning Plan**, where your instructor is able to view them.

Personalized Learning at a Glance

Advantage Assignments: Average

Average Score	Time Spent	Participation
	18 mins	15 / 63

Performance Summary

Congratulations! You have demonstrated competency in Bipolar & Related Disorders

The following topics could use further study and review. Focus study time on:

Neurocognitive Disorders

Bereaved Individual

Edge Assignments

Average Score	Time Spent	Participation
	15 mins	13 / 63

Your dashboard provides a snapshot of your **performance at a glance** as you work through your assignments.

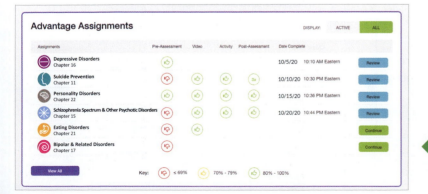

Advantage Assignments

DISPLAY: ACTIVE   ALL

Assignments	Pre-Assessment	Video	Activity	Post-Assessment	Date Complete	
Depressive Disorders Chapter 16					10/5/20 10:10 AM Eastern	Review
Suicide Prevention Chapter 11				3x	10/10/20 10:30 PM Eastern	Review
Personality Disorders Chapter 22					10/15/20 10:36 PM Eastern	Review
Schizophrenia Spectrum & Other Psychotic Disorders Chapter 15					10/20/20 10:44 PM Eastern	Review
Eating Disorders Chapter 21						Continue
Bipolar & Related Disorders Chapter 17						Continue

View All

Key: ≤ 69%   70% - 79%   80% - 100%

Your **Personalized Learning Plan** is mapped to your needs and tracks your progress by topic to identify the exact areas that require additional study.

Online content subject to change upon publication.

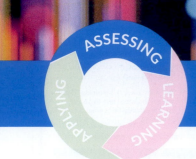
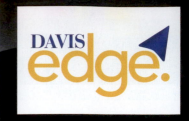

As you complete the **Davis Edge assignments** created by your instructor, your **Personalized Learning Plan** identifies your strengths and weaknesses topic by topic.

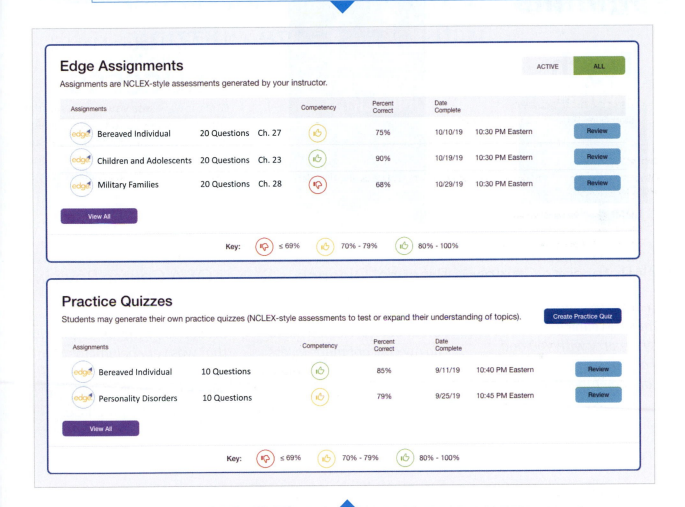

Edge Assignments

Assignments are NCLEX-style assessments generated by your instructor.

ACTIVE   ALL

Assignments			Competency	Percent Correct	Date Complete		
edge Bereaved Individual	20 Questions	Ch. 27	👍	75%	10/10/19	10:30 PM Eastern	Review
edge Children and Adolescents	20 Questions	Ch. 23	👍	90%	10/19/19	10:30 PM Eastern	Review
edge Military Families	20 Questions	Ch. 28	👎	68%	10/29/19	10:30 PM Eastern	Review

View All

Key: 👎 ≤ 69%   👍 70% - 79%   👍 80% - 100%

Practice Quizzes

Students may generate their own practice quizzes (NCLEX-style assessments to test or expand their understanding of topics).

Create Practice Quiz

Assignments		Competency	Percent Correct	Date Complete		
edge Bereaved Individual	10 Questions	👍	85%	9/11/19	10:40 PM Eastern	Review
edge Personality Disorders	10 Questions	👍	79%	9/25/19	10:45 PM Eastern	Review

View All

Key: 👎 ≤ 69%   👍 70% - 79%   👍 80% - 100%

Create your own **practice quizzes** to focus on topic areas where you are struggling, or use as a study tool to review for an upcoming exam.

GET STARTED TODAY!

Use the access code on the inside front cover to redeem access.

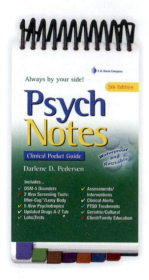
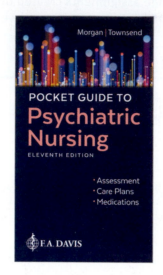
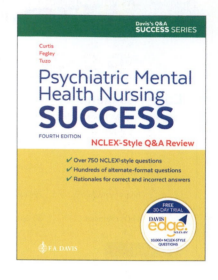

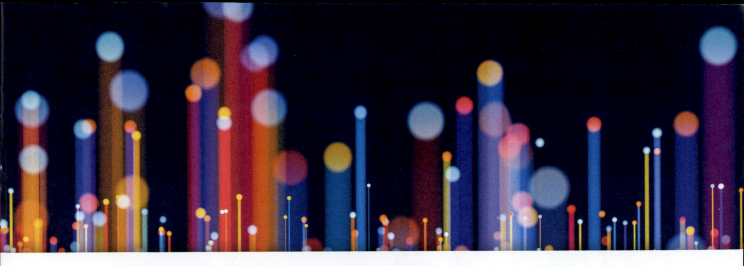

ESSENTIALS OF
Psychiatric Mental Health Nursing EIGHTH EDITION

Karyn I. Morgan, RN, MSN, APRN-CNS

Psychiatric Clinical Nurse Specialist
    Professor of Instruction, Mental Health Nursing
    The University of Akron
    Akron, Ohio

Mary C. Townsend, DSN, PMHCNS-BC-Retired

Clinical Specialist Adult Psychiatric Mental Health Nursing
    Former Assistant Professor and Coordinator, Mental Health Nursing
    Kramer School of Nursing
    Oklahoma City University
    Oklahoma City, Oklahoma

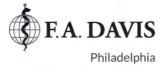

F.A. DAVIS

Philadelphia

F. A. Davis Company
1915 Arch Street
Philadelphia, PA 19103
www.fadavis.com

Printed in the United States of America

Last digit indicates print number: 10 9 8 7 6 5 4 3 2

Senior Acquisitions Editor, Nursing: Susan R. Rhyner
Senior Content Project Manager: Amy M. Romano
Design and Illustrations Manager: Carolyn O'Brien

As new scientific information becomes available through basic and clinical research, recommended treatments and drug therapies undergo changes. The author(s) and publisher have done everything possible to make this book accurate, up to date, and in accord with accepted standards at the time of publication. The author(s), editors, and publisher are not responsible for errors or omissions or for consequences from application of the book, and make no warranty, expressed or implied, in regard to the contents of the book. Any practice described in this book should be applied by the reader in accordance with professional standards of care used in regard to the unique circumstances that may apply in each situation. The reader is advised always to check product information (package inserts) for changes and new information regarding dose and contraindications before administering any drug. Caution is especially urged when using new or infrequently ordered drugs.

Library of Congress Cataloging-in-Publication Data

Names: Townsend, Mary C., 1941- author. | Morgan, Karyn I., author.
Title: Essentials of psychiatric mental health nursing : concepts of care in
  evidence-based practice / Karyn I. Morgan, Mary C. Townsend.
Description: 8th edition. | Philadelphia : F.A. Davis Company, [2020] |
  Authors' names reversed on the previous edition. | Includes
  bibliographical references and index.
Identifiers: LCCN 2018059540 (print) | LCCN 2018060748 (ebook) | ISBN
  9780803699175 | ISBN 9780803676787 (paper cover)
Subjects: | MESH: Psychiatric Nursing–methods | Mental Disorders–nursing |
  Nursing Process | Evidence-Based Nursing
Classification: LCC RC440 (ebook) | LCC RC440 (print) | NLM WY 160 | DDC
  616.89/0231–dc23
LC record available at https://lccn.loc.gov/2018059540

Contributors

Lois Angelo, MSN, APRN, BC
ED Care Manager
Newton Wellesley Hospital
Newton, Massachusetts

Cathy Melfi Curtis, MSN, RN-BC
Nursing Educator Consultant
Charleston, South Carolina

Tona Leiker, PhD, APRN, CNE
Assistant Dean, Nursing Curriculum and Assessment
American Sentinel University
Aurora, Colorado

Mary Jean Thompson, RN, BN, MHS, MPC
Instructor, MHC
University of Calgary
Medicine Hat, Alberta, Canada

Carol Norton Tuzo, MSN, RN-BC
Nursing Educator Consultant
Charleston, South Carolina

Reviewers

Lois Angelo, MSN, APRN, BC
ED Care Manager
Newton Wellesley Hospital
Newton, Massachusetts

Linda Blair, BSN, RN
Nursing Instructor
Central Carolina Community College
Sanford, North Carolina

Debra DeVoe, RN, MSN, NE-BC
Nursing Instructor
Thomas Edison State University
Trenton, New Jersey

Donna A. Enrico, MBS, BSN, RN
Clinical Instructor
College of Southern Nevada
Las Vegas, Nevada

Elizabeth Fife, MSN, RN, CNS, CPN
Associate Professor
Louisiana Tech University
Ruston, Louisiana

Wanda Golden, RN, MSN, CCRN, PhD(c)
Dean and Associate Professor of Nursing
Abraham Baldwin Agricultural College
Tifton, Georgia

Sandra Gustafson, MA, RN, CNE
Nursing Faculty
Hibbing Community College
Hibbing, MN

Patricia J. Hefner, MSN, RN-BC
Faculty; Course Coordinator of Psychiatric
    Mental Health Nursing
Heritage Valley Sewickley
Moon, Pennsylvania

Sharon A. Henle, EdD, ANP, RHIA, CNE
Assistant Professor of Nursing
Farmingdale State College
Farmingdale, New York

Jennifer E. Herrold, RN, MSN, CRNP
Instructor
Thomas Jefferson University
Danville, Pennsylvania

Beverly J. Howard, MSN, RN, FNP
Instructor
Alvin Community College
Alvin, Texas

Katherine M. Howard, MS, RN-BC
Nursing Instructor
Middlesex County College Nursing Program,
    Raritan Bay Medical Center
Edison, New Jersey

JoAnna Johns, MSN, RN, BA
Assistant Professor of Nursing
Atlantic Cape Community College
Mays Landing, NJ

Janet K. Johnson, MBA, MSN, RN
Nursing Coordinator
Fort Berthold Community College
New Town, North Dakota

Rebecca King, RN, MSN, PMHCNS-BC
Division Chair for Nursing and Allied Health
University of Arkansas, Community College
    of Batesville
Batesville, Arkansas

Brenda Kucirka, PhD, RN, PMHCNS-BC, CNE
Clinical Instructor
Widener University
Chester, Pennsylvania

Jan E. Lawrenz Blasi, MSN, RN
Nursing Instructor
Chandler School of Nursing and Allied Health,
    Pratt Community College
Pratt, Kansas

Anne Marie Leveille, RN, MSN, MPH
Assistant Professor
Medgar Evers College
Brooklyn, New York

Mark Longshore, JD, MSN, RN
Nursing Department Chair
Front Range Community College
Fort Collins, Colorado

Dimitra Loukissa, PhD, RN
Professor
North Park University
Chicago, Illinois

Tamar Lucas, Ed.D, MSN, RN-BC
Nursing Instructor
Itawamba Community College
Tupelo, Mississippi

Jana S. Martin, MS, RN, CNE
Division Chair, Allied Health Services
OSU Institute of Technology
Okmulgee, Oklahoma

Renee Menkens, RN, MS

Assistant Professor
Southwestern Oregon Community College
Coos Bay, Oregon

Bonnie Parker, DNP, RN, CRRN

Assistant Professor of Nursing, Malek School
of Health Professions
Marymount University
Arlington, Virginia

Norma Perez, MSN/Ed, RN

Assistant Professor
Ivy Tech Community College Northwest
Valparaiso, Indiana

Larry Purnell, PhD, RN, FAAN

Professor Emeritus, University of Delaware
Adjunct Professor, Florida International University
Adjunct Professor, Excelsior College

Susan M. Reading-Martin, MS, RN, CS, FNP,
ARNP-BC

Nursing Faculty
Western Nebraska Community College
Scottsbluff, Nebraska

Donna F. Rye, MSN, RN

Assistant Professor
Cox College
Springfield, Missouri

Karen B. Silva, RN, MSN, MFN, BC

Nursing Faculty
Keiser University
Sarasota, Florida

Alexandra Winter, RN, MSN

Assistant Director of Nursing
Metropolitan Community College
Omaha, Nebraska

Acknowledgments

Sincere thanks go to:

Susan Rhyner, for your skills, your integrity, and your gift of encouragement.

Amy Romano and, Kathleen Scogna, and Lori Bradshaw for all your support, accessibility, and assistance in preparing the manuscript.

The nursing educators, students, and clinicians, who provide critical information about the usability of the textbook and offer suggestions for improvements. Many changes have been made based on your input.

The individuals who critiqued the manuscript for this edition and shared your ideas, opinions, and suggestions for enhancement. I sincerely appreciate your contributions to the final product.

Special thanks also to Erin Barnard, Alan Brunner, Vic Farracone, Fred Frese, Bridget Hutchens, Myrle Weems, and the others who courageously allowed their stories to be told and to Jennifer Feldman for research assistance.

I appreciate each of you more than I can say.

Karyn I. Morgan

To the Instructor

The impact of the COVID-19 global pandemic put a spotlight on psychiatric and mental health concerns in ways we could not even imagine a mere six months ago. The need for confident nurses—well-versed in assessment and intervention across a broad spectrum of mental health disorders—has perhaps never been higher. To that end, in this edition of *Essentials of Psychiatric Mental Health Nursing*, we felt it was imperative to present a new chapter, **Caring for Patients with Mental Illness and Substance Use Disorders in General Practice Settings,** to highlight why every nurse—regardless of the care setting—needs the knowledge and skills necessary to support and treat clients with mental health disorders, wherever they are encountered.

Additionally, the onset of COVID-19 challenged faculty and students across the globe to migrate almost overnight from in-person, "brick-and-mortar" classroom settings to online and distance education. Recognizing those challenges, with this edition of the textbook we are pleased to provide a complete teaching and learning package, including an exciting new online resource, *Davis Advantage for Essentials of Psychiatric Mental Health Nursing*. Davis Advantage provides a wide array of online activities, animations, and assessments, designed specifically for distance learning, with a dashboard of metrics delivered seamlessly to faculty and students alike.

Prior to Covid-19, as faculty we were already aware of dangerous trends related to suicide and addiction, especially opioids. Current federally endorsed initiatives, such as the Zero Suicide Initiative (2012) and HEAL (Helping to End Addiction Long-term) (2018), underscore the magnitude of these two mental health issues and make clear that nurses practicing in any arena need a strong foundation in psychiatric mental health nursing care. Perhaps as never before, many nurse leaders see this period of mental healthcare reform as an opportunity for nurses to expand their roles and assume key positions in education, prevention, assessment, and referral. Nurses are, and will continue to be, in key positions to assist individuals to attain, maintain, or regain optimal emotional wellness.

As it has been with each new edition of *Essentials of Psychiatric Mental Health Nursing: Concepts of Care in Evidence-Based Nursing*, the goal of this eighth edition is to bring to practicing nurses and nursing students the most up-to-date information related to neurobiology, psychopharmacology, and evidence-based nursing interventions. This edition includes changes associated with the latest (fifth) edition of the American Psychiatric Association's *Diagnostic and Statistical Manual of Mental Disorders (DSM-5)*.

How students learn is constantly evolving, as they consume and process information in new ways. As instructors, we can be no less prepared, and must be ready to provide instruction online, in ways that are engaging and dynamic. Relying on the textbook alone to support an active classroom leaves a gap. *Davis Advantage for Essentials of Psychiatric Mental Health Nursing* fills that gap with the following resources:

■ **A Strong Core Textbook** that provides the foundation of knowledge that today's nursing students need to pass the NCLEX and enter practice prepared for success.

- **Online Student Tools** to learn and practice the content in an engaging, interactive format. **Pre-Assessment Quizzes** test students on their comprehension of a key topic and then give them a **Personalized Learning Plan** to work through that is based on their strengths and weaknesses. Students are engaged in an interactive experience that uses multimedia content to help spark connections and bring concepts to life. Once they complete the interactive experience, **Post-Assessment Quizzes** assess their comprehension of the material.

- **Online Instructor Resources** create a dynamic classroom experience that is tailored to students' needs. Results from the pre-and-post-assessments are available to faculty, in aggregate or by student, and inform a **Personalized Teaching Plan** that faculty can use to deliver a targeted classroom experience. Faculty will know students' strengths and weaknesses *before* they come to class and can spend class time focusing on where students are struggling. Turn-key, easy to implement in-class activities are provided to help create an active, hands-on learning environment that helps students connect more deeply with the content. NCLEX-style questions from the **Instructor Test Bank** and **PowerPoint** slides that correspond to the textbook chapters are referenced in the Personalized Teaching Plans.

- **Davis Edge** online quizzing assesses understanding, using an adaptive format with NCLEX-style questions. Faculty can set up a review and remediation system to take a constant pulse of classroom performance, with student results available in real-time to easily identify areas of weakness. Comprehensive rationales for all answer options are provided for students and explain why an answer is correct or incorrect.

Updated or New Content in the 8th Edition text

All content has been updated to reflect the current state of the discipline of nursing.

- All nursing diagnoses are current with the NANDA-I *Nursing Diagnoses: Definitions and Classification 2018–2020.*
- A new chapter, Chapter 12, Caring for Patients with Mental Illness and Substance Use Disorders in General Practice Settings, reinforces the need for generalist nurses to be skilled in adequate screening and referral of patients with mental health issues.

- "Real People, Real Stories" appear in Chapter 11, Suicide Prevention; Chapter 14, Substance Use and Addiction Disorders; Chapter 15, Schizophrenia Spectrum and Other Psychotic Disorders; Chapter 16, Depressive Disorders; Chapter 17, Bipolar and Related Disorders; Chapter 21, Eating Disorders; Chapter 23, Children and Adolescents; Chapter 25, Survivors of Abuse or Neglect; Chapter 28, Military Families; and Chapter 32 (online), Issues Related to Human Sexuality and Gender Dysphoria. This recent addition includes an interview format with real individuals conducted by our author, Karyn Morgan. They provide examples of a therapeutic communication process, promote an understanding of the experience of having a mental illness from the individual's perspective, and real patient perspectives on what is needed from the nurses they encounter. They may be used by the instructor as exercises geared toward destigmatizing those with mental illnesses.

- Chapters 31, Cultural and Spiritual Concepts Relevant to Psychiatric Mental Health Nursing, and Chapter 32, Issues Related to Human Sexuality and Gender Dysphoria, have been moved from the text to online chapters.

- Content has been added to several chapters to integrate concepts on trauma-informed care.

- The term *patient* is used to refer to the recipient of nursing care and the term *client* is used to describe individuals in a broader concept of the individual who accesses a variety of mental health-related services. The purpose is to add consistency, particularly with concepts such as "patient-centered care," one of the six Quality and Safety Education for Nurses (QSEN) criteria.

- QSEN icons in many chapters highlight when specific content represents an application of one of the six QSEN criteria.

Features That Have Been Retained in the Eighth Edition

The concept of holistic nursing is retained in the eighth edition of *Essentials of Psychiatric Mental Health Nursing*. An attempt has been made to ensure that the physical aspects of psychiatric mental health nursing are not overlooked. In all relevant situations, the mind/body connection is addressed.

Nursing process is retained in the eighth edition as the tool for delivery of care to the individual with a psychiatric disorder or to assist in the primary prevention or exacerbation of mental illness symptoms. The six steps of the nursing process, as described in the American Nurses Association *Standards of Clinical Nursing Practice,* are used to provide guidelines for the nurse. These standards of care are included for the *DSM-5* diagnoses featured in specific chapters as well as for the aging individual, the bereaved individual, victims of abuse and neglect, and as examples in several of the therapeutic approaches. The six steps are:

- **Assessment:** Background assessment data, including a description of symptomatology, provides an extensive knowledge base from which the nurse may draw when performing an assessment. Several assessment tools are also included.
- **Diagnosis:** Analysis of the data is included from which nursing diagnoses common to specific psychiatric disorders are derived.
- **Outcome identification:** Outcomes are derived from the nursing diagnoses and stated as measurable goals.
- **Planning:** A plan of care is presented with selected nursing diagnoses for the selected *DSM-5* diagnoses as well as for the elderly client, the bereaved individual, survivors of abuse and neglect, the elderly homebound client, and the primary caregiver of the client with a chronic mental illness. The planning standard also includes tables that list topics for educating clients and families about mental illness. Concept map care plans are included for all major psychiatric diagnoses.
- **Implementation:** The interventions that have been identified in the plan of care are included along with rationale for each. Case studies at the end of each *DSM-5* chapter assist the student in the practical application of theoretical material. Also included as a part of this particular standard is Unit 2 of the textbook, Psychiatric Mental Health Nursing Interventions. This section of the textbook addresses psychiatric nursing intervention in depth and frequently speaks to the differentiation in scope of practice between the basic psychiatric nurse and advanced-practice psychiatric nurse.
- **Evaluation:** The evaluation standard includes a set of questions that the nurse may use to assess whether the nursing actions have been successful in achieving the objectives of care.

Other Features

- QSEN teaching strategies in many chapters provide activities that can be used by students and guided by instructors to focus on one of the six criteria: patient-centered care, safety, teamwork and collaboration, informatics, quality improvement, and evidence-based practice.
- All psychiatric diagnostic content is reflective of the American Psychiatric Association's *Diagnostic and Statistical Manual of Mental Disorders, 5th edition* (2013).
- Communication Exercises boxes are presented in Chapter 10, The Recovery Model; Chapter 13, Neurocognitive Disorders; Chapter 14, Substance Use and Addiction Disorders; Chapter 15, Schizophrenia Spectrum and Other Psychotic Disorders; Chapter 16, Depressive Disorders; Chapter 17, Bipolar and Related Disorders; Chapter 21, Eating Disorders; Chapter 22, Personality Disorders; Chapter 25, Survivors of Abuse or Neglect; Chapter 27, The Bereaved Individual; and Chapter 32, Issues Related to Human Sexuality and Gender Dysphoria, These exercises portray clinical scenarios that allow the student to practice communication skills with clients. Answers appear in Appendix D at the back of the book.
- A list of movies at the end of most diagnostic chapters may be used to visually reinforce material discussed in the textbook. These movies may be used as learning tools to allow students to see on-screen the behaviors that they may only read about.
- Tables that list topics for patient and family education are included in the clinical chapters.
- Boxes that highlight current research studies with implications for evidence-based nursing practice are included in the clinical chapters.
- Additional Web site resources, formerly at the end of selected chapters, are now available on DavisPlus as Internet Resources.
- Assigning nursing diagnoses to patient behaviors is addressed in the disorder-specific chapters found in Unit 3, Care of Patients With Psychiatric Disorders.
- Taxonomy and diagnostic criteria from the *DSM-5* (2013) are used throughout the text.
- References throughout the text have been updated, and classical references are distinguished from general references.
- Boxes with definitions of core concepts are presented throughout the text.
- Appendix B provides a comprehensive glossary.
- Answers to end-of-chapter review questions are presented in Appendix C.
- Answers to communication exercises are presented in Appendix D.

- Web site. DavisPlus contains additional nursing care plans that do not appear in the text, links to psychotropic medications, and concept map care plans.
- Premium Content on DavisPlus includes learning activities, concept map care plans, client teaching guides, and interactive clinical scenarios (six new for this edition).

Davis Edge Online Progressive Quizzing

Davis Edge is an online platform which affords faculty and students access to over 1,000 NCLEX-style questions, with complete and detailed rationales for all correct answers and incorrect distractors. Davis Edge provides faculty with a powerful assessment tool that seamlessly integrates with learning management systems and gradebooks. As students take quizzes in Davis Edge, the system provides data back to faculty as well, tracking student progress and reporting on areas of student strength and weakness (as individuals and at the cohort level) to assist with remediation. These tools empower instructors to continuously take the vital signs of their students' performance – Davis Edge's real-time analysis helps indicate when students are struggling with course content, so faculty can more quickly and easily identify, monitor, and support at-risk individuals as well as track overall class trends. All questions in Davis Edge are completely different from those in the faculty test bank, so that quizzing and exams are separate experiences.

For students, the Davis Edge platform offers nearly endless opportunities to ensure that they comprehend and retain the information presented in the textbook. The program also provides integrated access to the e-book version of the text, so students can quickly look up and refresh their knowledge base as a part of their quizzing experience.

Additional Educational Resources

Faculty may also find the following teaching aids that accompany this textbook helpful. Instructor materials on DavisPlus include the following:

- Faculty test bank, with hundreds of multiple choice questions (including new format questions reflecting the latest NCLEX blueprint)
- Lecture outlines for all chapters
- Learning activities for all chapters (including answer key)
- Answers to the Test Your Critical Thinking Skills exercises from the textbook
- PowerPoint Presentation to accompany all chapters in the textbook
- Answers to the Homework Assignment questions from the textbook

It is hoped that the revisions and additions to this eighth edition of *Essentials of Psychiatric Mental Health Nursing* continue to satisfy a need in psychiatric mental health nursing practice. The mission of this textbook has been, and continues to be, to provide both students and clinicians with up-to-date information about psychiatric mental health nursing. The user-friendly format and easy-to-understand language, for which we have received many positive comments, have been retained in this edition. We hope that this eighth edition continues to promote and advance the commitment to psychiatric mental health nursing.

Mary C. Townsend and Karyn Morgan

Contents in Brief

Contents

UNIT 4
Psychiatric Mental Health Nursing of Special Populations   597

Ebook Bonus Chapters

Contents

Introduction to Psychiatric Mental Health Concepts

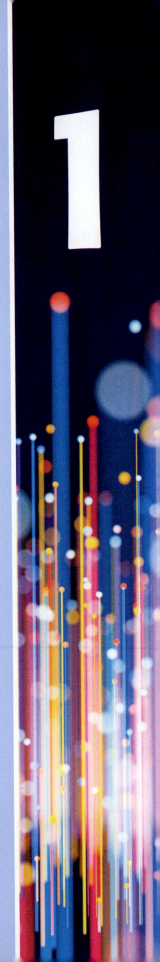

1

Mental Health and Mental Illness

CHAPTER OUTLINE

KEY TERMS

OBJECTIVES

After reading this chapter, the student will be able to:

1. Define *mental health* and *mental illness*.
2. Discuss cultural elements that influence attitudes toward mental health and mental illness.
3. Identify physiological responses to stress.
4. Discuss the concepts of anxiety and grief as psychological responses to stress.

HOMEWORK ASSIGNMENT

Please read the chapter and answer the following questions:

1. Explain the concepts of incomprehensibility and cultural relativity.
2. Describe some symptoms of panic anxiety.
3. Jane was involved in an automobile accident in which both her parents were killed. When you ask her about it, she says she has no memory of the accident. What ego defense mechanism is she using?
4. An individual with delayed or inhibited grief is fixed in what stage of the grieving process?

Introduction

The concepts of mental health and mental illness are rooted in the culture of one's society. Some cultures are quite liberal in the range of behaviors that are considered acceptable, whereas others have very little tolerance for behaviors that deviate from the cultural norms (Abdullah & Brown, 2011). A study of the history of psychiatric care reveals some shocking truths about past treatment of mentally ill individuals.

Many were kept in control by means that were cruel and inhumane because of erroneous views of mental illness that we now know to be incorrect.

Older beliefs regarding mental disturbances took several views. Some thought that an individual with mental illness had been dispossessed of his or her soul and that the only way wellness could be achieved was if the soul returned. Others believed that evil spirits or supernatural or magical powers had entered the body. The "cure" for these individuals involved a ritualistic exorcism that often consisted of brutal beatings, starvation, or other harsh means to purge the body of these unwanted forces. Still others considered that the mentally ill individual may have broken a taboo or sinned against another individual or God, for which ritualistic purification was required or various types of retribution were demanded. The correlation of mental illness to demonology or witchcraft led to some mentally ill individuals being executed.

This chapter defines *mental health* and *mental illness* and describes physical and psychological responses to stress. Symptoms associated with anxiety and grief are presented as major psychological responses in the adaptation to stress.

Mental Health

A number of theorists have attempted to define the concept of mental health. Many of these concepts focus on how well the individual is able to function. Maslow (1970) emphasized that mental health is associated with an individual's motivation toward self-actualization. He identified a "hierarchy of needs," the lower needs requiring fulfillment before those at higher levels can be achieved, with self-actualization being fulfillment of one's highest potential. An individual's position within the hierarchy may fluctuate on the basis of life circumstances. For example, an individual facing major surgery who has been working on tasks to achieve self-actualization may become preoccupied, if only temporarily, with the need for physiological safety. A representation of this needs hierarchy is presented in Figure 1–1.

Maslow described self-actualization as the state of being "psychologically healthy, fully human, highly evolved, and fully mature." He believed that healthy, or self-actualized, individuals possessed the following characteristics:

- An appropriate perception of reality
- The ability to accept oneself, others, and human nature

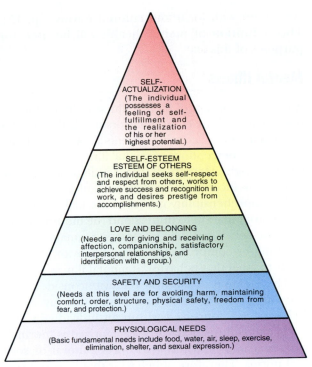

FIGURE 1–1 Maslow's hierarchy of needs.

- The ability to manifest spontaneity
- The capacity for focusing concentration on problem-solving
- A need for detachment and desire for privacy
- Independence, autonomy, and a resistance to enculturation
- An intensity of emotional reaction
- A frequency of "peak" experiences that validate the worthwhileness, richness, and beauty of life
- An identification with humankind
- The ability to achieve satisfactory interpersonal relationships
- A democratic character structure and strong sense of ethics
- Creativity
- A degree of nonconformance

Black and Andreasen (2014) describe mental health as a state of being that is relative rather than absolute but marked by the successful performance of mental functions such as adapting to change, coping with stressors, fulfilling relationships with others, and accomplishing productive activities.

Townsend & Morgan (2018) define *mental health* as "the successful adaptation to stressors from the internal or external environment, evidenced by thoughts, feelings, and behaviors that are age appropriate and congruent with local and cultural norms" (p. 15). This definition of mental health will be used for purposes of this text.

Mental Illness

A universal concept of mental illness is difficult to define because of the cultural factors that influence this concept. However, certain elements are associated with individuals' perceptions of mental illness regardless of cultural origin. Horwitz (2010) identifies two of these elements as incomprehensibility and cultural relativity.

Incomprehensibility relates to the inability of the general population to understand the motivation behind the behavior. When observers are unable to find meaning or comprehensibility in behavior, they are likely to label that behavior as mental illness.

The element of cultural relativity considers that the rules, conventions, and understanding about behavior are conceived within an individual's own particular culture. Behavior is categorized as "normal" or "abnormal" according to one's cultural or societal norms. Therefore, a behavior that is recognized as evidence of mental illness in one society may be viewed as normal in another society and vice versa.

> The American Psychiatric Association (APA, 2013) defines a mental disorder as a syndrome characterized by clinically significant disturbance in an individual's cognitions, emotional regulation, or behavior that reflects a dysfunction in the psychological, biological, or developmental processes underlying mental functioning. Mental disorders are usually associated with significant distress or disability in social, occupational, or other important activities. An expected or culturally approved response to a common stressor or loss such as the death of a loved one is not a mental disorder (p. 20).

Townsend & Morgan (2018) define *mental illness* as "maladaptive responses to stressors from the internal or external environment, evidenced by thoughts, feelings, and behaviors that are incongruent with the local and cultural norms, and interfere with the individual's social, occupational, and/or physical functioning" (p. 16). This definition of mental illness will be used for purposes of this text.

Physical and Psychological Responses to Stress

Physical Responses

In 1956, Hans Selye published the results of his research concerning the physiological response of a biological system to a change imposed on it. After the initial publication of his findings, he revised his definition of stress to "the state manifested by a specific syndrome which consists of all the nonspecifically-induced changes within a biologic system" (Selye, 1976, p. 64). This syndrome of symptoms has come to be known as the **fight-or-flight syndrome.** Selye called this general reaction of the body to stress the general adaptation syndrome. He described the reaction in three distinct stages:

1. **Alarm reaction stage.** During this stage, the responses of the fight-or-flight syndrome are initiated.
2. **Stage of resistance.** The individual uses the physiological responses of the first stage as a defense in an attempt to adapt to the stressor. If adaptation occurs, the third stage is prevented or delayed. Physiological symptoms may disappear.
3. **Stage of exhaustion.** This stage occurs when there is a prolonged exposure to the stressor to which the body has become adjusted. The adaptive energy is depleted, and the individual can no longer draw from the resources for adaptation described in the first two stages. Diseases of adaptation (e.g., headaches, mental disorders, coronary artery disease, ulcers, colitis) may occur. Without intervention for reversal, exhaustion and even death ensues (Selye, 1956, 1974).

Biological responses associated with the fight-or-flight syndrome include the following:

- **The immediate response:** The hypothalamus stimulates the sympathetic nervous system, which results in the following physical effects:
  - The adrenal medulla releases norepinephrine and epinephrine into the bloodstream.
  - The pupils of the eye dilate.
  - Secretion from the lacrimal (tear) glands is increased.
  - In the lungs, the bronchioles dilate, and the respiration rate is increased.
  - The force of cardiac contraction increases, as does cardiac output, heart rate, and blood pressure.
  - Gastrointestinal motility and secretions decrease, and sphincters contract.
  - In the liver, there is increased glycogenolysis and gluconeogenesis and decreased glycogen synthesis.
  - The bladder muscle contracts, and the sphincter relaxes; there is increased ureter motility.

- Secretion from the sweat glands is increased.
- Lipolysis occurs in the fat cells.
- **The sustained response:** When the stress response is not relieved immediately and the individual remains under stress for a long period, the hypothalamus stimulates the pituitary gland to release hormones that produce the following effects:
  - Adrenocorticotropic hormone stimulates the adrenal cortex to release glucocorticoids and mineralocorticoids, resulting in increased gluconeogenesis and retention of sodium and water and decreased immune and inflammatory responses.
  - Vasopressin (antidiuretic hormone) increases fluid retention and also increases blood pressure through constriction of blood vessels.
  - Growth hormone has a direct effect on protein, carbohydrate, and lipid metabolism, resulting in increased serum glucose and free fatty acids.
  - Thyrotropic hormone stimulates the thyroid gland to increase the basal metabolic rate.
  - Gonadotropins cause a decrease in secretion of sex hormones, resulting in decreased libido and impotence.

This fight-or-flight response undoubtedly served our ancestors well. When *Homo sapiens* had to face the giant grizzly bear or the saber-toothed tiger as part of their struggle for survival, these adaptive resources were advantageous. The response was elicited in emergencies, used in the preservation of life, and followed by restoration of the compensatory mechanisms to the pre-emergent condition (homeostasis).

Selye performed his extensive research in a controlled setting with laboratory animals as subjects. He elicited physiological responses with physical stimuli, such as exposure to heat or extreme cold, electric shock, injection of toxic agents, restraint, and surgical injury. Since the publication of Selye's original research, it has become apparent that the fight-or-flight syndrome occurs in response to psychological or emotional stimuli just as it does to physical stimuli. The psychological or emotional stressors are often not resolved as rapidly as some physical stressors; therefore, the body may be depleted of its adaptive energy more readily than it is from physical stressors. The fight-or-flight response may be inappropriate or even dangerous to the lifestyle of today, wherein stress has been described as a psychosocial state that is pervasive, chronic, and relentless. It is this chronic response that maintains the body in the aroused condition for extended periods that promotes susceptibility to diseases of adaptation.

Psychological Responses

Anxiety and grief have been described as two major, primary psychological response patterns to stress. A variety of thoughts, feelings, and behaviors are associated with each of these response patterns. Adaptation is determined by the degree to which the thoughts, feelings, and behaviors interfere with an individual's functioning.

CORE CONCEPT
Anxiety
A feeling of discomfort and apprehension related to fear of impending danger. The individual may be unaware of the source of his or her anxiety, but it is often accompanied by feelings of uncertainty and helplessness.

Anxiety

Feelings of anxiety are so common in our society that they are almost considered universal. Anxiety arises from the chaos and confusion that exists in the world today. Fears of the unknown and conditions of ambiguity offer a perfect breeding ground for anxiety to take root and grow. Low levels of anxiety are adaptive and can provide the motivation required for survival. Anxiety becomes problematic when the individual is unable to prevent the anxiety from escalating to a level that interferes with the ability to meet basic needs.

Peplau (1963) described four levels of anxiety: mild, moderate, severe, and panic. Nurses must be able to recognize the symptoms associated with each level to plan for appropriate intervention with anxious individuals:

- **Mild anxiety:** This level of anxiety is seldom a problem for the individual. It is associated with the tension experienced in response to the events of day-to-day living. Mild anxiety prepares people for action. It sharpens the senses, increases motivation for productivity, increases the perceptual field, and results in a heightened awareness of the environment. Learning is enhanced, and the individual is able to function at his or her optimal level.
- **Moderate anxiety:** As the level of anxiety increases, the extent of the perceptual field diminishes.

The moderately anxious individual is less alert to events occurring within the environment. The individual's attention span and ability to concentrate decrease, although he or she may still attend to needs with direction. Assistance with problem-solving may be required. Increased muscular tension and restlessness are evident.

■ **Severe anxiety:** The perceptual field of the severely anxious individual is so greatly diminished that concentration centers on one particular detail only or on many extraneous details. Attention span is extremely limited, and the individual has much difficulty completing even the simplest task. Physical symptoms (e.g., headaches, palpitations, insomnia) and emotional symptoms (e.g., confusion, dread, horror) may be evident. Discomfort is experienced to the degree that virtually all overt behavior is aimed at relieving the anxiety.

■ **Panic anxiety:** In this most intense state of anxiety, the individual is unable to focus on even one detail within the environment. Misperceptions are common, and a loss of contact with reality may occur. The individual may experience hallucinations or delusions. Behavior may be characterized by wild and desperate actions or extreme withdrawal. Human functioning and communication with others are ineffective. Panic anxiety is associated with a feeling of terror, and individuals may be convinced that they have a life-threatening illness or fear that they are "going crazy," are losing control, or are emotionally weak. Prolonged panic anxiety can lead to physical and emotional exhaustion and can be life threatening.

A variety of behavioral adaptation responses occur at each level of anxiety. Figure 1–2 depicts these behavioral responses on a continuum of anxiety ranging from mild to panic.

Mild Anxiety

At the mild level, individuals may use a number of behaviors that satisfy their needs for comfort. Menninger (1963) described the following types of coping mechanisms that individuals use to relieve anxiety in stressful situations:

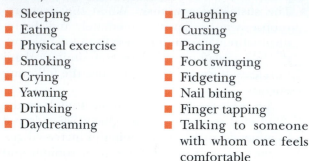

- Sleeping
- Eating
- Physical exercise
- Smoking
- Crying
- Yawning
- Drinking
- Daydreaming
- Laughing
- Cursing
- Pacing
- Foot swinging
- Fidgeting
- Nail biting
- Finger tapping
- Talking to someone with whom one feels comfortable

Undoubtedly, there are many more coping mechanisms, too numerous to mention here, considering that each individual develops his or her own unique ways to relieve anxiety at the mild level. Some of these behaviors are more adaptive than others. The term **coping skills** is used to describe those coping behaviors that enhance one's adaptation. These include enhancing knowledge, social affiliation with others, and problem-solving.

Mild to Moderate Anxiety

Sigmund Freud (1961) identified the ego as the reality component of the personality that governs problem-solving and rational thinking. As the level of anxiety increases, the strength of the ego is tested, and energy is mobilized to confront the threat. Anna Freud (1953) identified a number of defense mechanisms employed by the ego in the face of threat to biological or psychological integrity (Table 1–1). Some of these **ego defense mechanisms** are more adaptive than others, but all are used either consciously or unconsciously as protective devices for the ego in an effort to relieve mild to moderate anxiety. They become maladaptive when an individual uses them to such a degree that the defense mechanism interferes with the ability to deal with reality, with interpersonal relations, or with occupational performance.

Moderate to Severe Anxiety

Anxiety at the moderate to severe level that remains unresolved over an extended period can contribute to a number of physiological disorders. The *Diagnostic and Statistical Manual of Mental Disorders, Fifth Edition* (DSM-5) (APA, 2013) describes these disorders under the category "Psychological Factors Affecting Other Medical Conditions." The psychological factors may exacerbate symptoms of, delay recovery from, or interfere with treatment of the medical condition.

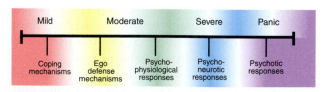

FIGURE 1–2 Adaptation responses on a continuum of anxiety.

TABLE 1–1 Ego Defense Mechanisms

DEFENSE MECHANISM	EXAMPLE	DEFENSE MECHANISM	EXAMPLE
COMPENSATION Covering up a real or perceived weakness by emphasizing a trait one considers more desirable	A physically disabled boy is unable to participate in football, so he compensates by becoming a great scholar.	**RATIONALIZATION** Attempting to make excuses or formulate logical reasons to justify unacceptable feelings or behaviors	John tells the rehab nurse, "I drink because it's the only way I can deal with my bad marriage and my worse job."
DENIAL Refusing to acknowledge the existence of a real situation or the feelings associated with it	A woman drinks alcohol every day, cannot stop, and does not acknowledge that she has a problem.	**REACTION FORMATION** Preventing unacceptable or undesirable thoughts or behaviors from being expressed by exaggerating opposite thoughts or types of behaviors	Jane hates nursing. She attended nursing school to please her parents. During career day, she speaks to prospective students about the excellence of nursing as a career.
DISPLACEMENT The transfer of feelings from one target to another that is considered less threatening or that is neutral	A client is angry at his doctor and does not express it but becomes verbally abusive with the nurse.	**REGRESSION** Responding to stress by retreating to an earlier level of development and the comfort measures associated with that level of functioning	When 2-year-old Jay is hospitalized for tonsillitis, he will drink only from a bottle, although his mother states he has been drinking from a cup for 6 months.
IDENTIFICATION An attempt to increase self-worth by acquiring certain attributes and characteristics of an individual one admires	A teenager who required lengthy rehabilitation after an accident decides to become a physical therapist as a result of his experiences.	**REPRESSION** Involuntarily blocking unpleasant feelings and experiences from one's awareness	A trauma victim is unable to remember anything about the traumatic event.
INTELLECTUALIZATION An attempt to avoid expressing actual emotions associated with a stressful situation by using the intellectual processes of logic, reasoning, and analysis	Susan's husband is being transferred with his job to a city far away from her parents. She hides anxiety by explaining to her parents the advantages associated with the move.	**SUBLIMATION** Rechanneling of drives or impulses that are personally or socially unacceptable into activities that are constructive	A mother whose son was killed by a drunk driver channels her anger and energy into being the president of the local chapter of Mothers Against Drunk Drivers.
INTROJECTION Integrating the beliefs and values of another individual into one's own ego structure	Children integrate their parents' value system into the process of conscience formation. A child says to a friend, "Don't cheat. It's wrong."	**SUPPRESSION** The voluntary blocking of unpleasant feelings and experiences from one's awareness	Scarlett says, "I don't want to think about that now. I'll think about that tomorrow."
ISOLATION Separating a thought or memory from the feeling, tone, or emotion associated with it	A young woman describes being attacked and raped without showing any emotion.	**UNDOING** Symbolically negating or canceling out an experience that one finds intolerable	Joe is nervous about his new job and yells at his wife. On his way home, he stops and buys her some flowers.
PROJECTION Attributing feelings or impulses unacceptable to one's self to another person	Sue feels a strong sexual attraction to her track coach and tells her friend, "He's coming on to me!"		

The condition may be initiated or exacerbated by an environmental situation that the individual perceives as stressful. Measurable pathophysiology can be demonstrated. It is thought that psychological and behavioral factors may affect the course of almost every major category of disease, including, but not limited to, cardiovascular, gastrointestinal, neoplastic, neurological, and pulmonary conditions.

Severe Anxiety

Extended periods of repressed severe anxiety can result in neurotic patterns of behaving. Neurosis is no longer considered a separate category of mental disorder. However, the term sometimes is still used in the literature to further describe the symptomatology of certain disorders and to differentiate them from behaviors that occur at the more serious level of psychosis. **Neuroses** are psychiatric disturbances characterized by excessive anxiety that is expressed directly or altered through defense mechanisms. It appears as a symptom, such as an obsession, a compulsion, a phobia, or a sexual dysfunction (Sadock, Sadock, & Ruiz, 2015). The following are common characteristics of people with neuroses:

■ They are aware that they are experiencing distress.
■ They are aware that their behaviors are maladaptive.
■ They are unaware of any possible psychological causes of the distress.
■ They feel helpless to change their situation.
■ They experience no loss of contact with reality.

The following disorders are examples of psychoneurotic responses to severe anxiety as they appear in the DSM-5:

■ Anxiety disorders: Disorders in which the characteristic features are symptoms of anxiety and avoidance behavior (e.g., phobias, panic disorder, generalized anxiety disorder, and separation anxiety disorder)
■ Somatic symptom and related disorders: Disorders in which the characteristic feature is a preoccupation with distressing somatic symptoms for which there is no demonstrable organic pathology; psychological factors are judged to play a significant role in the onset, severity, exacerbation, or maintenance of the symptoms (e.g., somatic symptom disorder, illness anxiety disorder, conversion disorder, and factitious disorder)
■ Dissociative disorders: Disorders in which the characteristic feature is a disruption in the usually integrated functions of consciousness, memory, identity, or perception of the environment (e.g., dissociative amnesia, dissociative identity disorder, and depersonalization-derealization disorder)

Panic Anxiety

At this extreme level of anxiety, an individual is not capable of processing what is happening in the environment and may lose contact with reality. **Psychosis** is defined as a significant thought disturbance in which reality testing is impaired, resulting in delusions, hallucinations, disorganized speech, or catatonic behavior. The following are common characteristics of people with psychoses:

■ They exhibit minimal distress (emotional tone is flat, bland, or inappropriate).
■ They are unaware that their behavior is maladaptive.
■ They are unaware of any psychological problems (**anosognosia**).
■ They are exhibiting a flight from reality into a less stressful world or into one in which they are attempting to adapt.

Examples of psychotic responses to anxiety include the schizophrenic, schizoaffective, and delusional disorders.

CORE CONCEPT
Grief
Grief is a subjective feeling of sorrow and sadness accompanied by emotional, physical, and social responses to the loss of a loved person or thing.

Grief

Most individuals experience intense emotional anguish in response to a significant personal loss. A loss is anything that is perceived as such by the individual. Losses may be real, in which case they can be substantiated by others (e.g., death of a loved one, loss of personal possessions), or they may be perceived by the individual alone and unable to be shared or identified by others (e.g., loss of the feeling of femininity following a mastectomy). Any situation that creates change for an individual can be identified as a loss. Failure (either real or perceived) can be viewed as a loss.

The loss, or anticipated loss, of anything of value to an individual can trigger the grief response. This period of grief-related emotions and behaviors is called mourning. The "normal" mourning process, which may include feelings of sadness, guilt, anger, helplessness, hopelessness, and despair, is adaptive. Indeed, an absence of mourning after a loss may be considered maladaptive.

Stages of Grief

Kübler-Ross (1969), in extensive research with terminally ill patients, identified five stages of feelings and behaviors that individuals experience in response to a real, perceived, or anticipated loss:

- **Stage 1—Denial:** This is a stage of shock and disbelief. The response may be one of "No, it can't be true!" The reality of the loss is not acknowledged. Denial is a protective mechanism that allows the individual to cope within an immediate time frame while organizing more effective defense strategies.
- **Stage 2—Anger:** "Why me?" and "It's not fair!" are comments often expressed during the anger stage. Envy and resentment toward individuals not affected by the loss are common. Anger may be directed at the self or displaced on loved ones, caregivers, and even God. There may be a preoccupation with an idealized image of the lost entity.
- **Stage 3—Bargaining:** "If God will help me through this, I promise I will go to church every Sunday and volunteer my time to help others." During this stage, which is usually not visible or evident to others, a "bargain" is made with God in an attempt to reverse or postpone the loss. Sometimes the promise is associated with feelings of guilt for not having performed satisfactorily, appropriately, or sufficiently.
- **Stage 4—Depression:** During this stage, the full impact of the loss is experienced. The sense of loss is intense, and feelings of sadness and depression prevail. This is a time of quiet desperation and disengagement from all association with the lost entity. This stage differs from pathological depression in that it represents advancement toward resolution rather than the fixation in an earlier stage of the grief process.
- **Stage 5—Acceptance:** The final stage brings a feeling of peace regarding the loss that has occurred. It is a time of quiet expectation and resignation. The focus is on the reality of the loss and its meaning for the individuals affected by it.

Not all individuals experience each of these stages in response to a loss, nor do they necessarily experience them in this order. Some individuals' grieving behaviors may fluctuate, and even overlap, among the stages.

Anticipatory Grief

When a loss is anticipated, individuals often begin the work of grieving before the actual loss occurs. This is called **anticipatory grief.** Most people reexperience the grieving behaviors once the loss occurs, but having this time to prepare for the loss can facilitate the process of mourning, actually decreasing the length and intensity of the response. Problems arise, particularly in anticipating the death of a loved one, when family members experience anticipatory grieving and the mourning process is completed prematurely. They disengage emotionally from the dying person, who then may feel rejected by loved ones at a time when this psychological support is so important.

Resolution

The grief response can last from weeks to years. It cannot be hurried, and individuals must be allowed to progress at their own pace. After the loss of a loved one, grief work usually lasts for at least a year, during which time the grieving person experiences each significant "anniversary" date for the first time without the loved one present. Norms for the duration of grief tend to be defined by one's society, but current research supports that bereavement does not end within a prescribed period and, in fact, certain aspects may continue indefinitely in individuals who are otherwise healthy and functioning well (Sadock et al., 2015).

The grief process may be complicated or prolonged by a number of factors. If the relationship with the lost entity had been marked by ambivalence or if there had been an enduring "love–hate" association, reaction to the loss may be burdened with guilt. Guilt lengthens the grief reaction by promoting feelings of anger toward the self for having committed a wrongdoing or behaved in an unacceptable manner toward that which is now lost. It may even lead to feeling that one's behavior has contributed to the loss.

Anticipatory grieving is thought to shorten the grief response in some individuals who are able to work through some of the feelings before the loss occurs. If the loss is sudden and unexpected, mourning may take longer than it would if individuals were able to grieve in anticipation of the loss.

Length of the grieving process is also affected by the number of recent losses experienced by an individual and whether he or she is able to complete one grieving process before another loss occurs. This is particularly true for elderly individuals who may be experiencing numerous losses—such as spouse, friends, other relatives, independent functioning, home, personal possessions, and pets—in a relatively short time. As grief accumulates, a type of **bereavement overload** occurs, which for some individuals presents an impossible task of grief work.

The process of mourning may be considered resolved when an individual is able to regain a sense of organization, redefine his or her life in the absence of the lost person or object, and pursue new interests and relationships. Disorganization and emotional pain have been experienced and tolerated. Preoccupation with the lost entity has been replaced with a renewed energy and new resolve about ways to keep the memory of the lost one alive. Most grief, however, does not permanently disappear but will reemerge from time to time in response to triggers such as anniversary dates (Sadock et al., 2015).

Maladaptive Grief Responses

Maladaptive responses to loss occur when an individual is unable to progress satisfactorily through the stages of grieving to achieve resolution. Usually in such situations, an individual becomes fixed in the denial or anger stage of the grief process. Several types of grief responses have been identified as pathological, including those that are prolonged, delayed or inhibited, or distorted. The prolonged response is characterized by an intense preoccupation with memories of the lost entity for many years after the loss has occurred. Behaviors associated with the stages of denial or anger are manifested, and disorganization of functioning and intense emotional pain related to the lost entity are evidenced.

In the delayed or inhibited response, the individual becomes fixed in the denial stage of the grieving process. The emotional pain associated with the loss is not experienced, but anxiety disorders (e.g., phobias, somatic symptom disorders) or sleeping and eating disorders (e.g., insomnia, anorexia) may be evident. The individual may remain in denial for many years until the grief response is triggered by a reminder of the loss or even by another, unrelated loss. The individual who experiences a distorted response is fixed in the anger stage of grieving. In the distorted response, all the normal behaviors associated with grieving, such as helplessness, hopelessness, sadness, anger, and guilt, are exaggerated out of proportion to the situation. The individual turns the anger inward on the self, is consumed with overwhelming despair, and is unable to function in normal activities of daily living. Distorted grief reactions may culminate in pathological depression.

Summary and Key Points

- For purposes of this text, mental health is defined as "the successful adaptation to stressors from the internal or external environment evidenced by thoughts, feelings, and behaviors that are age appropriate and congruent with local and cultural norms" (Townsend & Morgan, 2018).
- Mental illness is defined as "maladaptive responses to stressors from the internal or external environment, evidenced by thoughts, feelings, and behaviors that are incongruent with the local and cultural norms, and interfere with the individual's social, occupational, and/or physical functioning" (Townsend & Morgan, 2018).
- Most cultures label behavior as mental illness on the basis of incomprehensibility and cultural relativity.
- When observers are unable to find meaning or comprehensibility in behavior, they are likely to label that behavior as mental illness. The meaning of behaviors is determined within individual cultures.
- Selye, who has become known as the founding father of stress research, defined stress as "the state manifested by a specific syndrome which consists of all the nonspecifically-induced changes within a biologic system" (Selye, 1976).
- Selye determined that physical beings respond to stressful stimuli with a predictable set of physiological changes. He described the response in three distinct stages: (1) the alarm reaction stage, (2) the stage of resistance, and (3) the stage of exhaustion. Many illnesses, or diseases of adaptation, have their origin in this aroused state, which is the preparation for fight or flight.
- Anxiety and grief have been identified as the two primary responses to stress.
- Peplau (1963) defined anxiety by levels of symptom severity: mild, moderate, severe, and panic.
- Behaviors associated with levels of anxiety include coping mechanisms, ego defense mechanisms, psychophysiological responses, psychoneurotic responses, and psychotic responses.
- Grief is described as a response to loss of a valued entity.
- Stages of normal mourning, as identified by Kübler-Ross (1969), are denial, anger, bargaining, depression, and acceptance.
- Anticipatory grief is grief work that is begun, and sometimes completed, before the loss occurs.
- Resolution of grief is thought to occur when an individual is able to remember and accept both the positive and negative aspects associated with the lost entity.
- Grieving is thought to be maladaptive when the mourning process is prolonged or delayed or inhibited or becomes distorted and exaggerated out of proportion to the situation.
- Distorted grief reactions may contribute to the development of pathological depression.

Additional information is available at davisplus.fadavis.com.

Review Questions
Self-Examination/Learning Exercise

Select the answer that is most appropriate for each of the following questions:

1. Three years ago, Anna's dog Lucky, whom she had had for 16 years, was run over by a car and killed. Anna's daughter reports that since that time, Anna has lost weight, rarely leaves her home, and just sits and talks about Lucky. Anna's behavior would be considered maladaptive for which of the following reasons?
   a. It has been more than 3 years since Lucky died.
   b. Her grief is too intense over just the loss of a dog.
   c. Her grief is interfering with her functioning.
   d. Cultural norms typically don't comprehend grief over the loss of a pet.

2. Anna states that Lucky was her closest friend, and since his death, there is no one who could ever replace the relationship they had. According to Maslow's hierarchy of needs, which level of need is not being met?
   a. Physiological needs
   b. Self-esteem needs
   c. Safety and security needs
   d. Love and belonging needs

3. Anna's daughter notices that Anna appears to be listening to another voice when just the two of them are in a room together. When questioned, Anna admits that she hears someone telling her that she was a horrible caretaker for Lucky and did not deserve to ever have a pet. Which of the following best describes what Anna is experiencing?
   a. Neurosis
   b. Psychosis
   c. Depression
   d. Bereavement

4. Anna, who is 72 years old, is of an age when she may have experienced many losses coming close together. She is at risk for which of the following?
   a. Bereavement overload
   b. Normal mourning
   c. Isolation
   d. Cultural relativity

5. Anna, age 72, has been grieving the death of her dog, Lucky, for 3 years. She is not able to take care of her activities of daily living and wants only to make daily visits to Lucky's grave. What is the most likely reason her daughter has put off seeking help for Anna?
   a. Women are less likely than men to seek help for emotional problems.
   b. Relatives often try to "normalize" the behavior rather than label it mental illness.
   c. She knows that all older people are expected to be a little depressed.
   d. She is afraid that the neighbors "will think her mother is crazy."

6. Anna's dog Lucky got away from her while they were taking a walk. He ran into the street and was hit by a car. Anna cannot remember any of these circumstances of his death. This is an example of what defense mechanism?
   a. Rationalization
   b. Suppression
   c. Denial
   d. Repression

Continued

Review Questions—cont'd
Self-Examination/Learning Exercise

7. Lucky sometimes refused to obey Anna and indeed did not come back to her when she called to him on the day he was killed. But Anna continues to insist, "He was the very best dog. He always minded me. He always did everything I told him to do." Which of the following is the correct term for this defense mechanism?
   a. Sublimation
   b. Compensation
   c. Reaction formation
   d. Undoing

8. Anna has been a widow for 20 years. Her maladaptive grief response to the loss of her dog may be attributed to which of the following? (Select all that apply.)
   a. Unresolved grief over loss of her husband
   b. Loss of several relatives and friends over the last few years
   c. Repressed feelings of guilt over the way in which Lucky died
   d. Inability to prepare in advance for the loss

9. When Anna's daughter expresses concern about her mother's reports of hearing troubling voices and recommends she see a counselor, Anna declares, "I'm fine. There is nothing wrong with me!" Which of the following best describes Anna's response?
   a. Grief resolution
   b. Somatic disorder
   c. Anosognosia
   d. Intellectualization

10. Which of the following statements by Anna might suggest that she is achieving resolution of her grief over Lucky's death?
    a. "I never cry when I think about Lucky."
    b. "It's true. Lucky didn't always mind me. Sometimes he ignored my commands, but he was also a good companion."
    c. "I remember how it happened now. I should have held tighter to his leash! I didn't deserve to have a dog."
    d. "I won't ever have another dog. It's just too painful to lose them."

References

Abdullah, T., & Brown, T. L. (2011). Mental illness stigma and ethnocultural beliefs, values, and norms: An integrative review. *Clinical Psychology Review, 31*(6), 934–948.

American Psychiatric Association (APA). (2013). *Diagnostic and statistical manual of mental disorders* (5th ed.). Washington, DC: Author.

Black, D. W., & Andreasen, N. C. (2014). *Introductory textbook of psychiatry* (6th ed.). Washington, DC: American Psychiatric Association.

Horwitz, A. V. (2010). *The social control of mental illness.* Clinton Corners, NY: Percheron Press.

Sadock, B. J., Sadock, V. A., & Ruiz, P. (2015). *Synopsis of psychiatry: Behavioral sciences/clinical psychiatry* (11th ed.). Philadelphia, PA: Wolters Kluwer.

Townsend, M. C., & Morgan, K. (2018). *Psychiatric/mental health nursing: Concepts of care in evidence-based practice* (9th ed.). Philadelphia, PA: F.A. Davis.

Classical References

Freud, A. (1953). *The ego and mechanisms of defense.* New York, NY: International Universities Press.

Freud, S. (1961). *The ego and the id.* In Standard edition of the complete psychological works of Freud, Vol. XIX. London, England: Hogarth Press.

Kübler-Ross, E. (1969). *On death and dying.* New York, NY: Macmillan.

Maslow, A. (1970). *Motivation and personality* (2nd ed.). New York, NY: Harper & Row.

Menninger, K. (1963). *The vital balance.* New York, NY: Viking Press.

Peplau, H. (1963). A working definition of anxiety. In S. Burd & M. Marshall (Eds.), *Some clinical approaches to psychiatric nursing.* New York, NY: Macmillan.

Selye, H. (1956). *The stress of life.* New York, NY: McGraw-Hill.

Selye, H. (1974). *Stress without distress.* New York, NY: Signet Books.

Selye, H. (1976). *The stress of life* (Rev. ed.). New York, NY: McGraw-Hill.

Biological Implications 2

CORE CONCEPTS

Genetics
Neuroendocrinology
Psychobiology
Psychoneuroimmunology
Psychopharmacology

KEY TERMS

axon
cell body
circadian rhythms
dendrites
genotype
limbic system

neuron
neurotransmitters
phenotype
receptor sites
synapse

OBJECTIVES
After reading this chapter, the student will be able to:

1. Identify gross anatomical structures of the brain and describe their functions.
2. Discuss the physiology of neurotransmission in the central nervous system.
3. Describe the role of neurotransmitters in human behavior.
4. Discuss the association of endocrine functioning with the development of psychiatric disorders.
5. Describe the role of genetics in the development of psychiatric disorders.
6. Discuss the correlation of alteration in brain functioning to various psychiatric disorders.
7. Identify various diagnostic procedures used to detect alteration in biological functioning that may be contributing to psychiatric disorders.
8. Discuss the influence of psychological factors on the immune system.
9. Describe the biological mechanisms of psychoactive drugs at neural synapses.
10. Recognize various theorized influences in the development of psychiatric disorders, including brain physiology, genetics, endocrine function, immune system, and psychosocial and environmental factors.
11. Discuss the implications of psychobiological concepts for the practice of psychiatric mental health nursing.

Introduction

In recent years, a greater emphasis has been placed on the study of the organic basis for psychiatric illness. This "neuroscientific revolution," with its focus on the biological basis of behavior, has led to several mental illnesses now being considered neurodevelopmental disorders resulting from malfunctions and/or malformations of the brain.

That some behaviors and psychiatric illnesses can be traced to biological causes does not imply that psychosocial and sociocultural influences do not play a role in mental health disorders. For example, there is evidence that *psychological* interventions have an influence on brain activity that is similar to psychopharmacological intervention (Furmark et al., 2002), and evidence exists that lifestyle choices, such as marijuana use, can precipitate mental illness (psychosis) in individuals with genetic vulnerability (National Institutes of Health [NIH], 2015). Ongoing research will build a better understanding of the complex interplay of neural activities within the brain and in interaction with one's environment.

The systems of biology, psychology, and sociology are not mutually exclusive—they are interacting systems. This interaction is clearly indicated by the fact that individuals experience biological changes in response to various environmental events. Indeed, one or several of these systems may, at various times, explain behavioral phenomena.

This chapter focuses on the role of neurophysiological, neurochemical, genetic, and endocrine influences on psychiatric illness. An introduction to psychopharmacology is included (discussed in more detail in Chapter 4), and various diagnostic procedures used to detect alteration in biological function that may contribute to psychiatric illness are identified. The implications for psychiatric mental health nursing are discussed.

CORE CONCEPT

Psychobiology

The study of the biological foundations of cognitive, emotional, and behavioral processes.

The Nervous System: An Anatomical Review

The Brain

The brain has three major divisions subdivided into five major parts:

1. Forebrain
   a. Cerebrum
   b. Diencephalon
2. Midbrain (Mesencephalon)
3. Hindbrain
   a. Pons
   b. Medulla
   c. Cerebellum

Each of these structures is discussed individually. A summary is presented in Table 2–1.

Cerebrum

The cerebrum consists of a right and left hemisphere and constitutes the largest part of the human brain. The right and left hemispheres are separated by a deep groove but remain connected to each other by a band of 200 million axons (nerve fibers) called the *corpus callosum*. Because each hemisphere controls different functions, information is processed through the corpus callosum so that each hemisphere is aware of the activity of the other.

The surface of the cerebrum consists of gray matter and is called the *cerebral cortex*. The gray matter is composed of neuron cell bodies that appear gray to the eye. These structures are thought to be the actual "thinking" structures of the brain. The *basal ganglia*, four subcortical nuclei of gray matter (the striatum,

TABLE 2–1	**Structure and Function of the Brain**
STRUCTURE	**PRIMARY FUNCTION**
I. THE FOREBRAIN	
A. Cerebrum	Composed of two hemispheres connected by a band of nerve tissue that houses a band of 200 million axons called the *corpus callosum*. The outer layer is called the *cerebral cortex*. It is extensively folded and consists of billions of neurons. The left hemisphere appears to deal with logic and solving problems. The right hemisphere may be called the "creative" brain and is associated with affect, behavior, and spatial-perceptual functions. Each hemisphere is divided into four lobes:
1. Frontal lobes	Voluntary body movement, including movements that permit speaking, thinking and judgment formation, and expression of feelings.
2. Parietal lobes	Perception and interpretation of most sensory information (including touch, pain, taste, and body position).
3. Temporal lobes	Hearing, short-term memory, and sense of smell; expression of emotions through connection with limbic system.*
4. Occipital lobes	Visual reception and interpretation.
B. Diencephalon	Connects cerebrum with lower brain structures.
1. Thalamus	Integrates all sensory input (except smell) on way to cortex; some involvement with emotions and mood.
2. Hypothalamus	Regulates anterior and posterior lobes of pituitary gland; exerts control over actions of the autonomic nervous system; regulates appetite and temperature. Regulates visceral responses to emotional situations and body rhythms such as mood changes and sleep–wake cycles.
*Limbic system	Consists of medially placed cortical and subcortical structures and the fiber tracts connecting them with one another. Two of these structures are the thalamus and hypothalamus. It is sometimes called the "emotional brain"—associated with feelings of fear and anxiety; anger and aggression; love, joy, and hope; and with sexuality and social behavior. As research has advanced our understanding of the connectivity in brain structures, it has become harder to define the boundaries of the limbic system.
II. THE MIDBRAIN (mesencephalon)	Responsible for visual, auditory, and balance ("righting") reflexes.
III. THE HINDBRAIN	
A. Pons	Regulation of respiration and skeletal muscle tone; ascending and descending tracts connect brainstem with cerebellum and cortex.
B. Medulla	Pathway for all ascending and descending fiber tracts; contains vital centers that regulate heart rate, blood pressure, and respiration; reflex centers for swallowing, sneezing, coughing, and vomiting.
C. Cerebellum	Regulates muscle tone and coordination and maintains posture and equilibrium.

pallidum, substantia nigra, and subthalamic nuclei) are found deep within the cerebral hemispheres. They are responsible for certain subconscious aspects of voluntary movement, such as swinging the arms when walking, gesturing while speaking, and regulating muscle tone (Scanlon & Sanders, 2015).

The cerebral cortex is identified by numerous folds, called *gyri*, and deep grooves between the folds, called *sulci*. This extensive folding extends the surface area of the cerebral cortex and thus permits the presence of millions more neurons than would be possible without it (as is the case in the brains of some animals, such as dogs and cats). Each hemisphere of the cerebral cortex is divided into the frontal lobe, parietal lobe, temporal lobe, and occipital lobe. These lobes, which are named for the overlying bones in the cranium, are identified in Figure 2–1.

The Frontal Lobes

Voluntary body movement is controlled by the impulses through the frontal lobes. The right frontal lobe controls motor activity on the left side of the body, and the left frontal lobe controls motor activity on the right side of the body. The frontal lobe may also play a role in emotional experience, as evidenced by changes in mood and character after damage to this area.

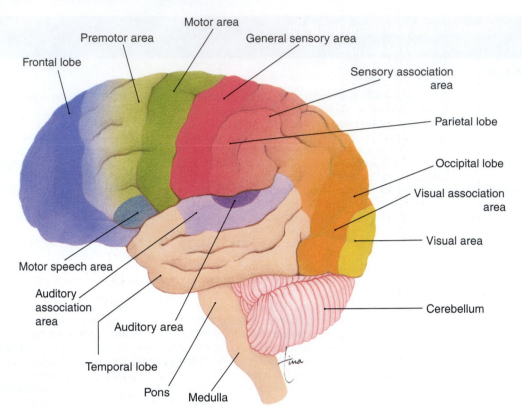

FIGURE 2–1   Left cerebral hemisphere showing some of the functional areas that have been mapped. (From *Essentials of Anatomy and Physiology* [7th ed.], by V. C. Scanlon and T. Sanders, 2015, Philadelphia, PA: F.A. Davis Company. Reprinted with permission.)

Particularly, the prefrontal cortex (the front part of the frontal lobe) plays an essential role in the regulation and adaptation of our emotions to new situations and may have implications in moral and spiritual responses (Sadock, Sadock, & Ruiz, 2015). Neuroimaging tests suggest that there may be some structural abnormalities in the frontal lobes (as well as temporal, parietal, and subcortical structures) in people with chronic schizophrenia (Lyall, Kubicki, & Shenton, 2017).

The Parietal Lobes

The parietal lobes manage somatosensory input, including touch, pain and pressure, taste, temperature, perception of joint and body position, and visceral sensations. The parietal lobes also contain association fibers linked to the primary sensory areas through which interpretation of sensory-perceptual information is made. Language interpretation is associated with the left hemisphere of the parietal lobe.

The Temporal Lobes

The upper anterior temporal lobe is concerned with auditory functions, and the lower part is dedicated to short-term memory. The sense of smell has a

connection to the temporal lobes because the impulses carried by the olfactory nerves end in this area of the brain. The temporal lobes also play a role in the expression of emotions through an interconnection with the limbic system. The left temporal lobe, along with the left parietal lobe, is involved in language interpretation.

The Occipital Lobes

The occipital lobes are the primary area of visual reception and interpretation. Visual perception, which gives individuals the ability to judge spatial relationships such as distance and to see in three dimensions, is also processed in this area. Language interpretation is influenced by the occipital lobes through an association with the visual experience.

Diencephalon

The second part of the forebrain is the diencephalon, which connects the cerebrum with lower structures of the brain. The major components of the diencephalon include the thalamus and the hypothalamus, which are part of a neuroanatomical loop of structures known as the **limbic system.** These structures are identified in Figures 2–1 and 2–2.

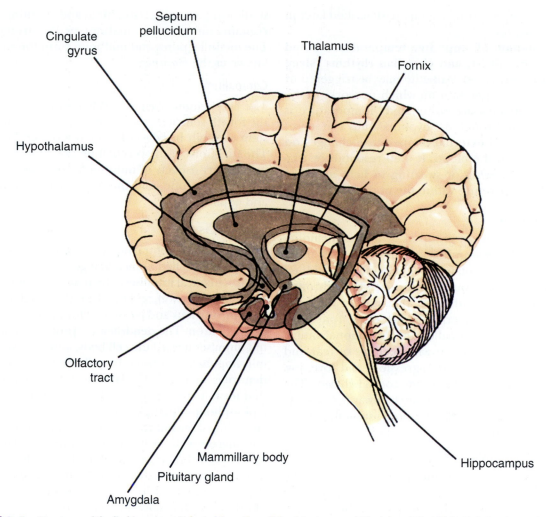

FIGURE 2–2 Structures of the limbic system. (Adapted from *Essentials of Anatomy and Physiology* [7th ed.], by V. C. Scanlon and T. Sanders, 2015, Philadelphia, PA: F.A. Davis Company. Reprinted with permission.)

Thalamus

The thalamus integrates all sensory input (except smell) on its way to the cortex. This helps the cerebral cortex interpret the whole picture very rapidly rather than experiencing each sensation individually. The thalamus is also involved in temporarily blocking minor sensations so that an individual can concentrate on one important event when necessary. For example, an individual who is studying for an examination may be unaware of the clock ticking in the room, or even of another person walking into the room, because the thalamus has temporarily blocked these incoming sensations from the cortex. The impact of dopamine in the thalamus is associated with several neuropsychiatric disorders.

Hypothalamus

The hypothalamus is located just below the thalamus and just above the pituitary gland and has the following diverse functions:

1. **Regulation of the pituitary gland.** Many hormones are regulated by "releasing factors" from the hypothalamus. When the hormones are required by the body, the releasing factors stimulate the release of the hormone from the anterior pituitary, and the hormone in turn stimulates its target organ to carry out its specific functions.
2. **Direct neural control over the actions of the autonomic nervous system.** The hypothalamus regulates the appropriate visceral responses during various emotional states. The actions of the

autonomic nervous system are described later in this chapter.

3. **Regulation of appetite, temperature, blood pressure, thirst, and circadian rhythms (sleep and wakefulness).** Appetite may be triggered or inhibited depending on which networks in the hypothalamus are stimulated. Temperature is regulated through the hypothalamus as it senses internal and external temperature changes on skin and in the blood. It then responds by triggering shivering or sweating to help maintain body temperature within the normal range.

Limbic System

The limbic system is a group of structures including the amygdala, mammillary body, olfactory tract, hypothalamus, cingulate gyrus, septum pellucidum, thalamus, hippocampus, and fornix, which, through communication with the hypothalamus, control several autonomic, endocrine, and somatic functions. This system has been called the "emotional brain" because of its association with feelings of fear and anxiety; anger, rage, and aggression; and love, joy, and hope and with sexuality and social behavior. The amygdala seems to be a primary gateway for processing novel and ambiguous emotional stimuli, particularly related to fear, anxiety, and panic.

Mesencephalon (Midbrain)

The mesencephalon extends from the pons to the hypothalamus and is responsible for integration of various reflexes, including visual reflexes (e.g., automatically turning away from a dangerous object when it comes into view), auditory reflexes (e.g., automatically turning toward a sound that is heard), and righting reflexes (e.g., automatically keeping the head upright and maintaining balance).

Pons

The pons is part of the brainstem that acts as a relay station transmitting messages between various parts of the nervous system, including the cerebrum and cerebellum. It contains the central connections of cranial nerves V through VIII and centers for respiration and skeletal muscle tone. The pons is also associated with sleep and dreaming.

Medulla

The medulla is the connecting structure between the spinal cord and the pons, and all of the ascending and descending fiber tracts pass through it. The vital centers are contained in the medulla, and it is responsible for regulation of heart rate, blood pressure, and respiration. In the medulla are reflex centers for swallowing, sneezing, coughing, and vomiting. It also contains nuclei for cranial nerves IX through XII. The medulla, pons, and midbrain form the structure known as the *brainstem*.

Cerebellum

The cerebellum is separated from the brainstem by the fourth ventricle but has connections to the brainstem through bundles of fiber tracts (see Fig. 2–1). The functions of the cerebellum are concerned with involuntary aspects of movement, such as coordination, muscle tone, and the maintenance of posture and equilibrium.

Nerve Tissue

The tissue of the central nervous system (CNS) consists of nerve cells called *neurons* that generate and transmit electrochemical impulses. The **neuron** is composed of a cell body, an axon, and dendrites. The **cell body** contains the nucleus and is essential for the continued life of the neuron. The **dendrites** are processes that transmit impulses toward the cell body, and the **axon** transmits impulses away from the cell body. The axons and dendrites are covered by layers of cells called *neuroglia* that form a coating, or "sheath," of myelin. *Myelin* is a phospholipid that provides insulation against shortcircuiting of the neurons during their electrical activity and increases the velocity of the impulse. The white matter of the brain and spinal cord is so called because of the whitish appearance of the myelin sheath over the axons and dendrites. The gray matter is composed of cell bodies that contain no myelin.

Classes of Neurons

The three classes of neurons include afferent (sensory), efferent (motor), and interneurons. The *afferent neurons* carry impulses from receptors in the internal and external periphery to the CNS, where they are then interpreted into various sensations. The *efferent neurons* carry impulses from the CNS to *effectors* in the periphery, such as muscles (that respond by contracting) and glands (that respond by secreting).

Interneurons exist entirely within the CNS, and 99% of all nerve cells belong to this group. They may carry only sensory or motor impulses, or they may serve as integrators in the pathways between afferent and efferent neurons. They account in large part for thinking, feelings, learning, language, and memory.

Synapses

Information is transmitted through the body from one neuron to another. Some messages may be processed through only a few neurons, whereas others may require thousands of neuronal connections. The neurons that transmit the impulses do not actually touch each other. The junction between two neurons is called a **synapse.** The small space between the axon terminals of one neuron and the cell body or dendrites of another is called the *synaptic cleft.* Neurons conducting impulses toward the synapse are called *presynaptic neurons,* and those conducting impulses away are called *postsynaptic neurons.*

Chemicals that act as **neurotransmitters** are stored in the axon terminals of the presynaptic neuron. An electrical impulse through the neuron causes the release of this neurotransmitter into the synaptic cleft. The neurotransmitter then diffuses across the synaptic cleft and combines with **receptor sites** that are situated on the cell membrane of the postsynaptic neuron. The type of neurotransmitter determines whether or not another electrical impulse is generated at the receptor site. Excitatory neurotransmitters, when combined at the receptor site, generate an *excitatory response* and the electrical impulse moves on to the next synapse, where the same process recurs.

Inhibitory neurotransmitters generate an *inhibitory response* at the receptor site, and synaptic transmission is terminated. Activity at the neural synapse is relevant in the study of psychiatric disorders because excessive or deficient activity of neurotransmitters influences a variety of cognitive and emotional symptoms and the synapse is believed to be the primary site of activity for psychotropic drugs.

The cell body or dendrite of the postsynaptic neuron also contains a chemical *inactivator* that is specific to the neurotransmitter that has been released by the presynaptic neuron. When the synaptic transmission has been completed, the chemical inactivator quickly inactivates the neurotransmitter to prevent unwanted, continuous impulses until a new impulse from the presynaptic neuron releases more neurotransmitter. Continuous impulses can result in excessive activity of neurotransmitters such as dopamine, which is believed to be responsible for symptoms such as hallucinations and delusions seen in people with schizophrenia. A schematic representation of a synapse is presented in Figure 2–3.

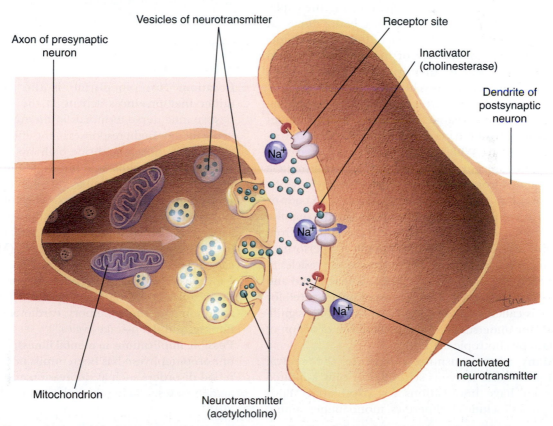

FIGURE 2–3   Impulse transmission at a synapse. The arrow indicates the direction of electrical impulses. (From *Essentials of Anatomy and Physiology* [7th ed.], by V. C. Scanlon and T. Sanders, 2015, Philadelphia, PA: F.A. Davis Company. Reprinted with permission.)

Autonomic Nervous System

The autonomic nervous system (ANS) is considered part of the peripheral nervous system. Its regulation is modulated by the hypothalamus, and emotions exert a great deal of influence over its functioning. For this reason, the ANS has been implicated in the etiology of a number of psychophysiological disorders.

The ANS has two divisions: the sympathetic and the parasympathetic. The sympathetic division is dominant in stressful situations and prepares the body for the fight-or-flight response (discussed in Chapter 1, Mental Health and Mental Illness). The fight-or-flight response causes an increase in heart rate and respirations and a decrease in digestive secretions and peristalsis. Blood is shunted to the vital organs and to skeletal muscles to ensure adequate oxygenation.

The parasympathetic division dominates when an individual is in a relaxed, nonstressful condition. The heart and respirations are maintained at a normal rate, and secretions and peristalsis increase for normal digestion. Elimination functions are promoted. A schematic representation of the ANS is presented in Figure 2–4.

Neurotransmitters

Neurotransmitters were described during the explanation of synaptic activity. They are being discussed separately and in detail because of the essential function they play in the role of human emotion and behavior and because they are central to the therapeutic action of many psychotropic medications.

Neurotransmitters are chemicals that convey information across synaptic clefts to neighboring target cells. They are stored in small vesicles in the axon terminals of neurons. When the action potential, or electrical impulse, reaches this point, the neurotransmitters are released from the vesicles. They cross the synaptic cleft and bind with receptor sites on the cell body or dendrites of the adjacent neuron to allow the impulse to continue its course or to prevent the impulse from continuing. After the neurotransmitter has performed its function in the synapse, it returns to the vesicles to be stored and used again, or else it is inactivated and dissolved by enzymes. The process of being stored for reuse is called *reuptake,* a function that holds significance for understanding the mechanism of action of certain psychotropic medications.

Many neurotransmitters exist in the central and peripheral nervous systems, but only a limited number have implications for psychiatry. Major categories include cholinergics, monoamines, amino acids, and neuropeptides. Each of these is discussed separately and summarized in Table 2–2.

Cholinergics

Acetylcholine

■ **Location:** Acetylcholine was the first chemical to be identified and proven as a neurotransmitter. It is a major effector chemical in the ANS, producing activity at all sympathetic and parasympathetic presynaptic nerve terminals and all parasympathetic postsynaptic nerve terminals. It is highly significant in the neurotransmission that occurs at the junctions of nerve and muscles. Acetylcholinesterase is the enzyme that destroys acetylcholine or inhibits its activity. In the CNS, acetylcholine neurons innervate the cerebral cortex, hippocampus, and limbic structures. The pathways are especially dense through the area of the basal ganglia in the brain.

■ **Functions:** Functions of acetylcholine are numerous and include sleep, arousal, pain perception, motor control, learning, and memory.

■ **Possible implications in mental illness:** Cholinergic mechanisms may have some role in certain disorders of motor behavior and memory, such as Parkinson's disease, Huntington's disease, and Alzheimer's disease.

Monoamines

Norepinephrine

■ **Location:** Norepinephrine is the neurotransmitter that produces activity at the sympathetic postsynaptic nerve terminals in the ANS, resulting in the fight-or-flight responses in the effector organs. In the CNS, norepinephrine pathways originate in the pons and medulla and innervate the thalamus, dorsal hypothalamus, limbic system, hippocampus, cerebellum, and cerebral cortex. When norepinephrine is not returned for storage in the vesicles of the axon terminals, it is metabolized and inactivated by the enzymes monoamine oxidase (MAO) and catechol-*O*-methyl-transferase (COMT).

■ **Functions:** The functions of norepinephrine include the regulation of mood, cognition, perception, attention, vigilance, memory, cardiovascular functioning, and sleep–wake cycles.

■ **Possible implications in mental illness:** The activity of norepinephrine has been implicated in certain mood disorders such as depression and mania, in anxiety states, and in schizophrenia (Sadock et al., 2015).

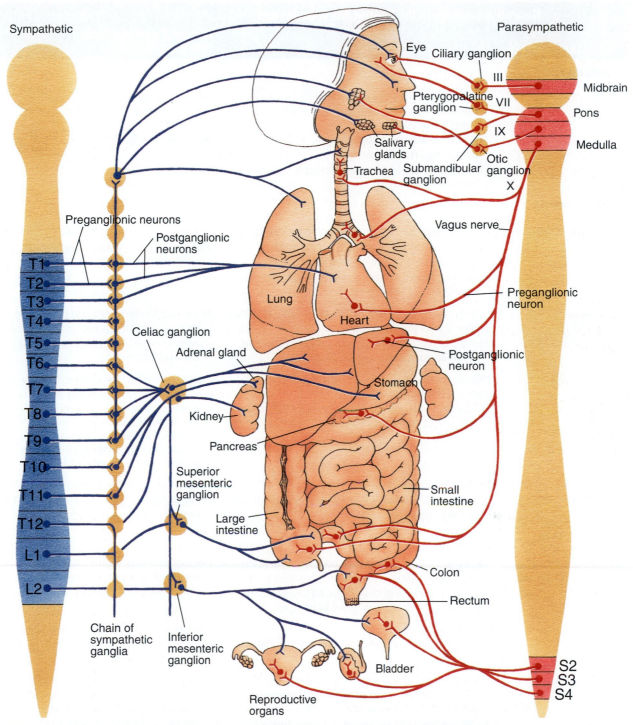

Sympathetic

Parasympathetic

Eye
Ciliary ganglion
III
Midbrain
Pterygopalatine ganglion
VII
Pons
IX
Medulla
Salivary glands
Submandibular ganglion
Otic ganglion
X
Trachea

Preganglionic neurons

Postganglionic neurons

Vagus nerve

T1
T2
T3
T4
T5
T6
T7
T8
T9
T10
T11
T12
L1
L2

Lung

Heart

Preganglionic neuron

Celiac ganglion

Adrenal gland

Postganglionic neuron

Stomach

Kidney

Pancreas

Superior mesenteric ganglion

Large intestine

Small intestine

Colon

Rectum

Chain of sympathetic ganglia

Inferior mesenteric ganglion

Bladder

Reproductive organs

S2
S3
S4

FIGURE 2–4   The autonomic nervous system. The sympathetic division is shown on the left, and the parasympathetic division is shown on the right (both divisions are bilateral). (From *Essentials of Anatomy and Physiology* [7th ed.], by V. C. Scanlon and T. Sanders, 2015, Philadelphia, PA: F.A. Davis Company. Reprinted with permission.)

TABLE 2–2 Neurotransmitters in the Central Nervous System

NEUROTRANSMITTER	LOCATION/FUNCTION	POSSIBLE IMPLICATIONS FOR MENTAL ILLNESS
I. CHOLINERGICS		
A. Acetylcholine	*ANS:* Sympathetic and parasympathetic presynaptic nerve terminals; parasympathetic postsynaptic nerve terminals *CNS:* Cerebral cortex, hippocampus, limbic structures, and basal ganglia *Functions:* Sleep, arousal, pain perception, movement, memory	*Decreased levels:* Alzheimer's disease, Huntington's disease, Parkinson's disease *Increased levels:* Depression
II. MONOAMINES		
A. Norepinephrine	*ANS:* Sympathetic postsynaptic nerve terminals *CNS:* Thalamus, hypothalamus, limbic system, hippocampus, cerebellum, cerebral cortex *Functions:* Mood, cognition, perception, locomotion, cardiovascular functioning, and sleep and arousal	*Decreased levels:* Depression *Increased levels:* Mania, anxiety states, schizophrenia
B. Dopamine	Frontal cortex, limbic system, basal ganglia, thalamus, posterior pituitary, and spinal cord *Functions:* Movement and coordination, emotions, voluntary judgment, release of prolactin	*Decreased levels:* Parkinson's disease, depression, Tourette syndrome, and ADHD *Increased levels:* Mania, schizophrenia, and addictions
C. Serotonin	Hypothalamus, thalamus, limbic system, cerebral cortex, cerebellum, spinal cord *Functions:* Sleep and arousal, libido, appetite, mood, aggression, pain perception, coordination, judgment	*Decreased levels:* Depression, anxiety *Increased levels:* Anxiety states (of the seven different types of serotonin receptors, increased levels of some [5HT1A] have an antianxiety effect, and increased levels of others [5HT3] may increase anxiety [Elsworth & Roth, 2017])
D. Histamine	Hypothalamus *Functions:* Wakefulness; pain sensation and inflammatory response	*Decreased levels:* Depression *Increased levels:* Sleep disorders, anxiety, Alzheimer's disease, psychosis
III. AMINO ACIDS		
A. Gamma-amino-butyric acid (GABA)	Hypothalamus, hippocampus, cortex, cerebellum, basal ganglia, spinal cord, retina *Functions:* Slowdown of body activity, reduces the activity of neurons to which it binds	*Decreased levels:* Huntington's disease, anxiety disorders, schizophrenia, and various forms of epilepsy
B. Glycine	Spinal cord and brainstem *Function:* Recurrent inhibition of motor neurons	*Toxic levels:* "Glycine encephalopathy" *Decreased levels:* Correlated with spastic motor movements
C. Glutamate and aspartate	Pyramidal cells of the cortex, cerebellum, and the primary sensory afferent systems; hippocampus, thalamus, hypothalamus, spinal cord *Functions:* Relay of sensory information and in the regulation of various motor and spinal reflexes	*Increased levels:* Huntington's disease, temporal lobe epilepsy, spinal cerebellar degeneration, anxiety disorders, depressive disorders *Decreased levels:* Schizophrenia
D. D-Serine	Cerebral cortex, forebrain, hippocampus, cerebellum, striatum, thalamus *Functions:* Binds at NMDA receptors and with glutamate, is a coagonist whose functions include mediating NMDA receptor transmission, synaptic plasticity, neurotoxicity	*Decreased levels:* Schizophrenia

TABLE 2–2 Neurotransmitters in the Central Nervous System—cont'd

NEUROTRANSMITTER	LOCATION/FUNCTION	POSSIBLE IMPLICATIONS FOR MENTAL ILLNESS
IV. NEUROPEPTIDES		
A. Endorphins and enkephalins	Hypothalamus, thalamus, limbic structures, midbrain, and brainstem; enkephalins are also found in the gastrointestinal tract *Functions:* Modulation of pain and reduced peristalsis (enkephalins)	Modulation of dopamine activity by opioid peptides may indicate some link to the symptoms of schizophrenia
B. Substance P	Hypothalamus, limbic structures, midbrain, brainstem, thalamus, basal ganglia, and spinal cord; also found in gastrointestinal tract and salivary glands *Function:* Regulation of pain	*Decreased levels:* Huntington's disease and Alzheimer's disease *Increased levels:* Depression
C. Somatostatin	Cerebral cortex, hippocampus, thalamus, basal ganglia, brainstem, and spinal cord *Functions:* Depending on part of the brain being affected, stimulates release of dopamine, serotonin, norepinephrine, and acetylcholine, and inhibits release of norepinephrine, histamine, and glutamate. Also acts as a neuromodulator for serotonin in the hypothalamus	*Decreased levels:* Alzheimer's disease *Increased levels:* Huntington's disease

Dopamine

- **Location:** Dopamine pathways arise from the midbrain and hypothalamus and terminate in the frontal cortex, limbic system, basal ganglia, and thalamus. As with norepinephrine, the inactivating enzymes for dopamine are MAO and COMT.
- **Functions:** Dopamine functions include regulation of movements and coordination, emotions, reward signals, learning, memory, voluntary decision-making ability, and because of dopamine's influence on the pituitary gland, it inhibits the release of prolactin (Sadock et al., 2015).
- **Possible implications in mental illness:** Increased levels of dopamine are associated with mania and schizophrenia. Decreased levels of dopamine have been associated with Parkinson's disease and depression. Dopamine has been implicated in contributing to addictions.

Serotonin

- **Location:** Serotonin pathways originate from cell bodies located in the pons and medulla and project to areas including the hypothalamus, thalamus, limbic system, cerebral cortex, cerebellum, and spinal cord. Serotonin that is not returned to be stored in the axon terminal vesicles is catabolized by the enzyme MAO.
- **Functions:** Serotonin may play a role in the sleep–wake cycle, sexual behavior, appetite, mood, anxiety,

aggression, and pain perception. The fact that both too much and too little serotonin have been associated with anxiety has led to the hypothesis that serotonin may modulate intense emotional states rather than influencing one kind of mood disruption. Further, there are seven different subgroups of serotonin receptors, which, when activated result in different effects (Elsworth & Roth, 2017).
- **Possible implications in mental illness:** The serotonergic system has been implicated in anxiety states, depression, and schizophrenia (Sadock et al., 2015).

Histamine

- **Location:** The role of histamine in mediating allergic and inflammatory reactions has been well documented. Its role in the CNS as a neurotransmitter is the subject of ongoing research. The highest concentrations of histamine are found within various regions of the hypothalamus.
- **Functions:** Brain histamine regulates many physiological functions: neuroendocrine, circadian rhythms (the sleep–wake cycle), psychomotor activity, mood, learning, cognition, appetite, and eating behavior (Cacabelos, Torrellas, Fernández-Novoa, & López-Muñoz, 2016). The enzyme that catabolizes histamine is MAO.
- **Possible implications in mental illness:** Alterations in brain histamine are associated with several pathological conditions, such as epilepsy,

stroke, anxiety, depression, psychosis, neurode-generation, and neuroinflammatory processes (Cacabelos et al., 2016).

Amino Acids

Inhibitory Amino Acids

Gamma-Aminobutyric Acid

- **Location:** Gamma-aminobutyric acid (GABA) has a widespread distribution in the CNS, with high concentrations in the hypothalamus, hippocampus, cortex, cerebellum, and basal ganglia of the brain; the gray matter of the dorsal horn of the spinal cord; and the retina. GABA is catabolized by the enzyme GABA transaminase.
- **Functions:** Inhibitory neurotransmitters, such as GABA, prevent postsynaptic excitation, interrupting the progression of the electrical impulse at the synaptic junction. This function is significant when slowdown of body activity is advantageous. Enhancement of the GABA system is the mechanism of action by which the benzodiazepines produce their calming effect.
- **Possible implications in mental illness:** Alterations in the GABA system have been implicated in anxiety disorders, movement disorders (e.g., Huntington's disease), and various forms of epilepsy. GABA levels, in a complex interaction with other neurotransmitters such as dopamine, have also been implicated in substance use disorders and addiction.

Glycine

- **Location:** The highest concentrations of glycine in the CNS are found in the spinal cord and brainstem. Little is known about the possible enzymatic metabolism of glycine.
- **Functions:** Glycine appears to be the neurotransmitter of recurrent inhibition of motor neurons within the spinal cord and is possibly involved in the regulation of spinal and brainstem reflexes.
- **Possible implications in mental illness:** Glycine has been implicated in the pathogenesis of certain types of spastic disorders and in "glycine encephalopathy," which is known to occur with toxic accumulation of the neurotransmitter in the brain and cerebrospinal fluid (Van Hove, Coughlin, & Sharer, 2013).

Excitatory Amino Acids

Glutamate and Aspartate

- **Location:** Glutamate and aspartate appear to be primary excitatory neurotransmitters in the pyramidal cells of the cortex, the cerebellum, and the primary sensory afferent systems. They are also found in the hippocampus, thalamus, hypothalamus, and spinal cord. Glutamate and aspartate are inactivated by uptake into the tissues and through assimilation in various metabolic pathways.
- **Functions:** Glutamate and aspartate function in the relay of sensory information and in the regulation of various motor and spinal reflexes. Glutamate also plays a role in memory and learning.
- **Possible implications in mental illness:** Alterations in these systems have been implicated in the etiology of certain neurodegenerative disorders, such as Huntington's disease, temporal lobe epilepsy, and spinal cerebellar degeneration. Increases in glutamate have been associated with neuron degeneration in Alzheimer's disease (Coyle, 2017). Problems in making or using glutamate have been linked to many mental disorders, including autism, obsessive-compulsive disorder (OCD), schizophrenia, and depression (National Institute of Mental Health [NIMH], no date).

Neuropeptides

Neuropeptides act as signaling molecules in the CNS. Their activities include regulating processes related to sex, sleep, stress, pain, emotion, and social cognition, and they may contribute to symptoms and behaviors associated with psychosis, mood disorders, dementias, and autism spectrum disorders (Sadock et al., 2015). Hormonal neuropeptides are discussed in the "Neuroendocrinology" section of this chapter.

Opioid Peptides

- **Location:** Opioid peptides, which include the endorphins and enkephalins, have been widely studied. Opioid peptides are found in various concentrations in the hypothalamus, thalamus, limbic structures, midbrain, and brainstem. Enkephalins are also found in the gastrointestinal tract.
- **Functions:** With their natural morphine-like properties, opioid peptides are thought to have a role in pain modulation. They are released in response to painful stimuli and may be responsible for producing the analgesic effect following acupuncture. Opioid peptides alter the release of dopamine and affect the spontaneous activity of the dopaminergic neurons.
- **Possible implications in mental illness:** Modulation of dopamine activity by opioid peptides may be associated with addiction and some symptoms of schizophrenia.

Substance P

- **Location:** Substance P was the first neuropeptide to be discovered. It is present in high concentrations in the hypothalamus, limbic structures, midbrain, and brainstem and is also found in the thalamus, basal ganglia, and spinal cord.
- **Functions:** Substance P plays a role in sensory transmission, particularly in the regulation of pain.
- **Possible implications in mental illness:** Recent studies demonstrated that people with depression and post-traumatic stress disorder (PTSD) had elevated levels of substance P in their cerebral spinal fluid (Sadock et al., 2015).

Somatostatin

- **Location:** Somatostatin (also called *growth hormone—inhibiting*) is found in the cerebral cortex, hippocampus, thalamus, basal ganglia, brainstem, and spinal cord.
- **Functions:** Somatostatin has been shown to stimulate dopamine, serotonin, norepinephrine, and acetylcholine and to inhibit norepinephrine, histamine, and glutamate. It also acts as a neuromodulator for serotonin in the hypothalamus, thereby regulating its release (i.e., controlling whether it is stimulated or inhibited). It is possible that somatostatin may serve this function for other neurotransmitters as well.
- **Possible implications in mental illness:** High concentrations of somatostatin have been reported in brain specimens of clients with Huntington's disease and low concentrations in those with Alzheimer's disease.

CORE CONCEPT

Neuroendocrinology

Study of the interaction between the nervous system and the endocrine system and of the effects of various hormones on cognitive, emotional, and behavioral functioning.

Neuroendocrinology

Human endocrine functioning has a strong foundation in the CNS under the direction of the hypothalamus, which has direct control over the pituitary gland. The pituitary gland has two major lobes—the anterior lobe (also called the *adenohypophysis*) and the posterior lobe (also called the *neurohypophysis*). The pituitary gland is only about the size of a pea, but despite its size and because of the powerful control it exerts over endocrine functioning in humans, it is sometimes called the "master gland." (Figure 2–5 shows the hormones of the pituitary gland and their target organs.) Many of the hormones subject to hypothalamus-pituitary regulation may have implications for behavioral functioning. Discussion of these hormones is summarized in Table 2–3.

Pituitary Gland

The Posterior Pituitary (Neurohypophysis)

The hypothalamus has direct control over the posterior pituitary through efferent neural pathways. Two hormones are found in the posterior pituitary: vasopressin (antidiuretic hormone) and oxytocin. They are actually produced by the hypothalamus and stored in the posterior pituitary. Their release is mediated by neural impulses from the hypothalamus (Fig. 2–6).

Antidiuretic Hormone

The main function of antidiuretic hormone (ADH) is to conserve body water and maintain normal blood pressure. The release of ADH is stimulated by pain, emotional stress, dehydration, increased plasma concentration, and decreases in blood volume. An alteration in the secretion of this hormone is related to the polydipsia seen in patients with diabetes and may be one of many factors contributing to the polydipsia, or water intoxication, observed in about 10% to 20% of patients with severe mental illness, particularly those with schizophrenia. Other factors correlated with excessive thirst include adverse effects of psychotropic medications and features of the behavioral disorder itself. There are probably many factors that influence excessive intake of water in patients with severe psychiatric illness, and polydipsia can be severe enough to result in electrolyte imbalance and death (Gill & McCauley, 2015). ADH also may play a role in learning and memory, in alteration of the pain response, and in the modification of sleep patterns.

Oxytocin

Oxytocin stimulates contraction of the uterus at the end of pregnancy and stimulates release of milk from the mammary glands. It is also released in response to stress and during sexual arousal. Oxytocin functions to promote mother-infant bonding and bonding between sexes and has been used experimentally with children with autism to increase socialization (Sadock et al., 2015). Increases in oxytocin demonstrate antianxiety effects (in interaction with ACTH) and may facilitate

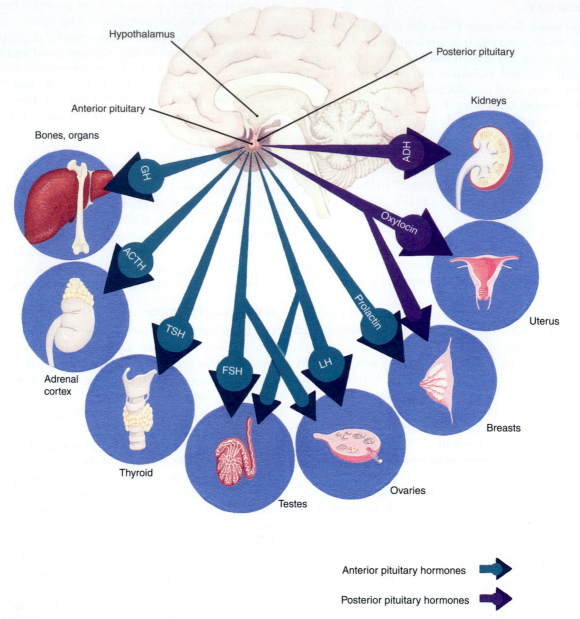

FIGURE 2–5   Hormones of the pituitary gland and their target organs. (From *Essentials of Anatomy and Physiology* [6th ed.], by V. C. Scanlon and T. Sanders, 2014, Philadelphia, PA: F.A. Davis Company. Reprinted with permission.)

development of substance use disorders, especially with "party drugs" (MDMA and GBH) often used to facilitate social interaction (Harris, Wolkowitz, & Reus, 2017). Decreased levels have been reported in patients with autism and anorexia.

The Anterior Pituitary (Adenohypophysis)

The hypothalamus produces *releasing hormones* that pass through capillaries and veins of the hypophyseal portal system to capillaries in the anterior pituitary, where they stimulate secretion of specialized hormones. This pathway is presented in Figure 2–6. The hormones of the anterior pituitary gland regulate multiple body functions and include growth hormone, thyroid-stimulating hormone, ACTH, prolactin, gonadotropin-stimulating hormone, and melanocyte-stimulating hormone. Most of these hormones are regulated by a *negative feedback mechanism.* Once the hormone has exerted its effects, the information is "fed back" to the anterior pituitary, which

TABLE 2–3 Hormones of the Neuroendocrine System

HORMONE	LOCATION AND STIMULATION OF RELEASE	TARGET ORGAN	FUNCTION	POSSIBLE BEHAVIORAL CORRELATION TO ALTERED SECRETION
Antidiuretic hormone (ADH)	Posterior pituitary; release stimulated by dehydration, pain, stress	Kidney (causes increased reabsorption)	Conservation of body water and maintenance of blood pressure	Polydipsia; altered pain response; modified sleep pattern
Oxytocin	Posterior pituitary; release stimulated by end of pregnancy; stress; during sexual arousal	Uterus; breasts	Contraction of the uterus for labor; release of breast milk	May play role in stress response by stimulation of ACTH
Growth hormone (GH)	Anterior pituitary; release stimulated by growth hormone-releasing hormone from hypothalamus	Bones and tissues	Growth in children; protein synthesis in adults	Anorexia nervosa
Thyroid-stimulating hormone (TSH)	Anterior pituitary; release stimulated by thyrotropin-releasing hormone from hypothalamus	Thyroid gland	Stimulation of secretion of needed thyroid hormones for metabolism and regulation of temperature	*Increased levels of thyroid hormones (decreased secretion of TSH):* Insomnia, anxiety, emotional lability *Decreased levels of thyroid hormones (increased secretion of TSH):* Fatigue, depression
Adrenocorticotropic hormone (ACTH)	Anterior pituitary; release stimulated by corticotropin-releasing hormone from hypothalamus	Adrenal cortex	Stimulation of secretion of cortisol, which plays a role in response to stress	*Decreased levels:* Depression, apathy, fatigue *Increased levels:* Mood disorders, psychosis
Prolactin	Anterior pituitary; release stimulated by prolactin-releasing hormone from hypothalamus	Breasts	Stimulation of milk production	*Increased levels:* Depression, anxiety, decreased libido, irritability
Gonadotropic hormones	Anterior pituitary; release stimulated by gonadotropin-releasing hormone from hypothalamus	Ovaries and testes	Stimulation of secretion of estrogen, progesterone, and testosterone; role in ovulation and sperm production	*Decreased levels:* Depression and anorexia nervosa *Increased testosterone:* Increased sexual behavior and aggressiveness
Melanocyte-stimulating hormone	Anterior pituitary; release stimulated by onset of darkness	Pineal gland	Stimulation of secretion of melatonin	*Increased levels:* Depression

inhibits the release, and ultimately decreases the effects, of the stimulating hormones.

Growth Hormone

The release of growth hormone (GH), also called somatotropin, is stimulated by growth hormone-releasing hormone (GHRH) from the hypothalamus. Its release is inhibited by growth hormone-inhibiting hormone (GHIH), or somatostatin, also from the hypothalamus. It is responsible for growth in children as well as for continued protein synthesis throughout life. During periods of fasting, it stimulates the release of fat from the adipose tissue to be used for increased energy. The release of GHIH is stimulated in response

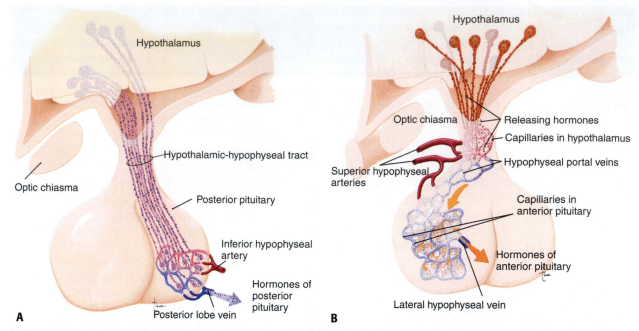

FIGURE 2–6   Structural relationships of hypothalamus and pituitary gland. (A) Posterior pituitary stores hormones produced in the hypothalamus. (B) Releasing hormones of the hypothalamus circulate directly to the anterior pituitary and influence its secretions. Notice the two networks of capillaries. (From *Essentials of Anatomy and Physiology* [7th ed.], by V. C. Scanlon and T. Sanders, 2015, Philadelphia, PA: F.A. Davis Company. Reprinted with permission.)

to periods of hyperglycemia. GHRH is stimulated in response to hypoglycemia and to stressful situations. During prolonged stress, GH has a direct effect on protein, carbohydrate, and lipid metabolism, resulting in increased serum glucose and free fatty acids to be used for increased energy. GH deficiency has been noted in many patients with major depressive disorder, and several GH abnormalities have been noted in patients with anorexia nervosa.

Thyroid-Stimulating Hormone

Thyrotropin-releasing hormone (TRH) from the hypothalamus stimulates the release of thyroid-stimulating hormone (TSH), or thyrotropin, from the anterior pituitary. TSH stimulates the thyroid gland to secrete triiodothyronine (T_3) and thyroxine (T_4). Thyroid hormones are integral to metabolism and the regulation of temperature.

A correlation between thyroid dysfunction and altered behavioral functioning has been well documented. Common symptoms of hyperthyroidism include irritability, insomnia, anxiety, restlessness, weight loss, emotional lability, and, in some instances, progression to delirium or psychosis. Symptoms of fatigue, decreased libido, memory impairment, depression, and suicidal ideations have been associated with chronic hypothyroidism. Studies have correlated various forms of thyroid dysfunction with mood disorders, anxiety, eating disorders, psychosis, and dementia.

Adrenocorticotropic Hormone

Corticotropin-releasing hormone (CRH) from the hypothalamus stimulates the release of ACTH from the anterior pituitary. ACTH stimulates the adrenal cortex to secrete cortisol. CRH, ACTH, and cortisol levels all rise in response to stress. Disorders of the adrenal cortex have been associated with mood disorders, PTSD, Alzheimer's dementia, and substance use disorders.

Addison's disease is the result of hyposecretion of the hormones of the adrenal cortex. Behavioral symptoms of hyposecretion include mood changes with apathy, social withdrawal, impaired sleep, decreased concentration, and fatigue. Hypersecretion of cortisol results in Cushing's disease and is associated with behaviors that include depression, mania, psychosis, and suicidal ideation. Cognitive impairments also have been commonly observed.

Prolactin

Prolactin is mainly involved in reproductive functions and milk production in the mammary glands during pregnancy. First generation antipsychotic medication increases prolactin levels and may be responsible for the undesired side effect of lactation in patients on these medications. High prolactin levels are also associated with depression, decreased libido, anxiety, irritability, and the negative symptoms of schizophrenia. Prolactin levels in psychotic patients have been positively correlated with severity of tardive dyskinesia (Sadock et al., 2015).

Gonadotropic Hormones

The gonadotropic hormones are so called because they produce an effect on the gonads—the ovaries and the testes. The gonadotropins include follicle-stimulating hormone (FSH) and luteinizing hormone (LH). In women, FSH initiates maturation of ovarian follicles into the ova and stimulates their secretion of estrogen. LH is responsible for ovulation and the secretion of progesterone from the corpus luteum. In men, FSH initiates sperm production in the testes, and LH increases secretion of testosterone by the interstitial cells of the testes.

Limited evidence exists to correlate gonadotropins to behavioral functioning, although some observations have been made to warrant hypothetical consideration. Studies have indicated decreased levels of testosterone, LH, and FSH in men with depression. Increased sexual behavior and aggressiveness have been linked to elevated testosterone levels in both men and women. Decreased plasma levels of LH and FSH commonly occur in patients with anorexia nervosa. Supplemental estrogen therapy has resulted in improved mentation and mood in some women with depression.

Melanocyte-Stimulating Hormone

Melanocyte-stimulating hormone from the hypothalamus stimulates the pineal gland to secrete melatonin. The release of melatonin appears to depend on the onset of darkness and is suppressed by light. Studies of this hormone have indicated that environmental light can affect neuronal activity and influence *circadian rhythms*. Correlation between abnormal secretion of melatonin and symptoms of depression has led to the implication of melatonin in the etiology of seasonal affective disorder, in which individuals become depressed only during the fall and winter months when the amount of daylight decreases.

Circadian Rhythms

Human biological rhythms are largely determined by genetic coding with input from the external environment influencing the cyclic effects. **Circadian**
 rhythms in humans follow a near-24-hour cycle and may influence a variety of regulatory functions, including the sleep–wakefulness cycle, body temperature regulation, patterns of activity such as eating and drinking, and hormone secretion. The 24-hour rhythms in humans are affected to a large degree by the cycles of lightness and darkness.

Other Biological Rhythms

Most of the biological rhythms of the body operate over a period of about 24 hours, but cycles of longer lengths have been studied. For example, women of menstruating age show monthly cycles of variable progesterone levels.

Some rhythms may last as long as a year. These circannual rhythms may influence the effectiveness of laboratory tests results and some medications. Clinical studies have shown that chemotherapy, when administered during the appropriate circadian phase, can significantly increase its efficacy and decrease the toxic effects of certain cytotoxic agents (Garlapow, 2016; Lis et al., 2003).

The Role of Circadian Rhythms in Psychopathology

Circadian rhythms may play a role in psychopathology. Abnormal circadian rhythms have been associated with a variety of mental illnesses including depression, bipolar disorder, and seasonal affective disorder. Because many hormones have been implicated in behavioral functioning, it is reasonable to believe that peak secretion times could be influential in predicting certain behaviors. The association of depression with increased secretion of melatonin during darkness hours has already been discussed. External manipulation of the light–dark cycle and removal of external time cues often have beneficial effects on mood disorders.

Symptoms that occur in the premenstrual cycle have been linked to disruptions in biological rhythms. A number of the symptoms associated with premenstrual dysphoric disorder (PMDD) strongly resemble those attributed to depression, and hormonal changes have been implicated in the etiology. The sleep–wakefulness cycle is probably the most fundamental of biological rhythms, and sleep disturbances are common in both depression and PMDD. Neurochemicals such as serotonin and norepinephrine appear to be most active during non–rapid eye movement (REM) sleep, whereas the neurotransmitter acetylcholine is activated during REM sleep (Skudaev, 2018). Several studies have revealed information about the sleep-inducing characteristics of serotonin. L-tryptophan, the amino acid precursor to serotonin, has been used for many years as an effective sedative-hypnotic to induce sleep in individuals with sleep-onset disorder.

CORE CONCEPT

Genetics

Study of the biological transmission of certain characteristics (physical and/or behavioral) from parent to offspring.

Genetics

Human behavioral genetics seeks to understand both genetic and environmental contributions to individual variations in human behavior. This type of study is complicated by the fact that behaviors, like all complex traits, involve *multiple genes.*

The term **genotype** refers to the total set of genes present in an individual and coded in the DNA. The physical manifestations of a particular genotype are designated by characteristics that specify a specific **phenotype**. Examples of phenotypes include eye color, height, blood type, language, and hair type. As evident by the examples presented, phenotypes are not *only* genetic but may also be acquired (i.e., influenced by the environment) or a combination of both. Many psychiatric disorders are likely the result of a combination of genetics and environmental influences.

Investigators who study the etiological implications for psychiatric illness may explore several risk factors. Studies to determine if an illness is *familial* compare the percentages of family members with the illness to those in the general population or within a control group of unrelated individuals. These studies estimate the prevalence of psychopathology among relatives and make predictions about the predisposition to an illness based on familial risk factors. Schizophrenia, bipolar disorder, major depressive disorder, anorexia nervosa, panic disorder, somatic symptom disorder, antisocial personality disorder, and alcoholism are examples of psychiatric illness in which familial tendencies have been indicated.

Studies that are purely genetic in nature search for a specific gene that is responsible for an individual having a particular illness. A number of disorders exist in which the mutation of a specific gene or change in the number or structure of a chromosome has been associated with the etiology. Examples include Huntington's disease, cystic fibrosis, phenylketonuria, Duchenne's muscular dystrophy, and Down syndrome.

The search for pure genetic links to certain psychiatric disorders continues. Risk factors for early-onset Alzheimer's disease have been linked to mutations on chromosomes 21, 14, and 1 (National Institute on Aging, 2015). Other studies have linked a gene in the region of chromosome 19 that produces apolipoprotein E with late-onset Alzheimer's disease. One large study (Cross-Disorder Group of the Psychiatric Genomics Consortium, 2013) found similar genetic variations in five mental health disorders that were previously considered completely distinct. These disorders—autism, attention deficit-hyperactivity disorder (ADHD), bipolar disorder, major depression, and schizophrenia—all showed some common gene variations, including differences in two genes that regulate the flow of calcium into cells. Although these findings are intriguing, they do not explain all the genetic risks for mental illness, the nongenetic risks, or the interaction between the two. Future research will continue to search for answers with the ultimate goal of improving diagnosis and treatment and perhaps uncovering the keys to prevention of mental illness.

In addition to familial and purely genetic investigations, other types of studies have been conducted to estimate the existence and degree of genetic and environmental contributions to the etiology of certain psychiatric disorders. Twin studies and adoption studies have been successfully employed for this purpose.

Twin studies examine the frequency of a disorder in monozygotic (genetically identical) and dizygotic (fraternal; not genetically identical) twins. Twins are called *concordant* when both members have the same disorder in question. Concordance in monozygotic twins is considered stronger evidence of genetic involvement than it is in dizygotic twins. Twin studies have supported genetic vulnerability in the etiology of several mental illnesses including adjustment disorders, PTSD, substance abuse, schizophrenia, bipolar disorder, major depression, obsessive-compulsive disorder, risk for suicide, and others (Sadock et al., 2015). *Adoption studies* allow comparisons to be made between the influences of genetics and environment on the development of a psychiatric disorder. Knowles (2003) describes the following four types of adoption studies that have been conducted:

1. The study of adopted children whose biological parent(s) had a psychiatric disorder but whose adoptive parent(s) did not
2. The study of adopted children whose adoptive parent(s) had a psychiatric disorder but whose biological parent(s) did not

3. The study of adoptive and biological relatives of adopted children who developed a psychiatric disorder

4. The study of monozygotic twins reared apart by different adoptive parents

Disorders in which adoption studies have suggested a possible genetic link include alcoholism, schizophrenia, major depression, bipolar disorder, ADHD, and antisocial personality disorder (Sadock et al., 2015).

A summary of various psychiatric disorders and the possible biological influences discussed in this chapter is presented in Table 2–4. Various diagnostic procedures used to detect alteration in biological functioning that may contribute to psychiatric disorders are presented in Table 2–5.

CORE CONCEPT

Psychoneuroimmunology
The study of the relationship between the immune system, the nervous system, and psychological processes such as thinking and behavior.

Psychoneuroimmunology (PNI)

Normal Immune Response

Cells responsible for *nonspecific* immune reactions include neutrophils, monocytes, and macrophages. They work to destroy the invasive organism and initiate and facilitate healing of damaged tissue. If these cells are not effective in accomplishing a satisfactory healing response, *specific* immune mechanisms take over.

Cytokines are molecules that regulate immune and inflammatory responses. They are active when an individual is fighting an infection and the inflammatory processes that accompany these illnesses. Recent research has also demonstrated that cytokines are active in mood disorders such as depression and bipolar disorder. Current research focuses on the impact of cytokines as part of an essential and complex system of responses that are crucial for reducing inflammation and bolstering the immune response. Studies are also attempting to identify what happens when inflammation is not resolved and when cytokines remain active or cross the blood-brain barrier; there is evidence that these maladaptations may trigger a multitude of illnesses (Ratnayake et al., 2013).

Implications of the Immune System in Psychiatric Illness

In studies of the biological response to stress, it has been hypothesized that individuals become more susceptible to physical illness following exposure to a stressful stimulus or life event (see Chapter 1). This response is thought to be due to the effect of increased glucocorticoid release from the adrenal cortex following stimulation from the hypothalamic-pituitary-adrenal axis during stressful situations. The result is a suppression in lymphocyte proliferation and function.

Studies have shown that nerve endings exist in tissues of the immune system. The CNS has connections in both bone marrow and the thymus, where immune system cells are produced, and in the spleen and lymph nodes, where those cells are stored.

GH, which may be released in response to certain stressors, may enhance immune functioning, whereas testosterone is thought to inhibit immune functioning. Increased production of epinephrine and norepinephrine occurs in response to stress and may decrease immunity. Serotonin has been described as an immunomodulatory because it has demonstrated both enhancing and inhibitory effects on inflammation and immunity (Arreola et al., 2015). Studies have correlated a decrease in lymphocyte functioning with periods of grief, bereavement, and depression, associating the degree of altered immunity with severity of the depression. A number of research studies have been conducted attempting to correlate the onset of schizophrenia to abnormalities of the immune system. These studies have considered autoimmune responses, viral infections, and immunogenetics (Sadock et al., 2015). The role of these factors in the onset and course of schizophrenia remains unclear. Attempts to identify a neurotoxic virus that triggers the manifestations of schizophrenia have not been successful; however, there is clear evidence of higher incidence of schizophrenia following viral epidemics. Immunological abnormalities have also been investigated in a number of other psychiatric illnesses, including alcoholism, autism spectrum disorder, and neurocognitive disorder.

Evidence exists to support a correlation between psychosocial stress and the onset of illness. Research is still required to determine the specific processes involved in stress-induced modulation of the immune system.

TABLE 2–4	**Biological Implications of Psychiatric Disorders**			
ANATOMICAL BRAIN STRUCTURES INVOLVED	**NEUROTRANSMITTER HYPOTHESIS**	**POSSIBLE ENDOCRINE CORRELATION**	**IMPLICATIONS OF CIRCADIAN RHYTHMS**	**POSSIBLE GENETIC LINK**
SCHIZOPHRENIA				
Frontal cortex, temporal lobes, limbic system	Dopamine hyperactivity; decreased glutamate	Decreased prolactin levels	May correlate antipsychotic medication administration to times of lowest level	Twin, familial, and adoption studies suggest genetic link
DEPRESSIVE DISORDERS				
Frontal lobes, limbic system, temporal lobes	Decreased levels of norepinephrine, dopamine, and serotonin; increased glutamate	Increased cortisol levels, thyroid hormone hyposecretion, increased melatonin	DST* used to predict effectiveness of antidepressants; melatonin linked to depression during periods of darkness	Twin, familial, and adoption studies suggest a genetic link
BIPOLAR DISORDER				
Frontal lobes, limbic system, temporal lobes	Increased levels of norepinephrine and dopamine in acute mania	Elevated thyroid hormones may manifest as manic symptoms	Abnormal circadian rhythms have been associated with bipolar disorder	Twin, familial, and adoption studies suggest a genetic link
PANIC DISORDER				
Limbic system, midbrain	Increased levels of norepinephrine; decreased gamma amino butyric acid (GABA) activity	Elevated levels of thyroid hormones	May have some application for times of medication administration	Twin and familial studies suggest a genetic link
ANOREXIA NERVOSA				
Limbic system, particularly the hypothalamus	Decreased levels of norepinephrine, serotonin, and dopamine	Decreased levels of gonadotropins and growth hormone; increased cortisol levels	DST* often shows same results as in depression	Twin and familial studies suggest a genetic link
OBSESSIVE-COMPULSIVE DISORDER				
Limbic system, basal ganglia (specifically caudate nucleus)	Decreased levels of serotonin	Increased cortisol levels	DST* often shows same results as in depression	Twin studies suggest a possible genetic link
ALZHEIMER'S DISEASE				
Temporal, parietal, and occipital regions of cerebral cortex; hippocampus	Decreased levels of acetylcholine, norepinephrine, serotonin, and somatostatin	Decreased corticotropin-releasing hormone	Decreased levels of acetylcholine and serotonin may inhibit hypothalamic-pituitary axis and interfere with hormonal releasing factors	Familial studies suggest a genetic predisposition; late-onset disorder linked to marker on chromosome 19; early-onset to chromosomes 21, 14, and 1

*DST, dexamethasone suppression test. Dexamethasone is a synthetic glucocorticoid that suppresses cortisol secretion via the feedback mechanism. In this test, 1 mg of dexamethasone is administered at 11:30 p.m., and blood samples are drawn at 8:00 a.m., 4:00 p.m., and 11:00 p.m. on the following day. A plasma value greater than 5 mcg/dL suggests that the individual is not suppressing cortisol in response to the dose of dexamethasone. This is a positive result for depression and may have implications for other disorders as well.

TABLE 2–5	Diagnostic Procedures Used to Detect Altered Brain Functioning	
EXAM	**TECHNIQUE USED**	**PURPOSE AND POSSIBLE FINDINGS**
Electroencephalography (EEG)	Electrodes are placed on the scalp in a standardized position. Amplitude and frequency of beta, alpha, theta, and delta brain waves are graphically recorded on paper by ink markers for multiple areas of the brain surface.	Measures brain electrical activity; identifies dysrhythmias, asymmetries, or suppression of brain rhythms; used in the diagnosis of epilepsy, neoplasm, stroke, metabolic or degenerative disease.
Computerized EEG mapping	EEG tracings are summarized by computer-assisted systems in which various regions of the brain are identified and functioning is interpreted by color coding or gray shading.	Measures brain electrical activity; used largely in research to represent statistical relationships between individuals and groups or between two populations of subjects (e.g., patients with schizophrenia vs. control subjects).
Computed tomographic (CT) scan	CT scan may be used with or without contrast medium. X-rays are taken of various transverse planes of the brain while a computerized analysis produces a precise reconstructed image of each segment.	Measures accuracy of brain structure to detect possible lesions, abscesses, areas of infarction, or aneurysm. CT has also identified various anatomical differences in patients with schizophrenia, organic mental disorders, and bipolar disorder.
Magnetic resonance imaging (MRI)	Within a strong magnetic field, the nuclei of hydrogen atoms absorb and reemit electromagnetic energy that is computerized and transformed into image information. No radiation or contrast medium is used.	Measures anatomical and biochemical status of various segments of the brain; detects brain edema, ischemia, infection, neoplasm, trauma, and other changes such as demyelination. Morphological differences have been noted in brains of patients with schizophrenia as compared with control subjects.
Positron emission tomography (PET)	The patient receives an IV injection of a radioactive substance (type depends on brain activity to be visualized). The head is surrounded by detectors that relay data to a computer that interprets the signals and produces the image.	Measures specific brain functioning, such as glucose metabolism, oxygen utilization, blood flow, and, of particular interest in psychiatry, neurotransmitter-receptor interaction.
Single photon emission computed tomography (SPECT)	The technique is similar to PET, but longer-acting radioactive substance must be used to allow time for a gamma-camera to rotate about the head and gather the data, which are then computer assembled into a brain image.	Measures various aspects of brain functioning, as with PET; has also been used to image activity of cerebrospinal fluid circulation.

Psychopharmacology and the Brain

Understanding the brain and the biological processes involved in thinking, feeling, and behaving has far more ramifications and benefits than simply better understanding of psychopharmacological treatment options. As mentioned earlier, future research may continue to demonstrate the impact of psychological interventions on brain activity and neurotransmitters, which would open opportunities to hone psychological treatments and avoid some of the troubling side effects that accompany many medications.

Furthermore, continued research in areas such as psychoneuroimmunology may reveal causes of mental illness, which would provide the opportunity for primary prevention.

Despite these potential opportunities, psychopharmacology remains a primary treatment modality for mental disorders. Understanding, as best we can with current evidence, the biological mechanisms at work in psychoactive drugs is essential to nursing practice. See Chapter 4, Psychopharmacology, for further discussion of the influence of psychoactive drugs on neurosynaptic transmission.

Implications for Nursing

The discipline of psychiatric mental health nursing has always spoken of its role in holistic healthcare, but historical review reveals that emphasis has been placed on treatment approaches that focus on psychological and social factors. Psychiatric nurses must integrate knowledge of the biological sciences into their practices if they are to ensure safe and effective care to people with mental illness. Much progress has been made in understanding the biochemical, neuroanatomical, and genetic influences in mental illness but much remains theoretical. Further, there is evidence that psychosocial influences, particularly history of traumas such as abuse and neglect, interact significantly with an individual's biological vulnerabilities in the development of these illnesses.

To ensure a smooth transition from a strictly psychosocial focus to one of *bio*psychosocial emphasis, nurses must have a clear understanding of the following:

- **Neuroanatomy and neurophysiology:** The structure and functioning of the various parts of the brain and their correlation to human behavior and psychopathology.
- **Neuronal processes:** The various functions of the nerve cells, including the role of neurotransmitters, receptors, synaptic activity, and informational pathways.
- **Neuroendocrinology:** The interaction of the endocrine and nervous systems and the role that the endocrine glands and their respective hormones play in behavioral functioning.
- **Circadian rhythms:** The regulation of biochemical functioning over periods of rhythmic cycles and its influence in predicting certain behaviors.
- **Genetic influences:** The hereditary factors that predispose individuals to certain psychiatric disorders.
- **PNI:** The influence of stress on the immune system and its role in the susceptibility to illness.
- **Trauma:** Both physical trauma (traumatic brain injury) and psychosocial trauma (especially early childhood trauma such as abuse, neglect, and abandonment) are influential in the development of several mental illnesses.
- **Psychopharmacology:** The increasing use of psychotropic drugs in the treatment of mental illness, demanding greater knowledge of psychopharmacological principles and nursing interventions necessary for safe and effective management.
- **Diagnostic technology:** The importance of keeping informed about the latest in technological procedures for diagnosing alterations in brain structure and function.

Why are these concepts important to the practice of psychiatric mental health nursing? The interrelationship between psychosocial adaptation and physical functioning has been established. Integrating biological and behavioral concepts into psychiatric nursing practice is essential for nurses to meet the complex needs of clients with mental illness. Psychobiological perspectives must be incorporated into nursing practice, education, and research to attain the evidence-based outcomes necessary for the delivery of competent care.

Summary and Key Points

- It is important for nurses to understand the interaction between biological and behavioral factors in the development and management of mental illness.
- Psychobiology is the study of the biological foundations of cognitive, emotional, and behavioral processes.
- The limbic system has been called the "emotional brain." It is associated with feelings of fear and anxiety; anger, rage, and aggression; love, joy, and hope; and sexuality and social behavior.
- The three classes of neurons include afferent (sensory), efferent (motor), and interneurons. The junction between two neurons is called a synapse.
- Neurotransmitters are chemicals that convey information across synaptic clefts to neighboring target cells. Many neurotransmitters have implications in the etiology of emotional disorders and in the pharmacological treatment of those disorders.
- Major categories of neurotransmitters include cholinergics, monoamines, amino acids, and neuropeptides.
- The endocrine system plays an important role in human behavior through the hypothalamic-pituitary axis.
- Hormones and their circadian rhythm of regulation significantly influence a number of physiological and psychological life-cycle phenomena, such as moods, sleep and arousal, stress response, appetite, libido, and fertility.

■ Research continues to validate the role of genetics in psychiatric illness.

■ Familial, twin, and adoption studies suggest that genetics may be implicated in the etiology of schizophrenia, bipolar disorder, depressive disorder, panic disorder, anorexia nervosa, alcoholism, and obsessive-compulsive disorder.

■ Psychoneuroimmunology (PNI) examines the impact of psychological factors on the immune system.

■ Evidence exists to support a link between psychosocial stressors and suppression of the immune response.

■ Technologies such as magnetic resonance imaging (MRI), computed tomographic (CT) scan, positron emission tomography (PET), and electroencephalography (EEG) are used as diagnostic tools for detecting alterations in psychobiological functioning.

■ Psychotropic medications have given many individuals a chance to function effectively.

■ Integrating knowledge of the expanding biological focus into psychiatric nursing is essential if nurses are to meet the changing needs of today's psychiatric clients.

Review Questions
Self-Examination/Learning Exercise

Select the answer that is most appropriate for each of the following questions:

1. Which of the following parts of the brain is associated with multiple feelings and behaviors and is sometimes referred to as the "emotional brain"?
   a. Frontal lobe
   b. Thalamus
   c. Hypothalamus
   d. Limbic system

2. Which of the following parts of the brain is concerned with visual reception and interpretation?
   a. Frontal lobe
   b. Parietal lobe
   c. Temporal lobe
   d. Occipital lobe

3. Which of the following parts of the brain is associated with voluntary body movement, thinking and judgment, and expression of feeling?
   a. Frontal lobe
   b. Parietal lobe
   c. Temporal lobe
   d. Occipital lobe

4. Which of the following parts of the brain integrates all sensory input (except smell) on the way to the cortex?
   a. Temporal lobe
   b. Thalamus
   c. Limbic system
   d. Hypothalamus

5. Which of the following parts of the brain deals with sensory perception and interpretation?
   a. Hypothalamus
   b. Cerebellum
   c. Parietal lobe
   d. Hippocampus

Continued

Review Questions—cont'd
Self-Examination/Learning Exercise

6. Which of the following parts of the brain is concerned with hearing, short-term memory, and sense of smell?
   a. Temporal lobe
   b. Parietal lobe
   c. Cerebellum
   d. Hypothalamus

7. Which of the following parts of the brain has control over the pituitary gland and autonomic nervous system as well as regulation of appetite and temperature?
   a. Temporal lobe
   b. Parietal lobe
   c. Cerebellum
   d. Hypothalamus

8. At a synapse, the determination of further impulse transmission is accomplished by means of which of the following?
   a. Potassium ions
   b. Interneurons
   c. Neurotransmitters
   d. The myelin sheath

9. A decrease in which of the following neurotransmitters has been implicated in depression?
   a. GABA, acetylcholine, and aspartate
   b. Norepinephrine, serotonin, and dopamine
   c. Somatostatin, substance P, and glycine
   d. Glutamate, histamine, and opioid peptides

10. Which of the following hormones has been implicated in the etiology of mood disorder with seasonal pattern?
   a. Increased levels of melatonin
   b. Decreased levels of oxytocin
   c. Decreased levels of prolactin
   d. Increased levels of thyrotropin

11. Psychotropic medications may act at the neural synapse to accomplish which of the following? (Select all that apply.)
   a. Inhibit the reuptake of certain neurotransmitters, creating more availability.
   b. Inhibit catabolic enzymes, promoting more availability of a neurotransmitter.
   c. Block receptors, resulting in less neurotransmitter activity.
   d. Add synthetic neurotransmitters found in the drug.

12. Psychoneuroimmunology is a branch of science that involves which of the following? (Select all that apply.)
   a. The impact of psychoactive medications at the neural synapse.
   b. The relationship among the immune system, the nervous system, and psychological processes, including mental illness.
   c. The correlation between psychosocial stress and the onset of illness.
   d. The potential role of viruses in the onset of schizophrenia.
   e. The genetic factors that influence prevention of mental illness.

References

Arreola, R., Becerril-Villanueva, E., Cruz-Fuentes, C., Velasco-Velázquez, M. A., Garcés-Alvarez, M. E., Hurtado-Alvarado, G., . . . Pavón, L. (2015). Immunomodulatory effects mediated by serotonin. *Journal of Immunology Research.* doi:http://dx.doi. org/10.1155/2015/354957

Cacabelos, R., Torrellas, C., Fernandez-Novoa, L., & Lopez-Munoz, F. (2016). Histamine and immune biomarkers in CNS disorders. *Mediators of Inflammation,* 2016, 1924603. Retrieved from https://www.ncbi.nlm.nih.gov/pmc/articles/PMC4846752/

Coyle, J. T. (2017). Amino acid neurotransmitters. In B. J. Sadock, V. A. Sadock, & P. Ruiz (Eds.), *Comprehensive textbook of psychiatry* (10th ed., pp. 76–84). Philadelphia, PA: Wolters Kluwer.

Cross-Disorder Group of the Psychiatric Genomics Consortium. (2013). Identification of risk loci with shared effects on five major psychiatric disorders: A genome-wide analysis. *Lancet, 381*(9875),1371–1379. doi: 10.1016/S0140-6736(12)62129-1

Elsworth, J. D., & Roth, R. H. (2017). Biogenic amine transmitters. In B. J. Sadock, V. A. Sadock, & P. Ruiz (Eds.), *Comprehensive textbook of psychiatry* (10th ed., pp. 61–75). Philadelphia, PA: Wolters Kluwer.

Furmark, T., Tilfors, M., Martiensdottir, I., Fischer, H., Pissiota, A., Langstrom, B., & Fredrikson, M. (2002). Common changes in cerebral blood flow in patients with social phobia treated with citalopram or cognitive behavior therapy. *Archives of General Psychiatry, 59*(5), 425–433.

Garlapow, M. (2016). Timing chemotherapy administration to circadian rhythm improves drug effectiveness. *Oncology Nurse Advisor.* Retrieved from https://www.oncologynurseadvisor.com/side-effect-management/chemotherapy-more-effective-when-synced-with-circadian-rhythm/article/504455/

Gill, M., & McCauley, M. (2015). Psychogenic polydipsia: The result, or cause of, deteriorating psychotic symptoms? A case report of the consequences of water intoxication. *Case Reports in Psychiatry.* doi: 10.1155/2015/846459

Harris, D. S., Wolkowitz, M. D., & Reus, V. I. (2017). Psychoneuro-endocrinology. In B. J. Sadock, V. A. Sadock, & P. Ruiz (Eds.), *Comprehensive textbook of psychiatry* (10th ed., pp. 164–178). Philadelphia, PA: Wolters Kluwer.

Knowles, J. A. (2003). Genetics. In R. E. Hales & S. C. Yudofsky (Eds.), *Textbook of psychiatry* (2nd ed.). Washington, DC: American Psychiatric Association.

Lis, C. G., Grutsch, J. F., Wood, P., You, M., Rich, I., & Hrushesky, W. J. (2003). Circadian timing in cancer treatment: The biological foundation for an integrative approach. *Integrative Cancer Therapies, 2*(2), 105–111.

Lyall, A. E., Kubicki, M., & Shenton, M. E. (2017) Structural brain imaging in schizophrenia. In B. J. Sadock, V. A. Sadock, & P. Ruiz (Eds.), *Comprehensive textbook of psychiatry* (10th ed., pp. 1463–1475). Philadelphia, PA: Wolters Kluwer.

National Institutes of Health (NIH). (2015). *Is there a link between marijuana and mental illness?* Retrieved from http://www.drugabuse.gov/publications/research-reports/marijuana/there-link-between-marijuana-use-mental-illness

National Institute of Mental Health (NIMH). (no date.) *Brain basics.* Retrieved from https://www.nimh.nih.gov/brainbasics/index.html

National Institute on Aging. (2015). *Alzheimer's disease genetics fact sheet.* Retrieved from https://www.nia.nih.gov/health/alzheimers-disease-genetics-fact-sheet

Ratnayake, U., Quinn, T., Walker, D. W., & Dickinson, H. (2013). Cytokines and the neurodevelopmental basis of mental illness. *Frontiers in Neuroscience, 7.* doi: 10.3389/fnins.2013.00180

Sadock, B. J., Sadock, V. A., & Ruiz, P. (2015). *Synopsis of psychiatry: Behavioral sciences/clinical psychiatry* (11th ed.). Philadelphia, PA: Wolters Kluwer.

Scanlon, V. C., & Sanders, T. (2015). *Essentials of anatomy and physiology* (7th ed.). Philadelphia, PA: F.A. Davis.

Skudaev, S. (2018). *The neurophysiology and neurochemistry of sleep* (review). Retrieved from https://www.scribd.com/document/25882706/1022170-Neurophysiology-and-Neurochemistry-of-Sleep

Van Hove, J., Coughlin, C., & Sharer, G. (2013). Glycine enceph-alopathy. In R. A. Pagon, M. P. Adam, H. H. Ardinger, et al. (Eds.), *GeneReviews®* [Internet]. National Library of Medicine. Retrieved from http://www.ncbi.nlm.nih.gov/books/NBK1357

3

Ethical and Legal Issues

CORE CONCEPTS

Bioethics
Ethics
Moral behavior
Right
Values
Values clarification

CHAPTER OUTLINE

Objectives
Homework Assignment
Introduction
Ethical Considerations

Legal Considerations
Summary and Key Points
Review Questions

KEY TERMS

advocacy
assault
autonomy
battery
beneficence
bioethics
Christian ethics
civil law
common law
criminal law
defamation of character
ethical dilemma
ethical egoism
ethics
false imprisonment
informed consent
justice

Kantianism
libel
malpractice
moral behavior
natural law theory
negligence
nonmaleficence
privileged communication
right
slander
statutory law
tort
utilitarianism
values
values clarification
veracity

OBJECTIVES

After reading this chapter, the student will be able to:

1. Differentiate among *ethics, morals, values,* and *rights*.
2. Discuss ethical theories, including utilitarianism, Kantianism, Christian ethics, natural law theories, and ethical egoism.
3. Define *ethical dilemma*.
4. Discuss the ethical principles of autonomy, beneficence, nonmaleficence, justice, and veracity.
5. Use an ethical decision-making model to make an ethical decision.

6. Describe ethical issues relevant to psychiatric mental health nursing.
7. Define *statutory law* and *common law*.
8. Differentiate between civil and criminal law.
9. Discuss legal issues relevant to psychiatric mental health nursing.
10. Differentiate between *malpractice* and *negligence*.
11. Identify behaviors relevant to the psychiatric mental health setting for which specific malpractice action could be taken.

HOMEWORK ASSIGNMENT
Please read the chapter and answer the following questions:

1. Malpractice and negligence are examples of what kind of law?
2. What charges may be brought against a nurse for confining a client against his or her wishes (outside of an emergency situation)?
3. Which ethical theory espouses that what is right and good is what is best for the individual making the decision? Which quality and safety in nursing education competency may be, at least in part, consistent with ethical egoism?
4. Name the three major elements of informed consent.

Introduction

Nurses are constantly faced with the challenge of making difficult decisions regarding good and evil or life and death. Complex situations frequently arise in caring for individuals with mental illness, and nurses are held to the highest level of legal and ethical accountability in their professional practice. This chapter presents basic ethical and legal concepts and their relationship to psychiatric mental health nursing. A discussion of ethical theory is presented as a foundation upon which ethical decisions may be made. The American Nurses Association (ANA) has established a code of ethics for nurses to use as a framework within which to make ethical choices and decisions (ANA, 2015) (Box 3–1). These recently revised provisions and interpretive guidelines have been expanded to address some of the complexities of the current healthcare environment and include ethical principles regarding the nurse's duty not only to the patient but also to himself or herself and to all persons with whom the nurse interacts; all relationships should be conducted within a culture of respect and civility.

The ANA Code of Ethics interpretive guidelines include a discussion of the importance of teamwork and collaboration, which is consistent with one of the recommendations of the Institute of Medicine (2003) [now renamed The National Academy of Medicine] for improving the future of healthcare and has become one of the Quality and Safety in Education for Nurses competencies.

The ANA, in cooperation with the American Psychiatric Nurses Association and the International Society of Psychiatric-Mental Health Nurses (2014), has published a scope and standards of practice manual specifically for psychiatric mental health nursing, which maintains consistency with the ANA code of ethics and applies those provisions to psychiatric mental health nursing issues. Knowledge about the ANA's *Code of Ethics for Nurses with Interpretive Statements* (ANA, 2015) and the *Psychiatric-Mental Health Nursing: Scope and Standards of Practice* (American Nurses Association, American Psychiatric Nurses Association, & International Society of Psychiatric-Mental Health Nurses, 2014) is essential for guiding practice because these documents clarify the accepted expectations of the nurse in this field.

Because legislation determines what is *right* or *good* within a society, legal issues pertaining to psychiatric mental health nursing are also discussed in this chapter. Definitions are presented along with a description of the generally accepted and legal rights of psychiatric clients. Nursing competency and client care accountability are compromised when the nurse has inadequate knowledge about the laws, rules, and guidelines that govern the practice of nursing.

Knowledge of the legal and ethical concepts presented in this chapter promotes quality care in psychiatric mental health nursing practice and promotes legal accountability. The right to practice nursing carries with it the responsibility to maintain a

BOX 3–1 American Nurses Association Code of Ethics for Nurses

1. The nurse practices with compassion and respect for the inherent dignity, worth, and unique attributes of every person.
2. The nurse's primary commitment is to the patient whether an individual, family, group, community, or population.
3. The nurse promotes, advocates for, and strives to protect the health, safety, and rights of the patient.
4. The nurse has authority, accountability, and responsibility for nursing practice; makes decisions; and takes action consistent with the obligation to promote health and to provide optimal care.
5. The nurse owes the same duties to self as to others, including the responsibility to promote health and safety, preserve wholeness of character and integrity, maintain competence, and continue personal and professional growth.
6. The nurse, through individual and collective effort, establishes, maintains, and improves the ethical environment of the work setting and conditions of employment that are conducive to safe, quality health care.
7. The nurse, in all roles and settings, advances the profession through research and scholarly inquiry, professional standards development, and the generation of both nursing and health policy.
8. The nurse collaborates with other health professionals and the public to protect human rights, promote health diplomacy, and reduce health disparities.
9. The profession of nursing, collectively through its professional organizations, must articulate nursing values, maintain the integrity of the profession, and integrate principles of social justice into nursing and health policy.

Source: Reprinted with permission from American Nurses Association (ANA), Code of Ethics for Nurses with Interpretive Statements, © 2015 Nursebooks, Silver Spring, MD: ANA.

CORE CONCEPTS

Ethics is a branch of philosophy that deals with systematic approaches to distinguishing right from wrong behavior (Butts & Rich, 2016). **Bioethics** is the term applied to these principles when they refer to concepts within the scope of medicine, nursing, and allied health.

Moral behavior is conduct that results from serious critical thinking about how individuals ought to treat others. Moral behavior reflects the way a person interprets basic respect for other persons, such as the respect for autonomy, freedom, justice, honesty, and confidentiality.

Values are personal beliefs about what is important and desirable (Butts & Rich, 2016). **Values clarification** is a process of self-exploration through which individuals identify and rank their own personal values. This process increases awareness about why individuals behave in certain ways. Values clarification is important in nursing to increase understanding about why certain choices and decisions are made over others and how values affect nursing outcomes. A **right** is defined as "a valid, legally recognized claim or entitlement, encompassing both freedom from government interference or discriminatory treatment and an entitlement to a benefit or service" (Levy & Rubenstein, 1996). A right is *absolute* when there is no restriction whatsoever on the individual's entitlement. A *legal right* is one on which the society has agreed and formalized into law. Both the National League for Nursing and the American Hospital Association (AHA) have established guidelines of patients' rights. Although these are not considered legal documents, nurses and hospitals are considered responsible for upholding these rights of patients.

specific level of competency and to practice in accordance with certain ethical and legal standards of care.

Ethical Considerations

Theoretical Perspectives

An *ethical theory* is a moral principle or a set of moral principles that can be used in assessing what is morally right or morally wrong. These principles provide different frameworks for ethical decision making.

Utilitarianism

The basis of **utilitarianism** is "the greatest-happiness principle." This principle holds that actions are right to the degree that they tend to promote happiness and wrong as they tend to produce the reverse of happiness. Thus, the good is happiness and the right is that which promotes the good. Conversely, the wrongness of an action is determined by its tendency to bring about unhappiness. An ethical decision based on the utilitarian view looks at the end results of the decision. Action is taken on the basis of the end results that produced the most good (happiness) for the most people.

Kantianism

Named for philosopher Immanuel Kant, **Kantianism** is directly opposed to utilitarianism. Kant argued that it is not the consequences or end results that make an action right or wrong; rather it is the principle or motivation on which the action is based that is the morally decisive factor. Kantianism suggests that our actions are bound by a sense of duty. This theory is often called *deontology* (from the Greek word *deon*, which means "that which is binding; duty"). Kantian-directed ethical decisions are made out of respect for moral law. For example, "I make this choice because it is morally right and my duty to do so" (not because of consideration for a possible outcome).

Christian Ethics

This approach to ethical decision making is focused on the way of life and teachings of Jesus Christ. It advances the importance of virtues such as love, forgiveness, and honesty. One basic principle often associated with Christian ethics is known as the golden rule: "Do unto others as you would have them do unto you." The imperative demand of **Christian ethics** is that all decisions about right and wrong should be centered in love for God and in treating others with the same respect and dignity with which we would expect to be treated.

Natural Law Theory

Natural law theory is based on the writings of St. Thomas Aquinas. It advances the idea that decisions about right versus wrong are self-evident and determined by human nature. The theory espouses that, as rational human beings, we inherently know the difference between good and evil (believed to be knowledge that is given to man from God), and this knowledge directs our decision making.

Ethical Egoism

Ethical egoism espouses that what is right and good is what is best for the individual making the decision. An individual's actions are determined by what is to his or her own advantage. The action may not be best for anyone else involved, but consideration is only for the individual making the decision.

Providing patient-centered care, an important health professions education competency identified in the IOM report (2013), speaks to some elements of ethical egoism. This competency promotes listening to and respecting the patient's values, preferences, and expressed needs in care management decisions.

Ethical Dilemmas

An **ethical dilemma** is a situation that requires an individual to make a choice between two equally unfavorable alternatives (Catalano, 2015). Evidence exists to support both moral "rightness" and moral "wrongness" related to a certain action. The individual who must make the choice experiences conscious conflict regarding the decision.

Not all ethical issues are dilemmas. An ethical dilemma arises when there is no clear reason to choose one action over another. Ethical dilemmas generally create a great deal of emotion. Often, the reasons supporting each side of the argument for action are logical and appropriate. The actions associated with both sides are desirable in some respects and undesirable in others. In most situations, taking no action is considered an action taken. For example, consider a patient who refuses to take a prescribed cardiac medication, claiming that he does not believe it is necessary. Although each patient has the right to refuse medication under ordinary circumstances, if the same patient is known to be depressed and suicidal, might he be intending self-harm by his refusal to take such a medication? And, if so, what is the best course of action? Many healthcare settings have established guidelines for how to proceed should an ethical question or dilemma arise. Hospitals typically have a formal committee to explore and analyze ethical issues from several vantage points. Nurses can improve their critical thinking and clinical judgment skills by identifying such issues and seeking clarification through collaborative exploration with others and through ethics committee involvement.

Ethical Principles

Ethical principles are fundamental guidelines that influence decision making. The ethical principles of autonomy, beneficence, nonmaleficence, veracity, and justice are helpful and used frequently by healthcare workers to assist with ethical decision making.

Autonomy

The principle of **autonomy** arises from the Kantian view of persons as independent moral agents whose right to determine their own destinies should always be respected. Autonomy presumes that individuals are always capable of making independent choices for themselves. Healthcare workers know that this is not always the case. Children, comatose individuals, and people with serious mental illness are examples of clients who are incapable of making informed choices. In these instances, a representative for the individual is usually asked to intervene and give consent. However, healthcare workers must ensure that respect for an individual's autonomy is not disregarded in favor of what another person may view as best for the client.

Beneficence

Beneficence refers to one's duty to benefit or promote the good of others. Healthcare workers who act in their clients' interests are beneficent, provided their actions really do serve the client's best interest. In fact, some duties seem to take preference over other duties. For example, the duty to respect the autonomy of an individual may be overridden when that individual has been deemed harmful to self or others. "Doing good" for the patient should not be confused with "doing whatever the patient wants" (What do I do now?, 2013). Good care must include a holistic focus that considers the patient's beliefs, feelings, and wishes; the wishes of the family and significant others; and considerations about competent nursing care (Catalano, 2015). Despite these guidelines, it is not always clear which action *is* in the best interest of the patient. When such dilemmas occur, nurses should reach out to available resources such as supervisors and ethics committees to build confidence that decisions about patient care have explored various vantage points.

Peplau (1991) recognized client **advocacy** as an essential role for the psychiatric nurse. The term *advocacy* means acting in another's behalf—being a supporter or defender. Being a client advocate in psychiatric nursing means helping clients fulfill needs that, without assistance and because of their illness, may go unfulfilled. Individuals with mental illness are not always able to speak for themselves. Nurses serve in this manner to protect the clients' rights and interests. Strategies include educating clients and their families about their legal rights, ensuring that clients have sufficient information to make informed decisions or to give informed consent, and assisting clients to consider alternatives and supporting them in the decisions they make. Additionally, nurses may act as advocates by speaking on behalf of individuals with mental illness to secure essential mental health services.

Nonmaleficence

Nonmaleficence is the requirement that healthcare providers do no harm to their clients, either intentionally or unintentionally. Some philosophers suggest that this principle is more important than beneficence; that is, they support the notion that it is more important to avoid doing harm than it is to do good. In any event, ethical dilemmas often arise when a conflict exists between an individual's rights and what is thought to best represent the welfare of the individual. An example of this conflict might occur when a psychiatric client refuses antipsychotic medication (consistent with his or her rights), and the nurse must then decide how to maintain client safety while psychotic symptoms continue.

Justice

The principle of **justice** has been referred to as the "justice as fairness" principle. It is sometimes called *distributive justice,* and its basic premise lies with the right of individuals to be treated equally and fairly regardless of race, sex, marital status, medical diagnosis, social standing, economic level, or religious beliefs (Catalano, 2015). When applied to healthcare, this principle suggests that all resources within the society (including healthcare services) ought to be distributed evenly without respect to socioeconomic status. Thus, according to this principle, the vast disparity in the quality of care dispensed to the various classes within our society would be considered unjust. *Retribution* or *restorative* justice refers to the rules for responding when expectations for fairness are violated. *Social* justice can be summarized as the principle that rules for both distribution and rules for retribution should be fair and people should play by the rules (Maiese, 2017). It is important for nurses to recognize that in the latest revision of the Code of Ethics for Nurses (ANA, 2015), a new focus in one of the provisions states that nursing should integrate principles of social justice both in practice and in developing health policy.

Veracity

The principle of **veracity** refers to one's duty to always be truthful. Catalano (2015) states that veracity "requires the health care provider to tell the truth and not intentionally deceive or mislead clients" (p. 126). There are times when limitations must be placed on this principle, such as when the truth would knowingly produce harm or interfere with the recovery process. Being honest is not always easy, but rarely is lying justified. Clients have the right to know about their diagnosis, treatment, and prognosis.

A Model for Making Ethical Decisions

The following is a set of steps that may be used in making an ethical decision. These steps closely resemble the steps of the nursing process:

1. **Assessment:** Gather the subjective and objective data about a situation. Consider personal values

as well as values of others involved in the ethical dilemma.

2. **Problem identification:** Identify the conflict between two or more alternative actions.
3. **Planning:**
   a. Explore the benefits and consequences of each alternative.
   b. Consider principles of ethical theories.
   c. Select an alternative.
4. **Implementation:** Act on the decision made and communicate the decision to others.
5. **Evaluation:** Evaluate outcomes.

A schematic of this model is presented in Figure 3–1. A case study using this decision-making model is presented in Box 3–2. If the outcome is acceptable, action continues in the manner selected. If the outcome is unacceptable, benefits and consequences of the remaining alternatives are reexamined, and steps 3 through 7 in Box 3–2 are repeated.

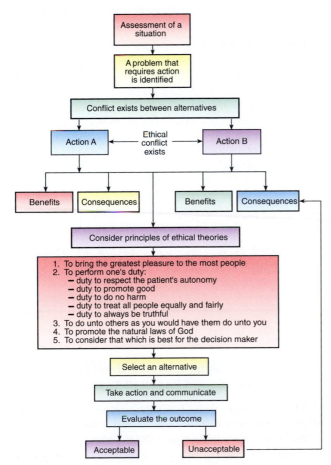

FIGURE 3–1   Ethical decision-making model.

Ethical and Legal Issues in Psychiatric Mental Health Nursing

The Right to Treatment

Anyone who is admitted to a hospital has the right to treatment. For example, a psychiatric patient cannot legally be hospitalized and then denied appropriate treatment. The AHA, although not having the authority of law, has also identified the rights of any hospitalized patient. The AHA patient bill of rights was historically written with an emphasis on protecting the patient from a breach of reasonable standards while hospitalized. These rights were revised in 2003 to create an emphasis on the importance of the collaborative relationship between the client and the hospital healthcare team. Titled "The Patient Care Partnership," this brochure informs patients that they have a right to high-quality care while hospitalized, to a clean and safe environment, to be involved in their care, to have their privacy protected, to get help when leaving the hospital, and to get help with their billing claims (AHA, 2003). In 2010, federal law expanded patient rights to include insurability in spite of pre-existing conditions. However, federal healthcare law continues to be a debated issue and will no doubt continue to see changes depending on the prevailing political climate. Nurses practicing in hospital settings need to be aware of and adhere to legal statutes, accepted standards of practice, and organizational policies with regard to a client's rights during hospital treatment.

The Right to Refuse Treatment (Including Medication)

Legally, patients have the right to refuse treatment unless the treatment requires immediate intervention to prevent death or serious harm to the patient or another person (Sadock, Sadock, & Ruiz, 2015). The U.S. Constitution and several of its amendments affirm this right (e.g., the First Amendment, which addresses the rights of speech, thought, and expression; the Eighth Amendment, which grants the right to freedom from cruel and unusual punishment; and the Fifth and Fourteenth Amendments, which grant due process of law and equal protection for all). In psychiatry, however, there are both ethical and legal issues that must be considered. Sometimes patients are involuntarily hospitalized because they are at risk of harming themselves or others and do not recognize the dangerousness of their symptoms. In emergency cases, sedative medication may be administered without the patient's consent in order to protect patients from harming themselves

BOX 3–2 Ethical Decision Making—A Case Study

STEP 1. ASSESSMENT

Tonja is a 17-year-old girl who is currently on the psychiatric unit with a diagnosis of conduct disorder. Tonja reports that she has been sexually active since she was 14. She had an abortion when she was 15 and a second one just 6 weeks ago. She states that her mother told her she has "had her last abortion" and that she has to start taking birth control pills. She asks her nurse, Kimberly, to give her some information about the pills and to tell her how to go about getting some. Kimberly believes Tonja desperately needs information about birth control pills, as well as other types of contraceptives, but the psychiatric unit is part of a Catholic hospital, and hospital policy prohibits distributing this type of information.

STEP 2. PROBLEM IDENTIFICATION

A conflict exists between the client's need for information, the nurse's desire to provide that information, and the institution's policy prohibiting the provision of that information.

STEP 3. ALTERNATIVES—BENEFITS AND CONSEQUENCES

Alternative 1: Give the client information and risk losing job.

Alternative 2: Do not give client information and compromise own values of holistic nursing.

Alternative 3: Refer the client to another source outside the hospital and risk reprimand from supervisor.

STEP 4. CONSIDER PRINCIPLES OF ETHICAL THEORIES

Alternative 1: Giving the client information would certainly respect the client's autonomy and would benefit the client by decreasing her chances of becoming pregnant again. It would not be to the best advantage of Kimberly, in that she would likely lose her job. And according to the beliefs of the Catholic hospital, the natural laws of God would be violated.

Alternative 2: Withholding information restricts the client's autonomy. It has the potential for doing harm, in that without the use of contraceptives, the client may become pregnant again (and she implies that this is not what she wants). Kimberly's Christian ethic is violated in that this action is not what she would want "done unto her."

Alternative 3: A referral would respect the client's autonomy, would promote good, would do no harm (except perhaps to Kimberly's ego from the possible reprimand), and this decision would comply with Kimberly's Christian ethic.

STEP 5. SELECT AN ALTERNATIVE

Alternative 3 is selected on the basis of the ethical theories of utilitarianism (does the most good for the greatest number), Christian ethics (Kimberly's belief of "Do unto others as you would have others do unto you"), Kantianism (to perform one's duty), and the ethical principles of autonomy, beneficence, and nonmaleficence. The success of this decision depends on the client's follow-through with the referral and compliance with use of the contraceptives.

STEP 6. TAKE ACTION AND COMMUNICATE

Taking action involves providing information in writing for Tonja, perhaps making a phone call and setting up an appointment for her with Planned Parenthood. Communicating involves sharing the information with Tonja's mother. Communication also includes documentation of the referral in the client's chart.

STEP 7. EVALUATE THE OUTCOME

An acceptable outcome might indicate that Tonja did indeed keep her appointment at Planned Parenthood and is complying with the prescribed contraceptive regimen. It might also include Kimberly's input into the change process in her institution to implement these types of referrals to other clients who request them.

An unacceptable outcome might be indicated by Tonja's lack of follow-through with the appointment at Planned Parenthood or lack of compliance in using the contraceptives, resulting in another pregnancy. Kimberly may also view a reprimand from her supervisor as an unacceptable outcome, particularly if she is told that she must select other alternatives should this situation arise in the future. This may motivate Kimberly to make another decision—that of seeking employment in an institution that supports a philosophy more consistent with her own.

---

or others. Because laws vary from state to state, it is important for nurses to know the laws that pertain in their local jurisdiction. Organizational policies in the nurse's practice setting should also guide decision making.

Although many courts support a client's right to refuse medications in the psychiatric area, exceptions do exist. When making a decision about forced medication, Weiss-Kaffie and Purtell (2001) state:

The treatment team must determine that three criteria be met to force medication without client consent. The client must exhibit behavior that is dangerous to self or others; the medication ordered by the physician must have a reasonable chance of providing help to the client; and clients who refuse medication must be judged incompetent to evaluate the benefits of the treatment in question. (p. 361)

Evidence supports the long-term benefits of involuntary medication, particularly for patients with schizophrenia and bipolar disorders (Mental Illness Policy Org., 2017) and current research demonstrating the particular benefits of treating a first episode of psychosis as important in decreasing long-term negative consequences may increase acceptability of involuntary medication as an early intervention when needed.

More recently, some states have adopted laws that allow a court to mandate outpatient treatment for people with mental illness who have a history of violent behavior. In New York City, this law (known as *Kendra's law*) also includes a provision for ordering an individual to take medication as part of the treatment plan.

The Right to the Least Restrictive Treatment Alternative

The right to the least restrictive treatment alternative means that clients who can be adequately treated in an outpatient setting should not be hospitalized, and if they are hospitalized, they should not be sedated, restrained, or secluded unless other less restrictive measures were found to be unsuccessful. In other words, clients have a right to whatever level of treatment is effective and least restricts their freedom. The "restrictiveness" of psychiatric therapy can be described in the context of a continuum based on severity of illness. Clients may be treated on an outpatient basis, in day hospitals, or through voluntary or involuntary hospitalization. Symptoms may be treated with verbal rehabilitative techniques and move successively to behavioral techniques, chemical interventions, mechanical restraints, or electroconvulsive therapy. However, ethical issues arise in selecting the least restrictive means among involuntary chemical intervention, seclusion, and mechanical restraints. Sadock and colleagues (2015) state that

distinguishing among these interventions on the basis of restrictiveness proves to be a purely subjective exercise fraught with personal bias. Moreover, each of these three interventions is both more and less restrictive than each of the other two. Nevertheless, the effort should be made to think in terms of restrictiveness when deciding how to treat patients. (p. 1386)

Although these rights may seem reasonable and expected, it is important to recognize that clients with mental illness have historically been hospitalized against their will simply because they had a mental illness. In the case of *O'Connor v. Donaldson* (1976), the Supreme Court ruled that harmless mentally ill individuals cannot be confined against their will if they are able to remain safe outside of a hospital setting. Only if they are considered dangerous to themselves or others or are so unable to care for themselves that their safety and survival are at risk may they be confined involuntarily. In 1981, the case of *Roger v. Oken* culminated in the ruling that all patients, even those involuntarily hospitalized, are competent to refuse treatment, but a legal guardian may authorize treatment (Sadock et al., 2015). These laws and policies have attempted to better protect the rights of clients with mental illness while still recognizing that, at times, individuals with acute mental illness may be unable to make decisions in the interest of their safety and survival.

Ideally, it is hoped that the person with mental illness recognizes his or her need for treatment and agrees voluntarily to be hospitalized if this measure is recommended by the healthcare provider. The client who is voluntarily hospitalized typically signs a consent to treatment upon admission, but it remains the client's right, as a voluntary patient, to revoke that consent and to be discharged from the hospital if he or she so chooses.

Legal Considerations

The Patient Self-Determination Act, as part of the Omnibus Budget Reconciliation Act of 1990, went into effect on December 1, 1991. Cady (2010) states:

The Patient Self-determination Act requires healthcare facilities to provide clear written information for every patient concerning his/her legal rights to make healthcare decisions, including the right to accept or refuse treatment. (p. 118)

Box 3–3 lists the rights of patients affirmed by this law.

Nurse Practice Acts

The legal parameters of professional and practical nursing are defined within each state by the state's nurse practice act. These documents are passed by the state legislature and in general are concerned with such provisions as the following:

- The definition of important terms, including the definition of *nursing* and the various types of nurses recognized
- A statement of the education and other training or requirements for licensure and reciprocity

---

BOX 3–3 Patient Self-Determination Act–Patient Rights

1. The right to appropriate treatment and related services in a setting and under conditions that are the most supportive of such person's personal liability, and restrict such liberty only to the extent necessary consistent with such person's treatment needs, applicable requirements of law, and applicable judicial orders.

2. The right to an individualized, written treatment or service plan (such plan to be developed promptly after admission of such person), the right to treatment based on such plan, the right to periodic review and reassessment of treatment and related service needs, and the right to appropriate revision of such plan, including any revision necessary to provide a description of mental health services that may be needed after such person is discharged from such program or facility.

3. The right to ongoing participation, in a manner appropriate to a person's capabilities, in the planning of mental health services to be provided (including the right to participate in the development and periodic revision of the plan).

4. The right to be provided with a reasonable explanation, in terms and language appropriate to a person's condition and ability to understand the person's general mental and physical (if appropriate) condition, the objectives of treatment, the nature and significant possible adverse effects of recommended treatment, the reasons why a particular treatment is considered appropriate, and reasons why access to certain visitors may not be appropriate, and any appropriate and available alternative treatments, services, and types of providers of mental health services.

5. The right not to receive a mode or course of treatment in the absence of informed, voluntary, written consent to treatment except during an emergency situation or as permitted by law when the person is being treated as a result of a court order.

6. The right not to participate in experimentation in the absence of informed, voluntary, written consent (includes human subject protection).

7. The right to freedom from restraint or seclusion, other than as a mode or course of treatment or restraint or seclusion during an emergency situation with a written order by a responsible mental health professional.

8. The right to a humane treatment environment that affords reasonable protection from harm and appropriate privacy with regard to personal needs.

9. The right to access, on request, to such person's mental healthcare records.

10. The right, in the case of a person admitted on a residential or inpatient care basis, to converse with others privately, to have convenient and reasonable access to the telephone and mail, and to see visitors during regularly scheduled hours. (For treatment purposes, specific individuals may be excluded.)

11. The right to be informed promptly and in writing at the time of admission of these rights.

12. The right to assert grievances with respect to infringement of these rights.

13. The right to exercise these rights without reprisal.

14. The right of referral to other providers upon discharge.

Source: Adapted from the U.S. Code, Title 42, Section 10841, The Public Health and Welfare, 1991.

■ Broad statements that describe the scope of practice for various levels of nursing (APN, RN, LPN)

■ Conditions under which a nurse's license may be suspended or revoked, and instructions for appeal

■ The general authority and powers of the state board of nursing

Most nurse practice acts are general in their terminology and do not provide specific guidelines for practice. Nurses must understand the scope of practice that is protected by their license and should seek assistance from legal counsel if they are unsure about the proper interpretation of a nurse practice act.

Types of Law

There are two general categories of law that are of most concern to nurses: statutory law and common law. These laws are identified by their source or origin.

Statutory Law

A **statutory law** is a law that has been enacted by a legislative body, such as a county or city council, state legislature, or the U.S. Congress. An example of statutory law is the nurse practice acts.

Common Law

Common laws are derived from decisions made in previous cases. These laws apply to a body of principles that evolve from court decisions resolving various controversies. Because common law in the United States has been developed on a state basis, the law on specific subjects may differ from state to state. An example of a common law might be how different states deal with a nurse's refusal to provide care for a specific client.

Classifications Within Statutory and Common Law

Broadly speaking, there are two kinds of unlawful acts: civil and criminal. Both statutory law and common law have civil and criminal components.

Civil Law

Civil law protects the private and property rights of individuals and businesses. Private individuals or groups may bring a legal action to court for breach of civil law. These legal actions are of two basic types: torts and contracts.

Torts

A **tort** is a violation of a civil law in which an individual has been wronged. In a tort action, one party asserts that wrongful conduct on the part of the other has caused harm, and the first party seeks compensation for harm suffered. A tort may be *intentional* or *unintentional*. Examples of unintentional torts are malpractice and negligence actions. An example of an intentional tort is the touching of another person without that person's consent. Intentional touching (e.g., a medical treatment) without the client's consent can result in a charge of battery, an intentional tort.

Contracts

In a contract action, one party asserts that the other party, in failing to fulfill an obligation, has breached the contract, and either compensation or performance of the obligation is sought as remedy. An example is an action by a mental health professional whose clinical privileges have been reduced or terminated in violation of an implied contract between the professional and a hospital.

Criminal Law

Criminal law provides protection from conduct deemed injurious to the public welfare. It provides for punishment of those found to have engaged in such conduct, which commonly includes imprisonment, parole conditions, a loss of privilege (such as a license), a fine, or any combination of these (Ellis & Hartley, 2012). An example of a violation of criminal law is the theft by a hospital employee of supplies or drugs.

Legal Issues in Psychiatric Mental Health Nursing

Confidentiality and Right to Privacy

The Fourth, Fifth, and Fourteenth Amendments to the U.S. Constitution protect an individual's privacy. Most states have statutes protecting the confidentiality of client records and communications. Nurses must recognize that the only individuals who have a right to observe a client or have access to medical information are those involved in his or her medical care. The patient must provide written consent for healthcare information to be shared with anyone outside the current treatment team.

HIPAA

Until 1996, client confidentiality in medical records was not protected by federal law. In August 1996, President Clinton signed the Health Insurance Portability and Accountability Act (HIPAA) into law. This federal privacy rule pertains to data called *protected health information* (PHI) and applies to most individuals and institutions involved in healthcare. Notice of privacy policies must be provided to clients upon entry into the healthcare system. PHI is individually identifiable health information indicators that "relate to past, present, or future physical or mental health or condition of the individual, or the past, present, or future payment for the provision of health care to an individual; and (1) that identifies the individual; or (2) with respect to which there is a reasonable basis to believe the information can be used to identify the individual" (U.S. Department of Health & Human Services, 2003). These specific identifiers are listed in Box 3–4.

Under HIPAA, individuals have the rights to access their medical records, to have corrections made to their medical records, and to decide with whom their medical information may be shared. The actual document belongs to the facility or the therapist, but the information contained therein belongs to the client. The passage of HIPAA increased the level of control clients have over the information maintained in their medical records.

In 2013, HIPAA privacy and security rules were expanded to afford more rights to patients with regard to their medical information and to ensure greater security of a person's health information. In some cases, patients, for example, when they are paying out of pocket for care, can tell a provider that they do not want treatment information shared with their health insurance provider (U.S. Department of Health & Human Services, 2013). Nurses in any practice setting need to be aware of these HIPAA laws and of any new provisions in law that will impact the conduct of their practice.

Pertinent medical information may be released without consent in a life-threatening situation. If information is released in an emergency, the following

BOX 3–4 Protected Health Information (PHI): Individually Identifiable Indicators

1. Names
2. Postal address information (except state), including street address, city, county, precinct, and zip code
3. All elements of dates (except year) for dates directly related to an individual, including birth date, admission date, discharge date, date of death; and all ages over 89 and all elements of dates (including year) indicative of such age, except that such ages and elements may be aggregated into a single category of age 90 or older
4. Telephone numbers
5. Fax numbers
6. Electronic mail addresses
7. Social Security numbers
8. Medical record numbers
9. Health plan beneficiary numbers
10. Account numbers
11. Certificate/license numbers
12. Vehicle identifiers and serial numbers, including license plate numbers
13. Device identifiers and serial numbers
14. Web Universal Resource Locators (URLs)
15. Internet protocol (IP) address numbers
16. Biometric identifiers, including finger and voice prints
17. Full face photographic images and any comparable images
18. Any other unique identifying number, characteristic, or code

Source: U.S. Department of Health and Human Services (USDHHS). (2003). *Standards for privacy of individually identifiable health information. Washington, DC: USDHHS.*

information must be recorded in the client's record: date of disclosure, person to whom information was disclosed, reason for disclosure, reason written consent could not be obtained, and the specific information disclosed.

Most states have statutes that pertain to the doctrine of **privileged communication.** Although the codes differ markedly from state to state, most grant certain professionals privileges under which they may refuse to reveal information about, and communications with, clients. In most states, the doctrine of privileged communication applies to psychiatrists and attorneys; in some instances, psychologists, clergy, and nurses are also included.

In certain instances, nurses may be called on to testify in cases in which the medical record is used as evidence. In most states, the right to privacy of these records is exempted in civil or criminal proceedings. Therefore, it is important that nurses document with these possibilities in mind. Strict record-keeping using statements that are objective and nonjudgmental, care plans that are specific in their prescriptive interventions, and documentation that describes those interventions and their subsequent evaluation all serve the best interests of the client, the nurse, and the institution should questions regarding care arise. Documentation very often weighs heavily in malpractice case decisions.

The right to confidentiality is a basic one, and especially so in psychiatry. Although societal attitudes are improving, individuals have experienced discrimination in the past for no other reason than that they have a history of mental illness. Nurses working in psychiatric mental health nursing must guard the privacy of their clients with great diligence.

Exception: A Duty to Warn (Protection of a Third Party)

There are exceptions to the laws of privacy and confidentiality. One of these exceptions stems from the 1974 case of *Tarasoff v. Regents of the University of California.* The incident from which this case evolved came about in the late 1960s. Mr. P., a young man from Bengal, India, who was a graduate student at the University of California (UC), Berkeley, fell in love with another university student (Ms. Tarasoff). Because she was not interested in an exclusive relationship with Mr. P., he became very resentful and angry. He began to stalk her and to record some of their conversations in an effort to determine why she did not love him. He soon became very depressed and neglected his health, appearance, and studies.

Ms. Tarasoff spent the summer of 1969 in South America. During this time, Mr. P. entered therapy with a psychologist at UC. He confided in the psychologist that he intended to kill his former girlfriend (identifying her by name) when she returned from vacation. The psychologist recommended civil commitment for Mr. P., claiming that he was suffering from acute and severe paranoid schizophrenia. Mr. P. was picked up by the campus police but released a short time later because he appeared rational and promised to stay away from Ms. Tarasoff. Neither Ms. Tarasoff nor her parents received any warning of the threat of Mr. P.'s intention to kill her.

When Ms. Tarasoff returned to campus in October 1969, Mr. P. resumed his stalking behavior and eventually stabbed her to death. Ms. Tarasoff's parents sued the psychologist, several psychiatrists, and the university for failure to warn. The case was referred to the California Supreme Court, which ruled that a mental health professional has a duty not only to a client but also to individuals who are being threatened by that client. The Court stated:

> Once a therapist does in fact determine, or under applicable professional standards should have determined, that a patient poses a serious danger of violence to others, he bears a duty to exercise reasonable care to protect the foreseeable victim of that danger. While the discharge of this duty of due care will necessarily vary with the facts of each case, in each instance the adequacy of the therapist's conduct must be measured against the traditional negligence standard of reasonable care under the circumstances. (*Tarasoff v. Regents of University of California,* 1974a)

The defendants argued that warning the woman or her family would have breached professional ethics and violated the client's right to privacy. But the court ruled that "the confidential character of patient-psychotherapist communications must yield to the extent that disclosure is essential to avert danger to others. The protective privilege ends where the public peril begins" (*Tarasoff v. Regents of University of California,* 1974b).

In 1976, the California Supreme Court expanded the original case ruling (now referred to as *Tarasoff I*). The second ruling (known as *Tarasoff II*) broadened the ruling of "duty to warn" to include "duty to protect." They stated that, under certain circumstances, a therapist might be required to warn an individual, notify police, or take whatever steps are necessary to protect the intended victim from harm. This duty to protect can also occur in instances when patients must be protected by healthcare providers because they are vulnerable as a result of their inability to identify harmful situations (Guido, 2014).

The *Tarasoff* rulings created a great deal of controversy in the psychiatric community regarding breach of confidentiality and the subsequent negative impact on the client-therapist relationship. However, most states now recognize that therapists have ethical and legal obligations to prevent their clients from harming themselves or others. Many states have passed their own variations on the original "protect and warn" legislation, but in most cases, courts have outlined the following guidelines for therapists to

follow in determining their obligation to take protective measures:

1. Assessment of a threat of violence by a client toward another individual
2. Identification of the intended victim
3. Ability to intervene in a feasible, meaningful way to protect the intended victim

When these guidelines apply to a specific situation, it is reasonable for the therapist to notify the victim, law enforcement authorities, and/or relatives of the intended victim. The therapist may also consider initiating voluntary or involuntary commitment of the client in an effort to prevent potential violence.

Implications for Nursing Although the original decision in the *Tarasoff* ruling was directed toward psychotherapists, it has become more broadly applied since that time. Not all states identify registered nurses as having a duty to warn, but other statutes include a duty to warn for anyone from a licensed practical nurse to licensed certified advanced practice nurses. As of 2015, there are three states (Maine, Nevada, and North Dakota) that have not yet addressed the issue of duty to warn and one state (North Carolina) that does not recognize the duty to warn (Henderson, 2015; National Conference of State Legislatures, 2016). Even in states that do not address a duty to warn, practitioners still need to make an ethical decision about warning a potential victim. All nurses, not just those practicing in psychiatric nursing, need to be informed about the laws in their state regarding duty to warn. As Henderson (2015) notes, emergency nurses are often the frontline healthcare workers in a position to identify persons at risk for violence and to protect the safety of the patient and others. In psychiatric mental health nursing practice, if a client confides in the nurse the potential for harm to an intended victim, it is the duty of the nurse to report this information to the psychiatrist or to other team members. Doing so is not a breach of confidentiality, and the nurse may be considered negligent for failure to do so. All members of the treatment team must be made aware of the potential danger that the client poses to self or others. Detailed written documentation of the situation is also essential.

Exception: Suspected Child or Elder Abuse

Every state requires that healthcare professionals—and in many jurisdictions, every citizen—report suspicion of child abuse to legal authorities (Hartsell & Bernstein, 2013). Many jurisdictions also have statutes requiring that suspected elder abuse or neglect be reported. At times, healthcare professionals are worried that they may be liable for false allegations and therefore may be reluctant to report, but reporting statutes generally grant immunity to anyone making a good faith report about a reasonable suspicion, and in some jurisdictions, it is a criminal act *not* to report, "so declining to report should not be considered an option" (Hartsell & Bernstein, 2013, p. 170).

Implications for Nursing There is often an element of clinical judgment about whether a patient's communication raises a reasonable suspicion of abuse. For example, when a person is experiencing hallucinations or delusions, his or her perception about events may be distorted. The nurse has a responsibility to explore all of the patient's perceptions of abuse or mistreatment and discuss them with other healthcare team members to identify the most appropriate decision considering legal, ethical, and clinical factors.

Informed Consent

According to law, all individuals have the right to decide whether to accept or reject treatment. A healthcare provider can be charged with assault and battery for providing life-sustaining treatment to a client when the client has not agreed to it. The rationale for the doctrine of **informed consent** is the preservation and protection of individual autonomy in determining what will and will not happen to the person's body (Guido, 2014).

Informed consent is a client's permission granted to a physician to perform a therapeutic procedure, before information about the procedure has been presented to the client with adequate time given for consideration about the pros and cons. The client should receive information such as what treatment alternatives are available; why the physician believes this treatment is most appropriate; the possible outcomes, risks, and adverse effects; the possible outcome should the client select another treatment alternative; and the possible outcome should the client choose to have no treatment. An example of a treatment in the psychiatric area that requires informed consent is electroconvulsive therapy.

There are some conditions under which treatment may be performed without obtaining informed consent. A client's refusal to accept treatment may be challenged under the following circumstances (Guido, 2014; Levy & Rubenstein, 1996):

1. When a client is mentally incompetent to make a decision and treatment is necessary to preserve life or avoid serious harm

2. When refusing treatment endangers the life or health of another

3. During an emergency in which a client is in no condition to exercise judgment

4. When the client is a child (consent is obtained from parent or surrogate)

5. In the case of therapeutic privilege: Information about a treatment may be withheld if the physician can show that full disclosure would

   a. Hinder or complicate necessary treatment,

   b. Cause severe psychological harm, or

   c. Be so upsetting as to render a rational decision by the client impossible.

Although most clients in psychiatric and mental health facilities are competent and capable of giving informed consent, those with severe psychiatric illness do not possess the cognitive ability to do so. If an individual has been legally determined to be mentally incompetent, consent is obtained from the legal guardian. Difficulty arises when no legal determination has been made, but the individual's current mental state prohibits informed decision making (e.g., the person who is psychotic, unconscious, or inebriated). In these instances, informed consent is usually obtained from the individual's nearest relative, or if none exist and time permits, the physician may ask the court to appoint a conservator or guardian. When time does not permit court intervention, permission may be sought from the hospital administrator.

A client or guardian always has the right to withdraw consent after it has been given. When this occurs, the physician should inform (or re-inform) the client about the consequences of refusing treatment. If treatment has already been initiated, the physician should terminate treatment in a way least likely to cause injury to the client and inform the client or guardian of the risks associated with interrupted treatment (Guido, 2014).

The nurse's role in obtaining informed consent is usually defined by agency policy. A nurse may sign the consent form as witness for the client's signature. However, legal liability for informed consent lies with the physician. The nurse acts as client advocate ensuring that the following three major elements of informed consent have been addressed:

1. **Knowledge:** The client has received adequate information on which to base his or her decision.

2. **Competency:** The individual's cognition is not impaired to an extent that would interfere with decision making, but if cognition is so impaired, the individual has a legal representative.

3. **Free will:** The individual has given consent voluntarily without pressure or coercion from others.

Restraints and Seclusion

An individual's privacy and personal security are protected by the Patient Self-Determination Act of 1991. This legislation includes a set of patient rights, one of which is an individual's right to freedom from restraint and from seclusion except in an emergency situation. The use of seclusion and restraint as a therapeutic intervention for psychiatric patients has been controversial, and many efforts have been made through federal and state regulations and through standards set forth by accrediting bodies to minimize or eliminate its use. In addition, an element of moral decision making is involved when any kind of treatment is coerced, as is often the case with seclusion and restraint. Landeweer, Abma, and Widdershoven (2011) point out that although coercion may sometimes be necessary, it can be detrimental to the patient because it may produce trauma and mistrust. Most hospitals have a forum, such as an ethics committee, to discuss these ethical issues. One advantage of using such forums to guide moral decision making is that, by exploring issues (such as the use of seclusion and restraint) with a diverse group of people who have different vantage points, alternative treatments can be identified and explored.

Because injuries and deaths have been associated with restraint and seclusion, this treatment requires careful attention whenever it is used. Further, the laws, regulations, accreditation standards, and hospital policies are frequently revised, so it is important for anyone practicing in inpatient psychiatric settings to be well informed in each of these areas.

In psychiatry, the term *restraints* generally refers to a set of leather straps that are used to restrain the extremities of an individual whose behavior is out of control and who poses an immediate risk to the physical safety and psychological well-being of the individual and others. It is important to note, however, that the current generally accepted definition of restraint refers not only to leather restraints but also to any manual method or medication used to restrict a person's freedom of movement. Restraints are never to be used as punishment or for the convenience of staff. Other measures to decrease agitation, such as "talking down" (verbal intervention) and chemical restraints (tranquilizing medication) are the preferred first-line interventions. If these interventions are ineffective, mechanical restraints may be instituted (although some controversy exists as to whether chemical restraints are indeed less restrictive than mechanical restraints). *Seclusion* is another type of physical restraint in which the client is confined alone in a room from which he or she is unable to leave. The room is usually minimally furnished with items to promote the client's comfort and safety.

The Joint Commission, an association that accredits healthcare organizations, has established specific standards regarding the use of seclusion and restraint in behavioral healthcare. Some examples of current standards include the following (The Joint Commission, 2017):

1. Staff are trained and competent to minimize the use of restraint and seclusion and, when use is indicated, to use restraint and seclusion safely.

2. Seclusion or restraint is discontinued at the earliest possible time regardless of when the order is scheduled to expire.

3. Unless state law is more restrictive, written and verbal orders for restraint or seclusion must be renewed every 4 hours for adults ages 18 and older, every 2 hours for children and adolescents ages 9 to 17, and every hour for children younger than 9 years.

4. The initial assessment of an individual who is at risk for harming himself or herself, staff, or others includes identifying techniques to help the individual control his or her behavior; any pre-existing medical conditions, physical disabilities, or other limitations that might place the individual at greater risk during restraint or seclusion; history of physical or sexual abuse or other trauma; and their preferences about whether they would like family notified in the event of an episode of seclusion or restraint. Patients who are simultaneously restrained and secluded must be continuously monitored in person by trained staff. After the first hour a person in seclusion without restraints may be continuously monitored through simultaneous audio and video equipment if consistent with the individual's condition and wishes. Staff who are involved in restraint and seclusion are trained and competent to assess the patient at the initiation of restraint or seclusion and every 15 minutes thereafter including assessment for any signs of injury, nutrition and hydration, circulation and

range of motion, vital signs, hygiene and elimination, physical and psychological status and comfort, and readiness for discontinuation of restraint or seclusion.

The laws, regulations, accreditation standards, and hospital policies pertaining to restraint and seclusion share a common priority of maintaining patient safety for a procedure that has the potential to incur injury or death. The importance of close and careful monitoring cannot be overstated.

False imprisonment is the deliberate and unauthorized confinement of a person within fixed limits by the use of verbal or physical means (Ellis & Hartley, 2012). Healthcare workers may be charged with false imprisonment for restraining or secluding—against the wishes of the client—anyone having been admitted to the hospital voluntarily. Should a voluntarily admitted client decompensate to a point that restraint or seclusion for protection of self or others is necessary, court intervention to determine competency and involuntary commitment is required to preserve the client's rights to privacy and freedom.

Hospitalization

Voluntary Admissions

Each year, more than 1 million persons are admitted to healthcare facilities for psychiatric treatment; of these admissions, approximately two-thirds are considered voluntary. To be admitted voluntarily, an individual makes direct application to the institution for services and may stay as long as treatment is deemed necessary. He or she may sign out of the hospital at any time unless, following a mental status examination, the healthcare professional determines that the client may be harmful to self or others and recommends that the admission status be changed from voluntary to involuntary. Although these types of admissions are considered voluntary, it is important to ensure that the individual comprehends the meaning of his or her actions, has not been coerced in any manner, and is willing to proceed with admission.

Involuntary Commitment

Although the term *involuntary hospitalization* is preferred by some rather than the term *involuntary commitment*, it must be understood that this process needs to be conducted with respect to state and federal law. Because involuntary hospitalization results in substantial restrictions of the rights of an individual, the admission process is subject to the guarantee of the Fourteenth Amendment to the U.S. Constitution that provides citizens protection against loss of liberty and ensures due process rights (Weiss-Kaffie & Purtell, 2001). Involuntary hospitalizations are made for various reasons. Most states commonly cite the following criteria:

- The person is imminently dangerous to himself or herself (i.e., suicidal intent).
- The person is a danger to others (i.e., aggressive, violent, or homicidal).
- The person is unable to take care of basic personal needs (the "gravely disabled").

Under the Fourth Amendment, individuals are protected from unlawful searches and seizures without probable cause. Therefore, the individual recommending involuntary hospitalization must show probable cause for hospitalizing the client against his or her wishes; that is, the person must show that there is cause to believe that the client would be dangerous to self or others, is mentally ill and in need of treatment, or is gravely disabled.

Emergency Commitments

Emergency commitments are sought when an individual manifests behavior that is clearly and imminently dangerous to self or others. These admissions are usually instigated by relatives or friends of the individual, police officers, the court, or healthcare professionals. Emergency commitments are time-limited, and a court hearing for the individual is scheduled, usually within 72 hours. At that time, the court may decide that the client may be discharged; or, if deemed necessary, and voluntary admission is refused by the client, an additional period of involuntary hospitalization may be ordered. In most instances, another hearing is scheduled for a specified time (usually in 7 to 21 days).

The Mentally Ill Person in Need of Treatment

A second type of involuntary commitment is for the observation and treatment of mentally ill persons in need of treatment. These are typically longer than emergency commitments. Most states have established definitions of what constitutes "mentally ill" for purposes of state involuntary admission statutes. Some examples include individuals who, because of severe mental illness, are

- Unable to make informed decisions concerning treatment
- Likely to cause harm to self or others
- Unable to fulfill basic personal needs necessary for health and safety

In determining whether commitment is required, the court looks for substantial evidence of abnormal conduct—evidence that cannot be explained as the result of a physical cause. There must be "clear and convincing evidence" as well as "probable cause" to substantiate the need for involuntary hospitalization to ensure that an individual's rights under the Constitution are protected. As mentioned earlier, the U.S. Supreme Court, in *O'Connor v. Donaldson,* held that the existence of mental illness alone does not justify involuntary hospitalization. State standards require a specific impact or consequence to flow from the mental illness that involves danger or an inability to care for one's own needs. These clients are entitled to court hearings with representation, at which time determination of commitment and length of stay are considered. Legislative statutes governing involuntary commitments vary from state to state.

Involuntary Outpatient Commitment

Involuntary outpatient commitment (IOC) is a court-ordered mechanism used to compel a person with mental illness to submit to treatment on an outpatient basis. A number of eligibility criteria for commitment to outpatient treatment have been cited (Appelbaum, 2001; Csere, 2013; Maloy, 1996; Torrey & Zdanowicz, 2001). Some of these criteria include the following:

■ A history of repeated decompensation requiring involuntary hospitalization
■ Likelihood that without treatment the individual will deteriorate to the point of requiring inpatient commitment
■ Presence of severe and persistent mental illness (e.g., schizophrenia or bipolar disorder) and limited awareness of the illness or need for treatment
■ Presence of severe and persistent mental illness contributing to a risk for homelessness, incarceration, violence, or suicide.
■ Existence of an individualized treatment plan likely to be effective and a service provider who has agreed to provide the treatment

Most states have already enacted IOC legislation or currently have resolutions that speak to this topic on their agendas. Most commonly, clients who are committed into the IOC programs are those with severe and persistent mental illness, such as schizophrenia. The rationale behind the legislation is to improve preventive care and reduce the number of readmissions and lengths of hospital stays of these clients. The need for this kind of legislation arose after it

was recognized that individuals with schizophrenia who did not meet criteria for involuntary hospital treatment were, in some cases, ultimately dangerous to themselves or others. In New York, public attention to this need arose after a man with schizophrenia who had stopped taking his medication pushed a young woman into the path of a subway train. He would not have met criteria for involuntary hospitalization until he was deemed dangerous to others, but advocates for this legislation argued that there should be provisions to prevent violence rather than waiting until it happens. The subsequent law governing IOC in New York became known as Kendra's Law in reference to the woman who was pushed to her death. Opponents of this legislation fear that it may violate the individual rights of psychiatric clients without significant improvement in outcomes.

Research studies have attempted to evaluate whether IOC improves care, reduces lengths of stay in the hospital, and/or reduces episodes of violence. Some studies have shown positive outcomes with IOC, including a decrease in hospital readmissions (Ridgely, Borum, & Petrila, 2001; Swartz et al., 2001; Swartz & Swanson, 2008). But a Cochran literature review (Kisely, Campbell, & O'Reilly, 2017) concluded that compulsory community treatment resulted in no significant differences in service use, social functioning, mental state, or quality of life, although those in mandated outpatient treatment were less likely to be victims of crimes. The issues around whether IOC will improve treatment compliance and enhance quality of life in the community for individuals with severe and persistent mental illness will continue to be a focus of study and debate.

The Gravely Disabled Client

A number of states have statutes that specifically define the "gravely disabled" client. For those that do not use this label, the description of the individual who, because of mental illness, is unable to take care of basic personal needs is very similar.

Gravely disabled is generally defined as a condition in which an individual, as a result of mental illness, is in danger of serious physical harm resulting from inability to provide for basic needs such as food, clothing, shelter, medical care, and personal safety. Inability to care for oneself cannot be established by showing that an individual lacks the resources to provide the necessities of life. Rather, it is established by showing the individual's inability to make use of available resources.

Should it be determined that an individual is gravely disabled, a guardian, conservator, or committee is appointed by the court to ensure the management of the person and his or her estate. To legally restore competency requires another court hearing to reverse the previous ruling. The individual whose competency is being determined has the right to be represented by an attorney.

It is an ethical and legal duty to ensure that whenever coercive treatments are used, including involuntary hospitalizations, seclusion and restraint, involuntary outpatient commitments, mandated medication, and even prison commitments, the least restrictive intervention must first be considered. Sashadahran and Saraceno (2017) identified a concern that there is a current shift globally toward more coercive care similar to that which existed prior to the community mental health movement. They cite increasing numbers of involuntary hospitalizations and note, in addition, that in the United States there are currently three times as many individuals with mental illness in prisons as there are in hospitals, and that sexual predator laws in the United States allow indefinite hospital stays for serious sex offenders beyond their prison sentence completion. The authors raise the concern that if risk management supersedes the most appropriate level of care for treatment, stigmatization of this population will increase (Sashadahran & Saraceno, 2017).

Nursing Liability

Mental health practitioners—psychiatrists, psychologists, psychiatric nurses, and social workers—have a duty to provide appropriate care based on the standards of their professions and the standards set by law. The standards of practice for psychiatric mental health nursing are presented in Chapter 6, The Nursing Process in Psychiatric Mental Health Nursing.

Malpractice and Negligence

The terms **malpractice** and **negligence** are often used interchangeably. Negligence has been defined as failure to exercise the care toward others that a reasonable or prudent person would do in the circumstances, or taking action that such a reasonable person would not. Negligence is accidental as distinguished from "intentional torts" (assault or trespass, for example) or from crimes, but a crime can also constitute negligence, such as reckless driving (Hill & Hill, 2018). Any person may be negligent. In contrast, malpractice is a specialized form of negligence applicable only to professionals. Malpractice may be defined as an act or continuing conduct of a professional that does not meet the standard of professional

competence and results in provable damages to his or her client or patient. Such an error or omission may be through negligence, ignorance (when the professional should have known), or intentional wrongdoing (Hill & Hill, 2018). In the absence of any state statutes, common law is the basis of liability for injuries to clients caused by acts of malpractice and negligence of individual practitioners. In other words, most decisions of negligence in the professional setting are based on legal precedent (decisions that have previously been made about similar cases) rather than any specific action taken by the legislature.

To summarize, when the breach of duty is characterized as malpractice, the action is weighed against the professional standard. When it is brought forth as negligence, action is contrasted with what a reasonably prudent professional would have done in the same or similar circumstances.

Austin (2011) cites the following basic elements of a nursing malpractice lawsuit:

1. A duty to the patient existed based on the recognized standard of care.
2. A breach of duty occurred, meaning that the care rendered was not consistent with the recognized standard of care.
3. The client was injured.
4. The injury was directly caused by the breach of a standard of care.

For the client to prevail in a malpractice claim, each of these elements must be proved. Juries' decisions are generally based on the testimony of expert witnesses because members of the jury are laypeople and cannot be expected to know what nursing interventions should have been carried out. Without the testimony of expert witnesses, a favorable verdict usually goes to the defendant nurse.

Types of Lawsuits That Occur in Psychiatric Nursing

Most malpractice suits against nurses are civil actions; that is, they are considered breach of conduct actions on the part of the professional, for which compensation is being sought. The nurse in the psychiatric setting should be aware of the types of behaviors that may result in charges of malpractice.

Basic to the psychiatric client's hospitalization is his or her right to confidentiality and privacy. A nurse may be charged with *breach of confidentiality* for revealing aspects about a client's case, or even for revealing that an individual has been hospitalized, if that person can show that making this information known resulted in harm.

When shared information is detrimental to the client's reputation, the person sharing the information may be liable for **defamation of character.** When the information is in writing, the action is called **libel.** Oral defamation is called **slander.** Defamation of character involves communication that is malicious and false (Ellis & Hartley, 2012). Occasionally, libel arises out of critical, judgmental statements written in the client's medical record. Nurses need to be very objective in their charting, backing up all statements with factual evidence.

Invasion of privacy is a charge that may result when a client is searched without probable cause. Many institutions conduct body searches on clients with mental illness as a routine intervention. In these cases, there should be a physician's order and written rationale showing probable cause for the intervention. Many institutions are reexamining their policies regarding this procedure.

Assault is an act that results in a person's genuine fear and apprehension that he or she will be touched without consent. **Battery** is the unconsented touching of another person. These charges can result when a treatment is administered to a client against his or her wishes and outside of an emergency situation. Harm or injury need not have occurred for these charges to be legitimate.

For confining a client against his or her wishes, and outside of an emergency situation, the nurse may be charged with false imprisonment. Examples of actions that may invoke these charges include locking an individual in a room; taking a client's clothes for purposes of detainment against his or her will; and retaining in mechanical restraints a competent, voluntary client who demands to be released.

Avoiding Liability

Catalano (2015) suggests the following proactive nursing actions in an effort to avoid nursing malpractice and the risk of lawsuits:

1. *Effective communication* with patients and other caregivers. The SBAR model of reporting information, which stands for situation, background, assessment, and recommendations, has been identified as a useful tool for effective communication with caregivers. Establishing rapport with clients encourages open and honest communication.
2. *Accurate and complete documentation in the medical record.* The electronic health record (EHR) has been identified as the best way to document and share this information. The use of best sources for informatics is also identified as an important standard for quality and safety in nursing education (Institute of Medicine, 2003).

3. *Complying with standards of care,* including those established within the profession (such as ANA standards) and those identified by specific hospital policies.
4. *Knowing the client,* which includes helping the client become involved in his or her care as well as understanding and responding to aspects of care in which the client is dissatisfied.
5. *Practicing within the nurse's level of competence and scope of practice,* which includes not only adhering to professional standards (those of the ANA and state boards of nursing) but also keeping knowledge and nursing skills current through evidence-based literature, in-services, and continuing education.

Some clients appear to be more "suit prone" than others. Suit-prone clients are often very critical, complaining, uncooperative, and even hostile. A natural staff response to these clients is to become defensive or withdrawn. Either of these behaviors increases the likelihood of a lawsuit should an unfavorable event occur (Ellis & Hartley, 2012). No matter how high the nurse's technical competence and skill, his or her insensitivity to a client's complaints and failure to meet the client's emotional needs often influence whether or not a lawsuit is generated. A great deal depends on the psychosocial skills of the healthcare professional.

CLINICAL PEARL
- Always put the client's rights and welfare first.
- Develop and maintain a good interpersonal relationship with each client and his or her family.

Summary and Key Points

- *Ethics* is a branch of philosophy that addresses methods for determining the rightness or wrongness of one's actions.
- *Bioethics* is the term applied to these principles when they refer to concepts within the scope of medicine, nursing, and allied health.
- *Moral behavior* is conduct that results from serious critical thinking about how individuals ought to treat others.
- *Values* are personal beliefs about what is important or desirable.
- A *right* is "a valid, legally recognized claim or entitlement, encompassing both freedom from government interference or discriminatory treatment and an entitlement to a benefit or service" (Levy & Rubenstein, 1996).

■ The ethical theory of utilitarianism is based on the premise that what is right and good is that which produces the most happiness for the most people.

■ The ethical theory of Kantianism suggests that actions are bound by a sense of duty and that ethical decisions are made out of respect for moral law.

■ The code of Christian ethics is that all decisions about right and wrong should be centered in love for God and in treating others with the same respect and dignity with which we would expect to be treated.

■ The moral precept of the natural law theory is "do good and avoid evil." Good is viewed as that which is inscribed by God into the nature of things. Evil acts are never condoned, even if they are intended to advance the noblest of ends.

■ Ethical egoism espouses that what is right and good is what is best for the individual making the decision.

■ Ethical principles include autonomy, beneficence, nonmaleficence, veracity, and justice.

■ An ethical dilemma is a situation that requires an individual to make a choice between two equally unfavorable alternatives.

■ Ethical issues may arise in psychiatric mental health nursing around the client's right to refuse medication and the right to the least restrictive treatment alternative.

■ Statutory laws are those that have been enacted by legislative bodies, and common laws are derived from decisions made in previous cases. Both types of laws have civil and criminal components.

■ Civil law protects the private and property rights of individuals and businesses, and criminal law provides protection from conduct deemed injurious to the public welfare.

■ Legal issues in psychiatric mental health nursing center around confidentiality and the right to privacy, informed consent, restraints and seclusion, and commitment issues.

■ Nurses are accountable for their own actions in relation to legal issues, and violation can result in malpractice lawsuits against the physician, the hospital, and the nurse.

■ Developing and maintaining a good interpersonal relationship with the client and his or her family appears to be a positive factor when the question of malpractice is being considered.

Review Questions
Self-Examination/Learning Exercise

Select the answer that is most appropriate for each of the following questions:

1. The nurse decides to go against family wishes and tell the patient of his terminal status because that is what she would want if she were the patient. Which of the following ethical theories is considered in this decision?
   a. Kantianism
   b. Christian ethics
   c. Natural law theories
   d. Ethical egoism

2. The nurse decides to respect family wishes and not tell the patient of his terminal status because that would bring the most happiness to the most people. Which of the following ethical theories is considered in this decision?
   a. Utilitarianism
   b. Kantianism
   c. Christian ethics
   d. Ethical egoism

3. The nurse decides to tell the patient of his terminal status because she believes it is her duty to do so. Which of the following ethical theories is considered in this decision?
   a. Natural law theories
   b. Ethical egoism
   c. Kantianism
   d. Utilitarianism

Review Questions—cont'd
Self-Examination/Learning Exercise

4. The nurse assists the physician with electroconvulsive therapy on his patient who has refused to give consent. With which of the following legal actions might the nurse be charged because of this nursing action?
   a. Assault
   b. Battery
   c. False imprisonment
   d. Breach of confidentiality

5. A competent, voluntary client has stated that he wants to leave the hospital. The nurse hides his clothes in an effort to keep him from leaving. With which of the following legal actions might the nurse be charged because of this nursing action?
   a. Assault
   b. Battery
   c. False imprisonment
   d. Breach of confidentiality

6. Joe is very restless and is pacing a lot. The nurse says to Joe, "If you don't sit down in the chair and be still, I'm going to put you in restraints!" With which of the following legal actions might the nurse be charged because of this nursing action?
   a. Defamation of character
   b. Battery
   c. Breach of confidentiality
   d. Assault

7. An individual may be considered *gravely disabled* for which of the following reasons? (Select all that apply.)
   a. A person, because of mental illness, cannot fulfill basic needs.
   b. A mentally ill person is in danger of physical harm based on inability to care for self.
   c. A mentally ill person lacks the resources to provide the necessities of life.
   d. A mentally ill person is unable to make use of available resources to meet daily living requirements.

8. Which of the following statements is correct regarding the use of restraints? (Select all that apply.)
   a. Restraints may never be initiated without a physician's order.
   b. Orders for restraints must be reissued by a physician every 2 hours for children and adolescents.
   c. Clients in restraints must be observed and assessed every hour for issues regarding circulation, nutrition, respiration, hydration, and elimination.
   d. An in-person evaluation must be conducted within 1 hour of initiating restraints.

9. Guidelines relating to "duty to warn" state that a therapist should consider taking action to warn a third party when his or her client does which of the following? (Select all that apply.)
   a. Threatens violence toward another individual
   b. Identifies a specific intended victim
   c. Is having command hallucinations
   d. Reveals paranoid delusions about another individual

10. Attempting to calm an angry client by using "talk therapy" is an example of which of the following clients' rights?
    a. The right to privacy
    b. The right to refuse medication
    c. The right to the least restrictive treatment alternative
    d. The right to confidentiality

References

American Hospital Association (AHA). (2003). *The patient care partnership: Understanding expectations, rights, and responsibilities.* Retrieved from https://www.aha.org/system/files/2018-01/aha-patient-care-partnership.pdf

American Nurses Association (ANA). (2015). *Code of ethics for nurses with interpretive statements.* Silver Spring, MD: Author.

American Nurses Association (ANA), American Psychiatric Nurses Association, & International Society of Psychiatric-Mental Health Nurses. (2014). *Psychiatric-mental health nursing: Scope and standards of practice* (2nd ed.). Silver Spring, MD: American Nurses Association.

Appelbaum, P. S. (2001, March). Thinking carefully about outpatient commitment. *Psychiatric Services, 52*(3), 347–350.

Austin, S. (2011). Stay out of court with proper documentation. *Nursing, 41*(4), 25–29.

Butts, J., & Rich, K. (2016). *Nursing ethics: Across the curriculum and into practice* (4th ed.). Burlington, MA: Jones & Bartlett.

Cady, R. F. (2010). A review of basic patient rights in psychiatric care. *JONA's Healthcare Law, Ethics, and Regulation, 12*(4), 117–125.

Catalano, J. T. (2015). *Nursing now! Today's issues, tomorrow's trends* (7th ed.). Philadelphia, PA: F.A. Davis.

Csere, M. (2013). Updated report: Involuntary outpatient mental health treatment laws. *OLR Research Report.* Retrieved from https://www.cga.ct.gov/2013/rpt/2013-R-0105.htm

Ellis, J. R., & Hartley, C. L. (2012). *Nursing in today's world: Challenges, issues, and trends* (10th ed.). Philadelphia, PA: Lippincott Williams & Wilkins.

Guido, G. W. (2014). *Legal and ethical issues in nursing* (6th ed.). Upper Saddle River, NJ: Pearson.

Hartsell, T. L., & Bernstein, B. E. (2013). *The portable lawyer for mental health professionals: An A–Z guide to protecting your clients, your practice, and yourself* (3rd ed.). Hoboken, NJ: Wiley & Sons.

Henderson, E. (2015). Potentially dangerous patients: A review of the duty to warn. *Journal of Emergency Nursing, 41*(3), 193–200.

Hill, G., & Hill, K. (2018). *The people's law dictionary.* Retrieved from https://dictionary.law.com

Institute of Medicine. (2003). *Health professions education: A bridge to quality.* Washington, DC: Author.

The Joint Commission. (2017). *The comprehensive accreditation manual for behavioral health care (CAMBHC).* Oakbrook, IL: Author.

Kisely, S. R., Campbell, L. A., & O'Reilly, R. (2017). *Compulsory community and involuntary outpatient treatment for people with severe mental disorders.* Retrieved from http://www.cochrane.org/CD004408/SCHIZ_compulsory-community-and-involuntary-outpatient-treatment-people-severe-mental-disorders

Landeweer, E., Abma, T. A., & Widdershoven, G. (2011). Moral margins concerning the use of coercion in psychiatry. *Nursing Ethics, 18*(3), 304–316.

Maiese, M. (2017 [originally posted July 2003]). Principles of justice and fairness. *Beyond intractability.* Eds. C. Burgess & H. Burgess. Conflict Information Consortium, University of Colorado, Boulder. Retrieved from http://www.beyondintractability.org/essay/principles-of-justice

Maloy, K. A. (1996). Does involuntary outpatient commitment work? In B. D. Sales & S. A. Shah (Eds.), *Mental health and law: Research, policy and services* (pp. 41–74). Durham, NC: Carolina Academic Press.

Mental Illness Policy Org. (2017). *The effects of involuntary medication on individuals with schizophrenia and manic-depressive disorder.* Retrieved from https://mentalillnesspolicy.org/medical/involuntary-medication.html

National Conference of State Legislatures. (2016). *Mental health professionals' duty to warn.* Retrieved from http://www.ncsl.org/research/health/mental-health-professionals-duty-to-warn.aspx

Ridgely, M. S., Borum, R., & Petrila, J. (2001). *The effectiveness of involuntary outpatient treatment: Empirical evidence and the experience of eight states.* Santa Monica, CA: Rand Publications.

QSEN Institute. (2013). *Competencies.* Retrieved from http://qsen.org/competencies/

Sadock, B. J., Sadock, V. A., & Ruiz, P. (2015). *Synopsis of psychiatry: Behavioral sciences/clinical psychiatry* (11th ed.). Baltimore, MD: Lippincott Williams & Wilkins.

Sashadahran, S. P., & Saraceno, B. (2017). Is psychiatry becoming more coercive? *The British Medical Journal, 357.* doi:https://doi.org/10.1136/bmj.j2904

Swartz, M., Swanson, J., Hiday, V., Wagner, H. R., Burns, B., & Borum, R. (2001). A randomized controlled trial of outpatient commitment in North Carolina. *Psychiatric Services, 52*(3), 325–329.

Swartz, M. S., & Swanson, J. W. (2008). Outpatient commitment: When it improves patient outcomes. *Current Psychiatry, 7*(4), 25–35. doi:http://dx.doi.org/10.1176/appi.ps.52.3.325

Tarasoff v. Regents of University of California et al. (1974a), 551 P.d 345.

Tarasoff v. Regents of University of California et al. (1974b), 554 P.d 347.

Torrey, E. F., & Zdanowicz, M. (2001). Outpatient commitment: What, why, and for whom. *Psychiatric Services, 52*(3), 337–341.

U.S. Code, Title 42, Section 10841, The public health and welfare, 1991.

U.S. Department of Health & Human Services (USDHHS). (2003). *Standards for privacy of individually identifiable health information.* Washington, DC: Author.

U.S. Department of Health & Human Services. (2013, January 17). *New rule protects patient privacy, secures health information* [News release]. Washington, DC: Author.

Weiss-Kaffie, C. J., & Purtell, N. E. (2001). Psychiatric nursing. In M. E. O'Keefe (Ed.), *Nursing practice and the law: Avoiding malpractice and other legal risks* (pp. 352–371). Philadelphia, PA: F.A. Davis.

What do I do now? Ethical dilemmas in nursing and health care. (2013). *ISNA Bulletin, 13*(2), 5–12.

Classical References

Levy, R. M., & Rubenstein, L. S. (1996). *The rights of people with mental disabilities.* Carbondale: Southern Illinois University Press.

Patient Self-Determination Act—Patient Rights. (1991). U.S. Code, Title 42, Section 10841, The Public Health and Welfare.

Peplau, H. E. (1991). *Interpersonal relations in nursing: A conceptual frame of reference for psychodynamic nursing.* New York, NY: Springer.

Psychopharmacology 4

CORE CONCEPTS

Neurotransmitter
Psychotropic medication
Receptor

KEY TERMS

agranulocytosis
akathisia
akinesia
amenorrhea
dystonia
extrapyramidal side effects
gynecomastia
hypertensive crisis

neuroleptic malignant syndrome
neurotransmitter
oculogyric crisis
priapism
pseudoparkinsonism
retrograde ejaculation
serotonin syndrome
tardive dyskinesias

OBJECTIVES
After reading this chapter, the student will be able to:

1. Discuss historical perspectives related to psychopharmacology.
2. Describe indications, actions, contraindications, precautions, side effects, and nursing implications for the following classifications of drugs:
   a. Antianxiety agents
   b. Antidepressants
   c. Mood-stabilizing agents
   d. Antipsychotics and agents for the treatment of tardive dyskinesia
   e. Antiparkinsonian agents
   f. Sedative-hypnotics
   g. Agents for attention deficit-hyperactivity disorder
3. Apply the steps of the nursing process to the administration of psychotropic medications.

HOMEWORK ASSIGNMENT
Please read the chapter and answer the following questions:

1. Identify three priority safety concerns for each class of psychotropic medications.
2. Differentiate primary actions and side effects for traditional versus atypical antipsychotics.
3. Differentiate primary actions and side effects for tricyclic versus SSRI antidepressants.

Introduction

The middle of the 20th century represents a pivotal period in the treatment of individuals with mental illness. It was during this time that the phenothiazine class of antipsychotics was introduced in the United States. Before that time, phenothiazines had been used in France as preoperative medications. As Dr. Henri Laborit of the Hospital Boucicaut in Paris stated:

> It was our aim to decrease the anxiety of the patients to prepare them in advance for their postoperative recovery. With these new drugs, the phenothiazines, we were seeing a profound psychic and physical relaxation . . . a real indifference to the environment and to the upcoming operation. It seemed to me these drugs must have an application in psychiatry. (Sage, 1984)

Indeed, they have had a significant application in psychiatry. Not only have they helped many individuals to function effectively, but they have also provided researchers and clinicians with information to study the origins and etiologies of mental illness. Knowledge gained from learning how these drugs work has promoted advancement in understanding how behavioral disorders develop. Dr. Arnold Scheibel, director of the UCLA Brain Research Institute, stated:

> [When these drugs came out] there was a sense of disbelief that we could actually do something substantive for the patients . . . see them for the first time as sick individuals and not as something bizarre that we could literally not talk to. (Sage, 1984)

This chapter explores historical perspectives in the use of psychotropic medications in the treatment of mental illness. Eight classifications of medications are discussed: antianxiety agents, antidepressants, mood-stabilizing agents, antipsychotic agents, medications to treat extrapyramidal side effects, medications to treat tardive dyskinesia, sedative-hypnotics, and ADHD medications. Their implications for psychiatric nursing are presented in the context of the steps of the nursing process.

CORE CONCEPT
Psychotropic medication
Medication that affects the mind, behavior, or emotions.

Historical Perspectives

Historically, reaction to and treatment of individuals with mental illness has ranged from benign involvement to intervention that some would consider inhumane. Individuals with mental illness were feared because of common beliefs associating them with demons or the supernatural. They were looked upon as loathsome and often were mistreated.

Beginning in the late 18th century, a type of "moral reform" in the treatment of persons with mental illness began to occur. Community and state hospitals concerned with the needs of persons with mental illness were established. Considered a breakthrough in the humanization of care, these institutions, however well intentioned, fostered the concept of custodial care. Patients were ensured food and shelter but received little or no hope of change for the future. As they became increasingly dependent on the institution to fulfill their needs, the likelihood of their return to the family or community diminished.

The early part of the 20th century saw the advent of the somatic therapies in psychiatry. Individuals with mental illness were treated with insulin shock therapy, wet sheet packs, ice baths, electroconvulsive therapy, and psychosurgery. Before 1950, sedatives and amphetamines were the only significant psychotropic medications available. Even these drugs had limited use because of their toxicity and addictive effects. Since the 1950s, the development of psychopharmacology has expanded to include widespread use of antipsychotic, antidepressant, antianxiety, and mood stabilizer medications. Research into how these drugs work has provided an understanding of the biochemical influences in many psychiatric disorders.

Psychotropic medications are not a "cure" for mental illness. Most mental health practitioners who prescribe these medications for their patients use them as an adjunct to individual or group psychotherapy. Although their contribution to psychiatric care cannot be minimized, it must be emphasized that psychotropic medications relieve some physical and behavioral symptoms. They do not eliminate mental disorders.

The Role of the Nurse in Psychopharmacology

Ethical and Legal Implications

Nurses must understand the ethical and legal implications associated with the administration of psychotropic medications. Laws differ from state to state, but most adhere to the patient's right to refuse treatment. Exceptions exist in emergency situations when it has been determined that patients are likely to harm themselves or others. Many states have adopted laws that allow courts to order outpatient treatment, which may include medication, in circumstances in which an individual is not seeking treatment and has a history of violent, aggressive behavior. The original law, called Kendra's law, was enacted after a young woman, Kendra Webdale, was pushed in front of a New York City subway by a man who was living in the community but was not seeking treatment for his mental illness (New York State Office of Mental Health, 2012). This law is perhaps more developed in New York state than are similar laws in other states. It includes a medication grant clause that provides un-interrupted medication for those transitioning from hospitals or correctional facilities. Some states do not have these types of laws; therefore, it is important for nurses to be informed about local, state, and federal laws when they are working in any healthcare setting or correctional facility and providing care to patients with a psychiatric disorder.

Assessment

A thorough baseline assessment must be conducted before a patient is placed on a regimen of psycho-pharmacological therapy. A history and physical examination (see Chapter 6, The Nursing Process in Psychiatric Mental Health Nursing), ethnocultural assessment, and a comprehensive medication assessment (Box 4–1) are all essential components

---

BOX 4–1 Medication Assessment Tool

Date _____

Patient's Name _____ Age _____

Marital Status _____ Children _____

Occupation _____

Presenting Symptoms (subjective & objective) _____

_____

_____

Diagnosis (DSM-5) _____

Current Vital Signs: Blood Pressure: Sitting _____/_____ Standing _____/_____

Pulse _____

Respirations _____

Height _____ Weight _____

CURRENT/PAST USE OF PRESCRIPTION DRUGS (Indicate with "c" or "p" beside name of drug whether current or past use):

Name	Dosage	How Long Used	Why Prescribed	By Whom	Side Effects/Results
_____	_____	_____	_____	_____	_____
_____	_____	_____	_____	_____	_____
_____	_____	_____	_____	_____	_____

CURRENT/PAST USE OF OVER-THE-COUNTER DRUGS (Indicate with "c" or "p" beside name of drug whether current or past use):

Name	Dosage	How Long Used	Why Prescribed	By Whom	Side Effects/Results
_____	_____	_____	_____	_____	_____
_____	_____	_____	_____	_____	_____
_____	_____	_____	_____	_____	_____

CURRENT/PAST USE OF STREET DRUGS, ALCOHOL, NICOTINE, AND/OR CAFFEINE (Indicate with "c" or "p" beside name of drug whether current or past use):

Name	Amount Used	How Often Used	When Last Used	Effects Produced
_____	_____	_____	_____	_____
_____	_____	_____	_____	_____
_____	_____	_____	_____	_____

Continued

BOX 4–1 Medication Assessment Tool–cont'd

Any allergies to food or drugs?
_____

Any special diet considerations?
_____

Do you have (or have you ever had) any of the following? If yes, provide explanation on the back of this sheet.

Yes No

Difficulty swallowing _____
Delayed wound healing _____
Constipation problems _____
Urination problems _____
Recent change in elimination
patterns _____
Weakness or tremors _____
Seizures _____
Headaches _____
Dizziness _____
High blood pressure _____
Palpitations _____

Yes No

Chest pain _____
Blood clots/pain in legs _____
Fainting spells _____
Swollen ankles/legs/hands _____
Asthma _____
Varicose veins _____
Numbness/tingling (location?) _____
Ulcers _____
Nausea/vomiting _____
Problems with diarrhea _____
Shortness of breath _____
Sexual dysfunction _____

Yes No

Lumps in your breasts _____
Blurred or double vision _____
Ringing in the ears _____
Insomnia _____
Skin Rashes _____
Diabetes _____
Hepatitis (or other liver disease) _____
Kidney disease _____
Glaucoma _____

Are you pregnant or breastfeeding? _____ Date of last menses_____ Type of contraception used
_____

Describe any restrictions/limitations that might interfere with your use of medication for your current problem: _____
_____
_____

Prescription orders: Patient teaching related to medications prescribed:

Lab work or referrals prescribed:

Nurse's signature_____
Patient's signature_____

---

of this database. The ethnocultural assessment is necessary because genetic variations in selected populations and cultural factors, including dietary preferences, may influence response to some medications; CYP450 isoenzyme variations, for example, influence metabolism of some medications, and pharmacogenetic testing may be ordered to identify individuals at risk for being poor metabolizers of certain medications (see Table 4–1 for degrees of risk for poor metabolism of selected medications; and Chapter 31, Cultural and Spiritual Issues Relevant to Psychiatric Mental Health Nursing, available online at Davis*Plus*).

Medication Administration and Evaluation

For the patient in an inpatient setting, as well as for many others in partial hospitalization programs, day treatment centers, home healthcare, and other settings, the nurse is the key healthcare professional in direct contact with the individual receiving psychotropic medication. Medication administration is followed by a careful evaluation, which includes continuous monitoring for side effects and adverse reactions. The nurse also evaluates the therapeutic effectiveness of the medication. It is essential for the nurse to have a thorough knowledge of psychotropic medications to be able to anticipate potential problems and outcomes associated with their administration.

TABLE 4–1	**Variations in CYP 450 Enzymes and Response to Selected Psychotropic Medications***		
CYP 450 ISOENZYME	**% RISK FOR BEING POOR METABOLIZERS BY ETHNIC GROUP**	**SELECTED PSYCHOTROPIC MEDICATIONS AFFECTED**	**SELECTED POTENTIAL OUTCOMES**
2C19	Asian 12–23% African, African American 18% Caucasian 3–7%	Diazepam, tricyclics, citalopram	1. Higher blood levels and faster therapeutic response to tricyclic antidepressants. Experience more toxic side effects and more risk for tricyclic antidepressant delirium 2. Increased sensitivity to effects of alcohol
2D6	East Asian 0–2% African, African American 0–19% Caucasian 3–9%	Tricyclics, fluoxetine, paroxetine venlafaxine, sertraline, chlorpromazine, haloperidol, clozapine, risperidone	1. Higher incidence of extrapyramidal side effects with haloperidol 2. More sensitive to the effects of many psychotropic medications
3A4	Although results are inconsistent, poor metabolizers are rare (<1%) but drug–drug and drug–food interactions, such as interactions with grapefruit juice, may inhibit metabolism	mirtazapine, sertraline, haloperidol, clozapine, quetiapine, risperidone, ziprasidone, gabapentin, lamotrigine, clonazepam, diazepam, zolpidem, buspirone, lurasidone, pimozide, ketamine, fentanyl, oxycodone, alfentanil, dextromethorphan, triazolam	1. Higher risk for respiratory depression with alfentanil, fentanyl, ketamine, and oxycodone 2. Higher risk for torsade de pointes with lurasidone, pimozide, and ziprasidone 3. Risk for hallucinations and somnolence with dextromethorphan 4. Increased sedation with buspirone and triazolam

*CYP 450 enzymes are responsible for metabolizing many medications. Variations can occur due to genetic vulnerability or through drug–drug or drug–food interactions. CYP 450 induction increases the metabolism of selected drugs, thereby decreasing their effectiveness. Inhibition of CYP 450 enzymes decreases the metabolism of selected drugs, which can result in severe toxicity and several adverse effects.
Sources: Anderson, L. (2018). *Drug interactions with grapefruit juice*. Retrieved from https://www.drugs.com/article/grapefruit-drug-interactions.html; Horn, J. R. & Hansten, P. D. (2008). *Get to know an enzyme: CYP2C19*. Retrieved from https://www.pharmacytimes.com/publications/issue/2008/2008-05/2008-05-8538; Jones, D. S. (2006). Racial Profiling in Psychiatry: Does It Help Patients? *Psychiatric Times, 23*(14); Lynch, T. & Price, A. (2007). The Effect of Cytochrome P450 Metabolism on Drug Response, Interactions, and Adverse Effects. *American Family Physician, 76*(3): 391–396.

Patient Education

The information associated with psychotropic medications is copious and complex. An important role of the nurse is to translate that complex information into terms that can be easily understood by the patient. Patients must understand why the medication has been prescribed, when it should be taken, and what they may expect in terms of side effects and possible adverse reactions. They must know whom to contact when they have a question and when it is important to report to their physician. For women of childbearing age, pregnancy risk information is an important aspect of patient education. In 2015 a new FDA rule went into effect, which requires that drug labeling includes more specific narrative information on pregnancy-associated risks, lactation considerations, and reproductive potential. This new system replaces the lettered risk categories that were criticized for being overly simplistic although the implementation of the system is still in progress (Drugs.com, 2018). Nurses should use the latest informatics resources to provide current and relevant education on this and other medication-related topics. Medication education encourages patient cooperation and promotes accurate and effective management of the treatment regimen.

CORE CONCEPTS

Neurotransmitter
A chemical that is stored in the axon terminals of the presynaptic neuron. An electrical impulse through the neuron stimulates the release of the neurotransmitter into the synaptic cleft, which in turn determines whether another electrical impulse is generated.

Receptor
Molecules situated on the cell membrane that are binding sites for neurotransmitters.

How Do Psychotropics Work?

Most of the psychotropic medications have their effects at the neuronal synapse, producing changes in **neurotransmitter** release and the receptors to which they bind (Fig. 4–1). Researchers hypothesize that most antidepressants work by blocking the reuptake of neurotransmitters, specifically, serotonin and norepinephrine. *Reuptake* is the process of neurotransmitter inactivation by which the neurotransmitter is reabsorbed into the presynaptic neuron from which it had been released. Blocking the reuptake process allows more of the neurotransmitter to be available for neuronal transmission. This mechanism of action may also result in undesirable side effects (Table 4–2). Some antidepressants also block receptor sites that are unrelated to their mechanisms of action. These include α-adrenergic, histaminergic, and muscarinic cholinergic receptors. Blocking these receptors is also associated with the development of certain side effects. Individuals being treated with tricyclic antidepressants, for example, are at risk for developing postural hypotension. The specific type of receptor that a medication binds to is also relevant to the medication's level of antianxiety, antidepressant, and sedative properties (Table 4–2).

Antipsychotic medications block dopamine receptors, and some affect muscarinic cholinergic, histaminergic, and α-adrenergic receptors. The "atypical" (or second generation) antipsychotics focus primarily on blocking specific serotonin receptors. Benzodiazepines facilitate the transmission of the inhibitory neurotransmitter gamma-aminobutyric acid (GABA). The psychostimulants work by increasing norepinephrine, serotonin, and dopamine release.

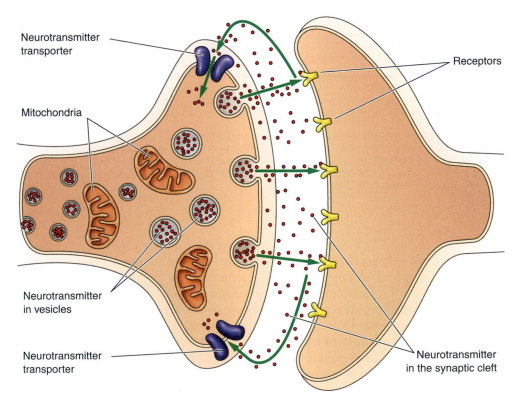

FIGURE 4–1 Area of synaptic transmission that is altered by drugs. The green arrows describe the movement of neurotransmitters at the synaptic cleft.

TABLE 4–2 Effects of Psychotropic Influence on Neurotransmitters

EXAMPLE OF MEDICATION	ACTION ON NEUROTRANSMITTER AND/OR RECEPTOR	PHYSIOLOGICAL EFFECTS	SIDE EFFECTS
SSRIs	Inhibit reuptake of serotonin (5-HT)	Reduce depression Control anxiety Control obsessions	Nausea, agitation, headache, sexual dysfunction
Tricyclic antidepressants	Inhibit reuptake of serotonin (5-HT) Inhibit reuptake of norepinephrine (NE) Block NE (α_1) receptor Block ACh receptor Block histamine (H_1) receptor	Reduce depression Relief of severe pain Prevent panic attacks	Sexual dysfunction (NE & 5-HT) Sedation, weight gain (H_1) Dry mouth, constipation, blurred vision, urinary retention (ACh) Postural hypotension and tachycardia (α_1)
MAO inhibitors	Increase NE and 5-HT by inhibiting the enzyme that degrades them (MAO-A)	Reduce depression Control anxiety	Sedation, dizziness Sexual dysfunction Hypertensive crisis (interaction with tyramine)
Trazodone and nefazodone	5-HT reuptake block 5-HT$_2$ receptor antagonism Adrenergic receptor blockade	Reduce depression Reduce anxiety	Nausea (5-HT) Sedation (5-HT$_2$) Orthostasis (α_1) Priapism (α_2)
SNRIs: venlafaxine, desvenlafaxine, duloxetine, and levomilnacipran	Potent inhibitors of serotonin and norepinephrine reuptake Weak inhibitors of dopamine reuptake	Reduce depression Relieve pain of neuropathy (duloxetine) Relieve anxiety (venlafaxine)	Nausea (5-HT) Increased sweating (NE) Insomnia (NE) Tremors (NE) Sexual dysfunction (5-HT)
Bupropion	Inhibits reuptake of NE and dopamine (D)	Reduces depression Aids in smoking cessation Decreases symptoms of ADHD	Insomnia, dry mouth, tremor, seizures
Antipsychotics: phenothiazines and haloperidol	Strong D$_2$ receptor blockade Weaker blockade of ACh, H$_1$, α_1-adrenergic, and 5-HT$_2$ receptors	Relief of psychosis Relief of anxiety (Some) provide relief from nausea and vomiting and intractable hiccoughs	Blurred vision, dry mouth, decreased sweating, constipation, urinary retention, tachycardia (ACh) EPS (D$_2$) Increases plasma prolactin (D$_2$) Sedation; weight gain (H$_1$) Ejaculatory difficulty (5-HT$_2$) Postural hypotension (α; H$_1$)
Antipsychotics (second generation, atypical): aripiprazole, asenapine, brexpiprazole, clozapine, iloperidone, lurasidone, olanzapine, paliperidone, quetiapine, risperidone, ziprasidone	Receptor antagonism of 5-HT$_1$ and 5-HT$_2$, D$_1$–D$_5$ (varies with drug), H$_1$, α_1-adrenergic, muscarinic (ACh)	Relief of psychosis (with minimal or no EPS) Relief of anxiety Relief of acute mania	Potential with some of the drugs for mild EPS (D$_2$) Sedation, weight gain (H$_1$), hyperglycemia/diabetes Orthostasis and dizziness (α-adrenergic) Blurred vision, dry mouth, decreased sweating, constipation, urinary retention, tachycardia (ACh)

Continued

TABLE 4–2	Effects of Psychotropic Influence on Neurotransmitters—cont'd		
EXAMPLE OF MEDICATION	**ACTION ON NEUROTRANSMITTER AND/ OR RECEPTOR**	**PHYSIOLOGICAL EFFECTS**	**SIDE EFFECTS**
Antianxiety: benzodiazepines	Bind to BZ receptor sites on the GABA$_A$ receptor complex; increase receptor affinity for GABA	Relief of anxiety Sedation	Dependence (with long-term use) Confusion; memory impairment; motor incoordination
Antianxiety: buspirone	5-HT$_{1A}$ agonist D$_2$ agonist D$_2$ antagonist	Relief of anxiety	Nausea, headache, dizziness, restlessness

ACh, acetylcholine; ADHD, attention deficit-hyperactivity disorder; BZ, benzodiazepine; D, dopamine; EPS, extrapyramidal symptoms; GABA, gamma-aminobutyric acid; H, histamine; 5-HT, 5-hydroxytryptamine (serotonin); MAO, monoamine oxidase; NE, norepinephrine; SNRI, serotonin-norepinephrine reuptake inhibitor; SSRI, selective serotonin reuptake inhibitor.

Although each psychotropic medication affects neurotransmission, the specific drugs within each class have varying neuronal effects. Their exact mechanisms of action are unknown. Many of the neuronal effects occur rapidly; however, the therapeutic effects of some medications, such as antidepressants and atypical antipsychotics, may take weeks to become apparent. Acute alterations in neuronal function do not fully explain how these medications work. Sadock et al. (2015) note that

if merely raising or lowering levels of neurotransmitter activity is associated with the clinical effects of a drug, then all drugs that cause these changes should produce equivalent benefits [and] this is not the case. (p. 911)

Long-term neuropharmacological reactions to increased norepinephrine and serotonin levels may better explain their mechanisms of action. Recent research suggests that the therapeutic effects are related to the nervous system's adaptation to increased levels of neurotransmitters. These adaptive changes result from a homeostatic mechanism, much like a thermostat, that regulates the cell and maintains equilibrium.

Applying the Nursing Process in Psychopharmacological Therapy

An assessment tool for obtaining a drug history is provided in Box 4–1. This tool may be adapted for use by staff nurses admitting patients to the hospital or by nurse practitioners with prescriptive privileges.

One of the Quality and Safety in Nursing Education (QSEN) culminating from the Institute of Medicine (IOM) (2003) report on essential competencies of healthcare professionals, stresses that the patient must be at the center of decisions about treatment, and an assessment tool such as that provided in Box 4–1 provides an opportunity to actively engage the patient in describing what medications have been effective or ineffective and identifying side effects that may impact their willingness to adhere to a medication regimen.

Antianxiety Agents

Background Assessment Data

Indications

Antianxiety drugs are also called *anxiolytics* and historically were referred to as *minor tranquilizers*. They are used in the treatment of anxiety disorders, anxiety symptoms, acute alcohol withdrawal, skeletal muscle spasms, convulsive disorders, status epilepticus, and preoperative sedation. They are most appropriate for the treatment of acute anxiety states rather than for long-term treatment. Their use and efficacy for periods greater than 4 months has not been substantiated. For longer-term management of anxiety disorders, antidepressants are often used as the first line of treatment because they are not addictive. (A table of antianxiety agents currently approved by the U.S. Food and Drug Administration [FDA], half-life, and daily dosage ranges can be found online at Davis*Plus* and in Chapter 18, Anxiety, Obsessive-Compulsive, and Related Disorders.)

Action

Antianxiety drugs depress subcortical levels of the central nervous system (CNS), particularly the limbic system and reticular formation. They may potentiate the effects of the powerful inhibitory neurotransmitter GABA in the brain, thereby producing a calmative effect. All levels of CNS depression can be affected, from mild sedation to hypnosis to coma. The most commonly prescribed antianxiety agents are benzodiazepines, including clonazepam (Klonopin), diazepam (Valium), and alprazolam (Xanax). Benzodiazepines are much like alcohol in their effects on GABA receptors, which explains why benzodiazepines may be used for the management of alcohol withdrawal.

The antianxiety agent buspirone (BuSpar) is not a benzodiazepine and thus does not depress the CNS. Although its action is unknown, the drug is believed to produce the desired effects through interactions with serotonin, dopamine, and other neurotransmitter receptors. Patients should be instructed that this drug has a lag period of 7 to 10 days before improvement is seen and full therapeutic benefits take 3 to 4 weeks of treatment. It does not have the addiction potential that some of the other antianxiety agents have. Consequently, it may be a better option for patients with anxiety disorders who also have substance use disorders.

Some medications from other classes, such as antidepressants (SSRIs and SNRIs), beta blockers (propranolol), and antihistamines (hydroxyzine) have also demonstrated benefits in relieving anxiety.

Interactions

- Increased effects of antianxiety agents can occur when they are taken concomitantly with alcohol, barbiturates, narcotics, antipsychotics, antidepressants, antihistamines, neuromuscular blocking agents, cimetidine, or disulfiram.
- The FDA (2016a) recently added a boxed warning (its strongest warning) related to the serious risks and possible death associated with combining benzodiazepines with opioid pain or cough medicines.
- Increased effects can also occur with herbal depressants (e.g., kava, valerian, lemon verbena, L-tryptophan, melatonin, and chamomile).
- Decreased effects can be noted with cigarette smoking and caffeine consumption.

Diagnosis

The following nursing diagnoses may be considered for patients receiving therapy with antianxiety agents:

1. Risk for injury related to seizures; panic anxiety; acute agitation from alcohol withdrawal (indications); abrupt withdrawal from the medication after long-term use; effects of medication intoxication or overdose
2. Anxiety (specify) related to threat to physical integrity or self-concept
3. Risk for activity intolerance related to side effects of sedation, confusion, and/or lethargy
4. Disturbed sleep pattern related to situational crises, physical condition, or severe level of anxiety

Safety Issues in Planning and Implementing Care for Patients Taking Antianxiety Agents

The Institute of Medicine (IOM) (2003) identified *ensuring safety* as a core competency for nursing education. With that goal in mind, the following are some of the significant safety issues to be considered for patients taking antianxiety agents. Nursing interventions related to each side effect are noted to the right of each safety issue in Table 4–3.

One trend noted by Olfson, King, and Schoenbaum (2015) is an increased use of benzodiazepines in the older adult population despite known safety concerns, including psychomotor impairment, impaired cognitive function, and paradoxical increase in anxiety. The researchers add that 33% of benzodiazepine prescriptions are for long-term use in older adults, a practice that has not been supported in evidence and one that increases risks for side effects and dependence. Nurses are in a position to assess safety risks and, in collaboration with the patient, physician, and other healthcare team members, explore all viable options for treatment of anxiety and insomnia.

Outcome Criteria and Evaluation

The following criteria may be used for evaluating the effectiveness of therapy with antidepressant medications.

The patient:

- Demonstrates a reduction in anxiety, tension, and restless activity.
- Experiences no seizure activity.
- Experiences no physical injury.
- Is able to tolerate usual activities without excessive sedation.
- Exhibits no evidence of confusion.
- Tolerates the medication without gastrointestinal distress.
- Verbalizes understanding of the need for, side effects of, and regimen for self-administration.
- Verbalizes possible consequences of abrupt withdrawal from the medication.

TABLE 4–3 Safety Issues and Nursing Interventions for Patients Taking Antianxiety Agents

SAFETY ISSUES	NURSING INTERVENTIONS
Tolerance and physical dependence may develop. **Abrupt withdrawal can be life threatening** (except with buspirone); signs include sweating, agitation, tremors, nausea and vomiting, delirium, seizures	Instruct patient not to stop taking the drug abruptly. Assess the patient for signs of developing tolerance (requiring higher doses of medication to achieve effects). Educate the patient about symptoms of withdrawal. Contact the doctor immediately if symptoms of withdrawal are assessed.
Drowsiness, confusion, lethargy are the most common side effects.	Instruct patient not to drive or operate dangerous machinery while taking this medication.
Effect of other CNS depressants is increased.	Instruct the patient not to drink alcohol or take other CNS depressants, as well as antihistamines, cimetidine, antidepressants, neuromuscular blocking agents, and disulfiram, while taking antianxiety agent.
Antianxiety agents may **aggravate symptoms of depression.**	Assess the patient's mood and assess for suicide risk.
Orthostatic hypotension may occur.	Instruct the patient to rise slowly from a sitting to standing position to minimize risks for falls. Monitor lying and standing blood pressures to assess for orthostatic hypotension.
Paradoxical excitement (opposite from the desired effect) may occur. Especially the elderly may be at higher risk for agitation and increased anxiety. In general, safety risks associated with benzodiazepines may be greater for the older adult (especially with long-acting benzodiazepines and long-term use), including impaired cognitive function, reduced mobility, risk for falls, and chemical dependence (Olfson, King, & Schoenbaum, 2015).	Hold the medication and notify the doctor. Assess for other side effects and safety issues including impaired cognition and impaired mobility. Use a patient-centered, collaborative team approach to explore options in safe management of anxiety and insomnia (lower dose, shorter-acting benzodiazepines; psychological interventions, etc.).
Blood dyscrasias, although rare, can be serious or life threatening.	Assess for sore throat, fever, bruising, or unusual bleeding. Hold medication and report these symptoms immediately to the doctor.
Congenital malformations have been associated with use of these drugs during the first trimester of pregnancy.	Instruct the female patient who is pregnant or of childbearing age while on these medications to explore alternative treatment options with her physician.

Antidepressants

Sorting out information on antidepressant medication can be particularly confusing because there are several types, and some antidepressant medications are also prescribed in the treatment of anxiety disorders. The first "antidepressant" drug was the monoamine oxidase inhibitor (MAOI) isoniazid, which was initially used to treat tuberculosis. When patients began describing their increased feelings of well-being while taking these drugs, MAOIs were developed specifically for the treatment of depression. However, they were also associated with potentially deadly side effects in individuals who ate foods high in tyramine and they were found to have several serious interactions with other drugs. Because MAOIs increase the availability of norepinephrine, researchers have focused on developing drugs that affect norepinephrine without the need for food restrictions, leading to the introduction of the *tricyclic antidepressants (TCAs)*.

Tricyclics were the first-line treatment for depression for many years but were effective for only about 70% of those treated. In addition, because all neurotransmitters bind to various receptor sites, increasing the availability of norepinephrine, they also have anticholinergic effects and increase the risk for postural hypotension, which limited their use in the elderly and for those with cardiovascular problems.

In the late 1980s, serotonin, an antianxiety hormone and neurotransmitter, was identified as a potential biochemical target for treatment of depression and anxiety without significant anticholinergic side effects. These second generation antidepressants, *selective serotonin reuptake inhibitors (SSRIs)* and *serotonin/norepinephrine reuptake inhibitors (SNRIs),* are now the preferred first-line treatment for depression.

The most recent additions to the pharmacological treatments for depression and anxiety are atypical antipsychotics that increase the availability of serotonin and dopamine. These medications, such as aripiprazole (Abilify) and quetiapine (Seroquel), are being promoted as adjunctive to antidepressant therapy. In a recent large study sponsored by the National Institute of Mental Health, the combination of Abilify with venlafaxine demonstrated 44% improvement in elderly adults who were not responding to antidepressants alone. This finding is important for treatment of elderly clients because over one-half of older adults with clinical depression do not respond to antidepressants alone (Lenze et al., 2015).

Despite these developments and client-subjective reports of improvement with antidepressant medications, our understanding of the exact mechanisms of action remains theoretical. Currently, levels of neurotransmitters in the brain cannot be directly measured. In the STAR*D study (a large study funded by the National Institute of Mental Health), it was found that two-thirds of patients on antidepressant medication do not experience full recovery (Tartakovsky, 2016).

Research continues with the goal of identifying broadly effective antidepressant therapies. Several of the newest drugs on the market for treatment of depression are not significantly different from existing products. For example, a "new" antidepressant approved by the FDA in 2016, Oleptro, is simply a reformulation of trazodone. But new mechanisms are being explored, some of which are in clinical trials. Glutamate receptors (NMDA) are being studied for potential antidepressant effects; ketamine and midazolam (a benzodiazepine with transient effects similar to those of ketamine) are being explored as potentially faster acting than traditional antidepressants. Intranasal application of esketamine, currently in phase II clinical trials, is demonstrating effectiveness in reducing depressive symptoms within 4 hours and it is hoped that this may offer a treatment that will bridge the gap before which traditional antidepressants begin to demonstrate therapeutic effects (Canuso et al., 2018). More research is needed to substantiate this claim. Despite the lack of FDA approval, ketamine is increasingly being used for management of treatment-resistant depression for this indication (Johnston, 2017), and there are concerns about the risk for dependence. Drugs that act on melatonin receptors are currently in clinical trials for use in depression (one is already approved for use in Europe); and a new group of antidepressants called triple reuptake inhibitors (TRIs) that block reuptake of serotonin, norepinephrine, and dopamine simultaneously are in preliminary phases of research (Tartakovsky, 2016).

Current research also continues to explore genetic testing to identify factors that may influence whether an individual is more likely to respond to one kind of antidepressant than to another. If reliability is established, the research will provide a valuable resource for making decisions about which antidepressant to prescribe first.

Background Assessment Data

Indications

In addition to the indications for antidepressant medications in the treatment of major depressive and dysthymic disorders, some of the newer drugs, such as SSRIs, have received FDA approval for the treatment of most anxiety disorders, bulimia nervosa and other eating disorders, premenstrual dysphoric disorder, borderline personality disorder, obesity, and smoking cessation (Sadock et al., 2015).

A hallmark review of the research on antidepressants (Fournier et al., 2010) found that the benefits of antidepressant therapy for clients with mild to moderate symptoms of depression may be minimal or nonexistent but that for clients with severe depression, the benefits, when compared to placebo effects, are substantial. Therefore, these medications are particularly indicated when an individual is identified as having severe levels of depression. (A table of current FDA-approved antidepressants, pregnancy categories, half-life, and daily dosage ranges can be found online at Davis*Plus* and in Chapter 16, Depressive Disorders.)

Action

These drugs ultimately work to increase the concentration of norepinephrine, serotonin, and/or dopamine through a complex series of interactions in the body. This is accomplished in the brain by blocking the reuptake of these neurotransmitters by the neurons (TCAs, tetracyclics, SSRIs, and SNRIs). It also occurs when the enzyme monoamine oxidase (MAO), which is known to inactivate norepinephrine, serotonin, and dopamine, is *inhibited* at various sites in the nervous system (MAOIs).

> **CLINICAL PEARL** All antidepressants carry an FDA black-box warning for increased risk of suicidality in children and adolescents.

Interactions

Tables 4–4, 4–5, 4–6, and 4–7 identify some of the significant, dangerous drug interactions with antidepressant medications. It is important to recognize that new information about drug interactions is being discovered and published frequently. To fully understand safety issues related to medication administration,

nurses need to access the most current, evidence-based informatics on drug interaction information.

> **CLINICAL PEARL** As antidepressants begin to take effect, the individual may have increased energy with which to implement a suicide plan. The nurse should be particularly alert to sudden or dramatic changes in mood.

Atypical Antidepressants

Atypical antidepressants are a group of drugs that work differently and do not fit into the previously mentioned classes. These include bupropion (Wellbutrin), mirtazapine (Remeron), nefazodone (Serzone), vortioxetine (Trintellix), vilazodone (Viibryd), and trazodone (Desyrel). Drug interactions vary widely within these groups. Concomitant use with MAOIs results in serious, sometimes fatal, effects resembling **neuroleptic malignant syndrome.** Coadministration is contraindicated.

TABLE 4–4 Drug Interactions With SSRIs

INTERACTING DRUGS	ADVERSE EFFECTS
Buspirone (Buspar), tricyclic antidepressants (especially clomipramine), selegiline (Eldepryl), St. John's wort	Serotonin syndrome[a]
Monoamine oxidase inhibitors	Hypertensive crisis
Warfarin, NSAIDs	Increased risk of bleeding
Alcohol, benzodiazepines	Increased sedation
Antiepileptics	Lowered seizure threshold

[a] **Serotonin syndrome** is a potentially fatal syndrome of serotonin overstimulation with rapid onset that progresses from diarrhea, restlessness, agitation, hyperreflexia, and fluctuations in vital signs to later symptoms of myoclonus, seizures, hyperthermia, uncontrolled shivering, and muscle rigidity, and ultimately it can lead to delirium, coma, status epilepticus, cardiovascular collapse, and death. Immediate cessation of offending drugs and comprehensive supportive intervention are essential (Sadock et al., 2015).

TABLE 4–5 Drug Interactions With Tricyclic Antidepressants (TCAs)

INTERACTING DRUGS	ADVERSE EFFECTS
Monoamine oxidase inhibitors	High fever, convulsions, death
St. John's wort, tramadol (Ultram)	Seizures, serotonin syndrome
Clonidine (Catapres), epinephrine	Severe hypertension
Acetylcholine blockers	Paralytic ileus
Alcohol and carbamazepine (Tegretol)	Blocks antidepressant action; increases sedation
Cimetidine (Tagamet), bupropion (Wellbutrin)	Increased TCA blood levels and increased side effects

TABLE 4–6 Drug Interactions With Monoamine Oxidase Inhibitors (MAOIs)

INTERACTING DRUGS	ADVERSE EFFECTS
SSRIs, TCAs, atomoxetine (Strattera), duloxetine (Cymbalta), dextromethorphan (an ingredient in many cough syrups), venlafaxine (Effexor), St. John's wort, ginkgo	Serotonin syndrome
Morphine and other narcotic pain relievers, antihypertensives	Hypotension
All other antidepressants, pseudoephedrine, amphetamines, cocaine cyclobenzaprine (Flexeril), dopamine, methyldopa, levodopa, epinephrine, buspirone (Buspar)	Hypertensive crisis (these side effects can occur even if taken within 2 weeks of stopping MAOIs)
Buspirone (Buspar)	Psychosis, agitation, seizures
Antidiabetics	Hypoglycemia
Tegretol	Fever, hypertension, seizures

TABLE 4–7 Diet Restrictions for Clients on MAOI Therapy

FOODS CONTAINING TYRAMINE		
HIGH TYRAMINE CONTENT (AVOID WHILE ON MAOI THERAPY)	MODERATE TYRAMINE CONTENT (MAY EAT OCCASIONALLY WHILE ON MAOI THERAPY)	LOW TYRAMINE CONTENT (LIMITED QUANTITIES PERMISSIBLE WHILE ON MAOI THERAPY)
Aged cheeses (cheddar, Swiss, Camembert, blue cheese, Parmesan, provolone, Romano, brie)	Gouda cheese, processed American cheese, mozzarella	Pasteurized cheeses (cream cheese, cottage cheese, ricotta)
Raisins, fava beans, flat Italian beans, Chinese pea pods	Yogurt, sour cream	Figs
Red wines (Chianti, burgundy, cabernet sauvignon)	Avocados, bananas	Distilled spirits (in moderation)
Liqueurs	Beer, white wine, coffee, colas, tea, hot chocolate	
Smoked and processed meats (salami, bologna, pepperoni, summer sausage)	Meat extracts, such as bouillon	
Caviar, pickled herring, corned beef, chicken or beef liver	Chocolate	
Soy sauce, brewer's yeast, meat tenderizer (MSG)		
Sauerkraut (Krakus)		

Sources: Sadock, B. J., Sadock, V. A., & Ruiz, P. (2015). Synopsis of psychiatry: Behavioral sciences/clinical psychiatry (11th ed.). Baltimore: Lippincott Williams & Wilkins; and Vallerand, A. H, Sanoski, C. A., & Deglin, J. H. (2017). Davis drug guide for nurses (15th ed.). Philadelphia: F.A. Davis.

The following are examples of possible drug interactions that can occur with use of SSRIs, SNRIs, and other atypical antidepressants:

■ Serotonin syndrome may occur when any of the following are used together: St. John's wort, sumatriptan, sibutramine, trazodone, nefazodone, venlafaxine, duloxetine, levomilnacipran, SSRIs, 5-HT-receptor agonists (triptans).

■ Increased effects of haloperidol, clozapine, and desipramine may occur with concomitant use of venlafaxine.

■ Increased effects of levomilnacipran may occur with concomitant use of CYP3A4 inhibitors.

■ Increased effects of venlafaxine may occur with concomitant use of cimetidine.

■ Increased effects of duloxetine may occur with concomitant use of CYP1A2 inhibitors (e.g., fluvoxamine, quinolone antibiotics) or CYP2D6 inhibitors (e.g., fluoxetine, quinidine, paroxetine).

■ Risk of liver injury is increased with concomitant use of alcohol and duloxetine.

■ Risk of toxicity or adverse effects from drugs extensively metabolized by CYP2D6 (e.g., flecainide, phenothiazines, propafenone, tricyclic antidepressants, thioridazine) is increased when these drugs are used concomitantly with duloxetine or bupropion.

■ Decreased effects of bupropion and trazodone may occur with concomitant use of carbamazepine.
■ The anticoagulant effect of warfarin may be altered with concomitant use of bupropion, venlafaxine, desvenlafaxine, duloxetine, levomilnacipran, or trazodone.
■ SNRIs increase risks of bleeding in combination with aspirin, warfarin, or other blood thinners.
■ Risk of seizures is increased when bupropion is coadministered with drugs that lower the seizure threshold (e.g., antidepressants, antipsychotics, systemic steroids, theophylline, tramadol).
■ Effects of midazolam are decreased with concomitant use of desvenlafaxine.
■ Effects of desvenlafaxine and levomilnacipran are increased with concomitant use of potent CYP3A4 inhibitors (e.g., ketoconazole).

Diagnosis

The following nursing diagnoses may be considered for patients receiving therapy with antidepressant medications:

1. Risk for suicide related to depressed mood
2. Risk for injury related to side effects of sedation, lowered seizure threshold, orthostatic hypotension, **priapism,** photosensitivity, arrhythmias, **hypertensive crisis,** or serotonin syndrome
3. Social isolation related to depressed mood
4. Risk for constipation related to side effects of the medication
5. Insomnia related to depressed mood and elevated level of anxiety

Safety Issues in Planning and Implementing Care for Patients Taking Antidepressant Medication

Some of the common but manageable side effects of antidepressant medications include dry mouth, sedation, and nausea. General nursing interventions such as offering hard candies, ice, and frequent sips of water are helpful in alleviating dry mouth. Clients may find that sedation is less bothersome if they take the daily dose of antidepressant at bedtime. They should be encouraged to discuss this side effect with the prescribing physician or nurse practitioner. Taking antidepressant medication with food may be helpful in minimizing the common side effect of nausea.

Some individuals taking SSRIs or SNRIs complain of sexual dysfunction while on these medications. Men may report abnormal ejaculation or impotence, and women may report loss of orgasm. Because of these side effects, clients sometimes stop the medication abruptly, which may put them at risk for discontinuation syndrome and worsen their symptoms of depression. Nurses must develop an open attitude regarding discussion and assessment of patient sexual concerns, and patients who are particularly troubled by this side effect can be encouraged to discuss their concerns with their physician or nurse practitioner to explore an alternative medication.

Other side effects or adverse reactions may be dangerous or even fatal. Many are related to drug–drug or drug–food interactions, as discussed previously.

Because of the large amount of information and because new drug development is ongoing, practicing nurses should ensure that they are accessing evidence-based informatics to keep up to date on side effects as well. Many healthcare organizations provide online medication resources to employees, and mobile device applications may also provide a readily available resource for up-to-date drug information. Some important safety issues and nursing interventions are listed in Table 4–8.

Outcome Criteria and Evaluation

The following criteria may be used for evaluating the effectiveness of therapy with antidepressant medications.

The patient:

■ Has not harmed self.
■ Has not experienced injury caused by side effects.
■ Exhibits vital signs within normal limits.
■ Manifests symptoms of improvement in mood (brighter affect, interaction with others, improvement in hygiene, clear thought, expressing hopefulness, ability to make decisions).
■ Willingly participates in activities and interacts appropriately with others.

Mood-Stabilizing Agents

Background Assessment Data

For many years, the drug of choice for treatment and management of bipolar mania was lithium carbonate. However, in recent years, several other medications have demonstrated effectiveness either alone or in combination with lithium. Most notably are many drugs in the class of anticonvulsant medications, which are now FDA approved as indicated for mood stabilization. Second generation, atypical antipsychotics have also demonstrated benefits for management of this disorder.

TABLE 4–8 **Safety Issues and Nursing Interventions for Patients Taking Antidepressants**	
SAEFTY ISSUES	**NURSING INTERVENTIONS**
Drug interactions (multiple, as discussed in the text)	Instruct patients to inform their physician or nurse practitioner of *all* medications they are taking, including herbal preparations, over-the-counter (OTC) drugs, and any medications they have stopped taking within the previous 2 weeks. Notify the physician immediately when any symptoms of serotonin syndrome are assessed. Do not administer the offending agent. ■ Monitor vital signs. ■ Protect from injury secondary to muscle rigidity or change in mental status. ■ Cooling blankets for temperature regulation. ■ Monitor intake and output. The condition usually resolves when the offending agent is promptly discontinued but can be fatal without intervention (Cooper & Sejnowski, 2013).
Increased risk for suicide	Assess frequently for presence or worsening of suicide ideation. Initiate suicide precautions as needed. Monitor patient's use of medication as prescribed, because these medications can be lethal in overdose.
Sedation	Instruct patient not to drive or operate dangerous machinery when experiencing sedation.
Discontinuation syndrome: SSRIs— tremor, akathisia, Parkinsonism, dizziness, lethargy, headache, nausea TCAs—hypomania, tremor, akathisia, Parkinsonism, cardiac arrhythmias, GI upset, panic attacks MAOIs—myoclonic jerks, catatonia, flu-like symptoms, confusion, hypomania	Instruct patient that all antidepressants have some potential for discontinuation syndrome and should not be stopped abruptly but rather should be tapered off. Paroxetine is associated with the highest risk for discontinuation syndrome (Janicak & Hussain, 2017).
Photosensitivity	Instruct patient of vulnerability to severe sunburn and recommend sunscreen.
Orthostatic hypotension (TCAs)	Instruct patient to rise slowly from sitting to standing. Monitor blood pressure to assess for symptoms.
Tachycardia, arrhythmias (TCAs)	Monitor vital signs, especially in elderly patients with pre-existing cardiovascular disorders.
Hyponatremia (SSRIs), especially among the elderly[a]	Instruct patient to report any symptoms of nausea, malaise, lethargy, muscle cramps. Assess for disorientation or restlessness. Monitor sodium levels: ■ <120 mEq/L risk for seizure, coma, respiratory arrest ■ Withhold medication, contact physician, restrict water intake ■ Take a detailed history of antidepressant therapy, particularly the duration of new antidepressant use (Lien, 2018)
Blurred vision (TCAs, SSRIs, and SNRIs)	Instruct patient to avoid driving and reassure patient that this side effect usually resolves within 3 weeks. Monitor blood pressure to rule out symptoms of hypertension.
Constipation	Recommend a high-fiber diet and regular exercise and instruct patient to report any symptoms of ongoing difficulty with bowel movements.

[a] Potentially life threatening.

Bipolar disorder is characterized by cycles of depression and manic episodes that may manifest as grandiose thinking and behavior, rapid thoughts, hyperactivity, and/or impulsive agitation. The effective medication treatment for this disorder is one that reduces the rollercoaster of "ups and downs" often described by clients; thus, the name "mood stabilizer" is an apt description of their purpose. Lithium was first identified as an antimanic but was later recognized as successful for stabilizing the mood swings of bipolar disorder as well.

Lithium is a salt that is present in mineral springs and popularly added to spa baths. Although it also was used for other medicinal purposes, in 1949, John Cade, a physician in Australia, reported that he was using lithium to treat manic excitement and found that it was so successful for some that they became symptom free and were able to be discharged after years of institutionalization (Shorter, 2009). It remains true today that people who respond to lithium and remain on the medication may show no evidence of bipolar mood swings. Although lithium is not a cure for bipolar disorder, it is often described as "like insulin to a diabetic" in that proper use and response can reduce or eliminate symptoms. Unfortunately, not everyone responds to lithium with the same degree of success, and too much lithium can be fatal. Today, we are able to measure specifically the blood levels of lithium and can be confident of its safety when maintained within the specified therapeutic range (0.6–1.2 mEq/L). The exact mechanism of action remains unknown, but it is believed to have an impact on the same neurotransmitters (serotonin, norepinephrine, glutamate, GABA, and dopamine) as previously discussed.

In 1995, the FDA approved valproate (Depakote) as a mood stabilizer, and since then, a shift toward this group of anticonvulsant/mood stabilizers (including carbamazepine, clonazepam, topiramate, and lamotrigine) and away from lithium has occurred (Shorter, 2009). The mechanism of action for these drugs, as with lithium, is also unclear. Impact on cellular sodium transport, GABA modulation, and raising the seizure threshold have all been advanced as possible explanations for their effectiveness. Both first generation and second generation antipsychotics have been used alone or as adjuncts to other medication treatment for bipolar mania. Because lithium has a lag period of 7 to 10 days, first generation antipsychotics such as haloperidol may be helpful in that their sedative effects are more immediate and may bring some relief from manic symptoms before lithium reaches therapeutic levels. It also increases the effects of lithium, so monitoring blood serum levels is especially important in the initial phase of treatment when these two drugs are used in combination. (A table of current FDA-approved mood stabilizer medication agents, pregnancy categories, half-life, and daily dosage ranges can be found online at Davis*Plus* and in Chapter 17, Bipolar and Related Disorders.)

Interactions

Many drugs either increase or decrease the effectiveness of mood stabilizers (Table 4–9). Understanding that lithium is a salt is relevant in explaining some of these interactions. Because lithium is an imperfect substitute for sodium, anything that depletes sodium will make more receptor sites available to lithium and increase the risk for lithium toxicity. This is also the rationale for advising patients to maintain their usual dietary sodium and fluid intake, because major fluctuations impact lithium levels. For example, significant increases in dietary sodium intake may reduce the effectiveness of lithium because sodium will bind at more receptor sites and lithium will be excreted. Other drugs that increase serum sodium levels will also have an impact on lithium levels.

Diagnosis

The following nursing diagnoses may be considered for patients receiving therapy with mood-stabilizing agents:

1. Risk for injury related to manic hyperactivity
2. Risk for self-directed or other-directed violence related to unresolved anger turned inward on the self or outward on the environment
3. Risk for injury related to lithium toxicity
4. Risk for injury related to adverse effects of mood-stabilizing drugs
5. Risk for activity intolerance related to side effects of drowsiness and dizziness

Planning and Implementing Care for Patients Taking Mood Stabilizers

One of the primary safety issues with lithium has to do with its narrow therapeutic range. A description of lithium toxicity, other safety concerns with mood-stabilizing agents, and relevant nursing interventions are discussed in Table 4–10.

Lithium Maintenance

Patients who respond to lithium will typically remain on the medication indefinitely. To ensure safe maintenance and prevent lithium toxicity, patient education and regular monitoring are essential. Monitoring the

TABLE 4-9 Drug Interactions With Mood-Stabilizing Agents

THE EFFECTS OF	ARE INCREASED BY	ARE DECREASED BY	CONCURRENT USE MAY RESULT IN
Antimanic: Lithium	Carbamazepine, fluoxetine, haloperidol, loop diuretics, methyldopa, NSAIDs, and thiazide diuretics	Acetazolamide, osmotic diuretics, theophylline, and urinary alkalinizers	Increased effects of neuromuscular blocking agents and TCAs; decreased pressor sensitivity of sympathomimetics; neurotoxicity may occur with phenothiazines or calcium channel blockers
Anticonvulsants: Clonazepam	CNS depressants, cimetidine, hormonal contraceptives, disulfiram, fluoxetine, isoniazid, ketoconazole, metoprolol, propranolol, valproic acid, probenecid	Rifampin, theophylline (↓ sedative effects), phenytoin	Increased phenytoin levels; decreased efficacy of levodopa
Carbamazepine	Verapamil, diltiazem, propoxyphene, erythromycin, clarithromycin, SSRIs, TCAs, cimetidine, isoniazid, danazol, lamotrigine, niacin, acetazolamide, dalfopristin, valproate, nefazodone	Cisplatin, doxorubicin, felbamate, rifampin, barbiturates, hydantoins, primidone, theophylline	Decreased levels of corticosteroids, doxycycline, quinidine, warfarin, estrogen-containing contraceptives, cyclosporine, benzodiazepines, theophylline, lamotrigine, valproic acid, bupropion, haloperidol, olanzapine, tiagabine, topiramate, voriconazole, ziprasidone, felbamate, levothyroxine, or antidepressants; increased levels of lithium; life-threatening hypertensive reaction with MAOIs
Valproic Acid	Chlorpromazine, cimetidine, erythromycin, felbamate, salicylates	Rifampin, carbamazepine, cholestyramine, lamotrigine, phenobarbital, ethosuximide, hydantoins	Increased effects of TCAs, carbamazepine, CNS depressants, ethosuximide, lamotrigine, phenobarbital, warfarin, zidovudine, hydantoins
Lamotrigine	Valproic acid	Primidone, phenobarbital, phenytoin, rifampin, succinimides, oral contraceptives, oxcarbazepine, carbamazepine, acetaminophen	Decreased levels of valproic acid; increased levels of carbamazepine and topiramate
Topiramate	Metformin, hydrochlorothiazide	Phenytoin, carbamazepine, valproic acid, lamotrigine	Increased risk of CNS depression with alcohol or other CNS depressants; increased risk of kidney stones with carbonic anhydrase inhibitors; increased effects of phenytoin, metformin, amitriptyline; decreased effects of oral contraceptives, digoxin, lithium, risperidone, and valproic acid
Oxcarbazepine	Carbamazepine, phenobarbital, phenytoin, valproic acid, verapamil		Increased concentrations of phenobarbital and phenytoin; decreased effects of oral contraceptives, felodipine, and lamotrigine
Calcium Channel Blocker: Verapamil	Amiodarone, beta blockers, cimetidine, ranitidine, and grapefruit juice	Barbiturates, calcium salts, hydantoins, rifampin, and antineoplastics	Increased effects of beta blockers, disopyramide, flecainide, doxorubicin, benzodiazepines, buspirone, carbamazepine, digoxin, dofetilide, ethanol, imipramine, nondepolarizing muscle relaxants, prazosin, quinidine, sirolimus, tacrolimus, and theophylline; altered serum lithium levels

Continued

TABLE 4–9 Drug Interactions With Mood-Stabilizing Agents—cont'd

THE EFFECTS OF	ARE INCREASED BY	ARE DECREASED BY	CONCURRENT USE MAY RESULT IN
Antipsychotics: Olanzapine	Fluvoxamine and other CYP1A2 inhibitors, fluoxetine	Carbamazepine and other CYP1A2 inducers, omeprazole, rifampin	Decreased effects of levodopa and dopamine agonists; increased hypotension with antihypertensives; increased CNS depression with alcohol or other CNS depressants
Aripiprazole	Ketoconazole and other CYP3A4 inhibitors; quinidine, fluoxetine, paroxetine, or other potential CYP2D6 inhibitors	Carbamazepine, famotidine, valproate	Increased CNS depression with alcohol or other CNS depressants; increased hypotension with antihypertensives
Chlorpromazine	Beta blockers, paroxetine	Centrally acting anticholinergics	Increased effects of beta blockers; excessive sedation and hypotension with meperidine; decreased hypotensive effect of guanethidine; decreased effect of oral anticoagulants; decreased or increased phenytoin levels; increased orthostatic hypotension with thiazide diuretics; increased CNS depression with alcohol or other CNS depressants; increased hypotension with antihypertensives; increased anticholinergic effects with anticholinergic agents
Quetiapine	Cimetidine; ketoconazole, itraconazole, fluconazole, erythromycin, or other CYP3A4 inhibitors	Phenytoin, thioridazine	Decreased effects of levodopa and dopamine agonists; increased CNS depression with alcohol or other CNS depressants; increased hypotension with antihypertensives
Risperidone	Clozapine, fluoxetine, paroxetine, or ritonavir	Carbamazepine	Decreased effects of levodopa and dopamine agonists; increased effects of clozapine and valproate; increased CNS depression with alcohol or other CNS depressants; increased hypotension with antihypertensives
Ziprasidone	Ketoconazole and other CYP3A4 inhibitors	Carbamazepine	Life-threatening prolongation of QT interval with quinidine, dofetilide, other class Ia and III antiarrhythmics, pimozide, sotalol, thioridazine, chlorpromazine, pentamidine, arsenic trioxide, mefloquine, dolasetron, tacrolimus, droperidol, gatifloxacin, or moxifloxacin; decreased effects of levodopa and dopamine agonists; increased CNS depression with alcohol or other CNS depressants; increased hypotension with antihypertensives
Asenapine	Fluvoxamine, imipramine, valproate	Carbamazepine, cimetidine, paroxetine	Increased effects of paroxetine and dextromethorphan; increased CNS depression with alcohol or other CNS depressants; increased hypotension with antihypertensives; additive effects of QT interval prolongation with quinidine, dofetilide, other class Ia and III antiarrhythmics, pimozide, sotalol, thioridazine, chlorpromazine, pentamidine, arsenic trioxide, mefloquine, dolasetron, tacrolimus, droperidol, gatifloxacin, or moxifloxacin

TABLE 4–10 Safety Issues and Nursing Interventions for Patients Taking Mood Stabilizers

SAFETY ISSUES	NURSING INTERVENTIONS
Lithium toxicity: blood levels >1.2 mEq/L (or <1.2 in elderly or debilitated but most common at or above 1.5 mEq/L) ■ Early signs: vomiting, diarrhea ■ Over 2 mEq/L: tremors, sedation, confusion ■ Levels over 3.5 mEq/L: delirium, seizures, coma, cardiovascular collapse, death ■ Chlorpromazine may mask early signs of lithium toxicity (Vallerand, Sanoski, & Deglin, 2017)	Instruct patient to report all medications, herbals, and caffeine use to physician or nurse practitioner to evaluate for drug interactions. Encourage patient to maintain fluid intake at 2,000–3,000 mL/day and to avoid activities that cause excessive sweating or fluid loss because decreases in sodium levels increase lithium absorption and the potential for lithium toxicity. Instruct patient about the importance of regular monitoring of serum lithium levels. Blood levels should be drawn 12 hours after the last dose.
Increased risk of suicide for all antiepileptics (FDA, 2008)	Assess for suicide risk regularly and instruct patient of risks associated with anticonvulsants.
Hyponatremia (lithium, carbamazepine)	Instruct patient to maintain usual dietary intake of sodium. Assess for and educate patient to report any episodes of nausea, vomiting, headache, muscle weakness, confusion, seizures; these may be signs of hyponatremia and/or lithium toxicity.
Stevens-Johnson syndrome (especially with lamotrigine and carbamazepine) This toxic skin necrolysis can be life threatening	Assess for and educate the patient to report any signs of rash or unusual skin breakdown.
Hypotension, arrhythmias (lithium)	Monitor vital signs and instruct patient to report any symptoms of dizziness or palpitations.
Blood dyscrasias (valproic acid, carbamazepine)	Educate patient to report infections or other illness while on these medications. Ensure that platelet counts and bleeding time are determined before initiation of therapy. Monitor for spontaneous bleeding or bruising.
Increased risk of birth defects (anticonvulsant/ mood stabilizers)	Instruct female patients on the risks of birth defects and provide education about contraception as desired.
Drowsiness (lithium and all anticonvulsants)	Instruct patient to avoid driving or operating dangerous machinery when experiencing this side effect. Assess patients' mental status for level of alertness.

patient includes evaluating serum lithium levels to ensure that they remain within the therapeutic range.

The usual ranges of therapeutic serum concentrations are different for initiation of treatment in an acute manic state and are as follows (Vallerand et al., 2017):

■ For acute mania: 1 to 1.5 mEq/L
■ For maintenance: 0.6 to 1.2 mEq/L

Serum lithium levels should be monitored once or twice a week after initial treatment until dosage and serum levels are stable, then monthly during maintenance therapy. Blood samples should be drawn 12 hours after the last dose.

Some clients complain that they miss the "high" feeling of being in a manic or hypomanic state once they begin mood-stabilizing medications. They may be at risk for self-adjusting medication or discontinuing it altogether.

 Open discussion and exploring the benefits versus disadvantages of medication treatment promotes patient-centered care and enables the nurse to troubleshoot with the patient ways to minimize risks.

Another generally undesirable side effect of lithium is weight gain. Patients should be educated about this potential, and weight should be monitored at regular intervals. It may be helpful to discuss low-calorie diets while stressing the importance of not making large changes in sodium intake because of its impact on serum blood levels of lithium.

CLINICAL PEARL The FDA requires that all antiepileptic (anticonvulsant) drugs carry a warning label indicating that use of the drug increases risk for suicidal thoughts and behaviors. Patients being treated with these medications should be monitored for the emergence or worsening of depression, suicidal thoughts or behavior, or any unusual changes in mood or behavior.

Outcome Criteria and Evaluation

The following criteria may be used for evaluating the effectiveness of therapy with mood-stabilizing agents. The patient:

- Is maintaining stability of mood.
- Has not harmed self or others.
- Has experienced no injury from hyperactivity.
- Is able to participate in activities without excessive sedation or dizziness.
- Is maintaining appropriate weight.
- Exhibits no signs of lithium toxicity.
- Verbalizes importance of taking medication regularly and reporting for regular laboratory blood tests.

Antipsychotic Agents

Background Assessment Data

Antipsychotic medications are also called *neuroleptics*. Historically, they have been referred to as *major tranquilizers*, and they do clearly have sedative effects. The term *antipsychotics* is most descriptive because the primary benefit over time is the alleviation of psychotic symptoms such as hallucinations and delusions. Antipsychotic medications were introduced in the United States in the 1950s with the phenothiazines. Other drugs in this classification soon followed. Unfortunately, this group of medications has the potential for **extrapyramidal side effects** that interfere with normal movements, including acute dystonias (muscle spasms), which can be life threatening; parkinsonian-like symptoms; and **tardive dyskinesias** (later-onset involuntary movement disorders primarily in the tongue, lips, and jaw that may also involve other movement disturbances). These side effects may be permanent even after the drug is discontinued.

Second generation antipsychotic medications have since been developed that have less potential for extrapyramidal symptoms (EPS). These drugs have become the first-line treatment for clients with psychotic disorders such as schizophrenia. This group of drugs is used to alleviate the positive symptoms of schizophrenia such as hallucinations, delusions, and agitation and may also be effective for treating some negative symptoms. More recently, the atypical antipsychotic aripiprazole (Abilify) has been described as a third generation antipsychotic because of its unique functional profile with dopamine receptors, and it has been identified as having minimal risk for EPS (Brust et al., 2015). In 2017, the FDA approved a novel (and controversial) formulation of Abilify (called Abilify MyCite) that includes a sensor device embedded in the pill that enables the patient (and others) to track whether they are taking the medication.

Typical antipsychotics include the phenothiazines, haloperidol, loxapine, pimozide, and thiothixene. Atypical antipsychotics include aripiprazole, asenapine, clozapine, olanzapine, quetiapine, risperidone, paliperidone, iloperidone, lurasidone, ziprasidone, and the new drugs brexpiprazole (Rexulti), cariprazine (Vraylar), and pimavanserin (Nuplazid). Pimavanserin is indicated for the treatment of hallucinations and delusions associated with Parkinson's disease psychosis.

Indications

Antipsychotics are used to treat schizophrenia and other psychotic disorders. Selected agents are used in the treatment of bipolar mania (see previous section "Mood-Stabilizing Agents"). Others are used as antiemetics (chlorpromazine, perphenazine, prochlorperazine) in the treatment of intractable hiccoughs (chlorpromazine) and for the control of tics and vocal utterances in Tourette's disorder (haloperidol, pimozide). Selected atypical antipsychotics, including aripiprazole, are being used as adjuncts in the treatment of major depressive disorders. (A table of current FDA-approved antipsychotics, pregnancy categories, half-life, and daily dosage ranges and medications used to treat extrapyramidal side effects of antipsychotic medications can be found online at Davis*Plus* and in Chapter 15, Schizophrenia Spectrum and Other Psychotic Disorders.)

Action

Typical antipsychotics work by blocking postsynaptic dopamine receptors in the basal ganglia, hypothalamus, limbic system, brainstem, and medulla. They also demonstrate varying affinity for cholinergic, alpha$_1$-adrenergic, and histaminic receptors. Antipsychotic effects may also be related to inhibition of dopamine-mediated transmission of neural impulses at the synapses.

Atypical antipsychotics are weaker dopamine receptor antagonists than the conventional antipsychotics, but they are more potent antagonists of serotonin type 2A (5-HT$_{2A}$) receptors. They also exhibit antagonism for cholinergic, histaminic, and adrenergic receptors. As mentioned previously, aripiprazole is a dopamine receptor antagonist but seems to have a unique way of accomplishing this action and thus has a minimal risk of EPS.

Contraindications and Precautions

Certain individuals may be at greater risk for experiencing side effects associated with antipsychotic agents. The elderly have been identified as an at-risk population because of accounts of stroke and sudden death while taking antipsychotic medication. Studies have indicated that elderly patients with neurocognitive-related psychosis who are treated with antipsychotic drugs are at increased risk of death compared with those taking a placebo (Steinberg & Lyketsos, 2012). Causes of death are most commonly related to infections or cardiovascular problems. All antipsychotic drugs now carry black-box warnings about these potential effects. They are not approved for treatment of elderly patients with neurocognitive disorder (NCD)-related psychosis.

Typical antipsychotics are contraindicated in clients with known hypersensitivity (cross sensitivity may exist among phenothiazines). They should not be used in patients in comatose states or when CNS depression is evident; when blood dyscrasias exist; in clients with Parkinson's disease or narrow-angle glaucoma; in those with liver, renal, or cardiac insufficiency; in individuals with poorly controlled seizure disorders; or in elderly clients with dementia-related psychosis. Caution should be used when administering these drugs to patients who are elderly, severely ill, or debilitated and to patients with diabetes, respiratory insufficiency, prostatic hypertrophy, or intestinal obstruction. The risk for metabolic disturbances such as weight gain can be particularly dangerous in the elderly.

Atypical antipsychotics are contraindicated in hypersensitivity, comatose or severely depressed patients, elderly patients with dementia-related psychosis, and lactation. Ziprasidone, risperidone, paliperidone, asenapine, and iloperidone are contraindicated in patients with a history of QT prolongation or cardiac arrhythmias, recent myocardial infarction (MI), or uncompensated heart failure, and concurrent use with other drugs that prolong the QT interval is also contraindicated. Clozapine is contraindicated in patients with myeloproliferative disorders, with a history of clozapine-induced agranulocytosis or severe granulocytopenia, and in uncontrolled epilepsy. Lurasidone and cariprazine are contraindicated in concomitant use with strong inhibitors of cytochrome P450 isozyme 3A4 (CYP3A4) (e.g., ketoconazole, an antifungal) and strong CYP3A4 inducers (e.g., rifampin, an antitubercular).

Caution should be used when administering these drugs to elderly or debilitated patients; patients with cardiac, hepatic, or renal insufficiency; those with a history of seizures; patients with diabetes or risk factors for diabetes; patients exposed to temperature extremes; to pregnant patients or children (safety not established); under conditions that cause hypotension (dehydration, hypovolemia, treatment with antihypertensive medication). The risk for metabolic disturbances such as weight gain can be particularly dangerous in the elderly.

Interactions

Table 4–11 highlights some drug interactions that warrant monitoring and assessment by nurses.

Diagnosis

The following nursing diagnoses may be considered for patients receiving antipsychotic therapy:

1. Risk for other-directed violence related to panic anxiety and mistrust of others
2. Risk for injury related to medication side effects of sedation, photosensitivity, reduction of seizure threshold, agranulocytosis, extrapyramidal symptoms, tardive dyskinesia, neuroleptic malignant syndrome, and/or QT prolongation
3. Risk for activity intolerance related to medication side effects of sedation, blurred vision, and/or weakness
4. Nonadherence with medication regimen related to suspiciousness and mistrust of others

Safety Issues in Planning and Implementing Care for Patients Taking Antipsychotic Medication

Table 4–12 defines some significant safety issues to consider and relevant nursing interventions for patients taking antipsychotic medication.

Additional Issues for Patient Education

■ Smoking increases the metabolism of antipsychotics, requiring an adjustment in dosage to achieve a therapeutic effect; nicotine decreases the effectiveness of these medications. Encourage the patient to discuss this issue with the prescribing physician or nurse practitioner.
■ Advise patients to dress warmly in cold weather and avoid extended exposure to very high or low temperatures. Body temperature is harder to maintain with this medication.

TABLE 4–11 **Drug Interactions With Antipsychotic Medications**	
DRUG INTERACTION	**ADVERSE EFFECT**
Antihypertensives, CNS depressants Epinephrine or dopamine in combination with haloperidol or phenothiazines	Additive and potentially severe hypotension
Oral anticoagulants with phenothiazines	Less effective anticoagulant effects
Drugs that prolong QT intervals	Additive effects
Drugs that trigger orthostatic hypotension	Additive hypotension
Drugs with anticholinergic effects, prescription and OTC drugs	Additive anticholinergic effects, including anticholinergic toxicity, signs of which are as follows: ■ Flushing ■ Dry mouth ■ Mydriasis ■ Altered mental status ■ Tachycardia ■ Urinary retention ■ Tremulousness ■ Hypertension

Source: Ramnarine & Ahmed, 2015.

■ Alcohol and antipsychotic medications potentiate each other's effects, so patients should be advised to avoid drinking alcohol while on antipsychotic therapy. Many medications contain substances that interact with antipsychotics in a way that may be harmful. Patients should avoid taking other medications (including over-the-counter products) before consulting with the physician.

■ A significant number of patients on clozapine report excessive salivation. Sugar-free gum and medications (anticholinergic or alpha$_2$ adrenoceptor agonists) may alleviate symptoms. Patients should be encouraged to discuss these options with the prescribing physician or nurse practitioner.

■ Safe use during pregnancy has not been established. Antipsychotics are thought to readily cross the placental barrier and may therefore affect the fetus. Advise patients of possible risks of taking antipsychotics during pregnancy. Patients should inform the physician immediately if pregnancy occurs, is suspected, or is planned.

Issues in Antipsychotic Maintenance Therapy

The nurse must understand the side effects associated with antipsychotic medication in order to conduct a thorough assessment and minimize risks. In addition, some of these side effects can be difficult for patients to manage or to understand, particularly when they are struggling with impaired mental status including psychosis and cognitive deficits. Three of these side effects are discussed next.

Clozapine (Clozaril) and the Risk for Agranulocytosis

Some medications, because of the risks associated with their use, are required to be monitored more closely. Clozaril is one such drug. Due to the risk of agranulocytosis, the FDA requires that clozapine be part of a risk evaluation and mitigation strategy (REMS) program to ensure that risk for agranulocytosis is monitored, managed, and reported. **Agranulocytosis** is a potentially fatal blood disorder in which the patient's absolute neutrophil count (ANC) drops to extremely low levels (less than or equal to 500 µL). This condition is called *neutropenia*. An ANC must be assessed before initiation of treatment with clozapine and weekly for the first 6 months of treatment. Initially, only a 1-week supply of medication is dispensed at a time. If the ANC remains within the acceptable levels (i.e., ANC at least 1,500 µL) during the first 6 months, blood counts may be monitored biweekly for another 6 months and monthly thereafter. Some darker skinned ethnic groups, particularly those of African and Middle Eastern descent, have normally lower ANC (benign ethnic neutropenia) than other ethnic groups and in such cases the parameters for identifying clinically significant neutropenia are altered (Clozapine REMS, 2015).

TABLE 4–12 Safety Issues in Planning and Implementing Care for Patients Taking Antipsychotic Medication

SAFETY ISSUES	NURSING INTERVENTIONS
Extrapyramidal side effects[a] (More common with typical antipsychotic agents)	Instruct patient to report any signs of muscle stiffness or spasms; hold the medication if signs occur. Administer antiparkinsonian agents as ordered and immediately when signs of acute dystonia are present. Assess the patient for abnormal involuntary movements (see Box 4–2). (See next section, "Extrapyramidal Side Effects," for further discussion.)
Hyperglycemia, weight gain, and diabetes (More common with atypical antipsychotic agents)	Assess for history of diabetes. Evaluate blood sugars. Instruct patient in these risks and the importance of diet and exercise. Assess for signs of hyperglycemia, including polydipsia, polyphagia, polyuria, and weakness.
Hypotension	Educate patient about risk for hypotension. Monitor blood pressure.
Orthostatic hypotension	Instruct patient to rise slowly from sitting to standing. Monitor blood pressure lying and then standing to assess for postural changes.
Lower seizure threshold (especially with Clozapine)	Assess patient for history of seizure disorder. Monitor patient for evidence of seizure activity, and report to prescribing physician or nurse practitioner.
Prolonged QT interval[b] Especially ziprasidone, thioridazine, pimozide, haloperidol, paliperidone, iloperidone, asenapine, and clozapine	Assess for history of arrhythmias, recent myocardial infarction, or heart failure, and report to prescribing physician or nurse practitioner because these events are contraindications. Assess for other medications the patient is taking that prolong QT interval (there are many; online resources such as www.crediblemeds.org provide a composite list for comparison). Instruct patient to report any rapid heartbeat, dizziness, or fainting. Check baseline electrocardiogram before beginning treatment.
Anticholinergic effects	Instruct patient about additive effects of other anticholinergic drugs in combination with antipsychotics and to report any other medications being taken, including over-the-counter and herbal remedies. For minor symptoms such as dry mouth, recommend hard candies, sips of water. Instruct patient regarding the importance of good oral hygiene. Assess for, and instruct patient to report, any evidence of urinary retention, tachycardia, tremulousness, or hypertension, because these may be signs of anticholinergic toxicity.
Sedation	Educate patient about this side effect and instruct patient not to drive or operate dangerous machinery if experiencing sedation.
Photosensitivity	Instruct patient to use sunblock and sunglasses and to wear protective clothing when in the sun because of the increased risk for severe sunburn while on these medications.
Agranulocytosis (more common with typical antipsychotics but especially with the atypical antipsychotic agent clozapine)[b]	Instruct patient receiving clozapine that regular monitoring of white blood cell and absolute neutrophil blood levels is essential. Instruct patient to report any signs of sore throat, fever, or malaise. (See additional guidelines below.)
Neuroleptic malignant syndrome (NMS)[c]	Instruct patient to report immediately any fever, muscle rigidity, diaphoresis, tachycardia. Assess vital signs regularly, including temperature. Assess for deteriorating mental status or any other sign of NMS; presence of any of these signs requires holding the medication and contacting the prescribing physician or nurse practitioner immediately and monitoring vital signs and intake and output.

Continued

TABLE 4–12	Safety Issues in Planning and Implementing Care for Patients Taking Antipsychotic Medication—cont'd
SAFETY ISSUES	**NURSING INTERVENTIONS**
Drug reaction with eosinophilia and systemic symptoms (DRESS) (olanzapine)[d] (FDA, 2016b)	Assess for symptoms of DRESS including fever, rash, swollen lymph glands, swelling in the face. Hold medication and contact physician immediately.
New impulse control problems such as compulsive or uncontrollable urges to gamble, binge eat, shop, and have sex (aripiprazole) (FDA, 2016 c)	Assess for newly developing impulse control problems for patients taking aripiprazole. Closely monitor patients who may be at increased risk for impulse control problems such as those with personal or family history of obsessive-compulsive disorder, bipolar disorder, impulsive personality, alcohol, drug, or other addictive behaviors.

[a] Acute dystonias can be life threatening.
[b] Potentially life threatening.
[c] Rare but potentially life-threatening side effect characterized by muscle rigidity, severe hyperthermia, and cardiac effects, which can be rapidly progressive over 24–72 hours and is potentially fatal.
[d] Rare but serious; can lead to organ injury and even death.

Although the benefits of clozapine can be profound, this medication is typically used when patients fail to respond to other antipsychotics because of the strict protocols for adherence. If the patient agrees to this option, the nurse can be a vital link in ensuring that support services, both professional and personal (such as family members or peers), are engaged to assist the patient with follow-through as needed.

Extrapyramidal Side Effects

Several distinct types of extrapyramidal side effects may occur with antipsychotics, and the nurse must be familiar with them to conduct a thorough assessment:

■ **Pseudoparkinsonism** (tremor, shuffling gait, drooling, rigidity): Symptoms may appear 1 to 5 days following initiation of antipsychotic medication; occurs most often in women, the elderly, and dehydrated patients.
■ **Akinesia** absence or impairment in voluntary movement.
■ **Akathisia** (continuous restlessness and fidgeting): This side effect occurs most frequently in women; symptoms may occur 50 to 60 days after therapy begins.
■ **Dystonia:** This side effect is characterized by involuntary muscle spasms in the face, arms, legs, and neck and occurs most often in men and in people younger than 25 years of age. If untreated, it can progress to laryngospasms and can be fatal. Dystonia should be treated as an emergency situation and the physician should be contacted

immediately. Dystonia is typically treated with intramuscular or intravenous benztropine (Cogentin). Stay with the patient and offer reassurance and support; these adverse effects can be very frightening.
■ **Oculogyric crisis (uncontrolled rolling back of the eyes):** This side effect may appear as part of the syndrome described as dystonia and may be mistaken for seizure activity. As with other symptoms of acute dystonia, this side effect should be treated as a medical emergency.
■ **Tardive dyskinesia:** This later-onset adverse effect is characterized by bizarre facial and tongue movements, stiff neck, and difficulty swallowing; it may occur with all classifications but is more common with first generation antipsychotics. All patients receiving long-term (months or years) antipsychotic therapy are at risk, and the symptoms are potentially irreversible. Nurses should immediately report any early signs of tardive dyskinesia (usually abnormal tongue movements) to the prescribing physician or nurse practitioner. The Abnormal Involuntary Movement Scale (AIMS) is a rating scale that was developed in the 1970s by the National Institute of Mental Health to measure involuntary movements associated with tardive dyskinesia. The AIMS aids in early detection of movement disorders and provides a means for ongoing surveillance (see Box 4–2). A decision may be made to change to a different drug, adjust the dosage, or discontinue the drug. In 2017 the

BOX 4–2 Abnormal Involuntary Movements Scale (AIMS)

Name _____ Rater Name _____ Date _____

Instructions: Complete the examination procedure before making ratings. For movement ratings, circle the highest severity observed. Rate movements that occur upon activation one *less* than those observed spontaneously. Circle movement as well as code number that applies.

Code:
- 0 = None
- 1 = Minimal, may be normal
- 2 = Mild
- 3 = Moderate
- 4 = Severe

Facial and Oral Movements	1. **Muscles of Facial Expression** (e.g., movements of forehead, eyebrows, periorbital area, cheeks, including frowning, blinking, smiling, grimacing)	0 1 2 3 4
	2. **Lips and Perioral Area** (e.g., puckering, pouting, smacking)	0 1 2 3 4
	3. **Jaw** (e.g., biting, clenching, chewing, mouth opening, lateral movement)	0 1 2 3 4
	4. **Tongue** (Rate only increases in movement both in and out of mouth. NOT inability to sustain movement. Darting in and out of mouth.)	0 1 2 3 4
Extremity Movements	5. **Upper (arms, wrists, hands, fingers)** Include choreic movements (i.e., rapid, objectively purposeless, irregular, spontaneous) and athetoid movements (i.e., slow, irregular, complex serpentine). *Do not include tremor* (i.e., repetitive, regular, rhythmic)	0 1 2 3 4
	6. **Lower (legs, knees, ankles, toes)** (e.g., lateral knee movement, foot tapping, heel dropping, foot squirming, inversion and eversion of foot)	0 1 2 3 4
Trunk Movements	7. **Neck, shoulders, hips** (e.g., rocking, twisting, squirming, pelvic gyrations)	0 1 2 3 4
Global Judgments	8. **Severity of abnormal movements overall**	0 1 2 3 4
	9. **Incapacitation due to abnormal movements**	0 1 2 3 4
	10. **Patient's awareness of abnormal movements** (Rate only the patient's report) No awareness Aware, no distress Aware, mild distress Aware, moderate distress Aware, severe distress	0 1 2 3 4
Dental Status	11. **Current problems with teeth and/or dentures?**	No Yes
	12. **Are dentures usually worn?**	No Yes
	13. **Edentia?**	No Yes
	14. **Do movements disappear in sleep?**	No Yes

Either before or after completing the examination procedure, observe the patient unobtrusively, at rest (e.g., in waiting room). The chair to be used in this examination should be a hard, firm one without arms.

1. Ask patient to remove shoes and socks.
2. Ask patient whether there is anything in his/her mouth (e.g., gum, candy), and if so, to remove it.
3. Ask patient about the current condition of his/her teeth. Ask patient if he/she wears dentures. Do teeth or dentures bother patient now?

Continued

BOX 4–2 **Abnormal Involuntary Movements Scale (AIMS)—cont'd**

4. Ask patient whether he/she notices any movements in mouth, face, hands, or feet. If yes, ask to describe and to what extent movements currently bother patient or interfere with his/her activities.
5. Have patient sit in chair with both hands on knees, legs slightly apart, and feet flat on floor. (Look at entire body for movements while in this position.)
6. Ask patient to sit with hands hanging unsupported. If male, between legs, if female and wearing a dress, hanging over knees. (Observe hands and other body areas.)
7. Ask patient to open mouth. (Observe tongue at rest within mouth.) Do this twice.
8. Ask patient to protrude tongue. (Observe abnormalities of tongue movement.) Do this twice.
9. Ask patient to tap thumb with each finger as rapidly as possible for 10 to 15 seconds; separately with right hand, then with left hand. (Observe facial and leg movements.)
10. Flex and extend patient's left and right arms (one at a time). (Note any rigidity.)
11. Ask patient to stand up. (Observe in profile. Observe all body areas again, hips included.)
12. Ask patient to extend both arms outstretched in front with palms down. (Observe trunk, legs, and mouth.)
13. Have patient walk a few paces, turn, and walk back to chair. (Observe hands and gait.) Do this twice.

INTERPRETATION OF AIMS SCORE
Add patient scores and note areas of difficulty.
Score of:

0 to 1 = Low risk
2 in only ONE of the areas assessed = borderline/observe closely
2 in TWO or more of the areas assessed *or* 3 to 4 in ONLY ONE area = indicative of TD

From U.S. Department of Health and Human Services. Available for use in the public domain.

FDA approved the first drugs for treating tardive dyskinesia: valbenazine (Ingrezza) and deutetrabenazine (Austedo). Although their mechanism of action is unknown, both drugs are believed to inhibit monoamine uptake. In clinical trials, there were significant reductions in abnormal involuntary movements.

Some extrapyramidal side effects can be life threatening and those that are not can sometimes be permanent. The abnormal movements in the tongue and lips can be very visible and even severe enough to interfere with a person's ability to speak or swallow.

The nurse's empathic approach in listening to the patient's wishes with regard to medication and advocating for exploring other options for management of symptoms is one way to promote patient-centered care (IOM, 2003) and to promote a recovery model that empowers patients to make decisions about management of their illness. There is evidence (Haddad, Brain, & Scott, 2014) that remaining on antipsychotic medication can reduce the frequency of hospitalizations, and early treatment at the first psychotic episode may reduce some longer term consequences of illness, so educating patients about these facts is important in assisting them to make an informed decision about medication treatment.

In addition to the drugs used to treat tardive dyskinesia, there are several medications that may be used to treat acute extrapyramidal side effects. These include anticholinergics such as benztropine (Cogentin), antihistamines such as diphenhydramine (Benadryl), or dopaminergic agents such as amantadine (Symmetrel). A list of these agents, their actions, contraindications, side effects, half-life, and daily dosages can be found in Chapter 15, Schizophrenia Spectrum and Other Psychotic Disorders.

Hormonal Side Effects

Following are sexual side effects that may accompany these medications:

■ Decreased libido, **retrograde ejaculation** (the discharge of seminal fluid into the bladder rather than through the urethra); **gynecomastia** (men)
■ **Amenorrhea galactorrhea** (women)

These side effects can be very troubling for anyone, and for a patient struggling with thought disturbances, they can become the foundation for delusions. A male patient with gynecomastia, for example, might begin to believe that external forces are taking over his body and turning him into a woman. An amenorrheic woman may begin to believe that she has been divinely impregnated. It is important for the nurse to be clear that these are side effects of the medication and to offer reassurance that they are reversible. Women with amenorrhea should be instructed that this side effect does not indicate cessation of ovulation, so use of contraception should continue as usual. Patients should be encouraged to explore alternative treatment if these side effects are deemed intolerable.

Current Developments in Psychopharmacological Treatment of Schizophrenia

One of the identified limitations of medication treatments available for schizophrenia is that there are several cognitive deficits that are core symptoms of this illness, including deficits in working memory, long-term memory, reduced processing speed, verbal fluency, and executive functions. Some atypical antipsychotics have demonstrated efficacy in lessening cognitive deficits but not eliminating residual effects. A drug recently approved by the FDA, cariprazine (Vraylar), has demonstrated efficacy in treating some negative symptoms of schizophrenia, which include flat affect, social withdrawal, and apathy (Harrison, 2015). Although cariprazine is similar to other atypical antipsychotics, its particular affinity for certain dopamine receptors (D3) is believed to be associated with its superior impact on negative symptoms, particularly improving social behavior and self-care. In addition, cariprazine demonstrated effectiveness in reducing substance use, a common comorbidity in patients with schizophrenia, and its long half-life enables it to maintain efficacy even when a few doses are missed (Scarff, 2017). All of these negative symptoms can complicate the prognosis in treatment of schizophrenia and as Scarff (2017) points out, the evidence supports "cautious optimism" that this may become a treatment of choice for patients with "disabling negative symptoms or impairment in self-care and interpersonal relationships" (p. 237).

Outcome Criteria and Evaluation

The following criteria may be used for evaluating the effectiveness of therapy with antipsychotic medications.

The patient:

- Has not harmed self or others.
- Has not experienced injury caused by side effects of lowered seizure threshold or photosensitivity.
- Maintains an ANC within normal limits.
- Exhibits no symptoms of extrapyramidal side effects, neuroleptic malignant syndrome, or hyperglycemia.
- Maintains weight within normal limits.

- Tolerates activity unaltered by the effects of sedation or weakness.
- Takes medication willingly.
- Verbalizes understanding of medication regimen and the importance of regular administration.
- Demonstrates improvement in self-care and prosocial behavior.

Sedative-Hypnotics

Background Assessment Data

Indications

Sedative-hypnotics are used in the short-term management of various anxiety states and to treat insomnia. Selected agents are used as anticonvulsants (pentobarbital, phenobarbital) and preoperative sedatives (pentobarbital, secobarbital) and to reduce anxiety associated with alcohol withdrawal (phenobarbital). (A table of current FDA-approved sedative-hypnotics, pregnancy categories, half-life, and daily dosage ranges can also be found online at Davis*Plus*.)

Action

Sedative-hypnotics cause generalized CNS depression. They may produce tolerance with chronic use and have the potential for psychological or physical dependence. **EXCEPTION:** Ramelteon (Rozerem) is not a controlled substance. It does not produce tolerance or physical dependence. Its sleep-promoting properties are due to its agonist activity on selective melatonin receptors.

Contraindications and Precautions

Sedative-hypnotics are contraindicated in individuals with hypersensitivity to the drug or to any drug within the chemical class; during pregnancy (exceptions based on assessment of the benefit-to-risk ratio may be made in certain cases); during lactation; in clients with severe hepatic, cardiac, respiratory, or renal disease; in children younger than age 15 (flurazepam); and in children younger than age 18 (estazolam, quazepam, temazepam, triazolam). Triazolam is contraindicated with concurrent use of medications that impair the metabolism of triazolam by cytochrome P4503A (CYP3A), including ketoconazole, itraconazole, and nefazodone, and with concurrent use of fluvoxamine. Zolpidem, zaleplon, eszopiclone, and ramelteon are contraindicated in children.

Caution should be used in administering sedative-hypnotics to patients with cardiac, hepatic, renal, or respiratory insufficiency and in patients who may be suicidal or who have a history of substance use

TABLE 4–13 **Sedative-Hypnotic Agents**			
CHEMICAL CLASS	**GENERIC (TRADE) NAME**	**CATEGORIES**	**DAILY DOSAGE RANGE (MG)**
Barbiturates	Amobarbital	CII	60–200
	Butabarbital (Butisol)	CIII	45–120
	Pentobarbital (Nembutal)	CII	150–200
	Phenobarbital (Luminal; Solfoton)	CIV	30–200
	Secobarbital (Seconal)	CII	100 (hypnotic) 200–300 (preop sedation)
Benzodiazepines	Estazolam	CIV	1–2
	Flurazepam	CIV	15–30
	Quazepam (Doral)	CIV	7.5–15 mg
	Temazepam (Restoril)	CIV	15–30 mg
	Triazolam (Halcion)	CIV	0.125–0.5
Miscellaneous	Eszopiclone (Lunesta)	CIV	1–3
	Ramelteon (Rozerem)	CIV	8
	Zaleplon (Sonata)	CIV	5–20
	Zolpidem (Ambien)	CIV	5–10 (immediate release), 12.5 (extended release)

disorders. Hypnotics should be used for short-term treatment: for an acute episode of insomnia or for several days. Elderly patients may be more sensitive to CNS depressant effects, and dosage reduction may be required. Chloral hydrate should be used with caution in patients susceptible to acute intermittent porphyria (Table 4–13).

Interactions

Barbiturates The effects of barbiturates are increased with concomitant use of alcohol, other CNS depressants, MAOIs, or valproic acid. The effects of barbiturates may be decreased with rifampin. Possible decreased effects of the following drugs may occur when used concomitantly with barbiturates: anticoagulants, beta blockers, carbamazepine, clonazepam, oral contraceptives, corticosteroids, digitoxin, doxorubicin, doxycycline, felodipine, fenoprofen, griseofulvin, metronidazole, phenylbutazone, quinidine, theophylline, and verapamil. Concomitant use with methoxyflurane may enhance renal toxicity.

Benzodiazepines The effects of the benzodiazepine hypnotics are increased with concomitant use of alcohol or other CNS depressants, cimetidine, oral contraceptives, disulfiram, isoniazid, or probenecid. The effects of the benzodiazepine hypnotics are decreased with concomitant use of rifampin, theophylline, carbamazepine, or St. John's wort and with cigarette smoking. The effects of digoxin or phenytoin are increased when used concomitantly with

benzodiazepines. There is increased bioavailability of triazolam with concurrent use of macrolides.

Eszopiclone Additive effects of eszopiclone occur with alcohol or other CNS depressants. Decreased effects of eszopiclone occur with CYP3A4 inducers (e.g., rifampin, phenytoin, carbamazepine, phenobarbital), with lorazepam, or following a high-fat or heavy meal. Increased effects of eszopiclone occur with CYP3A4 inhibitors (e.g., ketoconazole, clarithromycin, nefazodone, ritonavir). There are decreased effects of lorazepam with concomitant use.

Zaleplon Additive effects of zaleplon occur with alcohol or other CNS depressants. Decreased effects of zaleplon occur with CYP3A4 inducers (e.g., rifampin, phenytoin, carbamazepine, phenobarbital) or following a high-fat or heavy meal. There are increased effects of zaleplon with cimetidine.

Zolpidem Increased effects of zolpidem occur with alcohol or other CNS depressants, azole antifungals, ritonavir, or SSRIs. Decreased effects of zolpidem occur with flumazenil, rifampin, and with food. There is a risk of life-threatening cardiac arrhythmias with concomitant use of amiodarone.

Ramelteon Increased effects of ramelteon occur with alcohol, ketoconazole (and other CYP3A4 inhibitors), or fluvoxamine (and other CYP1A2 inhibitors). Decreased effects of ramelteon occur with rifampin (and other CYP3A4 inducers) and following a heavy or high-fat meal.

Diagnosis

The following nursing diagnoses may be considered for patients receiving therapy with sedative hypnotics:

1. Risk for injury related to abrupt withdrawal from long-term use or decreased mental alertness caused by residual sedation
2. Disturbed sleep pattern/insomnia related to situational crises, physical condition, or severe level of anxiety
3. Risk for activity intolerance related to side effects of lethargy, drowsiness, and dizziness
4. Risk for acute confusion related to action of the medication on the central nervous system

Safety Issues in Planning and Implementing Care for Patients Taking Sedative-Hypnotics

Refer to the earlier discussion of safety issues in the section "Antianxiety Agents." In addition to the side effects listed there abnormal thinking and behavioral changes including aggressiveness, hallucinations, and suicidal ideation have also been noted in some individuals taking sedative-hypnotics.

Certain complex behaviors, such as sleep-driving, preparing and eating food, and making phone calls with no memory of the behavior, have occurred. Although a direct correlation to the behavior with the use of sedative-hypnotics cannot be made, the emergence of any new behavioral sign or symptom of concern requires careful and immediate evaluation.

Outcome Criteria and Evaluation

The following criteria may be used for evaluating the effectiveness of therapy with sedative-hypnotic medications:

The patient:

■ Demonstrates a reduction in anxiety, tension, and restless activity.
■ Falls asleep within 30 minutes of taking the medication and remains asleep for 6 to 8 hours without interruption.
■ Is able to participate in usual activities without residual sedation.
■ Experiences no physical injury.
■ Exhibits no evidence of confusion.
■ Verbalizes understanding of taking the medication on a short-term basis.
■ Verbalizes understanding of potential for development of tolerance and dependence with long-term use.

Agents for Attention Deficit-Hyperactivity Disorder (ADHD)

Background Assessment Data

Indications

The medications in this section are used for ADHD in children and adults. Amphetamines are also used in the treatment of narcolepsy and exogenous obesity. Bupropion is also used in the treatment of major depression and for smoking cessation (Zyban only). Clonidine and guanfacine are also used to treat hypertension. (A table of current FDA-approved agents for ADHD, pregnancy categories, half-life, and daily dosage ranges can be found online at Davis*Plus* and in Chapter 23, Children and Adolescents.)

Action

CNS stimulants increase levels of neurotransmitters (probably norepinephrine, dopamine, and serotonin) in the CNS. They produce CNS and respiratory stimulation, dilated pupils, increased motor activity and mental alertness, diminished sense of fatigue, and enhanced mood. The CNS stimulants discussed in this section include dextroamphetamine sulfate, methamphetamine, lisdexamfetamine, amphetamine mixtures, methylphenidate, and dexmethylphenidate. Action in the treatment of ADHD is unclear. However, recent research indicates that their effectiveness in the treatment of hyperactivity disorders is based on the activation of dopamine D_4 receptors in the basal ganglia and thalamus, which depress, rather than enhance, motor activity (Erlij et al., 2012).

Atomoxetine inhibits the reuptake of norepinephrine, and bupropion blocks the neuronal uptake of serotonin, norepinephrine, and dopamine. Clonidine and guanfacine stimulate central alpha-adrenergic receptors in the brain, resulting in reduced sympathetic outflow from the CNS. The exact mechanism by which these nonstimulant drugs produce the therapeutic effect in ADHD is unclear.

Contraindications and Precautions

CNS stimulants are contraindicated in individuals with hypersensitivity to sympathomimetic amines. They should not be used in advanced arteriosclerosis, cardiovascular disease, hypertension, hyperthyroidism, glaucoma, agitated or hyperexcitability states, in patients with a history of drug abuse, during or within 14 days of receiving therapy with MAOIs, in children younger than 3 years of age, or in pregnancy and lactation. Atomoxetine and bupropion are contraindicated in clients with hypersensitivity to the drugs or their components, during lactation, and in concomitant use with or within 2 weeks of using MAOIs. Atomoxetine is contraindicated in clients with narrow-angle glaucoma. Bupropion is contraindicated in individuals with known or suspected seizure disorder, in the acute phase of myocardial infarction, and in clients with bulimia or anorexia nervosa. Alpha agonists are contraindicated in clients with known hypersensitivity to the drugs.

Caution is advised in using CNS stimulants in children with psychosis; in Tourette disorder; in clients with anorexia or insomnia; in elderly, debilitated, or asthenic clients; and in clients with a history of suicidal or homicidal tendencies. Prolonged use may result in tolerance and physical or psychological dependence. Use atomoxetine and bupropion cautiously in clients with urinary retention; hypertension; hepatic, renal, or cardiovascular disease; in suicidal clients; in clients who are pregnant; and in elderly and debilitated clients. Alpha agonists should be used with caution in clients with coronary insufficiency, recent myocardial infarction, or cerebrovascular disease; in clients with chronic renal or hepatic failure; in the elderly; and during pregnancy and lactation.

Interactions

CNS Stimulants (Amphetamines) Effects of amphetamines are increased with furazolidone or urinary alkalinizers. Hypertensive crisis may occur with concomitant use of (and up to several weeks after discontinuing) MAOIs. Increased risk of serotonin syndrome occurs with coadministration of SSRIs. Decreased effects of amphetamines occur with urinary acidifiers, and decreased hypotensive effects of guanethidine occur with amphetamines.

Dexmethylphenidate and Methylphenidate Effects of antihypertensive agents and pressor agents (e.g., dopamine, epinephrine, phenylephrine) are decreased with concomitant use of the methylphenidates. Effects of coumarin anticoagulants, anticonvulsants (e.g., phenobarbital, phenytoin, primidone), tricyclic antidepressants, and SSRIs are increased with the methylphenidates. Hypertensive crisis may occur with coadministration of MAOIs.

Atomoxetine Effects of atomoxetine are increased with concomitant use of CYP2D6 inhibitors (e.g., paroxetine, fluoxetine, quinidine). Potentially fatal reactions may occur with concurrent use of (or within 2 weeks of discontinuation of) MAOIs. Risk of cardiovascular effects is increased with concomitant use of albuterol or vasopressors.

Bupropion Effects of bupropion (Wellbutrin, Zyban) are increased with amantadine, levodopa, or ritonavir. Effects of bupropion are decreased with carbamazepine. There is increased risk of acute toxicity with MAOIs. Increased risk of hypertension may occur with nicotine replacement agents, and adverse neuropsychiatric events may occur with alcohol. Increased anticoagulant effects of warfarin, as well as increased effects of drugs metabolized by CYP2D6 (e.g., nortriptyline, imipramine, desipramine, paroxetine, fluoxetine, sertraline, haloperidol, risperidone, thioridazine, metoprolol, propafenone, and flecainide), occur with concomitant use.

Alpha Agonists Synergistic pharmacological and toxic effects, possibly causing atrioventricular block, bradycardia, and severe hypotension, may occur with concomitant use of calcium channel blockers or beta blockers. Additive sedation occurs with CNS depressants, including alcohol, antihistamines, opioid analgesics, and sedative-hypnotics. Effects of clonidine may be decreased with concomitant use of tricyclic antidepressants and prazosin. Decreased effects of levodopa may occur with clonidine, and effects of guanfacine are decreased with barbiturates or phenytoin.

Diagnosis

The following nursing diagnoses may be considered for patients receiving therapy with agents for ADHD:

1. Risk for injury related to overstimulation and hyperactivity (CNS stimulants) or seizures (possible side effect of bupropion)
2. Risk for suicide secondary to major depression related to abrupt withdrawal after extended use (CNS stimulants)
3. Risk for suicide (children and adolescents) as a side effect of atomoxetine and bupropion (black-box warning)
4. Imbalanced nutrition, less than body requirements, related to side effects of anorexia and weight loss (CNS stimulants)
5. Insomnia related to side effects of overstimulation
6. Nausea related to side effects of atomoxetine or bupropion
7. Pain related to side effect of abdominal pain (atomoxetine, bupropion) or headache (all agents)

8. Risk for activity intolerance related to side effects of sedation and dizziness with atomoxetine or bupropion

Planning and Implementation

The plan of care should include monitoring for the following side effects from agents for ADHD.

■ Overstimulation, restlessness, insomnia (CNS stimulants)
  ▪ Assess mental status for changes in mood, level of activity, degree of stimulation, and aggressiveness.
  ▪ Ensure that the patient is protected from injury.
  ▪ Keep stimuli low and environment as quiet as possible to discourage overstimulation.
  ▪ To prevent insomnia, administer the last dose at least 6 hours before bedtime. Administer sustained-release forms in the morning.
■ Palpitations, tachycardia (CNS stimulants, atomoxetine, bupropion, clonidine), or bradycardia (clonidine, guanfacine)
  ▪ Monitor and record vital signs at regular intervals (two or three times a day) throughout therapy. Report significant changes to the physician immediately.

NOTE: The FDA has issued warnings associated with CNS stimulants and atomoxetine of the risk for sudden death in patients who have cardiovascular disease. A careful personal and family history of heart disease, heart defects, or hypertension should be obtained before these medications are prescribed. Careful monitoring of cardiovascular function during administration must be ongoing.

■ Anorexia, weight loss (CNS stimulants, atomoxetine, bupropion)
  ▪ To reduce anorexia, the medication may be administered immediately after meals.
  ▪ Weigh the patient regularly (at least weekly) when receiving therapy with CNS stimulants, atomoxetine, or bupropion because of the potential for anorexia and weight loss and temporary interruption of growth and development.
■ Tolerance, physical and psychological dependence (CNS stimulants)
  ▪ Assess for signs of tolerance, which can develop rapidly.
  ▪ In children with ADHD, a drug "holiday" should be attempted periodically under direction of the physician to determine the effectiveness of the medication and the need for continuation.

■ Do not abruptly discontinue CNS stimulants. To do so could initiate the following syndrome of symptoms: nausea, vomiting, abdominal cramping, headache, fatigue, weakness, mental depression, suicidal ideation, increased dreaming, and psychotic behavior.
■ Nausea and vomiting (atomoxetine and bupropion)
  ▪ Recommend taking medication with food to minimize gastrointestinal (GI) upset.
■ Constipation (atomoxetine, bupropion, clonidine, guanfacine)
  ▪ Recommend increasing fiber and fluid in diet if not contraindicated.
■ Dry mouth (clonidine and guanfacine)
  ▪ Offer the patient sugarless candy, ice, frequent sips of water.
  ▪ Reinforce the importance of strict oral hygiene.
■ Sedation (clonidine and guanfacine)
  ▪ Warn patient that sedation is increased by concomitant use of alcohol and other CNS drugs.
  ▪ Warn patients to refrain from driving or performing hazardous tasks until response has been established.
■ Potential for seizures (bupropion)
  ▪ Protect patient from injury if seizure should occur. Instruct family and significant others of patients on bupropion therapy how to protect patient during a seizure if one should occur. Ensure that doses of the immediate-release medication are administered at least 4 to 6 hours apart and doses of the sustained-release medication are administered at least 8 hours apart.
■ Severe liver damage (with atomoxetine)
  ▪ Monitor for the following side effects and report to physician immediately: itching, dark urine, right upper quadrant pain, yellow skin or eyes, sore throat, fever, malaise.
■ New or worsened psychiatric symptoms (with CNS stimulants and atomoxetine)
  ▪ Monitor for psychotic symptoms (e.g., hearing voices, paranoid behaviors, delusions).
  ▪ Monitor for manic symptoms, including aggressive and hostile behaviors.
■ Rebound syndrome (with clonidine and guanfacine)
  ▪ The patient should be instructed not to discontinue therapy abruptly. To do so may result in symptoms of nervousness, agitation, headache, and tremor and a rapid rise in blood pressure. Dosage should be tapered gradually under the supervision of the physician.

Patient and Family Education

Instruct the patient that he or she should:

- Use caution in driving or operating dangerous machinery. Drowsiness, dizziness, and blurred vision can occur.
- Not stop taking CNS stimulants abruptly. To do so could produce serious withdrawal symptoms.
- Avoid taking CNS stimulants late in the day to prevent insomnia. Take no later than 6 hours before bedtime.
- Not take other medications (including over-the-counter drugs) without physician's approval. Many medications contain substances that, in combination with agents for ADHD, can be harmful.
- Monitor blood sugar two or three times a day or as instructed by the physician if the patient is diabetic. Be aware of the need for possible alteration in insulin requirements because of changes in food intake, weight, and activity.
- Avoid consumption of large amounts of caffeinated products (coffee, tea, colas, chocolate), as they may enhance the CNS stimulant effect.
- Notify the physician if restlessness, insomnia, anorexia, or dry mouth becomes severe or if rapid, pounding heartbeat becomes evident.
- Report any of the following side effects to the physician immediately: shortness of breath, chest pain, jaw/left arm pain, fainting, seizures, sudden vision changes, weakness on one side of the body, slurred speech, confusion, itching, dark urine, right upper quadrant pain, yellow skin or eyes, sore throat, fever, malaise, increased hyperactivity, believing things that are not true, or hearing voices.
- Be aware of possible risks of taking agents for ADHD during pregnancy. Safe use during pregnancy and lactation has not been established. Inform the physician immediately if pregnancy is suspected or planned.
- Be aware of potential side effects of agents for ADHD. Refer to written materials furnished by healthcare providers for safe self-administration.
- Carry a card or other identification at all times describing medications being taken.

Outcome Criteria and Evaluation

The following criteria may be used for evaluating the effectiveness of therapy with agents for ADHD.

The patient:

- Does not exhibit excessive hyperactivity.
- Has not experienced injury.

- Is maintaining expected parameters of growth and development.
- Verbalizes understanding of safe self-administration and the importance of not discontinuing medication abruptly.

Summary and Key Points

- Psychotropic medications are intended to be used as adjunctive therapy to individual or group psychotherapy.
- *Antianxiety agents* are used in the treatment of anxiety disorders and to alleviate acute anxiety symptoms. The benzodiazepines are the most commonly used group. They are CNS depressants and have a potential for physical and psychological dependence. They should not be discontinued abruptly following long-term use because they can produce a life-threatening withdrawal syndrome. The most common side effects are drowsiness, confusion, and lethargy.
- *Antidepressants* elevate mood and alleviate other symptoms associated with moderate-to-severe depression. These drugs work to increase the concentration of norepinephrine and serotonin in the body.
- The tricyclics and related drugs are believed to accomplish this action by blocking the reuptake of these chemicals by the neurons.
- Another group of antidepressants inhibits MAO, an enzyme that is known to inactivate norepinephrine and serotonin. They are called MAO inhibitors (MAOIs). MAOIs can cause hypertensive crisis if foods or other products containing tyramine are consumed while taking these medications.
- A third category of antidepressant drugs blocks neuronal reuptake of serotonin and has minimal or no effect on reuptake of norepinephrine or dopamine. They are called selective serotonin reuptake inhibitors (SSRIs).
- Antidepressant medications may take up to 4 weeks to produce full therapeutic benefits. The most common side effects are anticholinergic effects, such as orthostatic hypotension (especially TCAs) and sedation. They can also reduce the seizure threshold.
- Lithium carbonate is widely used as a *mood-stabilizing agent.* Its mechanism of action is not fully understood, but it is thought to enhance the reuptake of norepinephrine and serotonin in the brain, thereby lowering the levels in the body, resulting in decreased hyperactivity. The most common side effects are dry mouth, GI upset, polyuria, and weight gain.

- There is a very narrow margin between the therapeutic and toxic levels of lithium. Serum levels must be drawn regularly to monitor for toxicity. Symptoms of lithium toxicity may begin to appear at serum levels above 1.2 mEq/L but are more pronounced at levels above 1.5 mEq/L. If left untreated, lithium toxicity can be life threatening.
- Several other medications are used as mood-stabilizing agents. Two groups, anticonvulsants (carbamazepine, clonazepam, valproic acid, lamotrigine, oxcarbazepine, and topiramate) and the calcium channel blocker verapamil, have been used with some effectiveness. Their action in the treatment of bipolar mania is unknown.
- Most recently, a number of atypical antipsychotic medications have been used with success in the treatment of bipolar mania. These include olanzapine, aripiprazole, quetiapine, risperidone, asenapine, and ziprasidone. The phenothiazine chlorpromazine has also been used effectively. The action of antipsychotics in the treatment of bipolar mania is not understood.
- *Antipsychotic drugs* are used in the treatment of acute and chronic psychoses. The action of typical antipychotics is related to blocking postsynaptic dopamine receptors in the basal ganglia. Their most common side effects include anticholinergic effects, sedation, weight gain, reduction in seizure threshold, photosensitivity, and extrapyramidal symptoms.
- A newer generation of antipsychotic medications (atypical or second generation), which includes clozapine, risperidone, paliperidone, olanzapine, quetiapine, aripiprazole, asenapine, iloperidone, lurasidone, and ziprasidone, may have an effect on dopamine, serotonin, and other neurotransmitters. They show promise of greater efficacy with fewer side effects.
- *Antiparkinsonian agents* are used to counteract the extrapyramidal symptoms associated with antipsychotic medications. Antiparkinsonian drugs work to restore the natural balance of acetylcholine and dopamine in the brain. The most common side effects of these drugs are the anticholinergic effects. They may also cause sedation and orthostatic hypotension.
- *Agents for treatment of tardive dyskinesia* are used to reduce movement disturbances associated with antipsychotic medications. Their action is unknown but believed to be associated with inhibition of monoamine transport. Valbenazine (Ingrezza) and deutetrabenazine (Austeda) were both FDA approved for this indication in 2017.
- *Sedative-hypnotics* are used in the management of anxiety states and to treat insomnia. These CNS depressants (with the exception of ramelteon) have the potential for physical and psychological dependence. They are indicated for short-term use only. Side effects and nursing implications are similar to those described for antianxiety medications.
- Several medications have been designated as *agents for treatment of ADHD*. These include CNS stimulants, which have the potential for physical and psychological dependence. Tolerance develops quickly with CNS stimulants, and they should not be discontinued abruptly because they can produce serious withdrawal symptoms. The most common side effects are restlessness, anorexia, and insomnia. Other medications that have been shown to be effective with ADHD include atomoxetine, bupropion, and the alpha-adrenergic agonists clonidine and guanfacine. Their mechanism of action in the treatment of ADHD is not clear.

Review Questions
Self-Examination/Learning Exercise

Select the answer that is most appropriate for each of the following questions:

1. How do antianxiety medications, such as benzodiazepines, produce a calming effect by which of the following actions?
   a. Depressing the CNS
   b. Decreasing levels of norepinephrine and serotonin in the brain
   c. Decreasing levels of dopamine in the brain
   d. Inhibiting production of the enzyme MAO

Continued

Review Questions—cont'd
Self-Examination/Learning Exercise

2. Tam has a new diagnosis of panic disorder. Dr. S has written a prn order for alprazolam (Xanax) for when Tam is feeling anxious. She says to the nurse, "Dr. S prescribed buspirone for my friend's anxiety. Why did he order something different for me?" The nurse's answer is based on which of the following?
   a. Buspirone is not an antianxiety medication.
   b. Alprazolam and buspirone are essentially the same medication, so either one is appropriate.
   c. Buspirone has delayed onset of action and cannot be used on a prn basis.
   d. Alprazolam is the only medication that really works for panic disorder.

3. Education for the patient who is taking an MAOI should include which of the following?
   a. Fluid and sodium replacement when appropriate, frequent drug blood levels, signs and symptoms of toxicity
   b. Lifetime of continuous use, possible tardive dyskinesia, advantages of an injection every 2 to 4 weeks
   c. Short-term use, possible tolerance to beneficial effects, careful tapering of the drug at end of treatment
   d. Tyramine-restricted diet, prohibitive concurrent use of over-the-counter medications without physician notification

4. There is a very narrow margin between the therapeutic and toxic levels of lithium carbonate. Symptoms of toxicity are most likely to appear if the serum levels exceed which of the following levels?
   a. 0.15 mEq/L
   b. 1.5 mEq/L
   c. 15 mEq/L
   d. 150 mEq/L

5. Initial symptoms of lithium toxicity include which of the following?
   a. Constipation, dry mouth
   b. Dizziness, thirst
   c. Vomiting, diarrhea
   d. Anuria, arrhythmias

6. Antipsychotic medications are thought to decrease psychotic symptoms by which of the following actions?
   a. Blocking reuptake of norepinephrine and serotonin
   b. Blocking the action of dopamine in the brain
   c. Inhibiting production of the enzyme MAO
   d. Depressing the CNS

7. Part of the nurse's continual assessment of the patient taking antipsychotic medications is to observe for extrapyramidal symptoms. Examples include which of the following?
   a. Muscular weakness, rigidity, tremors, facial spasms
   b. Dry mouth, blurred vision, urinary retention, orthostatic hypotension
   c. Amenorrhea, gynecomastia, retrograde ejaculation
   d. Elevated blood pressure, severe occipital headache, stiff neck

8. If extrapyramidal symptoms should occur, which of the following would be a priority nursing intervention?
   a. Notify the physician immediately.
   b. Administer prn trihexyphenidyl (Artane) as ordered.
   c. Withhold the next dose of antipsychotic medication.
   d. Explain to the patient that these symptoms are only temporary and will disappear shortly.

Review Questions—cont'd
Self-Examination/Learning Exercise

9. Which of the following is a concern with children on long-term therapy with CNS stimulants for ADHD?
   a. Addiction
   b. Weight gain
   c. Substance abuse
   d. Growth suppression

10. What is the reason that doses of bupropion should be administered at least 4 to 6 hours apart and never doubled when a dose is missed?
    a. To prevent orthostatic hypotension
    b. To prevent seizures
    c. To prevent hypertensive crisis
    d. To prevent extrapyramidal symptoms

11. Clozapine (Clozaril) is an antipsychotic required to have an approved risk evaluation and mitigation strategy (REMS) program. Which of the following actions are included in that program? (Select all that apply.)
    a. Absolute neutrophil counts are assessed before initiation of treatment.
    b. Initially only 1-week supply of clozapine is dispensed at a time.
    c. Acceptable ANC levels for continuation of treatment are identified as 1,500 µL.
    d. Patients are not permitted to smoke cigarettes while on clozapine.

References

Anderson, L. (2018). *Drug interactions with grapefruit juice.* Retrieved from https://www.drugs.com/article/grapefruit-drug-interactions.html

Brust, T. F., Hayes, M. P., Roman, D. L., & Watts, V. J. (2015). New functional activity of aripiprazole revealed: Robust antagonism of D2 dopamine receptor-stimulated Gβγ signaling. *Biochemical Pharmacology, 93*(1), 85–91. doi:10.1016/j.bcp.2014 10.014

Canuso, C. M., Singh, J. B., Fedgchin, M., Alphs, L., Lane, R., Lim, P., . . . Drevets, W. C. (2018, April). Efficacy and safety of intranasal esketamine for the rapid reduction of symptoms of depression and suicidality in patients at imminent risk for suicide: Results of a double-blind, randomized, placebo-controlled study. *American Journal of Psychiatry.* Retrieved from https://doi.org/10.1176/appi.ajp.2018.17060720

Clozapine REMS. (2015). *Clozapine and the risk of neutropenia: A guide for healthcare providers.* Retrieved from https://www.clozapinerems.com/CpmgClozapineUI/rems/pdf/resources/Clozapine_REMS_HCP_Guide.pdf

Cooper, B. E., & Sejnowski, C. A. (2013). Serotonin syndrome: Recognition and treatment. *AACN Advanced Critical Care, 24*(1), 15–20.

Drugs.com. (2018). *FDA pregnancy categories: FDA pregnancy risk information: An update.* Retrieved from https://www.drugs.com/pregnancy-categories.html

Erlij, D., Acosta-Garcia, J., Rojas-Marquez, M., Gonzalez-Hernandez, B., Escartin-Perez, E., Aceves, J., & Floran, B. (2012). Dopamine D4 receptor stimulation in GABAergic projections of the globus pallidus to the reticular thalamic nucleus and the substantia nigra reticulate of the rat decreases locomotor activity. *Neuropharmacology, 62*(2), 1111–1118.

Food and Drug Administration (FDA). (2008). *FDA requires warnings about risk of suicidal thoughts and behavior for antiepileptic medications.* Retrieved from http://www.fda.gov/Drugs/DrugSafety/PostmarketDrugSafetyInformationforPatientsandProviders/ucm100197.htm

Food and Drug Administration (FDA). (2016a). *FDA Drug Safety Communication: FDA warns about serious risks and death when combining opioid pain or cough medicines with benzodiazepines; requires its strongest warning.* Retrieved from http://www.fda.gov/Drugs/DrugSafety/ucm518473.htm.

Food and Drug Administration (FDA). (2016b). *FDA Drug Safety Communication: FDA warns about rare but serious skin reactions with mental health drug olanzapine (Zyprexa, Zyprexa Zydis, Zyprexa Relprevv, and Symbyax).* Retrieved from https://www.fda.gov/Drugs/DrugSafety/ucm499441.htm

Food and Drug Administration (FDA). (2016c). *FDA Drug Safety Communication: FDA warns about new impulse-control problems associated with mental health drug aripiprazole (Abilify, Abilify Maintena, Aristada).* Retrieved from https://www.fda.gov/Drugs/DrugSafety/ucm498662.htm

Fournier, J. C., DeRubeis, R. J., Hollon, S. D., Dimidjian, S., Amsterdam, J. D., Shelton, R. C., & Fawcett, J. (2010). Antidepressant drug effects and depression severity: A patient-level meta-analysis. *Journal of the American Medical Association, 303*(1), 47–53. doi: 10.1001/jama.2009.1943

Haddad, P. M., Brain, C., & Scott, J. (2014). *Nonadherence with antipsychotic medication in schizophrenia: Challenges and management strategies.* Retrieved from http://www.ncbi.nlm.nih.gov/pmc/articles/PMC4085309/

Harrison, P. (2015). *Novel drug first to treat negative symptoms in schizophrenia.* Retrieved from http://www.medscape.com/viewarticle/850701

Horn, J. R., & Hansten, P. D. (2008). *Get to know an enzyme: CYP2C19*. Retrieved from https://www.pharmacytimes.com/publications/issue/2008/2008-05/2008-05-8538

Institute of Medicine. (2003). *Health professions education: A bridge to quality*. Washington, DC: Author.

Janicak, P. G., & Hussain, K. (2017). Medication induced movement disorders. In B. J. Sadock, V. A. Sadock, & P. Ruiz (Eds), *Comprehensive textbook of psychiatry* (10th ed., pp. 2936–2944). Philadelphia, PA: Wolters Kluwer.

Johnston, G. (2017). *Ketamine for depression: A Q&A with psychiatrist Alexander Papp, MD*. UC San Diego Health Newsroom. Retrieved from https://health.ucsd.edu/news/features/Pages/2018-01-03-q-and-a-ketamine-for-depression.aspx

Jones, D. S. (2006). Racial profiling in psychiatry: Does it help patients? *Psychiatric Times, 23*(14).

Lenze, E. J., Mulsant, B. H., Blumberger, D. M., Karp, J. F., Newcomer, J. W., Anderson, S. J., & Reynolds, C. F. (2015). Efficacy, safety, and tolerability of augmentation pharmacotherapy with aripiprazole for treatment resistant depression in late life: A randomized placebo-controlled study. *Lancet, 386*(10011), 2404–2412.

Lien, Y. H. H. (2018). Antidepressants and hyponatremia. *American Journal of Medicine, 131*(1), 7–8. doi.org/10.1016/j.amjmed.2017.09.002

Lynch, T., & Price, A. (2007). The effect of cytochrome P450 metabolism on drug response, interactions, and adverse effects. *American Family Physician, 76*(3), 391–396.

New York State Office of Mental Health. (2012). *An explanation of Kendra's law*. Retrieved from http://www.omh.ny.gov/omhweb/Kendra_web/Ksummary.htm

Olfson, M., King, M., & Schoenbaum, M. (2015). Benzodiazepine use in the United States. *JAMA Psychiatry, 72*(2), 136–142. doi:10.1001/jamapsychiatry.2014.1763

Ramnarine, M., & Ahmed, D. (2015). *Anticholinergic toxicity*. Retrieved from http://medicine.medscape.com/article/812644-overview

Sadock, B. J., Sadock, V. A., & Ruiz, P. (2015). *Synopsis of psychiatry: Behavioral sciences/clinical psychiatry* (11th ed.). Baltimore, MD: Lippincott Williams & Wilkins.

Sage, D. L. (Producer). (1984). *The brain: Madness*. Washington, DC: Public Broadcasting Company.

Scarff, J. R. (2017). The prospects of cariprazine in the treatment of schizophrenia. *Therapeutic Advances in Psychopharmacology, 7*(11), 237–239. doi: 10.1177/2045125317727260

Shorter, E. (2009). The history of lithium therapy. *Bipolar Disorders, 11*(2), 4–9. doi: 10.1111/j.1399-5618.2009.00706.x

Steinberg, M., & Lyketsos, C. G. (2012). Atypical antipsychotic use in patients with dementia: Managing safety concerns. *American Journal of Psychiatry, 169*(9), 900–906. doi: 10.1176/appi.aip.2012.12030342

Tartakovsky, M. (2016). Depression: New medications on the horizon. *Psych Central*. Retrieved from http://psychcentral.com/lib/depression-new-medications-on-the-horizon/

Vallerand, A. H., Sanoski, C. A., & Deglin, J. H. (2017). *Davis drug guide for nurses* (15th ed.). Philadelphia, PA: F.A. Davis.

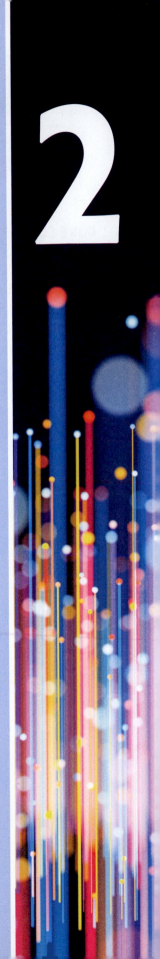

UNIT **2**

Psychiatric Mental Health Nursing Interventions

5

Relationship Development and Therapeutic Communication

KEY TERMS

concrete thinking

confidentiality

countertransference

density

empathy

genuineness

intimate distance

motivational interviewing

paralanguage

personal distance

public distance

rapport

social distance

sympathy

territoriality

transference

unconditional positive regard

OBJECTIVES

After reading this chapter, the student will be able to:

1. Describe the relevance and dynamics of a therapeutic nurse-patient relationship.
2. Identify types of pre-existing conditions that influence the outcome of the communication process.
3. Define *territoriality, density,* and *distance* as components of the environment.
4. Identify components of nonverbal expression.
5. Describe therapeutic and nontherapeutic verbal communication techniques.
6. Describe motivational interviewing as a communication strategy.
7. Describe active listening.
8. Discuss therapeutic feedback.
9. Identify and discuss essential conditions for a therapeutic relationship to occur.
10. Describe the phases of relationship development and the tasks associated with each phase.

Introduction

The nurse-patient relationship is the foundation on which psychiatric nursing is established. It is a relationship in which both participants must recognize each other as unique and important human beings. It is also a relationship in which mutual learning occurs. In today's healthcare environment, patient-centered care is being promoted as central to quality and safety, and the therapeutic relationship remains at the foundation. Concepts that were developed over 50 years ago (Peplau, 1952) and have been the core of nursing practice to the present day are now being recognized by the larger medical community as not only still relevant but also critical to improving quality and safety in the future of healthcare. Peplau (1991) describes the foundation for therapeutic relationship development (and the accomplishment of nursing care) as follows:

> Shall a nurse do things *for* a patient or can participant relationships be emphasized so that a nurse comes to do things *with* a patient as her share of an agenda of work to be accomplished in reaching a goal—health. *It is likely that the nursing process is educative and therapeutic when nurse and patient can come to know and to respect each other, as persons who are alike, and yet, different, as persons who share in the solution of problems.* (p. 9)

Hays and Larson (1963) stated, "To relate therapeutically with a patient, it is necessary for the nurse to understand his or her role and its relationship to the patient's illness." They describe the role of the nurse as providing the patient with the opportunity to

■ Identify and explore problems in relating to others.
■ Discover healthy ways of meeting emotional needs.
■ Experience a satisfying interpersonal relationship.

The *therapeutic interpersonal relationship* is the process by which nurses provide care for patients in need of psychosocial intervention. *Therapeutic use of self* is the instrument for delivery of that care. *Interpersonal communication techniques* (both verbal and nonverbal) are the "tools" of psychosocial intervention.

This chapter describes the phases of development of a therapeutic nurse-patient relationship. Therapeutic use of self and techniques of interpersonal communication are discussed.

CORE CONCEPT
Therapeutic relationship
An interaction between two people (usually a caregiver and a care receiver) in which input from both participants contributes to a climate of healing, growth promotion, and/or illness prevention.

The Therapeutic Nurse-Patient Relationship

Travelbee (1971), who expanded on Peplau's theory of interpersonal relations in nursing, stated that it is only when each individual in the interaction perceives the other as a human being that a relationship is possible. She refers not to a nurse-patient relationship but to a human-to-human relationship, which she describes as a "mutually significant experience." That is, both the nurse and the recipient of care have needs met when each views the other as a unique human being, not as "an illness," "a room number," or "all nurses" in general.

Therapeutic relationships are goal oriented. Ideally, the nurse and patient decide together what the goal of the relationship will be. Most often, the goal is directed at learning and growth promotion in an effort to bring about some type of change in the patient's life. In general, the goal of a therapeutic relationship may be based on a problem-solving model.

EXAMPLE

Goal

The patient will demonstrate more adaptive coping strategies for dealing with (specific life situation).

Intervention

- Identify what is troubling the patient at this time.
- Encourage the patient to discuss changes he or she would like to make.
- Discuss with the patient which changes are possible and which are not possible.
- Have the patient explore feelings about aspects that cannot be changed and alternative ways of coping more adaptively.
- Discuss alternative strategies for creating changes the patient desires to make.
- Weigh the benefits and consequences of each alternative.
- Assist the patient to select an alternative.
- Encourage the patient to implement the change.
- Provide positive feedback for the patient's attempts to create change.
- Assist the patient to evaluate outcomes of the change and make modifications as required.

Therapeutic Use of Self

Travelbee (1971) described the instrument for delivery of the process of interpersonal nursing as the *therapeutic use of self,* which she defined as "the ability to use one's personality consciously and in full awareness in an attempt to establish relatedness and to structure nursing interventions" (p. 19).

Use of the self in a therapeutic manner requires that the nurse have a great deal of self-awareness and self-understanding, having arrived at a philosophical belief about life, death, and the overall human condition. The nurse must understand that the ability to, and the extent to which one can, effectively help others in time of need is strongly influenced by this internal value system—a combination of intellect and emotions.

Conditions Essential to Development of a Therapeutic Relationship

Several characteristics that enhance the achievement of a therapeutic relationship have been identified. These concepts are highly significant to the use of self as the therapeutic tool in interpersonal relationship development.

Rapport

Getting acquainted and establishing rapport is the primary task in relationship development. **Rapport** implies special feelings on the part of both the patient and the nurse based on acceptance, warmth, friendliness, common interest, a sense of trust, and a nonjudgmental attitude. Establishing rapport may be accomplished by discussing non–health-related topics. Travelbee (1971) states,

> [To establish rapport] is to create a sense of harmony based on knowledge and appreciation of each individual's uniqueness. It is the ability to be still and experience the other as a human being—to appreciate the unfolding of each personality one to the other. The ability to truly care for and about others is the core of rapport. (pp. 152, 155)

Trust

To trust another, one must feel confidence in that person's presence, reliability, integrity, veracity, and sincere desire to provide assistance when requested. As discussed in Chapter 29, Concepts of Personality Development, available online in Davis*Plus*, trust is the initial developmental task described by Erikson. If the task has not been achieved, this component of relationship development becomes more difficult. That is not to say that trust cannot be established but only that additional time and patience may be required on the part of the nurse.

> **CLINICAL PEARL** The nurse must convey an aura of trustworthiness, which requires that he or she possess a sense of self-confidence. Confidence in the self is derived out of knowledge gained through achievement of personal and professional goals as well as the ability to integrate these roles and to function as a unified whole.

Trust cannot be presumed; it must be earned. Trustworthiness is demonstrated through nursing interventions that convey a sense of warmth and caring to the patient. These interventions are initiated simply and concretely and are directed toward activities that address the patient's basic needs for physiological and psychological safety and security. Psychiatric patients with thought disorders, such as schizophrenia, may also have difficulty thinking abstractly (a symptom called **concrete thinking**) so it becomes even more important that the nurse communicate and behave in a simple, concrete manner to promote the development of trust. Examples of nursing interventions that would promote trust in an individual who is thinking concretely include the following:

■ Providing a blanket when the patient is cold
■ Providing food when the patient is hungry
■ Keeping promises
■ Being honest (e.g., saying, "I don't know the answer to your question, but I'll try to find out") and then following through
■ Simply and clearly providing reasons for certain policies, procedures, and rules
■ Providing a written, structured schedule of activities
■ Attending activities with the patient if he or she is reluctant to go alone
■ Being consistent in adhering to unit guidelines
■ Listening to the patient's preferences, requests, and opinions and making collaborative decisions concerning his or her care
■ Ensuring **confidentiality;** providing reassurance that what is discussed will not be repeated outside the boundaries of the healthcare team

Trust is the basis of a therapeutic relationship. The nurse working in psychiatry must perfect the skills that foster the development of trust. Trust must be established in order for the nurse-patient relationship to progress beyond the superficial level of tending to the patient's immediate needs.

Respect

To show respect is to believe in the dignity and worth of an individual regardless of his or her unacceptable behavior. The psychologist Carl Rogers called this **unconditional positive regard** (Raskin, Rogers, & Witty, 2014). The attitude is nonjudgmental, and the respect is unconditional in that it does not depend on the behavior of the patient to meet certain standards. The nurse, in fact, may not approve of the patient's lifestyle or pattern of behaving. However, with unconditional positive regard, the patient is accepted and respected for no other reason than that he or she is considered to be a worthwhile and unique human being.

Many psychiatric patients have very little self-respect. Lack of self-respect may be related to the low self-esteem that accompanies illnesses such as clinical depression or it may be related to rejection and stigmatization by others. Recognition that patients are being accepted and respected as unique individuals on an unconditional basis can serve to elevate feelings of self-worth and self-respect. The nurse can convey an attitude of respect in the following ways:

■ Calling the patient by name (and title, if he or she prefers)
■ Spending time with the patient

■ Allowing for sufficient time to answer the patient's questions and concerns
■ Promoting an atmosphere of privacy during therapeutic interactions with the patient or when the patient may be undergoing physical examination or therapy
■ Always being open and honest with the patient, even when the truth may be difficult to discuss
■ Listening to the patient's ideas, preferences, and requests, and making collaborative decisions concerning his or her care whenever possible
■ Striving to understand the motivation behind the patient's behavior, regardless of how unacceptable it may seem

Genuineness

The concept of **genuineness** refers to the nurse's ability to be open, honest, and "real" in interactions with the patient. To be real is to be aware of what one is experiencing internally and to allow the quality of this inner experiencing to be apparent in the therapeutic relationship. When one is genuine, there is congruence between what is felt and what is being expressed (Raskin et al., 2014). The nurse who possesses the quality of genuineness responds to the patient with truth and honesty rather than with responses that he or she may consider more "professional" or that merely reflect the "nursing role."

Genuineness may call for a degree of self-disclosure on the part of the nurse. This is not to say that the nurse must disclose to the patient everything he or she is feeling or all personal experiences that may relate to what the patient is going through. On the contrary, care must be taken when using self-disclosure to avoid reversing the roles of the nurse and patient.

When the nurse uses self-disclosure, a quality of "humanness" is revealed to the patient, creating a role for the patient to model in similar situations. The patient may then feel more comfortable revealing personal information to the nurse.

Most individuals have an uncanny ability to detect other people's artificiality. When the nurse does not bring the quality of genuineness to the relationship, a reality base for trust cannot be established. These qualities are essential to helping the patient actualize their potential within the nurse-patient relationship and for change and growth to occur (Raskin et al., 2014).

Empathy

Empathy is the ability to see beyond outward behavior and to understand the situation from the patient's point of view. With empathy, the nurse can accurately perceive and understand the meaning and relevance of the patient's thoughts and feelings. The nurse must also be able to communicate this perception to the patient by attempting to translate words and behaviors into feelings.

It is not uncommon for the concept of empathy to be confused with that of **sympathy.** The major difference is that with empathy the nurse "accurately perceives or understands" what the patient is feeling and encourages the patient to explore these feelings. With sympathy the nurse actually "shares" what the patient is feeling and experiences a need to alleviate distress. Schuster (2000) stated,

> Empathy means that you remain emotionally separate from the other person, even though you can see the patient's viewpoint clearly. This is different from sympathy. Sympathy implies taking on the other's needs and problems as if they were your own and becoming emotionally involved to the point of losing your objectivity. To empathize rather than sympathize, you must show feelings but not get caught up in feelings or overly identify with the patient's and family's concerns. (p. 102)

Empathy is considered to be one of the most important characteristics of a therapeutic relationship. Accurate empathetic perceptions on the part of the nurse assist the patient to identify feelings that may have been suppressed or denied. Positive emotions are generated as the patient realizes that he or she is truly understood by another. As the feelings surface and are explored, the patient learns aspects about self of which he or she may have been unaware. This insight contributes to the process of personal identification and the promotion of positive self-concept.

With empathy, while understanding the patient's thoughts and feelings, the nurse is able to maintain sufficient objectivity to allow the patient to achieve problem resolution with minimal assistance. With sympathy, the nurse actually feels what the patient is feeling, objectivity is lost, and the nurse may become focused on relief of personal distress rather than on helping the patient resolve the problem at hand. The following example describes an empathetic and sympathetic response to the same situation.

EXAMPLE

Situation: BJ is a patient on the psychiatric unit with a diagnosis of dysthymic disorder. She is 5 ft 5 in. tall and weighs 295 lb. BJ has been overweight all of her life. She is single, has no close friends, and has never had an intimate relationship with another person. It is her first day on the unit, and she is refusing to come out of her room. When she appeared for lunch in the dining room following admission, she was embarrassed when several of the other patients laughed out loud and call her "fatso."

Sympathetic response: Nurse: "I can certainly identify with what you are feeling. I've been overweight most of my life, too. I just get so angry when people act like that. They are so insensitive! It's just so typical of skinny people to act that way. You have a right to want to stay away from them. We'll just see how loud they laugh when you get to choose what movie is shown on the unit after dinner tonight."

Empathetic response: Nurse: "You feel angry and embarrassed by what happened at lunch today." As tears fill BJ's eyes, the nurse encourages her to cry if she feels like it and to express her anger at the situation. She stays with BJ but does not dwell on her own feelings about what happened. Instead she focuses on BJ and what the patient perceives are her most immediate needs.

Rapport, trust, respect, genuineness, and empathy all are essential to forming therapeutic relationships, and they can certainly be assets in social relationships, too. The primary differences between social and therapeutic relationships are that therapeutic relationships always remain focused on the healthcare needs of the patient, they are never for the purpose of addressing the nurse's personal needs, and they progress through identified phases of development for the purpose of helping the patient to solve health-related problems.

Phases of a Therapeutic Nurse-Patient Relationship

Psychiatric nurses use interpersonal relationship development as the primary intervention with patients in various psychiatric mental health settings. Developing an interpersonal relationship with the patient is congruent with Peplau's (1962) identification of *counseling* as the major subrole of nursing in psychiatry. Sullivan (1953), from whom Peplau patterned her own interpersonal theory of nursing, strongly believed that many emotional problems were closely related to difficulties with interpersonal relationships. With this concept in mind, this role of the nurse in psychiatry becomes especially meaningful and purposeful—an integral part of the total therapeutic regimen.

The therapeutic interpersonal relationship is the means by which the nursing process is implemented. Through the relationship, problems are identified and resolution is sought. Tasks of the relationship have been categorized into four phases:

1. Preinteraction phase
2. Orientation (introductory) phase
3. Working phase
4. Termination phase

Although each phase is presented as specific and distinct from the others, some tasks may overlap,

TABLE 5–1	Phases of Relationship Development and Major Nursing Goals
PHASE	**GOALS**
1. Preinteraction	Explore self-perceptions
2. Orientation (introductory)	Establish trust and formulate contract for intervention
3. Working	Promote patient change
4. Termination	Evaluate goal attainment and ensure therapeutic closure

particularly when the interaction is limited. The major goals during each phase of the nurse-patient relationship are listed in Table 5–1.

The Preinteraction Phase

The preinteraction phase involves preparation for the first encounter with the patient. Tasks include the following:

■ Obtaining available information about the patient from his or her chart, significant others, or other health team members. From this information, the initial assessment is begun. This initial information may also allow the nurse to become aware of personal responses to knowledge about the patient.
■ Examining one's feelings, fears, and anxieties about working with a particular patient. For example, the nurse may have been reared in an alcoholic family and have ambivalent feelings about caring for a patient who is alcohol dependent. All individuals bring attitudes and feelings from prior experiences to the clinical setting. The nurse needs to be aware of how these preconceptions may affect his or her ability to care for individual patients.

The Orientation (Introductory) Phase

During the orientation phase, the nurse and patient become acquainted. Tasks include the following:

■ Creating an environment for the establishment of trust and rapport
■ Establishing a contract for intervention that details the expectations and responsibilities of both the nurse and patient
■ Gathering assessment information to build a strong database
■ Identifying the patient's strengths and limitations
■ Formulating nursing diagnoses
■ Setting goals that are mutually agreeable to the nurse and patient

■ Developing a plan of action that is realistic for meeting the established goals
■ Exploring feelings of both the patient and nurse in terms of the introductory phase

Introductions often are uncomfortable, and the participants may experience some anxiety until a degree of rapport has been established. Interactions may remain on a superficial level until anxiety subsides. Several interactions may be required to fulfill the tasks associated with this phase.

The Working Phase

The therapeutic work of the relationship is accomplished during this phase. Tasks include the following:

■ Maintaining the trust and rapport that was established during the orientation phase
■ Promoting insight and perception of reality
■ Problem-solving using the model presented earlier in this chapter
■ Overcoming resistance behaviors as the level of anxiety rises in response to discussion of painful issues
■ Continuously evaluating progress toward goal attainment

Transference and Countertransference

Transference and countertransference are common phenomena that often arise during the course of a therapeutic relationship.

Transference

Transference occurs when the patient unconsciously displaces (or "transfers") to the nurse feelings formed toward a person from his or her past (Sadock, Sadock, & Ruiz, 2015). These feelings toward the nurse may be triggered by something about the nurse's appearance or personality that reminds the patient of the person. Transference can interfere with the therapeutic interaction when the feelings being expressed include anger and hostility. Anger toward the nurse can be manifested by uncooperativeness and resistance to the therapy.

Transference can also take the form of overwhelming affection for the nurse or excessive dependency on the nurse. The nurse is overvalued, and the patient forms unrealistic expectations of the nurse. When the nurse is unable to fulfill those expectations or meet the excessive dependency needs, the patient may become angry and hostile.

Interventions for Transference Hilz (2013) stated,

In cases of transference, the relationship does not usually need to be terminated, except when the transference poses a serious barrier to therapy or safety. The nurse should work with the patient in sorting out the past from the present, assist the patient into identifying the transference, and reassign a new and more appropriate meaning to the current nurse-patient relationship. The goal is to guide the patient to independence by teaching them to assume responsibility for their own behaviors, feelings, and thoughts, and to assign the correct meanings to the relationships based on present circumstances instead of the past.

Countertransference

Countertransference refers to the nurse's behavioral and emotional response to the patient. These responses may be related to unresolved feelings toward significant others from the nurse's past, or they may be generated in response to transference feelings on the part of the patient. It is not easy to refrain from becoming angry when the patient is consistently antagonistic, to feel flattered when showered with affection and attention by the patient, or even to feel quite powerful when the patient exhibits excessive dependency on the nurse. These feelings can interfere with the therapeutic relationship when they initiate the following types of behaviors:

- The nurse overidentifies with the patient's feelings because they remind him or her of problems from the nurse's past or present.
- The nurse and patient develop a social or personal relationship.
- The nurse begins to give advice or attempts to "rescue" the patient.
- The nurse encourages and promotes the patient's dependence.
- The nurse's anger engenders feelings of disgust toward the patient.
- The nurse feels anxious and uneasy in the presence of the patient.
- The nurse is bored and apathetic in sessions with the patient.
- The nurse has difficulty setting limits on the patient's behavior.
- The nurse defends the patient's behavior to other staff members.

The nurse may be completely unaware or only minimally aware of the countertransference as it is occurring (Hilz, 2013).

Interventions for Countertransference Hilz (2013) states,

> The relationship usually should not be terminated in the presence of countertransference. Rather, the nurse or staff member experiencing the countertransference should be supportively assisted by other staff members to identify his or her feelings and behaviors

and recognize the occurrence of the phenomenon. It may be helpful to have evaluative sessions with the nurse after his or her encounter with the patient, in which both the nurse and other staff members (who are observing the interactions) discuss and compare the exhibited behaviors in the relationship.

The Termination Phase

Termination of the relationship may occur for a variety of reasons: the mutually agreed-on goals may have been reached; the patient may be discharged from the hospital; or, in the case of a student nurse, it may be the end of a clinical rotation. Termination can be a difficult phase for both the patient and nurse. The main task involves bringing a therapeutic conclusion to the relationship. This occurs when

- Progress has been made toward attainment of mutually set goals.
- A plan for continuing care or for assistance during stressful life experiences is mutually established by the nurse and patient.
- Feelings about termination of the relationship are recognized and explored. Both the nurse and patient may experience feelings of sadness and loss. The nurse should share his or her feelings with the patient. Through these interactions, the patient learns that it is acceptable to have these feelings at a time of separation. Through this knowledge, the patient experiences growth during the process of termination. This is also a time when both nurse and patient may evaluate and summarize the learning that occurred as an outgrowth of their relationship.

CLINICAL PEARL When the patient feels sadness and loss, behaviors to delay termination may become evident. If the nurse experiences the same feelings, he or she may allow the patient's behaviors to delay termination. For therapeutic closure, the nurse must establish the reality of the separation and resist being manipulated into repeated delays by the patient.

Boundaries in the Nurse-Patient Relationship

A boundary indicates a border or a limit. It determines the extent of acceptable limits. Many types of boundaries exist. Examples include the following:

- **Material boundaries:** These are physical property that can be seen, such as fences that border land.
- **Social boundaries:** These boundaries are established within a culture and define how individuals are expected to behave in social situations.

- **Personal boundaries:** These are boundaries that individuals define for themselves. These include *physical distance boundaries,* or just how close individuals will allow others to invade their physical space; and *emotional boundaries,* or how much individuals choose to disclose of their most private and intimate selves to others.

- **Professional boundaries:** These boundaries limit and outline expectations for appropriate professional relationships with patients. "Professional boundaries are the spaces between a nurse's power and the patient's vulnerability" (National Council of State Boards of Nursing [NCSBN], 2014). Nurses must recognize that they have an imbalance of power with their patients by virtue of their role and the patient information to which they have access. They must be consistently conscientious in avoiding any circumstance in which they might achieve personal gain within that relationship.

Concerns regarding professional boundaries are commonly related to the following issues:

1. **Self-disclosure:** Self-disclosure on the part of the nurse may be appropriate when it is judged that the information may therapeutically benefit the patient. It should never be undertaken for the purpose of meeting the nurse's needs.

2. **Gift giving:** Individuals who are receiving care often feel indebted toward healthcare providers. Gift giving may even be part of the therapeutic process for people who receive care (College and Association of Registered Nurses of Alberta [CARNA], 2011). Cultural belief and values may also enter into the decision of whether to accept a gift from a patient. In some cultures, failure to do so would be interpreted as an insult (Pie, 2012). Accepting financial gifts is never appropriate, but in some instances, nurses may be permitted to suggest instead a donation to a charity of the patient's choice. If acceptance of a small gift of gratitude is deemed appropriate, the nurse may choose to share it with other staff members who have been involved in the patient's care. In all instances, nurses should exercise professional judgment when deciding whether to accept a gift from a patient. Attention should be given not only to what the gift giving means to the patient but also to institutional policy, the American Nurses Association's (ANA) *Code of Ethics for Nurses,* and the ANA's *Scope and Standards of Practice.*

3. **Touch:** Nursing by its very nature involves touching patients. Touching is required to perform the many therapeutic procedures involved in the physical care of patients. Caring touch is the touching of patients when there is no physical need. Touching or hugging can be beneficial when it is implemented with therapeutic intent and patient consent. When using caring touch, make sure it is appropriate, supportive, and welcomed (College of Registered Nurses of British Columbia, 2015). Caring touch may provide comfort or encouragement, but some vulnerable patients may misinterpret the meaning of touch. In some cultures, touch is not considered acceptable unless the parties know each other very well (Purnell, 2014). The nurse must be sensitive to these cultural nuances and aware when touch is crossing a personal boundary. Additionally, patients who are experiencing high levels of anxiety, suspiciousness, or psychosis. These are times when touch should be avoided or considered with extreme caution.

4. **Friendship or romantic association:** When a nurse is acquainted with a patient, the relationship must move from one of a personal nature to professional. If the nurse is unable to accomplish this separation, he or she should withdraw from the nurse-patient relationship. Likewise, nurses must guard against personal relationships developing as a result of the nurse-patient relationship. Romantic, sexual, or similar personal relationships are never appropriate between nurse and patient.

Certain warning signs exist that indicate that professional boundaries of the nurse-patient relationship may be in jeopardy. Some of these include the following (Coltrane & Pugh, 1978):

- Favoring one patient's care over that of another
- Keeping secrets with a patient
- Changing dress style for working with a particular patient
- Swapping patient assignments to care for a particular patient
- Giving special attention or treatment to one patient over others
- Spending free time with a patient
- Frequently thinking about the patient when away from work
- Sharing personal information or work concerns with the patient
- Receiving gifts from or continuing communication with the patient after discharge

Boundary crossings can threaten the integrity of the nurse-patient relationship. Nurses must gain self-awareness and insight to be able to recognize when professional integrity is being compromised. Although some variables such as the care setting, community influences, patient needs, and the nature of therapy affect how boundaries are delineated, "any action that oversteps the established boundaries to meet the needs of the nurse are boundary violations" (NCSBN, 2014).

CORE CONCEPT
Communication
An interactive process of transmitting information between two or more entities.

Interpersonal Communication

It has been said that individuals "cannot *not* communicate." Every word that is spoken, every movement that is made, and every action that is taken or is not taken gives a message to someone. Interpersonal communication is a transaction between the sender and the receiver. In the transactional model of communication, both participants simultaneously perceive each other, listen to each other, and mutually are involved in creating meaning in a relationship.

The Impact of Pre-existing Conditions

In all interpersonal transactions, both the sender and receiver bring certain pre-existing conditions to the exchange that influence both the intended message and the way in which it is interpreted. Examples of these conditions include one's value system, internalized attitudes and beliefs, culture or religion, social status, gender, background knowledge and experience, and age or developmental level. The type of environment in which the communication takes place also may influence the outcome of the transaction.

Values, Attitudes, and Beliefs

Values, attitudes, and beliefs are learned ways of thinking. Children generally adopt the value systems and internalize the attitudes and beliefs of their parents. Children may retain this way of thinking into adulthood or develop a different set of attitudes and values as they mature.

Values, attitudes, and beliefs can influence communication in numerous ways. For example, prejudice is expressed verbally through negative stereotyping.

One's value system may be communicated with behaviors that are more symbolic in nature. For example, an individual who values youth may dress and behave in a manner that is characteristic of one who is much younger. Persons who value freedom and the American way of life may fly the U.S. flag in front of their homes each day. In each of these situations, a message is being communicated.

Culture and Religion

Communication has its roots in culture. Cultural mores, norms, ideas, and customs provide the basis for our way of thinking. Cultural values are learned and differ from society to society. For example, in some European countries (e.g., Italy, Spain, and France), men may greet each other with hugs and kisses; in the United States or England, shaking hands is a more culturally accepted style of greeting among men.

Religion also can influence communication. Priests and ministers who wear clerical collars publicly communicate their mission in life. The collar also may influence the way in which others relate to them, either positively or negatively. Other symbolic gestures, such as wearing a cross around the neck or hanging a crucifix on the wall, also communicate an individual's religious beliefs.

Social Status

Studies of nonverbal indicators of social status or power have suggested that high-status persons are associated with gestures that communicate their higher-power position. For example, they use less eye contact, have a more relaxed posture, use louder voice pitch, place hands on hips more frequently, are "power dressers," have greater height, and maintain more distance when communicating with individuals considered to be of lower social status.

Gender

Gender influences the manner in which individuals communicate. Most cultures have *gender signals* that are recognized as either masculine or feminine and provide a basis for distinguishing between members of each gender. Examples include differences in posture, both standing and sitting, between many men and women in the United States. Men usually stand with thighs 10 to 15 degrees apart, the pelvis rolled back, and the arms slightly away from the body. Women often are seen with legs close together, the pelvis tipped forward, and the arms close to the body. When sitting, men may lean back in the chair with legs apart or may rest the ankle of one leg over the knee of the other. Women tend to sit more upright in the chair with legs together, perhaps crossed at the ankles, or one leg crossed over the other at thigh level.

Roles have historically been identified as either male or female. For example, in the United States, masculinity typically was communicated through such roles as husband, father, breadwinner, doctor, lawyer, and engineer. Traditional female roles included wife, mother, homemaker, nurse, teacher, and secretary.

Gender signals are changing in U.S. society as gender roles become less distinct. Behaviors that once were considered typically masculine or feminine may now be generally accepted in members of both genders. Words such as *unisex* communicate a desire by some individuals to diminish the distinction between the genders and minimize the discrimination of either. Gender roles are changing as both women and men enter professions that once were dominated by members of the opposite gender.

Age or Developmental Level

Age influences communication, and it is especially evident during adolescence. In their struggle to separate from parental confines and establish their own identity, adolescents generate a unique pattern of communication that changes from generation to generation. Words such as *dude, groovy, clueless, awesome, cool,* and *wasted* have had special meaning for different generations of adolescents. The technological age has produced a whole new language for today's adolescents. Communication by text messaging includes such acronyms as BRB ("be right back"), BFF ("best friends forever"), and MOS ("mom over shoulder").

Developmental physiological alterations may also influence communication. For people who are deaf or hearing impaired, American Sign Language may be their preferred method of communication. Individuals who are blind at birth never learn the subtle nonverbal gestures that typically accompany language and can totally change the meaning of the spoken word.

Environment in Which the Transaction Takes Place

The place where the communication occurs influences the outcome of the interaction. Some individuals who feel uncomfortable and refuse to speak during a group therapy session may be open and willing to discuss problems privately on a one-to-one basis with the nurse.

Territoriality, density, and distance are aspects of environment that communicate messages. **Territoriality** is the innate tendency to own space. Individuals lay claim to areas around them as their own. This influences communication when an interaction takes place in the territory "owned" by one or the other. Interpersonal communication can be more successful if the interaction takes place in a "neutral" area. For example, with the concept of territoriality in mind, the nurse may choose to conduct the psychosocial assessment in an interview room rather than in his or her office or in the patient's room.

Density refers to the number of people within a given environmental space. It has been shown to influence interpersonal interaction. Some studies indicate that a correlation exists between prolonged high-density situations and certain behaviors, such as aggression, stress, criminal activity, hostility toward others, and a deterioration of mental and physical health.

Distance is the means by which various cultures use space to communicate. Hall (1966) identified four kinds of spatial interaction, or distances, that people maintain from each other in their interpersonal interactions and the kinds of activities in which people engage at these various distances. **Intimate distance** is the closest distance that individuals will allow between themselves and others. In the United States, this distance, which is restricted to interactions of an intimate nature, is 0 to 18 inches. **Personal distance** is approximately 18 to 40 inches and is reserved for interactions that are personal in nature, such as close conversations with friends or colleagues. **Social distance** is about 4 to 12 feet away from the body. Interactions at this distance include conversations with strangers or acquaintances, such as at a cocktail party or in a public building. A **public distance** is one that exceeds 12 feet. Examples include speaking in public or yelling to someone some distance away. This distance is considered public space, and communicants are free to move about in it during the interaction.

Nonverbal Communication

It has been estimated that about 70 to 80 percent of all effective communication is nonverbal (Khan, 2014). Some aspects of nonverbal expression were discussed in the previous section on pre-existing conditions that influence communication. Other components of nonverbal communication include physical appearance and dress, body movement and posture, touch, facial expressions, eye behavior, and vocal cues or *paralanguage.* These nonverbal messages vary from culture to culture.

Physical Appearance and Dress

Physical appearance and dress are part of the total nonverbal stimuli that influence interpersonal responses, and, under some conditions, they are the primary determinants of such responses. Body coverings—both dress and hair—are manipulated by the wearer in a manner that conveys a distinct message to the receiver. Dress can be formal or casual, stylish or unkempt. Hair can be long or short, and even the presence or absence of hair conveys a message about the person. Other body adornments that are considered potential communicative stimuli include tattoos, masks, cosmetics, badges, jewelry, and eyeglasses. Some jewelry worn in specific ways can give special messages (e.g., a gold band or diamond ring worn on the fourth finger of the left hand, a pin bearing Greek letters worn on the lapel, or the wearing of a ring that is inscribed with the insignia of a college or university). Some individuals convey a specific message with the total absence of any type of body adornment.

Body Movement and Posture

The way in which an individual positions his or her body communicates messages regarding self-esteem, gender identity, status, and interpersonal warmth or coldness. The individual whose posture is slumped, with head and eyes pointed downward, conveys a message of low self-esteem. Specific ways of standing or sitting are considered to be either feminine or masculine within a defined culture. To stand straight and tall with head high and hands on hips indicates a superior status over the person being addressed.

Reece and Whitman (1962) identified response behaviors that were used to designate individuals as either "warm" or "cold" persons. Individuals who were perceived as warm responded to others with a shift of posture toward the other person, a smile, direct eye contact, and hands that remained still. Individuals who responded to others with a slumped posture, by looking around the room, drumming fingers on the desk, and not smiling were perceived as cold.

Touch

Touch is a powerful communication tool. It can elicit both negative and positive reactions, depending on the people involved and the circumstances of the interaction. It is a very basic and primitive form of communication, and the appropriateness of its use is culturally determined.

Touch can be categorized according to the message communicated (Knapp & Hall, 2014):

- ■ **Functional-professional:** This type of touch is impersonal and businesslike. It is used to accomplish a task.

EXAMPLE

A tailor measuring a customer for a suit or a physician examining a patient

- ■ **Social-polite:** This type of touch is still rather impersonal, but it conveys an affirmation or acceptance of the other person.

EXAMPLE

A handshake

- ■ **Friendship-warmth:** Touch at this level indicates a strong liking for the other person—a feeling that he or she is a friend.

EXAMPLE

Laying one's hand on the shoulder of another

- ■ **Love-intimacy:** This type of touch conveys an emotional attachment or attraction to another person.

EXAMPLE

Engaging in a strong, mutual embrace

- ■ **Sexual arousal:** Touch at this level is an expression of physical attraction only.

EXAMPLE

Caressing or touching another with intent to create sexual arousal

Some cultures encourage more touching of various types than do others. Individuals in "contact cultures" (e.g., France, Latin America, Italy) use a greater frequency of touch cues than do those in "noncontact cultures" (e.g., Germany, United States, Canada) (Givens, 2016a). The nurse should understand the cultural meaning of touch before using this method of communication in specific situations.

Facial Expressions

Next to human speech, facial expression is the primary source of communication. Facial expressions primarily reveal an individual's emotional states, such as happiness, sadness, anger, surprise, and fear. The face is a complex multimessage system. Facial expressions serve to complement and qualify other communication behaviors and at times even take the place of verbal messages. A summary of feelings associated with various facial expressions is presented in Table 5–2.

Eye Behavior

Eyes have been called the "windows of the soul." It is through eye contact that individuals view and are viewed by others in a revealing way. An interpersonal

TABLE 5–2 **Summary of Facial Expressions**	
FACIAL EXPRESSION	**ASSOCIATED FEELINGS**
NOSE	
Nostril flare	Anger; arousal
Wrinkling up	Dislike; disgust
LIPS	
Grin; smile	Happiness; contentment
Grimace	Fear; pain
Compressed	Anger; frustration
Canine-type snarl	Disgust
Pouted; frown	Unhappiness; discontent; disapproval
Pursing	Disagreement
Sneer	Contempt; disdain
BROWS	
Frown	Anger; unhappiness; concentration
Raised	Surprise; enthusiasm
TONGUE	
Stuck out	Dislike; disagree
EYES	
Widened	Surprise; excitement
Narrowed; lids squeezed shut	Threat; fear
Stare	Threat
Stare, blink, look away	Dislike; disinterest
Eyes downcast; lack of eye contact	Submission; low self-esteem
Eye contact (generally intermittent as opposed to a stare)	Self-confidence; interest

Source: Adapted from Givens, D. B. (2016b). Facial expression. In *The nonverbal dictionary of gestures, signs, and body language.* Retrieved from http://center-for-nonverbal-studies.org/htdocs/6101.html.

connectedness occurs through eye contact. In American culture, eye contact conveys a personal interest in the other person. Eye contact indicates that the communication channel is open, and it is often the initiating factor in verbal interaction between two people.

Eye behavior is regulated by social rules. These rules dictate where, when, for how long, and at whom we may look. Staring is often used to register disapproval of the behavior of another. People are extremely sensitive to being looked at, and if the gazing or staring behavior violates social rules, they often assign meaning to it, such as the following statement implies: "He kept staring at me, and I began to wonder if I was dressed inappropriately or had mustard on my face!"

Gazing at another's eyes arouses strong emotions. Thus, eye contact rarely lasts longer than 3 seconds before one or both viewers experience a powerful urge to glance away. Breaking eye contact lowers stress levels (Givens, 2016c).

Vocal Cues or Paralanguage

Paralanguage is the vocal component of the spoken word. It consists of pitch, tone, and loudness of spoken messages, the rate of speaking, expressively placed pauses, and emphasis assigned to certain words. These vocal cues greatly influence the way individuals interpret verbal messages. A normally soft-spoken individual whose pitch and rate of speaking increases may be perceived as being anxious or tense. Paralanguage may also include facial expressions and gestures that accompany vocal components and contribute to the interpretation of the message.

Different vocal emphases can alter interpretation of the message. For example,

- "I felt SURE you would notice the change."
  Interpretation: I was SURE you would, but you didn't.
- "I felt sure YOU would notice the change."
  Interpretation: I thought YOU would, even if nobody else did.
- "I felt sure you would notice the CHANGE."
  Interpretation: Even if you didn't notice anything else, I thought you would notice the CHANGE.

Verbal cues play a major role in determining responses in human communication situations. *How* a message is verbalized can be as important as *what* is verbalized.

CORE CONCEPT

Therapeutic communication

Caregiver verbal and nonverbal techniques that focus on the care receiver's needs and advance the promotion of healing and change. Therapeutic communication encourages exploration of feelings and fosters understanding of behavioral motivation. It is nonjudgmental, discourages defensiveness, and promotes trust.

Therapeutic Communication Techniques

Hays and Larson (1963) identified a number of techniques to assist the nurse in interacting more therapeutically with patients. These are important "technical procedures" carried out by the nurse working in psychiatry, and they should serve to enhance development of a therapeutic nurse-patient relationship. Table 5–3 includes a list of these techniques, a

TABLE 5–3 **Therapeutic Communication Techniques**		
TECHNIQUE	**EXPLANATION/RATIONALE**	**EXAMPLES**
Using silence	Silence encourages the patient to organize thoughts and put them into words and allows the patient time to think about the significance of events, thoughts, and feelings. Allowing the patient to break the silence often provides the nurse with important information about the patient's foremost concerns.	Pt: "My husband divorced me so I must be undesirable." Nurse: (silence) Pt: "You know, when I think about it, no matter what my husband does I always assume it's my fault or it's something wrong with me."
Accepting	Acceptance conveys an attitude of understanding and willingness to interact.	"Yes, I understand what you said." Eye contact; nodding
Giving recognition	Acknowledging and indicating awareness is better than complimenting, which reflects the nurse's judgment.	"Hello, Mr. J. I notice that you made a ceramic ash tray in OT." "I see you made your bed."
Offering self	Willingness to spend time with the patient and show interest on an unconditional basis helps to increase the patient's feelings of self-worth.	"I'll stay with you awhile." "How are you feeling today?" "I'm interested in hearing your thoughts about the group you just attended."
Giving broad openings	Broad openings allow the patient to direct the focus of the interaction and emphasize the importance of the patient's role in the communication process.	"What would you like to talk about today?" "Is there anything you want to discuss?"
Offering general leads	General leads offer the patient encouragement to continue with minimal input from the nurse.	"Go on." "And after that?"
Placing the event in time or sequence	Encouraging the patient to identify the sequence of events and when they occurred in time facilitates organizing one's thoughts about their experiences.	"What happened first?" "What happened next?" "Was this before or after . . . ?" "When did this happen?"
Making observations	Verbalizing observations about a patient's behavior or appearance encourages the patient to develop awareness of how they are perceived by others and promotes exploration of issues that may be problematic.	"You appear sad today." "I notice you are pacing a lot." "I notice that when I ask you about whether you have thoughts of suicide you change the subject."
Encouraging description of perceptions	Asking the patient to verbalize his or her perceptions facilitates the patient's ability to develop awareness and understanding. For the patient experiencing hallucinations, it can facilitate both nurse's and patient's clarification about what the patient's perceptual experiences are communicating.	"Tell me more about the voices you said you are hearing." "What was it that increased your agitation during the group activity?" "Are these voices you hear directing you to take some action?"
Encouraging comparison	Asking the patient to compare similarities and differences in ideas, experiences, or interpersonal relationships helps the patient recognize life experiences that tend to recur and those aspects of life that are changeable.	"Was this episode similar to . . . ?" "How does this compare with the time when . . . ?" "What was your response the last time this situation occurred?"

TABLE 5–3	Therapeutic Communication Techniques–cont'd	
TECHNIQUE	**EXPLANATION/RATIONALE**	**EXAMPLES**
Restating	Repeating the main idea of what the patient has said lets the patient know whether an expressed statement has been understood and gives him or her the chance to continue, or to clarify if necessary.	Pt: "I can't study. My mind keeps wandering." Nurse: "You have trouble concentrating." Pt: "I can't take that new job. What if I can't do it?" Nurse: "You're afraid you will fail in this new position."
Reflecting	Questions and feelings are referred back to the patient so that the patient is empowered to actively engage in problem-solving rather than simply asking the nurse for advice.	Pt: "Don't you think I should tell my boss I'm not putting up with that?" Nurse: "What do *you* think you should do?" Pt: "She makes me so upset!" Nurse: "So you're feeling angry at your boss?"
Focusing	Taking notice of a single idea or even a single word encourages specific discussion about a relevant issue and is especially helpful with patients who are moving rapidly from one thought to another. However, focusing is very difficult for a patient with severe anxiety so in this case the nurse should not pursue focusing until the anxiety level lessens.	"Tell me more about this specific point."
Exploring	When the nurse hears the patient mention an issue or theme that seems relevant, the nurse asks the patient to explore this further. Exploring facilitates the patient's development of awareness and understanding about events, thoughts, and feelings. However, if the patient chooses not to disclose further information, the nurse should refrain from pushing or probing in an area that obviously creates discomfort.	"Please explain that situation in more detail." "Tell me more about that particular situation." "You mentioned feeling like no one cares about you. Tell me more about those feelings."
Seeking clarification and validation	Striving to explain that which is vague or incomprehensible and searching for mutual understanding facilitates and increases understanding for both patient and nurse.	"I'm not sure that I understand. Would you please explain?" "Tell me if my understanding agrees with yours." "Do I understand correctly that you said . . . ?"
Presenting reality	When the patient has a misperception of the environment, the nurse defines reality by expressing his or her perception of the situation without challenging the patient's perceptions.	"I understand that the voices seem real to you, but I do not hear any voices." "I don't see anyone else in the room but you and me."
Voicing doubt	Expressing uncertainty about the validity of the patient's perceptions is a technique often used with patients experiencing delusional thinking.	"It's difficult to believe that the president of the United States would be listening to all of your phone calls." "I find that hard to believe [or accept]." "That seems rather doubtful to me."

Continued

TABLE 5–3	Therapeutic Communication Techniques–cont'd	
TECHNIQUE	**EXPLANATION/RATIONALE**	**EXAMPLES**
Verbalizing the implied	Putting into words what the patient has only implied or said indirectly is a technique that can be helpful with patients experiencing impaired verbal communication.	Pt: "I can't talk about this . . . you haven't been where I've been." Nurse: "Does it seem like no one could understand your thoughts and feelings unless they've had the same experiences you've had?" Pt: "I . . . I don't know where to begin." Nurse: "So it feels overwhelming to think about sharing the details of this experience."
Attempting to translate words into feelings	When the patient has difficulty identifying feelings or feelings are expressed indirectly, the nurse tries to "desymbolize" what has been said and to find clues to the underlying true feelings.	Pt: "I'm just an empty pit." Nurse: "It sounds like you are feeling hopeless, is that right?"
Formulating a plan of action	Encouraging the patient to identify a plan for behavior change promotes developing better coping skills.	"What could you do differently if you are faced with this situation in the future?" "What are some steps you could take to manage your anger without punching someone?" "What is one thing you might be willing to try to decrease your anxiety instead of using alcohol?"

Source: Hays, J. S., & Larson, K. H. (1963). *Interacting with patients.* New York, NY: Macmillan; Engard, B. (2018). *17 therapeutic communication techniques.* Retrieved from https://online.rivier.edu/therapeutic-communication-techniques/; Sullivan, H. S. (1954). *The psychiatric interview.* New York, NY: Norton.

short explanation of their usefulness, and examples of each.

Nontherapeutic Communication Techniques

Several approaches are considered to be barriers to open communication between the nurse and patient. Hays and Larson (1963) identified a number of these techniques, which are presented in Table 5–4. Nurses should recognize and eliminate the use of these patterns in their relationships with patients. Avoiding these communication barriers will maximize the effectiveness of communication and enhance the nurse-patient relationship.

Active Listening

To listen actively is to be attentive and to really desire to hear and understand what the patient is saying, both verbally and nonverbally. Attentive listening creates a climate in which the patient can communicate; the nurse communicates acceptance and respect for the patient, and trust is enhanced. A climate is established in the relationship that promotes openness and honest expression.

Several nonverbal behaviors have been designated as facilitative skills for attentive listening. Those listed here can be identified by the acronym SOLER:

S: Sit squarely facing the patient. This gives the message that the nurse is there to listen and is interested in what the patient has to say.

O: Observe an open posture. Posture is considered "open" when arms and legs remain uncrossed. This posture suggests that the nurse is "open" to what the patient has to say. With a "closed" posture, the nurse can convey a somewhat defensive stance, possibly invoking a similar response in the patient.

L: Lean forward toward the patient. This nonverbal behavior conveys to the patient that you are involved in the interaction, interested in what is being said, and making a sincere effort to be attentive.

E: Establish eye contact. Direct eye contact is another behavior that conveys the nurse's involvement and willingness to listen to what the patient has to say. The absence of eye contact, or the constant shifting of eye contact, gives the message that the nurse is not really interested in what is being said.

TABLE 5–4	Nontherapeutic Communication Techniques	
TECHNIQUE	**EXPLANATION/RATIONALE**	**EXAMPLES**
Giving false reassurance	False reassurance conveys that the nurse already knows the outcome of a situation and minimizes the patient's expressed concerns. It may discourage the patient from further expression of feelings if he or she believes the feelings will be downplayed or ridiculed.	Patient: "My husband doesn't love me anymore. I think he wants a divorce." Nurse: "I'm sure he must still love you. Everything will be fine." **Better alternative:** "Tell me more about what's been happening in your relationship with your husband."
Rejecting	Refusing to consider or showing contempt for the patient's ideas or behavior may cause the patient to discontinue interaction with the nurse for fear of further rejection.	Patient: "Since I started taking this medication I can't be intimate with my girlfriend." Nurse: "Let's not talk about that right now." **Better alternative:** "Tell me more about what you mean by not being able 'to be intimate' with your girlfriend."
Approving or disapproving	Sanctioning or denouncing the patient's ideas or behavior implies that the nurse's role is to pass judgment on whether the patient's ideas or behaviors are "good" or "bad" and that the patient is expected to please the nurse. The nurse's acceptance of the patient is then seen as conditional depending on the patient's behavior.	"It's good that you confronted your wife about her behavior." "You shouldn't yell at your wife." **Better alternative:** "What happened after you confronted your wife in a loud voice?"
Agreeing or disagreeing	Indicating accord with or opposition to the patient's ideas or opinions implies that the nurse has the right to pass judgment on whether the patient's ideas or opinions are "right" or "wrong." Agreement prevents the patient from later modifying his or her point of view without the risk of displeasing the nurse. Disagreement may provoke defensiveness on the part of the patient.	Patient: "I think my doctor doesn't care about me." Nurse: "I disagree. You shouldn't think that way." or "I can't believe that's true." **Better alternative:** "Tell me more about why you think your doctor doesn't care."
Giving advice	Telling the patient what to do or how to behave implies that the nurse knows what is best and nurtures the patient in the dependent role by discouraging independent thinking.	"You need to do deep breathing exercises when you become anxious." "You should stop drinking alcohol and start going to Alcoholics Anonymous meetings." **Better alternative:** "What do *you* think you should do?" or "Let's explore some options for solving this problem."
Probing	Persistent questioning of the patient and pushing for answers to issues the patient does not wish to discuss or does not know the answers to may contribute to the patient feeling used only for what information the nurse is seeking and may place the patient on the defensive.	"Why was your family angry with you?" "How many times did you receive poor evaluations before you got fired?" "How many girlfriends were you lying to?" **Better alternative:** The nurse should actively listen to the patient's response and discontinue the interaction at the first sign of discomfort.
Defending	Defending someone or something the patient has criticized minimizes or completely ignores the patient's concerns. Defending may cause the patient to think the nurse is taking sides against him or her.	"None of the nurses here would lie to you." "You have a very capable physician." "Your children want only what's best for you." **Better alternative:** "Tell me more about these concerns you've expressed."

Continued

TABLE 5-4 Nontherapeutic Communication Techniques—cont'd

TECHNIQUE	EXPLANATION/RATIONALE	EXAMPLES
Requesting an explanation	This technique involves asking the patient why he or she has certain thoughts, feelings, and behaviors. Asking "why" a patient did something or feels a certain way can be very intimidating and implies that the patient must defend his or her behavior or feelings.	"Why do you think people are out to get you?" "Why do you feel depressed?" "Why were you taking drugs?" **Better alternative:** "Describe what you were feeling just before that happened."
Indicating the existence of an external source of power	Attributing the source of thoughts, feelings, and behavior to something or someone other than the patient encourages the patient to project blame for his or her thoughts or behaviors on others rather than accepting the responsibility personally.	"What made you go on a drinking binge?" "What made you say that you are a worthless person?" **Better alternative:** "What was happening just before you started binge drinking?" "What do you mean when you say you are 'a worthless person'?"
Belittling feelings expressed	When the nurse minimizes the degree of the patient's discomfort, a lack of empathy and understanding may be conveyed. When the nurse tells the patient to "cheer up" or "everybody feels that way," the patient may feel that his or her concerns are insignificant or unimportant.	Patient: "I don't even have the energy to go to work." Nurse: "We've all felt like that at times. You've just got to 'perk up' and get moving." **Better alternative:** "Tell me more about what you are feeling right now."
Making stereotyped comments	Trite expressions are meaningless in a nurse-patient relationship. When the nurse uses meaningless expressions, it encourages a similar response from the patient.	"How are you?" "Hang in there." "It'll all work out." **Better alternative:** Choose words, sentences, and nonverbal language that convey a sincere interest in encouraging the patient to share more about the patient's thoughts, feelings, and behaviors.
Using denial	Denying that a problem exists blocks discussion with the patient and avoids helping the patient identify and explore areas of difficulty.	Patient: "I have a problem interacting with people." Nurse: "You're doing fine." **Better alternative:** "Tell me more about that."
Interpreting	Interpreting attempts to tell the patient the meaning of his or her experience. Erroneous interpretations may leave the patient feeling that the nurse doesn't understand him or her, or that the nurse is being smug.	"What you really mean is. . . ." "You're angry because. . . ." **Better alternative:** The nurse must leave interpretation of the patient's behavior to a therapist who is trained to use interpretation in the context of specialized therapy.
Introducing an unrelated topic	When the nurse prematurely changes the subject, it conveys to the patient that the nurse does not want to discuss the original topic any further. This may occur in order to get to something that the nurse wants to discuss with the patient or to get away from a topic that he or she would prefer not to discuss.	Patient: "I don't have anything to live for." Nurse: "How well did you sleep last night?" **Better alternative:** "Tell me more." Sometimes silence may be appropriate to convey that the nurse is willing to hear all of what the patient wants to say before moving on to a different topic.

Source: Adapted from: Hays, J. S., & Larson, K. H. (1963). *Interacting with patients.* New York, NY: Macmillan; Engard, B. (2018). *17 therapeutic communication techniques.* Retrieved from https://online.rivier.edu/therapeutic-communication-techniques/; Sullivan, H. S. (1954). *The psychiatric interview.* New York, NY: Norton.

R: Relax. Whether sitting or standing during the interaction, the nurse should communicate a sense of being relaxed and comfortable with the patient. Restlessness and fidgetiness communicate a lack of interest and may convey a feeling of discomfort that is likely to be transferred to the patient.

> **CLINICAL PEARL** Ensure that eye contact conveys warmth, is accompanied by smiling and intermittent nodding of the head, and does not come across as staring or glaring, which can create intense discomfort in the patient.

MOTIVATIONAL INTERVIEWING

Motivational interviewing is an evidence-based, patient-centered style of communication that promotes behavior change by guiding patients to explore their own motivation for change and the advantages and disadvantages of their decisions. Patient-centered care has been identified as an important focus in the quest to improve the quality of communication and therapeutic relationships with patients (Institute of Medicine, 2003).

This style of communication incorporates active listening and therapeutic communication techniques, but it is focused on what the patient wants to do rather than what the nurse thinks *should* be the next steps in behavior change. Motivational interviewing was originally developed for use with patients who were struggling with substance use disorders, primarily because this style of communication is more likely to decrease defensive patient responses. It has since gained widespread acceptance as a patient-centered communication strategy that promotes behavior change for patients with many different healthcare issues. See the "Real People, Real Stories" feature for an example of motivational interviewing described in a process recording format.

Real People, Real Stories: A Sample of Motivational Interviewing in a Process Recording Format

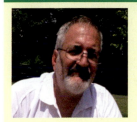

The following is part of an interaction with Alan, incorporating motivational interviewing communication strategies in a process recording format. Learn more about Alan's story in the chapter on substance use disorders.

Interaction	Nurse's Thoughts and Feelings	Communication Technique/ Evaluation
Karyn: You mentioned that you were at an event and you commented that you "needed a drink." Tell me more about what was happening. (SOLER)	I wasn't sure if Alan was willing to talk about this, but I thought it was important to facilitate his looking at his behavior in response to this experience.	Technique: **Exploring** Evaluation: This approach was effective. Alan talked more about the event and was able to articulate some thoughts and feelings as well.
Alan: (nodding) I was perturbed. I felt like I was stuck at this event. There was supposed to be entertainment, but it got cancelled due to rain, and suddenly I noticed people were drinking and smoking. It brought back a lot of memories. (looks down)	I was glad that Alan was open to discussing this experience, but he said so many things in this short statement that I had to be thoughtful about what to follow up on.	

Continued

Real People, Real Stories: A Sample of Motivational Interviewing in a Process Recording Format--cont'd

Interaction	Nurse's Thoughts and Feelings	Communication Technique/ Evaluation
Karyn: So you felt perturbed and stuck. . . . (looking up, not making direct eye contact)	I was thinking that I don't usually explore feelings right off the bat because I believe it's better to help someone fully describe events and thoughts first (or at least it's less threatening), but I've interacted with Alan many times, he's been through rehab, sober for seven years, and he's pretty comfortable talking about feelings.	Technique: **Reflecting** Evaluation: This technique was effective. Alan began to process his thoughts about why he might be feeling perturbed and stuck. I think I may have been not making direct eye contact because of my perception that feelings can be a little more threatening for some people to talk about.
Alan: Yeah, but it didn't last long. Maybe it had something to do with the fact that there was nothing else going on and it seemed like the whole thing became about drinking. But then I just blacked it out.	My immediate thought was that I want to tell him to go to an AA meeting or call his sponsor, but I was trying to incorporate a motivational interviewing strategy, and that meant it would be better to help him explore his motivation for how to respond to this experience. I didn't know what he meant by "blacked it out," but I felt uncomfortable when he said that.	
Karyn: What do you mean when you say you blacked it out? (SOLER)	I thought this was an important statement to clarify, since it might help him explore how he behaved in response to this event.	Technique: **Clarifying** Evaluation: Asking this question was effective. Alan talked at length about his thoughts and feelings.
Alan: (silent for several seconds) I do need to go back to an AA meeting. I mean, am I different than other people? I know there are other people out there that have to be struggling with the same kind of things. When I was in rehab, my mom and her boyfriend were always there taking me to meetings. My sister went, too. . . . (silent for several more seconds) I know it's important (silence) . . . about 75 percent of the people I went to rehab with are back out there using again.	Alan seemed to be thinking a lot about this and was responding with several different thoughts, so I felt like it was important to just use silence and facilitate his reflection. I thought Alan seemed to be genuinely considering a behavior change.	
Karyn: You said that you need to go back to a meeting and that they are important. Is it more helpful to go to meetings when you just start thinking about needing a drink, or do you think that meetings are only necessary after you actually take a drink?	I knew that Alan had not been going to meetings regularly for the last couple of years, even though he acknowledges their importance, so I wanted to know more about whether he thought behavior change (such as going to AA meetings) was necessary at this point.	Technique: **Restating, focusing** Evaluation: Restatement was effective. The way I chose to focus was probably leading Alan to choose the "right" answer, and that makes it harder to evaluate whether he is just telling me what I want to hear or is really motivated. It might have been better to use the technique of formulating a plan of action.

Real People, Real Stories: A Sample of Motivational Interviewing in a Process Recording Format—cont'd

Interaction	Nurse's Thoughts and Feelings	Communication Technique/ Evaluation
Alan: Oh no, you've got to go long before you take that first drink. (silence) People told me when I was in rehab that they could tell I was really listening in meetings . . . the meetings were helpful (silence), and I just reconnected with my sponsor on Facebook, so I need to get back to a meeting to see him.	Alan seemed like he was thinking about what is important to him, so I continued to remain silent to facilitate that process.	
Karyn: You've identified three reasons why you believe you need to go to a meeting: because they are helpful to you, because you want to find out if others are struggling with the same kinds of thoughts that you are, and because you need to reconnect with your sponsor. Do you have a plan in mind for how to follow through with that?	I was thinking that he talks about needing to go to AA, and *I* was feeling anxious about wanting him to commit to that, but at the same time, I recognized that the motivation for change and commitment to a plan of action has to come from him.	Technique: **Summarizing, formulating a plan of action** Evaluation: I think the techniques were effective, although Alan may not be ready to formulate an action plan at present.
Alan: Well, I haven't done it yet. I guess I'm still just thinking about it.	I was appreciating his honesty and thinking that this is the challenge of motivational interviewing: accepting where the patient is while continuing to explore and facilitate his or her motivations for behavior change.	

Process Recordings

Process recordings are written reports of verbal interactions with patients. They are verbatim (to the extent that this is possible) accounts written by the nurse or student as a tool for improving interpersonal communication techniques. The process recording can take many forms but usually includes the verbal and nonverbal communication of both nurse and patient. The exercise provides a means for the nurse to analyze the content and pattern of the interaction. The process recording, which is not considered documentation, is intended to be used as a learning tool for professional development. An example of one type of process recording is presented in Table 5–5.

Feedback

Feedback is a method of communication that helps the patient consider a modification of behavior by providing information about how he or she is perceived by others. Feedback can be useful to the patient if presented with objectivity by a trusted individual in a manner that discourages defensiveness.

Characteristics of useful feedback include the following:

■ Feedback should be descriptive rather than evaluative and focused on the behavior rather than on the person. Avoiding evaluative language reduces the need for the patient to react defensively. Objective descriptions allow patients to take the information and use it in whatever way they choose. When the focus is on the person, rather than the behavior, the patient may perceive that they are being judged as "good" or "bad."

EXAMPLE

Descriptive and focused on behavior: "Jane was very upset in group today when you called her 'fatty' and laughed at her in front of the others."
Evaluative: "You were very rude and inconsiderate to Jane in group today."
Focused on patient: "You are a very insensitive person."

■ Feedback should be specific rather than general. Information that gives details about the patient's behavior can be used more easily than a generalized description for modifying the behavior.

TABLE 5–5 Sample Process Recording

NURSE VERBAL (NONVERBAL)	PATIENT VERBAL (NONVERBAL)	NURSE'S THOUGHTS AND FEELINGS CONCERNING THE INTERACTION	ANALYSIS OF THE INTERACTION
"Do you still have thoughts about harming yourself?" (Sitting facing patient; looking directly at patient.)	"Not really. I still feel sad, but I don't want to die." (Looking at hands in lap.)	Felt a little uncomfortable. Always a hard question to ask.	**Therapeutic:** *Asking a direct, closed-ended question* about suicidal intent to elicit specific information
"Tell me what you were feeling before you took all the pills the other night." (Using SOLER techniques of active listening.)	"I was just so angry! To think that my husband wants a divorce now that he has a good job. I worked hard to put him through college." (Fists clenched. Face and neck reddened.)	Beginning to feel more comfortable. She seems willing to talk, and I think she trusts me.	**Therapeutic:** *Exploring.* Delving further into patient's feelings to help patient better understand her experience
"You wanted to hurt him because you felt betrayed." (SOLER)	"Yes! If I died, maybe he'd realize that he loved me more than that other woman." (Tears starting to well up in her eyes.)	Starting to feel sorry for her.	**Therapeutic:** *Attempting to translate words into feelings* to convey active listening
"Seems like a pretty drastic way to get your point across." (Small frown.)	"I know. It was a stupid thing to do." (Wiping eyes.)	Trying hard to remain objective.	**Nontherapeutic:** Sounds disapproving. Better to have focused on the patient's feelings such as "How are you feeling about that now?"
"How are you feeling about the situation now?" (SOLER)	"I don't know. I still love him. I want him to come home. I don't want him to marry her." (Starting to cry again.)	Wishing there was an easy way to help relieve some of her pain.	**Therapeutic:** *Focusing* on her current feelings to assess current mental status
"Yes, I can understand that you would like things to be the way they were before." (Offer patient a tissue.)	(Silence. Continues to cry softly.)	I'm starting to feel some anger toward her husband. Sometimes it's so hard to remain objective!	**Therapeutic:** *Conveying empathy* to support caring and connectedness
"What do you think are the chances of your getting back together?" (SOLER)	"None. He's refused marriage counseling. He's already moved in with her. He says it's over." (Wipes tears. Looks directly at nurse.)	Relieved to know that she isn't using denial about the reality of the situation.	**Therapeutic:** *Reflecting* on the patient's expressed desires to encourage her to recognize and clarify her perceptions
"So how are you preparing to deal with this inevitable outcome?" (SOLER)	"I'm going to do the things we talked about: join a divorced women's support group; increase my job hours to full-time; do some volunteer work; and call the suicide hotline if I feel like taking pills again." (Looks directly at nurse. Smiles.)	Positive feeling to know that she remembers what we discussed earlier and plans to follow through.	**Therapeutic:** *Formulating a plan of action* to set the foundation for problem-solving
"It won't be easy. But you have come a long way, and you've gained strength in your ability to cope." (Standing. Looking at patient. Smiling.)	"Yes, I know I will have hard times. But I also know I have support, and I want to go on with my life and be happy again." (Standing, smiling at nurse.)	Feeling confident that the session has gone well; hopeful that she will succeed in what she wants to do with her life.	**Therapeutic:** *Presenting reality, making observations, and giving recognition* to support her progress in problem-solving

EXAMPLE

Specific: "You were talking to Joe when we were deciding on the issue. Now you want to argue about the outcome."
General: "You just don't pay attention."

■ Feedback should be directed toward behavior that the patient has the capacity to modify. To provide feedback about a characteristic or situation that the patient cannot change will only provoke frustration.

EXAMPLE

Can modify: "I noticed that you did not want to hold your baby when the nurse brought her to you."
Cannot modify: "Your baby daughter is mentally retarded because you took drugs when you were pregnant."

■ Feedback should impart information rather than offer advice. Giving advice fosters dependence and may convey the message to the patient that he or she is not capable of making decisions and solving problems independently. It is the patient's right and privilege to be as self-sufficient as possible.

EXAMPLE

Imparting information: "There are various methods of assistance for people who want to lose weight, such as Overeaters Anonymous, Weight Watchers, regular visits to a dietitian, and the Physician's Weight Loss Program. You can decide what is best for you."
Giving advice: "You obviously need to lose a great deal of weight. I think the Physician's Weight Loss Program would be best for you."

■ Feedback should be well timed. Feedback is most useful when given at the earliest appropriate opportunity following the specific behavior.

EXAMPLE

Prompt response: "I saw you hit the wall with your fist just now when you hung up the phone from talking to your mother."
Delayed response: "You need to learn some more appropriate ways of dealing with your anger. Last week after group I saw you pounding your fist against the wall."

Summary and Key Points

■ Nurses who work in the psychiatric mental health field use special skills of relationship development and therapeutic communication to assist patients in adapting to difficulties or changes in life experiences.
■ Therapeutic nurse-patient relationships are goal oriented. Ideally, the goal is mutually agreed on by the nurse and patient and is directed at learning and growth promotion.
■ The instrument of delivery for the process of interpersonal nursing is the therapeutic use of self, which requires that the nurse possess a strong sense of self-awareness and self-understanding.
■ Several characteristics that enhance the achievement of a therapeutic relationship have been identified. They include rapport, trust, respect, genuineness, and empathy.
■ The tasks associated with the development of a therapeutic interpersonal relationship have been categorized into four phases: preinteraction phase, orientation (introductory) phase, working phase, and termination phase.
■ Interpersonal communication is a transaction between the sender and the receiver.
■ In all interpersonal transactions, both the sender and receiver bring certain pre-existing conditions to the exchange that influence both the intended message and the way in which it is interpreted. Examples of these conditions include one's value system, internalized attitudes and beliefs, culture or religion, social status, gender, background knowledge and experience, age or developmental level, and the type of environment in which the communication takes place.
■ Nonverbal expression is a primary component of communication in which meaning is assigned to various gestures and patterns of behavior.
■ Some components of nonverbal communication include physical appearance and dress, body movement and posture, touch, facial expressions, eye behavior, and vocal cues or paralanguage. The meaning of each of these nonverbal components is culturally determined.
■ Active listening is described as attentiveness to what the patient is saying through both verbal and nonverbal cues. Skills associated with active listening include **SOLER**; sitting **S**quarely facing the patient, maintaining an **O**pen posture, **L**eaning forward toward the patient, establishing **E**ye contact, and being **R**elaxed. The nurse must be aware of and avoid techniques that are barriers to effective communication.
■ Motivational interviewing is an evidence-based, patient-centered style of communication that facilitates patients' exploration of their own motivations for behavior change and guides the patient to explore the advantages and disadvantages of their decisions.

■ Process recordings are written analyses of the interaction between nurse and patient. They are used as tools for critical thinking and professional development.

■ The nurse must be aware of the therapeutic or nontherapeutic value of the communication techniques used with the patient because they are the primary tools of psychosocial intervention.

■ Feedback is a method of communication for helping the patient to develop self-awareness and consider modification of his or her behavior.

Additional information is available at davisplus. fadavis.com.

Review Questions
Self-Examination/Learning Exercise

Select the answer that is most appropriate for each of the following questions:

1. On Tom's day of discharge from the hospital, his wife brings a bouquet of flowers and box of chocolates to give to his primary care nurse. Tom presents these gifts to the nurse saying, "Thank you for taking care of me." What is a correct response by the nurse?
   a. "I don't want a gift from you!"
   b. "Thank you so much! I think you're really extra special, too!"
   c. "Thank you. I will share these with the rest of the staff."
   d. "I love chocolate but let me pay you for them!"

2. Chelsea says to the nurse, "I worked as a secretary to put my husband through college, and as soon as he graduated, he left me. I hate him! I hate all men!" Which is an empathetic response by the nurse?
   a. "You are very angry now. This is a normal response to your loss."
   b. "I know what you mean. Men can be very insensitive."
   c. "I understand completely. My husband is a jerk, too."
   d. "You are depressed now, but you will feel better in time."

3. Which of the following behaviors suggests a possible breach of professional boundaries? (Select all that apply.)
   a. The nurse repeatedly requests to be assigned to a specific patient.
   b. The nurse shares the details of her divorce with the patient.
   c. The nurse makes arrangements to meet the patient outside of the therapeutic environment.
   d. The nurse shares how she dealt with a similar difficult situation.

4. A patient states, "I refuse to shower in this room. I must be very cautious. The FBI has placed a camera in here to monitor my every move." Which of the following is the most therapeutic response?
   a. "That's not true."
   b. "I have a hard time believing that is true."
   c. "Surely you don't really believe that."
   d. "Let's search the room together to see if we can find a camera."

5. Nancy, a depressed patient who has been unkempt and untidy for weeks, today comes to group therapy wearing makeup and a clean dress and having washed and combed her hair. Which of the following responses by the nurse is most therapeutic?
   a. "Nancy, I see you have put on a clean dress and combed your hair."
   b. "Nancy, you look wonderful today!"
   c. "Nancy, I'm sure everyone will appreciate that you have cleaned up for the group today."
   d. "Now that you see how important it is, I hope you will do this every day."

Review Questions—cont'd
Self-Examination/Learning Exercise

6. Dorothy was involved in an automobile accident while under the influence of alcohol. She swerved her car into a tree and narrowly missed hitting a child on a bicycle. She is in the hospital with multiple abrasions and contusions. She is talking about the accident with the nurse. Which of the following statements by the nurse is most appropriate?
    a. "Now that you know what can happen when you drink and drive, I'm sure you won't let it happen again."
    b. "You know that was a terrible thing you did. That child could have been killed."
    c. "I'm sure everything is going to be okay now that you understand the possible consequences of such behavior."
    d. "How are you feeling about what happened?"

7. Judy has been in the hospital for 3 weeks. She has used Valium "to settle her nerves" for the past 15 years. She was admitted by her psychiatrist for safe withdrawal from the drug. She has passed the physical symptoms of withdrawal at this time but states to the nurse, "I don't know if I will make it without Valium after I go home. I'm already starting to feel nervous. I have so many personal problems." Which is the most appropriate response by the nurse?
    a. "Why do you think you have to have drugs to deal with your problems?"
    b. "Everybody has problems, but not everybody uses drugs to deal with them. You'll just have to do the best that you can."
    c. "Let's explore some things you can do to decrease your anxiety without resorting to drugs."
    d. "Just hang in there. I'm sure everything is going to be okay."

8. Mrs. S. asks the nurse, "Do you think I should tell my husband about my affair with my boss?" Which is the most appropriate response by the nurse?
    a. "What do you think would be best for you to do?"
    b. "Of course you should. Marriage has to be based on truth."
    c. "Of course not. That would only make things worse."
    d. "I can't tell you what to do. You have to decide for yourself."

9. Abbey, an adolescent, just returned from group therapy and is crying. She says to the nurse, "All the other kids laughed at me! I try to fit in, but I always seem to say the wrong thing. I've never had a close friend. I guess I never will." Which is the most appropriate response by the nurse?
    a. "Why will you never have any friends?"
    b. "You're feeling pretty down on yourself right now."
    c. "I'm sure they didn't mean to hurt your feelings."
    d. "You don't need friends to be happy."

10. Which of the following tasks are associated with the orientation phase of relationship development? (Select all that apply.)
    a. Promoting the patient's insight and perception of reality.
    b. Creating an environment for the establishment of trust and rapport.
    c. Using the problem-solving model toward goal fulfillment.
    d. Obtaining available information about the patient from various sources.
    e. Formulating nursing diagnoses and setting goals.

Continued

Review Questions—cont'd
Self-Examination/Learning Exercise

11. Joe has been in rehabilitation for alcohol dependence. When he returns from a visit to his home, he tells the nurse, "We were having a celebration and I did have one drink, but it really wasn't a problem." The nurse notices that his breath smells of alcohol. Which of the following responses by the nurse demonstrates a motivational interviewing style of communication?
    a. "You are obviously not motivated to change so perhaps we should discuss your discharge from the treatment program."
    b. "You need to abstain from alcohol in order to recover, so let me talk to your doctor about the consequences for your behavior."
    c. "Why would you destroy everything you've worked so hard to achieve?"
    d. "What do you mean when you say, 'it really wasn't a problem'?"

12. Bill, who has been diagnosed with schizophrenia and has been on medication for several months, states, "I'm not taking that stupid medication anymore!" Which of the following responses demonstrates a motivational interviewing style of communication?
    a. "Don't you know that if you don't take your medication you will never recover?"
    b. "Why won't you cooperate with the treatment your doctor prescribed?"
    c. "Bill, the medication is not stupid."
    d. "Tell me more about why you don't want to take the medication."

References

College and Association of Registered Nurses of Alberta (CARNA). (2011). *Professional boundaries for registered nurses: Guidelines for the nurse-client relationship.* Edmonton, Alberta, Canada: Author. Retrieved from http://www.nurses.ab.ca/content/dam/carna/pdfs/DocumentList/Guidelines/RN_ProfessionalBoundaries_May2011.pdf

College of Registered Nurses of British Columbia (CRNBC). (2015). *Boundaries in the nurse-client relationship.* Vancouver, BC, Canada: Author. Retrieved from https://www.crnbc.ca/Standards/PracticeStandards/Pages/boundaries.aspx

Engard, B. (2018). *17 therapeutic communication techniques.* Retrieved from https://online.rivier.edu/therapeutic-communication-techniques/

Givens, D. B. (2016a). Touch cue. In *The nonverbal dictionary of gestures, signs, and body language.* Retrieved from http://www.center-for-nonverbal-studies.org/touch.htm

Givens, D. B. (2016b). Facial expression. In *The nonverbal dictionary of gestures, signs, and body language.* Retrieved from http://www.center-for-nonverbal-studies.org/facialx.htm

Givens, D. B. (2016c). Eye contact. In *The nonverbal dictionary of gestures, signs, and body language.* Retrieved from http://www.center-for-nonverbal-studies.org/eyecon.htm

Hilz, L. M. (2013). Transference and countertransference. *Kathi's Mental Health Review.* Retrieved from http://www.toddlertime.com/mh/terms/countertransference-transference-3.htm

Institute of Medicine, Board on Health Care Services and Committee on the Health Professions Education Summit. (2003). *Health professions education: A bridge to quality.* Washington, DC: National Academies Press.

Khan, A. (2014). *Principles for personal growth.* Bellevue, WA: YouMeWorks.

Knapp, M. L., & Hall, J. A. (2014). *Nonverbal communication in human interaction* (8th ed.). Boston, MA: Wadsworth.

National Council of State Boards of Nursing (NCSBN). (2014). *A nurse's guide to professional boundaries.* Retrieved from https://www.ncsbn.org/ProfessionalBoundaries_Complete.pdf

Pie, R. W. (2012). The patient gift conundrum. *Medscape psychiatric and mental health.* Retrieved from http://www.medscape.com/viewarticle/775575

Raskin, N. J., Rogers, C. R., & Witty, M. C. (2014). Client-centered therapy. In D. Wedding & R. J. Corsini (Eds.), *Current psychotherapies* (10th ed., pp. 95–145). Belmont, CA: Brooks/Cole.

Sadock, B. J., Sadock, V. A., & Ruiz, P. (2015). *Synopsis of psychiatry: Behavioral sciences/clinical psychiatry* (11th ed.). Philadelphia, PA: Wolters Kluwer.

Schuster, P. M. (2000). *Communication: The key to the therapeutic relationship.* Philadelphia, PA: F.A. Davis.

Classical References

Coltrane, F., & Pugh, C. (1978). Danger signals in staff/patient relationships. *Journal of Psychiatric Nursing & Mental Health Services, 16*(6), 34–36.

Hall, E. T. (1966). *The hidden dimension.* Garden City, NY: Doubleday.

Hays, J. S., & Larson, K. H. (1963). *Interacting with patients.* New York, NY: Macmillan.

Peplau, H. E. (1952). *Interpersonal relations in nursing.* New York, NY: G.P. Putnam.

Peplau, H. E. (1962). Interpersonal techniques: The crux of psychiatric nursing. *American Journal of Nursing, 62*(6), 50–54.

Peplau, H. (1991). *Interpersonal relations in nursing: A conceptual frame of reference for psychodynamic nursing.* New York, NY: Springer.

Reece, M., & Whitman, R. (1962). Expressive movements, warmth, and verbal reinforcement. *Journal of Abnormal and Social Psychology, 64*(3), 234–236.

Sullivan, H. S. (1953). *The interpersonal theory of psychiatry.* New York, NY: Norton.

Sullivan, H. S. (1954). *The psychiatric interview.* New York, NY: Norton.

Travelbee, J. (1971). *Interpersonal aspects of nursing* (2nd ed.). Philadelphia, PA: F.A. Davis.

The Nursing Process in Psychiatric Mental Health Nursing

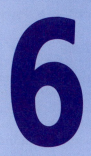

6

CHAPTER OUTLINE

Objectives
Homework Assignment
Introduction
The Nursing Process
Why Nursing Diagnosis?
Nursing Case Management

Applying the Nursing Process in the Psychiatric Setting
Concept Mapping
Documentation of the Nursing Process
Summary and Key Points
Review Questions

CORE CONCEPTS

Assessment
Nursing diagnosis
Outcomes
Planning
Implementation
Evaluation

KEY TERMS

case management
case manager
concept mapping
critical pathways of care (CPCs)
Focus Charting
interdisciplinary

managed care
Nursing Interventions Classification (NIC)
Nursing Outcomes Classification (NOC)
nursing process
PIE charting
problem-oriented recording

OBJECTIVES
After reading this chapter, the student will be able to:

1. Define the nursing process.
2. Identify six steps of the nursing process and describe nursing actions associated with each.
3. Describe the benefits of using nursing diagnosis.
4. Discuss the list of nursing diagnoses approved by NANDA International for clinical use and testing.
5. Define and discuss the use of case management and critical pathways of care in the clinical setting.
6. Apply the six steps of the nursing process in the care of a client in the psychiatric setting.
7. Document client care that validates use of the nursing process.

HOMEWORK ASSIGNMENT
Please read the chapter and answer the following questions:

1. Nursing outcomes (sometimes referred to as *goals*) are derived from the nursing diagnosis. Name two essential aspects of an acceptable outcome or goal.
2. Define *managed care*.
3. The American Nurses Association identifies certain interventions that may

be performed only by psychiatric nurses in advanced practice. What are they?
4. Identify three common elements that form the foundation for each of the documentation methods discussed in the chapter.

Introduction

For many years, the **nursing process** has provided a systematic framework for the delivery of nursing care. It is nursing's means of fulfilling the requirement for a *scientific methodology* in order to be considered a profession.

This chapter examines the steps of the nursing process as they are set forth by the American Nurses Association (ANA) in *Nursing: Scope and Standards of Practice* (ANA, 2015). The landmark Institute of Medicine report (2003) identifies six critical areas of focus (patient-centered care, safety, teamwork and collaboration, evidence-based practice, informatics, and quality improvement) that are needed to shape the future and improve quality of healthcare. The six critical areas are incorporated as an important model for implementing nursing care. These have become known as quality and safety education for nurses (QSEN) competencies (Cronenwett et al., 2007). This chapter explains the implementation of case management and the critical pathways tool used in the delivery of care with this methodology. A description of concept mapping is included, and documentation that validates the use of the nursing process is discussed.

The Nursing Process

Definition

The nursing process consists of six steps (Fig. 6–1) and uses a problem-solving approach that has come

to be accepted as nursing's scientific methodology. It is goal-directed with the objective being delivery of quality client care.

The nursing process is dynamic, not static. It is an ongoing process that continues for as long as the nurse and patient have interactions directed toward change in the patient's physical or behavioral responses. Figure 6–1 presents a schematic of the ongoing nursing process.

Standards of Practice

The ANA, in collaboration with the American Psychiatric Nurses Association (APNA) and the International Society of Psychiatric-Mental Health Nurses (ISPN) (2014), has delineated a set of standards that psychiatric nurses are expected to follow as they provide care for their patients. The ANA (2015) describes a *standard of practice* as an authoritative statement that is defined and promoted by the profession and which provides the foundation for evaluating quality of nursing practice. The nursing process is a critical-thinking model that integrates professional standards of practice to assess, diagnose, identify outcomes, plan, implement, and evaluate nursing care.

Following are the standards of practice for psychiatric mental health nurses as set forth by the ANA, APNA, and ISPN (2014). Three changes in the current standards of practice reflect issues and trends that have evolved more recently.

First, patients are now referred to as *healthcare consumers*. This change reflects the trend toward patient-centered care and conceptualizing that relationship as a collaborative partnership.

The second change is a differentiation of counseling interventions (performed by the psychiatric mental health registered nurse) from psychotherapy (performed by the psychiatric mental health *advanced practice* registered nurse). The third change, in Standard 5G: Therapeutic Relationship and Counseling, adds the phrase "assisting healthcare consumers in their individual recovery journeys." This language supports the recovery model of intervention, which is a current trend toward focusing intervention on a collaborative recovery process rather than on healthcare provider–prescribed treatment alone. (See Chapter 10, The Recovery Model, for more information.)

Standard 1. Assessment

The Psychiatric–Mental Health Registered Nurse collects and synthesizes comprehensive health data that are pertinent to the healthcare consumer's health and/or situation (ANA et al., 2014, p. 44).

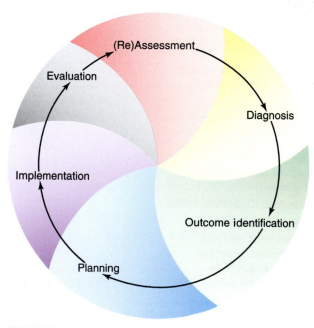

FIGURE 6–1   The ongoing nursing process.

CORE CONCEPT

Assessment

A systematic, dynamic process by which the registered nurse, through interaction with the patient, family, groups, communities, populations, and healthcare providers, collects and analyzes data. Assessment may include the following dimensions: physical, psychological, sociocultural, spiritual, cognitive, functional abilities, developmental, economic, and lifestyle (ANA et al., 2014, p. 87).

In this first step, information is gathered from which to establish a database for determining the best possible care for the patient. Information for this database is gathered from a variety of sources, including interviews with the patient and/or family, observation of the patient and his or her environment, consultation with other health team members, review of the patient's records, and a nursing physical examination. A biopsychosocial assessment tool based on the stress-adaptation framework is included in Box 6–1.

BOX 6–1 Nursing History and Assessment Tool

I. General Information

Patient name: _____   Allergies: _____

Room number: _____   Diet: _____

Doctor: _____   Height/weight: _____

Age: _____   Vital signs: TPR/BP _____

Sex: _____   Name and phone no. of significant other: _____

Race: _____

Dominant language: _____   City of residence: _____

Marital status: _____   Diagnosis (admitting & current): _____

Chief complaint: _____

_____

Conditions of admission:

Date: _____   Time: _____

Accompanied by: _____

Route of admission (wheelchair; ambulatory; cart): _____

Admitted from: _____

II. Predisposing Factors

  A. *Genetic Influences*

    1. Family configuration (use genograms):

      Family of origin: Present family:

      Family dynamics (describe significant relationships between family members): _____

_____

_____

_____

    2. Medical/psychiatric history:

      a. Patient: _____

_____

_____

      b. Family members: _____

_____

_____

    3. Other genetic influences affecting present adaptation. This might include effects specific to gender, race, appearance, such as genetic physical defects, or any other factor related to genetics that is affecting the client's adaptation that has not been mentioned elsewhere in this assessment.

_____

_____

Continued

BOX 6–1 Nursing History and Assessment Tool–cont'd

B. *Past Experiences*
   1. Cultural and social history:
      a. Environmental factors (family living arrangements, type of neighborhood, special working conditions): _____
      _____
      _____
      _____

      b Health beliefs and practices (personal responsibility for health; special self-care practices): _____
      _____
      _____

      c. Religious beliefs and practices: _____
      _____
      _____

      d. Educational background: _____
      _____
      _____

      e. Significant losses/changes (include dates): _____
      _____
      _____

      f. Peer/friendship relationships: _____
      _____
      _____

      g. Occupational history: _____
      _____
      _____

      h. Previous pattern of coping with stress: _____
      _____
      _____

      i. Other lifestyle factors contributing to present adaptation: _____
      _____
      _____

C. *Existing Conditions*
   1. Stage of development (Erikson):
      a. Theoretically: _____
      b. Behaviorally: _____
      c. Rationale: _____
      _____
      _____

   2. Support systems: _____
      _____

   3. Economic security: _____
      _____

   4. Avenues of productivity/contribution:
      a. Current job status: _____
      _____

      b. Role contributions and responsibility for others: _____
      _____

BOX 6–1 Nursing History and Assessment Tool–cont'd

III. Precipitating Event
Describe the situation or events that precipitated this illness/hospitalization: _____
_____
_____

IV. Patient's Perception of the Stressor
Patent's or family member's understanding or description of stressor/illness and expectations of hospitalization:
_____
_____
_____
_____

V. Adaptation Responses
   A. *Psychosocial*
      1. Anxiety level (circle one of the 4 levels and check the behaviors that apply):
         mild moderate severe panic
         calm _____ friendly _____ passive _____ alert _____ perceives environment correctly _____
         cooperative _____ impaired attention _____ "jittery" _____ unable to concentrate _____
         hypervigilant _____ tremors _____ rapid speech _____ withdrawn _____ confused _____
         disoriented _____ fearful _____ hyperventilating _____ misinterpreting the environment
         (hallucinations or delusions) _____ depersonalization _____ obsessions _____ compulsions _____
         somatic complaints _____ excessive hyperactivity _____ other _____
         _____

      2. Mood/affect (circle as many as apply):
         happiness sadness dejection despair elation euphoria suspiciousness apathy (little emotional tone)
         anger/hostility

      3. Ego defense mechanisms (describe how used by patient):
         Projection _____
         Suppression _____
         Undoing _____
         Displacement _____
         Intellectualization _____
         Rationalization _____
         Denial _____
         Repression _____
         Isolation _____
         Regression _____
         Reaction formation _____
         Splitting_____
         Religiosity _____
         Sublimation _____
         Compensation _____

      4. Level of self-esteem (circle one): low moderate high
         Things patient likes about self _____
         _____
         Things patient would like to change about self _____
         _____
         Objective assessment of self-esteem:
         Eye contact _____
         General appearance _____
         _____
         Personal hygiene _____
         Participation in group activities and interactions with others _____
         _____

Continued

BOX 6–1 Nursing History and Assessment Tool—cont'd

5. Stage and manifestations of grief (circle one):
Denial Anger Bargaining Depression Acceptance
Describe the patient's behaviors that are associated with this stage of grieving in response to loss or change.

_____
_____
_____

6. Thought processes (circle as many as apply):
clear logical easy to follow relevant confused blocking delusional rapid flow of thoughts slowness in thought suspicious

Recent memory (circle one):   loss   intact
Remote memory (circle one):   loss   intact
Other: _____
_____

7. Communication patterns (circle as many as apply):
clear coherent slurred speech incoherent
neologisms loose associations flight of ideas aphasic perseveration rumination
tangential speech loquaciousness slow, impoverished speech
speech impediment (describe): _____
Other: _____
_____

8. Interaction patterns (describe patient's pattern of interpersonal interactions with staff and peers on the unit, e.g., manipulative, withdrawn, isolated, verbally or physically hostile, argumentative, passive, assertive, aggressive, passive-aggressive, other): _____
_____
_____
_____

9. Reality orientation (check those that apply):
Oriented to: Time _____ Person _____
Place _____ Situation _____

10. Ideas of destruction to self/others?   Yes   No
If yes, consider plan; available means: _____
_____
_____
_____

B. *Physiological*
1. Psychosomatic manifestations (describe any somatic complaints that may be stress-related):
_____
_____
_____

2. Drug history and assessment:
Use of prescribed drugs:

Name	Dosage	Prescribed for	Results
_____	_____	_____	_____
_____	_____	_____	_____
_____	_____	_____	_____
_____	_____	_____	_____

Use of over-the-counter drugs:

Name	Dosage	Used for	Results
_____	_____	_____	_____
_____	_____	_____	_____
_____	_____	_____	_____

BOX 6–1 **Nursing History and Assessment Tool—cont'd**

Use of street drugs or alcohol:

Name	Amount Used	How Often Used	When Last Used	Effects Produced
_____	_____	_____	____	_____
_____	_____	_____	____	_____
_____	_____	_____	____	_____
_____	_____	_____	____	_____

3. Pertinent physical assessments:
   a. Respirations: normal _____ labored _____
      Rate_____ Rhythm_____
   b. Skin: warm _____ dry _____ moist _____ cool _____ clammy _____ pink _____
      cyanotic _____ poor turgor _____ edematous _____
      Evidence of: rash _____ bruising _____ needle tracks _____ hirsutism _____
      loss of hair _____ other _____
      _____
   c. Musculoskeletal status: weakness _____ tremors _____
      Degree of range of motion (describe limitations) _____
      _____
      Pain (describe) _____
      _____
      Skeletal deformities (describe) _____
      Coordination (describe limitations) _____
   d. Neurological status:
      History of (check all that apply): seizures _____ (describe method of control) _____
      _____
      headaches (describe location and frequency) _____
      fainting spells _____ dizziness _____
      tingling/numbness (describe location) _____
   e. Cardiovascular: B/P _____ Pulse _____
      History of (check all that apply):
      hypertension _____ palpitations _____
      heart murmur _____ chest pain _____
      shortness of breath _____ pain in legs _____
      phlebitis _____ ankle/leg edema _____
      numbness/tingling in extremities _____
      varicose veins _____
   f. Gastrointestinal:
      Usual diet pattern: _____
      Food allergies: _____
      Dentures? Upper _____ Lower _____
      Any problems with chewing or swallowing? _____
      Any recent change in weight? _____
      Any problems with:
      Indigestion/heartburn? _____
        Relieved by _____
        Nausea/vomiting? _____
        Relieved by _____
      History of ulcers? _____
      Usual bowel pattern _____
        Constipation? _____ Diarrhea? _____
        Type of self-care assistance provided for either of the above problems _____
        _____

Continued

BOX 6–1 **Nursing History and Assessment Tool—cont'd**

g. Genitourinary/Reproductive:
Usual voiding pattern _____
Urinary hesitancy? _____ Frequency? _____
Nocturia? _____ Pain/burning? _____
Incontinence? _____
Any genital lesions? _____
   Discharge? _____ Odor? _____
History of sexually transmitted disease? _____
   If yes, please explain: _____
   _____

Any concerns about sexuality/sexual activity? _____
   _____

Method of birth control used _____
Females:
   Date of last menstrual cycle _____
   Length of cycle _____
   Problems associated with menstruation? _____
   _____

Breasts: Pain/tenderness?
   Swelling? _____ Discharge? _____
   Lumps? _____ Dimpling? _____
Practice breast self-examination? _____
   Frequency? _____

Males:
   Penile discharge? _____
   Prostate problems? _____

h. Eyes:

	YES	NO	EXPLAIN
Glasses?	____	____	_____
Contacts?	____	____	_____
Swelling?	____	____	_____
Discharge?	____	____	_____
Itching?	____	____	_____
Blurring?	____	____	_____
Double vision?	____	____	_____

i. Ears

	YES	NO	EXPLAIN
Pain?	____	____	_____
Drainage?	____	____	_____
Difficulty hearing?	____	____	_____
Hearing aid?	____	____	_____
Tinnitus?	____	____	_____

j. Medication side effects:
What symptoms is the patient experiencing that may be attributed to current medication usage?
_____
_____

k. Altered lab values and possible significance: _____
_____
_____

BOX 6–1 Nursing History and Assessment Tool—cont'd

l. Activity/rest patterns:
Exercise (amount, type, frequency): _____

_____

Leisure time activities: _____

_____

Patterns of sleep: Number of hours per night _____
    Use of sleep aids? _____
    Pattern of awakening during the night? _____

    _____
    Feel rested upon awakening? _____
m. Personal hygiene/activities of daily living:
Patterns of self-care: independent _____
Requires assistance with:
    mobility _____
    hygiene _____
    toileting _____
    feeding _____
    dressing _____
    other _____
Statement describing personal hygiene and general appearance: _____

_____

_____

n. Other pertinent physical assessments: _____

_____

_____

VI. Summary of Initial Psychosocial/Physical Assessment:

Knowledge Deficits Identified:

Nursing Diagnoses Indicated:

An example of a simple and quick mental status evaluation is presented in Table 6–1. Sometimes the term *mental status assessment* is used to describe an assessment of strictly the cognitive aspects of functioning. This is the case with tools such as Folstein's Mini-Mental status evaluation (Folstein, Folstein, & McHugh, 1975). Likewise, the tool in Table 6–1 focuses solely on a brief assessment of cognitive aspects of mental functioning. In psychiatry and psychiatric mental health nursing, mental status assessment assumes a much broader definition and includes assessment of mood, affect, behavior, relationships, speech, perceptual disturbances, insight, and judgment in addition to an assessment of cognitive functioning. A comprehensive mental status assessment guide, with explanations and selected sample interview questions, is provided in Appendix A, Mental Status Assessment.

CORE CONCEPT

Nursing diagnosis
Clinical judgments about individual, family, or community experiences and responses to actual or potential health problems and life processes. A nursing diagnosis provides the basis for selection of nursing interventions to achieve outcomes for which the nurse has accountability (NANDA, 2018a).

Standard 2. Diagnosis

The Psychiatric–Mental Health Registered Nurse analyzes the assessment data to determine diagnoses, problems, and areas of focus for care and treatment, including level of risk (ANA et al., 2014, p. 46).

In the second step, data gathered during the assessment are analyzed. Diagnoses and potential

TABLE 6–1 **Brief Mental Status Evaluation**	
AREA OF MENTAL FUNCTION EVALUATED	**EVALUATION ACTIVITY**
Orientation to time	"What year is it? What month is it? What day is it?" (3 points)
Orientation to place	"Where are you now?" (1 point)
Attention and immediate recall	"Repeat these words now: bell, book, and candle." (3 points) "Remember these words, and I will ask you to repeat them in a few minutes."
Abstract thinking	"What does this mean: No use crying over spilled milk." (3 points)
Recent memory	"Say the three words I asked you to remember earlier." (3 points)
Naming objects	Point to eyeglasses and ask, "What is this?" Repeat with one other item (e.g., calendar, watch, pencil). (2 points possible)
Ability to follow simple verbal command	"Tear this piece of paper in half and put it in the trash container." (2 points)
Ability to follow simple written command	Write a command on a piece of paper (e.g., TOUCH YOUR NOSE), give the paper to the patient, and say, "Do what it says on this paper." (1 point for correct action)
Ability to use language correctly	Ask the patient to write a sentence. (3 points if sentence has a subject, a verb, and valid meaning)
Ability to concentrate	"Say the months of the year in reverse, starting with December." (1 point each for correct answers from November through August; 4 points possible)
Understanding spatial relationships	Instruct client to draw a clock; put in all the numbers; and set the hands on 3 o'clock. (clock circle = 1 point; numbers in correct sequence = 1 point; numbers placed on clock correctly =1 point; two hands on the clock =1 point; hands set at correct time =1 point) (5 points possible)

Scoring: 30–21 = normal; 20–11 = mild cognitive impairment; 10–0 = severe cognitive impairment. (Scores are not absolute and must be considered within the comprehensive diagnostic assessment.)
Sources: Folstein, M. F., Folstein, S. E., & McHugh, P. R. (1975). Mini-mental state: A practical method for grading the cognitive state of patients for the clinician. *Journal of Psychiatric Research, 12*(3), 189–198; Kaufman, D. M., & Zun, L. (1995). A quantifiable, brief mental status examination for emergency patients. *Journal of Emergency Medicine, 13*(4), 440–456; Kokman, E., Smith, G. E., Petersen, R. C., Tangalos, E., & Ivnik, R. C. (1991). The short test of mental status: Correlations with standardized psychometric testing. *Archives of Neurology, 48*(7), 725–728; Pfeiffer, E. (1975). A short portable mental status questionnaire for the assessment of organic brain deficit in elderly patients. *Journal of the American Geriatric Society, 23*(10), 433–441.

problem statements are formulated and prioritized. Diagnoses are congruent with available and accepted classification systems (e.g., *NANDA International Nursing Diagnosis Classification* [see Appendix A]).

Standard 3. Outcomes Identification

The Psychiatric–Mental Health Registered Nurse identifies expected outcomes and the healthcare consumer's goals for a plan individualized to the healthcare consumer or to the situation (ANA et al., 2014, p. 48).

CORE CONCEPT

Outcomes

Client behaviors and responses that are collaboratively agreed upon, measurable, desired results of nursing interventions.

Expected outcomes are derived from the diagnosis. They must be measurable and include a time estimate for attainment. They must be realistic for the client's capabilities and are most effective when formulated cooperatively by the interdisciplinary team members, the client, and significant others.

Nursing Outcomes Classification (NOC)

The **Nursing Outcomes Classification (NOC)** is a comprehensive, standardized classification of patient/client outcomes developed to evaluate the effects of nursing interventions (Moorhead et al., 2013). The outcomes have been linked to NANDA International (NANDA-I) diagnoses and to the **Nursing Interventions Classification (NIC).** NANDA-I, NIC, and NOC represent all domains of nursing and can be used together or separately (Moorhead & Dochterman, 2012). Each of the NOC outcomes has

> ## CORE CONCEPT
> **Planning**
> Selection of nursing interventions directed toward helping the patient achieve identified outcomes.

a label name, a definition, a list of indicators to evaluate client status in relation to the outcome, and a five-point Likert scale to measure client status (Moorhead et al., 2013).

Standard 4. Planning

The Psychiatric–Mental Health Registered Nurse develops a plan that prescribes strategies and alternatives to assist the healthcare consumer in attainment of expected outcomes (ANA et al., 2014, p. 50).

The care plan is individualized to the mental health problems, condition, or needs and is developed in collaboration with the patient, significant others, and interdisciplinary team members if possible. For each diagnosis identified, the most appropriate interventions, based on current psychiatric mental health nursing practice, standards, relevant statutes, and research evidence, are selected. Patient education and necessary referrals are included. Thorough and ongoing assessment is an important intervention to ensure that referrals are appropriate and timely. Priorities for delivery of nursing care are determined on the basis of physiological safety needs and risk for harm to self or others. The plan should be prioritized with input from the patient, the family, and others as appropriate (ANA et al., 2014).

Nursing Interventions Classification (NIC)

NIC is a comprehensive, standardized language describing treatments that nurses perform in all settings and in all specialties (Bulechek, Butcher, Dochterman, & Wagner, 2013). NIC includes both physiological and psychosocial interventions as well as interventions for illness treatment, illness prevention, and health promotion. NIC interventions are comprehensive, based on research, and reflect current clinical practice. They were developed inductively on the basis of existing practice.

Each NIC intervention has a definition and a detailed set of activities that describe what a nurse does to implement the intervention. The use of a

> ## CORE CONCEPT
> **Implementation**
> Execution of identified nursing interventions.

standardized language is thought to enhance continuity of care and facilitate communication among nurses and between nurses and other providers.

Standard 5. Implementation

The Psychiatric–Mental Health Registered Nurse implements the identified plan (ANA et al., 2014, p. 52).

Interventions selected during the planning stage are executed, taking into consideration the nurse's level of practice, education, and certification. The care plan serves as a blueprint for delivery of safe, ethical, and appropriate interventions. Documentation of interventions also occurs at this step in the nursing process.

Several specific interventions, described in standards 5A through 5H, are included in the standards of psychiatric mental health clinical nursing practice (ANA et al., 2014).

Standard 5A. Coordination of Care

The Psychiatric–Mental Health Registered Nurse coordinates care delivery (ANA et al., 2014, p. 54).

> One of the QSEN competencies, teamwork and collaboration, is related to this ANA standard of practice. In order for the nurse to coordinate care, it is critical that he or she understands the roles of other healthcare team members and develops strategies for effectively collaborating to meet the client's needs.

Standard 5B. Health Teaching and Health Promotion

The Psychiatric–Mental Health Registered Nurse employs strategies to promote health and a safe environment (ANA et al., 2014, p. 55). For the psychiatric patient, this often includes education about medications and strategies to manage side effects. It may also include teaching and health promotion from a recovery-oriented approach so that the patient has information about various treatment options and available community resources.

Standard 5C. Consultation

The Psychiatric–Mental Health Advanced Practice Registered Nurse provides consultation to influence the identified plan, enhance the abilities of other clinicians to provide services for healthcare consumers, and effect change (ANA et al., 2014, p. 57).

Standard 5D. Prescriptive Authority and Treatment

The Psychiatric–Mental Health Advanced Practice Registered Nurse uses prescriptive authority, procedures, referrals, treatments, and therapies in accordance with state and federal laws and regulations (ANA et al., 2014, p. 58).

Standard 5E. Pharmacological, Biological, and Integrative Therapies

The Psychiatric–Mental Health Registered Nurse incorporates knowledge of pharmacological, biological, and complementary interventions with applied clinical skills to restore the healthcare consumer's health and prevent further disability (ANA et al., 2014, p. 59).

Standard 5F. Milieu Therapy

The Psychiatric–Mental Health Registered Nurse provides, structures, and maintains a safe, therapeutic, recovery-oriented environment in collaboration with healthcare consumers, families, and other healthcare clinicians (ANA et al., 2014, p. 60).

Several models have been developed to identify what constitutes a therapeutic environment, and these are discussed further in Chapter 7, Milieu Therapy—The Therapeutic Community. Incorporation of the healthcare environment and the community of clients, their families, and healthcare providers is a unique aspect of treatment for the client with a psychiatric mental health disorder.

Standard 5G. Therapeutic Relationship and Counseling

The Psychiatric–Mental Health Registered Nurse uses the therapeutic relationship and counseling interventions to assist healthcare consumers in their individual recovery journeys by improving and regaining their previous coping abilities, fostering mental health and preventing mental disorder and disability (ANA et al., 2014, p. 62).

As mentioned previously, therapeutic relationship and counseling interventions are part of the role of registered nurses practicing in psychiatric mental health settings. These are basic psychoeducational and problem discussion interventions and are differentiated from psychotherapy that requires advanced practice education and competency.

Standard 5H. Psychotherapy

The Psychiatric–Mental Health Advanced Practice Registered Nurse conducts individual, couples, group, and family psychotherapy using evidence-based psychotherapeutic frameworks and the nurse-client therapeutic relationship (ANA et al., 2014, p. 63).

CORE CONCEPT
Evaluation
The process of determining the healthcare consumer's progress toward attainment of expected outcomes and the effectiveness of the registered nurse's care and interventions (ANA et al., 2014, p. 88).

Standard 6. Evaluation

The Psychiatric–Mental Health Registered Nurse evaluates progress toward attainment of expected outcomes (ANA et al., 2014, p. 65).

During the evaluation step, the nurse measures the success of the interventions in meeting the outcome criteria. The client's response to treatment is documented, validating use of the nursing process in the delivery of care. The diagnoses, outcomes, and plan of care are reviewed and revised as need is determined by the evaluation.

Why Nursing Diagnosis?

The concept of nursing diagnosis is not new. For centuries, nurses have identified specific unhealthy responses to healthcare problems for which nursing interventions were used in an effort to improve the patient's quality of life. Historically, however, the autonomy of practice to which nurses were entitled by virtue of their licensure was lacking in the provision of nursing care. Nurses assisted physicians as required and performed a group of specific tasks that were considered within their scope of responsibility.

The term *diagnosis* in relation to nursing first began to appear in the literature in the early 1950s. The formalized organization of the concept, however, was initiated only in 1973 with the convening of the First Task Force to Name and Classify Nursing Diagnoses. The Task Force of the National Conference Group on the Classification of Nursing Diagnoses was developed during this conference. These individuals were charged with the task of identifying and classifying nursing diagnoses.

Also in the 1970s, the ANA began to write standards of practice around the steps of the nursing process, of which nursing diagnosis is an inherent part. This format encompassed both the general and specialty standards outlined by the ANA.

From this progression a statement of policy was published in 1980 and included a definition of nursing. The ANA defined *nursing* as "the diagnosis and treatment of human responses to actual or potential health problems" (ANA, 2010). This definition has been expanded to describe more appropriately nursing's commitment to society and to the profession itself. The ANA (2018) defines *nursing* as follows:

> Nursing is the protection, promotion, and optimization of health and abilities, prevention of illness and injury, alleviation of suffering through the diagnosis and treatment of human response, and advocacy in the care of individuals, families, communities, and populations.

Nursing diagnosis is an inherent component of both the original and expanded definitions.

Decisions regarding professional negligence are made on the basis of standards of practice defined by the ANA and the individual state nursing practice acts. A number of states have incorporated the steps of the nursing process, including nursing diagnosis, into the scope of nursing practice described in their nursing practice acts. When this is the case, it is the legal duty of the nurse to show that nursing process and nursing diagnosis were accurately implemented in the delivery of nursing care.

NANDA-I evolved from the original task force that was convened in 1973 to name and classify nursing diagnoses. The major purpose of NANDA-I is "to develop, refine and promote terminology that accurately reflects nurses' clinical judgments. NANDA-I will be a global force for the development and use of nursing's standardized terminology to ensure patient safety through evidence-based care, thereby improving the health care of all people" (NANDA-I, 2018b). A list of nursing diagnoses approved by NANDA-I for use and testing is presented in Appendix A. This list is by no means exhaustive or all-inclusive. In an effort to maintain a common language within nursing and to encourage clinical testing of what is available, most of the nursing diagnoses used in this text come from the 2018–2020 list approved by NANDA-I (NANDA-I, 2018a). However, in a few instances, nursing diagnoses that have been retired by NANDA-I for various reasons will continue to be used because of their appropriateness and suitability in describing specific behaviors.

The use of nursing diagnosis affords a degree of autonomy that historically has been lacking in the practice of nursing. Nursing diagnosis describes the patient's condition, facilitating the prescription of interventions and establishment of parameters for outcome criteria based on what is uniquely nursing. The ultimate benefit is to the client, who receives effective and consistent nursing care based on knowledge of the problems that he or she is experiencing and of the most beneficial nursing interventions to resolve them.

Nursing Case Management

The concept of **case management** evolved with the advent of diagnosis-related groups (DRGs) and shorter hospital stays. Case management is a model of care delivery that can result in improved patient care. In this model, clients are assigned a manager who negotiates with multiple providers to obtain diverse services. This type of healthcare delivery process serves to decrease fragmentation of care while striving to contain cost of services.

Case management in the acute care setting strives to organize client care through an episode of illness so that specific clinical and financial outcomes are achieved within an allotted time frame. Commonly, the allotted time frame is determined by the established protocols for length of stay as defined by the DRGs.

Case management has been shown to be an effective method of treatment for individuals with a severe and persistent mental illness. This type of care strives to improve functioning by assisting the individual to solve problems, improve work and socialization skills, promote leisure-time activities, and enhance overall independence.

Ideally, case management incorporates concepts of care at the primary, secondary, and tertiary levels of prevention. Various definitions have emerged and should be clarified, as follows.

Managed care refers to a strategy employed by purchasers of health services who make determinations about various types of services in order to maintain quality and control costs. In a managed care program, individuals receive healthcare based on need, as assessed by coordinators of the providership. Managed care exists in many settings, including (but not limited to) the following:

- Insurance-based programs
- Employer-based medical providerships
- Social service programs
- The public health sector

Managed care may exist in virtually any setting in which medical providership is a part of the service; that is, in any setting in which an organization (whether private or government based) is responsible for payment of healthcare services for a group of people. Examples of managed care are health maintenance organizations (HMOs) and preferred provider organizations (PPOs).

Case management is the method used to achieve managed care. It is the actual coordination of services required to meet the needs of a client within the fragmented healthcare system. Case management strives to help at-risk clients prevent avoidable episodes of illness. Its goal is to provide these services while attempting to control healthcare costs to the consumer and third-party payers.

Types of clients who benefit from case management include (but are not limited to) the following:

- The frail elderly
- Individuals with developmental disabilities
- Individuals with physical disabilities

- Individuals with severe mental disabilities
- Individuals with long-term medically complex problems that require multifaceted, costly care (e.g., high-risk infants, those with human immunodeficiency virus [HIV] or acquired immunodeficiency syndrome [AIDS], and transplant clients)
- Individuals who are severely compromised by an acute episode of illness or an acute exacerbation of a severe and persistent illness (e.g., schizophrenia)

The **case manager** is responsible for negotiating with multiple healthcare providers to obtain a variety of services for the client. Nurses are exceptionally qualified to serve as case managers. The very nature of nursing, which incorporates knowledge about the biological, psychological, and sociocultural aspects related to human functioning, makes nurses highly appropriate as case managers. Several years of experience as a registered nurse are usually required for employment as a case manager. Some case management programs prefer advanced practice registered nurses who have experience working with the specific populations for whom the case management service will be rendered.

Critical Pathways of Care

Critical pathways of care (CPCs) may be used as the tools for provision of care in a case management system. A critical pathway is a type of abbreviated plan of care that provides outcome-based guidelines for goal achievement within a designated length of stay. A sample CPC is presented in Table 6–2. Only one nursing diagnosis is used in this sample. A CPC may have nursing diagnoses for several individual problems.

CPCs are intended to be used by the entire interdisciplinary team, which may include a nurse, case manager, clinical nurse specialist, social worker, psychiatrist, psychologist, dietitian, occupational therapist, recreational therapist, chaplain, and others. The team decides what categories of care are to be performed, by what date, and by whom. Each member of the team is then expected to carry out his or her functions according to the timeline designated on the CPC.

Unlike a nursing care plan, CPCs have the benefit of describing what an episode of care will look like when implemented by team members in collaboration with one another. Clarity about how team members collaborate is important not only for providing efficient patient care but also for improving quality and maintaining safety.

As a case manager, the nurse is ultimately responsible for ensuring that each of the assignments is carried out. If variations occur at any time in any of the categories of care, rationale must be documented in the progress notes. For example, with the sample CPC presented, the nurse case manager may admit the client into the detoxification center. The nurse contacts the psychiatrist to inform him or her of the admission. The psychiatrist performs additional assessments to determine if other consultations are required. The psychiatrist also writes the orders for the initial diagnostic work-up and medication regimen. Within 24 hours, the interdisciplinary team meets to decide on other categories of care, to complete the CPC, and to make individual care assignments from the CPC. The sample CPC in Table 6–2 relies heavily on nursing care of the client through the critical withdrawal period. However, other problems for the same client, such as imbalanced nutrition, impaired physical mobility, or spiritual distress, may involve other members of the team to a greater degree. Each member of the team stays in contact with the case manager regarding individual assignments. Ideally, team meetings are held daily or every other day to review progress and modify the plan as required.

CPCs can be standardized, as they are intended to be used with uncomplicated cases. A CPC can be viewed as protocol for clients who have specific problems for which a designated outcome can be predicted.

Applying the Nursing Process in the Psychiatric Setting

Based on the definition of *mental health* set forth in Chapter 1, Mental Health and Mental Illness the role of the nurse in psychiatry focuses on helping the patient successfully adapt to stressors in the environment. Goals are directed toward changes in thoughts, feelings, and behaviors that are age appropriate and congruent with local and cultural norms.

Therapy within the psychiatric setting is very often team oriented, or **interdisciplinary.** Therefore, it is important to delineate nursing's involvement in the treatment regimen. Nurses are valuable members of the team, providing services that are defined within the scope of nursing practice. Nursing diagnosis helps to define these nursing boundaries and provides a degree of autonomy and professionalism.

TABLE 6–2 Sample Critical Pathway of Care for Patient in Alcohol Withdrawal

Estimated Length of Stay: 7 days—variations from designated pathway should be documented in progress notes.

NURSING DIAGNOSES AND CATEGORIES OF CARE	TIME DIMENSION	GOALS AND/OR ACTIONS	TIME DIMENSION	GOALS AND/OR ACTIONS	TIME DIMENSION	DISCHARGE OUTCOME
Risk for injury related to CNS agitation					Day 7	Patient shows no evidence of injury sustained during ETOH withdrawal
Referrals	Day 1	Psychiatrist Assess need for neurologist, cardiologist, internist			Day 7	Discharge with follow-up appointments as required
Diagnostic studies	Day 1	Blood alcohol level Drug screen (urine and blood) Complete blood count with MCV Clotting screen Liver function test (with albumin and GGT) Urea/electrolytes Blood glucose Folate/B_{12}, magnesium, and phosphate levels	Day 4	Repeat of selected diagnostic studies as necessary		
Additional assessments	Day 1 Day 1–5 Ongoing	VS q4h I&O Assess withdrawal symptoms: tremors, nausea/vomiting, tachycardia, sweating, high blood pressure, seizures, insomnia, hallucinations	Day 2–3 Day 6 Day 4	VS q8h if stable DC I&O Marked decrease in objective withdrawal symptoms	Day 4–7 Day 7	VS bid; remain stable Discharge; absence of objective withdrawal symptoms
Medications	Day 1 Day 2 Day 1–6 Day 1–7	Chlordiazepoxide* 200 mg in divided doses Chlordiazepoxide 160 mg in divided doses Chlordiazepoxide prn (maximum of 250 mg total daily dose including regular and prn doses) Maalox pc & hs	Day 3 Day 4	Chlordiazepoxide 120 mg in divided doses Chlordiazepoxide 80 mg in divided doses	Day 5 Day 6 Day 7	Chlordiazepoxide 40 mg DC chlordiazepoxide Discharge; no withdrawal symptoms
Client education			Day 5	Discuss goals of AA and need for outpatient therapy	Day 7	Discharge with information regarding AA attendance or outpatient treatment

*Some physicians may elect to use Serax or Tegretol in the detoxification process.

AA, Alcoholics Anonymous; bid, twice a day; DC, discontinue; ECT, electrocardiogram; ETOH, alcohol; hs, bedtime; GGT, gamma-glutamyl transferase; I&O, intake and output; MCV, mean corpuscular volume; pc, after meals; prn, as needed; q4h, every 4 hours; q8h, every 8 hours; VS, vital signs.

For example, a newly admitted patient with the medical diagnosis of schizophrenia may be demonstrating the following behaviors:

- Inability to trust others
- Verbalizing hearing voices
- Refusing to interact with staff and peers
- Expressing a fear of failure
- Poor personal hygiene

From these assessments, the treatment team may determine that the patient has the following problems:

- Paranoid delusions
- Auditory hallucinations
- Social withdrawal
- Developmental regression

Team goals would be directed toward the following:

- Reducing suspiciousness
- Minimizing or eliminating auditory hallucinations
- Increasing feelings of self-worth

From this team treatment plan, nursing may identify the following nursing diagnoses:

- Disturbed sensory perception, auditory (evidenced by hearing voices)[1]
- Disturbed thought processes (evidenced by delusions)
- Low self-esteem (evidenced by fear of failure and social withdrawal)
- Self-care deficit (evidenced by poor personal hygiene)
- Social isolation (evidenced by suspiciousness and social withdrawal)

Nursing diagnoses are prioritized according to life-threatening potential. Maslow's hierarchy of needs is a good model to follow in prioritizing nursing diagnoses. In this instance, disturbed sensory perception (auditory) is identified as the priority nursing diagnosis because the client may be hearing voices that command him or her to harm self or others. Psychiatric nursing, regardless of the setting—hospital (inpatient or outpatient), office, home, community—is goal-directed care. The goals (or expected outcomes) are patient-oriented, measurable, and focus on resolution of the problem (if resolution is realistic) or on a more short-term outcome (if resolution is unrealistic). For example, in the previous situation, expected outcomes for the identified nursing diagnoses might be as follows:

The Patient

1. Demonstrates trust in one staff member within 3 days.
2. Verbalizes understanding that the voices are not real (not heard by others) within 5 days.
3. Completes one simple craft project within 5 days.
4. Takes responsibility for own self-care and performs activities of daily living independently by time of discharge.

Nursing's contribution to the interdisciplinary treatment regimen will focus on establishing trust on a one-to-one basis (thus reducing the level of anxiety that may be promoting hallucinations), giving positive feedback for small day-to-day accomplishments in an effort to build self-esteem, and assisting with and encouraging independent self-care. These interventions describe *independent nursing* actions and goals that are evaluated apart from, while also being directed toward achievement of, the *team's* treatment goals.

In this manner of collaboration with other team members, nursing provides a unique service based on sound knowledge of psychopathology, scope of practice, and legal implications of the role. Although there is no dispute that "following doctor's orders" continues to be accepted as a priority of care, nursing interventions that enhance achievement of the overall goals of treatment are important as well. The nurse who administers a medication prescribed by the physician to decrease anxiety may also choose to stay with the anxious client and offer reassurance of safety and security, thereby providing an independent nursing action that is distinct from, yet complementary to, the medical treatment.

Concept Mapping[2]

Concept mapping is a diagrammatic teaching and learning strategy that allows students and faculty to visualize interrelationships between medical diagnoses, nursing diagnoses, assessment data, and treatments. In general, it is a diagram of client problems and interventions. Compared with the commonly used column format care plans, concept map care plans are more succinct. They are practical, realistic, and time saving, and they serve to enhance critical-thinking skills and clinical reasoning ability by

---

[1] Disturbed sensory perception and Disturbed thought processes (see next list item) were removed from the NANDA-I list of approved nursing diagnoses in 2012. However, they will continue to be used in this textbook because of their appropriateness to certain behaviors.

[2] Content in this section is adapted from Doenges, Moorhouse, and Murr (2016) and Schuster (2015).

creating a holistic picture of various problems and their interconnectedness to one another.

The nursing process is foundational to developing and using the concept map care plan, just as it is with all types of nursing care plans. Client data are collected and analyzed, nursing diagnoses are formulated, outcome criteria are identified, nursing actions are planned and implemented, and the success of the interventions in meeting the outcome criteria is evaluated.

The concept map care plan may be presented in its entirety on one page, or the assessment data and nursing diagnoses may appear in diagram format on one page, with outcomes, interventions, and evaluation written on a second page. Alternatively, the diagram may appear in circular format, with nursing diagnoses and interventions branching off the "client" in the center of the diagram. Or, it may begin with the "client" at the top of the diagram, with branches emanating in a linear fashion downward. Whichever format is chosen to visualize the concept map, the diagram should reflect the nursing process in a stepwise fashion, beginning with the client and his or her reason for needing care, nursing diagnoses with subjective and objective clinical evidence for each, nursing interventions, and outcome criteria for evaluation.

Figure 6–2 presents one example of a concept map care plan. It is assembled for the hypothetical client with schizophrenia discussed in the previous section, "Applying the Nursing Process in the Psychiatric Setting." Different colors may be used in the diagram to designate various components of the care plan. Connecting lines are drawn between components to indicate any relationships that exist. For example, there may be a relationship between two nursing diagnoses (e.g., between the nursing diagnoses of pain or anxiety and disturbed sleep pattern). A line between these nursing diagnoses should be drawn to show the relationship.

Concept map care plans allow for a great deal of creativity on the part of the user and permit viewing the "whole picture" without generating a great deal of paperwork. Because they reflect the steps of the nursing process, concept map care plans also are valuable guides for documentation of client care. Doenges, Moorhouse, and Murr (2016) describe how the shortcoming of traditional care plans is that they fail to clarify how all of the client's identified needs are related to each other, and consequently the user may not develop a holistic view. The concept map clarifies those linkages. Whether these care-planning strategies are used for learning or in actual practice, both the concept map and traditional care plan are useful tools for developing and visualizing the critical-thinking process that goes into planning patient care.

> 🔷 The concept map can be expanded to visualize an episode of care that not only includes various client needs and associated nursing care but also visualizes how other disciplines within the treatment team are collaborating to address those needs. In this presentation the concept map informs about teamwork and collaboration, one of the six QSEN competencies.

Documentation of the Nursing Process

Equally important as using the nursing process in the delivery of care is the written documentation that it has been used. Some contemporary nursing leaders are advocating that with solid standards of practice and procedures in place within the institution, nurses need only chart when there has been a deviation in the care as outlined by that standard. This method of documentation, known as *charting by exception*, is not widely accepted because many legal decisions are still based on the precept that "if it was not charted, it was not done." While carefully designed flow sheets are part of "a good charting by exception system . . . this form of documentation should also call for notes concerning any significant indicator of the patient's condition or change in status, any subsequent interventions and the patient's response" (Nurses Service Organization [NSO], 2018).

Because nursing process and nursing diagnosis are mandated by nursing practice acts in some states, documentation of their use is being considered in those states as evidence in determining certain cases of negligence by nurses. Some healthcare organization accrediting agencies also require that nursing process be reflected in the delivery of care. Therefore, documentation must bear written testament to the use of the nursing process.

Types of Documentation Methods

A variety of documentation methods can be used to reflect use of the nursing process in the delivery of nursing care. Three examples are presented here: problem-oriented recording (POR); Focus Charting; and the problem, intervention, evaluation (PIE) system of documentation.

Problem-Oriented Recording

Problem-oriented recording follows the subjective, objective, assessment, plan, implementation, and evaluation (SOAPIE) format. It has as its basis a list of problems. When it is used in nursing, the problems (nursing diagnoses) are identified on a written

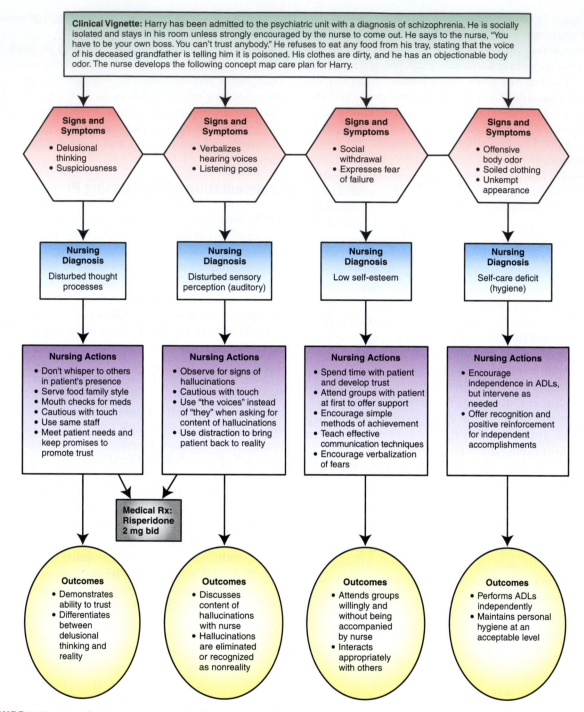

Clinical Vignette: Harry has been admitted to the psychiatric unit with a diagnosis of schizophrenia. He is socially isolated and stays in his room unless strongly encouraged by the nurse to come out. He says to the nurse, "You have to be your own boss. You can't trust anybody." He refuses to eat any food from his tray, stating that the voice of his deceased grandfather is telling him it is poisoned. His clothes are dirty, and he has an objectionable body odor. The nurse develops the following concept map care plan for Harry.

Signs and Symptoms
- Delusional thinking
- Suspiciousness

Signs and Symptoms
- Verbalizes hearing voices
- Listening pose

Signs and Symptoms
- Social withdrawal
- Expresses fear of failure

Signs and Symptoms
- Offensive body odor
- Soiled clothing
- Unkempt appearance

Nursing Diagnosis
Disturbed thought processes

Nursing Diagnosis
Disturbed sensory perception (auditory)

Nursing Diagnosis
Low self-esteem

Nursing Diagnosis
Self-care deficit (hygiene)

Nursing Actions
- Don't whisper to others in patient's presence
- Serve food family style
- Mouth checks for meds
- Cautious with touch
- Use same staff
- Meet patient needs and keep promises to promote trust

Nursing Actions
- Observe for signs of hallucinations
- Cautious with touch
- Use "the voices" instead of "they" when asking for content of hallucinations
- Use distraction to bring patient back to reality

Nursing Actions
- Spend time with patient and develop trust
- Attend groups with patient at first to offer support
- Encourage simple methods of achievement
- Teach effective communication techniques
- Encourage verbalization of fears

Nursing Actions
- Encourage independence in ADLs, but intervene as needed
- Offer recognition and positive reinforcement for independent accomplishments

Medical Rx: Risperidone 2 mg bid

Outcomes
- Demonstrates ability to trust
- Differentiates between delusional thinking and reality

Outcomes
- Discusses content of hallucinations with nurse
- Hallucinations are eliminated or recognized as nonreality

Outcomes
- Attends groups willingly and without being accompanied by nurse
- Interacts appropriately with others

Outcomes
- Performs ADLs independently
- Maintains personal hygiene at an acceptable level

FIGURE 6–2 Example: Concept map care plan for a patient with schizophrenia.

plan of care, with appropriate nursing interventions described for each. Documentation written in the SOAPIE format includes the following:

S = Subjective data: Information gathered from what the client, family, or other source has said or reported.

O = Objective data: Information gathered through direct observation by the person performing the assessment; may include a physiological measurement such as blood pressure or a behavioral response such as affect.

A = Assessment: The nurse's interpretation of the subjective and objective data.

P = Plan: The actions or treatments to be carried out (may be omitted in daily charting if the plan is clearly explained in the written nursing care plan and no changes are expected).

I = Intervention: Those nursing actions that were actually carried out.

E = Evaluation: An appraisal of the problem following nursing intervention (some nursing interventions cannot be evaluated immediately, so this section may be optional).

Table 6–3 shows how POR corresponds to the steps of the nursing process.

The following is an example of a three-column documentation in the POR format.

EXAMPLE

Date/Time	Problem	Progress Notes
9-12-19 1000	Social isolation	**S:** States he does not want to sit with or talk to others; "They frighten me." **O:** Stays in room alone unless strongly encouraged to come out; no group involvement; at times listens to group conversations from a distance but does not interact; some hypervigilance and scanning noted. **A:** Inability to trust; panic level of anxiety; delusional thinking. **I:** Initiated trusting relationship by spending time alone with patient; discussed his feelings regarding interactions with others; accompanied patient to group activities; provided positive feedback for voluntarily participating in assertiveness training.

Focus Charting

Another type of documentation that reflects use of the nursing process is **Focus Charting.** Focus Charting differs from POR in that the main perspective is "focus" instead of "problem," and a data, action, and response (DAR) format replaces SOAPIE.

Lampe (1985) suggested that a focus for documentation can be any of the following:

- Nursing diagnosis
- Current client concern or behavior
- Significant change in the client's status or behavior
- Significant event in the client's therapy

The focus cannot be a medical diagnosis. The documentation is organized in the format of DAR. These categories are defined as follows:

D = Data: Information that supports the stated focus or describes pertinent observations about the client

A = Action: Immediate or future nursing actions that address the focus and evaluation of the present care plan along with any changes required

R = Response: Description of the client's responses to any part of the medical or nursing care

Table 6–4 shows how Focus Charting corresponds to the steps of the nursing process.

The following is an example of a three-column documentation in the DAR format.

EXAMPLE

Date/Time	Focus	Progress Notes
9-12-19 1000	Social isolation related to mistrust, panic anxiety, delusions	**D:** States he does not want to sit with or talk to others; they "frighten" him; stays in room alone unless strongly encouraged to come out; no group involvement; at times listens to group conversations from a distance but does not interact; some hypervigilance and scanning noted. **A:** Initiated trusting relationship by spending time alone with patient; discussed his feelings regarding interactions with others; accompanied patient to group activities; provided positive feedback for voluntarily participating in assertiveness training. **R:** Cooperative with therapy; still acts uncomfortable in the presence of a group of people; accepted positive feedback from nurse.

TABLE 6–3 Validation of the Nursing Process With Problem-Oriented Recording

PROBLEM-ORIENTED RECORDING	WHAT IS RECORDED	NURSING PROCESS
S and O (Subjective and Objective data)	Verbal reports to, and direct observation and examination by, the nurse	Assessment
A (Assessment)	Nurse's interpretation of S and O	Diagnosis and outcome identification
P (Plan) (Omitted in charting if written plan describes care to be given)	Description of appropriate nursing actions to resolve the identified problem	Planning
I (Intervention)	Description of nursing actions actually carried out	Implementation
E (Evaluation)	A reassessment of the situation to determine results of nursing actions implemented	Evaluation

TABLE 6–4 Validation of the Nursing Process With Focus Charting

FOCUS CHARTING	WHAT IS RECORDED	NURSING PROCESS
D (Data)	Information that supports the stated focus or describes pertinent observations about patient	Assessment
Focus	A nursing diagnosis; current patient concern or behavior; significant change in patient status; significant event in patient's therapy (*Note:* If outcome appears on written care plan, it need not be repeated in daily documentation unless a change occurs.)	Diagnosis and outcome identification
A (Action)	Immediate or future nursing actions that address the focus; appraisal of the care plan along with any changes required	Plan and implementation
R (Response)	Description of patient responses to any part of the medical or nursing care	Evaluation

The PIE Method

The PIE method, sometimes referred to as "APIE" (assessment, problem, intervention, evaluation), is a systematic approach to documenting the nursing process and nursing diagnosis. A problem-oriented system, **PIE charting** uses accompanying flow sheets that are individualized by each institution. Criteria for documentation are organized in the following manner:

A = Assessment: A complete patient assessment is conducted at the beginning of each shift. Results are documented under this section in the progress notes. Some institutions elect instead to use a daily patient assessment sheet designed to address specific assessment needs within particular units. Explanation of any deviation from the norm is included in the progress notes.

P = Problem: A problem list, or list of nursing diagnoses, is an important part of the APIE method of charting. The name or number of the problem being addressed is documented in this section.

I = Intervention: Nursing actions are performed, directed at resolution of the problem.

E = Evaluation: Outcomes of the implemented interventions are documented, including an evaluation of patient responses to determine the effectiveness of nursing interventions and the presence or absence of progress toward resolution of a problem.

Table 6–5 shows how APIE charting corresponds to the steps of the nursing process.

The following is an example of a three-column documentation in the APIE format.

EXAMPLE

Date/Time	Focus	Progress Notes
9-12-19 1000	Social isolation	**A:** States he does not want to sit with or talk to others; they "frighten" him; stays in room alone unless strongly encouraged to come out; no group involvement; at times listens to group conversations from a distance but does not interact; some hypervigilance and scanning noted. **P:** Social isolation related to inability to trust, panic level of anxiety, and delusional thinking. **I:** Initiated trusting relationship by spending time alone with client; discussed his feelings regarding interactions with others; accompanied client to group activities; provided positive feedback for voluntarily participating in assertiveness training. **E:** Cooperative with therapy; still uncomfortable in the presence of a group of people; accepted positive feedback from nurse.

TABLE 6–5 Validation of the Nursing Process With APIE Method

APIE CHARTING	WHAT IS RECORDED	NURSING PROCESS
A (Assessment)	Subjective and objective data about the patient that are gathered at the beginning of each shift	Assessment
P (Problem)	Name (or number) of nursing diagnosis being addressed from written problem list and identified outcome for that problem (*Note:* If outcome appears on written care plan, it need not be repeated in daily documentation unless a change occurs.)	Diagnosis and outcome identification
I (Intervention)	Nursing actions performed, directed at problem resolution	Plan and implementation
E (Evaluation)	Appraisal of patient responses to determine effectiveness of nursing interventions	Evaluation

All three of the documentation methods discussed share in common a clear identification of important patient care problems, what the nurse did in response to those problems, and how the patient responded to those interventions. It is the nursing process that forms the foundation for critical thinking regardless of the method used to document patient care.

Electronic Documentation

Most healthcare facilities have implemented—or are in the process of implementing—some type of electronic health records (EHRs) or electronic documentation system. Federal regulations and programs promoted EHR system adoption by offering financial incentives to providers who installed or upgraded EHR systems and demonstrated meaningful use of EHRs by 2014; as of 2015, progressive reductions in reimbursement were initiated for healthcare providers who are not demonstrating meaningful use of EHRs.

The rationale for this move is that EHRs have been shown to improve both the quality of client care and the efficiency of the healthcare system (U.S. Government Accountability Office, 2010). In 2003, the U.S. Department of Health and Human Services commissioned the Institute of Medicine (IOM) to study the capabilities of EHR systems. The IOM identified a set of eight core functions that EHR systems should perform in the delivery of safer, higher quality, and more efficient healthcare (Institute of Medicine, 2003):

■ **Health information and data:** EHRs provide more rapid access to important patient information (e.g., allergies, laboratory test results, a medication list, demographic information, and clinical narratives) thereby improving care providers' ability to make sound clinical decisions in a timely manner.

■ **Results management:** Computerized results of all types (e.g., laboratory test results, radiology procedure result reports) can be accessed more easily by the provider at the time and place they are needed.

- **Order entry/order management:** Computer-based order entries improve workflow processes by eliminating lost orders and ambiguities caused by illegible handwriting, generating related orders automatically, monitoring for duplicate orders, and improving the speed with which orders are executed.
- **Decision support:** Computerized decision support systems enhance clinical performance for many aspects of healthcare. Using reminders and prompts, improvement in regular screenings and other preventive practices can be accomplished. Other aspects of healthcare support include identifying possible drug interactions and facilitating diagnosis and treatment.
- **Electronic communication and connectivity:** Improved communication among care associates, such as medicine, nursing, laboratory, pharmacy, and radiology, can enhance client safety and quality of care. Efficient communication among

providers improves continuity of care, allows for more timely interventions, and reduces the risk of adverse events.

- **Patient support:** Computer-based interactive client education, self-testing, and self-monitoring have been shown to improve control of chronic illnesses.
- **Administrative processes:** Electronic scheduling systems (e.g., for hospital admissions and outpatient procedures) increase the efficiency of healthcare organizations and provide more timely service to patients.
- **Reporting and population health management:** Healthcare organizations are required to report healthcare data to government and private sectors for patient safety and public health. Uniform electronic data standards facilitate this process at the provider level, reduce the associated costs, and increase the speed and accuracy of the data reported.

Table 6–6 lists some of the advantages and disadvantages of paper records and EHRs.

TABLE 6–6 **Advantages and Disadvantages of Paper Records and Electronic Health Records (EHRs)**	
PAPER*	**EHR**
■ Advantages	■ Advantages
■ People know how to use it.	■ Can be accessed by multiple providers from remote sites.
■ It is fast for current practice.	■ Facilitates communication between disciplines.
■ It is portable.	■ Provides reminders about completing information.
■ It is nonbreakable.	■ Provides warnings about incompatibilities of medications or variances from normal standards.
■ It accepts multiple data types, such as graphs, photographs, drawings, and text.	■ Reduces redundancy of information.
■ Legal issues and costs are understood.	■ Requires less storage space and more difficult to lose.
■ Disadvantages	■ Easier to research for audits, quality assurance, and epidemiological surveillance.
■ It can be lost.	■ Provides immediate retrieval of information (e.g., test results).
■ It is often illegible and incomplete.	■ Provides links to multiple databases of healthcare knowledge, thus providing diagnostic support.
■ It has no remote access.	■ Decreases charting time.
■ It can be accessed by only one person at a time.	■ Reduces errors due to illegible handwriting.
■ It is often disorganized.	■ Facilitates billing and claims procedures.
■ Information is duplicated.	■ Disadvantages
■ It is hard to store.	■ Expense to implement the system.
■ It is difficult to research, and continuous quality improvement is laborious.	■ Substantial learning curve involved for new users; training and retraining required.
■ Same client has separate records at each facility (physician's office, hospital, home care).	■ Stringent requirements to maintain security and confidentiality.
■ Records are shared only through hard copy.	■ Technical difficulties are possible.
	■ Involves legal and ethical issues regarding privacy and access to client information.
	■ Requires consistent use of standardized terminology to support information sharing across wide networks.

*From Young, K. M. (2015). Nursing informatics. In J. T. Catalano (Ed.), *Nursing now! Today's issues, tomorrow's trends* (7th ed.). Philadelphia, PA: F.A. Davis. With permission.

Summary and Key Points

- The nursing process provides a methodology by which nurses may deliver care using a systematic, scientific approach.
- The focus of nursing process is goal directed and based on a decision-making or problem-solving model consisting of six steps: assessment, diagnosis, outcome identification, planning, implementation, and evaluation.
- Assessment is a systematic, dynamic process by which the nurse, through interaction with the patient, significant others, and healthcare providers, collects and analyzes data about the patient.
- Nursing diagnoses are clinical judgments about individual, family, or community responses to actual or potential health problems and life processes.
- Outcomes are measurable, expected, patient-focused goals that translate into observable behaviors.
- Evaluation is the process of determining both the patient's progress toward the attainment of expected outcomes and the effectiveness of nursing care.
- The psychiatric nurse uses the nursing process to assist patients to adapt successfully to stressors within the environment.
- The nurse serves as a valuable member of the interdisciplinary treatment team, working both independently and cooperatively with other team members.
- Case management is a model of care delivery that serves to provide quality client care while controlling healthcare costs. Critical pathways of care (CPCs) serve as the tools for provision of care in a case management system.
- Nurses may serve as case managers, who are responsible for negotiating with multiple healthcare providers to obtain a variety of services for the client.
- Concept mapping is a diagrammatic teaching and learning strategy that allows students and faculty to visualize interrelationships among medical diagnoses, nursing diagnoses, assessment data, and treatments. It can be expanded to include a visual picture of how other disciplines are collaborating with nursing to meet specific patient needs. Nurses must document that the nursing process has been used in the delivery of care. Three methods of documentation that reflect use of the nursing process include POR, Focus Charting, and the PIE method.
- Many healthcare facilities have implemented the use of EHRs, or electronic documentation systems. EHRs have been shown to improve both the quality of client care and the efficiency of the healthcare system.

Review Questions
Self-Examination/Learning Exercise

Select the answer that is most appropriate for each of the following questions:

1. The nurse is using nursing process to care for a patient who is suicidal. Which of the following nursing actions is a part of the assessment step of the nursing process?
   a. Identifies the nursing diagnosis: Risk for suicide
   b. Notes that patient's family reports recent suicide attempt
   c. Prioritizes the necessity for maintaining a safe environment for the patient
   d. Obtains a commitment from the patient to work collaboratively to identify adaptive coping

2. The nurse is using nursing process to care for a patient who is suicidal. Which of the following nursing actions is a part of the diagnosis step of the nursing process?
   a. Identifies patient as "At risk for suicide"
   b. Notes that patient's family reports recent suicide attempt
   c. Prioritizes the necessity for maintaining a safe environment for the patient
   d. Obtains a commitment from the patient to work collaboratively to identify adaptive coping skills

3. The nurse is using nursing process to care for a patient who is suicidal. Which of the following nursing actions is a part of the outcome identification step of the nursing process?
   a. Prioritizes the necessity for maintaining a safe environment for the patient
   b. Determines if nursing interventions have been appropriate to achieve desired results
   c. Obtains a commitment from the patient to work collaboratively to identify adaptive coping skills
   d. Identifies that the "Patient will not harm self during hospitalization"

Continued

Review Questions—cont'd
Self-Examination/Learning Exercise

4. The nurse is using nursing process to care for a patient who is suicidal. Which of the following nursing actions is a part of the planning step of the nursing process?
   a. Prioritizes the necessity for maintaining a safe environment for the patient
   b. Determines if nursing interventions have been appropriate to achieve desired results
   c. Obtains a commitment from the patient to work collaboratively to identify adaptive coping skills
   d. Identifies that the "Patient will not harm self during hospitalization"

5. The nurse is using nursing process to care for a patient who is suicidal. Which of the following nursing actions is a part of the implementation step of the nursing process?
   a. Prioritizes the necessity for maintaining a safe environment for the patient
   b. Determines if nursing interventions have been appropriate to achieve desired results
   c. Collaborates with the patient to develop a plan for ongoing safety and suicide prevention
   d. Identifies that "Patient will not harm self during hospitalization"

6. The nurse is using nursing process to care for a patient who is suicidal. Which of the following nursing actions is a part of the evaluation step of the nursing process?
   a. Prioritizes the necessity for maintaining a safe environment for the patient
   b. Determines if nursing interventions have been appropriate to achieve desired results
   c. Obtains a commitment from the patient to collaboratively work to identify adaptive coping skills
   d. Identifies that the "Patient will not harm self during hospitalization"

7. S.T. is a 15-year-old girl who has just been admitted to the adolescent psychiatric unit with a diagnosis of anorexia nervosa. She is 5 ft 5 in. tall and weighs 82 lb. She was elected to the cheerleading squad for the fall but states that she is not as good as the others on the squad. The treatment team has identified the following problems: refusal to eat, occasional purging, refusing to interact with staff and peers, and fear of failure. Which of the following nursing diagnoses would be appropriate for S.T.? (Select all that apply.)
   a. Social isolation
   b. Disturbed body image
   c. Low self-esteem
   d. Imbalanced nutrition: Less than body requirements

8. S.T. is a 15-year-old girl who has just been admitted to the adolescent psychiatric unit with a diagnosis of anorexia nervosa. She is 5 ft 5in. tall and weighs 82 lb. She was elected to the cheerleading squad for the fall but states that she is not as good as the others on the squad. The treatment team has identified the following problems: refusal to eat, occasional purging, refusing to interact with staff and peers, and fear of failure. Which of the following nursing diagnoses would be the highest priority diagnosis for S.T.?
   a. Social isolation
   b. Disturbed body image
   c. Low self-esteem
   d. Imbalanced nutrition: Less than body requirements

9. Nursing diagnoses are prioritized according to which of the following?
   a. Degree of potential for resolution
   b. Legal implications associated with nursing intervention
   c. Life-threatening potential
   d. Client and family requests

Review Questions—cont'd
Self-Examination/Learning Exercise

10. Which of the following describe advantages of electronic health records (EHRs)? (Select all that apply.)
    a. They reduce redundancy of information.
    b. They reduce issues regarding privacy.
    c. They decrease charting time.
    d. They facilitate communication between disciplines.

References

American Nurses Association (ANA). (2010). *Nursing's social policy statement: The essence of the profession* (3rd ed.). Silver Spring, MD: Nursesbooks.org.

American Nurses Association (ANA). (2015). *Nursing: Scope and standards of practice* (3rd ed.). Silver Spring, MD: Nursesbooks.org.

American Nurses Association (ANA). (2018.) *What is nursing?* Retrieved from http://www.nursingworld.org/especially ForYou/What-is-Nursing

American Nurses Association (ANA), American Psychiatric Nurses Association (APNA), & International Society of Psychiatric-Mental Health Nurses (ISPN). (2014). *Psychiatric-mental health nursing: Scope and standards of practice* (2nd ed.). Silver Spring, MD: ANA.

Bulechek, G., Butcher, H., Dochterman, J., & Wagner, C. (Eds.). (2013). *Nursing interventions classification* (NIC) (6th ed.). St. Louis, MO: Elsevier.

Cronenwett, L., Sherwood, G., Barnsteiner, J., Disch, J., Johnson, J., Mitchell, P., . . . Warren, D. J. (2007). Quality and safety education for nurses. *Nursing Outlook, 55*(3), 122–131. doi:10.1016/j.outlook.2007.02.006

Doenges, M. E., Moorhouse, M. F., & Murr, A. C. (2016). *Nursing diagnosis manual: Planning, individualizing, and documenting client care* (4th ed.). Philadelphia, PA: F.A. Davis.

Institute of Medicine. (2003). *Key capabilities of an electronic health record system: Letter report.* Washington, DC: The National Academies Press. doi:http://doi.org/10.17226/10781

Kaufman, D. M., & Zun, L. (1995). A quantifiable, brief mental status examination for emergency patients. *Journal of Emergency Medicine, 13*(4), 440–456.

Kokman, E., Smith, G. E., Petersen, R. C., Tangalos, E., & Ivnik, R. C. (1991). The short test of mental status: Correlations with standardized psychometric testing. *Archives of Neurology, 48*(7), 725–728.

Lampe, S. S. (1985). Focus charting: Streamlining documentation. *Nursing Management, 16*(7), 43–46.

Moorhead, S., & Dochterman, J. M. (2012). Languages and development of the linkages. In M. Johnson, S. Moorhead, G. Bulechek, M. Butcher, M. Maas, & E. Swanson, *NOC and NIC linkages to NANDA-I and clinical conditions: Supporting critical reasoning and quality care* (3rd ed., pp. 1–10). Maryland Heights, MO: Mosby.

Moorhead, S., Johnson, M., Maas, M., & Swanson, E. (2013). *Nursing outcomes classification (NOC)* (5th ed.). St. Louis, MO: Mosby Elsevier.

NANDA International. (2018a). *Nursing diagnoses: Definitions and classification, 2018–2020* (11th ed.). New York, NY: Thieme.

NANDA International. (2018b). *About NANDA International.* Retrieved from http://www.nanda.org/AboutUs.aspx

Nurses Service Organization (NSO). (2018). *Charting by exception: The legal risks.* Retrieved from https://www.nso.com/Learning/Artifacts/Articles/Charting-by-exception-the-legal-risks

Pfeiffer, E. (1975). A short portable mental status questionnaire for the assessment of organic brain deficit in elderly patients. *Journal of the American Geriatric Society, 23*(10), 433–441.

Schuster, P. M. (2015). *Concept mapping: A critical-thinking approach to care planning* (4th ed.). Philadelphia, PA: F.A. Davis.

U.S. Government Accountability Office (GAO). (2010). *Features of integrated systems support patient care strategies and access to care, but systems face challenges.* Washington, DC: Author.

Young, K. M. (2015). Nursing informatics. In J. T. Catalano (Ed.), *Nursing now! Today's issues, tomorrow's trends* (7th ed., pp. 429–451). Philadelphia, PA: F.A. Davis.

Classical Reference

Folstein, M. F., Folstein, S. E., & McHugh, P. R. (1975). Mini-mental state: A practical method for grading the cognitive state of patients for the clinician. *Journal of Psychiatric Research, 12*(3), 189–198.

7

Milieu Therapy—
The Therapeutic Community

KEY TERMS

milieu
milieu therapy

therapeutic community

OBJECTIVES
After reading this chapter, the student will be able to:

1. Define *milieu therapy*.
2. Explain the goal of therapeutic community, or milieu therapy.
3. Identify seven basic assumptions of a therapeutic community.
4. Discuss conditions that characterize a therapeutic community.
5. Identify the various therapies that may be included in the program of the therapeutic community and identify the healthcare workers who make up the interdisciplinary treatment team.
6. Describe the role of the nurse on the interdisciplinary treatment team.

HOMEWORK ASSIGNMENT
Please read the chapter and answer the following questions:

1. How are unit expectations established in a therapeutic community setting?
2. Which member of the interdisciplinary treatment team has a focus on rehabilitation and vocational training?
3. Identify the five elements of a therapeutic milieu and give an example of how each one may be accomplished in an inpatient psychiatric unit.
4. What are the expected outcomes of establishing a therapeutic milieu?

Introduction

Standard 5F: Milieu Therapy from the *Psychiatric-Mental Health Nursing: Scope and Standards of Practice* (American Nurses Association [ANA], American Psychiatric Nurses Association, & International Society of Psychiatric Nurses, 2014) states, "The

Psychiatric–Mental Health Nurse provides, structures, and maintains a safe, therapeutic, and recovery-oriented environment in collaboration with healthcare consumers, families, and other healthcare clinicians" (p. 60).

This chapter defines and explains the goal of milieu therapy. The conditions necessary for a therapeutic environment are discussed, and the roles of the various healthcare workers who comprise the interdisciplinary team are delineated. An interpretation of the nurse's role in milieu therapy is included.

Milieu, Defined

The word **milieu** is French for "middle." The English translation of the word is "surroundings, or environment." In psychiatry, therapy involving the milieu, or environment, may be called milieu therapy, **therapeutic community,** or the therapeutic environment. The goal of milieu therapy is to manipulate the environment so that all aspects of the client's hospital experience are considered therapeutic. In this therapeutic community setting, the client is expected to learn adaptive coping, interaction, and relationship skills that can be generalized to other aspects of his or her life.

> ## CORE CONCEPT
> **Milieu therapy**
> A scientific structuring of the environment in order to effect behavioral changes and to improve the psychological health and functioning of the individual (Skinner, 1979).

Current Status of the Therapeutic Community

Milieu therapy came into its own during the 1960s through early 1980s. During this period, psychiatric inpatient treatment provided sufficient time to implement programs of therapy that were aimed at social rehabilitation. Lengths of stay averaged from 28 to 30 days for acute care hospitalizations and several months or years for long-term hospitalizations. Nursing's focus of establishing interpersonal relationships with patients fit well within this concept of therapy. Patients were encouraged to be active participants in their therapy, and individual autonomy was emphasized.

The current focus of inpatient psychiatric care has changed, and particularly acute care hospitalization lengths of stay now average 2 to 3 days. Hall (1995) states:

> Care in inpatient psychiatric facilities can now be characterized as short and biologically based. By the time patients have stabilized enough to benefit from the socialization that would take place in a milieu as treatment program, they [often] have been discharged. (p. 51)

Although strategies for milieu therapy are still used, they have been modified for use in short-term hospital stays or outpatient treatment programs. Some programs, especially residential treatment settings (e.g., those for children and adolescents, clients with substance addictions, and geriatric clients) have successfully incorporated the concepts of milieu therapy to the specialized needs of their client populations (Bowler, 1991; DeSocio, Bowllan, & Staschak, 1997; Jani & Fishman, 2004; Kvarnstrom, 2017; Menninger Clinic, 2018; Whall, 1991). Evidence has supported the benefits of therapeutic communities in prison settings for individuals with substance use disorders (National Institutes of Health [NIH], 2015). In this context, work assignments, peer support, formal treatment, and accepting responsibility for one's actions are key elements, and the therapeutic community treatment may last 12 months or more. Evidence has also supported the idea that milieu therapy for longer term treatment of patients with schizophrenia yields positive benefits at lower doses of antipsychotic medications, and the researchers conclude that it is the positive emotional experience of milieu therapy that is most impactful (Ciompi & Hoffman, 2004; Kvarnstrom, 2017).

Echternacht (2001) suggested that more emphasis should be placed on unstructured components of milieu therapy. She described the unstructured components as a multitude of complex interactions between patients, staff, and visitors that occur around the clock. Echternacht called these interactions "fluid group work." They involve spontaneous opportunities within the milieu environment for the psychiatric nurse to provide "on-the-spot therapeutic interventions designed to enhance socialization competency and interpersonal relationship awareness. Emphasis is on social skills and activities in the context of interpersonal interactions" (p. 40). With fluid group work, the nurse applies psychotherapeutic knowledge and skills to brief clinical encounters that occur spontaneously in the therapeutic milieu setting. Echternacht (2001) believes that by using these techniques, nurses can "reclaim their milieu therapy functions in the midst of a changing health care environment" (p. 40).

Many of the original concepts of milieu therapy are presented in this chapter. It is important to remember that a number of modifications to these concepts have been applied in practice for use in a variety of settings.

Basic Assumptions

Skinner (1979) outlined seven basic assumptions on which a therapeutic community is based:

1. **The health in each individual is to be realized and encouraged to grow.** All individuals are considered to have strengths as well as limitations. These healthy aspects of the individual are identified and serve as a foundation for personality growth and the ability to function more adaptively and productively in all aspects of life.
2. **Every interaction is an opportunity for therapeutic intervention.** Within the structured setting of a therapeutic community, it is virtually impossible to avoid interpersonal interaction. The ideal situation promotes the opportunity to improve communication and relationship development skills. Learning occurs from immediate feedback of personal perceptions.
3. **Each individual owns his or her own environment.** Patients should have the opportunity to make decisions and solve problems related to the environment (milieu) of the unit. In this way, personal needs for autonomy as well as needs that pertain to the group as a whole are fulfilled.
4. **Each individual owns his or her behavior.** Each individual in the therapeutic community is expected to take responsibility for his or her own behavior.
5. **Peer pressure is a useful and powerful tool.** Behavioral group norms are established through peer pressure. Feedback is direct and frequent, so that behaving in a manner acceptable toward the other members of the community becomes essential.
6. **Inappropriate behaviors are dealt with as they occur.** Individuals examine the significance of their behavior, look at how it affects other people, and discuss more appropriate ways of behaving in certain situations.
7. **Restrictions and punishment are to be avoided.** Destructive behaviors can usually be controlled with group discussion. However, if an individual requires external controls, temporary isolation is preferred over lengthy restriction or other harsh consequences.

Conditions That Promote a Therapeutic Community

In a therapeutic community setting, the setting is the foundation. Everything that happens to the client, or in the client's environment, is considered to be part of the treatment program. Community factors—such as social interactions, the physical structure of the treatment setting, and schedule of activities—may generate negative responses from some clients. These stressful experiences are used as examples to help the client learn how to manage stress more adaptively in real-life situations.

Under what conditions, then, is a hospital environment considered therapeutic? Gunderson (1978) identified five elements of a community environment that are necessary for therapeutic outcomes:

1. **Containment.** The environment is contained to create a sense of safety and security. Patients who are struggling with strong suicidal intentions, for example, often find that locked doors and lack of access to easy methods of self-harm provide the containment they need to resist self-destructive impulses.
2. **Structure.** The environment needs to have a structure that promotes the goals of treatment. This includes a schedule of activities so that patients know what, when, and where activities are taking place. Group therapies, for example, are scheduled at specific times so patients can structure their day to attend. Knowing to whom they should go (perhaps a primary nurse or team leader) to express concerns, ask for medication, or contact other team members is another aspect of unit structure that promotes therapeutic outcomes.
3. **Involvement.** The environment must encourage involvement so that patients develop a sense of social community. Common dining areas, small group seating arrangements, and community meetings to discuss aspects of community living are examples of elements that promote involvement.
4. **Support.** The environment must be supportive and affirming rather than rigid or punitive. The nurse plays an active role offering emotional support, reinforcing the expectations within the community environment to promote supportive interaction, and redirecting patients who are struggling to accomplish therapeutic interaction with others. Support also includes creating a sense that patients are not only involved in treatment but empowered in decision making and direction around their care.
5. **Validation.** The environment must support and affirm the needs of the individual both within and separate from the community. Active, empathic listening to the patient's perceptions and

concerns and promoting autonomy are examples of validation.

The Program of Therapeutic Community

Care for patients in the therapeutic community is directed by an interdisciplinary treatment (IDT) team. An initial assessment is made by the admitting psychiatrist, nurse, or other designated admitting agent who identifies the reason for admission and priorities for care. The IDT team, with patient involvement whenever possible, determines a comprehensive treatment plan and goals of therapy and assigns intervention responsibilities. (See Box 7–1 for a QSEN teaching strategy for promoting teamwork and collaboration among the interdisciplinary treatment team.)

All members sign the treatment plan and meet regularly to update the plan as needed. Depending on the size of the treatment facility and scope of the therapy program, members representing a variety of disciplines may participate in the promotion of a therapeutic community. For example, an IDT team may include a psychiatrist, case manager, clinical psychologist, psychiatric clinical nurse specialist or psychiatric nurse practitioner, psychiatric nurse, mental health technician, psychiatric social worker, occupational therapist, recreational therapist, art therapist, music therapist, dietitian, and chaplain.

Whenever possible, the client should be actively involved as the central member of the IDT team. This is foundational to accomplishing patient-centered care and promoting a therapeutic milieu. Circumstances that preclude patient involvement might include the patient's acuity level, lack of insight about the need for treatment, or refusal to attend IDT meetings. Table 7–1 provides an explanation of responsibilities and educational preparation required for these members of the IDT team.

BOX 7–1 QSEN TEACHING STRATEGY

Assignment: Interviewing Members of the Interdisciplinary Team
The Process of Teamwork and Collaboration

Competency Domain: Teamwork and Collaboration, Safety

Learning Objectives:

The student will:
• Explain the process for collaboration between nursing and other members of the interdisciplinary team.
• Identify different team members' responsibilities with regard to key safety issues, such as suicide prevention, reporting to outside individuals/agencies regarding suspicions of abuse and duty to warn, and managing safety within the therapeutic milieu.
• Evaluate the contributions of each discipline within the interdisciplinary team to elements of milieu therapy.

Strategy Overview

This assignment is meant to familiarize the student with the roles and responsibilities of various members of the interdisciplinary team and to evaluate the processes that promote teamwork and collaboration within milieu therapy. Students may be assigned to specific activities in preparation for a clinical conference discussion or asked to complete a reflective writing assignment on the function of the IDT team in the provision of milieu therapy.

1. Attend an IDT team meeting to evaluate individual disciplines' contributions and describe the process of collaboration.
2. Interview one or more members of the interdisciplinary team to identify their perceptions of how the process of collaboration works between their discipline and nursing. Sample questions might include the following:
   "In what ways does your discipline collaborate with nursing?"
   "How effective is collaboration between disciplines within the IDT team?"
   "What barriers exist to effective collaboration between disciplines?"
   "What is your discipline's role in
       suicide prevention within the milieu?"
       reporting to outside individuals or agencies?"
       managing safety within the milieu?"
3. Attend structured group activities to evaluate the contributions of various team members in promoting the therapeutic milieu.

TABLE 7–1 The Interdisciplinary Treatment Team in Psychiatry

TEAM MEMBER	RESPONSIBILITIES	CREDENTIALS
Psychiatrist	May serve as the leader of the team. Responsible for diagnosis and treatment of mental disorders. Prescribes medication and other somatic therapies. Performs ongoing assessment and medication management.	Medical degree with residency in psychiatry and license to practice medicine.
Case manager	May serve as the leader of the team. Collaborates with other members of the IDT to ensure that the IDT care plan is implemented effectively and efficiently. May coordinate referral needs and follow-up appointments post-discharge. Some case managers also conduct utilization review functions.	Bachelor's or master's degree in case management, nursing, health, education, or human services.
Clinical psychologist	Conducts individual, group, and family therapy. Administers, interprets, and evaluates psychological tests that assist in the diagnostic process.	Doctorate in clinical psychology with 2- to 3-year internship supervised by a licensed clinical psychologist. State license is required to practice.
Psychiatric clinical nurse specialist or psychiatric nurse practitioner	Conducts individual, group, and family therapy. Presents educational programs for nursing staff. Provides consultation services to nurses who require assistance in the planning and implementation of care for individual clients. May also prescribe and manage the medication regime.	Registered nurse with minimum of a master's degree in psychiatric nursing. Some institutions require certification by national credentialing association.
Psychiatric nurse	Provides ongoing assessment of client condition, both mentally and physically. Manages the therapeutic milieu on a 24-hour basis. Administers medications. Assists patients with all therapeutic activities as required. Focus is on one-to-one relationship development.	Registered nurse with hospital diploma, associate degree, or baccalaureate degree. Some psychiatric nurses have national certification.
Mental health technician (also called psychiatric aide or assistant or psychiatric technician)	Functions under the supervision of the psychiatric nurse. Provides assistance to patients in the fulfillment of their activities of daily living. Assists activity therapists as required in conducting their groups. May also participate in one-to-one relationship development.	Varies from state to state. Requirements include high school education, with additional vocational education or on-the-job training. Some hospitals hire individuals with baccalaureate degree in psychology in this capacity. Some states require a licensure examination to practice.
Psychiatric social worker	Conducts individual, group, and family therapy. Is concerned with client's social needs, such as placement, financial support, and community requirements. Conducts in-depth psychosocial history on which the needs assessment is based. Works with patient and family to ensure that requirements for discharge are fulfilled and needs can be met by appropriate community resources.	Minimum of a master's degree in social work. Some states require additional supervision and subsequent licensure by examination.
Occupational therapist	Works with patients to help develop (or redevelop) independence in performance of activities of daily living. Focus is on rehabilitation and vocational training in which patients learn to be productive, thereby enhancing self-esteem. Creative activities and therapeutic relationship skills are used.	Baccalaureate or master's degree in occupational therapy.

TABLE 7–1	The Interdisciplinary Treatment Team in Psychiatry—cont'd	
TEAM MEMBER	**RESPONSIBILITIES**	**CREDENTIALS**
Recreational therapist	Uses recreational activities to promote patients to redirect their thinking or to rechannel destructive energy in an appropriate manner. Patients learn skills that can be used during leisure time and during times of stress following discharge from treatment. Examples include bowling, volleyball, exercises, and jogging. Some programs include activities such as picnics, swimming, and group attendance at functions such as state fairs.	Baccalaureate or master's degree in recreational therapy.
Music therapist	Encourages patients in self-expression through music. Patients listen to music, play instruments, sing, dance, and compose songs that help them get in touch with feelings and emotions that they may not be able to experience in any other way.	Graduate degree with specialty in music therapy.
Art therapist	Uses patient's creative abilities to encourage expression of emotions and feelings through artwork. Helps patients to analyze their own work in an effort to recognize and resolve underlying conflict.	Graduate degree with specialty in art therapy.
Dietitian	Plans nutritious meals for all patients. Consults with patients with specific eating disorders, such as anorexia nervosa, bulimia nervosa, obesity, and pica.	Baccalaureate or master's degree with specialty in dietetics.
Chaplain	Assesses, identifies, and attends to the spiritual needs of individuals and their family members. Provides spiritual support and comfort as requested by the individual or family. May provide counseling if educational background includes this type of preparation.	College degree with advanced education in theology, seminary, or rabbinical studies.

The Role of the Nurse in Milieu Therapy

Milieu therapy can take place in a variety of inpatient and outpatient settings. In the hospital, nurses are generally the only members of the IDT team who spend time with the patients on a 24-hour basis, and they assume responsibility for management of the therapeutic milieu. In all settings, the nursing process is used for the delivery of nursing care. In the management of the therapeutic milieu, the same model (ongoing assessment, diagnosis, outcome identification, planning, implementation, and evaluation) of the environment is necessary for an effective therapeutic milieu. Nurses are involved in all day-to-day activities that pertain to patient care. Suggestions and opinions of nursing staff are given serious consideration in the planning of care for individual patients. Information from the initial nursing assessment is used to create the IDT plan. Nurses have input into therapy goals and participate in the regular updates and modification of treatment plans.

In some treatment facilities, a separate nursing care plan is required in addition to the IDT plan. In this case, the nursing care plan must reflect diagnoses that are specific to nursing and include problems and interventions from the IDT plan that have been assigned to the nurse. In the therapeutic milieu, nurses are responsible for ensuring that patients' physiological needs are met. Patients must be encouraged to perform as independently as possible in fulfilling activities of daily living. However, the nurse should make ongoing assessments to provide assistance for those who require it. Assessing physical status is an important nursing responsibility and a priority that must not be overlooked in a psychiatric setting.

Reality orientation for patients who have disorganized thinking or who are disoriented or confused is important in the therapeutic milieu. Clocks with large hands and numbers, calendars that give the day and date in large print, and orientation boards that discuss daily activities and news events can help keep patients oriented to reality. Nurses should ensure that patients have written schedules of activities to which they are assigned and that they arrive at those activities on schedule. Some patients may require an identification sign on their door to remind them which room is theirs. On short-term units, nurses who are dealing with patients experiencing psychosis usually rely on a basic activity or topic that helps keep people oriented: for example, showing pictures of the hospital where they are housed, introducing people who were admitted during the night, and providing name badges with their first name.

Nurses are responsible for the management of medication administration on inpatient psychiatric units. In some treatment programs, patients are expected to accept the responsibility and request their medication at the appropriate time. Although ultimate responsibility lies with the nurse, he or she must encourage patients to be self-reliant. Nurses must work with the patients to determine methods that result in achievement and provide positive feedback for successes.

A major focus of nursing in the therapeutic milieu is the one-to-one relationship that grows out of a developing trust between the patient and nurse. Many individuals with psychiatric disorders have never achieved the ability to trust. If this can be accomplished in a relationship with the nurse, the trust may be generalized to other relationships in the patient's life. In an atmosphere of trust, the patient is encouraged to express feelings and emotions and to discuss unresolved issues that are creating problems in his or her life.

One of the first nursing interventions in establishing a foundation for trust and maintaining a therapeutic milieu is orienting new patients to the environment, their rights and responsibilities within the unit milieu, the structured activities designed for their personal growth, and any limits or restrictions necessary to maintain safety. Availability to provide support and validation to patients throughout their treatment is also an essential nursing competency in milieu therapy (ANA et al., 2014), and this, too, is rooted in a trusting relationship. In acute care hospitalizations, the ability to establish trust quickly and to assess and collaborate with patients about their needs post-discharge has become an essential role for nurses, because many aspects of the recovery treatment plan occur in treatment settings other than inpatient hospitalization. Don't underestimate the importance of these short-term relationships. Clients in outpatient treatment often identify that it was something a nurse said or something they learned within the hospital milieu that planted the seeds for their ongoing recovery plan.

The nurse is responsible for setting limits on unacceptable behavior in the therapeutic milieu. Doing so requires stating to the patient in understandable terminology what behaviors are not acceptable and what the consequences will be should the limits be violated. These limits must be established, written, and carried out by all staff. Consistency in carrying out the consequences of violation of the established limits is essential if the learning is to be reinforced.

> **CLINICAL PEARL** Developing trust means keeping promises that have been made. It means total acceptance of the individual as a person, separate from behavior that is unacceptable. It means responding to the patient with concrete behaviors that are understandable to him or her (e.g., "If you are frightened, I will stay with you"; "If you are cold, I will bring you a blanket"; "If you are thirsty, I will bring you a drink of water").

The role of teacher is important in psychiatric nursing, as it is in all areas of nursing. This requires being able to assess learning readiness in individual patients. Do they want to learn? What is their level of anxiety? What is their level of ability to understand the information being presented? Topics for patient education in psychiatry include information about medical diagnoses, side effects of medications, the importance of continuing to take medications, and stress management, among others. Some topics must be individualized for specific patients, whereas others may be taught in group situations. Box 7–2 outlines various topics of nursing concern for patient education in psychiatry.

Echternacht (2001) stated:

> Milieu therapy interventions are recognized as one of the basic-level functions of psychiatric-mental health nurses as addressed [in the *Psychiatric-Mental Health Nursing: Scope and Standards of Practice* (ANA et al., 2014)]. Milieu therapy has been described as an excellent framework for operationalizing [Hildegard] Peplau's interpretation and extension of Harry Stack Sullivan's Interpersonal Theory for use in nursing practice. (p. 39)

Now is the time to rekindle interest in the therapeutic milieu concept and to reclaim nursing's traditional milieu intervention functions. Nurses need to identify the number of registered nurses necessary to carry out structured and unstructured milieu functions consistent with their Standards of Practice. (p. 43)

BOX 7–2 The Therapeutic Milieu–Topics for Patient Education

1. Ways to increase self-esteem
2. Ways to deal with anger appropriately
3. Stress-management techniques
4. How to recognize signs of increasing anxiety and intervene to stop progression
5. Normal stages of grieving and behaviors associated with each stage
6. Assertiveness techniques
7. Relaxation techniques
   a. Progressive muscle relaxation
   b. Imagery (selectively)
   c. Deep breathing
   d. Mindfulness meditation
8. Medications (specify)
   a. Reason for taking
   b. Harmless side effects
   c. Side effects to report to physician
   d. Importance of taking regularly
   e. Importance of not stopping abruptly
9. Effects of (substances) on the body
   a. Alcohol
   b. Other depressants
   c. Stimulants
   d. Hallucinogens
   e. Narcotics
   f. Cannabinols
10. Problem-solving skills
11. Thought-stopping/thought-switching techniques
12. Sex education including sexually transmitted infections
13. The essentials of good nutrition
14. Exploring spiritual needs
15. Management of leisure time
16. Strategies for goal setting and goal accomplishment
17. (For parents/guardians)
    a. Signs and symptoms of substance abuse
    b. Effective parenting techniques

Summary and Key Points

- In psychiatry, milieu therapy (or a therapeutic community) constitutes a manipulation of the environment in an effort to create behavioral changes and to improve the psychological health and functioning of the individual.
- The goal of therapeutic community is for the patient to learn adaptive coping, interaction, and relationship skills that can be generalized to other aspects of his or her life.
- The community environment itself serves as the primary tool of therapy.
- According to Skinner (1979), a therapeutic community is based on seven basic assumptions:
  - The health in each individual is to be realized and encouraged to grow.
  - Every interaction is an opportunity for therapeutic intervention.
  - The individual owns his or her own environment.
  - Each individual owns his or her behavior.
  - Peer pressure is a useful and powerful tool.
  - Inappropriate behaviors are dealt with as they occur.
  - Restrictions and punishment are to be avoided.
- Because the goals of milieu therapy relate to helping the patient learn to generalize that which is learned to other aspects of his or her life, the conditions that promote a therapeutic community in the psychiatric setting are similar to the types of conditions that exist in real-life situations.
- Conditions that promote a therapeutic community include the following:
  - Containment
  - Structure
  - Involvement
  - Support
  - Validation
- The program of therapy on the milieu unit is conducted by the interdisciplinary treatment (IDT) team.
- The team includes some, or all, of the following disciplines and may include others that are not specified here: psychiatrist, case manager, clinical psychologist, psychiatric clinical nurse specialist or psychiatric nurse practitioner, psychiatric nurse, mental health technician, psychiatric social worker, occupational therapist, recreational therapist, art therapist, music therapist, dietitian, and chaplain.
- Nurses play a crucial role in the management of a therapeutic milieu. They are involved in the assessment, diagnosis, outcome identification, planning, implementation, and evaluation of all treatment programs.
- Nurses have significant input into IDT plans, which are developed for all patients. They are responsible for ensuring that patients' basic needs are fulfilled; assessing physical and psychosocial status; administering medication; helping the patient develop trusting relationships; setting limits on unacceptable behaviors; educating patients; and, ultimately, helping patients, within the limits of their capability, to become productive members of society.

Review Questions
Self-Examination/Learning Exercise

Select the answer that is most appropriate for each of the following questions:

1. Which of the following are basic assumptions of milieu therapy? (Select all that apply.)
   a. Each individual owns his or her own environment.
   b. Each individual owns his or her behavior.
   c. Peer pressure is a useful and powerful tool.
   d. Inappropriate behaviors are punished immediately.

2. John tells the nurse, "I think lights out at ten o'clock on a weekend is stupid. We should be able to watch TV until midnight!" Which of the following is the most appropriate response from the nurse on the milieu unit?
   a. "John, you were told the rules when you were admitted."
   b. "You may bring it up before the others at the community meeting, John."
   c. "Some people want to go to bed early, John."
   d. "You are not the only person on this unit, John. You must think of others besides yourself."

3. In prioritizing care within the therapeutic environment, which of the following nursing interventions would receive the highest priority?
   a. Ensuring that the physical facilities are conducive to achievement of the goals of therapy
   b. Scheduling a community meeting for 8:30 each morning
   c. Attending to patients' physiological and safety needs
   d. Establishing contacts with community resources

4. In the community meeting, which of the following actions is most important for reinforcing the democratic posture of the therapy setting?
   a. Allowing each person a specific and equal amount of time to talk
   b. Reviewing group rules and behavioral limits that apply to all patients
   c. Reading the minutes from yesterday's meeting
   d. Waiting until all patients are present before initiating the meeting

5. One of the goals of therapeutic community is for patients to become more independent and accept self-responsibility. Which of the following approaches by staff best encourages fulfillment of this goal?
   a. Including patient input and decisions into the treatment plan
   b. Insisting that each patient take a turn as "president" of the community meeting
   c. Making decisions for the patient regarding plans for treatment
   d. Requiring that the patient be bathed and dressed and attend breakfast on time each morning

6. Patient teaching is an important nursing function in milieu therapy. Which of the following statements by the patient indicates the need for knowledge and a readiness to learn?
   a. "Get away from me with that medicine! I'm not sick!"
   b. "I don't need psychiatric treatment. It's my migraine headaches that I need help with."
   c. "I've taken Valium every day of my life for the last 20 years. I'll stop when I'm good and ready!"
   d. "The doctor says I have bipolar disorder. What does that really mean?"

7. Which of the following activities would be a responsibility of the clinical psychologist member of the IDT team?
   a. Locates halfway house and arranges living conditions for patient being discharged from the hospital
   b. Manages the therapeutic milieu on a 24-hour basis
   c. Administers and evaluates psychological tests that assist in diagnosis
   d. Conducts psychotherapy and administers electroconvulsive therapy treatments

Review Questions—cont'd
Self-Examination/Learning Exercise

8. Which of the following activities would be a responsibility of the psychiatric clinical nurse specialist on the IDT team?
   a. Manages the therapeutic milieu on a 24-hour basis
   b. Conducts group therapies and provides consultation and education to staff nurses
   c. Directs a group of patients in acting out a situation that is otherwise too painful for a patient to discuss openly
   d. Locates halfway house and arranges living conditions for patient being discharged from the hospital

9. On the milieu unit, duties of the staff psychiatric nurse include which of the following? (Select all that apply.)
   a. Medication administration
   b. Patient teaching
   c. Medical diagnosis
   d. Reality orientation
   e. Relationship development
   f. Group therapy

10. Sally was sexually abused as a child. She is a client on the milieu unit with a diagnosis of borderline personality disorder. She has refused to talk to anyone. Which of the following therapies might the IDT team recommend for Sally? (Select all that apply.)
    a. Music therapy
    b. Art therapy
    c. Seclusion
    d. Electroconvulsive therapy

References

American Nurses Association (ANA), American Psychiatric Nurses, & International Society of Psychiatric Nurses. (2014). *Psychiatric-mental health nursing: Scope and standards of practice* (2nd ed.). Silver Spring, MD: Nuresbooks.org

Bowler, J. B. (1991). Transformation into a healing healthcare environment: Recovering the possibilities of psychiatric/mental health nursing. *Perspectives in Psychiatric Care, 27*(2), 21–25.

Ciompi, L., & Hoffman, H. (2004). Soteria Berne: An innovative milieu therapeutic approach to acute schizophrenia based on the concept of affect-logic. *World Psychiatry, 3*(3), 140–146.

DeSocio, J., Bowllan, N., & Staschak, S. (1997). Lessons learned in creating a safe and therapeutic milieu for children, adolescents, and families: Developmental considerations. *Journal of Child and Adolescent Psychiatric Nursing, 10*(4), 18–26.

Echternacht, M. R. (2001). Fluid group: Concept and clinical application in the therapeutic milieu. *Journal of the American Psychiatric Nurses Association, 7*(2), 39–44.

Hall, B. A. (1995). Use of milieu therapy: The context and environment as therapeutic practice for psychiatric-mental health nurses. In C. A. Anderson (Ed.), *Psychiatric nursing 1974 to 1994: A report on the state of the art* (pp. 46–56). St. Louis, MO: Mosby-Year Book.

Jani, S., & Fishman, M. (2004). *Advances in milieu therapy for adolescent residential treatment.* Program presented at the American Academy of Child and Adolescent Psychiatry 2004 Annual National Meeting. Retrieved from http://www.milieu-therapy .com/Presentations.en.html

Kvarnstrom, E. (2017). *A social treatment: Mental health benefits of milieu therapy for people living with schizophrenia.* Retrieved from https://www.hanbleceya.com/blog/a-social-treatment-mental-health-benefits-of-milieu-therapy-for-people-living-with-schizophrenia/

Menninger Clinic. (2018). *Professionals in crisis program.* Retrieved from http://www.menningerclinic.com/patient-care/ inpatient-treatment/professionals-in-crisis-program/milieu-therapy

National Institutes of Health (NIH). (2015). *How are therapeutic communities integrated into the criminal justice system?* Retrieved from https://www.drugabuse.gov/publications/research-reports/ therapeutic-communities/how-are-therapeutic-communities-integrated-criminal-justice-system

Whall, A. L. (1991). Using the environment to improve the mental health of the elderly. *Journal of Gerontological Nursing, 17*(7), 39.

Classical References

Gunderson, J. G. (1978). Defining the therapeutic processes in psychiatric milieus. *Psychiatry: Interpersonal and Biological Processes, 41*(4), 327–335.

Maslow, A. (1968). *Towards a psychology of being* (2nd ed.). New York, NY: D. Van Nostrand.

Skinner, K. (1979, August). The therapeutic milieu: Making it work. *Journal of Psychiatric Nursing and Mental Health Services, 17*(8), 38–44.

8

Intervention in Groups

CHAPTER OUTLINE

KEY TERMS

OBJECTIVES

After reading this chapter, the student will be able to:

1. Define a group.
2. Discuss eight functions of a group.
3. Identify various types of groups.
4. Describe physical conditions that influence groups.
5. Discuss "therapeutic factors" that occur in groups.
6. Describe the phases of group development.
7. Identify various leadership styles in groups.
8. Identify various roles that members assume within a group.
9. Discuss psychodrama and family therapy as specialized forms of group therapy.
10. Describe the role of the nurse in group therapy.

HOMEWORK ASSIGNMENT

Please read the chapter and answer the following questions:

1. What is the difference between therapeutic groups and group therapy?
2. What are the expectations of the leader in the initial or orientation phase of group development?
3. How does an autocratic leadership style affect member enthusiasm and morale?
4. How does size of the group influence group dynamics?
5. What is the major goal of family therapy?

Introduction

Human beings are complex creatures who share their activities of daily living with various *groups* of people. As Forsyth (2019) stated, "The tendency to join with others in groups is perhaps the single most important characteristic of humans and the processes that unfold within these groups leave an indelible imprint on their members and on society" (p. 1).

Healthcare professionals encounter multiple group situations in their role as clinician. Team conferences, committee meetings, grand rounds, and in-service sessions are but a few instances in which this occurs. In psychiatry, work with patients and families often takes the form of groups. With group work, not only does the nurse have the opportunity to reach out to a greater number of people at one time, but the group members also assist each other by bringing to the group and sharing their feelings, opinions, ideas, and behaviors. Patients learn from each other in a group setting.

This chapter explores various types of therapeutic groups that can be used in psychiatric settings and the role of the nurse in group intervention.

CORE CONCEPT
Group

A *group* is a collection of individuals whose association is founded on shared interests, values, norms, or purpose. Membership in a group is generally by chance (born into the group), by choice (voluntary affiliation), or by circumstance (the result of life-cycle events over which an individual may or may not have control).

Functions of a Group

Sampson and Marthas (1990) contend that groups may serve more than one function and usually serve different functions for different members of the group. They outlined the following eight functions that groups serve for their members:

1. **Socialization.** The cultural group into which we are born begins the process of teaching social norms. This process continues throughout our lives as we interact with members of other groups with which we become affiliated.
2. **Support.** One's fellow group members are available in time of need. Individuals derive a feeling of security from group involvement.
3. **Task completion.** Group members provide assistance in endeavors that are beyond the capacity of one individual alone or when results can be achieved more effectively as a team.
4. **Camaraderie.** Members of a group provide the joy and pleasure that individuals seek from interactions with significant others.
5. **Information sharing.** Learning takes place within groups. Knowledge is gained when individual members learn how others in the group have resolved situations similar to those with which they are currently struggling.
6. **Normative influence.** This function relates to the ways in which groups enforce the established norms. As group members interact, they begin to influence each other regarding the expected norms for communication and behavior.
7. **Empowerment.** Groups help to bring about improvement in existing conditions by providing support to individual members who seek to bring about change. Groups have power that individuals alone do not.
8. **Governance.** An example of the governing function is that of rules being made by committees within a larger organization.

Types of Groups

The functions of a group vary depending on the reason the group was formed. Clark (2009) identified three types of groups in which nurses most often participate: task, teaching, and supportive-therapeutic groups.

Task Groups

The function of a task group is to accomplish a specific outcome or task. The focus is on solving problems and making decisions to achieve this outcome. Often a deadline is placed on completion of the task, and such importance is placed on a satisfactory outcome that conflict in the group may be smoothed over or ignored in order to focus on the priority at hand.

Teaching Groups

Teaching, or educational, groups exist to convey knowledge and information to a number of individuals. Nurses can be involved in teaching groups of many varieties, such as medication education, childbirth education, and effective parenting classes. These groups usually have a set time frame or a set number of meetings. Members learn from each other as well as from the designated instructor. The objective of teaching groups is verbalization or demonstration by the learner of the material presented by the end of the designated period.

Supportive-Therapeutic Groups

The primary concern of support groups is to teach participants effective ways to deal with emotional stress arising from situational or developmental crises.

> ### CORE CONCEPT
> #### Group therapy
> Group therapy is a form of psychosocial treatment in which a number of clients meet together with a therapist for purposes of sharing, gaining personal insight, and improving interpersonal coping strategies.

For the purposes of this text, it is important to differentiate between *therapeutic groups* and *group therapy*. Leaders of group therapy generally have advanced degrees in psychology, social work, nursing, or medicine. They often have additional training or experience under the supervision of an accomplished professional in conducting group psychotherapy based on various theoretical frameworks such as psychoanalytic, psychodynamic, interpersonal, and family dynamics. Approaches based on these theories are used by the group therapy leaders to encourage improvement in the ability of group members to function on an interpersonal level.

Therapeutic groups, on the other hand, are not designed to conduct psychotherapy; rather, the focus is on group relations, interactions among group members, and the consideration of a selected issue. Like group therapists, individuals who lead therapeutic groups must be knowledgeable in *group process;* that is, the *way* in which group members interact with each other. Interruptions, silences, judgments, glares, and scapegoating are examples of group processes (Clark, 2009). Group process will happen whether or not there is a designated group leader, but nurses who are acting as group leaders can guide the way in which members interact with one another to facilitate accomplishing the goals or tasks of the group. This is one reason that group leaders are often referred to as *group facilitators*. They must also have a thorough knowledge of *group content*, the topic or issue being discussed among the group, and

the ability to present the topic in language that can be understood by all group members. Many nurses who work in psychiatry lead supportive-therapeutic groups.

Self-Help Groups

An additional type of group, in which nurses may or may not be involved, is the self-help group. Self-help groups have grown in number and credibility in recent years. They allow clients to talk about their fears and relieve feelings of isolation while receiving comfort and advice from others undergoing similar experiences. Examples of self-help groups are the Alzheimer's Association (originally known as the Alzheimer's Disease and Related Disorders Association), the National Association of Anorexia Nervosa and Associated Disorders, Weight Watchers, Alcoholics Anonymous, Reach to Recovery, Parents Without Partners, Overeaters Anonymous, Adult Children of Alcoholics, and many others related to specific needs or illnesses. These groups may or may not have a professional leader or consultant. They are run by the members, and leadership often rotates from member to member.

Nurses may become involved with self-help groups either voluntarily or because their advice or participation has been requested by the members. The nurse may function as a referral agent, resource person, member of an advisory board, or leader of the group. Self-help groups are a valuable source of referral for clients with specific problems. However, nurses must be knowledgeable about the purposes of the group, membership, leadership, benefits, and problems that might threaten the success of the group before referring their clients to a specific self-help group. The nurse may find it necessary to attend several meetings of a particular group, if possible, to assess its effectiveness of purpose and appropriateness for client referral.

Physical Conditions That Influence Group Dynamics

Seating

The physical conditions for the group should be set up so that there is no barrier between the members. For example, a circle of chairs is better than chairs set around a table. Members should be encouraged to sit in different chairs at each meeting. This openness and change creates a feeling of discomfort that encourages anxious and unsettled behaviors that can then be explored within the group.

Size

Various authors have suggested different ranges of size as ideal for group interaction: 5 to 10 (Yalom & Leszcz, 2005), 2 to 15 (Sampson & Marthas, 1990), and 4 to 12 (Clark, 2009). Group size does make a difference in the interaction among members. The larger the group, the less time is available to devote to individual members. In larger groups, aggressive individuals are most likely to be heard, whereas quiet members may be left out of the discussions altogether. Understanding this dynamic informs the nurse group leader to be alert to this possibility and to facilitate interaction in ways that promote greater involvement for all members. Larger groups have the advantage that they provide more opportunities for individuals to learn from other members. The wider range of life experiences and knowledge provides a greater potential for effective group problem-solving. Ultimately, there is no single right answer in identifying optimal group size because it is influenced by several variables including the group's purpose, group members' functional abilities, and expected outcomes.

Membership

Whether the group is open ended or closed ended is another condition that influences the dynamics of group process. Open-ended groups are those in which members leave and others join at any time while the group is active. The continuous movement of members in and out of the group creates discomfort that encourages individual members to explore their feelings about their own progress. These are the most common types of groups held on short-term inpatient units, although they are used in outpatient and long-term care facilities as well. In outpatient groups, the movement of members in and out of the group can be therapeutic as seasoned members relate to new members about where they were when they entered the group and what things contributed to their benefiting from the group process.

Closed-ended groups usually have a predetermined, fixed time frame. All members join at the time the group is organized and terminate at the end of the designated time period. Closed-ended groups are often composed of individuals with common issues or problems they wish to address.

Therapeutic Factors

Why are therapeutic groups helpful? Yalom and Leszcz (2005) described 11 therapeutic factors that individuals can achieve through interpersonal interactions within the group, some of which are present in most groups in varying degrees:

1. **Instillation of hope.** By observing the progress of others in the group with similar problems, a group member garners hope that his or her problems can also be resolved.
2. **Universality.** Through **universality,** individuals come to realize that they are not alone in the problems, thoughts, and feelings they are experiencing. Anxiety is relieved by the support and understanding of others in the group who share similar (universal) experiences.
3. **Imparting of information.** Knowledge is gained through formal instruction as well as the sharing of advice and suggestions among group members.
4. **Altruism.** **Altruism** is mutual sharing and concern for each other. Providing assistance and support to others creates a positive self-image and promotes self-growth.
5. **Corrective recapitulation of the primary family group.** Group members are able to reexperience early family conflicts that remain unresolved. Attempts at resolution are promoted through feedback and exploration.
6. **Development of socializing techniques.** Through interaction with and feedback from other members of the group, individuals are able to correct maladaptive social behaviors and learn and develop new social skills.
7. **Imitative behavior.** In this setting, members who have mastered particular psychosocial skills or developmental tasks can be valuable role models for others. Individuals may imitate selected behaviors that they wish to develop in themselves.
8. **Interpersonal learning.** The group offers many and varied opportunities for interacting with other people. Insight is gained regarding how one perceives and is being perceived by others.
9. **Group cohesiveness.** Members develop a sense of belonging that separates the individual ("I am") from the group ("we are"). Out of this alliance emerges a common feeling that individual members and the total group are of value to each other.

10. **Catharsis.** Within the group, members are able to express both positive and negative feelings—perhaps feelings that have never been expressed before—in a nonthreatening atmosphere. This **catharsis,** or open expression of feelings, is beneficial for the individual within the group.

11. **Existential factors.** The group is able to help individual members take direction of their own lives and to accept responsibility for the quality of their existence.

It may be helpful for a group leader to explain these therapeutic factors to members of the group. Positive responses are experienced by individuals who understand and are able to recognize therapeutic factors as they occur within the group.

Phases of Group Development

Groups, like individuals, move through phases of life-cycle development. Ideally, groups progress from the phase of infancy to advanced maturity in an effort to fulfill the objectives set forth by the membership. Unfortunately, as with individuals, some groups become fixed in early developmental levels and never progress, or they experience periods of regression in the developmental process. Three phases of group development are discussed here.

Phase I. Initial or Orientation Phase

Group Activities

The leader and members work together to establish the rules that govern the group (e.g., when and where meetings will occur, the importance of confidentiality, how meetings will be structured). Goals of the group are established. Members are introduced to each other.

Leader Expectations

The leader is expected to orient members to specific group processes, encourage members to participate without disclosing too much too soon, promote an environment of trust, and ensure that rules established by the group do not interfere with fulfillment of the goals.

Member Behaviors

In phase I, members have not yet established trust and will respond to this lack of trust by being overly polite. There is a fear of not being accepted by the group. They may try to "get on the good side" of the leader with compliments and conforming behaviors.

A power struggle may ensue as members compete for their position in the "pecking order" of the group.

Phase II. Middle or Working Phase

Group Activities

Ideally, during the working phase, cohesiveness has been established within the group. This is when the productive work toward completion of the task is undertaken. Problem-solving and decision making occur within the group. In the mature group, cooperation prevails, and differences and disagreements are confronted and resolved.

Leader Expectations

The role of leader diminishes and becomes more one of facilitator during the working phase. Some leadership functions are shared by certain members of the group as they progress toward resolution. The leader helps to resolve conflict and continues to foster cohesiveness among the members while ensuring that they do not deviate from the intended task or purpose for which the group was organized.

Member Behaviors

At this point, trust has been established among the members. They turn more often to each other and less often to the leader for guidance. They accept criticism from each other, using it in a constructive manner to create change. Occasionally, subgroups will form in which two or more members conspire with each other to the exclusion of the rest of the group. To maintain group cohesion, these subgroups must be confronted and discussed by the entire membership. Conflict is managed by the group with minimal assistance from the leader.

Phase III. Final or Termination Phase

Group Activities

The longer a group has been in existence, the more difficult termination is likely to be for the members. Termination should be mentioned from the outset of group formation. It should be discussed in depth for several meetings prior to the final session. A sense of loss that precipitates the grief process may be in evidence, particularly in groups that have been successful in their stated purpose.

Leader Expectations

In the termination phase, the leader encourages the group members to reminisce about what has occurred within the group, to review the goals and discuss the actual outcomes, to provide feedback to each other about individual progress within the group, and to discuss feelings of loss associated with termination of the group.

Member Behaviors

Members may express surprise over the actual materialization of the end. This represents the grief response of denial, which may then progress to anger. Anger toward other group members or toward the leader may reflect feelings of abandonment (Sampson & Marthas, 1990). These feelings may lead to individual members' discussions of previous losses for which similar emotions were experienced. Successful termination of the group may help members develop the skills needed when losses occur in other dimensions of their lives.

Leadership Styles

Lippitt and White (1958) identified three of the most common group leadership styles: autocratic, democratic, and laissez-faire. Table 8–1 outlines various similarities and differences among the three leadership styles.

Autocratic

Autocratic leaders have personal goals for the group. They withhold information from group members, particularly issues that may interfere with achievement of their own objectives. The message that is conveyed to the group is: "We will do it my way. My way is best." The focus in this style of leadership is on the leader. Members are dependent on the leader for problem-solving, decision making, and permission to perform. The approach of the autocratic leader is one of persuasion, striving to persuade others in the group that his or her ideas and methods are superior. Productivity is high with this type of leadership, but often morale within the group is low because of lack of member input and creativity.

Democratic

The **democratic** leadership style focuses on the members of the group. Information is shared with members in an effort to allow them to make decisions regarding achieving the goals for the group. Members are encouraged to participate fully in problem-solving of issues that relate to the group, including taking action to effect change. The message that is conveyed to the group is: "Decide what must be done, consider the alternatives, make a selection, and proceed with the actions required to complete the task." The leader provides guidance and expertise as needed. Productivity is lower than it is with autocratic leadership, but morale is much higher because of the extent of input allowed all members of the group and the potential for individual creativity.

Laissez-Faire

This leadership style allows people to do as they please. There is no direction from the leader. In fact, the **laissez-faire** leader's approach is noninvolvement. Goals for the group are undefined. No decisions are made, no problems are solved, and no action is taken. Members become frustrated and confused, and productivity and morale are low.

TABLE 8–1	**Leadership Styles–Similarities and Differences**		
CHARACTERISTICS	**AUTOCRATIC**	**DEMOCRATIC**	**LAISSEZ-FAIRE**
1. Focus	Leader	Members	Undetermined
2. Task strategy	Members are persuaded to adopt leader ideas	Members engage in group problem-solving	No defined strategy exists
3. Member participation	Limited	Unlimited	Inconsistent
4. Individual creativity	Stifled	Encouraged	Not addressed
5. Member enthusiasm and morale	Low	High	Low
6. Group cohesiveness	Low	High	Low
7. Productivity	High	High (may not be as high as autocratic)	Low
8. Individual motivation and commitment	Low (tend to work only when leader is present to urge them to do so)	High (satisfaction derived from personal input and participation)	Low (feelings of frustration from lack of direction or guidance)

Member Roles

Benne and Sheats (1948) identified three major types of roles that individuals play within the membership of the group. These are roles that serve to

1. Complete the task of the group.
2. Maintain or enhance group processes.
3. Fulfill personal or individual needs.

Task roles and maintenance roles contribute to the success or effectiveness of the group. Personal roles satisfy needs of the individual members, sometimes to the extent of interfering with the effectiveness of the group.

Table 8–2 outlines specific roles within these three major types and the behaviors associated with each.

TABLE 8–2	**Member Roles Within Groups**
ROLE	**BEHAVIORS**
TASK ROLES	
Coordinator	Clarifies ideas and suggestions that have been made within the group; brings relationships together to pursue common goals
Evaluator	Examines group plans and performance, measuring against group standards and goals
Elaborator	Explains and expands upon group plans and ideas
Energizer	Encourages and motivates group to perform at its maximum potential
Initiator	Outlines the task at hand for the group and proposes methods for solution
Orienter	Maintains direction within the group
MAINTENANCE ROLES	
Compromiser	Relieves conflict within the group by assisting members to reach a compromise agreeable to all
Encourager	Offers recognition and acceptance of others' ideas and contributions
Follower	Listens attentively to group interaction; is a passive participant
Gatekeeper	Encourages acceptance of and participation by all members of the group
Harmonizer	Minimizes tension within the group by intervening when disagreements produce conflict
INDIVIDUAL (PERSONAL) ROLES	
Aggressor	Expresses negativism and hostility toward other members; may use sarcasm in effort to degrade the status of others
Blocker	Resists group efforts; demonstrates rigid and sometimes irrational behaviors that impede group progress
Dominator	Manipulates others to gain control; behaves in authoritarian manner
Help-seeker	Uses the group to gain sympathy from others; seeks to increase self-confidence from group feedback; lacks concern for others or for the group as a whole
Monopolizer	Maintains control of the group by dominating the conversation
Mute or silent member	Does not participate verbally; remains silent for a variety of reasons—may feel uncomfortable with self-disclosure or may be seeking attention through silence
Recognition seeker	Talks about personal accomplishments in an effort to gain attention for self
Seducer	Shares intimate details about self with group; is the least reluctant of the group to do so; may frighten others in the group and inhibit group progress with excessive premature self-disclosure

Source: Benne, K. D., & Sheats, P. (1948, Spring). Functional roles of group members. *Journal of Social Issues, 4*(2), 41–49; Hobbs, D. J., & Powers, R. C. (1981). *Group member roles: For group effectiveness.* Ames: Iowa State University, Cooperative Extension Service.

Psychodrama

A specialized type of therapeutic group, called **psychodrama,** was introduced by J. L. Moreno, a Viennese psychiatrist. Moreno's method employs a dramatic approach in which clients become "actors" in life-situation scenarios.

The group leader is called the *director,* group members are the *audience,* and the *set,* or *stage,* may be specially designed or may just be any room or part of a room selected for this purpose. Actors are members from the audience who agree to take part in the "drama" by role-playing a situation about which they have been informed by the director. Usually, the situation is an issue with which one individual client has been struggling. The client plays the role of himself or herself and is called the *protagonist.* In this role, the client is able to express true feelings toward individuals (represented by group members) with whom he or she has unresolved conflicts.

In some instances, the group leader may ask for a client to volunteer to be the protagonist for that session. The client may choose a situation he or she wishes to enact and select the audience members to portray the roles of others in the life situation. The psychodrama setting provides the client with a safer and less threatening atmosphere than the real situation in which to express true feelings. Resolution of interpersonal conflicts is facilitated.

When the drama has been completed, group members from the audience discuss the situation they have observed, offer feedback, express their feelings, and relate their own similar experiences. In this way, all group members benefit from the session, either directly or indirectly.

Nurses often serve as actors, or role players, in psychodrama sessions. Leaders of psychodrama have graduate degrees in psychology, social work, nursing, or medicine with additional training in group therapy and specialty preparation to become a psychodramatist.

The Family as a Group

In family therapy, the family is viewed as a system in which the members are interdependent; a change in one part (member) within the system affects or creates change in all other parts (members). Thus, the major goal is to facilitate system change rather than focus on any one individual as the one in need of treatment.

Because the primary goal of family therapy is to facilitate change within the family as a group, it is important for the family therapist to identify who the family perceives to be family members and, ideally, to conduct an assessment with the entire family. One assessment tool often used by family therapists is a **genogram**. The genogram is a visual presentation of the members, their relationships, and sometimes their health issues, across several generations. It provides a convenient way to visualize and summarize a great deal of information in a concise format.

Nurses who conduct family therapy are expected to possess a graduate degree and have considerable knowledge of family theories. However, it is within the realm of the generalist registered nurse in psychiatric settings to contribute to the assessment, planning, and interventions with families for the purpose of counseling and education. All nurses should have a basic understanding of family dynamics and the ability to distinguish between functional and dysfunctional behaviors within a family system.

The Role of the Nurse in Therapeutic Groups

Nurses participate in group situations on a daily basis. In healthcare settings, nurses serve on or lead task groups that create policy, describe procedures, and plan patient care. They are also involved in a variety of other groups aimed at the institutional effort of serving the healthcare consumer. Nurses are encouraged to use the steps of the nursing process as a framework for task group leadership.

In psychiatry, nurses may lead various types of therapeutic groups, such as patient education, assertiveness training, grief support, parenting, and transition to discharge groups, among others. To function effectively in the leadership capacity for these groups, nurses need to be able to recognize various processes that occur in groups, such as the phases of group development, the various roles that people play within group situations, and the motivation behind these behaviors. They also need to be able to select the most appropriate leadership style for the type of group.

Generalist nurses may develop these skills as part of their undergraduate education, or they may pursue additional study while serving and learning as the co-leader of a group with a more experienced nurse leader.

Generalist nurses in psychiatry should not serve as leaders of psychotherapy groups. The *Psychiatric–Mental Health Nursing Scope and Standards of Practice* (American Nurses Association, American Psychiatric Nurses Association, & International Society of Psychiatric Nurses, 2014) specifies that nurses who serve as group psychotherapists should have a minimum of a master's degree in psychiatric nursing. Educational preparation in group theory, extended practice as a group co-leader or leader under the supervision of an experienced psychotherapist, and participation in group therapy on an experiential level are also recommended. Additional specialist training is required beyond the master's level to prepare nurses to become family therapists or psychodramatists.

Leading therapeutic groups is within the realm of nursing practice. Because group work is such a common therapeutic approach in the discipline of psychiatry, nurses working in this field must continually strive to expand their knowledge and use of group process as a significant psychiatric nursing intervention.

> **CLINICAL PEARL** Knowledge of human behavior in general and the group process in particular is essential to effective group leadership.

Summary and Key Points

- A *group* is defined as a collection of individuals whose association is founded on shared interests, values, norms, or purpose.
- Eight group functions identified by Sampson and Marthas (1990) are socialization, support, task completion, camaraderie, information sharing, normative influence, empowerment, and governance.
- The three major types of groups are task groups, teaching groups, and supportive-therapeutic groups.
- The function of task groups is to solve problems, make decisions, and achieve a specific outcome.
- In teaching groups, knowledge and information are conveyed to a number of individuals.
- The function of supportive-therapeutic groups is to facilitate members' learning how to deal effectively with emotional stress in their lives.
- In self-help groups, members share the same type of problem and help each other to prevent decompensation related to that problem.
- Therapeutic groups differ from group therapy in that the focus is not on psychotherapy but on interaction and relationships among group members with regard to a selected issue. Group therapy is more focused on specific models of psychotherapy, and the leaders generally have advanced degrees in psychology, social work, nursing, or medicine.
- Placement of the seating and size of the group can influence group interaction.
- Groups can be open ended (when members leave and others join at any time while the group is active) or closed ended (when groups have a predetermined, fixed time frame and all members join at the same time and leave when the group disbands).
- Yalom and Leszcz (2005) describe the following therapeutic factors that individuals derive from participation in therapeutic groups: the instillation of hope, universality, the imparting of information, altruism, the corrective recapitulation of the primary family group, the development of socializing techniques, imitative behavior, interpersonal learning, group cohesiveness, catharsis, and existential factors.
- Groups progress through three phases: the initial (orientation) phase, the working phase, and the termination phase.
- Group leadership styles include autocratic, democratic, and laissez-faire.
- Members play various roles within groups. These roles are categorized according to task roles, maintenance roles, and personal roles.
- Psychodrama is a specialized type of group therapy that uses a dramatic approach in which clients become "actors" in life-situation scenarios.
- The psychodrama setting provides the client with a safer and less threatening atmosphere than the real situation in which to express and work through unresolved conflicts.
- Family therapy is a specialized form of group intervention in which the client is the whole family

rather than any one individual and the goal is to facilitate change in the family system.

■ Nurses lead various types of therapeutic groups in the psychiatric setting. Knowledge of human behavior in general and the group process in particular is essential to effective group leadership.

■ Specialized training, in addition to a master's degree, is required for nurses to serve as group psychotherapists or psychodramatists.

Review Questions
Self-Examination/Learning Exercise

Select the answer that is most appropriate for each of the following questions:

1. Nicole is the nurse leader of a childbirth preparation group. Each week, she shows various films and sets out various reading materials. She expects the participants to utilize their time on a topic of their choice or practice skills they have observed on the films. Two couples have dropped out of the group, stating, "This is a big waste of time." Which type of group and style of leadership is described in this situation?
   a. Task; democratic
   b. Teaching; laissez-faire
   c. Self-help; democratic
   d. Supportive-therapeutic; autocratic

2. Aisha is a psychiatric nurse who has been selected to lead a group for women who desire to lose weight. The criterion for membership is that they must be at least 20 pounds overweight. All have tried to lose weight on their own many times in the past without success. At their first meeting, Aisha provides suggestions as the members determine what their goals will be and how they plan to achieve those goals. They decide how often they want to meet and what they plan to do at each meeting. Which type of group and style of leadership is described in this situation?
   a. Task; autocratic
   b. Teaching; democratic
   c. Self-help; laissez-faire
   d. Supportive-therapeutic; democratic

3. Eric is a staff nurse on a surgical unit. He has been selected as leader of a newly established group of staff nurses organized to determine ways to decrease the number of medication errors occurring on the unit. Eric has definite ideas about how to bring this about. He has also applied for the position of Head Nurse on the unit and believes that if he is successful in leading the group toward achievement of its goals, he can also facilitate his chances for promotion. At each meeting, he addresses the group in an effort to convince the members to adopt his ideas. Which type of group and style of leadership is described in this situation?
   a. Task; autocratic
   b. Teaching; autocratic
   c. Self-help; democratic
   d. Supportive-therapeutic; laissez-faire

4. The nurse leader is explaining about group "therapeutic factors" to members of the group. She tells the members that group situations are beneficial because members can see that they are not alone in their experiences. This is an example of which therapeutic factor?
   a. Altruism
   b. Imitative behavior
   c. Universality
   d. Imparting of information

Continued

Review Questions—cont'd
Self-Examination/Learning Exercise

5. Carol is the nurse leader of a bereavement group for widows. Nancy is a new member. She listens to the group and learns that Jane has been a widow for 5 years. Jane has adjusted well, and Nancy thinks maybe she can too. This is an example of which therapeutic factor?
   a. Universality
   b. Imitative behavior
   c. Installation of hope
   d. Imparting of information

6. Paul is a member of an anger management group. He knew that people did not want to be his friend because of his violent temper. In the group, he has learned to control his temper and form satisfactory interpersonal relationships with others. This is an example of which therapeutic factor?
   a. Catharsis
   b. Altruism
   c. Imparting of information
   d. Development of socializing techniques

7. Benjamin is a member of an Alcoholics Anonymous group. He learned about the effects of alcohol on the body when a nurse from the chemical dependency unit spoke to the group. This is an example of which therapeutic factor?
   a. Catharsis
   b. Altruism
   c. Imparting of information
   d. Universality

8. Sandra is the nurse leader of a supportive-therapeutic group for individuals with anxiety disorders. In this group, Helen talks incessantly. When someone else tries to make a comment, Helen refuses to allow him or her to speak. What type of member role is Helen assuming in this group?
   a. Aggressor
   b. Monopolizer
   c. Blocker
   d. Seducer

9. Sandra is the nurse leader of a supportive-therapeutic group for individuals with anxiety disorders. On the first day the group meets, Valerie speaks first and begins by sharing the intimate details of her incestuous relationship with her father. What type of member role is Valerie assuming in this group?
   a. Aggressor
   b. Monopolizer
   c. Blocker
   d. Seducer

10. Sandra is the nurse leader of a supportive-therapeutic group for individuals with anxiety disorders. Violet, who lacks self-confidence, states to the group, "Maybe if I became a blond, my boyfriend would love me more." Larry responds, "Listen, dummy, you need more than blond hair to keep the guy around. A bit more in the brains department would help!" What type of member role is Larry assuming in this group?
   a. Aggressor
   b. Monopolizer
   c. Blocker
   d. Seducer

References

American Nurses Association (ANA), American Psychiatric Nurses Association, & International Society of Psychiatric Nurses. (2014). *Psychiatric-mental health nursing: Scope and standards of practice* (2nd ed.). Silver Spring, MD: Nursesbooks.org.

Clark, C. C. (2009). *Group leadership skills for nurses and health professionals* (5th ed.). New York, NY: Springer.

Forsyth, D. R. (2019). *Group dynamics* (7th ed.). Boston, MA: Cengage Learning.

Sampson, E. E., & Marthas, M. (1990). *Group process for the health professions* (3rd ed.). Albany, NY: Delmar.

Yalom, I. D., & Leszcz, M. (2005). *The theory and practice of group psychotherapy* (5th ed.). New York, NY: Basic Books.

Classical References

Benne, K. D., & Sheats, P. (1948, Spring). Functional roles of group members. *Journal of Social Issues, 4*(2), 41–49.

Hobbs, D. J., & Powers, R. C. (1981). *Group member roles: For group effectiveness.* Ames: Iowa State University, Cooperative Extension Service.

Lippitt, R., & White, R. K. (1958). An experimental study of leadership and group life. In E. E. Maccoby, T. M. Newcomb, & E. L. Hartley (Eds.), *Readings in social psychology* (3rd ed.). New York, NY: Holt, Rinehart & Winston.

9

Crisis Intervention

CORE CONCEPT
Crisis

KEY TERMS

crisis intervention
disaster

prodromal syndrome

OBJECTIVES
After reading this chapter, the student will be able to:

1. Define *crisis*.
2. Describe four phases in the development
   of a crisis.
3. Identify types of crises that occur in
   people's lives.
4. Discuss the goal of crisis intervention.
5. Describe the steps in crisis intervention.
6. Identify the role of the nurse in crisis
   intervention.
7. Apply the nursing process to care
   of victims of disasters.
8. Define and differentiate between anger
   and aggression.
9. Discuss predisposing factors to the
   maladaptive expression of anger.

HOMEWORK ASSIGNMENT
Please read the chapter and answer the following questions:

1. Name the three factors that determine
   whether or not a person experiences a
   crisis in response to a stressful situation.
2. What is the goal of crisis intervention?
3. Individuals in crisis need to develop more
   adaptive coping strategies. How does
   the nurse provide assistance with this
   process?
4. Describe behaviors common to preschool
   children following a traumatic event.

Introduction

Stressful situations are a part of everyday life. Any stressful situation can precipitate a crisis. Crises result in a disequilibrium from which many individuals require assistance to recover. Crisis intervention requires problem-solving skills that are often diminished by the level of anxiety accompanying disequilibrium. Assistance with problem-solving during the crisis period preserves self-esteem and promotes growth with resolution.

In recent years, individuals in the United States have been faced with a number of catastrophic events, including natural disasters such as tornados, earthquakes, hurricanes, and floods. Also, man-made disasters, such as the Oklahoma City and Boston Marathon bombings and the attacks on the World Trade Center and the Pentagon have created psychological stress of enormous proportions in populations around the world.

This chapter examines the phases in the development of a crisis and the types of crises that occur in people's lives. The methodology of crisis intervention, including the role of the nurse, is explored. A discussion of disaster nursing is also presented.

> ## CORE CONCEPT
> **Crisis**
> A sudden event in one's life that disturbs homeostasis, during which usual coping mechanisms cannot resolve the problem (Lagerquist, 2012, p. 795).

Characteristics of a Crisis

A number of characteristics have been identified that can be viewed as assumptions upon which the concept of crisis is based (Aguilera, 1998; Caplan, 1964; Winston, 2008). They include the following:

1. Crisis occurs in all individuals at one time or another and is not necessarily equated with psychopathology.
2. Crises are precipitated by specific identifiable events.
3. Crises are personal by nature. What may be considered a crisis situation by one individual may not be so for another.
4. Crises are acute, not chronic, and will be resolved in one way or another within a brief period.
5. A crisis situation contains the potential for psychological growth or deterioration.

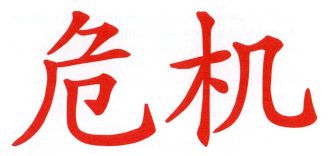

FIGURE 9–1   Chinese symbol for crisis.

Individuals who are in crisis feel helpless to change. They do not believe they have the resources to deal with the precipitating stressor. Levels of anxiety rise to the point that the individual becomes nonfunctional, thoughts become obsessional, and all behavior is aimed at relief of the anxiety being experienced. The feeling is overwhelming and may affect the individual physically as well as psychologically.

Bateman and Peternelj-Taylor (1998) stated:

> Outside Western culture, a crisis is often viewed as a time for movement and growth. The Chinese symbol for crisis consists of the characters for *danger* and *opportunity* [Fig. 9–1]. When a crisis is viewed as an opportunity for growth, those involved are much more capable of resolving related issues and more able to move toward positive changes. When the crisis experience is overwhelming because of its scope and nature or when there has not been adequate preparation for the necessary changes, the dangers seem paramount and overshadow any potential growth. The results are maladaptive coping and dysfunctional behavior. (pp. 144–145)

Phases in the Development of a Crisis

The development of a crisis situation follows a relatively predictable course. Caplan (1964) outlined four specific phases through which individuals progress in response to a precipitating stressor and that culminate in the state of acute crisis:

Phase 1. *The individual is exposed to a precipitating stressor.* Anxiety increases; previous problem-solving techniques are employed.

Phase 2. *When previous problem-solving techniques do not relieve the stressor, anxiety increases further.* The individual begins to feel a great deal of discomfort at this point. Coping techniques that have worked in the past are attempted, only to create feelings of helplessness when they are not successful. Feelings of confusion and disorganization prevail.

Phase 3. *All possible resources, both internal and external, are called on to resolve the problem and relieve the discomfort.* The individual may try to view the problem from a different perspective or even to overlook certain aspects of it. New problem-solving techniques may be used, and if effective, resolution may occur at this phase, with the individual returning to a higher, a lower, or the previous level of precrisis functioning.

Phase 4. *If resolution does not occur in previous phases, "the tension mounts beyond a further threshold or its burden increases over time to a breaking point. Major disorganization of the individual with drastic results often occurs"* (Caplan, 1998, p. 41). Anxiety may reach panic levels. Cognitive functions are disordered, emotions are labile, and behavior may reflect the presence of psychotic thinking.

These phases are congruent with the concept of "balancing factors" as described by Aguilera (1998). When individuals perceive a stressor as a threat to their well-being and they lack adaptive coping strategies or employ maladaptive strategies, crisis ensues. Similarly, Aguilera (1998) spoke of "balancing factors" that affect the way in which individuals perceive and respond to a precipitating stressor. A schematic of these balancing factors is illustrated in Figure 9–2.

The paradigm set forth by Aguilera suggests that whether or not an individual experiences a crisis in response to a stressful situation depends on the following three factors:

1. **The individual's perception of the event.** If the event is perceived realistically, the individual is more likely to draw upon adequate resources to restore equilibrium. If the perception of the event is distorted, attempts at problem-solving are likely to be ineffective, and equilibrium is not restored.

2. **The availability of situational supports.** Aguilera stated, "Situational supports are those persons who are available in the environment and who can be depended on to help solve the problem" (p. 37). Without adequate situational supports during a stressful situation, an individual is most likely to feel overwhelmed and alone.

3. **The availability of adequate coping mechanisms.** When a stressful situation occurs, individuals draw upon behavioral strategies that have been successful for them in the past. If these coping strategies work, a crisis may be diverted. If not, disequilibrium may continue, and tension and anxiety increase.

As previously stated, it is assumed that crises are acute, not chronic, situations that will be resolved in one way or another within a brief period. Winston (2008) stated, "Crises tend to be time limited, generally lasting no more than a few months; the duration depends on the stressor and on the individual's perception of and response to the stressor" (p. 1270).

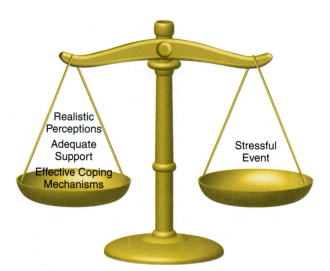

Stressful event is balanced by realistic perceptions, adequate support, effective coping mechanisms ➡ Equilibrium ➡ **No crisis**

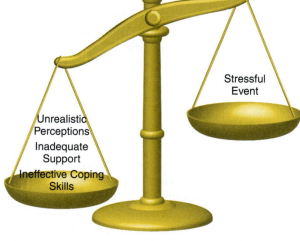

Problem unresolved ➡ Disequilibrium ➡ **Crisis**

FIGURE 9–2 The effect of balancing factors in a stressful event.

Crises can become growth opportunities when individuals learn new methods of coping that can be preserved and used when similar stressors recur.

Types of Crises

Baldwin (1978) identified six classes of emotional crises, which progress by degree of severity. As the measure of psychopathology increases, the source of the stressor changes from external to internal. The type of crisis determines the method of intervention selected.

Class 1: Dispositional Crises

Definition An acute response to an external situational stressor.

EXAMPLE

Brittany and Ethan have been married for 3 years and have a 1-year-old daughter. Ethan has been having difficulty with his boss at work. Twice during the past 6 months he has exploded in anger at home and become abusive with Brittany. Last night he became angry that dinner was not ready when he expected. He grabbed the baby from Brittany and tossed her, screaming, into her crib. He hit and punched Brittany until she feared for her life. This morning when he left for work, she took the baby and went to the emergency department of the city hospital, not knowing what else to do.

Intervention Physical care of wounds and screening for domestic violence issues should be conducted in the emergency department. The mental health counselor can provide support and guidance in terms of presenting alternatives to her. The emergency nurse should encourage and empower Brittany to clarify her needs and issues so that referrals for agency assistance can be made.

Class 2: Crises of Anticipated Life Transitions

Definition Normal life-cycle transitions that may be anticipated but over which the individual may feel a lack of control.

EXAMPLE

College student J.T. is placed on probationary status because of low grades this semester. His wife had a baby and had to quit her job. He increased his working hours from part time to full time to compensate and therefore had little time for studies. He presents himself to the student-health nurse practitioner and describes numerous vague physical complaints.

Intervention Physical examination should be performed (physical symptoms could be caused by depression) and ventilation of feelings encouraged. Reassurance and support should be provided as needed. J.T. should be referred to services that can provide financial and other types of needed assistance. Problematic areas should be identified and approaches to change discussed.

Class 3: Crises Resulting From Traumatic Stress

Definition Crisis precipitated by an unexpected external stressor over which the individual has little or no control and as a result of which he or she feels emotionally overwhelmed and defeated.

EXAMPLE

Ava is a waitperson whose shift ended at midnight. Two weeks ago, while walking to her car in the deserted parking lot, she was abducted by two men with guns, taken to an abandoned building, and raped and beaten. Since that time, her physical wounds have nearly healed. However, Ava cannot be alone, is constantly fearful, relives the experience in flashbacks and dreams, and is unable to eat, sleep, or work at her job in the restaurant. Her friend offers to accompany her to the mental health clinic.

Intervention The nurse should offer Ava the opportunity to talk about the experience and to express her feelings about the trauma when she demonstrates readiness. The nurse should offer reassurance and support; discuss stages of grief and how rape may precipitate feelings of loss, including loss of control, loss of power, and loss of a sense of self-worth, triggering the grief response; identify support systems that can help Ava to resume her normal activities; and explore new methods of coping with emotions arising from a situation with which she has had no previous experience. These interventions should be conducted in an environment that is sensitive to the impact of trauma on a person's sense of self and all interventions should convey dignity, respect, and hopefulness and promote the client's empowerment to make choices in his or her care (Substance Abuse and Mental Health Services Administration [SAMHSA], 2014)). See Chapter 19, Trauma- and Stressor-Related Disorders, for more information on trauma-informed care.

Class 4: Maturational and Developmental Crises

Definition Crises that occur in response to failed attempts to master developmental tasks associated with transitions in the life cycle.

EXAMPLE

Jada and Caleb have been married for 2 years, and their firstborn child is 4 months old. Jada's mother was recently diagnosed with cancer, and the prognosis is unclear. Over the past 3 weeks Jada has become increasingly anxious and disorganized. She has been calling the nurse practitioner 10 to 15 times each day with new fears that she is not addressing her child's health needs. Jada has been screaming at Caleb that he is never there when she needs help with the baby and states she is thinking of dropping their child off at the children's services agency because she believes they are both unable to be effective parents. She agrees to see a counselor at Caleb's insistence.

Intervention The primary intervention is to help Jada with anxiety reduction. When individuals have intense anxiety, their ability to gain insight about contributing factors and explore options for behavior change is impaired. The safety of their child should also be carefully assessed. Referrals and guidance in parenting skills may also lessen the anxiety associated with this new developmental phase. Anxiety and grief related to Jada's mother's illness could also be explored as a possible contributing factor to the current crisis.

Class 5: Crises Reflecting Psychopathology

Definition A crisis that is influenced or triggered by pre-existing psychopathology. Examples of psychopathology that may precipitate crises include personality disorders, anxiety disorders, bipolar disorder, and schizophrenia.

EXAMPLE

Sonja, age 29, was diagnosed with borderline personality disorder at age 18. This disorder is believed to be rooted in deep fear of abandonment. She has been in therapy on a weekly basis for 10 years with several hospitalizations for suicide attempts during that time. She has had the same therapist for the past 6 years. This therapist told Sonja today that she is to be married in 1 month and will be moving across the country with her new husband. Sonja is distraught, stating that no one cares about her and that she would be better off dead. She is found wandering in and out of traffic on a busy expressway, oblivious to her surroundings. Police bring her to the emergency department of the hospital.

Intervention The initial goal is to reduce Sonja's anxiety. She requires that someone stay with her and reassure her of her safety and security. After the feelings of panic and anxiety have subsided, she should be encouraged to verbalize her feelings of abandonment. Regressive behaviors should be discouraged. Positive reinforcement should be given for independent activities and accomplishments.

The primary therapist will need to pursue this issue of termination with Sonja and facilitate transfer of services to another therapist or treatment program. Hospitalization may be necessary to maintain patient safety.

Class 6: Psychiatric Emergencies

Definition Crisis situations in which general functioning has been severely impaired and the individual rendered incompetent or unable to assume personal responsibility for his or her behavior. Examples include acutely suicidal individuals, drug overdoses, reactions to hallucinogenic drugs, acute psychoses, uncontrollable anger, and alcohol intoxication.

EXAMPLE

Jennifer, age 14, had been dating Joe, the star high school football player, for 6 months. After the game on Friday night, Jennifer and Joe went to Jackie's house, where a number of high school students had gathered for an after-game party. No adults were present. About midnight, Joe told Jennifer that he did not want to date her anymore. Jennifer became hysterical, and Jackie was frightened by her behavior. She took Jennifer to her parent's bedroom and gave her a Valium from a bottle in her mother's medicine cabinet. She left Jennifer lying on her parent's bed and returned to the party downstairs. About an hour later, she returned to her parent's bedroom and found that Jennifer had removed the bottle of Valium from the cabinet and swallowed all of the tablets. Jennifer was unconscious, and Jackie could not awaken her. An ambulance was called, and Jennifer was transported to the local hospital.

Intervention Emergency medical care, including monitoring vital signs, ensuring maintenance of adequate airway, and initiating gastric lavage and/or activated charcoal, is the priority in this case. Jennifer is a minor, so notifying the parents is essential as well. Inpatient hospitalization is justifiable to ensure patient safety. Discussing feelings about self-esteem, rejection, and loss will help Jennifer explore more adaptive methods of dealing with stressful situations.

Crisis on the Inpatient Unit: Anger and Aggression Management

Assessment

Sometimes crises occur for hospitalized psychiatric patients when they become unable to manage personal responsibility for their behaviors in response to anger. Nurses must be aware of the symptoms associated with anger and aggression in order to make an accurate assessment. Because the best intervention is prevention, risk factors for assessing violence potential are also presented.

Symptoms Associated With Anger and Aggression

Anger

Anger is often manifested in the following ways:

- Anxious, tense, frowning, or angry facial expression (affect)
- Clenched fists
- Low-pitched verbalizations forced through clenched teeth
- Yelling and shouting
- Intense eye contact or avoidance of eye contact
- Hypersensitivity, easily offended
- Defensive response to criticism
- Passive-aggressive behaviors
- Lack of control or overcontrolled emotions
- Intense discomfort; continuous state of tension
- Flushed face

Anger is often described as a secondary emotion. For example, it may be a response to unresolved grief, depression, fear, anxiety, or unresolved post-traumatic stress. Anger is also one of the stages of the normal grief process and thus is an expected emotion. Because of the negative connotation to the word *anger,* some clients will not acknowledge that what they are feeling is anger. These individuals need assistance to recognize their true feelings and to understand that anger is a perfectly acceptable emotion when it is expressed appropriately; it is one's *behavior* in response to anger that may be unacceptable, such as when it results in aggression.

Aggression

Aggression can arise from a number of feeling states, including anger, anxiety, guilt, frustration, or suspiciousness. Aggressive behaviors can be classified as mild (e.g., sarcasm), moderate (e.g., slamming doors), severe (e.g., threats of physical violence against others), or extreme (e.g., physical acts of violence against others). Aggression may be evidenced in many behaviors, including (but not limited to) the following defining characteristics:

- Pacing, restlessness
- Threatening body language
- Verbal or physical threats
- Loud voice, shouting, use of obscenities, argumentativeness

- Threats of homicide or suicide
- Increase in agitation, with overreaction to environmental stimuli
- Panic anxiety, leading to misinterpretation of the environment
- Suspiciousness and defensive posturing
- Angry mood, often disproportionate to the situation
- Destruction of property
- Acts of physical harm toward another person

Kassinove (2016) states that aggression may include verbal and physical attacks that intend harm to another and often reflect a desire for dominance and control.

Aggression may be differentiated as reactive versus proactive. Reactive aggression is defined as fear-based and impulsive; proactive aggression is described as predatory and calculated. In both cases there is intent to harm another, but the motives differ. Intent is a requisite in the definition of aggression. It refers to behavior that is *intended* to inflict harm or destruction. Accidents that lead to *unintentional* harm or destruction are not considered aggression.

Assessing Risk Factors

Prevention is the key issue in the management of aggressive or violent behavior. The individual who becomes violent usually feels an underlying helplessness. Three factors have been identified as important considerations in assessing for potential violence:

1. Past history of violence
2. Client diagnosis
3. Current behavior

Past history of violence is widely recognized as a major risk factor for violence in a treatment setting. Assaultive behavior is also highly correlated with diagnosis. Substance abuse (alone or in combination with a mental illness) is the single largest risk factor for violence; the lifetime prevalence is 35 percent in individuals with substance abuse or dependence compared to 16 percent for those with schizophrenia or a major affective disorder and a notable 43.6 percent in those with a comorbid mental illness and substance abuse (Victoroff, 2017).

Novitsky, Julius, and Dubin (2009) stated:

The successful management of violence is predicated on an understanding of the dynamics of violence. A patient's threatening behavior is commonly an overreaction to feelings of impotence, helplessness, and perceived or actual humiliation. Aggression rarely occurs suddenly and unexpectedly. (p. 50)

Novitsky and associates describe a **prodromal syndrome** that is characterized by anxiety and tension, verbal abuse and profanity, and increasing hyperactivity. These escalating behaviors usually do not occur in stages but most often overlap and sometimes occur simultaneously. Behaviors associated with this prodromal stage include rigid posture; clenched fists and jaws; grim, defiant affect; talking in a rapid, raised voice; arguing and demanding; using profanity and threatening verbalizations; agitation and pacing; and pounding and slamming.

Most assaultive behavior is preceded by a period of increasing hyperactivity. Behaviors associated with the prodromal syndrome should be considered emergent and demand immediate attention. Keen observation skills and background knowledge for accurate assessment are critical factors in predicting potential for violent behavior. The Brøset

Violence Checklist (BVC) is presented in Box 9–1. It is a quick, simple, and reliable checklist that can be used as a risk assessment for potential violence. Testing has shown 63 percent accuracy for prediction of violence at a score of 2 or above (Almvik, Woods, & Rasmussen, 2000). De-escalation techniques are also included.

Diagnosis and Outcome Identification

NANDA International does not include a separate nursing diagnosis for anger, and in and of itself, anger is not an unhealthy response. Anger is one of a broad range of normal emotional responses but becomes an unhealthy response only when the behaviors that accompany anger are harmful to self or others. The nursing diagnosis of complicated grieving may be used when anger is related to a loss and is being expressed inappropriately.

BOX 9–1 The Brøset Violence Checklist

Behaviors	Score (Score 1 point for each behavior observed. At a score of ≥2, begin de-escalation techniques.)
Confusion Irritability Boisterousness Physical threats Verbal threats Attacks on objects Total Score	

De-escalation techniques:

Calm voice Helpful attitude Identify consequences Open hands and nonthreatening posture Allow phone call Offer food or drink Decrease waiting times and request refusals Distract with a more positive activity (e.g., soft music or a quiet room)	Walk outdoors or fresh air Reduction in demands Group participation Relaxation techniques Express concern Reduce stimulation and loud noise Verbal redirection and limit setting Time out, quiet time, open seclusion Offer prn medication

If de-escalation techniques fail:

Suggest prn medications

Time out or unlocked seclusion, which can progress to locked seclusion if all other de-escalation strategies and less restrictive measures have been unsuccessful

Source: Almvik, R., Woods, P., & Rasmussen, K. (2000). The Brøset violence checklist: Sensitivity, specificity, and interrater reliability. Journal of Interpersonal Violence, 15(12), *1284–1296. With permission. De-escalation techniques reprinted with permission from Barbara Barnes, Milwaukee County Behavioral Health Division.*

The following nursing diagnoses may be considered for clients demonstrating inappropriate behaviors in response to anger:

■ Ineffective coping related to anger and feelings of helplessness or negative role modeling evidenced by yelling, name calling, hitting others, and temper tantrums as expressions of anger
■ Risk for self-directed or other-directed violence related to inadequate anger management

Outcome Criteria

Outcome criteria include short- and long-term goals. Timelines are individually determined. The following criteria may be used for measurement of outcomes in the care of the patient needing assistance with management of anger and aggression.

The patient:

1. Recognizes when he or she is angry and seeks out staff to talk about his or her feelings.

2. Takes responsibility for his or her feelings of anger.
3. Demonstrates the ability to exert self-control over feelings of anger.
4. Demonstrates ability to diffuse anger before losing control.
5. Uses the tension generated by the anger in a constructive manner.
6. Causes no harm to self or others.
7. Uses steps of the problem-solving process rather than becoming violent as a means of seeking solutions.

Planning and Implementation

In Table 9–1, a plan of care is presented for the patient who expresses anger inappropriately. Outcome criteria and appropriate nursing interventions with rationales are included for each diagnosis.

TABLE 9–1 | CARE PLAN FOR THE INDIVIDUAL WHO EXPRESSES ANGER INAPPROPRIATELY

NURSING DIAGNOSIS: INEFFECTIVE COPING

RELATED TO: (Possible) negative role modeling, feelings of helplessness

EVIDENCED BY: Yelling, name calling, hitting others, and temper tantrums as expressions of anger

OUTCOME CRITERIA	NURSING INTERVENTION	RATIONALE
Patient recognizes anger in self and takes responsibility before losing control.	1. Remain calm when dealing with an angry patient. 2. Set verbal limits on behavior. Clearly delineate the consequences of inappropriate expression of anger, and always follow through.	1. Anger expressed by the nurse will most likely incite increased anger in patient. 2. Consistency in enforcing the consequences is essential if positive outcomes are to be achieved. Inconsistency creates confusion and encourages testing of limits.
	3. Have patient keep a diary of angry feelings, what triggered them, and how they were handled. 4. Avoid touching patient when he or she becomes angry. 5. Help patient determine the true source of the anger.	3. Journaling provides a more objective measure of the problem. 4. Patient may view touch as threatening and could become violent. 5. Often, anger is being displaced onto a safer object or person. If resolution is to occur, the first step is to identify the source of the problem.
	6. Help patient find alternative ways to release tension, such as physical outlets, and more appropriate ways to express anger, such as seeking out staff when feelings emerge. 7. Role model appropriate ways to express anger assertively, such as, "I dislike being called names. I get angry when I hear you saying those things about me."	6. Patient will likely need assistance to problem solve more appropriate ways of behaving. 7. Role modeling is one of the strongest methods of learning.

Continued

TABLE 9–1 | CARE PLAN FOR THE INDIVIDUAL WHO EXPRESSES ANGER INAPPROPRIATELY–cont'd

NURSING DIAGNOSIS: RISK FOR SELF-DIRECTED OR OTHER-DIRECTED VIOLENCE

RELATED TO: History of violence, inadequate management of anger, post-trauma stress

OUTCOME CRITERIA	NURSING INTERVENTION	RATIONALE
Patient does not harm self or others. Patient verbalizes anger rather than hit others.	1. Observe for escalation of anger (called the *prodromal syndrome*): increased motor activity, pounding, slamming, tense posture, defiant affect, clenched teeth and fists, arguing, demanding, and challenging or threatening staff.	1. Violence may be prevented if risks are identified in time.
	2. When these behaviors are observed, first ensure that sufficient staff are available to help with a potentially violent situation. Attempt to defuse the anger beginning with the least restrictive means.	2. The initial consideration must be having enough help to diffuse a potentially violent situation. Patient rights must be honored while preventing harm to patient and others.
	3. Techniques for dealing with aggression include:	3. Aggression control techniques promote safety and reduce risk of harm to patient and others:
	a. *Talking down*. For example, say, "John, you seem very angry. Let's sit down and talk about it." (Maintain safe distance and opportunity to leave the immediate area if needed.)	a. Promote a trusting relationship and may prevent patient's anxiety from escalating.
	b. *Physical outlets*. For example, say, "Maybe it would help if you did some walking or other exercise for a while to help you safely release this energy" or "I'll stay here with you if you want."	b. Provide effective way for patient to release tension associated with high levels of anger.
	c *Medication*. If agitation continues to escalate, offer patient choice of taking medication voluntarily. If he or she refuses, reassess the situation to determine if harm to self or others is imminent.	c. Tranquilizing medication may calm patient and prevent violence from escalating.
	d. *Call for assistance*. Remove self and other patients from the immediate area. Call violence code, push "panic" button, call for assault team, or institute measures established by the institution. Sufficient staff to indicate a show of strength may be enough to de-escalate the situation, and patient may agree to take the medication.	d. Patient and staff safety are of primary concern. Many states, accrediting bodies, and/or facilities require that staff members working with hospitalized psychiatric patients be trained and/or certified in psychiatric emergency interventions to ensure that the strategies used are in the best interest of staff and patient safety.
	e. *Seclusion or restraints*. If patient is not calmed by talking down or by medication, use of mechanical restraints and/or seclusion may be necessary. Be sure to have sufficient staff available to assist and appropriately deal with an out-of-control patient. Follow protocol for restraints/seclusion established by the institution. Restraints should be used as a last resort after all other interventions have been unsuccessful and patient is clearly at risk of harm to self or others.	e. Patients who do not have internal control over their own behavior may require external controls, such as mechanical restraints, in order to prevent harm to self or others.

TABLE 9–1 | CARE PLAN FOR THE INDIVIDUAL WHO EXPRESSES ANGER INAPPROPRIATELY—cont'd

OUTCOME CRITERIA	NURSING INTERVENTION	RATIONALE
	f. *Observation and documentation*. Hospital policy typically dictates the requirements for observation of patient in restraints. Basic safety principles include that patient in restraints should be observed throughout the period of restraint. Every 15 minutes, patient should be monitored to ensure that circulation to extremities is not compromised (check temperature, color, pulses). Assist patient with needs related to nutrition, hydration, and elimination. Position patient so that comfort is facilitated and aspiration can be prevented. (Patients should never be restrained in a prone position). Document all observations.	f. Patient and staff safety are of primary concern. Many state regulations, accrediting bodies (such as The Joint Commission), and/or facility policies require that staff members working with hospitalized psychiatric patients be trained and/or certified in psychiatric emergency interventions to ensure that the strategies used are in the best interest of staff and patient safety. Patient well-being is a nursing priority.
	g. *Ongoing assessment*. As agitation decreases, assess patient's readiness for restraint removal or reduction. With assistance from other staff members, remove one restraint at a time while assessing patient's response. This measure minimizes the risk of injury to patient and staff.	g. Gradual removal of the restraints allows for testing of patient's self-control. Patient and staff safety are of primary concern, as is ensuring that the patient is offered the least restrictive treatment option effective in maintaining safety.
	h. *Debriefing*. It is important when a patient loses control for staff to follow up with a discussion about the situation. This discussion should occur with patient and among other staff. The staff should discuss factors that necessitated the crisis intervention, factors that contributed to the failure of less restrictive interventions, and staff's thoughts about the safety and effectiveness of the intervention. When patient has regained control, a debriefing should occur in which patient is encouraged to discuss thoughts about what contributed to the crisis situation and about staff interventions and to explore strategies to avert a crisis situation in the future. It is also important to discuss the situation with other patients who witnessed the episode so they understand and process what happened. Some patients may fear that they could be at risk for experiencing a crisis or that they might be in danger when someone else's behavior becomes aggressive.	h. Debriefing helps to process the impact of the intervention. Mutual feedback is shared; staff and patient have an opportunity to process and learn from the event.

Evaluation

Evaluation consists of reassessment to determine if the nursing interventions have been successful in achieving the objectives of care. The following type of information may be gathered to determine the success of working with a patient exhibiting inappropriate expression of anger:

- Is the patient now able to recognize when he or she is angry?
- Can the patient take responsibility for these feelings and keep them in check without losing control?
- Does the patient seek out staff to talk about feelings when they occur?
- Is the patient able to transfer tension generated by the anger into constructive activities?
- Has harm to the patient and others been avoided?
- Is the patient able to solve problems adaptively without undue frustration and without becoming violent?

Crisis Intervention

Individuals experiencing crises have an urgent need for assistance. In **crisis intervention,** the therapist, or other intervener, becomes a part of the individual's life situation. Because of the individual's emotional state, he or she is unable to problem solve and so requires guidance and support from another to help mobilize the resources needed to resolve the crisis.

Lengthy psychological interpretations are not appropriate for crisis intervention. It is a time for doing what is needed to help the individual get relief and for calling into action all of the people and other resources required to do so. Aguilera (1998) stated:

> The goal of crisis intervention is the resolution of an immediate crisis. Its focus is on the supportive, with the restoration of the individual to his precrisis level of functioning or possibly to a higher level of functioning. The therapist's role is direct, supportive, and that of an active participant. (p. 24)

Crisis intervention takes place in inpatient settings, outpatient settings, and in the community. In the past few decades, people with mental illness have been increasingly involved with criminal justice personnel as first responders to manage mental health crisis situations. In 1988, the fatal shooting by police officers of a man with mental illness prompted the development of the *crisis intervention team (CIT) model* to ensure that select police officers are trained to identify mental illness and substance abuse, use de-escalation techniques, and divert individuals from criminal justice systems to mental health professionals (Watson & Fulambarker, 2012). Not all states have developed CIT training programs, but several studies have demonstrated improved safety outcomes for patients with mental illness where CIT-trained officers are available (National Alliance on Mental Illness [NAMI], 2018). Other resources that may be available for patients with mental illness who are experiencing an acute crisis include 24-hour crisis phone lines, walk-in crisis centers, mobile crisis teams, respite and residential services, and hospital services, including 23-hour observation beds. Nurses have a responsibility to know what resources exist in their community of practice. They can then become an important advocate for crisis intervention training in communities and can also be a support to families by encouraging them to ask for CIT-trained officers (where available) when they are faced with a family member's psychiatric crisis.

A more recent trend in some states, counties, and mental health facilities is to utilize *peer support specialists.* These are individuals who have personal experience with mental illness and who are trained and/or credentialed to help clients navigate everyday challenges of living with a mental illness. Evidence has demonstrated their effectiveness in diffusing psychiatric crises (Substance Abuse and Mental Health Services Administration [SAMHSA], 2015).

The basic methodology for crisis intervention work by healthcare professionals relies heavily on orderly problem-solving techniques and structured activities that are focused on change. Through adaptive change, crises are resolved and growth occurs. Because of the time limitation of crisis intervention, the individual must experience some degree of relief almost from the first interaction. Crisis intervention, then, is not aimed at major personality change or reconstruction (as may be the case in long-term psychotherapy) but rather at using a given crisis situation, at the very least, to restore functioning and, at most, to enhance personal growth.

Phases of Crisis Intervention: The Role of the Nurse

Nurses respond to crisis situations on a daily basis. Crises can occur on every unit in the general hospital, in the home setting, in the community healthcare setting, in schools and offices, and in private practice. Nurses may be called on to function as crisis helpers in virtually any setting committed to the practice of nursing.

Roberts and Ottens (2005) describe the clinical application of Roberts seven-stage model of crisis intervention. This model is summarized in Table 9–2. Aguilera (1998) described four specific phases in the technique of crisis intervention that are clearly comparable to the steps of the nursing process. These phases are discussed in the following paragraphs.

Phase 1. Assessment

In this phase, the nurse gathers information regarding the precipitating stressor and the resulting crisis that prompted the individual to seek professional help. A nurse in crisis intervention might perform some of the following assessments:

1. Ask the individual to describe the event that precipitated this crisis.
2. Determine when it occurred.
3. Assess the individual's mental *and* physical status.
4. Determine if the individual has experienced this stressor before. If so, what method of coping was used? Have these methods been tried this time?
5. If previous coping methods were tried, what was the result?
6. If new coping methods were tried, what was the result?
7. Assess suicide or homicide potential, plan, and means.
8. Assess the adequacy of support systems.
9. Determine level of precrisis functioning. Assess the usual coping methods, available support systems, and ability to problem solve.
10. Assess the individual's perception of personal strengths and limitations.
11. Assess the individual's use of substances.

TABLE 9–2 **Roberts' Seven-Stage Crisis Intervention Model**	
STAGE	**INTERVENTIONS**
Stage I. Psychosocial and lethality assessment	■ Conduct a rapid but thorough biopsychosocial assessment.
Stage II. Rapidly establish rapport	■ The counselor uses genuineness, respect, and unconditional acceptance to establish rapport with client. ■ Skills such as good eye contact, a nonjudgmental attitude, flexibility, and maintaining a positive mental attitude are important.
Stage III. Identify the major problems or crisis precipitants	■ Identify the precipitating event that led client to seek help at the present time. ■ Identify other situations that led to the precipitating event. ■ Prioritize major problems with which client needs help. ■ Discuss client's current style of coping and offer assistance in areas where modification would be helpful in resolving the present crisis and preventing future crises.
Stage IV. Deal with feelings and emotions	■ Encourage client to vent feelings. Provide validation. ■ Use therapeutic communication techniques to help client explain his or her story about the current crisis situation. ■ Eventually, and cautiously, begin to challenge maladaptive beliefs and behaviors, and help client adopt more rational and adaptive options.
Stage V. Generate and explore alternatives	■ Collaboratively explore options with client. ■ Identify coping strategies that have been successful for client in the past. ■ Help client problem solve strategies for confronting current crisis adaptively.
Stage VI. Implement an action plan	■ A shift from crisis to resolution occurs at this stage. ■ Develop a concrete plan of action to deal directly with the current crisis. ■ Having a concrete plan restores client's equilibrium and psychological balance. ■ Work through the meaning of the event that precipitated the crisis. How could it have been prevented? What responses may have aggravated the situation?
Stage VII. Follow up	■ Plan a follow-up visit with client to evaluate the postcrisis status of client. ■ Beneficial scheduling of follow-up visits includes 1-month and 1-year anniversaries of the crisis event.

Source: Adapted from Roberts, A. R., & Ottens, A. J. (2005). The seven-stage crisis intervention model: A road map to goal attainment, problem solving, and crisis resolution. *Brief Treatment and Crisis Intervention, 5*(4), 329–339.

Information from the comprehensive assessment is then analyzed, and appropriate nursing diagnoses reflecting the immediacy of the crisis situation are identified. Some nursing diagnoses that may be relevant include the following:

- Coping
- Anxiety (severe to panic)
- Disturbed thought processes (has been resigned from the NANDA-I list of approved diagnoses but is used for purposes of this textbook)
- Risk for self- or other-directed violence
- Rape-trauma syndrome
- Post-trauma syndrome
- Fear

Phase 2. Planning of Therapeutic Intervention

In the planning phase of crisis intervention, the nurse selects the appropriate nursing actions for the identified nursing diagnoses. In planning the interventions, the type of crisis, as well as the individual's strengths, desired choices, and available resources for support, are taken into consideration. Goals are established for crisis resolution and a return to, or increase in, the precrisis level of functioning.

Phase 3. Intervention

During phase 3, the actions that were identified in phase 2 are implemented. The following interventions are the focus of nursing in crisis intervention:

- Use a reality-oriented approach. The focus of the problem is on the here and now.
- Remain with the individual who is experiencing panic anxiety.
- Establish a rapid working relationship by showing unconditional acceptance, by active listening, and by attending to immediate needs.
- Discourage lengthy explanations or rationalizations of the situation; promote an atmosphere for verbalization of true feelings.
- Set firm limits on aggressive, destructive behaviors. At high levels of anxiety, behavior is likely to be impulsive and regressive. Establish at the outset what is acceptable and what is not and maintain consistency.
- Clarify the problem that the individual is facing. The nurse does this by describing his or her perception of the problem and comparing it with the individual's perception of the problem.
- Help the individual determine what he or she believes precipitated the crisis.

- Acknowledge feelings of anger, guilt, helplessness, and powerlessness without judgment.
- Guide the individual through a problem-solving process by which he or she may move in the direction of positive life change:
  - Help the individual confront the factors that are contributing to the experience of crisis.
  - Encourage the individual to discuss changes he or she would like to make. Jointly determine whether or not desired changes are realistic.
  - Encourage exploration of feelings about aspects that cannot be changed and explore alternative ways of coping more adaptively in these situations.
  - Discuss alternative strategies for creating changes that are realistically possible.
  - Weigh benefits and consequences of each alternative.
- Assist the individual to select alternative coping strategies that will help alleviate future crisis situations.
- Identify external support systems and new social networks from which the individual may seek assistance in times of stress.

> **CLINICAL PEARL** Coping mechanisms are highly individual and the choice ultimately must be made by the patient. The nurse may offer suggestions and provide guidance to help the patient identify coping mechanisms that are realistic for him or her, and that can promote positive outcomes in a crisis situation.

Phase 4. Evaluation of Crisis Resolution and Anticipatory Planning

To evaluate the outcome of crisis intervention, a reassessment is made to determine if the stated objective was achieved:

1. Have positive behavioral changes occurred?
2. Has the individual developed more adaptive coping strategies? Have they been effective?
3. Has the individual grown from the experience by gaining insight into his or her responses to crisis situations?
4. Does the individual believe that he or she could respond with healthy adaptation in future stressful situations to prevent crisis development?
5. Can the individual describe a plan of action for dealing with stressors similar to the one that precipitated this crisis?

During the evaluation period, the nurse and patient summarize what has occurred during the intervention. They review what the individual has learned and "anticipate" how he or she will respond in the future. A determination is made regarding follow-up therapy; if needed, the nurse provides referral information.

Disaster Nursing

Although there are many definitions of **disaster,** a common feature is that the event overwhelms local resources and threatens the function and safety of the community. A violent disaster, whether natural or man-made, may leave devastation to property or life. Such tragedies leave victims with a damaged sense of safety and well-being and varying degrees of emotional trauma. Often, spiritual distress is an issue as victims ask, "How could this have happened?" and "What is most important in life?" A care plan for responding to spiritual distress is included in Table 9–3. Children, who lack life experiences and coping skills, are particularly vulnerable. Their sense of order and security has been seriously disrupted, and they are unable to understand that the disruption is time-limited and that their world will eventually return to normal.

Application of the Nursing Process to Disaster Nursing

Background Assessment Data

Individuals respond to traumatic events in many ways. Grieving is a natural response following any loss, and it may be more extreme if the disaster is directly experienced or witnessed. The emotional effects of loss and disruption may show up immediately or may appear weeks or months later.

Psychological and behavioral responses common in adults following trauma and disaster include anger; disbelief; sadness; anxiety; fear; irritability; arousal; numbing; sleep disturbance; and increases in alcohol, caffeine, and tobacco use. Preschool children commonly experience separation anxiety, regressive behaviors, nightmares, and hyperactive or withdrawn behaviors. Older children may have difficulty concentrating, somatic complaints, sleep disturbances, and concerns about safety. Adolescents' responses are often similar to those of adults.

Traumatic bereavement is a term used to describe the grief process that accompanies unexpected losses resulting from traumatic events such as disasters. In such circumstances the survivor must come to grips not only with the loss but also the manner in which the loss occurred, and this can include powerful emotions ranging from guilt (at having survived when others lost their lives) to anger and rage (Assist Trauma Care, 2015). Ongoing assessment includes looking for signs of post-traumatic stress disorder (PTSD) and major depression that require additional intervention and treatment.

Nursing Diagnoses and Outcome Identification

Information from the assessment is analyzed, and appropriate nursing diagnoses reflecting the immediacy of the situation are identified. Some nursing diagnoses that may be relevant include the following:

1. Risk for injury (trauma, suffocation, poisoning)
2. Risk for infection
3. Anxiety (panic)
4. Fear
5. Spiritual distress
6. Risk for post-trauma syndrome
7. Ineffective community coping

The following criteria may be used for measurement of outcomes in the care of the patient having experienced a traumatic event. Timelines are individually determined.

The patient:

- Demonstrates behaviors necessary to protect self from further injury.
- Identifies interventions to prevent/reduce risk of infection.
- Maintains anxiety at a manageable level.
- Expresses beliefs and values about spiritual issues.
- Demonstrates ability to deal with emotional reactions in an individually appropriate manner.
- Demonstrates an increase in activities to improve community functioning.

Planning and Implementation

Table 9–3 provides a plan of care for the patient who has experienced a traumatic event. Selected nursing diagnoses are presented, along with outcome criteria, appropriate nursing interventions, and rationales for each.

Evaluation

In the final step of the nursing process, a reassessment is conducted to determine if the nursing actions have been successful in achieving the objectives of care. Evaluation of the nursing actions for the patient who

TABLE 9–3 | CARE PLAN FOR THE PATIENT WHO HAS EXPERIENCED A TRAUMATIC EVENT

NURSING DIAGNOSIS: **ANXIETY (PANIC)/FEAR**

RELATED TO: Real or perceived threat to physical well-being; threat of death; situational crisis; exposure to toxins; unmet needs

EVIDENCED BY: Persistent feelings of apprehension and uneasiness; sense of impending doom; impaired functioning; verbal expressions of having no control or influence over situation, outcome, or self-care; sympathetic stimulation; extraneous physical movements

OUTCOME CRITERIA	NURSING INTERVENTIONS	RATIONALE
Patient demonstrates that anxiety is at a manageable level. Patient demonstrates use of positive coping mechanisms to manage anxiety.	1. Determine degree of anxiety/fear present, associated behaviors (e.g., laughter, crying, calm or agitation, excited/hysterical behavior, expressions of disbelief and/or self-blame), and reality of perceived threat.	1. Clearly understanding patient's perception is pivotal to providing appropriate assistance in overcoming the fear. Individual may be agitated or totally overwhelmed. Panic state increases risk for harm to self or others in the environment.
	2. Note degree of disorganization.	2. Patient may be unable to handle activities of daily living or work requirements and may need more intensive intervention.
	3. Create as quiet an area as possible. Maintain a calm, confident manner. Speak in even tone using short, simple sentences.	3. Decreases sense of confusion or overstimulation; enhances sense of safety. Helps patient focus on what is said and reduces transmission of anxiety.
	4. Develop trusting relationship.	4. Trust is the basis of a therapeutic nurse-patient relationship and enables them to work effectively together.
	5. Identify whether incident has reactivated pre-existing or coexisting situations (physical or psychological).	5. Concerns and psychological issues are recycled every time trauma is re-experienced and affect how the individual views the current situation.
	6. Determine presence of physical symptoms (e.g., numbness, headache, tightness in chest, nausea, and pounding heart).	6. Physical problems need to be differentiated from anxiety symptoms so appropriate treatment can be given.
	7. Identify psychological responses (e.g., anger, shock, acute anxiety, panic, confusion, denial). Record emotional changes.	7. Although these are normal responses at the time of the trauma, they will recycle repeatedly until they are dealt with adequately.
	8. Discuss patient's perception of what is causing the anxiety.	8. Increases patient's ability to connect symptoms to subjective feeling of anxiety, providing opportunity to gain insight/control and make desired changes.
	9. Assist patient to correct any distortions being experienced. Share perceptions with patient.	9. Perceptions based on reality help to decrease fearfulness. How the nurse views the situation may help patient to see it differently.
	10. Explore with patient or significant other the manner in which patient has previously coped with anxiety-producing events.	10. May help patient regain sense of control and recognize significance of trauma.

TABLE 9–3 | CARE PLAN FOR THE PATIENT WHO HAS EXPERIENCED A TRAUMATIC EVENT—cont'd

OUTCOME CRITERIA	NURSING INTERVENTIONS	RATIONALE
	11. Engage patient in learning new coping behaviors (e.g., progressive muscle relaxation, thought-stopping)	11. Replacing maladaptive behaviors can enhance ability to manage and deal with stress. Interrupting obsessive thinking allows patient to use energy to address underlying anxiety, whereas continued rumination about the incident can retard recovery.
	12. Encourage use of techniques to manage stress and vent emotions such as anger and hostility.	12. Reduces the likelihood of eruptions that can result in abusive behavior.
	13. Give positive feedback when patient demonstrates better ways to manage anxiety and is able to calmly and realistically appraise the situation.	13. Provides acknowledgment and reinforcement, encouraging use of new coping strategies. Enhances patient's ability to deal with fearful feelings and gain control over situation, promoting future successes.
	14. Administer medications as indicated: Antianxiety—diazepam, alprazolam, oxazepam. Antidepressants—fluoxetine, paroxetine, bupropion.	14. Antianxiety medication provides temporary relief of anxiety symptoms, enhancing ability to cope with situation. Antidepressants lift mood and help suppress intrusive thoughts and explosive anger.

NURSING DIAGNOSIS: SPIRITUAL DISTRESS

RELATED TO: Physical or psychological stress; energy-consuming anxiety; loss(es), intense suffering; separation from religious or cultural ties; challenged belief and value system

EVIDENCED BY: Expressions of concern about disaster and the meaning of life and death or belief systems; inner conflict about current loss of normality and effects of the disaster; anger directed at deity; engaging in self-blame; seeking spiritual assistance

OUTCOME CRITERIA	NURSING INTERVENTIONS	RATIONALE
Patient expresses beliefs and values about spiritual issues.	1. Determine patient's religious/spiritual orientation, current involvement, and presence of conflicts.	1. Provides baseline for planning care and accessing appropriate resources.
	2. Establish environment that promotes free expression of feelings and concerns. Provide calm, peaceful setting when possible.	2. Promotes awareness and identification of feelings so they can be dealt with.
	3. Listen to patient's and significant other's expressions of anger, concern, alienation from God, belief that situation is a punishment for wrongdoing, and similar concerns.	3. It is helpful to understand patient's and significant other's points of view and how they are questioning their faith in the face of tragedy.
	4. Note sense of futility, feelings of hopelessness and helplessness, lack of motivation to help self.	4. These thoughts and feelings can result in patient feeling paralyzed and unable to move forward to resolve the situation.
	5. Listen to expressions of inability to find meaning in life and reason for living. Evaluate for suicidal ideation.	5. May indicate need for further intervention to prevent suicide attempt.
	6. Determine support systems available to patient.	6. Presence or lack of support systems can affect patient's recovery.

Continued

TABLE 9–3 | CARE PLAN FOR THE PATIENT WHO HAS EXPERIENCED A TRAUMATIC EVENT—cont'd

OUTCOME CRITERIA	NURSING INTERVENTIONS	RATIONALE
	7. Ask how you can be most helpful. Convey acceptance of patient's spiritual beliefs and concerns.	7. Promotes trust and comfort, encouraging patient to be open about sensitive matters.
	8. Make time for nonjudgmental discussion of philosophic issues and questions about spiritual impact of current situation.	8. Helps patient begin to look at basis for spiritual confusion. *Note:* There is a potential for care provider's belief system to interfere with patient finding own way. Therefore, it is most beneficial to remain neutral and not espouse own beliefs.
	9. Discuss difference between grief and guilt, and help patient to identify and deal with each, assuming responsibility for own actions, expressing awareness of the consequences of acting out of false guilt.	9. Blaming self for what has happened impedes dealing with the grief process and needs to be discussed and dealt with.
	10. Use therapeutic communication skills of reflection and active listening.	10. Helps patient find own solutions to concerns.
	11. Encourage patient to experience meditation, prayer, and forgiveness. Provide information that anger with God is a normal part of the grieving process.	11. This can help to heal past and present pain.
	12. Assist patient to develop goals for dealing with life situation.	12. Enhances commitment to goal, optimizing outcomes and promoting sense of hope.
	13. Identify and refer to resources that can be helpful, such as pastoral/parish nurse or religious counselor, crisis counselor, psychotherapy, Alcoholics Anonymous and/or Narcotics Anonymous.	13. Specific assistance may be helpful to recovery (e.g., relationship problems, substance abuse, suicidal ideation).
	14. Encourage participation in support groups.	14. Discussing concerns and questions with others can help patient resolve feelings.

NURSING DIAGNOSIS: RISK FOR POST-TRAUMA SYNDROME

RELATED TO: Events outside the range of usual human experience; serious threat or injury to self or loved ones; witnessing horrors or tragic events; exaggerated sense of responsibility; survivor's guilt or role in the event; inadequate social support

OUTCOME CRITERIA	NURSING INTERVENTIONS	RATIONALE
Patient demonstrates ability to deal with emotional reactions in an individually appropriate manner.	1. Determine involvement in event (e.g., survivor, significant other, rescue/aid worker, healthcare provider, family member).	1. All those concerned with a traumatic event are at risk for emotional trauma and have needs related to their involvement in the event. *Note:* Close involvement with victims affects individual responses and may prolong emotional suffering.
	2. Evaluate current factors associated with the event, such as displacement from home due to illness/injury, natural disaster, or terrorist attack. Identify how patient's past experiences may affect current situation.	2. Affects patient's reaction to current event and is basis for planning care and identifying appropriate support systems and resources.

TABLE 9–3 | CARE PLAN FOR THE PATIENT WHO HAS EXPERIENCED A TRAUMATIC EVENT—cont'd

OUTCOME CRITERIA	NURSING INTERVENTIONS	RATIONALE
	3. Listen for comments of taking on responsibility (e.g., "I should have been more careful or gone back to get her").	3. Statements such as these are indicators of "survivor's guilt" and blaming self for actions.
	4. Identify patient's current coping mechanisms.	4. Noting positive or negative coping skills provides direction for care.
	5. Determine availability and usefulness of patient's support systems, family, social contacts, and community resources.	5. Family and others close to patient may also be at risk and require assistance to cope with the trauma.
	6. Provide information about signs and symptoms of post-trauma response, especially if individual is involved in a high-risk occupation.	6. Awareness of these factors helps individual identify need for assistance when signs and symptoms occur.
	7. Identify and discuss patient's strengths as well as vulnerabilities.	7. Provides information to build on for coping with traumatic experience.
	8. Evaluate individual's perceptions of events and personal significance (e.g., rescue worker trained to provide lifesaving assistance but recovering only dead bodies).	8. Events that trigger feelings of despair and hopelessness may be more difficult to deal with and require long-term interventions.
	9. Provide emotional and physical presence by sitting with patient/significant other and offering solace.	9. Strengthens coping abilities.
	10. Encourage expression of feelings. Note whether feelings expressed appear congruent with events experienced.	10. It is important to talk about the incident repeatedly. Incongruencies may indicate deeper conflict and can impede resolution.
	11. Note presence of nightmares, reliving the incident, loss of appetite, irritability, numbness and crying, and family or relationship disruption.	11. These responses are normal in the early, post-incident time frame. If prolonged and persistent, they may indicate need for more intensive therapy.
	12. Provide a calm, safe environment.	12. Helps patient deal with the disruption in his or her life.
	13. Encourage and assist patient in learning stress-management techniques.	13. Promotes relaxation and helps individual exercise control over self and what has happened.
	14. Recommend participation in debriefing sessions that may be provided following major disaster events.	14. Dealing with the stresses promptly may facilitate recovery from the event or prevent exacerbation.
	15. Identify employment, community resource groups.	15. Provides opportunity for ongoing support to deal with recurrent feelings related to the trauma.
	16. Administer medications as indicated, such as antipsychotics (e.g., chlorpromazine, haloperidol, olanzapine, or quetiapine) or carbamazepine (Tegretol).	16. Low doses of antipsychotics may be used for reduction of psychotic symptoms when loss of contact with reality occurs, usually for patients with especially disturbing flashbacks. Carbamazepine may be used to alleviate intrusive recollections or flashbacks, impulsivity, and violent behavior.

Continued

TABLE 9–3 | CARE PLAN FOR THE PATIENT WHO HAS EXPERIENCED A TRAUMATIC EVENT—cont'd

NURSING DIAGNOSIS: INEFFECTIVE COMMUNITY COPING

RELATED TO: Natural or man-made disasters (earthquakes, tornados, floods, reemerging infectious agents, terrorist activity); ineffective or nonexistent community systems (e.g., lack of or inadequate emergency medical system, transportation system, or disaster planning systems)

EVIDENCED BY: Deficits of community participation; community does not meet its own expectations; expressed vulnerability; community powerlessness; stressors perceived as excessive; excessive community conflicts; high illness rates

OUTCOME CRITERIA	NURSING INTERVENTIONS	RATIONALE
Patient demonstrates an increase in activities to improve community functioning.	1. Evaluate community activities related to meeting collective needs within the community and between the community and the larger society. Note immediate needs, such as healthcare, food, shelter, funds.	1. Provides a baseline to determine community needs in relation to current concerns or threats.
	2. Note community reports of functioning, including areas of weakness or conflict.	2. Provides a view of how the community sees these areas.
	3. Identify effects of related factors on community activities.	3. In the face of a current threat, local or national, community resources need to be evaluated, updated, and given priority to meet the identified need.
	4. Determine availability and use of resources. Identify unmet demands or needs of the community.	4. Information is necessary to identify what else is needed to meet the current situation.
	5. Determine community strengths.	5. Promotes understanding of the ways in which the community is already meeting the identified needs.
	6. Encourage community members and groups to engage in problem-solving activities.	6. Promotes a sense of working together to meet community needs.
	7. Develop a plan jointly with the members of the community to address immediate needs.	7. Deals with deficits in support of identified goals.
	8. Create plans managing interactions within the community and between the community and the larger society.	8. Meets collective needs when the concerns or threats are shared beyond a local community.
	9. Make information accessible to the public. Provide channels for dissemination of information to the community as a whole (e.g., print media, radio and television reports and community bulletin boards, Internet sites, speaker's bureau, reports to committees, councils, advisory boards).	9. Readily available, accurate information can help citizens deal with the situation.

TABLE 9–3 | CARE PLAN FOR THE PATIENT WHO HAS EXPERIENCED A TRAUMATIC EVENT—cont'd

OUTCOME CRITERIA	NURSING INTERVENTIONS	RATIONALE
	10. Make information available in different modalities and geared to differing educational levels and cultures of the community.	10. Using languages other than English and making written materials accessible to all members of the community promotes understanding.
	11. Seek out and evaluate needs of underserved populations.	11. Homeless and those residing in lower income areas may have special requirements that need to be addressed with additional resources.

Source: Doenges, M. E., Moorhouse, M. F., & Murr, A. C. (2016). Nursing care plans: Guidelines for individualizing client care across the life span (14th ed.). Philadelphia, PA: F.A. Davis. With permission.

has experienced a traumatic event may be facilitated by gathering information utilizing the following types of questions.

Has the patient:

■ Been free from serious injury or infections or have they been resolved?

■ Been able to maintain anxiety at a manageable level?

■ Demonstrated appropriate problem-solving skills?

■ Discussed his or her beliefs about spiritual issues?

■ Demonstrated the ability to deal with emotional reactions in an individually appropriate manner?

■ Verbalized a subsiding of the physical manifestations (e.g., pain, nightmares, flashbacks, fatigue) associated with the traumatic event?

■ Recognized factors affecting the community's ability to meet its own demands or needs?

■ Demonstrated increased activities to improve community functioning?

■ Established and put in place a plan to deal with future contingencies?

Summary and Key Points

■ A *crisis* is defined as "a sudden event in one's life that disturbs homeostasis, during which usual coping mechanisms cannot resolve the problem" (Lagerquist, 2012, p. 795).

■ All individuals experience crises at one time or another. This does not necessarily indicate psychopathology. However, individuals with psychopathology are also vulnerable to crisis and may experience an exacerbation of psychiatric symptoms when in crisis.

■ Crises are precipitated by specific identifiable events and are determined by an individual's personal perception of the situation.

■ Crises are acute rather than chronic and generally last no more than a few weeks to a few months.

■ Crises occur when an individual is exposed to a stressor and previous problem-solving techniques are ineffective. This causes the level of anxiety to rise. Panic may ensue when new techniques are tried and resolution fails to occur.

■ Six types of crises have been identified: dispositional crises, crises of anticipated life transitions, crises resulting from traumatic stress, maturation and developmental crises, crises reflecting psychopathology, and psychiatric emergencies. The type of crisis determines the method of intervention selected.

■ Crisis intervention is designed to provide rapid assistance for individuals who have an urgent need.

■ The minimum therapeutic goal of crisis intervention is psychological resolution of the individual's immediate crisis and restoration to at least the level of functioning that existed before the crisis period. The ideal goal is improvement in functioning above the precrisis level.

■ Nurses regularly respond to individuals in crisis in all types of settings. Nursing process is the vehicle by which nurses assist individuals in crisis with a short-term problem-solving approach to change.

■ A four-phase technique of crisis intervention includes assessment and analysis, planning of therapeutic intervention, intervention, and evaluation of crisis resolution and anticipatory planning.

■ Through this structured method of assistance, nurses help individuals in crisis to develop more adaptive coping strategies for dealing with stressful situations in the future.

■ Nurses have many important skills that can assist individuals and communities in the wake of traumatic events. Nursing interventions presented in this chapter were developed for the nursing diagnoses of panic anxiety/fear, spiritual distress, risk for post-trauma syndrome, and ineffective community coping.

Review Questions
Self-Examination/Learning Exercise

Select the answer that is most appropriate for each of the following questions:

1. Which of the following is a correct assumption regarding the concept of crisis?
   a. Crises occur only in individuals with psychopathology.
   b. The stressful event that precipitates crisis is seldom identifiable.
   c. A crisis situation contains the potential for psychological growth or deterioration.
   d. Crises are chronic situations that recur many times during an individual's life.

2. Crises occur when an individual:
   a. Is exposed to a precipitating stressor.
   b. Perceives a stressor to be threatening.
   c. Has no support systems.
   d. Experiences a stressor and perceives coping strategies to be ineffective.

3. Amanda's mobile home was destroyed by a tornado. Amanda received only minor injuries but is experiencing disabling anxiety in the aftermath of the event. What is this type of crisis called?
   a. Crisis resulting from traumatic stress
   b. Maturational or developmental crisis
   c. Dispositional crisis
   d. Crisis of anticipated life transitions

4. The most appropriate crisis intervention with Amanda (from question 3) would be to:
   a. Encourage her to recognize how lucky she is to be alive.
   b. Discuss stages of grief and feelings associated with each.
   c. Identify community resources that can help Amanda.
   d. Suggest that she find a place to live that provides a storm shelter.

5. Jenny reported to the high school nurse that her mother drinks too much. She is drunk every afternoon when Jenny gets home from school. Jenny is afraid to invite friends over because of her mother's behavior. What is this type of crisis called?
   a. Crisis resulting from traumatic stress
   b. Maturational or developmental crisis
   c. Dispositional crisis
   d. Crisis reflecting psychopathology

6. The most appropriate nursing intervention with Jenny (from question 5) would be to:
   a. Make arrangements for her to start attending Alateen meetings.
   b. Help her identify the positive things in her life and recognize that her situation could be a lot worse than it is.
   c. Teach her about the effects of alcohol on the body and that it can be hereditary.
   d. Refer her to a psychiatrist for private therapy to learn to deal with her home situation.

7. Ginger, age 19 and an only child, left 3 months ago to attend a college of her choice 500 miles away from her parents. It is Ginger's first time away from home. She has difficulty making decisions and will not undertake anything new without first consulting her mother. They talk on the phone almost every day. Ginger has recently started having anxiety attacks. She consults the nurse practitioner in the student health center. What is this type of crisis called?
   a. Crisis resulting from traumatic stress
   b. Dispositional crisis
   c. Psychiatric emergency
   d. Maturational or developmental crisis

Review Questions—cont'd
Self-Examination/Learning Exercise

8. The most appropriate nursing intervention with Ginger (from question 7) would be to:
   a. Suggest she move to a college closer to home.
   b. Work with Ginger on unresolved dependency issues.
   c. Help her find someone in the college town from whom she could seek assistance rather than calling her mother regularly.
   d. Recommend that the college physician prescribe an antianxiety medication for Ginger.

9. Marie, age 56, is the mother of five children. Her youngest child, who had been living at home and attending the local college, recently graduated and accepted a job in another state. Marie has never worked outside the home and has devoted her life to satisfying the needs of her husband and children. Since the departure of her last child from home, Marie has become increasingly despondent. Her husband is very concerned and takes her to the local mental health center. What is this type of crisis called?
   a. Dispositional crisis
   b. Crisis of anticipated life transitions
   c. Psychiatric emergency
   d. Crisis resulting from traumatic stress

10. The most appropriate nursing intervention with Marie (from question 9) would be to:
    a. Refer her to her family physician for a complete physical examination.
    b. Suggest she seek outside employment now that her children have left home.
    c. Identify convenient support systems for times when she is feeling particularly despondent.
    d. Begin grief work and assist her to recognize areas of self-worth separate and apart from her children.

11. Which of the following is the desired outcome of working with an individual who has witnessed a traumatic event and is now experiencing panic anxiety?
    a. The individual will experience no anxiety.
    b. The individual will demonstrate hope for the future.
    c. The individual will identify that anxiety is at a manageable level.
    d. The individual will verbalize acceptance of self as worthy.

12. Andrew, a firefighter, and his entire unit responded to the aftermath of an earthquake. Working as a team, he and his best friend, Carlo, entered a building together to search for survivors. Carlo was killed when the building collapsed. Andrew was injured but survived. Since that time, Andrew has had frequent nightmares and anxiety attacks. He says to the mental health worker, "I don't know why Carlo had to die and I didn't!" This statement by Andrew suggests that he is experiencing:
    a. Spiritual distress.
    b. Night terrors.
    c. Survivor's guilt.
    d. Suicidal ideation.

13. Intervention with Andrew (from question 12) would include:
    a. Encouraging expression of feelings.
    b. Antianxiety medications.
    c. Participation in a support group.
    d. a and c.
    e. All of the above.

💬 **Communication Exercises**

1. A patient you have been working with for several days approaches you with apparent signs of agitation and yells in a loud voice, "I want out of this hospital right now! You don't listen to a thing I say, and my doctor just wants my money!"

   How will you respond?

2. Shelley enters the emergency department accompanied by a friend who reports that Shelley was raped after leaving a college campus party the night before. Shelley is staring off into space, exhibits a closed posture, and is mumbling inaudibly.

   How will you introduce yourself and begin to intervene in this crisis situation?

3. Thomas was secluded and restrained after punching another patient on the inpatient psychiatric unit. The next day he asks you what happened last night, stating he doesn't remember, and says he wants to know why he was arrested and tied up like an animal.

   What will you communicate to Thomas about the prior events and the crisis intervention process?

References

Aguilera, D. C. (1998). *Crisis intervention: Theory and methodology* (8th ed.). St. Louis, MO: C.V. Mosby.

Almvik, R., Woods, P., & Rasmussen, K. (2000). The Brøset violence checklist: Sensitivity, specificity, and interrater reliability. *Journal of Interpersonal Violence, 15*(12), 1284–1296.

Assist Trauma Care. (2015). *Traumatic bereavement.* Retrieved from http://assisttraumacare.org.uk/our-service/traumatic-bereavement/

Bateman, A., & Peternelj-Taylor, C. (1998). Crisis intervention. In C. A. Glod (Ed.), *Contemporary psychiatric-mental health nursing: The brain-behavior connection.* Philadelphia, PA: F.A. Davis.

Doenges, M. E., Moorhouse, M. F., & Murr, A. C. (2016). *Nurse's pocket guide: Diagnoses, prioritized interventions, and rationales* (14th ed.). Philadelphia, PA: F.A. Davis.

Kassinove, H. (2016). *How to recognize and deal with anger.* Retrieved from http://www.apa.org/helpcenter/recognize-anger.aspx

Lagerquist, S. L. (2012). *Davis's NCLEX-RN Success* (3rd ed.). Philadelphia, PA: F.A. Davis.

National Alliance on Mental Illness (NAMI). (2018). *What is CIT?* Retrieved from https://www.nami.org/Law-Enforcement-and-Mental-Health/What-Is-CIT

Novitsky, M. A., Julius, R. J., & Dubin, W. R. (2009). Nonpharmacologic management of violence in psychiatric emergencies. *Primary Psychiatry, 16*(9), 49–53.

Roberts, A. R., & Ottens, A. J. (2005). The seven-stage crisis intervention model: A road map to goal attainment, problem solving, and crisis resolution. *Brief Treatment and Crisis Intervention, 5*(4), 329–339.

Substance Abuse and Mental Health Services Administration (SAMHSA). (2014). *SAMHSA's concept of trauma and guidance for a trauma-informed approach.* Retrieved from https://store.samhsa.gov/shin/content//SMA14-4884/SMA14-4884.pdf

Substance Abuse and Mental Health Services Administration (SAMHSA). (2015). *Peer support and social inclusion.* Retrieved from https://www.samhsa.gov/recovery/peer-support-social-inclusion

Victoroff, J. (2017). The neuropsychiatry of human aggression. In B. A. Sadock, V. A. Sadock, & P. Ruiz (Eds.), *Comprehensive textbook of psychiatry* (10th ed.). Philadelphia, PA: Wolters Kluwer.

Watson, A. C., & Fulambarker, A. J. (2012). The crisis intervention team model of police response to mental health crisis: A primer for mental health practitioners. *Best Practices in Mental Health, 8*(2), 71.

Winston, A. (2008). Supportive psychotherapy. In R. E. Hales, S. C. Yudofsky, & G. O. Gabbard (Eds.), *Textbook of psychiatry* (5th ed., pp. 1257–1277). Washington, DC: American Psychiatric.

Classical References

Baldwin, B. A. (1978, July). A paradigm for the classification of emotional crises: Implications for crisis intervention. *American Journal of Orthopsychiatry, 48*(3), 538–551.

Caplan, G. (1964). *Principles of preventive psychiatry.* New York, NY: Basic Books.

The Recovery Model

CORE CONCEPT
Recovery

CHAPTER OUTLINE

Objectives

Homework Assignment

Introduction

What Is Recovery?

Guiding Principles of Recovery

Models of Recovery

Nursing Interventions That Assist
With Recovery

Summary and Key Points

Review Questions

Communication Exercises

KEY TERMS

hope

Psychological Recovery Model

purpose

Tidal Model

WRAP Model

OBJECTIVES
After reading this chapter, the student will be able to:

1. Define *recovery*.
2. Discuss the 10 guiding principles of recovery as delineated by the Substance Abuse and Mental Health Services Administration.
3. Describe three models of recovery: the Tidal Model, the WRAP Model,

and the Psychological Recovery Model.
4. Identify nursing interventions to assist individuals with mental illness in the process of recovery.

HOMEWORK ASSIGNMENT
Please read the chapter and answer the following questions:

1. What is the basic concept of a recovery model?
2. How is recovery supported by peer groups?
3. What is the focus of the Tidal Model of Recovery?
4. What is the intended outcome in the Psychological Recovery Model?

Introduction

For many years, the belief was that individuals with mental illnesses do not recover. Optimistically, the course of the illness was viewed in terms of maintenance, and pessimistically, with the expectation for deterioration. But research suggests that striving for and achieving recovery is in fact realistic for many individuals.

The concept of recovery is not new. It originally began in the addictions field, referring to a person recovering from a substance-related disorder. The term has recently been adopted by mental health professionals who believe that recovery from mental illness is also possible.

CORE CONCEPT

Recovery

A process of movement toward improvement in health and quality of life.

What Is Recovery?

A number of definitions of recovery as it applies to mental illness have been proposed. The Substance Abuse and Mental Health Services Administration (SAMHSA, 2017) suggests the following:

> Recovery [from mental health disorders and substance use disorders] is a process of change through which individuals improve their health and wellness, live a self-directed life, and strive to reach their full potential. Recovery is built on access to evidence-based clinical treatment and recovery support services for all populations.

Essential to understanding recovery definitions and models is the focus on recovery as an ongoing process rather than a set of interventions with a distinct endpoint.

SAMHSA suggests that a life in recovery is supported by four major dimensions:

1. **Health:** Overcoming or managing one's disease as well as living in a physically and emotionally healthy way
2. **Home:** A stable and safe place to live
3. **Purpose:** Meaningful daily activities, such as a job, school, volunteerism, family caretaking, or creative endeavors, and the independence, income, and resources to participate in society
4. **Community:** Relationships and social networks that provide support, friendship, love, and **hope**

SAMHSA (2017) adds that the process of recovery from mental illness and substance use disorders is highly personal and occurs via many pathways. It may include clinical treatment medications, faith-based approaches, peer support, family support, self-care, and other approaches. Recovery is characterized by continual growth and improvement in one's health and wellness that may involve setbacks. Because setbacks are a natural part of life, resilience becomes a key component of recovery.

The focus on recovery as a model for treatment is widely supported. The President's New Freedom Commission on Mental Health (2003) proposed to transform the mental health system by shifting the paradigm of care of persons with serious mental illness from traditional medical psychiatric treatment toward the concept of recovery, and the American Psychiatric Association has endorsed a recovery model from a psychiatric services perspective (Sharfstein, 2005).

In a systematic review and synthesis of the various approaches to what has become known as the recovery model, Leamy and associates (2011) identified six recovery processes that form a common foundation for this model: connectedness, hope, optimism about the future, identity, meaning in life, and empowerment. Empowerment means that the client takes primary control over decisions about his or her own care whenever possible. The National Association of Social Workers (NASW, 2006) suggests, "Consumers need to be as fully informed as possible about the potential benefits and consequences of each decision. They also need to know the possible results if they become a danger to themselves or others."

Guiding Principles of Recovery

As part of its Recovery Support Strategic Initiative, a year-long effort by SAMHSA and a wide range of partners in the behavioral healthcare community and other fields, a working definition of recovery from mental health and substance use disorders (previously stated) was developed. In addition, a set of guiding principles that support the recovery definition were delineated. These guiding principles include the following (SAMHSA, 2012):

■ **Recovery emerges from hope:** The belief that recovery is real provides the essential and motivating message of a better future—that people can and do overcome the internal and external challenges, barriers, and obstacles that confront them. Hope is internalized and can be fostered by peers, families, providers, allies, and others. Hope is the catalyst of the recovery process.

■ **Recovery is person-driven:** Self-determination and self-direction are the foundations for recovery as individuals define their own life goals and design their unique paths toward those goals. Individuals optimize their autonomy and independence to the greatest extent possible by leading, controlling, and exercising choice over the services and supports that assist their recovery and resilience. In so doing, they are empowered and provided the resources to make informed decisions, initiate recovery, build on their strengths, and gain or regain control over their lives.

■ **Recovery occurs via many pathways:** Individuals are unique with distinct needs, strengths, preferences, goals, culture, and backgrounds (including traumatic experiences) that affect and determine their pathways to recovery. Recovery is built on the multiple capacities, strengths, talents, coping abilities, resources, and inherent value of each individual. Recovery pathways are highly personalized. They may include professional clinical treatment, use of medications, support from families and in schools, faith-based approaches, peer support, and other approaches. Recovery is nonlinear, characterized by continual growth and improved functioning that may involve setbacks. Because setbacks are a natural, though not inevitable, part of the recovery process, it is essential to foster resilience for all individuals and families. Abstinence is the safest approach for those with substance use disorders. Use of tobacco and nonprescribed or illicit drugs is not safe for anyone. In some cases, recovery pathways can be enabled by creating a supportive environment. This is especially true for children, who may not have the legal or developmental capacity to set their own course.

■ **Recovery is holistic:** Recovery encompasses an individual's whole life, including mind, body, spirit, and community. A holistic approach to recovery addresses self-care practices, family, housing, employment, education, clinical treatment for mental disorders and substance use disorders, services and supports, primary healthcare, dental care, complementary and alternative services, faith, spirituality, creativity, social networks, transportation, and community participation. The array of services and supports available should be integrated and coordinated.

■ **Recovery is supported by peers and allies:** Mutual support and mutual aid groups, including the sharing of experiential knowledge and skills, as well as social learning, play an invaluable role in recovery. Peers encourage and engage other peers and provide each other with a vital sense of belonging, supportive relationships, valued roles, and community. Through helping others and giving back to the community, individuals also help themselves. Peer-operated supports and services provide important resources to assist people along their journeys of recovery and wellness. In addictions recovery, peer support has long been recognized as foundational, especially in 12-step programs such as Alcoholics Anonymous.

In mental health treatment, although formal peer support is a newer approach, the premises are similar. Sometimes called peer support specialists, individuals who facilitate peer-operated supports and services may be trained and/or certified in supportive skills; all participants share the experience of lived experience with mental illness and, as such, can provide a unique perspective for support and trust in ongoing relationships. In a fully implemented recovery model, peer support specialists should be considered equal members of the treatment team (Getty, 2015). Professionals can also play an important role in the recovery process by providing clinical treatment and other services that support individuals in their chosen recovery paths. Although peers and allies play an important role for many in recovery, their role for children and youth may be slightly different. Peer supports for families are very important for children with behavioral health problems and can also play a supportive role for youth in recovery.

■ **Recovery is supported through relationship and social networks:** An important factor in the recovery process is the presence and involvement of people who believe in the person's ability to recover; who offer hope, support, and encouragement; and who also suggest strategies and resources for change. Family members, peers, providers, faith groups, community members, and other allies form vital support networks. Through these relationships, people leave unhealthy and/or unfulfilling life roles behind and engage in new roles (e.g., partner, caregiver, friend, student, employee) that lead to a greater sense of belonging, personhood, empowerment, autonomy, social inclusion, and community participation.

■ **Recovery is culturally based and influenced:** Culture and cultural background in all of its diverse representations (including values, traditions, and beliefs) are keys in determining a person's journey and unique pathway to recovery. Services should be culturally grounded, attuned, sensitive, congruent, and competent as well as personalized to meet each individual's unique needs. SAMHSA (2017) stresses that mental health and substance addiction services must not only respect and actively address the cultural and linguistic needs of diverse populations but should also reduce disparities in access to care.

■ **Recovery is supported by addressing trauma:** The experience of trauma (such as physical or sexual abuse, domestic violence, war, disaster, and others) is often a precursor to or associated with alcohol and drug use, mental health problems, and related issues. Services and supports should be trauma-informed to foster safety (physical and emotional) and trust as well as promote choice, empowerment, and collaboration.

■ **Recovery involves individual, family, and community strengths and responsibility:** Individuals, families, and communities have strengths and resources that serve as a foundation for recovery. In addition, individuals have a personal responsibility for their own self-care and journeys of recovery. Individuals should be supported in speaking for themselves. Families and significant others have responsibilities to support their loved ones, especially for children and youth in recovery. Communities have responsibilities to provide opportunities and resources to address discrimination and to foster social inclusion and recovery. Individuals in recovery also have a social responsibility and should have the ability to join with peers to speak collectively about their strengths, needs, desires, and aspirations.

■ **Recovery is based on respect:** Acceptance and appreciation of people's lived experience with mental illness and substance use problems—by the community, systems, and society—is crucial in supporting recovery. Inherent in respecting individuals with mental health and substance use problems is protecting their rights and eliminating discrimination against them. There is a need to acknowledge that taking steps toward recovery may require great courage. Self-acceptance, developing a positive and meaningful sense of identity, and regaining belief in one's self are particularly important.

The recovery model integrates services provided by professionals (e.g., medication, therapy, case management), services provided by consumers (e.g., advocacy, peer support programs, hotlines, mentoring), and services provided in collaboration (e.g., recovery education, crisis planning, community integration, consumer rights education) (Jacobson & Greenley, 2001). Jacobson and Greenley state,

Although many of these services may sound similar to services currently being offered in many mental health systems, it is important to recognize that no service is recovery-oriented unless it incorporates the attitude that recovery is possible and has the goal of promoting hope, healing, empowerment, and connection. (p. 485)

The concepts of consumer-driven care and empowerment are closely related to the concept of patient-centered care that has been advanced by the Institute of Medicine (2003) as one of the key elements necessary to improve the quality of healthcare in the future. As this cultural shift evolves, nurses need to be thoughtful about language and attitudes that support patient-centered recovery models. For example, a traditional goal for a patient has been described as "Patient will comply with prescribed medication regime." In a patient-centered recovery model, a more appropriate goal might be stated as, "Patient will discuss preferences, advantages, and disadvantages of psychotropic medication in the management of his or her illness."

Models of Recovery

There are many different evidence-based models of recovery. SAMHSA lists these models in a database at the National Registry for Evidence-Based Programs and Practices (www.nrepp.samhsa.gov). Three models for recovery—the Tidal Model, the Wellness Action Recovery Plan (WRAP), and the Psychological Recovery Model—are discussed in the following sections.

The Tidal Model

The **Tidal Model** was developed in the late 1990s by Phil Barker and Poppy Buchanan-Barker of Newcastle, United Kingdom. It is a mental health nursing recovery model that may be used as the basis for interdisciplinary mental healthcare (Barker & Buchanan-Barker, 2012). The authors use the power of metaphor to engage with the person in distress. The metaphor of *water* is used to describe how individuals in distress can become emotionally, physically, and spiritually *shipwrecked* (Barker & Buchanan-Barker, 2005). The Tidal Model was the first recovery model to be developed by nurses in practice, drawing largely on nursing research and in collaboration with users and consumers of mental health services (Barker & Buchanan-Barker, 2005; Brookes, 2006).

The Tidal Model uses a person-centered approach to help people deal with their problems of human living. Focus is on the individual's personal story, which is where his or her problems first appeared and where any growth, benefit, or recovery will be found (Barker & Buchanan-Barker, 2000).

Barker and Buchanan-Barker (2005) developed a set of essential values upon which the model is based. These values, which they call the *10 Tidal Commitments,* provide practitioners with a philosophical focus for empowering people to make their own life changes rather than healthcare professionals trying to manage or control "patient symptoms" (Buchanan-Barker & Barker, 2008). From these commitments, the authors developed Tidal Competencies, which reflect the way the commitments are practiced in the clinical setting. These commitments and competencies include the following:

1. **Value the voice:** The person is encouraged to tell his or her story. "The person's story represents the beginning and endpoint of the helping encounter, embracing not only an account of the person's distress, but also the hope for its resolution" (p. 95). Practitioner competencies include a capacity to actively listen to the person's story and to help the person record the story in his or her own words.

2. **Respect the language:** Individuals are encouraged to speak their own words in their own unique way. "The language of the story— complete with its unusual grammar and personal metaphors—is the ideal medium for illuminating the way to recovery. We encourage people to speak their own words in their distinctive voice" (pp. 95–96). Practitioner competencies include helping individuals express in their own language their understanding of personal experiences through use of stories, anecdotes, and metaphors.

3. **Develop genuine curiosity:** Nurses and other caregivers "need to express genuine interest in the story so that they can better understand the storyteller and the story. Genuine curiosity reflects an interest in the person and the person's unique experience" (p. 96). Practitioner competencies include showing interest in the person's story, asking for clarification of certain points, and assisting the person to unfold the story at his or her own pace.

4. **Become the apprentice:** The individual is the expert on his or her life story, and he or she must be the leader in deciding what needs to be done. "Professionals may learn something of the power of that story, but only if they apply themselves diligently and respectfully to the task by becoming apprentice-minded" (p. 96). Practitioner competencies include developing a plan of care for the individual, based on his or her expressed needs or wishes, and helping the individual identify specific problems and ways to address them.

5. **Use the available toolkit:** Concentration is given to the individual's strengths, which are the major tools in the recovery process. "The story contains examples of 'what has worked' for the person in the past or beliefs about 'what might work' for this person in the future. These represent the main tools that need to be used to unlock or build the story of recovery" (p. 96). Practitioner competencies include helping individuals identify what efforts may be successful in relation to solving identified problems and which persons in the individual's life may be able to provide assistance.

6. **Craft the step beyond:** The individual and the practitioner decide together what needs to be done immediately. "Any 'first step' is a crucial step, revealing the power of change and potentially pointing towards the ultimate goal of recovery" (p. 96). Practitioner competencies include helping the individual determine what kind of change would represent a step toward recovery and what he or she needs to do to take that first step toward that goal.

7. **Give the gift of time:** Change happens when the individual and practitioner spend quality time in a therapeutic relationship. "The challenge is using time for things that are important" (Young, 2010, p. 573). Practitioner competencies include acknowledging (and helping the individual understand) the importance of time dedicated to addressing the needs of the individual and the planning and implementing of care.

8. **Reveal personal wisdom:** People often do not realize their own personal wisdom, strengths, and abilities. "A key task for the professional is to help the person reveal and come to value that wisdom, so that it might be used to sustain the person throughout the voyage of recovery" (Buchanan-Barker & Barker, 2008, p. 97). Practitioner competencies include helping individuals to identify personal strengths and weaknesses and to develop self-confidence in their ability to help themselves.

9. **Know that change is constant:** Because change is a constant in everyone's life, important decisions and choices must be made along the path to recovery in order for growth to occur. Professional competencies include helping the individual develop awareness of the changes that are occurring and how he or she has influenced these changes. "The task of the professional

helper is to develop awareness of how change is happening and to support the person in making decisions regarding the course of the recovery voyage" (p. 97).

10. **Be transparent:** Transparency is important in the teambuilding process between the individual and the professional helper. "Professionals are in a privileged position and should model confidence by being transparent at all times, helping the person understand exactly what is being done and why" (p. 97). Professional competencies include ensuring that the individual is aware of the significance of all interventions and that he or she receives copies of all documents related to the plan of care.

Young (2010) states,

> The Tidal Model is not a typical boxes-and-arrows diagram to use and follow. Instead, it is a way of thinking, a paradigm for giving person-centered care that is strength-based, empowering, and relational. (p. 574)

The Wellness Recovery Action Plan

The **WRAP Model** was developed in 1997 by a group of 30 individuals who were attending a mental health recovery skills seminar conducted by Mary Ellen Copeland in Vermont. This group (which included persons with psychiatric symptoms, family members, and care providers) determined the need for a system to incorporate into their everyday lives the skills and strategies they were learning during the seminar. Copeland (2001) states,

> [WRAP] is a structured system for monitoring uncomfortable and distressing symptoms and, through planned responses, reducing, modifying or eliminating those symptoms. It also includes plans for responses from others when a person's symptoms have made it impossible to continue to make decisions, take care of him/herself and keep him/herself safe. (p. 129)

Copeland suggests that all a person needs to begin the program is a system for storing information (e.g., a notebook, computer, or tape recorder) and possibly a friend, healthcare provider, or other supporter to give assistance and feedback. The program is a stepwise process through which an individual is able to monitor and manage distressing symptoms that occur in daily life. Individuals may be assisted in the process by others (e.g., healthcare professionals, significant others, friends), "but to be effective and empowering, the person experiencing the symptoms must develop

the plan for himself/herself" (p. 129). The WRAP process involves six steps:

Step 1. Developing a wellness toolbox: The individual creates a list of tools, strategies, and skills that he or she has used in the past (or has heard of in the past that he or she would like to try) to assist in relieving disturbing symptoms. Copeland (2001) offers a number of examples:

- Talking to a friend or healthcare professional
- Peer counseling or exchange listening
- Relaxation and stress reduction exercises
- Guided imagery
- Journaling
- Physical exercise
- Attending a support group
- Doing something special for someone else
- Listening to music

Step 2. Daily maintenance list: This list is divided into three parts. In part 1, the individual writes a description of how he or she feels (or would like to feel) when experiencing wellness (e.g., bright, cheerful, talkative, happy, optimistic, capable). This information is used as a reference point. In part 2, using the wellness toolbox as a reference, the individual makes a list of things he or she needs to do every day to maintain wellness. This is an important part of the plan and must be realistic so as not to set the individual up for failure or create additional frustration. Example items for part 2 may include the following (Copeland, 2001):

- Eat three healthy meals and three healthy snacks.
- Drink at least six 8-ounce glasses of water.
- Avoid caffeine, sugar, junk foods, and alcohol.
- Exercise for at least 30 minutes.
- Have 20 minutes of relaxation or meditation time.
- Write in my journal for at least 15 minutes.
- Take medications and vitamin supplements.
- Spend at least 30 minutes enjoying a fun, affirming, and/or creative activity.

In part 3 of this step, the individual keeps a list of things that need to be done. The individual reads this list daily as a reminder, and items may be considered for accomplishment on any given day at the individual's discretion. For part 3, Copeland (2001) suggests items such as the following:

- Spend time with my counselor or case manager.
- Make an appointment with my healthcare professional.

- Spend time with my friend or partner.
- Be in touch with my family.
- Spend time with children or pets.
- Buy groceries.
- Do the laundry.
- Write some letters.
- Remember someone's birthday or anniversary.

Step 3. Triggers: This step is divided into two parts. In part 1, the individual lists events or circumstances that, should they occur, would cause distress or discomfort. These triggers are situations to which the individual is susceptible or that have triggered or increased symptoms in the past. Copeland (2001) lists the following examples:

- The anniversary dates of losses or trauma
- Being overtired or exhausted
- Work stress
- Family friction
- A relationship ending
- Being judged, criticized, or teased
- Financial problems
- Physical illness
- Sexual harassment or inappropriate sexual behavior
- Substance abuse

In part 2, the individual uses items from the wellness toolbox to develop a plan for what to do if triggers interfere with wellness.

Step 4. Early warning signs: This step is divided into two parts. Part 1 involves identification of subtle signs that indicate a possible worsening of the situation. Copeland (2001) states, "Recognizing early warning signs and reviewing them regularly will help the person to become more aware of these early warning signs, allowing the person to take action before the signs worsen" (p. 136). Some types of early warning signs include anxiety, forgetfulness, lack of motivation, avoiding others or isolating, increased irritability, increase in smoking, using substances, or feeling worthless and inadequate. In part 2, the individual develops a plan for responding to the early warning signs that result in relief or in preventing them from escalating. The plan may include items such as consulting a supporter or counselor, increasing focus on peer counseling, increasing time spent in relaxation exercises, or utilizing other interventions from the wellness toolbox until warning signs diminish.

Step 5. Things are breaking down or getting worse: This step is divided into two parts. In part 1, the individual lists symptoms that are occurring that indicate that the situation has worsened. In this stage, the symptoms are producing great discomfort, but the individual is still able to take some action on his or her own behalf. Immediate action is required to prevent a crisis from developing. Symptoms at this stage differ greatly from person to person, and Copeland (2001) states, "What may mean 'things are breaking down' to one person may mean 'crisis' to another" (p. 137). She lists a number of examples of symptoms, which may include the following:

- Irrational responses to events and the actions of others
- Inability to sleep or sleeping all the time
- Headaches
- Not eating or overeating
- Social isolation
- Thoughts of self-harm
- Substance abuse or chain smoking
- Bizarre behaviors
- Seeing things that are not there
- Paranoia

In part 2, the individual makes a plan that he or she thinks will help when the symptoms have worsened to this degree. The plan must be very specific and direct, with clear instructions. Some examples include the following (Copeland, 2001):

- Call my healthcare professional; ask for and follow directions.
- Arrange for someone to stay with me around the clock until my symptoms subside.
- Take action so that I cannot hurt myself if my symptoms get worse, such as give my medication, checkbook, credit cards, and car keys to a previously designated friend for safe keeping.
- Make sure I do everything on my daily checklist.
- Have at least two peer counseling sessions daily.
- Increase use of items from wellness toolbox (e.g., relaxation exercises, physical exercises, creative activities).

Step 6. Crisis planning: This stage identifies symptoms indicating that individuals can no longer care for themselves, make independent decisions, or keep themselves safe. This stage is multifaceted and is meant for use by caregivers on behalf of the individual who developed the plan. It is composed of the following parts (Copeland, 2001, p. 130):

- Part 1. Gathers information that describes what the person is like when well.
- Part 2. Identifies the symptoms that indicate when others need to take responsibility for the person's care.

- Part 3. Provides names of supporters previously identified by the individual to speak on his or her behalf.
- Part 4. Includes the name of healthcare providers and phone numbers, medications currently being used, allergies to medications, medications the individual would prefer to take if additional medication is necessary, and medications that the individual refuses to take.
- Part 5. Includes the individual's preferred treatments and treatments that he or she wishes to be avoided.
- Part 6. Identifies the individual's preferences in treatment facilities (e.g., home, community care, respite center).
- Part 7. Identifies acceptable facilities if previous preferences cannot be executed. Facilities to be avoided are also indicated.
- Part 8. Includes an extensive description of what the individual expects from identified supporters who are acting on his or her behalf during a crisis situation.
- Part 9. Consists of a list of indicators, developed by the individual, that communicates to supporters when their services are no longer required. The individual should update this plan periodically when he or she learns new information or changes his or her mind about certain situations. Assurance of the use of the crisis plan may be increased if it is notarized and signed in the presence of two witnesses. To further increase its potential for use, the person may appoint a durable power of attorney, although because of the variability of the legality of these documents from state to state, there is no guarantee that the plan will be followed.

Copeland (2001) states,

> WRAP is a systematic method for developing skills in self-management and empowerment. It provides a means for individuals with a mental illness to work more collaboratively with healthcare providers. It is highly individualized and addresses the unique needs of the person and his/her situation. It is applicable to most any long-term illness/disability or problem situation. These benefits suggest that it can be used more widely and should be introduced as an option for individuals in need of a self-management system. (p. 149)

The Psychological Recovery Model

Andresen, Oades, and Caputi (2011) define *psychological recovery* as "the establishment of a fulfilling, meaningful life and a positive sense of identity founded on hopefulness and self-determination. Psychological recovery is necessary whether mental illness is biologically based or the result of the exacerbation of emotional problems caused by stress" (p. 40). The **Psychological Recovery Model** does not emphasize the absence of symptoms but focuses on the person's self-determination in the course of his or her recovery process.

In examining a number of studies, Andresen and associates (2011) identified four components that were consistently evident in the recovery process:

- **Hope:** Finding and maintaining hope that recovery can occur
- **Responsibility:** Taking responsibility for one's life and well-being
- **Self and identity:** Renewing the sense of self and building a positive identity
- **Meaning and purpose:** Finding **purpose** and meaning in life

Andresen and associates (2011) conceptualized a five-stage model of recovery, which they define by integrating into each stage the four components of the recovery process:

Stage 1. Moratorium: This stage is identified by dark despair and confusion. "It is called moratorium, because it seems 'life is on hold'" (p. 47).

- *Hope:* In the moratorium stage, hopelessness prevails. Clients may even perceive feelings of hopelessness from practitioners when treatment plans emphasize stabilization and maintenance, thereby conveying messages of no hope for recovery.
- *Responsibility:* In the moratorium stage, the individual feels out of control and powerless to change.
- *Self and identity:* In the moratorium stage, individuals feel "as though they no longer know who they are as a person" (p. 59). An individual's sense of identity as a valuable and functional member of society can be lost with a diagnosis of mental illness.
- *Meaning and purpose:* The diagnosis of severe mental illness is a traumatic event that can challenge an individual's fundamental beliefs, creating a loss of meaning and purpose in life.

Stage 2. Awareness: In this stage, the individual comes to a realization that a possibility for recovery exists. Andresen and associates state, "It involves an awareness of a possible self other than that of 'sick person': a self that is capable of recovery" (p. 47).

■ *Hope:* In the awareness stage, there is a dawn of hope that "life is not over." This feeling of hope may emanate from significant others, professionals, or family members. Individuals may also be inspired by others who have recovered. Hope may also be derived from strong inner determination and from personal faith and spirituality.

■ *Responsibility:* In this stage, the individual develops an awareness of the need to take control of his or her life. Feelings of control and responsibility lead to a sense of personal empowerment that paves the way for recovery.

■ *Self and identity:* In the awareness stage, the individual comes to realize that he or she is a person independent of the illness. "The person realizes that there still exists an 'intact self' capable of taking action on one's own behalf" (p. 72).

■ *Meaning and purpose:* In the awareness stage, the individual strives for a personal comprehension of the illness, why it occurred, and what the implications of the illness are for his or her future. "Seeking a meaning of the illness can be explained by theories of cognitive control, in which one tries to understand unexplainable negative events by finding a reason for them" (p. 74).

Stage 3. Preparation: This stage begins with the individual's resolve to begin the work of recovery.

■ *Hope:* In the preparation stage, hope is manifested in the mobilization of personal and external resources to foster self-care and find pathways to goals. The individual identifies strengths and weaknesses, gathers knowledge and information, and seeks out available support systems.

■ *Responsibility:* Taking responsibility in the preparation stage involves learning about the effects of the illness and how to recognize, monitor, and manage symptoms. Taking charge of one's life also includes the ability to be independent and take care of basic needs.

■ *Self and identity:* Andresen and associates state, "During the preparation stage, the person takes stock of his or her skills and strengths in order to build on them to rediscover a positive sense of identity" (p. 81). The person is willing to take risks and try new activities to re-establish a sense of self. Lost aspects of self are rediscovered, new aspects are identified, and both are incorporated into a new self-identity.

■ *Meaning and purpose:* The basis for a meaningful life lies in solid core values. "Living according to one's valued directions gives meaning to the work of recovery, and for this reason, some people hold on tenaciously to their goals" (p. 83). Each individual must live by certain tenets that make life personally valuable and enriching. Individuals living with a severe mental illness may require a reordering of priorities and setting of new goals as part of their recovery.

Stage 4. Rebuilding: The hard work of recovery takes place in the rebuilding stage. The individual "takes the necessary steps to work towards his or her goals in rebuilding a meaningful life" (p. 87).

■ *Hope:* In the rebuilding stage, the individual has hope for and looks forward to a more fulfilling life. Realistic goals are set, and the individual is encouraged to pursue the recovery process at his or her own pace. With each success, hope is renewed.

■ *Responsibility:* "Through setting and working towards goals, the person begins to actively take control of his or her life; not only management of symptoms, but also enlisting social support, improvement of self-image, handling social pressures, and building social competence" (p. 90). Assuming control of treatment decisions and illness management is an essential part of the recovery process.

■ *Self and identity:* The individual elaborates and enhances his or her sense of identity by having succeeded in previous stages in developing a positive self-identity separate from the illness and a new sense of self-confidence by succeeding at new activities. In the rebuilding stage, the work of examining core values and working toward value-congruent goals reinforce a positive sense of identity and a commitment to recovery.

■ *Meaning and purpose:* Having realistic goals and a positive sense of identity provides a sense of purpose in life. Individuals need a reason to start each day. Andresen and associates state, "Finding meaning [in life] is more than finding a valued occupation, but rather is more akin to finding a way to live. This may include, but is not limited to, vocational goals. It includes examining one's spirituality or philosophy of life. The journey is, in itself, a source of meaning for many" (p. 99).

Stage 5. Growth: The outcome of the psychological recovery process is growth. Although it is called the *final* stage of the psychological recovery model, it is important to remember that this is a dynamic stage and that personal growth is a continuing life process.

- *Hope:* In the growth stage, the individual feels a sense of optimism and hope of a rewarding future. Skills that have been nurtured in the previous stages are applied with confidence, and the individual strives for higher levels of well-being.
- *Responsibility:* "Achieving control requires sustained commitment in the face of set-backs" (p. 106). In the growth phase, individuals exhibit confidence in managing their illnesses and are resilient when relapses occur. They are empowered by personal input and decision making regarding their treatment.
- *Self and identity:* The individual in the growth stage has developed a strong, positive sense of self and identity. Andresen and associates state, "Many consumers have reported feeling that they are a better person as a result of their struggle with the illness. [In one research study] participants reported developing personal qualities, including strength and courage; more confidence in the self; resourcefulness and responsibility; a new philosophy of life; compassion and empathy; a sense of self-worth; and being happier and more carefree" (pp. 108–109).
- *Meaning and purpose:* Individuals who have reached the growth stage often report a more profound sense of meaning. Some describe having achieved a sense of serenity and peace, and for others it takes the form of a spiritual awakening. Some individuals find reward in educating others about the experience of mental illness and recovery.

Andresen and associates (2011) state,

> Recovery from serious mental illness is more than staying out of the hospital or a return to some arbitrary level of functioning. It is more than merely coping with the illness. In [the growth] stage, the notion of wellbeing replaces that of wellness. While wellness implies the absence of illness, wellbeing refers to a more holistic psychological experience of fulfilling life. Although we may not expect everyone (including those who do not have a mental illness) to reach the highest levels of self-actualization, we can expect that all people have the opportunity to develop a positive sense of self and identity and to live a meaningful life filled with purpose and hope for the future. (p. 113)

Nursing Interventions That Assist With Recovery

The President's New Freedom Commission on Mental Health (2003) proposed to transform the mental health system by shifting the paradigm of care of persons with serious mental illness from traditional medical psychiatric treatment toward the concept of recovery. It is within the scope of nursing to assist individuals in many aspects of the mental health recovery process. Caldwell and colleagues (2010) state,

> Professional nurses must play an active role in client recovery because they are employed in all aspects of service delivery systems, and most times professional nurses are responsible for the delivery and coordination of care. The professional nurse must be center stage in the development and implementation of any action plan involving client recovery. (p. 44)

Nurses have historically held as a primary goal the promotion of wellness within a collaborative nurse-client relationship. Peplau (1991) described nursing as "a human relationship between an individual who is sick, or in need of health services, and a nurse especially educated to recognize and to respond to the need for help" (pp. 5–6). As previously noted, recovery models are inherently collaborative in that services are provided by professionals, by consumers, and cooperatively by both. Examples of interventions and activities in which nurses and consumers may collaborate in the individual's journey to recovery are outlined in Table 10–1.

Advocates for the recovery model stress its positive, hopeful, and empowering aspects that have been lacking in traditional medical models of treatment. Critics argue that an individual's subjective perception of recovery does not necessarily validate the quality of healthcare interventions, particularly in cases where individuals (as in schizophrenia) may experience the symptom of anosognosia (in which they do not see themselves as having an illness despite apparent, significant symptoms). Duckworth (2015) promotes integrating recovery and medical models of treatment to ensure that scientific processes are used to validate outcomes associated with recovery models of intervention. He cites several examples of recovery-focused treatments that have been supported by research, such as the WRAP model (previously discussed); dialectical behavioral therapy (DBT) for borderline personality disorders; cognitive enhancement therapy (CET) for improving cognition problems in patients

TABLE 10–1 Nurse-Client Collaboration in the Mental Health Recovery Process

	TIDAL MODEL	WRAP MODEL	PSYCHOLOGICAL RECOVERY MODEL
Assessment	■ Client tells his or her personal story ■ Nurse actively listens and expresses interest in the story ■ Nurse helps client record story in client's own language ■ Client identifies specific problems he or she wishes to address ■ Nurse and client identify client's strengths and weaknesses	■ Client develops a wellness toolbox by creating a list of tools, strategies, and skills that have been helpful in the past ■ Client identifies strengths and weaknesses ■ Nurse provides assistance and feedback	■ Client is feeling hopeless and powerless ■ Client seeks meaning of the illness ■ Nurse helps by offering hope ■ Client begins to develop an awareness of the need to take control of and responsibility for his or her life

Interventions	■ Nurse and client determine what has worked in the past
	■ Client suggests new tools he or she would like to try
	■ Client decides what changes he or she would like to make and sets realistic goals
	■ Nurse and client decide what must be done as the first step
	■ Nurse gives positive feedback for client's efforts to make life changes and for successes achieved
	■ Nurse encourages client to be as independent as possible but offers assistance when required
	■ Nurse gives the "gift of time"
		■ Client creates a daily maintenance list:
		  - How he or she feels at best
		  - What must be done daily to maintain wellness
		  - Reminder list of other things that need to be accomplished
		■ Client identifies triggers that cause distress or discomfort and identifies what to do if triggers interfere with wellness
		■ Client identifies signs of worsening of symptoms and develops a plan to prevent escalation
		■ Client identifies when symptoms have worsened and help is needed
		■ Client identifies when he or she can no longer care for self and makes decisions (in writing) about treatment issues (what type, who will provide, who will represent client's interests)
		■ Nurse offers support and provides feedback and assistance when needed
			■ Client resolves to begin work of recovery
			■ Client and nurse identify strengths and weaknesses
			■ Nurse assists client to learn about effects of the illness and how to recognize, monitor, and manage symptoms
			■ Client identifies changes he or she wishes to occur and sets realistic goals to rebuild a meaningful life
			■ Client examines personal spirituality and philosophy of life in search of a meaning and purpose—one that gives him or her a "reason to start each day"

Outcomes	■ Client acknowledges that change has occurred and is ongoing ■ Client feels empowered to manage own self-care ■ Nurse is available for support	■ Client develops skills in self-management ■ Client develops self-confidence and hope for a brighter future	■ Client develops a positive self-identity separate from the illness ■ Client maintains commitment to recovery in the face of setbacks ■ Client feels a sense of optimism and hope of a rewarding future

with early-stage psychosis; and the National Alliance on Mental Health's (NAMI) Family-to Family Program, an education and peer support program for families experiencing mental illness.

Many nurse leaders see the current period of healthcare reform as an opportunity for nurses to expand their roles and assume key positions in education, prevention, assessment, and referral. Nurses are, and will continue to be, in key positions to assist individuals with mental illness to remain as independent as possible, to manage their illness within the community setting, and to strive to minimize the number of hospitalizations required. A vision of recovery from mental illness exists, and hope, trust, and self-determination should be incorporated into all treatment models.

Summary and Key Points

- Recovery is the restoration to a former and/or better state or condition.
- SAMHSA identifies four major dimensions that support a life in recovery: health, home, purpose, and community.
- The President's New Freedom Commission on Mental Health proposed to transform the mental health system by shifting the paradigm of care of persons with serious mental illness from traditional medical psychiatric treatment toward the concept of recovery.
- SAMHSA outlines 10 guiding principles that support recovery:
  - Recovery emerges from hope.
  - Recovery is person-driven.
  - Recovery occurs via many pathways.
  - Recovery is holistic.
  - Recovery is supported by peers and allies.
  - Recovery is supported through relationship and social networks.
  - Recovery is culturally based and influenced.
  - Recovery is supported by addressing trauma.
  - Recovery involves individual, family, and community strengths and responsibility.
  - Recovery is based on respect.
- Many models of recovery exist. Three models that are discussed in this chapter are the Tidal Model, the WRAP Model, and the Psychological Recovery Model.
- Nurses work in key positions to assist individuals with mental illness in the recovery process. Interventions based on the three previously mentioned recovery models are included in this chapter.

Review Questions
Self-Examination/Learning Exercise

Select the answer that is most appropriate for each of the following questions:

1. Which of the following is a true statement about mental health recovery? (Select all that apply.)
   a. Mental health recovery applies only to severe and persistent mental illnesses.
   b. Mental health recovery serves to provide empowerment to the consumer.
   c. Mental health recovery is based on the medical model.
   d. Mental health recovery is a collaborative process.

2. A nurse is assisting an individual with mental illness recovery using the Tidal Model. Which of the following is a component of this model?
   a. The wellness toolbox
   b. The daily maintenance list
   c. The individual's personal story
   d. Triggers

3. A nurse is assisting an individual with mental illness recovery using the Psychological Recovery Model. The patient states to the nurse, "I have schizophrenia. Nothing can be done. I might as well die." In which stage of the Psychological Recovery Model would the nurse assess this individual to be?
   a. The awareness stage
   b. The preparation stage
   c. The rebuilding stage
   d. The moratorium stage

Review Questions—cont'd
Self-Examination/Learning Exercise

4. A nurse who is helping a patient in the preparation stage of the Psychological Recovery Model might include which of the following interventions?
   a. Teach about effects of the illness and how to recognize, monitor, and manage symptoms.
   b. Help the patient identify "triggers" that cause distress or discomfort.
   c. Help the patient establish a daily maintenance list.
   d. Listen actively while the patient composes his or her personal story.

5. A nurse who is helping a patient with mental illness recovery using the WRAP Model says, "First you must create a wellness toolbox." She explains to the patient that a wellness toolbox is which of the following?
   a. A list of words that describe how the individual feels when he or she is feeling well
   b. A list of things the individual needs to do every day to maintain wellness
   c. A list of strategies the individual has used in the past that help relieve disturbing symptoms
   d. A list of the patient's favorite healthcare providers and phone numbers.

💬 Communication Exercises

1. Joshua comes to his appointment at the mental health clinic and states, "I can't sit still when I take those medications, so I don't want to take them anymore." Using principles of the recovery model, what are some options for responding to this patient?

2. Kelly is a war veteran who was admitted to inpatient hospitalization with depression, alcohol addiction, and complaints of troubling nightmares. She states, at the admission assessment, "I don't trust any 'mental health gurus.' You can't possibly understand what I've been through."

   How will you respond, and what principles of the recovery model will guide your response?

References

Andresen, R., Oades, L. G., & Caputi, P. (2011). *Psychological recovery: Beyond mental illness.* West Sussex, UK: John Wiley & Sons.

Barker, P. J., & Buchanan-Barker, P. (2000). *The Tidal Model: Reclaiming stories, recovering lives.* Retrieved from http://www.tidal-model.com

Barker, P. J., & Buchanan-Barker, P. (2005). *The Tidal Model: A guide for mental health professionals.* London, England: Brunner-Routledge.

Barker, P. J., & Buchanan-Barker, P. (2012). *Tidal Model of mental health nursing. Current Nursing.* Retrieved from http://www.currentnursing.com/nursing_theory/Tidal_Model.html

Brookes, N. (2006). Phil Barker: The Tidal Model of mental health recovery. In A. M. Tomey & M. R. Alligood (Eds.), *Nursing theorists and their work* (6th ed., pp. 696–725). New York, NY: Elsevier.

Buchanan-Barker, P., & Barker, P. J. (2008). The Tidal commitments: Extending the value base of mental health recovery. *Journal of Psychiatric and Mental Health Nursing, 15*(2), 93–100.

Caldwell, B. A., Sclafani, M., Swarbrick, M., & Piren, K. (2010). Psychiatric nursing practice and the recovery model of care. *Journal of Psychosocial Nursing, 48*(7), 42–48.

Copeland, M. E. (2001). Wellness recovery action plan: A system for monitoring, reducing and eliminating uncomfortable or dangerous physical symptoms and emotional feelings. In C. Brown (Ed.), *Recovery and wellness: Models of hope and empowerment for people with mental illness* (pp. 127–150). New York, NY: Haworth Press.

Duckworth, K. (2015). *Science meets the human experience: Integrating the medical and recovery models.* Retrieved from https://www.nami.org/blogs/nami-blog/april-2015/science-meets-the-human-experience-integrating-th

Getty, S. M. (2015). Implementing a mental health program using the recovery model. *OT Practice, 20*(3), 1–8.

Institute of Medicine. (2003). *Health professions education: A bridge to quality.* Washington, DC: Author.

Jacobson, N., & Greenley, D. (2001). What is recovery? A conceptual model and explication. *Psychiatric Services, 52*(4), 482–485.

Leamy, M., Bird, V., LeBoutillier, C., Williams, J., & Slade, M. (2011). Conceptual framework for personal recovery in mental health: Systematic review and narrative synthesis. *British Journal of Psychiatry, 199,* 445–452. doi:10.1192/bjp.bp.110.083733

National Association of Social Workers (NASW). (2006). *NASW Practice snapshot: The mental health recovery model.* Retrieved from http://www.socialworkers.org/practice/behavioral_health/0206snapshot.asp?

Peplau, H. E. (1991). *Interpersonal relations in nursing: A conceptual frame of reference for psychodynamic nursing.* New York, NY: Springer.

President's New Freedom Commission on Mental Health. (2003). *Achieving the promise: Transforming mental health care in America.* Retrieved from http://govinfo.library.unt.edu/mentalhealthcommission/index.htm

Sharfstein, S. (2005). Recovery model will strengthen psychiatrist-patient relationship. *Psychiatric News, 40*(20), 3.

Substance Abuse and Mental Health Services Administration (SAMHSA). (2012). *SAMHSA's working definition of recovery: 10 guiding principles of recovery* [Brochure]. Rockville, MD: Author.

Substance Abuse and Mental Health Services Administration (SAMHSA). (2017). *Recovery and recovery support.* Retrieved from https://www.samhsa.gov/recovery

Young, B. B. (2010). Using the Tidal Model of mental health recovery to plan primary health care for women in residential substance abuse recovery. *Issues in Mental Health Nursing, 31*(9), 569–575.

11

Suicide Prevention

CORE CONCEPTS

Suicide
Suicide risk assessment
Suicide prevention

KEY TERMS

altruistic suicide

egoistic suicide

anomic suicide

suicide risk factors

collaborative safety plan

suicide warning signs

OBJECTIVES

After reading this chapter, the student will be able to:

1. Discuss epidemiological statistics and risk factors related to suicide.
2. Describe predisposing factors implicated in the etiology of suicide.
3. Differentiate between facts and myths regarding suicide.
4. Apply the nursing process to individuals exhibiting suicidal behavior.

HOMEWORK ASSIGNMENT
Please read the chapter and answer the following questions:

1. How do age, race, and gender affect suicide risk?
2. Your neighbor tells you he is going to visit his sister-in-law in the hospital. The sister-in-law has been hospitalized after attempting suicide. Your neighbor asks, "What should I say when I go to visit Jane?" What suggestions might you give him?
3. John's father died by suicide when John was a teenager. John's wife, Mary, tells

the mental health nurse that she is afraid John "inherited" that predisposition from his father. How should the nurse respond to Mary?
4. The nurse notes that the mood of a patient being treated for depression and suicidal ideation suddenly brightens and the patient states, "I feel fine now. I don't feel depressed anymore." Why would this statement alert the nurse of a potential problem?

Introduction

Suicide is not a diagnosis or a disorder; it is a behavior. Specifically, it is the act of taking one's own life, and it derives from the Latin words for "one's own killing." Many religions hold that suicide is a sin and it is strictly forbidden. Canetto (American Psychiatric Association, 2010) states, "Everywhere, suicidal behavior is culturally scripted. Women and men adopt the self-destructive behaviors that are expected of them within their cultures." Yet, although some populations are considered at higher risk for suicide (such as American Indians and Alaska Natives; active and veteran military members; lesbian, gay, bisexual, or transgender individuals; and people in justice or child welfare settings) suicide touches the lives of all ages, ethnic, and racial groups in all parts of the country (Substance Abuse and Mental Health Services Administration [SAMHSA], 2017).

A recent, more secular view has influenced how some individuals view suicide in our society. Growing support for an individual's right to choose death over pain has been evidenced by a growing number of states that are considering or have adopted physician-assisted suicide laws. Some individuals are striving to advance the cause of physician-assisted suicides for the terminally ill. In 2008, Oregon was the only state in which physician-assisted suicide was legal. Since then, Montana, Vermont, Washington, California, and Colorado have adopted similar laws. New Mexico also adopted a similar law but it was overturned on appeal in August 2015. In 2018, Hawaii's state senate became the most recent to approve such a bill. Can suicide be a rational act? Most people in our society do not yet believe that it can.

In the field of psychiatry, suicide is considered an irrational act associated with mental illness and most commonly, but not exclusively, with depression. More than 90 percent of all persons who attempt or die by suicide have a diagnosed mental disorder (National Institute of Mental Health [NIMH], 2015). This chapter explores suicide from an epidemiological and etiological perspective. Care of the suicidal client is presented in the context of the nursing process.

Historical Perspectives

In ancient Greece, individuals were said to have "committed" suicide because it was an offense against the state, and individuals who did so were denied burial in community sites (Minois, 2001). In the culture of the imperial Roman army, individuals sometimes resorted to suicide to escape humiliation or abuse.

In the Middle Ages, suicide was viewed as a selfish or criminal act (Minois, 2001). Individuals who "committed suicide" were often denied cemetery burial and their property was confiscated and shared by the crown and the courts (MacDonald & Murphy, 1991). The issue of suicide changed during the Renaissance period. Although condemnation was still expected, the view became more philosophical, and intellectuals could discuss the issue more freely.

Most philosophers of the 17th and 18th centuries condemned suicide, but some writers recognized a connection between suicide and melancholy or other severe mental disturbances (Minois, 2001). Suicide was illegal in England until 1961, and only in 1993 was it decriminalized in Ireland. With the decriminalization of suicide, many have advanced the idea that the term "committed suicide" should be removed from our vocabulary because it is inaccurate and potentially maintains a stigmatizing attitude toward this population.

Most religions consider suicide as a sin. Judaism, Christianity, Islam, Hinduism, and Buddhism all condemn suicide. The Catholic Church still teaches that suicide is wrong, that it is in opposition to proper love of self and love of God, and that it wrongs others through the experience of loss and grief (Byron, 2016). But as Byron (2016) points out, some of the church's condemnation may have been rooted in a "denial of the responsibility to understand the pain that produces such an act," and he stresses the importance of encouraging those who "are hurting to open up," which, it is hoped, will remove some of the taboos of discussing suicide within the church. Likewise, replacing the term "committed suicide" may also help to reduce the stigma and taboo that has historically been associated with open conversation about suicide.

Epidemiological Factors

In 2017, the most recent year for which statistics have been recorded, 47,173 people died by suicide in the United States (American Foundation for Suicide Prevention, 2019). The numbers continue to climb despite nationwide attention to suicide prevention. These statistics have established suicide as the second-leading cause of death (behind unintentional injuries) among young Americans aged 10 to 34 years, the fourth-leading cause of death for individuals aged 35 to 54, the eighth-leading of death for individuals aged 55 to 64, and the 10th-leading cause of death overall (Centers for Disease Control and Prevention [CDC], 2016).

Many more people attempt suicide than succeed (about 12:1), and countless others seriously contemplate the act without carrying it out. With a steady incline in rates of suicide over the 12-year period from 2000 to 2017, suicide has become a major healthcare problem in the United States today. Not only are the number of suicides on the incline but the demographics have changed. Historically, the highest rates of suicide were among the elderly, but currently the highest rate of suicide occurs among middle-aged individuals and those 85 years and older. Historically, the suicide rate has been lower among military personnel than among the general population. However, in some time periods since the Iraq War began—including in 2010 and 2011—more soldiers died by suicide than died in combat (Nock et al., 2013). See Chapter 28, Military Families, for further discussion.

A wealth of research is being conducted to better understand the best methods for assessment of suicide risk, what differentiates those with suicidal ideation from those who attempt, and what kind of treatments and interventions are supported by evidence. The federal government, through SAMHSA, has endorsed the "Zero Suicide" movement (National Action Alliance for Suicide Prevention, 2015), an effort to identify evidence-based strategies for suicide prevention, so there is a great deal of national attention to this issue. Within the next several years, we may discover that our understanding of and approaches to treatment will dramatically change. We are certainly beginning to recognize that, with suicide rates on the rise, our conventional interventions have not adequately addressed the complex needs of this population.

Confusion exists over the reality of various notions regarding suicide. Some currently accepted facts and myths relating to suicide are presented in Table 11–1.

Risk Factors

Suicide risk factors are identified as factors that have statistically been correlated with a higher incidence of suicide. They should be differentiated from **suicide warning signs,** which are identified as factors suggesting a more immediate concern. Both are included as part of a comprehensive assessment of overall risk for suicide.

Marital Status

The suicide rate for single, never married persons is twice that for married persons, and divorce increases risk for suicide, particularly among men, who are three times more likely to take their own lives than are divorced women (Sadock, Sadock, & Ruiz, 2015). Widows and widowers, in some studies, have also been identified as high risk, but a longitudinal study (Kposowa, 2000) found that being single or widowed had no effect on suicide rates. However, their study did find that divorced men were twice as likely as married men to die by suicide.

For those who are divorced and widowed, the stresses associated with major life changes and loss are influential. Evidence has demonstrated that *change* in marital status increases risk for suicidal behavior, particularly in the first year after the change and particularly among older people (Roˇskar et al., 2011; Yamauchi et al., 2013). Again, it should be noted that demographics such as marital status, age, and gender may inform about populations that are statistically at higher risk, but none of these factors are predictive of immediate risk. A thorough assessment of variables, including risk factors, warning signs, and a host of other data, are essential to identifying individuals at acute risk for attempting suicide.

Gender

More women than men attempt suicide, but men succeed more often (about 70 percent of men and 30 percent of women). This rate reflects the lethality of the means. Women tend to overdose on drugs; men use more lethal means, such as firearms. These differences between men and women may also reflect differing societal expectations; women are more likely than men to seek and accept help from friends or professionals, whereas men often view help-seeking as a sign of weakness.

Transgender individuals are also a high-risk population for suicide with an alarming 41% lifetime prevalence (Stroumsa, 2014). Further research is needed to better understand whether this increased risk is associated with gender dysphoria versus environmental variables.

Age

Suicide risk and age are, in general, positively correlated, particularly with men. Although rates among women remain fairly constant throughout life, rates among men increase with age. The most recent statistics, according to the AFSP, revealed that in 2017, the highest rate of suicide occurred in the 45- to 54-year-old age group (with men at particular risk), and the second-highest rate was for those 85 or older (AFSP, 2019). A consistent high rate of suicide in both age groups was shown for the period 2000 to 2017, but the 45 to 54 age group showed a steady incline in suicide rates over the same period.

Although adolescents may statistically have a lower rate of suicide than some other age groups,

TABLE 11–1 **Facts and Myths About Suicide**	
MYTHS	**FACTS**
People who talk about suicide do not act on their ideas. Suicide happens without warning.	Eight out of 10 people who kill themselves have given definite clues and warnings about their suicidal intentions. Very subtle clues may be ignored or disregarded by others.
You cannot stop a suicidal person. He or she is fully intent on dying.	Most suicidal people are very ambivalent about their feelings regarding living or dying. Most are "gambling with death" and see it as a cry for someone to save them.
Once a person is suicidal, he or she is suicidal forever.	Suicidal ideation and risk fluctuate over time and may be time limited. If provided adequate support and resources, a suicidal person can go on to lead a normal life. However, multiple suicide attempts may reflect greater chronicity of suicidal ideation. Reassessment over time is important to identify current risks.
Improvement after severe depression means that the suicidal risk is over.	Most suicides occur within about 3 months after the beginning of "improvement," when the individual has the energy to carry out suicidal intentions.
Suicide is inherited, or "runs in families."	Family history and genetics may contribute to an increased risk for suicide. Many mental illnesses like depression, bipolar disorder, and substance abuse run in families and confer an increased risk but suicidal behavior is not inevitable in these populations. However, suicide by a close family member does increase the risk of similar behavior in other family members.
All suicidal individuals are mentally ill, and suicide is the act of a psychotic person.	Although a majority of people who attempt suicide are extremely unhappy, or clinically depressed, they are not necessarily psychotic. They are merely unable at that point in time to see an alternative solution to what they consider an unbearable problem.
Suicidal thoughts and attempts should be considered manipulative or attention-seeking behavior and should not be taken seriously.	All suicidal behavior must be approached with the gravity of the potential act in mind. Attention should be given to the possibility that the individual is issuing a cry for help.
People usually take their own lives by taking an overdose of drugs.	Gunshot wounds are the leading cause of death among suicide victims.
If an individual has attempted suicide, he or she will not do it again.	Between 50% and 80% of all people who ultimately kill themselves have a history of at least one previous attempt.
Suicide always happens in an impulsive moment.	People who are suicidal often contemplate, imagine, plan strategies, write notes, post things on the Internet. The importance of in-depth exploration and assessment cannot be overstated.
Young children (ages 5–12) cannot be suicidal.	Annually, 30 to 35 children younger than age 12 take their own lives and not all are clinically depressed.

Sources: Cardoza, K. (2016). *6 myths about suicide that every parent and educator should know*. Retrieved from https://www.npr.org/sections/ed/2016/09/02/478835539/6-myths-about-suicide-that-every-educator-and-parent-should-know. National Alliance on Mental Illness (NAMI). (2015). *Risks of suicide*. Retrieved from www.nami.org/Learn-More/Mental-Health-Conditions/Related-Conditions/Risk-of-Suicide; and The Samaritans. (2015). *Suicide myths and misconceptions*. Retrieved from http://samaritansnyc.org/myths-about-suicide

it is still important to note that it has been, over several years, the third-leading cause of death in this population, and in 2013 it jumped to the second-leading cause of death where it remained in 2014 (CDC, 2016). Several factors put adolescents at risk for suicide, including impulsive and high-risk behaviors, untreated mood disorders (e.g., major depression and bipolar disorder), access to lethal means (e.g., firearms), and substance abuse. One recent study (Reyes et al., 2015) found a link between some modes of anger expression in adolescents and suicide risk; in particular, hopelessness and hostility modes of anger expression were associated with an increase in suicidal tendency. The latest statistics from the CDC indicate that the most common method of completed suicide for adolescent males is by firearm; for adolescent females, it is suffocation (CDC, 2015a).

Among children younger than 10 years of age, the statistics demonstrate a low number of suicides, and some have argued that younger children do not have the capacity to intentionally consider and follow through with a suicide attempt. Anecdotal evidence has shown that this is not always the case, with some therapists identifying 5- to 9-year-olds actively talking about suicide (Jobes, 2015). Research is beginning to emerge that supports real risk in young children (Duran & McGuinness, 2016). Bridge and associates (2015) studied a large sample of children aged 5 to 11 and found that an average of 33 children per year die by suicide within this age group in the United States, predominately from suffocation and hanging. These researchers also noted that suicide was never coded as a cause of death for children under 5 years of age. When Whalen and associates (2015) studied children in the 3 to 7 age group, they found about 11% with suicidal ideation. This risk was correlated with male gender, psychiatric illness in their mothers, and psychiatric illness in the child. Over time, the incidence of self-inflicted harm in young males has remained stable, whereas steady increases have occurred in young females. In young girls aged 10 to 14 years, the incidence of self-inflicted injury has risen 18.8 percent every year between 2008 and 2015, and self-inflicted injury is one of the strongest risk factors for suicide (Mercado et al., 2017). Duran and McGuinness (2016) stress that the implications for nursing are clear; direct inquiry about suicide ideas is a "necessary component in healthcare encounters with children," including those in primary care, emergency departments, and with the school nurse.

Although the elderly comprise just over 13 percent of the population, they account for almost 15 percent of all suicides. In general, 70 percent of all suicides are among white males, but white males older than age 80 are at the greatest risk of all age, gender, and race groups. Almost 84 percent of elderly suicides are male, which is about five times greater than for females, and firearms are the most common means of completing suicide (American Association of Suicidology, 2015). The overall rate of suicide for females declines after age 65.

Religion

Historically, suicide rates among Protestants and Jews have been higher than among Roman Catholic or Muslim populations, but the degree of orthodoxy and affiliation with one's religion may be an important variable (Sadock et al., 2015). One study revealed that men and women who consider themselves affiliated with a religion are less likely than their non-religious counterparts to attempt suicide (Rasic et al., 2009). The authors found that religious affiliation is associated with decreased suicide attempts in both the general population and in those with a mental illness, independent of the availability of social support systems.

Socioeconomic Status

Individuals in the very highest and lowest social classes have higher suicide rates than those in the middle classes (Sadock et al., 2015). Suicide rates are higher in rural areas and with a twofold greater use of firearms as the means (Ivey-Stephenson et al., 2017). Kim and associates (2016) studied the factors influencing a move from suicide ideation to suicide attempts and found that low education and unemployment significantly increased the prevalence of attempts among young adult men and women *with suicide ideation*. Since previous attempts are a leading risk factor for completed suicide, assessing for suicide ideation and socioeconomic status may be an important preventive measure.

Ethnicity

With regard to ethnicity, statistics show that whites are at highest risk for suicide, followed by American Indians/Alaska Natives, African Americans, Hispanic Americans, and Asian Americans (CDC, 2015b). Recent research has highlighted two trends that illuminate issues of concern within specific ethnic groups. First, although suicide rates among whites are higher in adults and the elderly, within the American Indian community, young adults have a higher risk for suicide than does any other ethnic group, and the rate is higher than for the general population (Almendrala, 2015). Almendrala relays the story of a psychiatrist called to a reservation where there had been 17 suicides in the previous 8 months, and the community members described themselves as "grieved out." The second trend of concern, as Almendrala reports, is that the rates of suicide may be underestimated in this population because death certificates do not always report accurately regarding ethnicity.

Another recent study examined suicide trends among school-aged children younger than age 12 (Bridge et al., 2015) and found that suicide rates for black children 5 to 11 years of age nearly doubled over the period from 1993 to 2012, while the overall suicide rate in this age group remained relatively stable during the same time period. The use of hanging and/or suffocation as a means of taking one's own life also significantly increased in this population. It is hard to imagine what causes children so young to take their own lives. The contributing factors to these recent trends are not well understood and will require further research, including a review of the impact of healthcare disparities for select communities or populations.

Other Risk Factors

As previously stated, more than 90% of people who kill themselves have a diagnosable mental disorder, most commonly a mood disorder or a substance use disorder (NIMH, 2018). Individuals who have been hospitalized for a psychiatric illness have a five to 10 times greater risk of suicide than those with psychiatric illness in the general population (Sadock et al., 2015). This higher risk may be a reflection of the severity of their mental illness. Other recent research supports an increased risk of suicide in the period following discharge from psychiatric hospitalization, especially for those not connected to a system of care (Olfson et al., 2016). Suicide risk may increase early during treatment with antidepressants. One possible reason is that as an individual's energy returns, he or she may have an increased ability to act out self-destructive wishes. Although suicide is often thought of as strictly related to depression, there is also a recognized risk of suicide among people with schizophrenia, bipolar disorders, personality disorders, eating disorders, anxiety disorders, and substance use disorders. The importance of good suicide risk assessment for anyone seeking mental health services cannot be overstated.

Severe insomnia is associated with increased suicide risk even in the absence of depression. Use of alcohol, and particularly a combination of alcohol and barbiturates, increases the risk of suicide. Withdrawal from stimulants increases suicide risk as the person begins to "crash." Psychosis, especially with command hallucinations (hearing voices telling one to harm or kill oneself), poses a higher risk. Affliction with a chronic painful or disabling illness also increases the risk of suicide.

Several studies have indicated a higher risk for suicide among gay men, lesbians, and transgender (LGBT) individuals (Cassels, 2011; Cochran & Mays, 2000; Eisenberg & Resnick, 2006; King et al., 2008; Medscape Psychiatry, 2011; Plöderl et al., 2013). It is thought that this increased risk may be a function of the social stigma and discrimination associated with being part of a marginalized group. Additional personal stressors, including isolation, victimization, and stressful interpersonal relationships with family,

peers, and community, are not uncommon. A report from the CDC (2015c) identified that in a study of youth in grades 7 to 12, lesbian, gay, and bisexual youth were two times more likely to attempt suicide than their heterosexual peers.

Higher risk is also associated with a family history of suicide, especially in a same-gender parent and with individuals who have made previous suicide attempts. About one-half of individuals who kill themselves have previously attempted suicide. Loss of a loved one through death or separation and lack of employment or increased financial burden also increase risk.

In recent years, a number of suicides have been reported in the media among young people who are the victims of bullying. Zweig and Dank (2013) reported that 41% of youth are victims of physical bullying (most often boys), 17% are victims of cyberbullying, and girls are more likely to be victims of psychological bullying. Clearly, bullying is a prevalent concern among youth. Klomek, Sourander, and Gould (2011) report:

> Studies among middle school and high school students show an increased risk of suicidal behavior among bullies and victims. Both perpetrators and victims are at the highest risk for suicidal ideation.

Being bullied via the Internet or e-mail (called *cyberbullying*) has also been associated with increased risk of depression and suicidal behavior among young people. Researchers found that both perpetrators and victims of cyberbullying had more suicidal ideation and were more likely to attempt suicide than those who had not experienced such forms of peer aggression (Bauman, Toomey, & Walker, 2013; Hinduja & Patchin, 2010). Edgerton and Limber (2013), in a research brief on suicide and bullying, caution that although research does show that those who are bullied have high levels of suicidal thoughts and attempts, there is not enough research to identify a cause-and-effect relationship. Other risk factors such as mental health problems appear to play a larger role.

Predisposing Factors: Theories of Suicide

Psychological Theories

Anger Turned Inward

Freud (1957) believed that suicide was a response to the intense self-hatred that an individual possessed. The anger is first directed toward a love object but is ultimately turned inward against the self.

Hopelessness and Other Symptoms of Depression

Hopelessness has long been identified as both a symptom of depression and an underlying factor in the predisposition to suicide. Although many of the symptoms that are identified in suicide assessment tools attempt to assess for seriousness of suicide ideation, current research is attempting to glean which symptoms might be more predictive of the move from ideation to attempts, and although hopelessness is identified as a contributing factor, the strength of the person's intention to die may be more significant in triggering an attempt (Jobes, 2015).

History of Aggression and Violence

A history of violent behavior or impulsive acts has been associated with increased risk for suicide (Sadock et al., 2015), although recent evidence suggests that impulsive traits are higher in individuals with suicide ideation but not necessarily associated with more attempts (Klonsky & May, 2015b).

Shame and Humiliation

Shame and humiliation have long been identified as potential psychological triggers for attempting suicide. Some individuals view suicide as a "face-saving" mechanism—a way to prevent public humiliation following a social defeat, such as a sudden loss of status or income. Both shame and humiliation may also interrupt one's sense of connectedness with others, and sense of belonging and connectedness are considered protective against suicide. Evidence supports that the experience of shame is pronounced in trauma survivors (Taylor, 2015) and in females with borderline personality disorder (Wiklander et al., 2012). This research helps us understand some of the influencing factors for increased risk of suicide in these populations.

Interpersonal Theory

Durkheim (1951) studied the individual's interaction with the society in which he or she lived. He believed that the more cohesive the society and the more that the individual felt an integrated part of society, the less likely he or she was to carry out suicide. Durkheim described three social categories of suicide:

Egoistic suicide is the response of the individual who feels separate and apart from the mainstream of society. Integration is lacking, and the individual does not feel a part of any cohesive group (such as a family or a church).

Altruistic suicide is the opposite of egoistic suicide. The individual who is prone to altruistic suicide is excessively integrated into the group. The group is often governed by cultural, religious, or political ties, and allegiance is so strong that the individual will sacrifice his or her life for the group.

Anomic suicide occurs in response to changes in an individual's life (e.g., divorce, loss of job) that disrupt feelings of relatedness to the group. An interruption in the customary norms of behavior instills feelings of "separateness" and fears of being without support from the formerly cohesive group.

Interpersonal-Psychological Theories

Thomas Joiner's (2005) interpersonal-psychological theory of suicide supports some of the same principles advanced by Durkheim, associating lack of a feeling of belonging with suicide risk. But Joiner identifies that both interpersonal and psychological factors are critical to understanding suicide risk and his theory introduces the concept that suicide ideation and suicide attempts need to be understood as distinct processes. He proposed that low connectedness and a high sense of one's being a burden interact with each other to increase suicide thoughts and desires, but those features in the presence of high capability for suicide are strongly associated with the move from ideation to lethal attempts. He advances the concept that people become less fearful (and therefore more capable) of self-destructive acts when they expose themselves repeatedly to painful or violent stimuli; a kind of "working up" to actually being capable of self-harm. The move from suicide ideation to attempts is not viewed as an impulsive act but rather a process of steps that, over time, create greater and greater risk.

The Three-Step Theory

Klonsky and May (2015a), inspired by Joiner's theory and based on their research finding that impulsivity is elevated both in people who have made suicide attempts and those who have thoughts and have never made an attempt, sought to identify the factors that elevate suicide ideation to an active risk for attempts. Their research supported the following three-step trajectory:

1. Pain (usually psychological pain) when combined with hopelessness significantly increases suicide ideation (for both men and women and across age groups).
2. Connectedness prevents suicide ideation from escalating in those at risk, but when pain and hopelessness exceed one's sense of connectedness to others, suicide ideation becomes active.
3. When strong, active suicide ideation is present, it leads to an attempt only if one has the capacity to make an attempt.

Biological Theories

Genetics

Twin studies have shown a much higher concordance rate for monozygotic twins than for dizygotic twins. Some studies with people who have attempted suicide have focused on the genotypic variations in the gene for tryptophan hydroxylase, with results indicating significant association to suicidality (Sadock et al., 2015). Tryptophan hydroxylase is an enzyme associated with the synthesis of serotonin, and diminished serotonin has implications for both depression and suicidal behavior. Other research has identified a genetic variation in prefrontal cortex tissue that may be a biomarker for suicide risk when vulnerable individuals are exposed to a significant stressor (Sudak, 2017). These findings suggest the potential for genetic predisposition toward suicidal behavior but more research is needed.

Neurochemical Factors

A number of studies have revealed a deficiency of serotonin (measured as a decrease in the levels of 5-hydroxyindole acetic acid [5-HIAA] in the cerebrospinal fluid) in depressed clients who attempted suicide (Sadock et al., 2015). These studies, as well as postmortem studies, have supported the hypothesis that deficiencies in central nervous system (CNS) serotonin are associated with suicide.

However, a recent meta-analysis examining biological factors found that they are, in general, weak predictors of a future suicide attempt or death by suicide (Chang et al., 2016). The only two biological factors that had statistical significance in this analysis were cytokines (anti-inflammatory response chemicals) and low levels of fish oil nutrients (including omega-3).

Application of the Nursing Process With the Suicidal Client

A multitude of research studies are being published that explore suicide from many different vantage points to identify demographics, risk factors, predictors of risk for suicide attempts, and strategies for prevention. Many of these studies are helping nurses become more aware of the phenomenon of suicide and understand the limitations of research in making a clinical judgment about a patient's actual risks versus statistical risks. Influential organizations across the nation are advancing the importance of improving the quality of care, documentation, and reporting of details around sentinel events related to acts of or deaths

by suicide. In addition to government-endorsed national strategies for suicide prevention, the Joint Commission (2016) has advanced standards that include requiring organizations to conduct risk assessments "identifying specific patient characteristics and environmental features that may increase or decrease the risk of suicide." It is nurses practicing in general medical settings, including emergency departments and primary care practices, who are frontline practitioners in the fight to prevent suicide so these assessment skills are critical wherever nurses are practicing. The American Psychiatric Nurses Association (APNA, 2018; Puntil et al., 2013) has taken a leadership role in identifying psychiatric mental health nurse essential competencies for assessment and management of individuals at risk for suicide. The CDC (2011) has advanced strategies for uniform definition and reporting about acts of self-directed violence to improve data collection and ultimately improve our understanding and prevention of suicide. At the heart of this wealth of information is the necessity for accurate, comprehensive assessment that includes collaboration with the patient and other clinicians and is rooted in strategies to form a therapeutic relationship of trust and open communication.

Assessment

When nurses assess a client's suicide ideation, it is important to identify and distinguish ideas (thoughts), plans (intentions), and attempts (behavior). Each of these assessment factors can provide information about level of risk. When the client has attempted self-injury, it is important to distinguish between *suicidal self-injury* and *nonsuicidal self-injury*. The latter injury is often used as a method to release emotions, but it may also be a way of communicating the severity of distress that the client is experiencing (Nock et al., 2013). Dr. David Satcher, as Surgeon General of the United States, in his "Call to Action to Prevent Suicide," spoke of risk factors and protective factors (U.S. Public Health Service [USPHS], 1999). This report initiated a national movement toward research designed to better understand predictors of suicide risk and develop more evidence-based interventions. Current models have clarified risk factors as different from warning signs that are associated with a greater potential for suicide and suicidal behavior. Protective factors have been identified that are associated with reduced potential for suicide. Examples of protective factors are outlined in Box 11–1. Figure 11–1 presents a model for differentiating low, high, and imminent suicide risk. The goal of such models is not to

BOX 11–1 Examples of Protective Factors

Resilient temperament

Social competency

Skills in problem-solving, coping, and conflict resolution

Perception of social support from adults and peers

Positive expectations, optimism for the future; identification of future goals

Connectedness to family, school, community

Presence and involvement of caring adults (for adolescents)

Integration in social networks

Cultural and religious beliefs that discourage suicide and encourage preservation of life

Access to quality social services and clinical healthcare for mental, physical, and substance use disorders

Support through ongoing medical and mental healthcare relationships

Restricted access to highly lethal means of suicide

Source: Crosby, A.E., Ortega, L., & Melanson, C. (2011). Self-directed Violence Surveillance: Uniform definitions and recommended data elements, Version 1.0. Atlanta (GA): Centers for Disease Control and Prevention, National Center for Injury Prevention and Control. Retrieved from http://www.cdc.gov/violenceprevention/pdf/Self-Directed-Violence-a.pdf

predict a suicide attempt but to identify the level of intervention needed to prevent an attempt.

Demographics

The following demographics are assessed when evaluating a client for suicide risk:

■ **Age:** Adolescents and the elderly have been generally identified as high-risk groups, but recent statistics demonstrating the highest incidence in the 45- to 54-year age group as well as increasing incidence among children suggests that nurses should pay close attention to assessing for suicide risk in all age groups.

■ **Gender:** Males are at higher risk for death by suicide than females, but females attempt suicide more frequently.

■ **Ethnicity/race:** The CDC reports highest rates of suicide among Caucasians followed by American Indians and Alaska Natives (CDC, 2015b).

■ **Marital status:** Single, divorced, and widowed individuals are at higher risk for suicide than are married people, particularly during periods of change in status.

■ **Socioeconomic status:** Individuals in the highest and lowest socioeconomic classes are at higher risk than those in the middle classes.

■ **Occupation:** Healthcare professionals (especially physicians), law enforcement officers, dentists, artists, mechanics, lawyers, and insurance agents have all been identified as occupational groups incurring greater risks for suicide (Sadock et al., 2015). Potential contributing factors include occupations that involve high stress, isolation, lack of access to healthcare resources, and repeated exposure to painful or violent stimuli.

■ **Method:** The lethality of the method identified by an individual with suicide ideation or by one who has already made an attempt provides meaningful information about the client's intent to die. Use of firearms, hanging, and suffocation, for example, are considered highly lethal methods.

■ **Religion:** People with a close religious affiliation may be at less risk for attempting suicide if they believe, for example, that suicide is an unforgivable sin or that within their religious affiliation suicide is strictly forbidden. Conversely, people *without* close affiliations that impose restrictions about suicide may be at greater risk.

■ **Family history:** A family history of suicide increases an individual's risk for suicide.

■ **Military history:** Suicide rates among military personnel now exceed those of the general population (Nock et al., 2013).

Presenting Symptoms and Medical-Psychiatric Diagnosis

Assessment data to screen for suicide risk must be gathered for all clients regardless of the psychiatric or physical condition for which he or she is being treated. Mood disorders (major depression and bipolar disorders) are the most common disorders that precede suicide. Individuals with substance use disorders are also at high risk. Other psychiatric disorders in which suicide risks have been identified include anxiety disorders, schizophrenia, bipolar disorders, substance use disorders, anorexia nervosa, and borderline and antisocial personality disorders. Other chronic and terminal physical illnesses have also been identified as potentiating risk factors.

Suicidal Ideas or Acts

How serious is the client's intent to die by suicide? Does the person have a plan? If so, does he or she have the means? How lethal are the means? Does he or she intend to carry out this plan? Has the individual ever attempted suicide before? These are all questions that must be asked by the person conducting the assessment of the client who is deemed at risk for suicide.

Individuals may provide both behavioral and verbal clues as to the intent of their act. Examples of

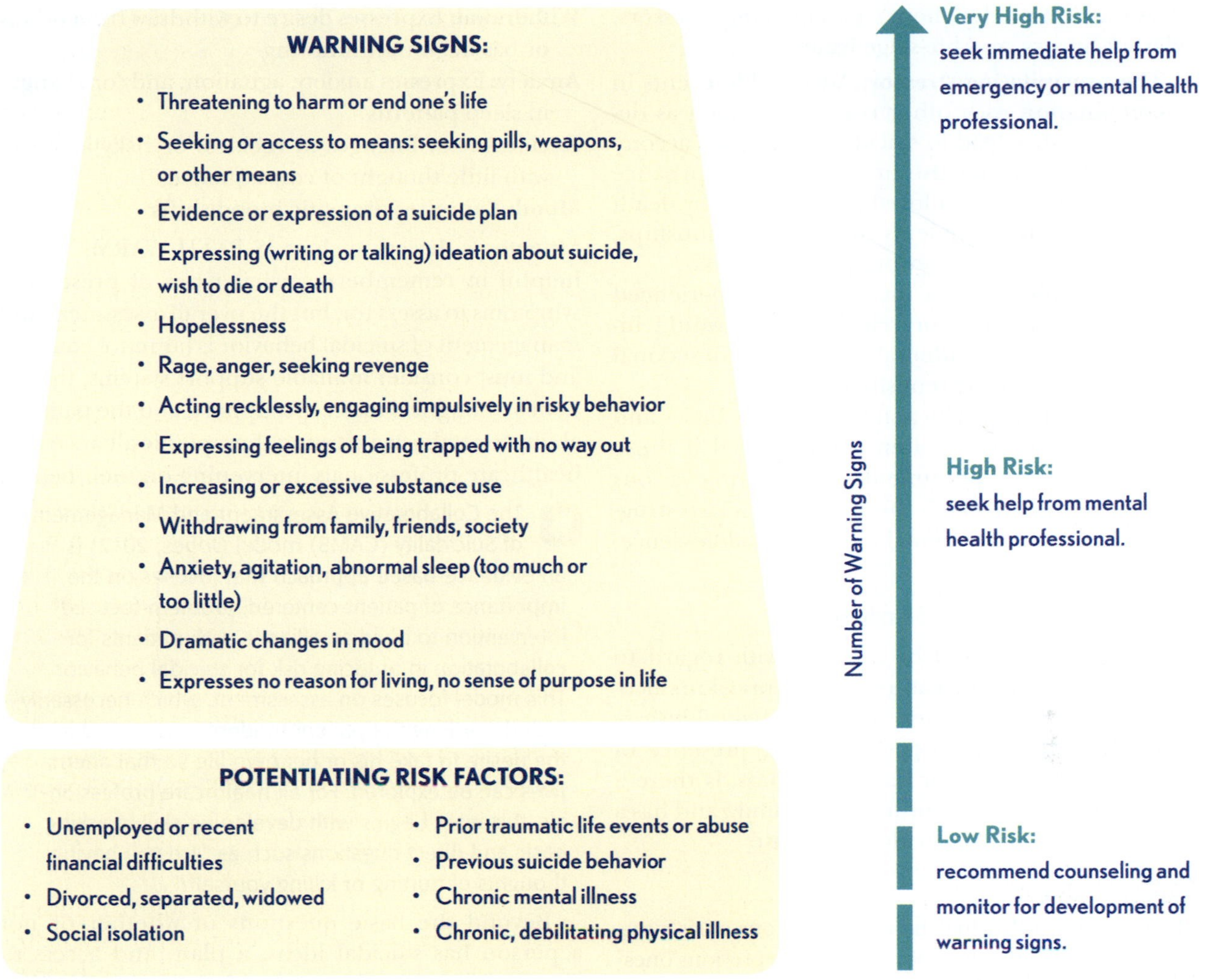

WARNING SIGNS:

- Threatening to harm or end one's life
- Seeking or access to means: seeking pills, weapons, or other means
- Evidence or expression of a suicide plan
- Expressing (writing or talking) ideation about suicide, wish to die or death
- Hopelessness
- Rage, anger, seeking revenge
- Acting recklessly, engaging impulsively in risky behavior
- Expressing feelings of being trapped with no way out
- Increasing or excessive substance use
- Withdrawing from family, friends, society
- Anxiety, agitation, abnormal sleep (too much or too little)
- Dramatic changes in mood
- Expresses no reason for living, no sense of purpose in life

POTENTIATING RISK FACTORS:

- Unemployed or recent financial difficulties
- Divorced, separated, widowed
- Social isolation
- Prior traumatic life events or abuse
- Previous suicide behavior
- Chronic mental illness
- Chronic, debilitating physical illness

Number of Warning Signs

Very High Risk: seek immediate help from emergency or mental health professional.

High Risk: seek help from mental health professional.

Low Risk: recommend counseling and monitor for development of warning signs.

FIGURE 11–1   Risk factors and warning signs for suicide. Reprinted with permission from the Ontario Hospital Association.

behavioral clues that may indicate a decision to carry out the intent include giving away prized possessions, getting financial affairs in order, writing suicide notes, and sudden lifts in mood.

Verbal clues may be both direct and indirect. Examples of direct statements include "I want to die" or "I'm going to kill myself." Examples of indirect statements include "This is the last time you'll see me," "I won't be around much longer for the doctor to have to worry about," or "I don't have anything worth living for anymore."

Assessment must include determining whether the individual has a plan, and if so, whether he or she has the means to carry out that plan. If the person states the suicide will be carried out with a gun, does he or she have access to a gun? Bullets? If pills are planned, what kind of pills? Are they accessible? The lethality of the method identified by an individual with suicide ideation provides meaningful information about the client's intent to die. Intent to use a firearm, for example, is a highly lethal method. Asking the client "How likely are you to carry out this plan?" may provide verbal confirmation of their level of intent.

Interpersonal Support System

Does the individual have support persons on whom he or she can rely during a crisis situation? Lack of a meaningful network of satisfactory relationships may implicate an individual as a high risk for suicide during an emotional crisis.

Analysis of the Suicidal Crisis

Three aspects of assessment that enhance understanding of the client's current suicidal crisis include an evaluation of the client's precipitating stressors, relevant history, and life-stage issues.

■ **The precipitating stressor:** Adverse life events in combination with other risk factors, such as depression, may lead to suicide. Life stresses accompanied by an increase in emotional disturbance include the loss of a loved person either by death or by divorce, problems in major relationships, changes in roles, or serious physical illness.

■ **Relevant history:** Has the individual experienced numerous failures or rejections that would increase his or her vulnerability for a dysfunctional response to the current situation?

■ **Life-stage issues:** The ability to tolerate losses and disappointments is often compromised if those losses and disappointments occur during various stages of life in which the individual is also struggling with developmental issues (e.g., adolescence, midlife, old age).

Psychiatric, Medical, and Family History

The individual should be assessed with regard to previous psychiatric treatment for depression, alcoholism, or previous suicide attempts. Medical history should be obtained to determine the presence of chronic, debilitating, or terminal illness. Is there a history of depressive disorder in the family, and has a close relative died by suicide in the past?

Coping Strategies

How has the individual handled previous crisis situations? How does this situation differ from previous ones?

Presenting Symptoms

Several acronyms have been developed as mnemonic devices to summarize important factors that may increase a person's risk for suicidal behavior. One of these is the acronym IS PATH WARM? (American Association of Suicidology, 2015; Juhnke, Granello, & Lebron-Striker, 2007). The assessment items and descriptors for each letter are as follows:

Ideation: Has suicide ideas that are current and active, especially with an identified plan

Substance abuse: Has current and/or excessive use of alcohol or other mood-altering drugs

Purposelessness: Expresses thoughts that there is no reason to continue living

Anger: Expresses uncontrolled anger or feelings of rage

Trapped: Expresses the belief that there is no way out of the current situation

Hopelessness: Expresses lack of hope and perceives little chance of positive change

Withdrawal: Expresses desire to withdraw from others or has begun withdrawing

Anxiety: Expresses anxiety, agitation, and/or changes in sleep patterns

Recklessness: Engages in reckless or risky activities with little thought of consequences

Mood: Expresses dramatic mood shifts

Mnemonic devices such as IS PATH WARM? can be helpful in remembering what types of presenting symptoms to assess for, but the overall assessment and management of suicidal behavior is far more complex and must consider available support systems, the patient's willingness to accept support, and the patient's ability to establish a trusting therapeutic alliance with healthcare professionals intervening on their behalf.

The Collaborative Assessment and Management of Suicidality (CAMS) model (Jobes, 2012) is an evidence-based approach that focuses on the importance of patient-centered, problem-focused intervention to build an alliance with patients for collaboration in reducing risk for suicidal behavior. This model focuses on assessment, which necessarily includes asking the patient to identify what is driving the desire to take his or her own life so that alternatives can be explored. For all healthcare professionals, this work begins with developing skill in asking basic and direct questions such as "Are you having thoughts of hurting or killing yourself?"

Beyond the basic questions of whether or not a person has suicidal ideas, a plan, and access to means, there must be recognition that patients are not always forthcoming or truthful in their answers to such questions. Several strategies for enhancing a collaborative, therapeutic relationship and communication about suicide assessment have been elaborated. Because nurses are often at the front line of this assessment in medical-surgical, emergency department, outpatient care, schools, and other healthcare settings, they must be thoughtful, comprehensive, and conscientious in this pursuit regardless of the practice setting and whether or not the patient has been identified as having mental health issues. Shea (2009) states that nurses need to assess not only what the client is directly stating about his or her suicidal intent (stated intent) but also the amount of thinking, planning, and behaviors associated with suicide ideation (reflected intent) and the suicide intent that is withheld from the nurse (withheld intent). A summary of guiding principles in suicide risk assessment is included in Table 11–2.

TABLE 11–2 Guiding Principles for Suicide Risk Assessment

PRINCIPLES	EXPLANATION
Screening for suicide risk should be conducted as an essential component of health assessment, and risk factors, warning signs, and threats should be taken seriously.	This includes identifying through detailed assessment the individual's unique situation to discern additional resources, consults, and interventions needed to ensure patient safety.
Establishment of a therapeutic relationship is foundational to effective suicide risk assessment.	This includes establishing trust through empathy and respect, which provides a safe environment for the client to tell his or her story.
Suicide risk assessment is complex and challenges the nurse to use many different communication strategies.	This includes exploring the client's thoughts, feelings, and behaviors from a variety of perspectives.
Suicide risk assessment is an ongoing process, and level of risk can increase or decrease over time.	This includes assessing over time for fluctuations in risk factors, changes in stress level, changes in intensity of ideation, changes in intention to act on suicide ideation, and changes in support systems.
Collaboration with the client and other sources of information facilitates confidence in clinical judgments.	This includes information provided by other people who are familiar with the client from home, work, or school and other clinical team members. Collaboration also implies that all those involved in the client's care are working together.
Suicide risk assessment uses direct rather than indirect language.	This includes using terminology such as "suicide" and "death" rather than "not happy with living" or other indirect statements. It also communicates to the client that these are acceptable topics to discuss.
Suicide risk assessment attempts to discern the underlying message.	This includes attempting to discern when the patient is communicating unbearable distress, feeling trapped, feeling hopeless, and/or feeling driven to avoid additional emotional or physical pain.
Suicide risk assessment considers cultural context.	This includes recognizing that anyone regardless of race, religion, or culture may be at risk for suicide. Some cultural or religious prohibitions may influence someone's willingness to openly discuss personal feelings.
Suicide risk assessment is documented in detail.	This includes risk factors, warning signs, underlying themes, level of risk, clinical judgments, and recommended interventions.

Source: Adapted from *Perlman, C.M., Neufeld, E., Martin, L., Goy, M., & Hirdes, J.P. (2011). Risk Assessment Inventory:* A resource guide for Canadian healthcare organizations. Toronto: Ontario Hospital Association and Canadian Patient Safety Institute.

One model for enhancing communication in suicide assessment is the CASE (Chronological Assessment of Suicide Events) approach. It is described as a flexible guide for interviewing that includes communication techniques designed to elicit and enhance detailed, valid feedback from clients about sensitive topics such as suicide. Several examples, as elaborated by Shea (2009), follow:

■ *Normalizing* communicates that the client is not the only one who experiences suicidal ideation. Example: "Sometimes when people are in a lot of emotional pain, they have thoughts of killing themselves. Have you had any thoughts like that?"

■ Asking about behavioral events rather than the client's opinions may elicit more concrete information. Example: "What did you do when you had those thoughts?" "How many pills did you take?" "What happened next?"

■ Gentle assumptions encourage further discussion by assuming there is more to tell. Example: "What other times have you attempted suicide?"

■ Denial of the specific is helpful when a client generally denies suicidal ideation. This strategy encourages more in-depth thought and response by asking questions that might trigger memories of specific events. Example: After the client denies suicidal ideation in response to a general question, the nurse asks more specifically, "Have you ever had thoughts of overdosing?" "Have you ever had thoughts about shooting yourself?"

■ Chronologically exploring the presenting suicide event, recent suicide events, past suicide events, and finally the immediate suicide events can broaden the nurse's understanding of the client's immediate suicidal intent in the context of his or her behavior over time.

Diagnosis and Outcome Identification

Nursing diagnoses for the suicidal patient may include the following:

■ Risk for suicide related to feelings of hopelessness and desperation
■ Hopelessness related to absence of support systems and perception of worthlessness

Outcome Criteria

Outcome criteria include short- and long-term goals. Timelines are individually determined. The criteria that follow may be used for measurement of outcomes in the care of the suicidal patient.

The patient

■ Has experienced no physical harm to self.
■ Sets realistic goals for self.
■ Expresses some optimism and hope for the future.

Planning and Implementation

Table 11–3 provides a plan of care for the hospitalized suicidal patient. Nursing diagnoses are presented, along with outcome criteria, appropriate nursing interventions, and rationales for each.

Intervention With the Suicidal Client Following Discharge (or Outpatient Suicidal Client)

In some instances, it may be determined that suicidal intent is low and that hospitalization is not required. Instead, the client with suicidal ideation may be treated in an outpatient setting. Guidelines for treatment of the suicidal client on an outpatient basis include the following:

■ The person should have immediate access to support systems and be tied to a system of care because the term following hospital discharge is a high-risk period. Arrangements must be made for the client to stay with family or friends. If this is not possible, hospitalization should be reconsidered.
■ A detailed safety plan should be developed that is an outgrowth of a comprehensive assessment and a collaborative problem-solving discussion with the client. This intervention explores with the client what he or she will do to stay safe if there is a repeat or increase in suicidal thoughts or urges. See

Box 11–2 for more on the essential components of a safety plan.
■ A safety plan should not be confused with a no-suicide contract See Boxes 11–3 and 11–4 to learn about issues associated with developing an appropriate safety plan.
■ Enlist the help of family or friends to ensure that the home environment is safe from dangerous items, such as firearms or stockpiled drugs. Give support persons the telephone number of the counselor or an emergency contact person in the event that the counselor is not available.
■ Appointments may need to be scheduled daily or every other day at first until the immediate suicidal crisis has subsided.
■ Establish rapport and promote a trusting relationship. It is important for the suicide counselor to become a key person in the client's support system at this time.
■ Accept the client's feelings in a nonjudgmental manner.

> **CLINICAL PEARL** Be direct. Talk openly and matter-of-factly about suicide. Listen actively and encourage expression of feelings, including anger.

■ Discuss the current crisis situation in the client's life. Use the problem-solving approach. Offer alternatives to suicide while at the same time empathizing with the client's pain that led to viewing suicide as an option (Jobes, 2012). An example of this kind of communication might be:

"I understand how this emotional pain you've been experiencing led you to consider suicide, but I'd like to explore with you some alternative ways to decrease your pain and to identify some reasons for continuing to live."

■ Help the client identify areas of the life situation that are within his or her control and those that the client does not have the ability to control. Discuss feelings associated with these control issues. It is important for the client to feel some control over his or her life situation in order to perceive a measure of self-worth.
■ The physician or nurse practitioner may prescribe antidepressants for an individual who is experiencing suicidal depression. It is wise to prescribe no more than a 3-day supply of the medication with no refills. The prescription can then be renewed at the client's next counseling session. **NOTE**: Sadock and associates (2015) have stated:

Patients with depressive disorders are at increased risk of suicide as they begin to improve and regain

TABLE 11–3 │ CARE PLAN FOR THE SUICIDAL PATIENT

NURSING DIAGNOSIS: RISK FOR SUICIDE

RELATED TO: Feelings of hopelessness and desperation

OUTCOME CRITERIA	NURSING INTERVENTIONS	RATIONALE
Patient will not harm self.	1. 💬 Ask directly: "Have you thought about harming yourself in any way? If so, what do you plan to do? Do you have the means to carry out this plan?"	1. The risk of suicide is greatly increased if patient has developed a plan and particularly if means are accessible for the patient to execute the plan.
	2. Create a safe environment for patient. Remove all potentially harmful objects from patient's access (sharp objects, straps, belts, ties, glass items, alcohol). Supervise closely during meals and medication administration. Perform room searches as deemed necessary.	2. Patient safety is a nursing priority.
	3. Maintain close observation of patient. Depending on level of suicide precaution, provide one-to-one contact, constant visual observation, or every-15-minute checks. Place in room close to nurse's station; do not assign to private room. Accompany to off-unit activities if attendance is indicated. May need to accompany to bathroom.	3. Close observation is necessary to ensure that patient does not harm self in any way. Being alert for suicidal and escape attempts facilitates being able to prevent or interrupt harmful behavior.
	4. Maintain special care in administration of medications.	4. Prevents saving up to overdose or discarding.
	5. Make rounds at frequent, *irregular* intervals (especially at night, toward early morning, at change of shift, or other predictably busy times for staff).	5. Prevents patient from saving up to overdose or discarding medication. Prevents staff surveillance from becoming predictable. To be aware of patient's location is important, especially when staff is busy and least available and observable.
	6. Encourage patient to express honest feelings, including anger. Provide activities for appropriate outlets for anger if needed.	6. Depression and suicidal behaviors may be viewed as anger turned inward on the self. If this anger can be verbalized in a nonthreatening environment, patient may be able to eventually resolve these feelings.
Patient develops a safety plan for management of suicidal thoughts and urges.	1. Establish a trusting, therapeutic relationship to encourage open discussion of suicide.	1. Establishing trust and open communications encourages client to share thoughts and feelings.
	2. Collaborate with patient to develop a safety plan that includes recognition of warning signs, coping strategies, supportive people and places, resources and contact information for crisis management, and plans to restrict access to lethal means.	2. Development of a comprehensive **collaborative safety plan** concretizes resources and management strategies. Actively engaging the patient in collaboration on the development of a safety plan promotes client ownership and investment in the process.

Continued

TABLE 11–3 | CARE PLAN FOR THE SUICIDAL PATIENT—cont'd

OUTCOME CRITERIA	NURSING INTERVENTIONS	RATIONALE
	3. Assess verbal and nonverbal clues to identify the likelihood that patient intends to follow through with the established safety plan and evaluate patient's follow-through with safety plan measures while still hospitalized.	3. Assessment of patient safety includes analyzing congruence of verbal communication, nonverbal communication, and behavior.

NURSING DIAGNOSIS: HOPELESSNESS

RELATED TO: Absence of support systems and perception of worthlessness

EVIDENCED BY: Verbal cues (despondent content, "I can't"); decreased affect; lack of initiative; suicidal ideas or attempts

OUTCOME CRITERIA	NURSING INTERVENTIONS	RATIONALE
Patient will verbalize a measure of hope and acceptance of life and situations over which he or she has no control.	1. Identify stressors in patient's life that precipitated current crisis. Include assessing the degree of emotional pain and hopelessness in relationship to feelings of connectedness or lack of connectedness with others.	1. It is important to identify causative or contributing factors in order to plan appropriate assistance.
	2. Determine coping behaviors previously used and patient's perception of effectiveness then and now.	2. It is important to identify patient's strengths and encourage their use in current crisis situation.
	3. Encourage patient to explore and verbalize feelings and perceptions related to reasons for wanting to die as well as reasons for wanting to live.	3. Identification of feelings underlying behaviors helps patient to begin process of taking control of own life and enables the nurse to help the patient focus on maximizing his or her reasons for wanting to live.
	4. 💬 Provide expressions of hope to patient in positive, low-key manner (e.g., "I know you feel you cannot go on, but I believe that things can get better for you. What you are feeling is temporary. It is okay if you don't see it just now." "You matter.")	4. Even though patient feels hopeless, it is helpful to hear positive expressions from others. Patient's current state of mind may prevent him or her from identifying anything positive in life. It is important to accept patient's feelings nonjudgmentally and to affirm the individual's personal worth and value.
	5. Help patient identify areas of life situation that are under own control.	5. Patient's emotional condition may interfere with ability to problem solve. Assistance may be required to perceive the benefits and consequences of available alternatives accurately.
	6. Identify sources that patient may use after discharge when crises occur or feelings of hopelessness and possible suicidal ideation prevail.	6. Patient should be made aware of local suicide hotlines or other local support services from which he or she may seek assistance following discharge from the hospital. A concrete plan provides hope in the face of a crisis situation.

BOX 11–2 Essential Components of a Safety Plan

According to Stanley and Brown (2008, pp. 3–4), the essential components of a safety plan include nursing support and assistance for the following:

1. Recognizing warning signs that precede suicide crises
2. Identifying and employing internal coping strategies that the client can implement without needing to contact additional support people
3. Identifying supportive family members and friends with whom he or she can discuss suicide and who may help resolve a potential crisis
4. Identifying people and healthy social settings that he or she can use for general support and distraction from suicidal thoughts and urges
5. Identifying resources and contact information for mental health professionals and agencies when needed in an escalating crisis situation
6. Problem-solving with the client ways to reduce the potential for access to and use of lethal means

Once the safety plan is elaborated with the client, an evaluation of the appropriateness of the plan and a collaborative assessment of the likelihood that the client will implement this plan should be conducted.

Assessment for suicidal risk and responsive intervention must be ongoing, because suicidal ideas and intent may change over hours, days, or longer time periods. The need for revision of the safety plan may become evident. Critical times for reassessment of risk and reevaluation of the safety plan (Hoffman, 2013) include the following:

1. When there is a change in the client's clinical presentation or worsening of symptoms
2. When medications or treatments are changed
3. When significant others identify an increase in concern
4. When a client stops treatment

BOX 11–3 The Issue of No-Suicide Contracts

A critical issue that needs to be understood is that of no-suicide contracts, sometimes called *safety contracts*, a strategy used by some clinicians in the context of a long-term, therapeutic relationship in which the client "promises" to contact the clinician before acting on suicidal ideation. No-suicide contracts are not the same as the development of a thorough safety plan. Contracting with a client is a controversial and often misused strategy (Hoffman, 2013; Shea, 2009). Evidence has not supported the efficacy of this method as a primary intervention (Drew, 2001; Freedenthal, 2013; Rudd, Mandrusiak, & Joiner, 2006). In fact, it may even be counterproductive in clients with borderline or passive-aggressive pathology (Shea, 2009). Such contracts should *never* be used in short-term encounters with clients, such as in emergency departments or during brief hospital stays, or with clients who are unknown, agitated, psychotic, impulsive, or under the influence of drugs and alcohol (Hoffman, 2013). They should never be used with the presumption that they will deter a client from attempting suicide. Shea adds that if clinicians use a safety contract with the belief that it will be a deterrent to suicide, they should understand that it not only "guarantees nothing [but also] may yield a false sense of security" among clinicians (2009, p. 21). The consequential danger is that clinicians may become less watchful or feel less need to reassess the client, thus missing critical signs of increasing suicide risk. Outside of practicing therapy in an advanced practice role, nurses should avoid no-suicide contracting altogether. Even in the conduct of therapy, it should be used with great caution and for limited, specific assessment purposes.

In general, it is important to recognize that not all suicidal individuals are alike, so interventions should be multifaceted and suicide prevention plans should be comprehensive. Many models and tools for suicide assessment have been developed. One such model, SAFE-T (Suicide Assessment Five-step Evaluation and Triage), summarizes the key elements in suicide assessment (see Box 11–4).

---

the energy needed to plan and carry out a suicide (paradoxical suicide). It is usually unwise to give a depressed patient a prescription for a large number of antidepressants, especially tricyclic drugs, at the time of their discharge from the hospital. (p. 366)

■ Psychological interventions that have demonstrated effectiveness in reducing suicidal behavior include dialectical behavior therapy (DBT), cognitive behavior therapy, and CAMS (Jobes, 2015).

Single interventions, including hospitalization, medication, and no-suicide contracts are not supported by evidence as effective in reducing suicides (Jobes, 2015). Clients need to be actively engaged as partners in every step of the assessment and intervention process.

Information for Family and Friends of the Suicidal Client

The following suggestions are made for family and friends of an individual who is suicidal:

■ Take any hint of suicide seriously. Anyone expressing suicidal feelings needs immediate attention.
■ Do not keep secrets. If a suicidal person says, "Promise you won't tell anyone," do not make that promise. Suicidal individuals are ambivalent about dying, and suicidal behavior is a cry for help. It is that ambivalence that leads the person to confide to you the suicidal thoughts. Get help for the

---

BOX 11–4 SAFE-T: Suicide Assessment Five-Step Evaluation and Triage

1. Identify risk factors
   Note those that can be modified to reduce risk.
2. Identify protective factors
   Note those that can be enhanced.
3. Conduct suicide inquiry
   Evaluate suicidal thoughts, plans, behavior, and intent.
4. Determine risk level and intervention
   Choose appropriate intervention to address and reduce level of risk.
5. Document
   Record assessment of risk, rationale, intervention, and follow-up.

---

person and for you. 1-800-SUICIDE is a national hotline that is available 24 hours a day.

- Be a good listener. If people express suicidal thoughts or feel depressed, hopeless, or worthless, be supportive. Let them know you are there for them and are willing to help them seek professional help.
- Many people find it awkward to put into words how another person's life is important for their own well-being, but it is important to stress that the person's life is important to you and to others. Emphasize in specific terms the ways in which the person's suicide would be devastating to you and to others.
- Express concern for individuals who express thoughts about suicide. The individual may make veiled comments or comments that sound as if he or she is joking, or the person may be withdrawn and reluctant to discuss what he or she is thinking. In each case ask questions, acknowledge the person's pain and feelings of hopelessness and encourage the individual to talk to someone else if he or she does not feel comfortable talking with you.
- Familiarize yourself with suicide intervention resources, such as mental health centers and suicide hotlines.
- Ensure that access to firearms or other means of self-harm is restricted.
- Communicate caring and commitment to provide support. Fleener (n.d.) offers the following suggestions for interacting with people who are suicidal:
  - Acknowledge and accept their feelings and be an active listener.
  - Try to give them hope and remind them that what they are feeling is temporary.
  - Stay with them. Do not leave them alone. Go to where they are, if necessary.

- Show love and encouragement. Hold them, hug them, touch them. Allow them to cry and express anger.
- Help the person seek professional help.
- Remove any items from the home with which the person may harm himself or herself.
- If there are children present, try to remove them from the home. Perhaps friends or relatives can assist by taking the children to their home. This type of situation can be extremely traumatic for children.
- DO NOT judge suicidal people, show anger toward them, provoke guilt in them, discount their feelings, or tell them to "snap out of it." This is a very real and serious situation to suicidal individuals. They are in real pain. They feel the situation is hopeless and that there is no other way to resolve it aside from taking their own life.

Intervention With Families and Friends of Suicide Victims

Suicide of a family member can induce a whole gamut of feelings in the survivors. It has long been recognized that the bereavement process for families in which a member has taken his or her own life is complicated and requires an understanding by healthcare providers of some unique burdens of this type of loss. Macnab (1993) identified the following symptoms, which may be evident in family and friends after the suicide of a loved one:

- A sense of guilt and responsibility
- Anger, resentment, and rage that can never find its "object"
- A heightened sense of emotionality, helplessness, failure, and despair
- A recurring self-searching: "If only I had done something," "If only I had not done something," "If only. . . ."
- A sense of confusion and search for an explanation: "Why did this happen?" "What does it mean?" "What could have stopped it?" "What will people think?"
- A sense of inner injury; family feels wounded; does not know how they will ever get over it and get on with life
- A severe strain placed on relationships; a sense of impatience, irritability, and anger possible between family members
- A heightened feeling of vulnerability to illness and disease possible with this added burden of emotional stress

Read "Real People, Real Stories" for a better understanding of one person's lived experience of losing a child to suicide.

Real People, Real Stories

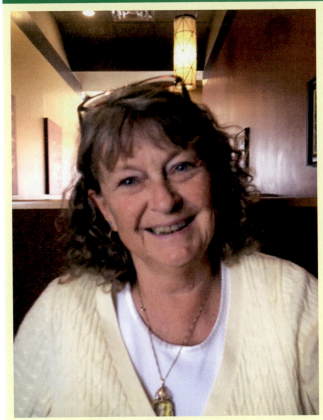

Losing a loved one to suicide results in a grief process often complicated by stigma, misinformation, lack of information, and sometimes a sense of alienation from others. Emmy's story describes her ongoing journey to grapple with the loss of her son to suicide.

Karyn: We've talked before but tell me more about your journey since Paul's death.

Emmy: My son Paul died in 1986 at age 17. The thing I remember most is that no one was talking about it. There were 10 students who died in his high school. Two others were known to be suicides.

Karyn: Do you mean no one was talking about it in the school system?

Emmy: Well, the students in Paul's class took up a collection that was for Paul, but the school couldn't decide how to use it, so it just sat there for the longest time. My other son heard they were going to use the money for supplies, so I went and talked to them to make sure that didn't happen. The school eventually built a memorial garden that became dedicated to all of the students who had died.

Paul died in June, and in August, when all the other students were returning to school, I got a call from a community suicide survivors counselor who told me she was holding a high school assembly to discuss suicide. I wanted her to talk to the ninth and tenth graders, but they wouldn't permit it. I thought the younger kids needed to talk about and learn about this too—they had been my younger son's classmates, and they were affected by it as well. When the suicide counselor intervened, the teachers were told to watch Paul's friends for any evidence of "copycat" behavior, but that was all. I felt the school administration thought there was a stigma in talking about the cause of his death. I found out later that the seniors were talking about and memorializing Paul in their study halls. They were remembering him as a friend who was missed.

Karyn: How has your family coped with Paul's death?

Emmy: We didn't talk about Paul for the longest time; it was as if he didn't exist. We were very separate; we all went in our own directions. My husband started taking long bicycle trips, and he worked on a suicide hotline. I got very involved with offering a program for high school students called Listening POST (people offering students time), which allowed students to talk about anything they wanted to.

Karyn: I know you've told me that you're still close to several of Paul's peers.

Emmy: Oh yes, and their children too. But our family just became very separate. I don't even know how my other son got through his freshman year of high school. We went to a suicide survivors group as a family, and it was important to me as an outlet to talk, but we didn't talk as a family . . . and then we just stopped going, and the people who knew Paul didn't talk to us. I *so* wanted to talk to people who knew Paul.

After we stopped going to the survivors group, I started going to CoDA [Co-Dependents Anonymous] meetings, even though I don't think I'm codependent. It was more because I needed to talk . . . to understand how this happened. I felt like I wasn't there for him. . . . I was busy with my job and maybe I wasn't tuned in to his moods. I was always taught that boys don't like to talk about feelings.

Karyn: Yes, I guess I've been taught that, too.

Emmy: I just remember that night he told his dad and I that he loved us, he went to bed, and the next morning we found him. I just couldn't make sense of it. Years later, one of Paul's peers, who now has a teenage son, said he could finally tell me what he remembered. And there were signs. Apparently, he had said to some friends (while they were drinking alcohol), "Have you ever thought of killing yourself?" and they all laughed about it and nothing more was said. I also found out that he told an older peer, whom he had met at church camp, that he didn't want to live. The peer smacked him and told him if he ever had thoughts like that again that he [Paul] needed to come talk to him first. But they never told anyone

Continued

Real People, Real Stories—cont'd

else; they kept it among their peers. They thought they were all-knowing, and never told an adult. He was hysterical when he found out what happened.

On that last weekend, he had been partying with his friends . . . there was alcohol involved . . . and the friend that was with him told me that someday he would tell me what went down that day. But it's 30 years later, and I still don't know. I know he was at the party with a girl, but I've never been able to find her or talk with her. She went to a different school.

Karyn: And much of this information that you do know came 10 or more years after his death?

Emmy: Yes.

Karyn: What a long journey you've been on trying to put all the pieces together.

Emmy: (tearful) That's exactly it. Trying to put the pieces together, sort it out . . . but it never gets solved. . . . It's like being in a maze and you can't get out, and I had a lot of guilt. . . . Now I recognize that he just made some tragic bad choices.

Karyn: Appreciating that we don't "get over" such tremendous loss but rather amend our lives with some different understanding of love and loss, what has been most helpful in your healing?

Emmy: Yes, I think there was a point when I realized it was okay to feel some happiness. Being with people who don't know me makes it easier. My faith and fellowship group has been an important part of healing. CoDA was helpful because we talked about how different people process things, and I could understand better how people can get stuck. I used to say that my

other son had lost his brother. I couldn't say that I had lost a son. When I had to fill out a health assessment at one point, and I had to respond to the question of how many pregnancies I'd had, that was the most difficult question . . . because I had to acknowledge . . . the reality. And I involved myself with all the boys who were on the track team with Paul and the Listening POST and just talked about everything.

Karyn: What is the most important thing that nurses need to know?

Emmy: By the time we would have had any contact with nurses, it was too late. There were no ER, medical, or mental health visits prior to that. If they were to have an impact, it would have been in prevention in the schools. For example, I didn't know at that time to ask questions like, "Are you having thoughts of hurting yourself?" and "Do you have a plan in mind?" And Paul put on a different face for me. He wasn't solitary; he had lots of friends; he was active on the track team. . . .

Karyn: I think you're not alone with not having been taught about things like suicide assessment. Because, as you've said, historically people haven't talked about it. There is an organization called Red Flags National that promotes mental health education for students, parents, and teachers as a standard part of health education in schools.

Emmy: Yes. It needs to be talked about. It's been helpful for me to talk about it even now. I've never had to try to explain the story before.

To learn more about Red Flags National, go to www.redflags.org.

Strategies for assisting survivors of suicide victims include the following:

- Encourage the clients to talk about the suicide, each responding to the others' viewpoints and reconstructing of events. Share memories.
- Be aware of any blaming or scapegoating of specific family members. Discuss how each person fits into the family situation, both before and after the suicide.
- Listen to feelings of guilt and self-persecution. Gently move the individuals toward the reality of the situation.
- Encourage the family members to discuss individual relationships with the lost loved one. Focus on both positive and negative aspects of the relationships. Gradually, point out the irrationality of any idealized concepts of the deceased

person. The family's recognition of both positive and negative aspects about the person may facilitate grief work. No two people grieve in the same way. It may appear that some family members are "getting over" the grief faster than others. All family members must be educated that if this occurs, it is not because those family members "care less"—it is just that they "grieve differently." Variables that enter into this phenomenon include individual past experiences, personal relationship with the deceased person, and individual temperament and coping abilities.

- Recognize how the suicide has caused disorganization in family coping. Reassess interpersonal relationships in the context of the event. Discuss coping strategies that have been successful in times of stress in the past, and work to reestablish these

---

BOX 11–5 Sources for Information Related to Issues of Suicide

National Suicide Hotline
1-800-SUICIDE (24/7)

National Suicide Prevention Lifeline
www.suicidepreventionlifeline.org
1-800-273-TALK (24/7)

American Association of Suicidology
www.suicidology.org
1-202-237-2280

Depression and Bipolar Support Alliance (DBSA)
www.dbsalliance.org/
1-800-826-3632

American Foundation for Suicide Prevention
www.afsp.org
1-888-333-AFSP

National Institute of Mental Health
www.nimh.nih.gov
1-866-615-6464

American Psychiatric Association
www.psychiatry.org
1-202-559-3900

Mental Health America
www.mentalhealthamerica.net
1-703-684-7722
1-800-969-6642

American Psychological Association
www.apa.org
1-800-374-2721

Screening for Mental Health

Stop a Suicide Today!
www.stopasuicide.org
1-781-239-0071

Boys Town
Cares for troubled boys and girls and families in crisis.
Staff is trained to handle calls related to violence and
   suicide.
www.boystown.org
1-800-448-3000 (24/7 national hotline)

Centre for Suicide Prevention
www.suicideinfo.ca
1-833-456-4566

Centers for Disease Control and Prevention
National Center for Injury Prevention and Control
Division of Violence Prevention
www.cdc.gov/injury/index.html
1-800-CDC-INFO

National Alliance on Mental Illness
www.nami.org
1-800-950-NAMI

---

strategies within the family. Identify new adaptive coping strategies that can be incorporated.

■ Identify resources that provide support: religious beliefs and spiritual counselors, close friends and relatives, support groups for survivors of suicide. One online connection that puts individuals in contact with survivors groups specific to each state is the American Foundation for Suicide Prevention at www.afsp.org. A list of resources that provide information and help for issues regarding suicide is presented in Box 11–5.

Evaluation

Evaluation of the client who is suicidal is an ongoing process accomplished through continuous reassessment of the client and determination of goal achievement. Once the immediate crisis has been resolved, extended psychotherapy may be indicated. The long-term goals of individual or group psychotherapy for the suicidal client would be for him or her to:

■ Develop and maintain a more positive self-concept.
■ Learn more effective ways to express feelings to others.
■ Achieve successful interpersonal relationships.
■ Feel accepted by others and achieve a sense of belonging.

A person contemplating suicide feels worthless, hopeless, and oftentimes numb. These goals serve to instill a sense of self-worth while offering a measure of hope and a meaning for living.

Summary and Key Points

■ More than 90% of all persons who commit, or attempt, or die by suicide have a diagnosed mental disorder.

■ Suicide is the second-leading cause of death among young Americans aged 15 to 34 years, the fourth-leading cause of death for those aged 35 to 44, and the fifth-leading cause of death for individuals aged 45 to 54. Based on recent statistics, the highest rates of suicide among all age groups occurred among those 45 to 54 years of age followed by those 85 years of age and older.

■ Single (never married), divorced, and widowed people are at greater risk for suicide than married people but evidence supports that recent change in status is a proximal risk factor.

■ More women than men attempt suicide, but men succeed more often.

■ Suicide and age are positively correlated.

■ Depressed men and women who consider themselves affiliated with a religion are less likely than their nonreligious counterparts to attempt suicide.

■ Individuals in the very highest and lowest social classes have higher suicide rates than those in the middle classes.

■ Whites are at highest risk for suicide, followed by American Indians/Alaska Natives, African Americans, Hispanic Americans, and Asian Americans.

■ Psychiatric disorders that predispose individuals to suicide include mood disorders, substance use disorders, schizophrenia, anorexia nervosa, borderline and antisocial personality disorders, and anxiety disorders.

■ Predisposing factors include internalized anger, hopelessness and other symptoms of severe depression, history of aggression and violence, shame and humiliation, developmental stressors, sociological influences, genetics, and neurochemical factors.

■ Suicide risk assessment should be a patient-centered, collaborative process in the context of a therapeutic relationship and should chronologically explore presenting suicide events, recent events, past events, and immediate intentions.

■ Assessment of the level of intervention needed includes identifying the number of proximal or potentiating risks as well as the number of warning signs.

■ It is important for the nurse to determine the seriousness of the patient's suicidal intentions, the existence of a plan, and the availability and lethality of the method.

■ The suicidal person should not be left alone.

■ A safety plan is developed with the patient following a comprehensive suicide risk assessment and includes assisting the patient to recognize warning signs, identify and employ coping strategies, engage family members and friends as available support persons, identify people and social settings that can be used to distract from suicidal thoughts or urges, identify resources and contact information for crisis intervention, and problem solve ways to restrict access to lethal means.

■ Once the crisis intervention is complete, the individual may require long-term psychotherapy, during which he or she works to
  ■ Develop and maintain a more positive self-concept.
  ■ Learn more effective ways to express feelings.
  ■ Improve interpersonal relationships.
  ■ Achieve a sense of belonging and a measure of hope for living.

■ Evidence-based psychological interventions include dialectical behavior therapy, cognitive behavior therapy, and the Collaborative Assessment and Management of Suicidality (CAMS) approach.

Review Questions
Self-Examination/Learning Exercise

Select the answer that is most appropriate for each of the following questions:

1. Which of the following individuals demonstrates the highest number of risk factors for suicide?
   a. John, who reports that he is in deep emotional pain, feels hopeless, and says "No one is there for me."
   b. Kelly, who has been seeing a doctor for chronic, intractable pain, verbalizes a deep commitment to her religious faith and is taking pain medication.
   c. Jim, an American Indian, who graduated from high school with honors but does not yet have a job.
   d. Mike, a physician, who reports feeling "burnt out" and is considering retirement.

Review Questions—cont'd
Self-Examination/Learning Exercise

2. The nurse in the emergency department encounters a patient, Niko, who is expressing suicide ideation. The nurse recognizes that which of the following considerations are important to good suicide risk assessment? (Select all that apply.)
   a. Collaborating with the patient
   b. Asking specific questions about leisure activities
   c. Establishing trust and open communication with the patient
   d. Asking the patient specific questions about the strength of his intention to die
   e. Identifying whether the patient has thought about a plan for trying to kill himself

3. Theresa, age 27, was admitted to the psychiatric unit from the medical intensive care unit where she was treated for taking a deliberate overdose of her antidepressant medication, trazodone (Desyrel). She says to the nurse, "My boyfriend broke up with me. We had been together for 6 years. I love him so much. I know I'll never get over him." Which is the best response by the nurse?
   a. "You'll get over him in time, Theresa."
   b. "Forget him. There are other fish in the sea."
   c. "You must be feeling very sad about your loss."
   d. "Why do you think he broke up with you, Theresa?"

4. The nurse identifies the primary nursing diagnosis for Theresa as "Risk for Suicide related to feelings of hopelessness from loss of relationship." Which is the outcome that would be most appropriate for this diagnosis?
   a. The patient has experienced no physical harm to herself.
   b. The patient sets realistic goals for herself.
   c. The patient expresses some optimism and hope for the future.
   d. The patient has reached a stage of acceptance in the loss of the relationship with her boyfriend.

5. Theresa is hospitalized following a suicide attempt after breaking up with her boyfriend. Klonsky and May's "Three-Step Theory" suggests that the nurse should assess which three issues to evaluate Theresa's active risk for a suicide attempt?
   a. Level of education, ethnic background, and current employment
   b. Relationships with previous boyfriends, coping mechanisms, and intent to have future boyfriends
   c. Self-esteem, grade point average, and physical attractiveness
   d. Degree of psychological pain, connectedness with others, and suicide ideation in combination with capacity to make an attempt

6. Theresa is hospitalized following a suicide attempt after breaking up with her boyfriend. Theresa says to the nurse, "When I get out of here, I'm going to try this again, and next time I'll choose a no-fail method." Which is the best response by the nurse?
   a. "You are safe here. We will make sure nothing happens to you."
   b. "You're just lucky your roommate came home when she did."
   c. "What exactly do you plan to do?"
   d. "I don't understand. You have so much to live for."

7. In determining degree of suicide risk with a suicidal patient, the nurse assesses the following behavioral manifestations: severely depressed, withdrawn, statements of worthlessness, difficulty accomplishing activities of daily living, no close support systems. The nurse identifies the patient's risk for suicide as which of the following?
   a. Low risk
   b. High risk
   c. Imminent risk
   d. Unable to be determined

Continued

Review Questions—cont'd
Self-Examination/Learning Exercise

8. Theresa, who has been hospitalized following a suicide attempt, is placed on suicide precautions on the psychiatric unit. She admits that she is still feeling suicidal. Which of the following interventions is most appropriate in this instance? (Select all that apply.)
   a. Restrict access to any item that might be harmful by placing the patient in a seclusion room.
   b. Check on Theresa every 15 minutes at irregular intervals or assign a staff person to stay with her on a one-to-one basis.
   c. Obtain an order from the physician to give Theresa a sedative to calm her and reduce suicide ideas.
   d. Do not allow Theresa to participate in any unit activities while she is on suicide precautions.
   e. Ask Theresa specific questions about her thoughts, plans, and intentions related to suicide.

9. Which of the following interventions are appropriate for a patient on suicide precautions? (Select all that apply.)
   a. Remove all sharp objects, belts, and other potentially dangerous articles from the patient's environment.
   b. Accompany the patient to off-unit activities.
   c. Reassess intensity of suicidal thoughts and urges on a regular basis.
   d. Put all of the patient's possessions in storage and explain to her that she may have them back when she is off suicide precautions.

10. Success of long-term psychotherapy with Theresa (who attempted suicide following a break-up with her boyfriend) could be measured by which of the following behaviors?
   a. Theresa has a new boyfriend.
   b. Theresa has an increased sense of self-worth.
   c. Theresa does not take antidepressants anymore.
   d. Theresa told her old boyfriend how angry she was with him for breaking up with her.

Communication Exercises

1. Mr. J was brought to the emergency department by his brother who is concerned about Mr. J's worsening depression. During the assessment, Mr. J tells the nurse, "None of this matters. There's nothing that can make this any better." What would be an appropriate response by the nurse?

2. Mr. J admits to the nurse that he has had suicide ideas for the last couple of weeks. How would the nurse intervene with Mr. J at this point?

3. Mr. J tells the nurse that ever since his wife died 3 months ago, he doesn't want to go on living. What would be an example of empathic communication in response to this statement by Mr. J?

References

Almendrala, A. (2015). *Native American youth suicide rates are at crisis levels.* Retrieved from http://www.huffingtonpost.com/entry/native-american-youth-suicide-rates-are-at-crisis-levels_us_560c3084e4b0768127005591

American Association of Suicidology. (2015). *Know the warning signs.* Retrieved from http://www.suicidology.org/resources/warning-signs

American Foundation for Suicide Prevention (AFSP). (2019). *Suicide statistics.* Retrieved from https://afsp.org/about-suicide/suicide-statistics

American Psychiatric Association. (2010). *Culture matters in suicidal behavior patterns and prevention, psychologist says.* Retrieved from http://www.apa.org/news/press/releases/2010/08/suicidal-behavior-patterns.aspx

American Psychiatric Nurses Association (APNA). (2018). *Psychiatric-mental health nurse essential competencies for assessment and management of individuals at risk for suicide.* Retrieved from https://www.apna.org/i4a/pages/index.cfm?pageid=5684

Bauman, S., Toomey, R. B., & Walker, J. L. (2013). Associations among bullying, cyberbullying, and suicide in high school students. *Journal of Adolescence, 36*(2), 341–350. doi:10.1016/j.adolescence.2012.12.001

Bridge, J. A., Asti, L., Horowitz, L. M., Greenhouse, J. B., Fontanella, C. A., Sheftall, A. H., & Campo, J. V. (2015). Suicide trends among elementary school-aged children in the United States from 1993 to 2012. *JAMA Pediatrics, 169*(7), 673–677. doi:10.1001/jamapediatrics.2015.0465

Byron, W. J. (2016). Do people who commit suicide go to hell? *Catholic Digest.* Retrieved from http://www.catholicdigest.com/articles/faith/knowledge/2007/04-01/do-people-whocommit-suicide-go-to-hell

Cardoza, K. (2016). *6 myths about suicide that every parent and educator should know.* Retrieved from http://www.npr.org/sections/ed/2016/09/02/478835539

Cassels, C. (2011). "Striking" risk for suicidality, depression in gay teens. *Medscape Medical News.* Retrieved from http://www.medscape.com/viewarticle/740429

Centers for Disease Control and Prevention (CDC). (2015a). *20 leading causes of death, United States*. National Center for Injury Prevention and Control. Retrieved from http://webappa.cdc .gov/sasweb/ncipc/leadcaus10_us.html

Centers for Disease Control and Prevention (CDC). (2015b). *Suicide facts at a glance: 2015*. Retrieved from http://www.cdc.gov/ violenceprevention/pdf/suicide-datasheet-a.pdf

Centers for Disease Control and Prevention (CDC). (2015c). *Gay and bisexual men's health*. Retrieved from http://www.cdc.gov/ msmhealth/suicide-violence-prevention.htm

Centers for Disease Control and Prevention. (2016). *Leading causes of death, national and regional, 1999–2014*. Retrieved from http://webappa.cdc.gov/sasweb/ncipc/leadcaus10_us.html

Chang, B. P., Franklin, J. C., Ribeiro, J. D., Fox, K. R., Bentley, K. H., Kleiman, E. M., & Nock, M. K. (2016). Biological risk factors for suicidal behaviors: A meta-analysis. *Translational Psychiatry, 6*(9), e887. doi:10.1038/tp.2016.165

Cochran, S. D., & Mays, V. M. (2000). Lifetime prevalence of suicide symptoms and affective disorders among men reporting same-sex sexual partners: Results from NHANES III. *American Journal of Public Health, 90*(4), 573–578.

Crosby, A. E., Ortega, L., & Melanson, C. (2011). *Self-directed violence surveillance: Uniform definitions and recommended data elements, version 1.0*. Atlanta, GA: Centers for Disease Control and Prevention, National Center for Injury Prevention and Control. Retrieved from http://www.cdc.gov/violenceprevention/ pdf/Self-Directed-Violence-a.pdf

Drew, B. (2001). Self-harm and no-suicide contract in psychiatric inpatient settings. *Archives of Psychiatric Nursing, 15*(3), 99–106.

Duran, S., & McGuinness, T. M. (2016). Suicide in childhood. *Journal of Psychosocial Nursing, 54*(10), 27–30.

Edgerton, E., & Limber, S. (2013). *Research brief: Suicide and bullying*. Retrieved from https://www.stopbullying.gov/blog/2013/02/27/ research-brief-suicide-and-bullying

Eisenberg, M. E., & Resnick, M. D. (2006). Suicidality among gay, lesbian and bisexual youth: The role of protective factors. *Journal of Adolescent Health, 39*(5), 662–668.

Fleener, P. (n.d.). How to help a suicidal person. *Mental Health Today*. Retrieved from http://www.mental-health-today.com/ suicide/sui2.htm

Freedenthal, S. (2013). *The use of no-suicide contracts*. Retrieved from http://www.speakingofsuicide.com/2013/05/15/ no-suicide-contracts

Hinduja, S., & Patchin, J. W. (2010). Bullying, cyberbullying, and suicide. *Archives of Suicide Research, 14*(3), 206–221.

Hoffman, R. (2013). Contracting for safety: A misused tool. *Pennsylvania Patient Safety Advisory, 10*(2), 82–84.

Ivey-Stephenson, A. Z., Crosby, A. E., Jack, S. P., Haileyesus, T., & Kresnow-Sedacca, M. (2017). Suicide trends among and within urbanization levels by sex, race/ethnicity, age group, and mechanism of death — United States, 2001–2015. *MMWR Surveillance Summary, 66*(SS-18), 1–16.

Jobes, D. A. (2012). The Collaborative Assessment and Management of Suicidality (CAMS): An evolving evidence-based clinical approach to suicide risk. *Suicide and Life Threatening Behavior, 42*(6), 640–653. doi:10.1111/j.1943-278X.2012.00119.x

Jobes, D. A. (2015, September). *Clinical suicidology: Innovations in assessment treatment of suicidal risk*. Presentation at Psychiatric Grand Rounds, Summa Health Systems, Akron, OH.

Joiner, T. E. (2005). *Why people die by suicide*. Cambridge, MA: Harvard University Press.

Juhnke, G. A., Granello, P. F., & Lebron-Striker, M. (2007). IS PATH WARM? A suicide assessment mnemonic for counselors. *ACA Professional Counseling Digest-03*. Retrieved from http://www.counseling.org/resources/library/ACA%20Digests/ACAPCD-03.pdf

Kim, J. L., Kim, J. M., Choi, Y., Lee, T., & Park, E. (2016). Effect of socioeconomic status on the linkage between suicidal ideation and suicide attempts. *Suicide and Life-Threatening Behavior 46*(5), 588–597. DOI: 10.1111/sltb.12242

King, M., Semlyen, J., Tai, S. S., Killaspy, H., Osborn, D., Popelyuk, D., & Nazareth, I. (2008). A systematic review of mental disorder, suicide, and deliberate self harm in lesbian, gay, and bisexual people. *BMC Psychiatry, 8*(70). Retrieved from http://www.biomedcentral.com/1471-244X/8/70

Klomek, A. B., Sourander, A., & Gould, M. S. (2011). Bullying and suicide: Detection and intervention. *Psychiatric Times, 28*(2). Retrieved from http://www.psychiatrictimes.com/suicide/ content/article/10168/1795797#

Klonsky, D. E., & May, A. M. (2015a). The three-step theory (3ST): A new theory of suicide rooted in the "ideation-to-action" framework. *International Journal of Cognitive Therapy, 8*(2), 114–129. doi:10.1521/ijct.2015.8.2.114

Klonsky, D. E., & May, A. M. (2015b). Impulsivity and suicide risk: Review and clinical implications. *Psychiatric Times, 32*(8). Retrieved from http://www.psychiatrictimes.com/specialreports/impulsivity-and-suicide-risk-review-and-clinicalimplications/page/0/2

Kposowa, A. (2000). Marital status and suicide in the National Longitudinal Mortality Study. *Journal of Epidemiology and Community Health, 54*(4), 254–261. doi:http://dx.doi.org/10.1136/ jech.54.4.254

Medscape Psychiatry. (2011). *Striking risk for suicidality, depression in gay teens*. Retrieved from http://www.medscape.com/ viewarticle/740429

Mercado, M. C., Holland, K., Leemis, R. W., Stone, D. M., & Wang, J. (2017). Trends in emergency department visits for nonfatal self-inflicted injuries among youth aged 10 to 24 years in the United States, 2001–2015. *Journal of the American Medical Association 318*(19), 1931–1933. doi:10.1001/ jama.2017.13317

National Action Alliance for Suicide Prevention. (2015). *What is zero suicide?* Retrieved from http://actionallianceforsuicideprevention.org/sites/actionallianceforsuicideprevention.org/ files/zero_suicide_final6.pdf

National Alliance on Mental Illness (NAMI). (2018). *Risk of suicide*. Retrieved from http://www.nami.org/Learn-More/ Mental-Health-Conditions/Related-Conditions/Risk-of-Suicide

National Institute of Mental Health (NIMH). (2015). *Director's blog: The under-recognized public health crisis of suicide*. Retrieved from http://www.nimh.nihgov/about/director/2010/the-under-recognized-public-health-crisis-of-suicide.shtml

Nock, M. K., Deming, C. A., Fullerton, C. S., Gilman, S. E., Goldenberg, M., Kessler, R. C., McCarroll, J. E., & Ursan, R. J. (2013). Suicide among soldiers: A review of psychosocial risk and protective factors. *Psychiatry, 76*(2), 97–125. Retrieved from http://www.ncbi.nlm.nih.gov/pmc/articles/PMC4060831 . doi: 10.1521/psyc.2013.76.2.97

Olfson, M., Wall, M., Wang, S., Crystal, S., Shang-Min Liu, S.-M., Gerhard, T., & Blanco, C. (2016). Short-term suicide risk after psychiatric hospital discharge. *JAMA Psychiatry, 73*(11), 1119–1126. doi:10.1001/jamapsychiatry.2016.2035

Perlman, C. M., Neufeld, E., Martin, L., Goy, M., & Hirdes, J. P. (2011). *Risk assessment inventory: A resource guide for Canadian healthcare organizations*. Toronto: Ontario Hospital Association and Canadian Patient Safety Institute.

Plöderl, M., Wagenmakers, E. J., Tremblay, P., Ramsay, R., Kralovek, K., Fartacek, C., & Fartacek, R. (2013). Suicide risk and sexual orientation: A critical review. *Archives of Sexual Behavior, 42*(5), 715–727.

Puntil, C., York, J., Limandri, B., Greene, P., Arauz, E., & Hobbs, D. (2013). Competency-based training for PMH nurse generalists: Inpatient intervention and prevention of suicide. *Journal of the American Psychiatric Nurses Association, 19*(4), 205–210. doi:10.1177/1078390313496275

Rasic, D. T., Belik, S. L., Elias, B., Katz, L. Y., Enns, M., & Sareen, J. (2009). Spirituality, religion, and suicidal behavior in a nationally representative sample. *Journal of Affective Disorders, 114*(1), 32–40.

Reyes, M. S., Cayubit, F. O., Angala, M. H., Bries, S. C., Capalungan, J. T., & McCutcheon, L. E. (2015). Exploring the link between adolescent anger expression and tendencies for suicide: A brief report. *North American Journal of Psychology, 17*(1), 113–118.

Ro˜skar, S., Podlesek, A., Kuzmani´c, M., Dem˜sar, L. O., Zaletel, M., & Maru˜si˜c, A. (2011). Suicide risk and its relationship to change in marital status. *Crisis, 32*(1), 24–30. doi:10.1027/0227-5910/a000054

Rudd, D. M., Mandrusiak, M., & Joiner, T. E. (2006). The case against no-suicide contract: The commitment to treatment statement as a practice alternative. *Journal of Clinical Psychology, 62*(2), 243–251.

Sadock, B. J., Sadock, V. A., & Ruiz, P. (2015). *Synopsis of psychiatry: Behavioral sciences/clinical psychiatry* (11th ed.). Philadelphia, PA: Wolters Kluwer.

Shea, S. C. (2009). Suicide assessment: Part 1: Uncovering suicidal intent: A sophisticated art; Part 2: Uncovering suicidal intent using the chronological assessment of suicide events. *Psychiatric Times, 26*(12), 1–26. Retrieved from http://www.psychiatrictimes.com/display/article/10168/1491291

Stanley, B., & Brown, G. K. (2008). *The safety plan treatment manual to reduce suicide risk: Veteran version.* Washington, DC: U.S. Department of Veterans Affairs.

Stroumsa, D. (2014). The state of transgender health care: Policy, law, and medical frameworks. *American Journal of Public Health, 104*(3), 31–37. doi:10.2105/AJPH.2013.301789

Substance Abuse and Mental Health Services Administration (SAMHSA). (2017). *Suicide prevention.* Retrieved from https://www.samhsa.gov/suicide-prevention

Sudak, H. S. (2017). Suicide treatment. In B.J. Sadock, Sadock, V.A., & Ruiz, P. (Eds.), *Comprehensive textbook of psychiatry* (pp. 2618–2622). Philadelphia, PA: Wolters Kluwer.

Taylor, T. F. (2015). The influence of shame on posttrauma disorders: Have we failed to see the obvious? *European Journal of Psychotraumatology, 6.* doi:10.3402/ejpt.v6.28847

The Joint Commission. (2016). *Sentinel Event Alert 56: Detecting and treating suicide ideation in all settings.* Retrieved from https://www.jointcommission.org/sea_issue_56

The Samaritans. (2015). *Suicide myths and misconceptions.* Retrieved from http://samaritansnyc.org/myths-about-suicide

Whalen, D., Dixon-Gordon, K., Belden, A., Barch, D., & Luby, J. (2015). Correlates and consequences of suicidal cognitions and behaviors in children ages 3 to 7 years. *Journal of the American Academy of Child & Adolescent Psychiatry, 54*(11), 926–937. doi:10.1016/j.jaac.2015.08.009

Wiklander, M., Samuelsson, M., Jokinen, J., Nilsonne, A., Wilczek, A., Rylander, G., & Åsberg, M. (2012). Shame-proneness in attempted suicide patients. *BMC Psychiatry, 12.* doi:10.1186/1471-244X-12-50

Yamauchi, T., Fujita, T., Tachimori, H., Takeshima, T., Inagaki, M., & Sudo, A. (2013). Age-adjusted relative suicide risk by marital and employment status over the past 25 years in Japan. *Journal of Public Health, 35*(1), 49–56. doi:10.1093/pubmed/fds054

Zweig, J., & Dank, M. (2013). *Technology, teen dating, violence and abuse, and bullying.* The Urban Institute. Retrieved from http://www.urban.org/sites/default/files/alfresco/publication-pdfs/412891

Classical References

Durkheim, E. (1951). *Suicide: A study of sociology.* Glencoe, IL: Free Press.

Freud, S. (1957). *Mourning and melancholia, Vol. 14* (standard ed.) London, England: Hogarth Press. (Original work published 1917)

MacDonald, M., & Murphy, T. R. (1991). *Sleepless souls: Suicide in early modern England.* New York, NY: Oxford University Press.

Macnab, F. (1993). *Brief psychotherapy: An integrative approach in clinical practice.* West Sussex, England: John Wiley & Sons.

Minois, G. (2001). *History of suicide: Voluntary death in Western culture.* Baltimore, MD: Johns Hopkins University Press.

U.S. Public Health Service (USPHS). (1999). *The Surgeon General's call to action to prevent suicide.* Washington, DC: Author.

UNIT 3

Care of Patients With Psychiatric Disorders

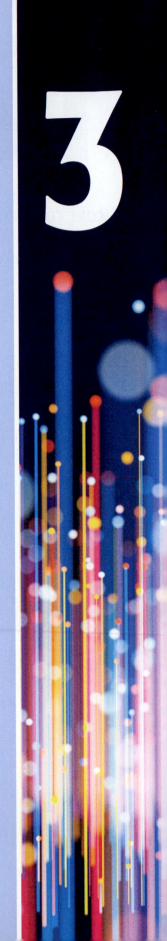

12

Caring for Patients With Mental Illness and Substance Use Disorders in General Practice Settings

KEY TERMS

diagnostic overshadowing

patient-centered care

SBIRT (screening, brief intervention, and referral to treatment)

screening

social distancing

stigmatization

suicide prevention

trauma-informed care

OBJECTIVES

After reading this chapter, the student will be able to:

1. Recognize the impact of inadequate assessment, treatment, and referral for the client with mental health and substance use disorders.
2. Discuss the evidence identifying the need for further mental health and substance use disorder education among healthcare providers in primary care and other nonpsychiatric settings.
3. Describe essential elements in appropriate screening and referral of mental health and substance abuse clients.
4. Analyze barriers that influence the screening, intervention, and referral process for clients with mental health and substance use concerns.
5. Describe essential aspects of the nurse's role in providing care for clients with psychiatric/mental health and substance use disorders in general practice.

HOMEWORK ASSIGNMENT

Please read the chapter and answer the following questions:

1. What are three outcomes associated with inadequate treatment of clients with mental health and substance use disorders?
2. What are two ways the nurse can access evidence-based psychiatric and substance use screening tools?
3. What is the definition of diagnostic overshadowing?
4. What is the definition of social distancing?
5. Describe the first step in accomplishing the nurse's role in caring for clients with mental health and substance use disorders and reflect on your own attitudes and beliefs about these clients.

Introduction

The client with mental illness has historically been misunderstood, misdiagnosed, and mistreated (see Chapter 1, Mental Health and Mental Illness). Current examples confirm that this problem is ongoing. In one case, a patient came into the emergency department setting with garbled speech that made her responses to questions difficult to comprehend. She was known to be a homeless person with chronic schizophrenia and was quickly transferred to a psychiatric hospital. Once there, her right-sided weakness, vital signs, and difficulty speaking were recognized as evidence of a cerebrovascular accident.

In another case, a hospitalized patient with schizophrenia reported to the nurse that there was a rock band playing music in his body and the drummer was playing in his chest; initially, these symptoms were identified as delusional thinking. However, after further assessment, it was determined that the patient was having a heart attack. Real examples of potentially fatal misdiagnoses like these are far too common.

Clients presenting with symptoms like pain, lack of energy, and feelings of helplessness could be experiencing a variety of medical conditions, but these can also be signs of depression. If effective screening is not conducted, the client may be at risk for worsening depression and suicide.

Nurses who choose to work in nonpsychiatric settings are *the* frontline responders in recognizing, intervening, and referring clients with neuropsychiatric illness for further treatment. Studies reveal, though, that attitudes, lack of education about the need for screening, and issues related to accessing services are all influential in lack of appropriate intervention to meet the needs of this population.

Clearly there are genetic, neurological, neurochemical, and environmental influences in the etiology of mental illness that differentiate clinical illness from the range of emotions and behavior that are a part of general human experience. However, without clear education and appreciation for these symptoms as distressing signs of neurological illness, clients will continue to remain at risk for lack of treatment or mistreatment of both psychiatric and physical illness. Nurses must take the lead in educating other healthcare professionals and the public, combating stigmatization of clients with mental illness, recognizing neuropsychiatric symptoms, conducting appropriate screening, and collaborating effectively with other healthcare providers to ensure appropriate referral when specialized mental health and addictions treatment are needed. This chapter explores the nurse's role and the evidence for education, screening, and referral needs in various nonpsychiatric settings.

The Need for Education of Healthcare Providers

Evidence supports that clients with significant mental illness die, on the average, 25 years earlier than the general population and that 60 percent of those deaths are related to preventable or treatable causes (Gomes, Duraes, & Lima, 2015). This may be related to **diagnostic overshadowing,** a phenomenon in which a person's physical symptoms are attributed to his or her mental illness. For example, Gomes and associates reviewed studies showing that patients with both mental illness and a cardiovascular condition received half as many follow-up interventions following a heart attack as those without a concurrent mental illness. This finding is significant because many patients with mental illnesses are at greater risk for cardiovascular disease due to genetic, lifestyle, or environmental issues or to adverse effects from psychotropic medications.

Other studies have demonstrated that clients with mental illness who present to general healthcare settings are at risk for lack of treatment or appropriate referral, which may be related to lack of knowledge about symptom detection (by patients and healthcare providers), stigmatization, and lack of awareness about counseling and referral services (Bay et al., 2016; Betz et al., 2013; Ndetei et al., 2011). These realities have led many people with mental illness to avoid seeking healthcare altogether. As we learn more about the progression and prognosis of illnesses like schizophrenia, it has become apparent that early intervention is critical because repeated psychotic episodes may have a cumulative damaging effect on the brain (see Chapter 15, Schizophrenia Spectrum and Other Psychotic Disorders, for further discussion). The barriers to early intervention are compounded for individuals with schizophrenia because one of the neurological symptoms in this disorder is *anosognosia* (a lack of awareness or recognition of symptoms). During acute psychotic episodes, these clients—who are suspicious of people and the surrounding environment and often unaware that they have a mental illness—may be brought to the emergency department against their will. It is not difficult to imagine how frightening this scenario might be for such an individual. Nurses in emergency settings play a key role in recognizing this patient as one who is experiencing significant neurological symptoms and requires immediate and ongoing care. Unfortunately, this patient may instead be stigmatized as one who is neither "really ill" nor requiring complex and compassionate intervention. The consequence of these attitudes for the patient is prolonged suffering and sometimes early death.

Nurses in any nonpsychiatric setting must also have a clear working knowledge of the impact of depressive disorders in treating other physical illnesses. Depression, a mental illness with multiple etiologies and symptoms, affects 1 in 5 women and 1 in 10 men during their lifetime, is increasingly being diagnosed in children and adolescents, and is demonstrating greater chronicity than previously thought (Akiskal, 2017) (see Chapter 16, Depressive Disorders, for further discussion). In addition, Akiskal (2017) notes that there is evidence that bipolar disorder, which is characterized by bouts of depression and mania, accounts for up to 50 percent of all cases of depression (see Chapter 17, Bipolar and Related Disorders, for further discussion of these disorders). Knowledge of the distinction between depressive disorder and bipolar disorder has important implications for medication management and ongoing treatment. With such a high prevalence, the potential disabling effects of untreated or mistreated illness, and the fact that suicide is a risk at all times in depressive illness, it seems apparent that all patients, in any encounter with healthcare professionals, should be screened for evidence of depression and risk for suicide. But this has not been the case.

In addition, there are links between depression and many other diseases. Depression not only increases risk for other illnesses but is associated with poorer outcomes when left untreated. Evidence has demonstrated that depression is a risk factor for cardiovascular disease, metabolic syndrome, diabetes, dementia, asthma, arthritis, and hyperlipidemia (Bica, Castelló, Toussaint, & Montesó-Curto, 2017). The risk of poorer outcomes has implications for both the medical condition and the depression and, ultimately, for the risk of suicide. Across the nation, the incidence of suicide has reached such epidemic proportions that it should be an assessment skill that every nurse is confident in performing (see Chapter 11, Suicide Prevention, for further discussion

of this topic). The importance of this knowledge base and appropriate screening may seem to be an obvious need in primary care and community settings but it is equally important in medical settings within hospitals. Suicide in hospital settings is a sentinel event that is frequently reported to the Joint Commission, an organization that accredits hospitals and healthcare systems. Horowitz and associates (2013) found that 25 percent of all inpatient suicides occur in nonbehavioral health settings and that in 80 percent the root cause was lack of adequate assessment.

Individuals affected by the national opioid epidemic and with other substance use disorders commonly seek care first in general medical and community practice settings before they are treated in psychiatric or substance abuse treatment settings. People often die of overdose before they ever reach an emergency department, which has prompted a nationwide effort to educate not only healthcare professionals but also the general public about how to recognize symptoms of overdose and administer treatment, such as naloxone and rescue breathing, to treat associated respiratory depression. Nurses play key educational, screening, and referral roles in community, primary, medical, and long-term care settings (see Chapter 14, Substance Use and Addictive Disorders, for further discussion of this topic).

Psychiatric nursing is an essential component of basic undergraduate nursing curricula. *Every* nurse needs education about recognition of mental illnesses to perform competently in *any* nursing role. Studies have shown that when healthcare professionals in nonpsychiatric settings are provided with education to feel confident in their ability to recognize the need for screening and utilize valid, reliable screening tools, rates of intervention and/or referral for mental health treatment improves. Although nurses typically enter general practice with a basic knowledge about mental illness recognition, communication strategies, and basic interventions, additional variables influence how these skills are put into practice. Three variables include availability of screening tools, knowledge and accessibility of referral sources, and attitudes about the patient with mental illness or substance use disorders.

CORE CONCEPT

Screening

Screening is the evaluation of the patient for conditions before they are known to be clinically significant. The purpose is for early diagnosis and treatment of illness.

Screening

Many valid and reliable screening tools exist for identifying mental illnesses and substance use disorders. The purpose of **screening** is to identify clinically significant symptoms that require further assessment and intervention. Tools that are completed by patient self-report are time efficient, but their use depends on the clinician's recognition of symptoms that support the need for screening and a belief that screening is essential for adequate identification and management of mental health and substance use issues.

Evidence supports that use of screening tools is better than clinical judgment alone in diagnosis of mental illness (Jackman, Honig, & Walter, 2016; Mitchell et al., 2011; Préville, Côté, & Hébert, 2004; Singer et al., 2011) and may help reduce situations in which an individual's illness is missed completely or incorrectly identified (i.e., a false-negative result).

In one study, Horowitz and associates (2013) developed a two-item nursing screen for suicide risk in any medical setting. The need was identified after the Joint Commission issued a "Sentinel Event" alert highlighting the importance of suicide risk assessment in all medical settings. The screen asked the patient two questions: "In the past month, have you had thoughts about suicide?" and "Have you ever made a suicide attempt?" A yes response to either question prompted a third question, "Are you having thoughts of suicide right now?" Their study demonstrated improvement in identification of medical-surgical patients who may be at risk for suicide (4 percent were referred for additional evaluation) and highlighted the time efficiency of such screening tools (this tool took about 2 minutes to complete). Again, critical to the success of any strategy is the nurse's belief that this kind of screening is essential. Endorsement for the necessity of this screening by accrediting bodies like the Joint Commission reinforces that this is an essential role for nurses.

Fortunately, more research is being done to identify the need for better screening for mental illness and substance abuse in nonpsychiatric settings. This has been particularly true with regard to screening for depression and anxiety. Roberge and associates (2016) conducted a qualitative study based on the recognition that depression and anxiety in patients seeking primary care for chronic diseases is linked to morbidity and mortality. Both patients and clinicians in this study identified a need for holistic care that includes screening and management of mental illness. Another study (Mollard, Brage Hudson, Ford, & Pullen, 2016) identified an increase in the incidence of postpartum depression among women in rural areas (a trend also seen internationally), and they concluded that nurses should be the lead change agents in improving policy around screening for depression in this population. The trend toward identifying the need for improvement in screening for depression and other neuropsychiatric illness has been echoed in many studies including those focused on home care, community care, long-term care, medical-surgical care, oncology, geriatric, and child-adolescent care (Bica et al., 2017; Grundberg, 2016; Koposov et al., 2017; Langdon et al., 2013; McGovern & Selwyn, 2014; Thompson, Lang, & Annells, 2008).

Integral in promoting the importance of screening are nursing managers who can equip their staff nurses with screening tools that are valid, reliable, time efficient, and user-friendly. Staff nurses must adopt an attitude that screening for mental illness is critical to their success in interventions for the physical illness that brought the patient to their nonpsychiatric setting and for referring patients to ongoing evaluation and treatment for the mental illness itself.

Many resources exist that identify valid and reliable screening tools for use in clinical practice settings. The Substance Abuse and Mental Health Services Administration (SAMHSA, no date) publishes a detailed list of available screening tools for identifying depression, bipolar disorder, drug and alcohol use, suicide risk, anxiety, and trauma. It stresses the importance and scope of this screening as such:

> Despite the high prevalence of mental health and substance use problems, too many Americans go without treatment—in part because their disorders go undiagnosed. Regular screenings in primary care and other healthcare settings enables earlier identification of mental health and substance use disorders, which translates into earlier care. Screenings should be provided to people of all ages, even the young and the elderly.

The American Academy of Pediatrics (2018) publishes a table of mental health screening and assessment tools for children, adolescents, and adults that were chosen because of their evidence-based reliability and accessibility. Many screening tools are free to use and widely accessible, whereas others are copyrighted, proprietary, and associated with a fee for use.

Priority Issues for Screening in Any Healthcare Setting

The importance of screening for depression has already been discussed with regard to its prevalence, its link to the development of other diseases, and its association with poorer outcomes. Other issues that arise as part of a general health assessment may trigger the need for screening and further assessment, but some issues are considered so prevalent and so high risk that they are priorities to screen for in all patients. Three of the most important issues to screen for are trauma, suicide risk, and substance use disorders.

Trauma History

Screening for violence and trauma history is now well-accepted as an essential psychosocial issue that should be conducted with patients when they first enter a healthcare setting. Even in the early 1990s, violence and trauma were identified in nursing literature as growing areas of concern that were linked to a high risk for injury, unhealthy coping mechanisms, and other illnesses such as arthritis, irritable bowel syndrome, and chronic pain (Hoff & Rosenbaum, 1994) as well as having implications in surgical outcomes (Schofferman et al., 1992). Hoff and Rosenbaum also noted that although violence and trauma cross gender boundaries (as well as race, ethnic, class, and national boundaries), most individuals affected by violence are women and children. Hoff and Ross (1993) estimate that up to 75 percent of female psychiatric patients have a current or past history of abuse. The classic study on adverse childhood events (ACEs) linked trauma in childhood to significant cognitive, social, psychological, and neurobiological changes that contribute to a host of physical and mental problems and to early death (Felitti et al., 1998). All of these important studies have clearly identified the critical importance of screening for trauma history. However, because many individuals with this history may be in denial, frightened about the consequences of sharing information, or experiencing guilt or shame, they may be reluctant to disclose information about their circumstances and history unless direct screening takes place. It is critical that nurses conduct screenings in private and communicate with a compassionate, nonjudgmental attitude. Pardee and associates (2017), in their review of ACE assessment tools, concluded that primary care nurse practitioners still need more education and more efficient assessment tools to ensure that this type of screening is accomplished in primary care settings. Even with a host of research behind the importance of screening, it is equally important to find feasible, efficient ways to promote its completion.

As research and nursing practice have focused more attention on the importance of screening for trauma and interpersonal violence history, we have also learned a great deal more about the importance of **trauma-informed care**—care that assesses for and demonstrates sensitivity to the impact of trauma history on current behavior and relationships in every aspect of nursing intervention. It is important that nurses recognize the risk for unwittingly retraumatizing a patient with a trauma history if there is lack of awareness or lack of sensitivity to the impact of that trauma on other aspects of the individual's everyday encounters (see Chapter 19, Trauma- and Stressor-Related Disorders, and Chapter 25, Survivors of Abuse and Neglect, for further discussion of these topics).

Risk for Suicide

National attention to the ever-alarming suicide rates across the life span, among military personnel, and within specific ethnic groups and communities has raised awareness of the critical needs for screening and intervention among laypeople and healthcare providers alike. Military personnel with post-traumatic stress disorder may present in medical settings with physical complaints, reports of nightmares, and/or substance use, but unless healthcare professionals specifically screen for suicide risk and warning signs, this potentially fatal risk may go undetected. The older adult with depression is another population that more often presents with physical complaints in primary care settings and may not even consider discussing depression, loneliness, or thoughts of suicide unless specifically asked. As with trauma victims, the fact that people at risk for suicide may not be forthcoming with this information; that it is a high-risk, potentially fatal problem; and that it is a highly prevalent concern reinforces the need for universal screening.

One very important caution about screening for suicide that we are learning from ongoing research in **suicide prevention** is that although brief screening may open a door for discussion with a client, it is not enough to prevent suicide in some individuals. In other words, just because a patient responds "no" to the question "Are you having thoughts of taking your own life?" does not mean that he or she is risk-free.

Jobes (2015) suggests that in spite of the numerous brief screening tools that are available, they have perhaps been more often used as defensive medicine than actually contributing to suicide prevention. Defensive medicine refers to doing the minimum number of interventions needed to "meet the letter of the law". In this case, it would mean asking the patient the preceding question, documenting that the patient denies suicidal ideation, and then assuming that we have "covered the necessary bases." Current research, as Jobes points out, has demonstrated that brief screening may be inadequate because of the many variables that influence a person's decision to take his or her own life and the fact that ideation (as well as the intent to act on ideation) can change in intensity over time. Patients in primary care settings with depression, substance abuse issues, and/or chronic pain should be recognized as having *identified risk factors* for suicide and should be screened carefully. In addition, given the current prevalence rates of suicide, nurses should develop the skill to carefully screen for suicide risk with every patient in every healthcare setting. Establishing trust with the patient, developing a collaborative relationship, and displaying a willingness to discuss this issue from various vantage points (such as past history, recent history, immediate risk, and strength of the individual's intent to harm him/herself) are all essential elements in identifying the need for referral and the level of care required for the patient's safety.

Nonsuicidal self-injuring behavior (NSSIB) is a related and complex phenomenon that is increasingly being seen in nonpsychiatric settings and challenges the nurse's skills to discern how to screen and when to refer for more intensive treatment. Kameg and associates (2013) report that although NSSIB is typically a nonlethal, repetitive act used to reduce distress rather than end one's life, the individual who uses NSSIB is more likely to consider or attempt suicide than non-self injurers. Individuals who exhibit NSSIB therefore require screening for suicide risk. The authors also state that a patient who is identified as having comorbid psychiatric symptoms such as labile mood, dysphoria, anxiety, depersonalization, anhedonia, or borderline personality disorder should be referred to specialized mental healthcare services. Those who exhibit NSSIB in response to command hallucinations should be considered in need of immediate medical attention. Several tools are available to screen for self-harm. Kameg and associates (2013) identify that The Self-Harm Inventory (Box 12–1) can be completed within 5 minutes and screens for borderline personality disorder symptoms as well as a variety of self-harm behaviors.

Substance Use Disorders

In the United States, rates of opioid abuse have reached epidemic levels, and rates of methamphetamine use have also increased significantly. Opioid addiction can lead to overdose, whereas methamphetamine withdrawal is associated with an increased risk for suicide. In addition, the numerous physical and psychological consequences of long-term alcohol use are well documented. All of these facts underscore the importance of screening for substance use disorders in nonpsychiatric settings. Although many tools exist to screen for substance abuse, the extent of their use in general practice settings varies. **Screening, brief intervention, and referral to treatment (SBIRT)** (SAMHSA, 2017) is an evidence-based approach that can be used in emergency departments, trauma centers, primary care, and other community settings. SAMHSA (2017) describes the SBIRT approach as follows:

■ Screening quickly assesses the severity of substance use and identifies the appropriate level of treatment.

■ Brief intervention focuses on increasing insight and awareness regarding substance use and motivation toward behavioral change.

■ Referral to treatment provides those identified as needing more extensive treatment with access to specialty care.

One study (Rahm et al., 2015) sought to identify why routine screening does not occur for an issue that has been so clearly identified as a public health concern. The authors, using SBIRT as the preferred model, asked primary care providers (including nurses, physicians, mental health specialists, and others) and patients to identify barriers to implementation of this approach. Although patients supported universal screening, they also noted that privacy concerns may be an issue. This is an important consideration for nurses who are screening patients for substances of abuse. Many patients may deny using substances, particularly illegal substances, because they fear legal consequences. For example, many states consider substance use during pregnancy to be child abuse with legal consequences, and 24 states and the District of Columbia require health professionals to report suspected prenatal drug use (Guttmacher Institute, 2018), which may deter some women from ever seeking prenatal care. Establishment of trust, clear communication about why this information is

BOX 12–1 The Self-Harm Inventory

Instructions: Please answer the following questions by checking either, "Yes," or "No." Check "yes" only to those items that you have intentionally, or on purpose, used to hurt yourself.

Yes	No	Have you ever intentionally, or on purpose, done any of the following:
___	___	1. Overdosed? (If yes, number of times _____)
___	___	2. Cut yourself on purpose? (If yes, number of times _____)
___	___	3. Burned yourself on purpose? (If yes, number of times _____)
___	___	4. Hit yourself? (if yes, number of times _____)
___	___	5. Banged your head on purpose? (If yes, number of times _____)
___	___	6. Abused alcohol?
___	___	7. Driven recklessly on purpose? (If yes, number of times _____)
___	___	8. Scratched yourself on purpose? (If yes, number of times _____
___	___	9. Prevented wounds from healing?
___	___	10. Made medical situations worse on purpose (e.g., skipped medication)?
___	___	11. Been promiscuous (i.e., had many sexual partners)? (If yes, how many? _____)
___	___	12. Set yourself up in a relationship to be rejected?
___	___	13. Abused prescription medication?
___	___	14. Distanced yourself from God as punishment?
___	___	15. Engaged in emotionally abusive relationships? (If yes, number of relationships? _____)
___	___	16. Engaged in sexually abusive relationships? (If yes, number of relationships? _____)
___	___	17. Lost a job on purpose? (If yes, number of times _____)
___	___	18. Attempted suicide? (If yes, number of times _____)
___	___	19. Exercised an injury on purpose?
___	___	20. Tortured yourself with self-defeating thoughts?
___	___	21. Starved yourself to hurt yourself?
___	___	22. Abused laxatives to hurt yourself? (If yes, number of times _____)

Have you engaged in any other self-destructive behaviors not asked about in this inventory? If so, please describe below.

_____

_____

Source: Used with permission from Sansone, R., & Sansone, L. (2010). Measuring self-harm behavior with the Self-Harm Inventory. Psychiatry, 7(4), 16–20.

being collected, and how it will be used are important first steps in the screening process.

The healthcare providers in Rahm and associates' study (2015) noted that another barrier to implementation of screening processes for mental health issues and substance use disorders is competing workload demands. This finding suggests that the success of screening may be tied, at least in part, to workload issues or lack of clarity about how to prioritize tasks. Nurses face these concerns in most areas of practice. Recognizing the vital importance of screening and creating the structure to ensure that it occurs requires multidisciplinary collaboration, commitment, and support from healthcare managers. Nurses are in a key position to educate others about the importance of screening for psychiatric and substance abuse issues in nonpsychiatric settings. Nurse leaders are in a key position to direct changes in screening requirements that address such critical public healthcare needs.

CORE CONCEPT

Referral

Referral entails sending a patient to another healthcare provider or specialty service for consultation or treatment.

Referral

Although structured screening of mental health issues has been identified as a critical first step in improving care for both mental illness and other medical illnesses, controversy exists over how much care can be provided in nonpsychiatric settings and when it is appropriate to refer to specialists for treatment. Grundberg (2016) concluded that if nonpsychiatric nurses are to be involved in early detection and interventions for mental health-related issues, these activities must be explicitly stated work objectives and there must be effective collaboration between care providers. If nurses lack clarity about their roles and responsibilities and the vital importance of this type of screening, referring the patient to needed services is unlikely to happen.

Several studies have found that providing training and education about evidence-based screening tools and referral pathways improved the referral process for mental health services (Allen et al., 2011; Brooker et al., 2007; Bruce et al., 2007; Hasche et al., 2013; Thompson, Lang, & Annells, 2008). The process for referral to specialized mental health services is one in which the nurse must collaborate effectively with physicians, social workers, and other healthcare providers within their practice setting and with the setting to which they are referring a patient.

CORE CONCEPT

Patient-centered care

Patient-Centered Care is an approach to care provision that intends to "identify, respect, and care about patients' differences, values, preferences, and expressed needs; relieve pain and suffering; coordinate continuous care; listen to, clearly inform, communicate with, and educate patients; share decision making and management: and continuously advocate disease prevention, wellness, and promotion of healthy lifestyles, including a focus on population health" (Institute of Medicine, 2003).

The process of referral also involves collaboration with the patient. This is the essence of **patient-centered care.** The Institute of Medicine (2003) has stressed, in its landmark study of deaths associated with medical errors, that we must improve our understanding and application of this concept to improve the safety and quality of healthcare in the future. To apply the concepts of patient-centered care requires that nurses and other healthcare professionals listen to the patient, empower them in decision making around their care, and establish a collaborative partnership.

Patients who are either strongly intent on hurting themselves or unaware that they have significant, life-threatening symptoms of mental illness need to be referred to a more restrictive environment even when it is against their own will. Essential elements in this process include collaboration with other healthcare professionals to increase confidence in the difficult clinical judgment to involuntarily hospitalize the patient and thoughtful communication with the patient about the reasons for this referral. Lauder and associates (2006), in their study of how nurses make clinical judgments about patients who are neglecting their self-care, caution that nurses need to be clear about the difference between severity of mental illness and capacity to make decisions. Just because a patient has a severe mental illness does not necessarily mean that the patient is incapable of making decisions. Nurses should only be making referral (or any other) decisions *for* patients when it is clear that they do not have the current capacity to make decisions in the interest of their personal safety and livelihood.

Two barriers to effective referral of patients with mental illness are lack of knowledge about available options for specialized treatment and difficulty accessing resources that are available. Some primary care settings and emergency departments have incorporated mental health specialists to either provide on-site intervention or to assist in the clinical judgment about needs for referral to more intensive treatment. Nurses in nonpsychiatric settings must be familiar with mental health services and facilities within the community in which they practice to effectively collaborate and refer patients appropriately for ongoing care. SAMHSA provides an online locator map to identify mental health and substance abuse treatment services in localities throughout the United States (https://findtreatment.samhsa.gov/locator). Box 12–2 lists some types of mental health and substance use disorder resources for referral.

CORE CONCEPT

Stigmatization

Stigmatization is the devaluing of a person because of a particular characteristic or illness. It is an attitude that is negative, discriminatory, and unethical. In the practice of health care, stigmatizing patients has the potential to inhibit the patient's ability to receive accurate diagnose and adequate treatment.

Stigma

Even with accessible, evidence-based screening tools and clear pathways for referral to mental health specialists, interventions can be derailed when the mental health client is stigmatized. **Stigmatization** has been identified as a barrier to effective mental

BOX 12-2 Types of Referral Resources for Mental Health and Substance Abuse Treatment

Self-Help Groups	12-step programs such as Alcoholics Anonymous, Emotions Anonymous, and others provide ongoing peer support and education. Location and availability of AA meetings can be found online (www.aa.org). Some meetings are also conducted online.
Mental Healthcare Professionals	Psychiatrists (MDs) and psych-mental health nurse practitioners (PMH NPs) provide diagnostic, medication management, and counseling services and may conduct psychotherapy. Licensed independent social workers (LISWs) provide counseling, case management, and advocacy. Psychologists (PhD) provide counseling, individual and group psychotherapy, and psychological testing services.
Community Mental Health Centers	Operated by community or county governments to provide public mental health services primarily to clients who cannot afford private services. Usually staffed with a broad range of mental health professionals and *peer support specialists* (individuals with mental illness who provide support in illness management and recovery), some of whom may have specialized training and certification. May provide a broad range of services for mental health and substance use disorders such as outpatient counseling, case management, intensive outpatient programs, and day programs. Often collaborate with and refer to area resources for support with employment, housing, and other care needs.
Substance Abuse and Addiction Treatment Centers	These treatment facilities usually have a broad range of mental health and addictions treatment health professionals including certified chemical dependency counselors and physicians certified in addictions medicine. Services usually include detoxification (for safe withdrawal from addictive substances), intensive outpatient services (intensive group therapy, 3 to 5 days per week, and support with establishing relapse prevention plans), and/or residential treatment (inpatient rehabilitation; lengths of stay may range from several weeks to several months).
Physician or Nurse Practitioner Primary Care	Some primary care practices have incorporated mental illness management within their practice settings, particularly in areas where specialists are not readily accessible.
Telemedicine	Some mental health organizations provide counseling and medication management via televideo interaction. Typically, these services are provided by psychiatrists and nurse practitioners.
General Hospital Inpatient Psychiatric Units	These units provide inpatient psychiatric care primarily for the purpose of assessment, monitoring and safety, medication management, and referral to outpatient mental health services for ongoing care. Typically staffed by a broad range of mental health professionals working as an interdisciplinary team that may include occupational or activities therapists, pastoral counselors, and mental health technicians in addition to psychiatrists, nurses, and social workers. Lengths of stay typically average 3 to 5 days.
State Psychiatric Hospitals	These are government-run inpatient treatment facilities with a broad range of mental health professionals, as listed previously. Provide public mental health services for those unable to afford private services. Lengths of stay vary from several days to months or even years depending on patient needs.

illness treatment in primary care, emergency departments, medical-surgical settings, and even at times in psychiatric settings.

One of the negative outcomes of stigma is that individuals with mental illnesses or addictions may not seek treatment at all, which can have devastating consequences on the progression of the illness and may leave many other physical illnesses undetected and untreated. This is an international problem, and in 2001, the World Health Organization (WHO) published a report recommending that mental healthcare be integrated in general healthcare settings, including primary care settings, based on the premise that clients with mental illness may avoid mental health services because of the associated stigma. Since then, research has informed us that there are several concerns to be addressed when the mental health client seeks help in a nonpsychiatric setting as well, particularly knowledge gaps, clinical skills, and stigma (Beaulieu et al., 2017; Gwaikolo, Kohrt, & Cooper, 2017; Li et al., 2014; Ng, Rashid, & O'Brien, 2017). In one study, it was found that clients, on the average, consulted more than three caregivers in a general hospital setting, and that 75 percent did not get a diagnosis or treatment (Li et al., 2014). Knowledge gaps about mental illnesses and attitudes toward the client manifesting symptoms of mental illness or substance addiction are primary influences. Ng and associates (2017) specifically studied nurses' attitudes and found that previous psychiatric training, a desire to learn about neuropsychiatric illnesses, and positive contact with people who have mental illnesses were associated with less stigmatizing attitudes. It is difficult to understand the lack of desire to be knowledgeable about a group of illnesses that have such a significant impact on all aspects of nursing care, but sometimes it is related to myths, fear, and stigma. Efforts to increase social contact and understand the *person* are important strategies to reduce stigma, but it first requires the nurse's willingness to engage meaningfully with people who have mental illnesses and addictions.

Social distancing is an aspect of stigma that refers to the tendency of healthcare workers and others to avoid people with mental illness or addiction. Symptoms like hallucinations, neglect of self-care, and agitation can be challenging symptoms for clinicians to manage when they feel frightened or ill-equipped to intervene effectively. Reavely and Jorm (2015) found that mental health clients reported similar avoidance behaviors among family and friends. These findings clarify the extent of the marginalization and disenfranchisement experienced by many individuals with mental illness and substance use disorders.

In a study of nurses in primary care settings (Ihalainen-Tamlander et al., 2016) researchers found that nurses' attitudes toward mental health clients were generally positive but that less experienced nurses or those without additional mental health training were more fearful and more likely to think that mental health patients should be segregated. The authors highlight the importance of ongoing on-the-job training, especially for less experienced nurses, to increase confidence, reduce fear, and prevent the development of stigmatizing and distancing attitudes. Several studies validate that education programs, consultation with mental health professionals to increase comfort and skill level, and exposure to individuals with mental illness or substance use disorders are effective tools in reducing negative stereotyping, social distancing, and other stigmatizing attitudes and behaviors (Beaulieu et al., 2017; Flanagan et al., 2016; Li, Li, Huang, & Thornicroft., 2014; Ng, Rashid, & O'Brien, 2017). Student nurses who have been educated about mental illnesses, communication, and intervention strategies; have developed an awareness of the problems associated with stigma; and have had encounters with patients in treatment for mental illness and/or substance use disorders enter the workforce in a unique position to spearhead culture change. Many chapters within this text, particularly those with the "Real People, Real Stories" features, provide important information to improve the nurse's knowledge and confidence in caring for clients with mental illness in any practice setting. To effectively apply those skills and knowledge requires that the nurse have a clear understanding of his or her role in this regard.

The Role of the Nurse in Caring for Patients With Psychiatric and Substance Use Disorders in Nonpsychiatric Settings

The nurse's role in caring for clients with psychiatric and substance use disorders in nonpsychiatric settings includes the following:

■ Examine one's personal beliefs and attitudes about clients with mental illness and substance use disorders, focusing on contributing factors such as fear or lack of confidence in managing the client's needs.
■ Develop awareness of the negative impact of stigmatization on provision of appropriate care and

actively seek knowledge and skills needed to increase confidence in patient care management.

■ Identify patients with potentially high-prevalence, high-risk mental health issues who require universal screening in any healthcare setting.

■ Utilize evidence-based screening tools to identify patients needing further evaluation and/or referral to mental health or substance use disorder services.

■ Provide for patient safety, up to and including continuous monitoring, while determinations are being made about referral needs.

■ Establish a working knowledge of available mental health services for referral and collaborate with physicians and other members of the healthcare team to identify the most appropriate resources.

■ Engage the patient throughout the assessment and referral process using a patient-centered approach that empowers the patient in decision making about care recommendations to the best of his or her ability.

It is clear that clients with mental illnesses and substance use disorders will be encountered in every healthcare setting where nurses practice. It is imperative that each nurse recognizes his or her role in reducing stigma personally and within the culture of the care team and provides the same attention to screening, intervention, and referral that is provided for patients with other chronic illnesses. This is the necessary foundation for nursing care that addresses priority healthcare needs, reduces poorer outcomes, improves individuals' quality of life, and minimizes the risks of premature death.

Summary and Key Points

■ In the United States and globally, clients with psychiatric illness and substance use disorders are vulnerable to lack of or inadequate treatment and this is associated with poorer outcomes with regard to the mental illness, undetected physical illnesses, and early death.

■ *Diagnostic overshadowing* is a process of wrongly assuming that the patient's medical symptoms are attributable to his or her mental illness.

■ Three variables that influence nurses' responses to the patient with mental health and substance use disorders are lack of education and recognition of symptoms, lack of appropriate screening, and nurses' attitudes about patients with these illnesses.

■ Many evidence-based screening tools exist for detection of mental illness or substance use disorders. Some are easily accessible, free to use, and time efficient.

■ Due to the high risk of morbidity and mortality, high prevalence, and risk that patients are not openly forthcoming about these issues, all patients should be screened for trauma history, substance use, and risk for suicide.

■ One of the identified barriers to adequate screening of mental health issues in nonpsychiatric settings is competing workload demands. Nurses and nurse managers have a responsibility to prioritize mental illnesses and substance abuse as critical public healthcare issues.

■ Another identified barrier to appropriate screening and intervention is *social distancing,* which refers to the nurses' avoidance of patients with mental illnesses because of fear, lack of knowledge, lack of confidence in clinical skills, and stigma.

■ Nurses in nonpsychiatric settings must have a working knowledge of available resources for referral when mental health and substance abuse are identified concerns. SAMHSA provides online information about available mental health and addictions services for every locality in the United States.

■ Referral is a collaborative process with members of the healthcare team, including the patient.

■ *Patient-centered care* requires that nurses listen to the patient, empower the patient in decision making around his or her care, develop a collaborative partnership, and only make decisions for the patient (such as involuntary hospitalization) when he or she is clearly unable to and when it is necessary to protect the patient's safety.

■ *Stigmatization* is the devaluing, marginalizing, and disenfranchising of certain patients because of symptoms or conditions. Stigmatizing patients with psychiatric and substance use disorders is an international concern contributing to patient neglect, inadequate treatment, avoidance of healthcare professionals and treatment settings, and risk of early death.

■ The first step for every nurse in accomplishing safe, effective care for the patient with mental health and substance use disorders is reflection on one's own beliefs, attitudes, and behaviors and actively making efforts to reduce stigma personally and within the culture of his or her practice setting.

Review Questions
Self-Examination/Learning Exercise

Select the answer that is most appropriate for each of the following questions:

1. Ellie presents in the emergency department loudly proclaiming with rapid speech, "If I don't get more pain medication right now, I'm going to call the attorney general and sue the entire health care network." Which of the following should be included in initial screening and assessment? (Select all that apply.)
   a. Substance use
   b. Pain
   c. Mental Illness
   d. Prior history of convictions
   e. Availability of an inpatient psychiatric bed

2. When Shelly enters the emergency department she reports, "My bed is on fire, and my stomach, and we're all dead." The nurse's initial response is to call the psychiatric unit to secure an inpatient bed for this patient. This is an example of:
   a. Prompt, appropriate referral
   b. Patient-centered care
   c. Stigma
   d. Collaboration

3. Adam was admitted to the ICU after a single car accident in which he struck a cement wall. He is now responsive and wants to be discharged within the next couple of days. Which of the following are priorities for screening? (Select all that apply.)
   a. Traumatic brain injury
   b. Chronic pain
   c. Sexual dysfunction
   d. Depression and risk for suicide

4. The nurse manager recognizes a need to improve mental health and substance use screening and referral services for their clients in the public health clinic. Which of the following is a priority to begin an effective process for implementation?
   a. Provide a list of referral sources that is readily available to staff.
   b. Educate staff about the importance of prioritizing these public health concerns.
   c. Explore the literature for evidence-based screening tools.
   d. Inform the staff that they have been stigmatizing patients and this will not be tolerated.

5. Mr. Li is a patient on a medical unit and is identified as having suicidal ideation. Which of the following is a priority in managing his immediate care?
   a. Screen for depression
   b. Provide sedative medication
   c. Refer him to another setting
   d. Continuous monitoring and observation

References

Akiskal, H. S. (2017). Mood disorders: Historical introduction and conceptual overview. In B. J. Sadock, V. A. Sadock, & P. Ruiz (Eds.), *Comprehensive textbook of psychiatry* (pp. 1599–1603). Philadelphia, PA: Wolters Kluwer.

Allen, J., Annells, M., Nunn, R., Petrie, E., Clark, E., Lang, L., & Robins, A. (2011). Evaluation of effectiveness and satisfaction outcomes of a mental health screening and referral clinical pathway for community nursing care. *Journal of Psychiatric and Mental Health Nursing, 18*(5), 375–385.

American Academy of Pediatrics. (2018). *Developmental, behavioral, psychosocial screening and assessment forms*. Retrieved from https://brightfutures.aap.org/materials-and-tools/tool-and-resource-kit/Pages/Developmental-Behavioral-Psychosocial-Screening-and-Assessment-Forms.aspx

Bay, N., Bjørnestad, J., Johannessen, J. O., Larsen, T. K., & Joa, I. (2016). Obstacles to care in first-episode psychosis patients with a long duration of untreated psychosis. *Early Intervention in Psychiatry, 10*(1), 71–76. doi:10.1111/eip.12152

Beaulieu, T., Patten, S., Knaak, S., Weinerman, R., Campbell, H., & Lauria-Horner, B. (2017). Impact of skill-based approaches in reducing stigma in primary care physicians: Results from a double-blind, parallel-cluster, randomized controlled trial. *The Canadian Journal of Psychiatry, 62*(5), 327–335.

Betz, M. E., Sullivan, A. F., Manton, A. P., Espinola, J. A., Miller, I., Camargo Jr, C. A., . . . ED-SAFE Investigators. (2013). Knowledge, attitudes, and practices of emergency department providers in the care of suicidal patients. *Depression & Anxiety, 30*(10), 1005–1012.

Bica, T., Castelló, R., Toussaint, L. L., & Montesó-Curto, P. (2017). Depression as a risk factor of organic diseases: An international integrative review. *Journal of Nursing Scholarship, 49*(4), 389–399.

Brooker, C., Ricketts, T., Bennett, S., & Lemme, F. (2007). Admission decisions following contact with an emergency mental health assessment and intervention service. *Journal of Clinical Nursing, 16*(7), 1313–1322.

Bruce, M. L., Brown, E. L., Raue, P. J., Mlodzianowski, A. E., Meyers, B. S., Leon, A. C., & Nassisi, P. (2007). A randomized trial of depression assessment intervention in home health care. *Journal of the American Geriatrics Society, 55*(11), 1793–1800.

Flanagan, E. H., Buck, T., Gamble, A., Hunter, C., Sewell, I., & Davidson, L. (2016). "Recovery speaks": A photovoice intervention to reduce stigma among primary care providers. *Psychiatric Services, 67*(5), 566–569. doi:10.1176/appi.ps.201500049

Gomes, J., Duraes, D., & Lima, G. (2015). Stigma kills. *European Psychiatry, 1*(30), 1863. doi: 10.1016/S0924-9338(15)31427-9

Grundberg, Å. (2016). District nurses' perspectives on detecting mental health problems and promoting mental health among community-dwelling seniors with multimorbidity. *Journal of Clinical Nursing, 25*(17/18), 2590–2599.

Guttmacher Institute. (2018). *Substance use during pregnancy.* Retrieved from https://www.guttmacher.org/state-policy/explore/substance-use-during-pregnancy

Gwaikolo, W. S., Kohrt, B. A., & Cooper, J. L. (2017). Health system preparedness for integration of mental health services in rural Liberia. *BMC Health Services Research, 17,* 1–10.

Hasche, L. K., Lee, M. J., Proctor, E. K., & Morrow-Howell, N. (2013). Does identification of depression affect community long-term care services ordered for older adults? *Social Work Research, 37*(3), 255–262.

Horowitz, L. M., Snyder, D., Ludi, E., Rosenstein, D. L., Kohn-Godbout, J., Lee, L., . . . Pao, M. (2013). Ask suicide-screening questions to everyone in medical settings: The asQ'em Quality Improvement Project. *Psychosomatics 54*(3), 239–247.

Ihalainen-Tamlander, N., Vähäniemi, A., Löyttyniemi, E., Suominen, T., & Välimäki, M. (2016). Stigmatizing attitudes in nurses towards people with mental illness: A cross-sectional study in primary settings in Finland. *Journal of Psychiatric and Mental Health Nursing, 23*(6–7), 427–437. doi:10.1111/jpm.12319

Institute of Medicine, Committee on the Health Professions Education Summit.(2003). *Health professions education: A bridge to quality.* Washington, DC: National Academy of Sciences.

Jackman, K., Honig, J., & Bockting, W. (2016). Nonsuicidal self-injury among lesbian, gay, bisexual and transgender populations: An integrative review. *Journal of Clinical Nursing, 25*(23/24), 3438–3453.

Jobes, D. A. (2015, September). *Clinical suicidology: Innovations in assessment treatment of suicidal risk.* Paper presented at Psychiatric Grand Rounds, Summa Health System, Akron, OH.

Kameg, K. M., Spencer Woods, A., Luther Szpak, J., & McCormick, M. (2013). Identifying and managing nonsuicidal self-injurious behavior in the primary care setting. *Journal of the American Association of Nurse Practitioners, 25*(4), 167–172.

Koposov, R., Fossum, S., Frodl, T., Nytrø, O., Leventhal, B., Sourander, A., . . . Skokauskas, N. (2017). Clinical decision support systems in child and adolescent psychiatry: A systematic

review. *European Child & Adolescent Psychiatry, 26*(11), 1309–1317.

Langdon, R., Johnson, M., Carroll, V., & Antonio, G. (2013). Assessment of the elderly: It's worth covering the risks. *Journal of Nursing Management, 21*(1), 94–105.

Lauder, W., Ludwick, R., Zeller, R., & Winchell, J. (2006). Factors influencing nurses' judgements about self-neglect cases. *Journal of Psychiatric & Mental Health Nursing, 13*(3), 279–287.

Li, J., Li, J., Huang, Y., & Thornicroft, G. (2014). Mental health training program for community mental health staff in Guangzhou, China: Effects on knowledge of mental illness and stigma. *International Journal of Mental Health Systems, 8*(1), 49.

Li, X., Zhang, W., Lin, Y., Zhang, X., Qu, Z., Wang, X., . . . Tian, D. (2014). Pathways to psychiatric care of patients from rural regions: A general-hospital-based study. *International Journal of Social Psychiatry, 60*(3), 280–289. doi:10.1177/0020764013485364

McGovern, A., & Selwyn, J. (2014). A quality improvement project: Improving recognition of low mood and depression in elderly inpatients. *Age & Ageing, 43* (Suppl. 2), ii7–ii7.

Mitchell, A. J., Hussain, N., Grainger, L., & Symonds, P. (2011). Identification of patient- reported distress by clinical nurse specialists in routine oncology practice: A multicentre UK study. *Psycho-Oncology, 20*(10), 1076–1083.

Mollard, E., Brage Hudson, D., Ford, A., & Pullen, C. (2016). An integrative review of postpartum depression in rural U.S. communities. *Archives of Psychiatric Nursing, 30*(3), 418–424.

Ndetei, D. M., Khasakhala, L. I., Mutiso, V., & Mbwayo, A. W. (2011). Knowledge, attitude and practice (KAP) of mental illness among staff in general medical facilities in Kenya: And policy implications. *African Journal of Psychiatry, 14*(3), 225–235.

Ng, Y. P., Rashid, A., & O'Brien, F. (2017). Determining the effectiveness of a video-based contact intervention in improving attitudes of Penang primary care nurses towards people with mental illness. *PLoS ONE, 12*(11), 1–19.

Pardee, M. L., Kuzma, E., Dahlem, C. H., Boucher, N., & Darling-Fisher, C. (2017). Current state of screening high-ACE youth and emerging adults in primary care: Screening of high-ACE youth in primary care settings. *Journal of the American Association of Nurse Practitioners, 29.* doi:10.1002/2327-6924.12531

Préville, M., Côté, G., Boyer, R., & Hébert, R. (2004). Detection of depression and anxiety disorders by home care nurses. *Aging & Mental Health, 8*(5), 400–409.

Rahm, A. K., Boggs, J. M., Martin, C., Price, D. W., Beck, A., Backer, T. E., & Dearing, J. W. (2015). Facilitators and barriers to implementing screening, brief intervention, and referral to treatment (SBIRT) in primary care in integrated health care settings. *Substance Abuse, 36*(3), 281–288.

Reavely, N. J., & Jorm, A. F. (2015). Experiences of discrimination and positive treatment in people with mental health problems: Findings from an Australian national survey. *Australian and New Zealand Journal of Psychiatry, 49*(10), 906–913. doi:10.1177/0004867415602068

Roberge, P., Hudon, C., Pavilanis, A., Beaulieu, M., Benoit, A., Brouillet, H., . . . Vanasse, A. (2016). A qualitative study of perceived needs and factors associated with the quality of care for common mental disorders in patients with chronic diseases: The perspective of primary care clinicians and patients. *BMC Family Practice, 17,* 1–14.

Sansone, R., & Sansone, L. (2010). Measuring self-harm behavior with the Self-Harm Inventory. *Psychiatry, 7*(4), 16–20.

Singer, S., Brown, A., Einenkel, J., Hauss, J., Hinz, A., Klein, A., . . . Brähler, E. (2011). Identifying tumor patients' depression. *Supportive Care in Cancer, 19*(11), 1697–1703.

Substance Abuse and Mental Health Services Administration (SAMHSA). (2017). *About screening, brief intervention, and referral to treatment (SBIRT).* Retrieved from https://www.samhsa.gov/sbirt/about

Substance Abuse and Mental Health Services Administration. (no date). *SAMHSA-HRSA Integrated Health Solutions: Screening Tools.*

Retrieved from https://www.integration.samhsa.gov/clinical-practice/screening-tools

Thompson, P., Lang, L., & Annells, M. (2008). A systematic review of the effectiveness of in-home community nurse led interventions for the mental health of older persons. *Journal of Clinical Nursing, 17*(11), 1419–1427.

Classical References

Felitti, V. J., Anda, R. F., Nordenberg, D., Williamson, D. F., Spitz, A. M., Edwards, V., . . . Marks, J. S. (1998). Relationship of childhood abuse and household dysfunction to many of the leading causes of death in adults—The adverse childhood experiences (ACE) study. *American Journal of Preventive Medicine, 14*, 245–258.

Hoff, L. A., & Rosenbaum, L. (1994). A victimization assessment tool: Instrument development and clinical implications. *Journal of Advanced Nursing, 20*, 627–634.

Hoff, L. A., & Ross, M. (1993). Curriculum guide for nursing: Violence against women and children. Ottawa, Canada: University of Ottawa, Faculty of Health Sciences, School of Nursing, Ottawa.

Schofferman, J., Anderson, D., Hines, R., Smith, G., & White, A. (1992). Childhood psychological trauma correlates with unsuccessful lumbar spine surgery. *Spine, 17*(Suppl.), 138–144.

World Health Organization (WHO). (2001). *The World* Health *Report 2001. Mental health: New understanding, new hope.* Geneva, Switzerland: Author. Retrieved from http://www.who.int/whr/2001/en/whr01_en.pdf

13

Neurocognitive Disorders

KEY TERMS

aphasia

apraxia

ataxia

confabulation

delirium

neurocognitive disorder (NCD)

pseudodementia

sundowning

OBJECTIVES

After reading this chapter, the student will be able to:

1. Define and differentiate among various neurocognitive disorders (NCDs).
2. Discuss predisposing factors implicated in the etiology of NCDs.
3. Describe clinical symptoms and use the information to assess patients with NCDs.
4. Identify nursing diagnoses common to patients with NCDs and select appropriate nursing interventions for each.
5. Identify topics for patient and family teaching relevant to NCDs.
6. Discuss criteria for evaluating nursing care of patients with NCDs.
7. Describe various treatment modalities relevant to care of patients with NCDs.

HOMEWORK ASSIGNMENT

Please read the chapter and answer the following questions:

1. Which biomarkers are associated with the development of Alzheimer's disease?
2. How does vascular neurocognitive disorder (NCD) differ from NCD due to Alzheimer's disease?
3. What is pseudodementia?
4. What is the primary concern for nurses working with patients with NCDs?

Introduction

Neurocognitive disorders include those in which a clinically significant deficit in cognition or memory exists, representing a significant change from a previous level of functioning. These disorders were previously identified in the *Diagnostic and Statistical Manual of Mental Disorders, Fourth Edition, Text Revision (DSM-IV-TR)* (American Psychiatric Association [APA], 2000) as delirium, dementia, and amnestic disorders. In the *DSM-5,* they include delirium and mild and major neurocognitive disorders (APA, 2013).

This chapter presents predisposing factors, clinical symptoms, and nursing interventions for care of patients with neurocognitive disorders. The objective is to provide these individuals with the dignity and quality of life they deserve while offering guidance and support to their families or primary caregivers.

CORE CONCEPT

Delirium

Delirium is a mental state characterized by an acute disturbance of cognition, which is manifested by short-term confusion, excitement, disorientation, and a clouding of consciousness. Hallucinations and illusions are common.

Delirium

Clinical Findings and Course

Delirium is characterized by a disturbance in attention and awareness and a change in cognition that develop rapidly over a short period (APA, 2013). Symptoms of delirium include difficulty sustaining and shifting attention. The person is extremely distractible and must be repeatedly reminded to focus attention. Disorganized thinking prevails and is reflected by speech that is rambling, irrelevant, pressured, and incoherent and that unpredictably switches from subject to subject. Reasoning ability and goal-directed behavior are impaired. Disorientation to time and place is common, and impairment of recent memory is invariably evident. Misperceptions of the environment, including illusions and hallucinations, prevail. Disturbances in the sleep–wake cycle occur.

The state of awareness may range from that of hypervigilance (heightened awareness to environmental stimuli) to stupor or semicoma. Sleep may fluctuate between hypersomnolence (excessive sleepiness) and insomnia. Vivid dreams and nightmares are common.

Psychomotor activity may fluctuate between agitated, purposeless movements (e.g., restlessness, hyperactivity, striking out at nonexistent objects) and a vegetative state resembling catatonic stupor. Various forms of tremor are frequently present.

Emotional instability may be manifested by fear, anxiety, depression, irritability, anger, euphoria, or apathy. These various emotions may be evidenced by crying, calls for help, cursing, muttering, moaning, acts of self-destruction, fearful attempts to flee, or attacks on others who are falsely viewed as threatening. Autonomic manifestations, such as tachycardia, sweating, flushed face, dilated pupils, and elevated blood pressure, are common.

The symptoms of delirium usually begin quite abruptly (e.g., following a head injury or seizure). At other times, they may be preceded by several hours or days of prodromal symptoms (e.g., restlessness, difficulty thinking clearly, insomnia or hypersomnolence, and nightmares). The slower onset is more common if the underlying cause is systemic illness or metabolic imbalance.

The duration of delirium is usually brief (e.g., 1 week; rarely more than 1 month) and, upon elimination of the underlying causes, symptoms usually diminish over a 3- to 7-day period but in some instances may take as long as 2 weeks (Sadock, Sadock, & Ruiz, 2015). The age of the client and duration of the delirium influence rate of symptom resolution. Delirium may transition into a more permanent cognitive disorder (e.g., major neurocognitive disorder) and is associated with a high mortality rate because of the seriousness of the medical conditions that precipitate delirium.

Predisposing Factors

Delirium

Individuals most predisposed to developing delirium include those with serious medical, surgical, or neurological conditions and sensory or cognitive impairments (such as dementia). People over 65 years of age are considered a high-risk group. Depression, falls, and elder abuse may also contribute to delirium. Other precipitating factors include the following (Fabian & Solai, 2017; Sadock et al., 2015):

■ Systemic infections
■ Febrile illness or hypothermia

- Metabolic disorders, such as electrolyte imbalances, hypercarbia, hypoglycemia, or hyponatremia
- Hypoxia and chronic obstructive pulmonary disease (COPD)
- Hepatic failure or renal failure
- Head trauma
- Seizures
- Migraine headaches
- Brain abscess or brain neoplasms
- Stroke
- Nutritional deficiency
- Uncontrolled pain
- Burns
- Heat stroke
- Orthopedic and cardiac surgeries
- Social isolation, emotional stress, physical restraints, admission to an intensive care unit

Other Etiological Implications

Substance Intoxication Delirium

In this subtype, the symptoms of delirium are attributed to intoxication from certain substances, such as alcohol, amphetamines, cannabis, cocaine, hallucinogens, inhalants, opioids, phencyclidine, sedative, hypnotic, and anxiolytics, or other (or unknown) substance (APA, 2013).

Substance Withdrawal Delirium

Withdrawal from certain substances can precipitate symptoms of delirium that are sufficiently severe to warrant clinical attention. These substances include alcohol, opioids, sedative-hypnotics and anxiolytics, and others.

Medication-Induced Delirium

Medications that have been known to precipitate delirium include anticholinergics, antihypertensives, corticosteroids, anticonvulsants, cardiac glycosides, analgesics, anesthetics, antineoplastic agents, antiparkinson drugs, H_2-receptor antagonists (e.g., cimetidine), and others (Fabian & Solai, 2017; Sadock et al., 2015). In addition, polypharmacy is, at times, implicated in precipitating delirium.

Delirium Due to Another Medical Condition or to Multiple Etiologies

There may be evidence from the history, physical examination, or laboratory findings that the symptoms of delirium are associated with another medical condition or can be attributable to more than one cause. The current evidence supports that delirium is usually the result of many factors rather than one (Fabian & Solai, 2017).

> ## CORE CONCEPT
> ### Neurocognitive
> A term that is used to describe cognitive functions closely linked to particular areas of the brain that have to do with thinking, reasoning, memory, learning, and speaking.

Neurocognitive Disorder

Neurocognitive disorder (NCD) is classified in the *DSM-5* (APA, 2013) as either *mild* or *major*, with the distinction primarily being one of severity of symptomatology. Mild NCD has been known in some settings as *mild cognitive impairment* and is particularly critical because it can be a focus of early intervention to prevent or slow progression of the disorder. Major NCD constitutes what was previously described as *dementia* in the *DSM-IV-TR* (APA, 2000). In progressive neurodegenerative conditions, these two diagnoses may serve to identify earlier and later stages of the same disorder. Either diagnosis may be appropriate (depending on severity of symptoms) for certain other NCDs that are the result of a reversible or temporary condition. Differentiation of these disorders is presented in Box 13–1.

> ## CORE CONCEPT
> ### Dementia (major neurocognitive disorder)
> A disease process in which there is progressive decline in cognitive ability in the presence of clear consciousness. It involves many cognitive deficits and significantly impairs social and occupational functioning (Sadock et al., 2015).

Clinical Findings, Epidemiology, and Course

NCD constitutes a large and growing public health problem. An estimated 5.7 million people in the United States currently have Alzheimer's disease (AD), the most common form of NCD, and the prevalence (the number of people with the disease at any one time) doubles for every 5-year age group beyond age 65 (Alzheimer's Association, 2018a; National Institute on Aging [NIA], 2017). For the period from 2000 to 2015 deaths from AD have increased 123 percent. The Alzheimer's Association (2018a) reports that of those with AD, an estimated 200,000 are under age 65. The incidence increases dramatically with age, affecting about 3 percent of individuals between

BOX 13–1 A Comparison of Diagnostic Criteria

Mild Neurocognitive Disorder	Major Neurocognitive Disorder
A. Evidence of modest cognitive decline from a previous level of performance in one or more cognitive domains (complex attention, executive function, learning and memory, language, perceptual-motor, or social cognition) based on: 1. Concern of the individual, a knowledgeable informant, or the clinician that there has been a mild decline in cognitive function; and 2. A modest impairment in cognitive performance, preferably documented by standardized neuropsychological testing, or, in its absence, another quantified clinical assessment. B. The cognitive deficits do not interfere with capacity for independence in everyday activities (i.e., complex instrumental activities of daily living such as paying bills or managing medications are preserved, but greater effort, compensatory strategies, or accommodation may be required). C. The cognitive deficits do not occur exclusively in the context of a delirium. D. The cognitive deficits are not better explained by another mental disorder (e.g., major depressive disorder, schizophrenia).	A. Evidence of significant cognitive decline from a previous level of performance in one or more cognitive domains (complex attention, executive function, learning and memory, language, perceptual-motor, or social cognition) based on: 1. Concern of the individual, a knowledgeable informant, or the clinician that there has been a significant decline in cognitive function; and 2. A substantial impairment in cognitive performance, preferably documented by standardized neuropsychological testing, or, in its absence, another quantified clinical assessment. B. The cognitive deficits interfere with independence in everyday activities (i.e., at a minimum, requiring assistance with complex instrumental activities of daily living such as paying bills or managing medications). C. The cognitive deficits do not occur exclusively in the context of a delirium. D. The cognitive deficits are not better explained by another mental disorder (e.g., major depressive disorder, schizophrenia).
Specify whether due to: • Alzheimer's disease • Frontotemporal lobar degeneration • Lewy body disease • Vascular disease • Traumatic brain injury • Substance/medication use • HIV infection • Prion disease • Parkinson's disease • Huntington's disease • Another medical condition • Multiple etiologies • Unspecified	Specify whether due to: • Alzheimer's disease • Frontotemporal lobar degeneration • Lewy body disease • Vascular disease • Traumatic brain injury • Substance/medication use • HIV infection • Prion disease • Parkinson's disease • Huntington's disease • Another medical condition • Multiple etiologies • Unspecified
Specify: **Without behavioral disturbance:** If the cognitive disturbance is not accompanied by any clinically significant behavioral disturbance. **With behavioral disturbance** (specify disturbance): If the cognitive disturbance is accompanied by a clinically significant behavioral disturbance (e.g., psychotic symptoms, mood disturbance, agitation, apathy, or other behavioral symptoms).	Specify: **Without behavioral disturbance:** If the cognitive disturbance is not accompanied by any clinically significant behavioral disturbance. **With behavioral disturbance** (specify disturbance): If the cognitive disturbance is accompanied by a clinically significant behavioral disturbance (e.g., psychotic symptoms, mood disturbance, agitation, apathy, or other behavioral symptoms). Specify current severity: **Mild:** Difficulties with instrumental activities of daily living (e.g., housework, managing money) **Moderate:** Difficulties with basic activities of daily living (e.g., feeding, dressing) **Severe:** Fully dependent

Source: Reprinted with permission from the Diagnostic and Statistical Manual of Mental Disorders, *Fifth Edition (Copyright 2013). American Psychiatric Association.*

65 and 74, 17 percent of individuals between 75 and 84, and 32 percent of individuals 85 and older. Despite these age-related increases, AD is not a normal part of aging (Alzheimer's Association, 2018a). Almost two-thirds of Americans with AD are women. It is projected that by 2050, the number of individuals aged 65 and older with AD will nearly triple if current population trends continue and no preventive treatments become available (Alzheimer's Association, 2018a). Healthcare costs for end-stage patients with dementia have now been identified as greater than the costs for any other disease (including cancer and heart disease), and the total annual costs are projected to increase from $277 billion in 2018 to $1.1 trillion by 2050 (Alzheimer's Association, 2018a).

This proliferation is not the result of an "epidemic." It has occurred because more people now survive into the high-risk period for NCD, which is middle age and beyond. Survival after diagnosis typically ranges from 3 to 12 years, with most of that time spent in the most severe stage (Mitchell, 2015). Despite the alarming statistics about AD, recent studies have indicated that dementia in general has declined in the United States over the past few years. This trend may be related to improved education and treatment for risk factors associated with heart disease and stroke (Langa et al., 2017).

NCDs can be classified as either primary or secondary. Primary NCDs are those, such as AD, in which the NCD itself is the major sign of some organic brain disease not directly related to any other organic illness. Secondary NCDs are caused by or related to another disease or condition, such as HIV disease or a cerebral trauma.

In NCD, impairment is evident in abstract thinking, judgment, and impulse control. The conventional rules of social conduct are often disregarded. Behavior may be uninhibited and inappropriate. Personal appearance and hygiene are often neglected. Language may or may not be affected. Some individuals may have difficulty naming objects, or the language may seem vague and imprecise. In severe forms of NCD, the individual may not speak at all (**aphasia**). The client may know his or her needs but may not know how to communicate those needs to a caregiver.

Personality change is common in NCD and may be manifested by either an alteration or accentuation of premorbid characteristics. For example, an individual who was previously very socially active may become apathetic and socially isolated. A previously neat person may become markedly untidy in his or her appearance. Conversely, an individual who may have had difficulty trusting others prior to the illness may exhibit extreme fear and paranoia as manifestations of the disorder.

The reversibility of NCD is dependent on the basic etiology of the disorder. Truly reversible NCD occurs in only a small percentage of cases and might be more appropriately termed *temporary* NCD. Reversible causes of NCD (dementia or dementia-like symptoms) include some brain tumors, subdural hematomas, depression, medication reactions, normal pressure hydrocephalus, vitamin/nutritional deficiencies (especially B_6 and B_{12}), central nervous system (CNS) infections, thyroid disorders, and metabolic disorders (hypoglycemia) (Mayo Clinic, 2018a). In most clients, NCD runs a progressive, irreversible course.

As the disease progresses, **apraxia,** the inability to carry out purposeful motor activities despite intact motor function and the inability to use objects properly, may develop. The individual may be irritable, moody, or exhibit sudden outbursts over trivial issues. The ability to work or care for personal needs independently will no longer be possible. These individuals can no longer be left alone because they do not comprehend their limitations and are therefore at serious risk for accidents. Wandering away from the home or care setting often becomes a problem. In advanced dementia, clinical features include profound memory deficits, minimal verbal communication, loss of ambulatory ability, inability to perform activities of daily living (ADLs), and incontinence. The most common clinical complications are eating problems and infections (Mitchell, 2015).

Several causes have been described for NCD (see section "Predisposing Factors"), but AD is the most common cause of dementia in older adults, accounting for 60 to 80 percent of all cases (Alzheimer's Association, 2018b). The progressive nature of symptoms associated with AD has been described in seven stages (NIA, 2017; WebMD, 2017):

Stage 1. No apparent symptoms. In the first stage of the illness, there is no apparent decline in memory despite changes that are beginning to occur in the brain; a positron emission tomography (PET) scan can be used to detect these changes.

Stage 2. Very mild change. The individual begins to lose things or forget names of people. Losses in short-term memory are common. The individual is aware of the intellectual decline and may feel ashamed, becoming anxious and depressed, which in turn may worsen the symptom. Maintaining organization with lists and a structured routine provides some compensation. These symptoms often are not noticed by others and do not interfere with the individual's ability to work or live independently.

Stage 3. Mild cognitive decline. In this stage there are changes in thinking and reasoning that interfere with work performance and become noticeable to coworkers. The individual may get lost when driving his or her car. Concentration may be interrupted. There is difficulty recalling names or words, which becomes noticeable to family and close associates. A decline occurs in the ability to plan or organize.

Stage 4. Moderate cognitive decline. At this stage, the individual may forget major events in personal history, such as his or her own child's birthday; experience declining ability to perform tasks, such as shopping, cooking, and managing personal finances; or be unable to understand current news events. He or she may deny that a problem exists by covering up memory loss with **confabulation** (creating imaginary events to fill in memory gaps). Depression and social withdrawal are common. At this stage the individual requires some assistance to maintain safety.

Stage 5. Moderately severe cognitive decline. At this stage, individuals lose the ability to perform some ADLs independently, such as hygiene, dressing, and grooming, and require some assistance to manage these tasks on an ongoing basis. They may forget addresses, phone numbers, and names of close relatives. They may become disoriented about place and time, but they maintain knowledge about themselves. Frustration, withdrawal, and self-absorption are common.

Stage 6. Severe cognitive decline. At this stage, individuals may be unable to recall the name of their spouse or may misidentify people (e.g., thinking a child is their spouse). Disorientation to surroundings is common, and the person may be unable to recall the day, season, or year. The person is unable to manage ADLs without assistance. Delusions often become apparent such as maintaining the belief that one must go to work even though the person is no longer employed. Urinary and fecal incontinence are common. Sleeping becomes a problem. Psychomotor symptoms include wandering, obsessiveness, agitation, and aggression. Symptoms seem to worsen in the late afternoon and evening—a phenomenon termed **sundowning.** Communication becomes more difficult with increasing loss of language skills. Institutional care is usually required at this stage.

Stage 7. Very severe decline. In the end stages of AD, the individual is unable to recognize family members. He or she most commonly is bedfast and aphasic. Problems of immobility, such as decubiti and contractures, may occur.

The NIA (2017) describes some specific symptoms of the latest stage of AD and associated care needs:

- Muscle immobility may require assistance from healthcare professionals to move, position, and exercise the patient with the goal of preventing contractures and pressure ulcers.
- The individual loses interest in food, lacks awareness of mealtimes, or can't remember if he or she has eaten and therefore will require assistance to maintain adequate nutrition. In addition, chewing and swallowing difficulties are common so supervision and assistance to prevent choking or aspiration pneumonia are important interventions.
- Body jerking (myoclonus) increases risk for injury; the physician may prescribe medication to ease these symptoms.

Predisposing Factors

NCDs are differentiated by their etiology, although they share a common symptom presentation. Categories include NCDs due to:

- Alzheimer's disease
- Vascular disease
- Frontotemporal lobar degeneration
- Traumatic brain injury
- Lewy body dementia
- Parkinson's disease
- HIV infection
- Substances/ medications
- Huntington's disease
- Prion disease
- Another medical condition
- Multiple etiologies
- Unspecified

Neurocognitive Disorder Due to Alzheimer's Disease

AD is characterized by the syndrome of symptoms identified as mild or major NCD and by those listed in the seven stages described previously. The onset of symptoms is slow and insidious, and the course of the disorder is generally progressive and deteriorating. Memory impairment is a prominent feature.

Refinement of diagnostic criteria now enables clinicians to use specific clinical features to identify the disease with considerable accuracy. Examination by computerized tomography (CT) scan or magnetic resonance imagery (MRI) reveals a degenerative pathology of the brain that includes atrophy, widened cortical sulci, and enlarged cerebral ventricles (Figs. 13–1 and 13–2). Diagnostic tests reveal specific biomarkers, tau neurofibrillary tangles and amyloid beta plaques, in the brains of clients with AD through

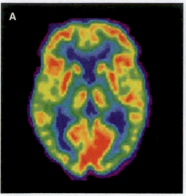

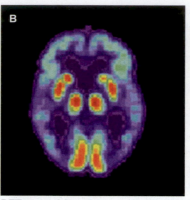

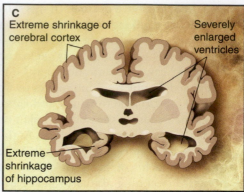

PET scan of normal brain

PET scan of Alzheimer's brain

FIGURE 13–1 Changes in the Alzheimer's brain. A. Metabolic activity in a healthy brain. B. Diminished metabolic activity in the Alzheimer's diseased brain. C. Late-stage Alzheimer's disease with generalized atrophy and enlargement of the ventricles and sulci. (Source: Alzheimer's Disease Education & Referral Center, A Service of the National Institute on Aging.)

specialized PET scans and in cerebrospinal fluid. These changes apparently occur as a part of the normal aging process. However, in clients with AD, they are found in dramatically increased numbers, and their profusion is concentrated in the hippocampus and certain parts of the cerebral cortex.

In 2018, the NIA and Alzheimer's Association redefined AD as identified by three specific biomarkers (amyloid beta plaques, tau neurofibrillary tangles, and neuronal damage) rather than by the progression of cognitive symptoms (Sullivan, 2018). It is believed that this redefinition will, in the short term, clarify research and clinical drug trials and in the long term may change the way AD is understood and treated. Because biomarkers are present before cognitive symptoms appear the potential for preventive interventions will, no doubt, be the focus of ongoing research.

Etiology

The etiology of AD is currently understood to be multifactorial; particularly in late-onset AD the risk is influenced by multiple genes and environmental factors and their interaction with amyloid beta proteins in the transition to AD (Graziane & Sweet, 2017). Several findings in research studies have led to hypotheses about contributing or causative factors, including the following:

■ **Neurotransmitter alterations.** Research indicates that in the brains of clients with AD, the enzyme required to produce acetylcholine is dramatically reduced. The reduction seems to be greatest in the nucleus basalis of the inferior medial forebrain area (Sadock et al., 2015). This decrease in production of acetylcholine reduces the amount of the neurotransmitter that is released to cells in the cortex and hippocampus, resulting in a disruption of the cognitive processes. Other neurotransmitters implicated in the pathology and clinical symptoms of AD include norepinephrine, serotonin, dopamine, and the amino acid glutamate. It has been proposed that in NCD, excess glutamate leads to overstimulation of the N-methyl-D-aspartate (NMDA) receptors, leading to increased intracellular calcium and subsequent neuronal degeneration and cell death. Decreased levels of somatostatin and corticotropin have also been found in individuals with AD.

■ **Plaques and tangles.** As mentioned previously, an overabundance of structures called *plaques* and *tangles* appear in the brains of individuals with AD. The plaques are made of a protein called amyloid beta (Aβ), which are fragments of a larger protein called amyloid precursor protein (APP). Plaques are formed when these fragments clump together and mix with molecules and other cellular matter. Tangles are formed from a special kind of cellular protein called *tau protein,* whose function is to provide stability to the neuron. In AD, the tau protein is chemically altered (NIA, 2011). Strands of the protein become tangled together, interfering with the neuronal transport system. It is thought that the plaques and tangles contribute to the destruction and death of neurons, leading to memory failure, personality changes, inability to carry out ADLs, and other features of the disease. The plaques themselves can cause space-occupying lesions in the cortex, which contribute to inflammatory processes, synapse loss, and neuronal death (Graziane & Sweet, 2017). The number

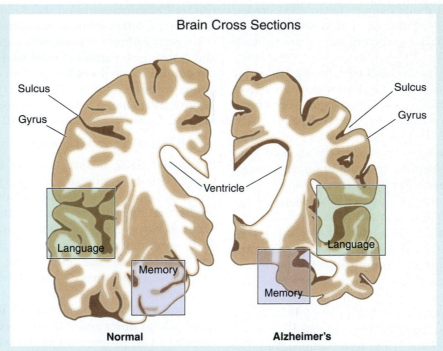

FIGURE 13–2   Neurobiology of Alzheimer's disease. Source: Copyright 2000 BrightFocus Foundation. https://www.brightfocus.org/alzheimers/infographic/brain-alzheimers-disease

NEUROTRANSMITTERS

A decrease in the neurotransmitter *acetylcholine* has been implicated in Alzheimer's disease. Cholinergic sources arise from the brainstem and the basal forebrain to supply areas of the basal ganglia, thalamus, limbic structures, hippocampus, and cerebral cortex.

Cell bodies of origin for the *serotonin* pathways lie within the raphe nuclei located in the brainstem. Those for *norepinephrine* originate in the locus ceruleus. Projections for both neurotransmitters extend throughout the forebrain, prefrontal cortex, cerebellum, and limbic system. *Dopamine* pathways arise from areas in the midbrain and project to the frontal cortex, limbic system, basal ganglia, and thalamus. Dopamine neurons in the hypothalamus innervate the posterior pituitary.

Glutamate, an excitatory neurotransmitter, has largely descending pathways, with highest concentrations in the cerebral cortex. It is also found in the hippocampus, thalamus, hypothalamus, cerebellum, and spinal cord.

AREAS OF THE BRAIN AFFECTED

Areas of the brain affected by Alzheimer's disease and associated symptoms include the following:

- Frontal lobe: Impaired reasoning ability; unable to solve problems and perform familiar tasks; poor judgment; inability to evaluate the appropriateness of behavior; aggressiveness.
- Parietal lobe: Impaired orientation ability; impaired visuospatial skills (unable to remain oriented within own environment).
- Occipital lobe: Impaired language interpretation; unable to recognize familiar objects.
- Temporal lobe: Inability to recall words; inability to use words correctly (language comprehension); in late stages, some clients experience delusions and hallucinations.
- Hippocampus: Impaired memory; short-term memory is affected initially; later, the individual is unable to form new memories.
- Amygdala: Impaired emotions: depression, anxiety, fear, personality changes, apathy, paranoia.
- Neurotransmitters: Alterations in acetylcholine, dopamine, norepinephrine, serotonin, and others may play a role in behaviors such as restlessness, sleep impairment, mood, and agitation.

MEDICATIONS AND THEIR EFFECTS ON THE BRAIN

1. Cholinesterase inhibitors (e.g., donepezil, rivastigmine, and galantamine) act by inhibiting acetylcholinesterase, which slows the degradation of acetylcholine, thereby increasing concentrations of the neurotransmitter in the brain. Most common side effects include dizziness, gastrointestinal upset, fatigue, and headache.
2. NMDA receptor antagonists (e.g., memantine) act by blocking NMDA receptors from excessive glutamate, preventing continuous influx of calcium into the cells, and ultimately slowing down neuronal degradation. Possible side effects include dizziness, headache, and constipation.

and density of senile plaques (also called *amyloid plaques*) found in postmortem studies has been correlated with the severity of the disease (Sadock et al., 2015).

■ **Head trauma.** Individuals who have a history of head trauma are at risk for AD. Studies have shown that some individuals who had experienced head trauma subsequently (after years) developed AD. There is evidence that head trauma can increase inflammatory mediators, causing amyloid beta plaques to be deposited in the brain, and the effects of traumatic brain injury on amyloid beta plaque development may also be mediated by genetic vulnerability (Graziane & Sweet, 2017).

■ **Genetic factors.** There is clearly a familial pattern for some forms of AD, with as many as 40 percent of AD patients having a family history for the disease and some families exhibiting a pattern of inheritance that suggests possible autosomal-dominant gene transmission (Sadock et al., 2015). Some studies indicate that early-onset cases are more likely than late-onset cases to be familial, and that from one-third to one-half of all cases may be of the genetic form. Research indicates that there is a link between AD and gene mutations found on chromosomes 21, 14, and 1 (Graziane & Sweet, 2017). Mutations on chromosome 21 cause the formation of abnormal APP. Mutations on chromosome 14 cause abnormal presenilin 1 *(PS-1)* to be made, and mutations on chromosome 1 leads to the formation of abnormal presenilin 2 *(PS-2)*. Each of these mutations results in an increased amount of the Aβ protein that is a major component of the plaques associated with AD. Individuals with Down syndrome (who carry an extra copy of chromosome 21) have been found to be unusually susceptible to AD.

Late-onset AD is influenced by a gene known as apolipoprotein E, but for individuals who do not have disease symptoms by the age of 65, only about 50 percent of those with this genotype will develop AD (Graziane & Sweet, 2017). As research has continued, 20 additional influential genes have been identified but their exact role in onset of AD is still unclear. Although much of the research has focused on toxic amyloid and tau proteins as correlated with AD, current research is exploring other molecular and cellular pathways that may be involved in the development of this disease, including glial cell activation, inflammation, glucose transport systems, and abnormal neuronal circuit activity. Because previous research has demonstrated that ketone bodies have a protective effect on neurons, some research is focused on the impact of ketones in improving memory and learning. A current clinical trial is investigating the potential benefits of ketone-rich diets in slowing or improving cognitive decline in AD since insulin resistance and abnormal glucose metabolism have been associated with this disease (NIA, 2015).

Vascular Neurocognitive Disorder

In vascular NCD, the syndrome of cognitive symptoms is due to significant cerebrovascular disease. When blood flow in the brain is impaired, progressive intellectual deterioration occurs. Impairment may occur in large vessels or in microvascular networks, so the symptoms vary depending on the type, extent, and location of vascular lesion (APA, 2013). Vascular NCD is the second most common form of NCD, ranking after AD (Sadock et al., 2015).

Vascular NCD differs from AD in that it has a more abrupt onset and a highly variable course. In vascular NCD, progression of the symptoms occurs in "steps" rather than as a gradual deterioration; that is, at times the symptoms seem to clear up and the individual exhibits fairly lucid thinking. Memory may seem better, and the client may become optimistic that improvement is occurring, only to experience further decline of functioning in a fluctuating pattern of progression. This irregular pattern of decline can be an intense source of anxiety for clients with this disorder.

In vascular NCD, clients may suffer the equivalent of small strokes that destroy many areas of the brain. The pattern of deficits is variable, depending on which regions of the brain have been affected. Certain focal neurological signs are commonly seen with vascular NCD, including weaknesses of the limbs, small-stepped gait, and difficulty with speech. The disorder is more common in men than in women.

Etiology

The cause of vascular NCD is directly related to an interruption of blood flow to the brain. Symptoms result from death of nerve cells in regions nourished by diseased vessels. Various diseases and conditions that interfere with blood circulation have been implicated.

High blood pressure is thought to be one of the most significant factors in the etiology of multiple small strokes or cerebral infarcts. Hypertension leads to damage to the lining of blood vessels. This damage can result in rupture of the blood vessel with subsequent hemorrhage or an accumulation of fibrin in the vessel with intravascular clotting and inhibited blood flow. NCD also can result from infarcts related to occlusion of blood vessels by particulate matter that travels through the bloodstream to the brain. These emboli may be solid (e.g., clots, cellular debris, platelet aggregates), gaseous (e.g., air, nitrogen), or liquid (e.g., fat, following soft tissue trauma or fracture of long bones).

Cognitive impairment can occur with multiple small infarcts (sometimes called "silent strokes") over time or with a single cerebrovascular insult that occurs in a strategic area of the brain. An individual may have both vascular NCD and AD simultaneously, referred to as a *mixed* disorder, the prevalence of which is likely to increase as the population ages.

Frontotemporal Neurocognitive Disorder

Symptoms from frontotemporal NCD (also referred to as frontotemporal dementia or FTD) occur as a result of shrinking of the frontal and temporal anterior lobes of the brain (National Institute of Neurological Disorders and Stroke [NINDS], 2017). This type of NCD was identified as Pick's disease in the *DSM-IV-TR*. The cause of frontotemporal NCD is unknown, but a genetic factor appears to be involved because this disorder often runs in families. Symptoms tend to fall into two clinical patterns: (1) behavioral and personality changes and (2) speech and language problems. Common behavioral changes include "behavior that can be either impulsive (disinhibited) or bored and listless (apathetic) and includes inappropriate social behavior; lack of social tact; lack of empathy; distractibility; loss of insight into the behaviors of oneself and others; an increased interest in sex; changes in food preferences; agitation or, conversely, blunted emotions; neglect of personal hygiene; repetitive or compulsive behavior, and decreased energy and motivation" (NINDS, 2017). Speech problems include impairment or loss of speech or increasing difficulty in using and understanding written and spoken language. Spatial skills and memory remain intact but the disease progresses steadily and often rapidly, ranging from less than 2 years in some individuals to more than 10 years in others (NINDS, 2017).

Neurocognitive Disorder Due to Traumatic Brain Injury

DSM-5 criteria state that this disorder "is caused by an impact to the head or other mechanisms of rapid movement or displacement of the brain within the skull, with one or more of the following: loss of consciousness, posttraumatic amnesia, disorientation and confusion, or neurological signs (e.g., positive neuroimaging demonstrating injury, a new onset of seizures or a marked worsening of a preexisting seizure disorder, visual field cuts, anosmia, hemiparesis)" (APA, 2013). Amnesia is the most common neurobehavioral symptom following head trauma. Other symptoms may include confusion and changes in speech, vision, and personality. Depending on the severity of the injury, these symptoms may eventually subside or may become permanent. Severe head injuries increase one's risk for AD or other dementias, especially in those who carry the apolipoprotein E *(APOE)* gene, which increases anyone's risk for AD (Graff-Radford, 2017). Repeated head trauma, such as the type experienced by boxers, can result in *dementia pugilistica,* a syndrome characterized by emotional lability, dysarthria, ataxia, and impulsivity (Sadock et al., 2015).

Neurocognitive Disorder Due to Lewy Body Dementia

Dementia with Lewy bodies is now identified as the second most common cause of dementia in the elderly after AD (Graziane & Sweet, 2017). Clinically, Lewy body NCD is fairly similar to AD; however, it tends to progress more rapidly, with earlier appearance of visual hallucinations and parkinsonian features. Depression and delusions are also common symptoms in this population. Lewy body dementia recently gained public attention when an autopsy of famous comedian Robin Williams revealed that he had this disease, and his widow reported that he had been seeking neurocognitive testing because he was aware of a decline in his mental capacities. He was also manifesting symptoms of depression and ultimately took his own life.

This disorder is distinguished by the presence of Lewy bodies—eosinophilic inclusion bodies—seen in the cerebral cortex and brainstem. Three core features include significant variations in alertness and attention, detailed visual hallucinations, and spontaneous motor features of parkinsonism (Graziane & Sweet, 2017). Acetylcholinesterase (ACh) concentrations are reduced in the brains of people with Lewy body NCD, and, consequently, cholinesterase inhibitors are likely to be more effective for this population than for those with Alzheimer's dementia (Crystal, 2017). These patients are highly sensitive to extrapyramidal effects of antipsychotic medications. The disease is progressive and irreversible, with a survival time of up to 10 years, and may account for as many as 25 percent of all NCD cases.

Neurocognitive Disorder Due to Parkinson's Disease

NCD is observed in as many as 75 percent of clients with Parkinson's disease (APA, 2013). In this disease, there is a loss of nerve cells located in the substantia nigra, and dopamine activity is diminished, resulting in involuntary muscle movements, slowness, and rigidity. Tremor in the upper extremities is characteristic. In some instances, the cerebral changes that occur in NCD due to Parkinson's disease closely resemble those of AD.

Neurocognitive Disorder Due to HIV Infection

Infection with the human immunodeficiency virus type 1 (HIV-1) can result in an NCD called *HIV-1-associated cognitive/motor complex*. A less severe form, HIV-1-associated minor cognitive/motor disorder, also occurs. The severity of symptoms is correlated to the extent of brain pathology. The immune dysfunction associated with HIV disease can lead to brain infections by other organisms, and HIV-1 also appears to cause NCD directly. In the early stages, neuropsychiatric symptoms may be manifested by barely perceptible changes in a person's normal psychological presentation. Severe cognitive changes, particularly confusion, changes in behavior, and sometimes psychoses, are not uncommon in the later stages.

With the advent of the highly active antiretroviral therapies (HAART), incidence rates of NCD due to HIV infection have been on the decline. However, Moore and Marquine (2017) note that several studies have observed elevated rates of NCDs in older adults who are HIV positive, suggesting that there may be additive negative effects for older HIV-positive individuals.

Substance or Medication-Induced Neurocognitive Disorder

NCD can occur as the result of substance reactions, overuse, or abuse. Symptoms are consistent with major or mild neurocognitive disorder and persist beyond the usual duration of intoxication and acute withdrawal (APA, 2013). Substances that have been associated with the development of NCDs include alcohol, sedatives, hypnotics, anxiolytics, and inhalants. Drugs that cause anticholinergic side effects and toxins such as lead and mercury have also been implicated.

Neurocognitive Disorder Due to Huntington's Disease

Huntington's disease is transmitted as a mendelian dominant gene. Damage is seen in the areas of the basal ganglia and the cerebral cortex. The onset of symptoms (i.e., involuntary twitching of the limbs or facial muscles, mild cognitive changes, depression or mood swings, and apathy) usually occurs between age 30 and 50 years. The client usually declines into a profound state of cognitive impairment and **ataxia** (muscular incoordination). The average duration of the disease is 10 to 25 years depending on the severity of symptoms. As the disease progresses, the weakened individual usually dies secondary to pneumonia, heart failure, choking, or other complications (Huntington's Disease Society of America [HDSA], 2018). About 10 percent of the cases occur in children and adolescents, and the progression is typically more rapid than it is in adult-onset Huntington's disease.

Neurocognitive Disorder Due to Prion Disease

Prion disease is a group of disorders caused by infectious agents called prions and characterized by insidious onset and rapid progression. Manifestations include problems with coordination and other movement disturbances along with rapidly progressing dementia. This type of NCD is diagnosed when there is evidence of characteristic biomarkers, including recognized lesions in the brain, specific types of proteins in the cerebrospinal fluid, and distinctive triphasic waves on electroencephalograms (APA, 2013). Five to 15 percent of cases of prion disease have a genetic component. Symptoms may develop at any age in adulthood but typically occur between ages 40 and 60 years. The clinical course is extremely rapid with progression from diagnosis to death in less than 2 years. The most common form of prion disease in humans is Creutzfeldt-Jakob's disease (Johns Hopkins Medicine, n.d.).

Neurocognitive Disorder Due to Another Medical Condition

A number of other general medical conditions can cause NCD. Some of these include structural lesions, hypothyroidism, hyperparathyroidism, pituitary insufficiency, uremia, hepatic or renal failure encephalitis, brain tumor, pernicious anemia, thiamine deficiency, pellagra, uncontrolled epilepsy, cardiopulmonary insufficiency, fluid and electrolyte imbalances, CNS and systemic infections such as neurosyphilis or cryptococcosis, systemic lupus erythematosus, and multiple sclerosis (APA, 2013).

The etiological factors associated with delirium and NCD are summarized in Box 13–2.

Application of the Nursing Process

Assessment

Nursing assessment of the patient with delirium or mild or major NCD is based on knowledge of the symptomatology associated with the various disorders previously described in this chapter. Subjective and objective data are gathered by various

---

BOX 13–2 Etiological Factors Implicated in the Development of Delirium and/or Mild or Major Neurocognitive Disorder

Biological Factors	Exogenous Factors
Hypoxia: Any condition leading to a deficiency of oxygen to the brain	Birth trauma: Prolonged labor, damage from use of forceps, other obstetric complications
Nutritional deficiencies: Vitamins (particularly B and C); protein; fluid and electrolyte imbalances	Cranial trauma: Concussion, contusions, hemorrhage, hematomas
Metabolic disturbances: Porphyria; encephalopathies related to hepatic, renal, pancreatic, or pulmonary insufficiencies; hypoglycemia	Volatile inhalant compounds: Gasoline, glue, paint, paint thinners, spray paints, cleaning fluids, typewriter correction fluid, varnishes, and lacquers
Endocrine dysfunction: Thyroid, parathyroid, adrenal, pancreas, pituitary	Heavy metals: Lead, mercury, manganese
Cardiovascular disease: Stroke, cardiac insufficiency, atherosclerosis	Other metallic elements: Aluminum
	Organic phosphates: Various insecticides
Primary brain disorders: Epilepsy, Alzheimer's disease, Pick's disease, Huntington's chorea, multiple sclerosis, Parkinson's disease	Substance abuse/dependence: Alcohol, amphetamines, caffeine, cannabis, cocaine, hallucinogens, inhalants, nicotine, opioids, phencyclidine, sedatives, hypnotics, anxiolytics
Infections: Encephalitis, meningitis, pneumonia, septicemia, neurosyphilis (dementia paralytica), HIV disease, acute rheumatic fever, Creutzfeldt-Jakob disease	Other medications: Anticholinergics, antihistamines, antidepressants, antipsychotics, antiparkinsonians, antihypertensives, steroids, digitalis
Intracranial neoplasms	
Congenital defects: Prenatal infections such as first-trimester maternal rubella	

---

members of the healthcare team. Clinicians report use of a variety of methods for obtaining assessment information.

Patient History

Nurses play a significant role in acquiring the patient history, including the specific mental and physical changes that have occurred and the age when the changes began. If the patient is unable to relate information adequately, the data should be obtained from family members or others who would be aware of the patient's physical and psychosocial history.

From the patient history, nurses should assess the following areas of concern: (1) type, frequency, and severity of mood swings; personality and behavioral changes; and catastrophic emotional reactions; (2) cognitive changes such as problems with attention span, thinking process, problem-solving, and memory (recent and remote); (3) language difficulties; (4) orientation to person, place, time, and situation; and (5) appropriateness of social behavior.

The nurse also should obtain information regarding current and past medication usage, history of other drug and alcohol use, and possible exposure to toxins. Knowledge regarding the history of related

symptoms or specific illnesses (e.g., Huntington's disease, AD, Pick's disease, or Parkinson's disease) in other family members might be useful.

Physical Assessment

Assessment of physical systems by both the nurse and the physician has two main emphases: (1) signs of damage to the nervous system and (2) evidence of diseases of other organs that could affect mental function. Diseases of various organ systems can induce confusion, loss of memory, and behavioral changes. These causes must be considered in diagnosing cognitive disorders. In the neurological examination, the patient is asked to perform maneuvers or answer questions that are designed to elicit information about the condition of specific parts of the brain or peripheral nerves. Testing will assess mental status and alertness, muscle strength, reflexes, sensory perception, language skills, and coordination. Physical assessment should include looking for signs of abuse or neglect and screening for hearing or vision impairments and conducting a mental status examination. An example of a mental status examination for a patient with NCD is presented in Box 13–3.

A battery of psychological tests may be ordered as part of the diagnostic examination. The results of

BOX 13-3 Mental Status Examination for Neurocognitive Disorder

Patient Name _____ Date _____
Age _____ Sex _____ Diagnosis _____

	Maximum	Patient's Score
1. VERBAL FLUENCY Ask patient to name as many animals as he/she can. (Time: 60 seconds) (Score 1 point/2 animals)	10 points	_____
2. COMPREHENSION		
a. Point to the ceiling	1 point	_____
b. Point to your nose and the window	1 point	_____
c. Point to your foot, the door, and ceiling	1 point	_____
d. Point to the window, your leg, the door, and your thumb	1 point	_____
3. NAMING AND WORD FINDING Ask the patient to name the following as you point to them:		
a. Watch stem (winder)	1 point	_____
b. Teeth	1 point	_____
c. Sole of shoe	1 point	_____
d. Buckle of belt	1 point	_____
e. Knuckles	1 point	_____
4. ORIENTATION		
a. Date	2 points	_____
b. Day of week	2 points	_____
c. Month	1 point	_____
d. Year	1 point	_____

5. NEW LEARNING ABILITY
Tell the patient: "I'm going to tell you four words, which I want you to remember."
Have the patient repeat the four words after they are initially presented, and then
say that you will ask him/her to remember the words later. Continue with the
examination, and at intervals of 5 and 10 minutes, ask the patient to recall the
words. Three different sets of words are provided here.

		5 min.	10 min.
a. Brown (Fun) (Grape)	2 points each:	_____	_____
b. Honesty (Loyalty) (Happiness)	2 points each:	_____	_____
c. Tulip (Carrot) (Stocking)	2 points each:	_____	_____
d. Eyedropper (Ankle) (Toothbrush)	2 points each:	_____	_____

6. VERBAL STORY FOR IMMEDIATE RECALL
Tell the patient: "I'm going to read you a short story, which   13 points   _____
I want you to remember. Listen closely to what I read
because I will ask you to tell me the story when I finish."
Read the story slowly and carefully, but without pausing
at the slash marks. After completing the paragraph, tell the
patient to retell the story as accurately as possible. Record
the number of correct memories (information within the slashes)
and describe confabulation if it is present. (1 point = 1 remembered item
[13 maximum points])

It was July / and the Rogers family, mom, dad, and four children / were packing up their station wagon /
to go on vacation.
They were taking their yearly trip / to the beach at Gulf Shores.
This year they were making a special 1-day stop / at The Aquarium in New Orleans.
After a long day's drive, they arrived at the motel / only to discover that in their excitement /
they had left the twins / and their suitcases / in the front yard.

BOX 13–3 Mental Status Examination for Neurocognitive Disorder—cont'd

7. VISUAL MEMORY (HIDDEN OBJECTS)

Tell the patient that you are going to hide some objects around the
office (desk, bed) and that you want him/her to remember where
they are. Hide four or five common objects (e.g., keys, pen, reflex hammer)
in various places in the patient's sight. After a delay of several minutes,
ask the patient to find the objects. (1 point per item found)

a. Coin	1 point	_____
b. Pen	1 point	_____
c. Comb	1 point	_____
d. Keys	1 point	_____
e. Fork	1 point	_____

8. PAIRED ASSOCIATE LEARNING

Tell the patient that you are going to read a list of words two at a time.
The patient will be expected to remember the words that go together
(e.g., big—little). When he/she is clear on the directions, read the first
list of words at the rate of one pair per second. After reading the first
list, test for recall by presenting the first recall list. Give the first word
of a pair and ask for the word that was paired with it. Correct incorrect responses
and proceed to the next pair. After the first recall has been completed, allow
a 10-second delay and continue with the second presentation and recall lists.

Presentation Lists

1	2
a. High—Low	a. Good—Bad
b. House—Income	b. Book—Page
c. Good—Bad	c. High—Low
d. Book—Page	d. House—Income

Recall Lists

1	2		
a. House _____	a. High _____	2 points	_____
b. Book _____	b. Good _____	2 points	_____
c. High _____	c. House _____	2 points	_____
d. Good _____	d. Book _____	2 points	_____

9. CONSTRUCTIONAL ABILITY

Ask patient to reconstruct this drawing and to draw the other two items: 3 points   _____

Draw a daisy in a flowerpot.   3 points   _____

Draw a clock with all the numbers and set the clock at 2:30.   3 points   _____

10. WRITTEN COMPLEX CALCULATIONS

a. Addition $\begin{array}{r} 108 \\ +79 \\ \hline \end{array}$ 1 point   _____

Continued

BOX 13–3 Mental Status Examination for Neurocognitive Disorder—cont'd

b. Subtraction	$\begin{array}{r} 605 \\ -86 \\ \hline \end{array}$	1 point	_____
c. Multiplication	$\begin{array}{r} 108 \\ \times 36 \\ \hline \end{array}$	1 point	_____
d. Division	$559 \div 43$	1 point	_____

11. PROVERB INTERPRETATION
Tell the patient to explain the following sayings. Record the answers.

a. Don't cry over spilled milk. 2 points _____
_____

b. Rome wasn't built in a day. 2 points _____
_____

c. A drowning man will clutch at a straw. 2 points _____
_____

d. A golden hammer can break down an iron door. 2 points _____
_____

e. The hot coal burns, the cold one blackens. 2 points _____
_____

12. SIMILARITIES
Ask the patient to name the similarity or relationship between each of the two items.

a. Turnip . . . . Cauliflower 2 points _____
b. Car . . . . Airplane 2 points _____
c. Desk. . . . . Bookcase 2 points _____
d. Poem . . . . Novel 2 points _____
e. Horse . . . . Apple 2 points _____

Maximum: 100 points _____

Normal Individuals		Patients with Alzheimer's Disease	
Age Group	**Mean Score (standard deviation)**	**Stage**	**Mean Score (standard deviation)**
40–49	80.9 (9.7)	I	57.2 (9.1)
50–59	82.3 (8.6)	II	37.0 (7.8)
60–69	75.5 (10.5)	III	13.4 (8.1)
70–79	66.9 (9.1)		
80–89	67.9 (11.0)		

Source: Adapted from Strub, R. L., & Black, F. W. (2000). The Mental Status Examination in Neurology, 4th ed., Philadelphia: F. A. Davis. With permission.

these tests may be used to make a differential diagnosis between NCD and **pseudodementia** (depression). Depression is the most common mental illness in the elderly, but it is often misdiagnosed and treated inadequately. Cognitive symptoms of depression may mimic NCD, and because of the prevalence of NCD in the elderly, diagnosticians are often too eager to make this diagnosis. A comparison of symptoms of NCD and pseudodementia (depression) is presented in Table 13–1. Nurses can assist in this assessment by carefully observing and documenting these sometimes subtle differences.

TABLE 13–1	**A Comparison of Neurocognitive Disorder (NCD) and Pseudodementia (Depression)**	
SYMPTOM ELEMENT	NCD	PSEUDODEMENTIA (DEPRESSION)
PROGRESSION OF SYMPTOMS	**SLOW**	**RAPID**
Memory	Progressive deficits; recent memory loss greater than remote; may confabulate for memory "gaps"; no complaints of loss	More like forgetfulness; no evidence of progressive deficit; recent and remote loss equal; complaints of deficits; no confabulation (will more likely answer "I don't know")
Orientation	Disoriented to time and place; may wander in search of the familiar	Oriented to time and place; no wandering
Task performance	Consistently poor performance but struggles to perform	Performance is variable; little effort is put forth
Symptom severity	Worse as the day progresses	Better as the day progresses
Affective distress	Appears unconcerned	Communicates severe distress
Appetite	Unchanged initially, but as dementia progresses there may be loss of appetite, inability to recognize hunger, or loss of interest in food	Diminished
Attention and concentration	Impaired	Generally intact but sometimes depressed patient has significant impairment in concentration and speed of processing information

Diagnostic Laboratory Evaluations

The nurse also may be required to help the patient fulfill the physician's orders for special diagnostic laboratory evaluations. Many of these tests are conducted to rule out other factors associated with dementia such as evaluation of blood and urine samples to test for various infections; liver function studies to rule out hepatic disease; glucose tests to rule out diabetes or hypoglycemia; electrolyte studies to rule out imbalances; thyroid tests to rule out hypothyroidism; vitamin B_{12} test to rule out nutritional deficiencies; and drug and alcohol screening to rule out the presence of toxic substances. A rapid plasma reagin (RPR) to test for syphilis and HIV testing should be included if the patient is at higher risk for these conditions.

CT scanning produces an image of the size and shape of the brain and MRI is used to obtain a computerized image of soft tissue in the brain. Both CT and MRI scans are useful in identifying areas of atrophy such as those seen in AD and may identify other pathological processes needed for differential diagnosis. A lumbar puncture may be performed to examine the cerebrospinal fluid for evidence of CNS infection or hemorrhage if this is suspected. PET is used to reveal the metabolic activity of the brain, an evaluation some researchers believe is important for early diagnosis of AD. New amyloid PET scan techniques are able to identify amyloid beta plaques and tau neurofibrillary tangles in the brain but these tests are primarily being used in research and clinical trials (Mayo Clinic, 2018b). "The Alzheimer's Association-sponsored Imaging Dementia–Evidence for Amyloid Scanning (IDEAS) study is assessing the clinical usefulness of amyloid PET scans and their impact on patient outcomes. The goal is to accumulate enough data to prove that amyloid scans are a cost-effective addition to the management of dementia patients. If federal payers agree and decide to cover amyloid scans, advocates hope that private insurers might follow suit" (Sullivan, 2018).

Nursing Diagnosis and Outcome Identification

Using information collected during the assessment, the nurse completes the patient database from which the selection of appropriate nursing diagnoses is determined. Table 13–2 presents a list of patient behaviors and the NANDA-I nursing diagnoses that correspond to those behaviors, which may be used in planning care for the patient with an NCD (Herdman & Kamitsuru, 2018).

Outcome Criteria

The following criteria may be used for measurement of outcomes in the care of the patient with an NCD.

TABLE 13–2 Assigning Nursing Diagnoses to Behaviors Commonly Associated With Neurocognitive Disorders

BEHAVIORS	NURSING DIAGNOSES
Falls, wandering, poor coordination, confusion, misinterpretation of the environment (illusions, hallucinations), lack of understanding of environmental hazards, memory deficits	Risk for trauma Risk for falls
Disorientation, confusion, memory deficits, inaccurate interpretation of the environment, suspiciousness, paranoia	Disturbed thought processes* Impaired memory
Having hallucinations (hears voices, sees visions, feels crawling sensation on skin)	Disturbed sensory perception*
Aggressiveness (hitting, scratching, or kicking)	Risk for other-directed violence
Inability to name objects/people, loss of memory for words, difficulty finding the right word, confabulation, incoherent, screaming and demanding verbalizations	Impaired verbal communication
Inability to perform activities of daily living (ADLs): feeding, dressing, hygiene, toileting	Self-care deficit (specify)
Expressions of shame and self-degradation, progressive social isolation, apathy, decreased activity, withdrawal, depressed mood	Situational low self-esteem; Grieving

*These nursing diagnoses have been resigned from the NANDA-I list of approved diagnoses but are used for purposes of this text.

The patient:
- Has not experienced physical injury.
- Has not harmed self or others.
- Maintains reality orientation to the best of his or her capability.
- Is able to communicate with a consistent caregiver.
- Fulfills ADLs with assistance (or for the patient who is unable, has needs met, as anticipated by the caregiver).
- Discusses positive aspects about self and life.

Planning and Implementation

Table 13–3 provides a plan of care for the patient with a cognitive disorder (irrespective of etiology). Selected nursing diagnoses are presented, along with outcome criteria, appropriate nursing interventions, and rationales for each.

Concept Care Mapping

The concept map care plan (see Chapter 6, The Nursing Process in Psychiatric Mental Health Nursing) is a diagrammatic teaching and learning strategy that allows visualization of interrelationships between medical diagnoses, nursing diagnoses, assessment data, and treatments. An example of a concept map care plan for a patient with an NCD is presented in Figure 13–3.

Patient and Family Education

The role of patient teacher is important in the psychiatric area, as it is in all areas of nursing. A list of topics for patient and family education relevant to NCDs is presented in Box 13–5.

Evaluation

In the final step of the nursing process, reassessment occurs to determine whether the nursing interventions have been effective in achieving the intended goals of care. Evaluation of the patient with an NCD is based on a series of short-term goals rather than on long-term goals. Resolution of identified problems is unrealistic for this client. Instead, outcomes must be measured in terms of slowing down the process rather than stopping or curing the problem. Evaluation questions may include the following:

- Has the patient experienced injury?
- Does the patient maintain orientation to time, person, place, and situation to the best of his or her cognitive ability?
- Is the patient able to fulfill basic needs? Have those needs unmet by the patient been fulfilled by caregivers?
- Is confusion minimized by familiar objects and structured, routine schedule of activities?
- Do the prospective caregivers have information regarding the progression of the patient's illness?
- Do caregivers have information regarding where to go for assistance and support in the care of their loved one?
- Have the prospective caregivers received instruction in how to promote the patient's safety, minimize confusion and disorientation, and cope with difficult client behaviors (e.g., hostility, anger, depression, agitation)?

Table 13–3 | CARE PLAN FOR THE PATIENT WITH A NEUROCOGNITIVE DISORDER (NCD)

NURSING DIAGNOSES: RISK FOR FALLS, RISK FOR TRAUMA

RELATED TO: Impairments in cognitive and psychomotor functioning

OUTCOME CRITERIA	NURSING INTERVENTIONS	RATIONALE

Short-Term Goals
■ Patient will call for assistance when ambulating or carrying out other activities (if it is within his or her cognitive ability).
■ Patient will maintain a calm demeanor, with minimal agitated behavior.
■ Patient will not experience physical injury.
 	
Long-Term Goal
■ Patient will not experience physical injury.
	1. The following measures may be instituted:
	  a. Arrange furniture and other items in the room to accommodate patient's disabilities.
	  b. Store frequently used items within easy access.
	  c. Do not keep bed in an elevated position. Pad siderails and headboard if client has history of seizures. Keep bedrails up when patient is in bed (if regulations permit).
	  d. Assign room near nurses' station; observe frequently.
	  e. Assist patient with ambulation.
	  f. Keep a dim light on at night.
	  g. If patient is a smoker, cigarettes and lighter or matches should be kept at the nurses' station and dispensed only when someone is available to stay with patient while he or she is smoking.
	  h. Frequently orient to place, time, and situation.
	  i. If patient is prone to wander, provide an area within which wandering can be carried out safely.
	  j. Soft restraints may be required if patient is very disoriented and hyperactive.
		To ensure patient safety.

NURSING DIAGNOSIS: DISTURBED THOUGHT PROCESSES; IMPAIRED MEMORY

RELATED TO: Cerebral degeneration

EVIDENCED BY: Disorientation, confusion, memory deficits, and inaccurate interpretation of the environment

OUTCOME CRITERIA	NURSING INTERVENTIONS	RATIONALE
Short-Term Goals ■ Patient will utilize measures provided (e.g., clocks, calendars, room identification) to maintain reality orientation. ■ Patient will experience fewer episodes of acute confusion. **Long-Term Goal** ■ Patient will maintain reality orientation to the best of his or her cognitive ability.	1. Frequently orient patient to reality. Use clocks and calendars with large numbers that are easy to read. Notes and large, bold signs may be useful as reminders. Allow patient to have personal belongings. 2. Keep explanations simple. Use face-to-face interaction. Speak slowly and do not shout.	1. All of these items serve to help maintain orientation and aid in memory and recognition. **Note:** Some believe that repeated reality orientation for individuals with NCD contributes to problems with mood and self-esteem (see Box 13–4, Validation Therapy, for an alternative or adjunctive intervention.) 2. These interventions facilitate comprehension. Shouting may create discomfort, and in some instances, may provoke anger.

Continued

Table 13–3 | CARE PLAN FOR THE PATIENT WITH A NEUROCOGNITIVE DISORDER (NCD)—cont'd

OUTCOME CRITERIA	NURSING INTERVENTIONS	RATIONALE
	3. Discourage rumination or delusional thinking. Talk about real events and real people. But remember that the patient's level of reality is different from the nurse's. Do not lie to the patient. May need to use validation therapy and redirection.	3. Rumination promotes disorientation. Reality orientation and validation therapy increase a sense of self-worth and personal dignity.
	4. Monitor for medication side effects.	4. Physiological changes in the elderly can alter the body's response to certain medications. Toxic effects may intensify altered thought processes.
	5. Encourage patient to view old photograph albums and utilize reminiscence therapy.	5. These are excellent ways to promote self-esteem and provide orientation to reality.

NURSING DIAGNOSIS: DISTURBED SENSORY PERCEPTION

RELATED TO: Cerebral degeneration

EVIDENCED BY: Auditory and visual hallucinations

OUTCOME CRITERIA	NURSING INTERVENTIONS	RATIONALE
Short-Term Goal ■ Patient will exhibit fewer manifestations of disturbed sensory perception. **Long-Term Goal** ■ Patient will maintain reality orientation to the best of his or her cognitive ability.	1. Do not ignore reports of hallucinations when it is clear that the patient is experiencing them. It is important for the nurse to hear an explanation of the hallucination from the patient.	1. These perceptions are very real and often very frightening to the patient. Unless they are appropriately managed, hallucinations can escalate into disturbing and even hostile behaviors.
	2. Rule out the disturbed sensory perception as a possible side effect of certain physical conditions or medications.	2. Physical changes in the elderly result in less ability to metabolize medications, causing an increased risk of side effects. Some infections are also known to cause hallucinations in the elderly.
	3. Check to ensure that hearing aid is working properly and that faulty sounds are not being emitted.	3. Faulty sounds from a hearing aid defect could be misinterpreted for auditory hallucinations.
	4. Check eyeglasses to ensure that the individual is indeed wearing his or her own glasses.	4. Wearing the wrong prescription eyeglasses could cause the individual to misinterpret visual perceptions.
	5. Try to determine from where the visual hallucination is emanating and correct the situation by moving or covering the item.	5. Patients often see faces in patterns on fabrics or in pictures on the wall. A mirror can also be the culprit when there are false perceptions.
	6. Provide distractions for the patient. Focus on real situations and real people	6. Hallucinations are less likely to occur when the person is occupied or involved in what is going on around them.

Table 13–3 | CARE PLAN FOR THE PATIENT WITH A NEUROCOGNITIVE DISORDER (NCD)—cont'd

OUTCOME CRITERIA	NURSING INTERVENTIONS	RATIONALE
	7. McShane (2000) suggests that, depending on the situation, it may be better at times to go along with the patient rather than attempting to distract him or her.	7. Not all hallucinations are upsetting, and there are times when trying to distract the person from the hallucination may incur increased stress and agitation in the individual.

NURSING DIAGNOSIS: SELF-CARE DEFICIT
RELATED TO: Disorientation, confusion, and memory deficits
EVIDENCED BY: Inability to fulfill ADLs

OUTCOME CRITERIA	NURSING INTERVENTIONS	RATIONALE

Short-Term Goal
■ Patient will participate in ADLs with assistance from caregiver.
 	
Long-Term Goals
■ Patient will accomplish ADLs to the best of his or her ability.
■ Unfulfilled needs will be met by caregivers.
	1. Provide a simple, structured environment:
	  a. Identify self-care deficits and provide assistance as required. Promote independent actions as able.
	  b. Allow plenty of time for patient to perform tasks.
	  c. Provide guidance and support for independent actions by talking the patient through the task one step at a time.
	  d. Provide a structured schedule of activities that does not change from day to day.
	  e. ADLs should follow usual routine as closely as possible.
	  f. Provide for consistency in assignment of daily caregivers.
	2. Perform ongoing assessment of patient's ability to fulfill nutritional needs, ensure personal safety, follow medication regimen, and communicate need for assistance with activities that he or she cannot accomplish independently.
	3. Assess prospective caregivers' ability to anticipate and fulfill patient's unmet needs. Provide information to assist caregivers with this responsibility. Ensure that caregivers are aware of available community support systems from which they may seek assistance when required. Examples include adult day care centers, housekeeping and homemaker services, respite care services, or the local chapter of a national support organization:
	  a. For Parkinson's disease information:
	     National Parkinson
	      Foundation Inc.
	     1501 NW 9th Ave.
	     Miami, FL 33136-1494
	     1-800-473-4636 1-800- 4PD-INFO
	     www.parkinson.org
	  b. For Alzheimer's disease information:
	     Alzheimer's Association
	     225 N. Michigan Ave., Fl. 17
	     Chicago, IL 60601-7633
	     1-800-272-3900
	     www.alz.org
		1. To minimize confusion.
		
		2. Patient safety and security are nursing priorities.
		
		3. To ensure provision and continuity of patient care.

Continued

Table 13–3 | CARE PLAN FOR THE PATIENT WITH A NEUROCOGNITIVE DISORDER (NCD)—cont'd

NURSING DIAGNOSIS: IMPAIRED VERBAL COMMUNICATION

RELATED TO: Impairments in cognitive and psychomotor functioning

OUTCOME CRITERIA	NURSING INTERVENTIONS	RATIONALE

Short-Term Goals
■ Patient will be able to make needs known to primary caregiver.
■ Patient is able to understand basic communications in interactions with primary caregiver.
 	
Long-Term Goal
■ Unfulfilled needs will be met by caregivers.
	1. The following communication techniques may be used:
	  a. Keep interactions with the patient calm and reassuring.
	  b. Use simple words, speak slowly and distinctly and maintain face-to-face contact with the patient.
	  c. Always identify yourself and call the patient by name at each meeting.
	  d. Use nonverbal gestures to help the patient understand what you want him or her to accomplish, if appropriate.
	  e. Ask only one question/give only one direction at a time and give the patient plenty of time to process the information and respond. Rephrase question only if it is clear that the patient has not understood the meaning of the direction.
		1. These interventions promote an effective communication process and facilitate the patient's comprehension.

	2. Approach the patient from the front whenever possible.	2. An unexpected approach/touch from behind may startle the patient and could promote aggressive behavior. When it is *clearly* appropriate, use touch and affection to communicate. Sometimes patients will respond to a hug or to a hand reaching for theirs when they will respond to nothing else.
	3. Provide for consistency in assignment of daily caregivers.	3. To minimize confusion and facilitate patient security.

Quality and Safety Education for Nurses (QSEN)

The Institute of Medicine (IOM), in its 2003 report *Health Professions Education: A Bridge to Quality,* challenged faculties of medicine, nursing, and other health professions to ensure that their graduates have achieved a core set of competencies in order to meet the needs of the 21st-century healthcare system. These competencies include *providing patient-centered care, maintaining safety, working in interdisciplinary teams, employing evidence-based practice, incorporating quality improvement,* and *utilizing informatics.* A QSEN teaching strategy is presented in Box 13–6. Several studies have demonstrated the positive outcomes associated with a *patient-centered care* approach for patients with dementia (Ballard et al., 2016; Ballard et al., 2018; Whitaker et al., 2014). This program, called "Well-Being and Health for People With Dementia (WHELD)," is a nonpharmacological, psychosocial intervention that focuses on tailored person-centered activities, exercise, and social interaction for patients with dementia in long-term care settings. The evidence supported that training staff and incorporating these patient-centered interventions reduced patient agitation, reduced the need for antipsychotic medication, and improved quality of life in this population. Lack of medications to improve dementia and the dangers associated with

BOX 13–4 Validation Therapy

Some people believe it is not helpful (and sometimes is even cruel) to try to insist that a person with moderate to severe NCD continually try to grasp what we know as the "real world." Allen (2000) states,

> There is no successful alternative but to accept whatever the dementia person claims as their reality, no matter how untrue it is to us. There is no successful way to "force" a person with dementia to join the "real" world. The most frustrated caregivers are the ones who do not accept this simple fact: the world of dementia is defined by the dementia victim.

Validation therapy (VT) was originated by Naomi Feil, a gerontological social worker, who describes the process as "communicating with a disoriented elderly person by validating and respecting their feelings in whatever time or place is real to them at the time, even though this may not correspond with our 'here and now' reality" (Day, 2013). Feil suggests that the validation principle is truthful to the person with NCD because people live on several levels of awareness (Feil, 2013). She suggests that if an individual asks to see his or her spouse, and the spouse has been dead for many years, that on some level of awareness, that person knows the truth. To keep reminding the person that the spouse is dead may only serve to cause repeated episodes of grief and distress, because he or she receives the information "anew" each time it is presented (Allen, 2000).

Validation therapy validates the feelings and emotions of a person with NCD. It often also integrates redirection techniques. Allen (2000) states, "The key is to 'agree' with what they want but by conversation and 'steering' get them to do something else without them realizing they are actually being redirected. This is both validation and redirection therapy."

EXAMPLES

 Mrs. W (agitated): "That old lady stole my watch! I know she did. She goes into people's rooms and takes our things. We call her 'sticky fingers!'"

Nurse: "That watch is very important to you. Have you looked around the room for it?"

Mrs. W: "My husband gave it to me. He will be so upset that it is gone. I'm afraid to tell him."

Nurse: "I'm sure you miss your husband very much. Tell me what it was like when you were together. What kinds of things did you do for fun?"

Mrs. W: "We did a lot of traveling. To Italy, and England, and France. We ate wonderful food."

Nurse: "Speaking of food, it is lunch time, and I will walk with you to the dining room."

Mrs. W: "Yes, I'm getting really hungry."

In this situation, the nurse validated Mrs. W's feelings about not being able to find her watch. She did not deny that it had been stolen, nor did she remind Mrs. W that her husband was deceased. (*Remember: A concept of VT is that on some level, Mrs. W knows that her husband is dead.*) The nurse validated the emotions Mrs. W was feeling about missing her husband. She brought up special times that Mrs. W and her husband had spent together, which served to elevate her mood and self-esteem. And lastly, she redirected Mrs. W to the dining room to have her lunch. (The watch was eventually found in Mrs. W's medicine cabinet, where she had hidden it for safekeeping.)

Feil (2013) presents another example:

> When a resident asks for his wife who is dead, caregivers reply, "She'll be here to see you later." The resident may not remember much, but he clings to that statement. He continues to ask for his wife on a daily basis, and the caregivers continue to lie. Eventually he loses trust in the caregivers, knowing that what they say is not true. With VT, the caregivers would encourage the resident to talk about his wife. They would validate his emotions and encourage him to express his needs, accepting the fact that there is a reason behind his behavior. He has not simply "forgotten that his wife died"; he needs to grieve for her. This is unfinished business. When the emotion is expressed and someone listens with empathy, it is relieved. The old man no longer needs to search for his wife. He feels safe with the caregiver, whom he trusts. He always knew on a deep level of awareness that his wife had died. (pp. 3, 4)

---

antipsychotic use in elderly patients with dementia make these evidence-based interventions an important tool for quality nursing care in this population.

Medical Treatment Modalities

Delirium

The first step in the treatment of delirium should be the determination and correction of the underlying causes. Additional attention must be given to fluid and electrolyte status, hypoxia, anoxia, and diabetic problems. Staff members should remain with the patient at all times to monitor behavior and provide reorientation and assurance. The room should maintain a low level of stimuli.

Some physicians prefer not to prescribe medications for the patient with delirium, reasoning that additional agents may only compound the syndrome of brain dysfunction. However, psychosis with agitation and aggression demonstrated by the patient with delirium may require chemical and/or mechanical restraint for his or her personal safety. Choice of specific therapy is made with consideration for the patient's clinical condition and the underlying cause of the delirium. Low-dose antipsychotics are

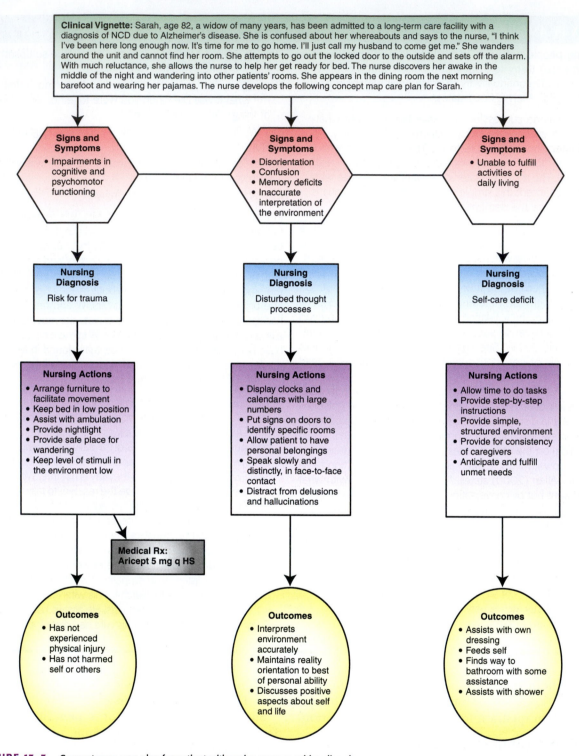

FIGURE 13–3 Concept map care plan for patient with major neurocognitive disorder.

the pharmacological treatment of choice in most cases. However, two recent meta-analyses have found mixed results. One analysis of 15 studies concluded that second generation antipsychotics are beneficial (and preferable to haloperidol) in the treatment of delirium (Kishi et al., 2015), but a second meta-analysis of 19 studies concluded that the evidence does not support use of antipsychotics for prevention or treatment of delirium (Neufeld et al., 2016). Haloperidol (Haldol) is commonly used to treat psychotic features,

---

BOX 13–5 Topics for Patient and Family Education Related to Neurocognitive Disorders

1. Nature of the illness
   a. Possible causes
   b. What to expect
   c. Symptoms
2. Management of the illness
   a. Ways to ensure patient safety
   b. How to maintain reality orientation
   c. Providing assistance with ADLs
   d. Nutritional information
   e. Difficult behaviors
   f. Medication administration
   g. Matters related to hygiene and toileting
3. Support services
   a. Financial assistance
   b. Legal assistance
   c. Caregiver support groups
   d. Respite care
   e. Home health care

---

but because it has been associated with prolongation of QT intervals, nurses should monitor the patient's cardiac status (Sadock et al., 2015). A benzodiazepine (e.g., lorazepam) is commonly used when the etiology is substance withdrawal. Melatonin, an over-the-counter supplement, and ramelteon (Rozerem), a prescription medication for treatment of insomnia, have both been identified as potentially beneficial in prevention and treatment of delirium, because melatonin levels were found to be altered in patients with delirium (Alagiakrishnan, 2016).

Neurocognitive Disorder (NCD)

Once a definitive diagnosis of NCD has been made, a primary consideration in the treatment of the disorder is the etiology. Focus must be directed to the identification and resolution of potentially reversible processes. Sadock and colleagues (2015) identify that once dementia is apparent, it is essential to complete a clinical workup to identify the syndrome and its causes because "approximately 15% of people with dementia have reversible illnesses if treatment is initiated before irreversible damage takes place" (p. 704).

The need for general supportive care, with provisions for security, stimulation, patience, and nutrition, has been recognized and accepted. A number of pharmaceutical agents have been tried, with varying degrees of success, in the treatment of clients with NCD. Some of these drugs are described in the following sections according to symptomatology for which they are indicated. A summary of medications for clients with NCD is provided in Table 13–4.

BOX 13–6 QSEN TEACHING STRATEGY

Assignment: Linking Evidence-Based Practice With a Nursing Procedure
Reality Orientation of Patients With Neurocognitive Disorder (NCD)

Competency Domain: Evidence-Based Practice
Learning Objectives: Student will:
- Locate an evidence-based practice article on a hospital protocol and compare and contrast this information with the facility's protocol.
- Identify whether evidence-based practice is utilized with this protocol and identify barriers or challenges with implementing evidence-based practice in the clinical setting.

Strategy Overview:
1. Research the nursing intervention of reality orientation of patients with NCD. Identify the pros and cons and ethical issues associated with this intervention (particularly with patients who have advanced NCD).
2. Find an evidence-based practice journal article about the intervention.
3. Locate the facility's protocol for reality orientation of patients with NCD.
4. Compare and contrast the facility's protocol with how unit staff carry out this intervention. If there are deviations from the written protocol, what are they, and why do they occur?
5. Compare and contrast the hospital's protocol with the information found in the evidence-based practice article.
6. At postconference, summarize the article on evidence-based practice to the clinical group, and report information gathered throughout the clinical day. Discuss any ethical dilemmas associated with the intervention.
7. Write a paper discussing personal reflections and feelings about this intervention.

Source: Adapted from teaching strategy submitted by Chris Tesch, Instructor, University of South Dakota, Sioux Falls, SD. © 2009 QSEN; http://qsen.org. With permission.

TABLE 13–4	**Selected Medications Used in the Treatment of Clients With NCD**			
MEDICATION	**CLASSIFICATION**	**FOR TREATMENT OF**	**DAILY DOSAGE RANGE (MG)**	**SIDE EFFECTS**
Donepezil (Aricept)	Cholinesterase inhibitor	Cognitive impairment	5–10	Insomnia, dizziness, gastrointestinal (GI) upset, headache
Rivastigmine (Exelon)	Cholinesterase inhibitor	Cognitive impairment	6–12	Dizziness, headache, GI upset, fatigue
Galantamine (Razadyne)	Cholinesterase inhibitor	Cognitive impairment	8–24	Dizziness, headache, GI upset
Memantine (Namenda)	NMDA receptor antagonist	Cognitive impairment	5–20	Dizziness, headache, constipation
Memantine, extended release + donepezil (Namzaric)	Anti-Alzheimer's agent	Moderate to severe Alzheimer's type dementia	Memantine ER 14–28 mg and donepezil 10 mg once daily	Headache, nausea, vomiting, dizziness, diarrhea, decreased appetite
Risperidone* (Risperdal)	Antipsychotic	Agitation, aggression, hallucinations, thought disturbances, wandering	1–4 (increase dosage cautiously)	Agitation, insomnia, headache, extrapyramidal symptoms
Olanzapine* (Zyprexa)	Antipsychotic	Agitation, aggression, hallucinations, thought disturbances, wandering	5 (increase dosage cautiously)	Hypotension, dizziness, sedation, constipation, weight gain, dry mouth
Quetiapine* (Seroquel)	Antipsychotic	Agitation, aggression, hallucinations, thought disturbances, wandering	Initial dose 25 (titrate slowly)	Hypotension, tachycardia, dizziness, drowsiness, headache, constipation, dry mouth
Haloperidol* (Haldol)	Antipsychotic	Agitation, aggression, hallucinations, thought disturbances, wandering	1–4 (increase dosage cautiously)	Dry mouth, blurred vision, orthostatic hypotension, extrapyramidal symptoms, sedation
Pimavanserin (Nuplazid)	Antipsychotic	Hallucinations and delusions specifically associated with Parkinson's disease psychosis. **Note:** Pimavanserin is not approved for dementia-related psychosis unrelated to Parkinson's disease psychosis	34 mg daily (17 mg, twice daily)	Peripheral edema, nausea, confusion, hallucinations, constipation, gait disturbance
Sertraline (Zoloft)	Antidepressant (SSRI)	Depression	50–100	Fatigue, insomnia, sedation, GI upset, headache, dizziness
Paroxetine (Paxil)	Antidepressant (SSRI)	Depression	10–40	Dizziness, headache, insomnia, somnolence, GI upset
Nortriptyline (Pamelor)	Antidepressant (Tricyclic)	Depression	30–50	Anticholinergic, orthostatic hypotension, sedation, arrhythmia
Lorazepam **(Ativan)	Antianxiety (Benzodiazepine)	Anxiety	1–2	Drowsiness, dizziness, GI upset, hypotension, tolerance, dependence

TABLE 13–4	Selected Medications Used in the Treatment of Clients With NCD—cont'd			
MEDICATION	**CLASSIFICATION**	**FOR TREATMENT OF**	**DAILY DOSAGE RANGE (MG)**	**SIDE EFFECTS**
Oxazepam** (Serax)	Antianxiety (Benzodiazepine)	Anxiety	10–30	Drowsiness, dizziness, GI upset, hypotension, tolerance, dependence
Temazepam** (Restoril)	Sedative-hypnotic (Benzodiazepine)	Insomnia	15	Drowsiness, dizziness, GI upset, hypotension, tolerance, dependence
Zolpidem (Ambien)	Sedative-hypnotic (Nonbenzodiazepine)	Insomnia	5	Headache, drowsiness, dizziness, GI upset
Zaleplon (Sonata)	Sedative-hypnotic (Nonbenzodiazepine)	Insomnia	5	Headache, drowsiness, dizziness, GI upset
Eszopiclone (Lunesta)	Sedative-hypnotic (Nonbenzodiazepine)	Insomnia	1–2	Headache, drowsiness, dizziness, GI upset, unpleasant taste
Ramelteon (Rozerem)	Sedative-hypnotic (Nonbenzodiazepine)	Insomnia	8	Dizziness, fatigue, drowsiness, GI upset
Trazodone	Antidepressant (Heterocyclic)	Depression and Insomnia	50	Dizziness, drowsiness, dry mouth, blurred vision, GI upset
Mirtazapine (Remeron)	Antidepressant (Tetracyclic)	Depression and insomnia	7.5–15	Somnolence, dry mouth, constipation, increased appetite

*Although clinicians may still prescribe these medications in low-risk patients, no antipsychotics have been approved by the FDA for the treatment of patients with NCD-related psychosis. All antipsychotics include black-box warnings about increased risk of death in elderly patients with NCD.
**Benzodiazepines should only be used for short-term treatment and NOT used in combination with opiate medication.

Cognitive Impairment

Cholinesterase inhibitors are often used for treatment of mild to moderate cognitive impairment in AD and have demonstrated efficacy in treating patients with Lewy body dementia (Crystal, 2017). (Higher-dose donepezil has also been approved for severe AD.) Some of the clinical manifestations of AD are thought to be the result of a deficiency of the neurotransmitter acetylcholine. In the brain, acetylcholine is inactivated by the enzyme acetylcholinesterase. Donepezil (Aricept), rivastigmine (Exelon), and galantamine (Razadyne) act by inhibiting acetylcholinesterase, which slows the degradation of acetylcholine, thereby increasing concentrations of the neurotransmitter in the cerebral cortex. Because their action relies on functionally intact cholinergic neurons, the effects of these medications may lessen as the disease process advances, and there is no evidence that these medications alter the course of the underlying degenerative process.

Another medication, an NMDA receptor antagonist, was approved by the Food and Drug Administration (FDA) in 2003. The medication, memantine (Namenda), was approved for the treatment of moderate to severe AD. Studies on the use of memantine for Parkinson's disease and dementia with Lewy bodies have been inconclusive (Schwarz, Froelich, & Burns, 2012). High levels of glutamate in the brains of AD patients are thought to contribute to the symptomatology and decline in functionality. These high levels are caused by a dysfunction in glutamate transmission. In normal neurotransmission, glutamate plays an essential role in learning and memory by triggering NMDA receptors to allow a controlled amount of calcium to flow into a nerve cell. This creates the appropriate environment for information processing. In AD, there is a sustained release of glutamate, which results in a continuous influx of calcium into the nerve cells. This increased intracellular calcium concentration ultimately leads to disruption and death of the neurons. Memantine may protect cells against excess glutamate by partially blocking NMDA receptors. Memantine has shown in clinical trials to be effective in improving cognitive function and the ability to perform ADLs in clients with moderate to severe AD. Although it does not stop or reverse the effects of the disease, it has been shown to slow down the progression of the decline in cognition and function. Because memantine's action differs from that of the cholinesterase inhibitors, consideration has been given to co-administration of these medications and one such medication (Namzaric) is currently approved for moderate to severe AD. However, combination therapy with ACh inhibitors and memantine remains controversial because research findings have demonstrated conflicting results (Schwarz et al., 2012).

Current drug trials are under way to test for a vaccine against AD. One recent study led by the Karolinska Institute in Sweden reported positive use with CAD106, a vaccine designed to trigger the body's immune defense against Aβ (Winblad et al., 2012). So far, active vaccines have not demonstrated effectiveness in humans and in some cases have proved harmful, which has redirected research efforts to a focus on passive vaccines (McDonald, 2014). Vaccine trials have continued for the last several years without major breakthroughs. However, in 2016, a group of American and Australian researchers reported a "very promising" vaccine that affects amyloid and tau proteins, both of which are implicated in AD. It is clear that interest in such research is high, with government funding for AD research exceeding $1 billion in 2016 (LaVigne, 2016). Since then, some drugs have failed to meet effectiveness standards in clinical trials. Aducanumab is one drug that is currently in Phase III clinical trials and has demonstrated ability to significantly reduce A-beta plaques in AD patients but no new drugs have yet been placed on the market (Hung & Fu, 2017).

In a study funded by the NIA and others, three drugs were evaluated for the prevention of a rare and aggressive form of autosomal-dominant AD (Bateman et al., 2012). This study includes individuals who are mutation carriers and are therefore genetically destined to develop AD at a young age, typically when they are in their 30s, 40s, or 50s. Because these individuals exhibit measurable biochemical and imaging changes up to 25 years before AD symptoms appear, the drugs will target these biomarkers to determine if the treatment can stop or slow the disease process. To date, there have been no medications clearly identified or approved as preventive for this condition. Genotyping and genetic counseling are available options for evaluation and management (National Center for Advancing Translational Sciences, 2015). Antipsychotics have been associated with increased mortality in patients with dementia, and Moussa (2016) recommends that prescribers use low doses of quetiapine or olanzapine only "in patients with severe, disabling symptoms after informing families of the mortality risk."

Gingko biloba is a popular over-the-counter supplement advanced as having benefits for improving cognitive impairment and symptoms of dementia. Its actions include dilating blood vessels, thinning blood, modifying neurotransmitters, and reducing the density of oxygen-free radicals (Birks & Grimley, 2009). But in a systematic review of 36 trials, Birks and Grimley conclude that evidence for benefits in cognitive impairment or dementia is inconsistent and unreliable.

More recent research has focused on the chemical resveratrol, found in grape skins, cacao, and other foods. It has been advanced as having anti-aging properties and neuroprotective functions as well as possibly reducing the buildup of amyloid plaques associated with AD. A recent study (Turner et al., 2015) found promising evidence that high doses of resveratrol (up to 2,000 mg daily) have CNS effects on biomarkers for AD. Kou and Chen (2017), in their review, report that "mounting evidence from in vitro and in vivo AD models has demonstrated that resveratrol, one of polyphenolic compounds, can exert neuroprotective role in neurodegenerative diseases especially AD." The researchers caution that more research is needed to fully understand the impact of these changes on the trajectory of AD.

With regard to nonpharmacological treatments for cognitive impairment in patients with NCD, cognitive rehabilitation (which includes education about cognitive strengths and weaknesses, cognitive retraining, and compensatory strategies) has demonstrated some evidence of modest improvement in cognitive domains, although research is in the early stages (Dancis & Cotter, 2015). Recent studies have also supported that mindfulness meditation results in observable changes in brain structures related to memory and emotional responses and therefore may have benefits in the treatment of NCDs (Sorrell, 2015). As previously mentioned, the WHELD Program of person-centered activities, social interaction, and exercise has demonstrated benefits for decreasing agitation, decreasing use of antipsychotic medication, and improving quality of life for patients with dementia in long-term care settings (Ballard, 2018).

Agitation, Aggression, Hallucinations, Thought Disturbances, and Wandering

Historically, physicians have prescribed antipsychotic medications to control agitation, aggression, hallucinations, thought disturbances, and wandering in clients with NCD. The atypical antipsychotic medications, such as risperidone, olanzapine, quetiapine, and ziprasidone, are often favored because of their lessened propensity to cause anticholinergic and extrapyramidal side effects. In 2005, however, following review of a number of studies, the FDA ordered black-box warnings on drug labels for all atypical antipsychotics, noting that the drugs are associated with an increased risk of death in elderly patients with psychotic behaviors associated with NCD. Most of the deaths appeared to be cardiovascular related. In July 2008, based on the results of several studies, the FDA extended this warning to include all first generation antipsychotics as well, such as haloperidol and perphenazine. This poses a clinical dilemma for physicians who have found these medications to be helpful to their clients, and some have chosen to continue to use them in clients without significant cerebrovascular disease, in whom previous behavioral programs have failed, and with consent from relatives or guardians who are clearly aware of the risks and benefits.

Many antipsychotic, antidepressant, and antihistaminic medications produce *anticholinergic side effects*, which include confusion, blurred vision, constipation, dry mouth, dizziness, and difficulty urinating. Older people, and especially those with NCD, are particularly sensitive to these effects because of decreased cholinergic reserves. Many elderly individuals are also at increased risk for developing an anticholinergic toxicity syndrome because of the additive anticholinergic effects of multiple medications.

Depression

It is estimated that up to 40 percent of people with AD also suffer from major depression (Alzheimer's Association, 2018c). Recognizing the symptoms of depression in these individuals is often a challenge. Depression—which affects thinking, memory, sleep, and appetite and interferes with daily life—is sometimes difficult to distinguish from NCD. Clearly, the presence of depression in the client with NCD complicates and worsens the individual's functioning.

Antidepressant medication is sometimes used in treatment of depression in NCD. The selective serotonin reuptake inhibitors (SSRIs) are considered by many to be the first-line drug treatment for depression in the elderly because of their favorable side effect profile. Although still used by some physicians, tricyclic antidepressants are often avoided because of cardiac and anticholinergic side effects. Trazodone may be a good choice, used at bedtime, for depression and insomnia. Dopaminergic agents (e.g., methylphenidate, amantadine, bromocriptine, and bupropion) may be helpful in the treatment of severe apathy.

Not only is depression common in AD, but evidence supports that individuals with depression—especially recurrent and chronic depression—are about two times more likely to develop AD than those who do not have depression (Herbert, 2016). Possible explanations for this increased risk have included common genetic links (which so far looks unlikely); disturbance in glucocorticoids that occurs in both AD and some forms of depression that inhibit hippocampal neurogenesis and plasticity; and cytokines, which are elevated in some forms of depression and are a known risk factor for AD (Herbert & Lucassen, 2016). The authors note that more research is needed to better understand subtypes of depression and their distinct connections to risk for AD.

Anxiety

The progressive loss of mental functioning is a significant source of anxiety in the early stages of NCD. It is important that clients be encouraged to verbalize their feelings and fears associated with this loss. These interventions may be useful in reducing the anxiety of clients with NCD.

Antianxiety medications may be helpful but should not be used routinely or for prolonged periods. The least toxic and most effective of the antianxiety medications are the benzodiazepines. Examples include diazepam (Valium), chlordiazepoxide (Librium), alprazolam (Xanax), lorazepam (Ativan), and oxazepam (Serax). The drugs with shorter half-lives (e.g., lorazepam and oxazepam) are preferred to those longer-acting medications (e.g., diazepam), which promote a higher risk of oversedation and falls. Barbiturates are not appropriate as antianxiety agents because they frequently induce confusion and paradoxical excitement in elderly individuals.

Sleep Disturbances

Sleep problems are common in clients with NCD and often intensify as the disease progresses. Wakefulness and nighttime wandering create much distress and anguish in family members who are charged with protection of their loved one. Sleep disturbances are among the problems that most frequently initiate the need for placement of the client in a long-term care facility.

Some physicians treat sleep problems with sedative-hypnotic medications. The benzodiazepines may be useful for some clients but are indicated for relatively brief periods only. Examples include flurazepam (Dalmane), temazepam (Restoril), and triazolam (Halcion). Daytime sedation and cognitive impairment, in addition to paradoxical agitation in elderly clients, are of particular concern with these medications. The nonbenzodiazepine sedative-hypnotics zolpidem (Ambien), zaleplon (Sonata), eszopiclone (Lunesta), and ramelteon (Rozerem) and the antidepressants trazodone (Desyrel) and mirtazapine (Remeron) are also prescribed. Daytime sedation may also be a problem with these medications. As previously stated, barbiturates should not be used in elderly clients. Sleep problems are usually ongoing, and most clinicians prefer to use medications only to help an individual through a short-term stressful situation. Rising at the same time each morning; minimizing daytime sleep; participating in regular physical exercise (but no later than 4 hours before bedtime); getting proper nutrition; avoiding alcohol, caffeine, and nicotine; and retiring at the same time each night are behavioral approaches to sleep problems that may eliminate the need for sleep aids, particularly in the early stages of NCD. Because of the tremendous potential for adverse drug reactions in the elderly, many of whom are already taking multiple medications, pharmacological treatment of insomnia should be considered only after attempts at nonpharmacological strategies have failed.

CASE STUDY AND SAMPLE CARE PLAN

NURSING HISTORY AND ASSESSMENT

Carmen is an 81-year-old widow who has lived in the same small town in the same house that she shared with her husband until his death 16 years ago. She and her husband reared two daughters, Joan and Nancy, who have been living with their husbands in a large city about 2 hours away from Carmen. They have always visited Carmen every 1 or 2 months. She has four grown grandchildren who live in distant states and who see their grandmother on holidays.

About a year ago, Carmen's daughters began to receive reports from friends and other family members about incidents in which Carmen was becoming forgetful (e.g., forgetting to go to a cousin's birthday party, taking a wrong turn and getting lost on the way to a niece's house [where she had driven many times], returning to church to search for something she thought she had forgotten [although she could not explain what it was], sending birthday gifts to people when it was not their birthday). During routine visits, the elder daughter, Joan, found bills left unpaid, sometimes months overdue. Housekeepers and yard workers reported to Joan that Carmen would forget she had paid them and try to pay them again and sometimes a third time. She became very confused when she would attempt to fill her weekly pillboxes, a task she had completed in the past without difficulty. Hundreds of dollars would disappear from her wallet, and she could not tell Joan what happened to them.

Joan and her husband subsequently moved to the small town where Carmen lived. They bought a home, and Joan visited her mother every day, took care of finances, and ensured that Carmen took her daily medications, although Joan worked at a job that required occasional out-of-town travel. As the months progressed, Carmen's cognitive abilities deteriorated. She burned food on the stove, left the house with the broiler-oven on, forgot to take her medication, got lost in her car, missed appointments, and forgot the names of her neighbors whom she had known for many years. She began to lose weight because she was forgetting to eat her meals.

Carmen was evaluated by a neurologist, who diagnosed her with Neurocognitive Disorder Due to Alzheimer's Disease. Because they believed that Carmen needed 24-hour care, Joan and Nancy made the painful decision to place Carmen in long-term care. In the nursing home, her condition has continued to deteriorate. Carmen wanders up and down the halls (day and night), and she has fallen twice, once while attempting to get out of bed. She requires assistance to shower and dress and has become incontinent of urine. The nurses found her attempting to leave the building, saying, "I'm going across the street to visit my daughter." One morning at breakfast she appeared in her pajamas in the communal dining room, not realizing that she had not dressed. She is unable to form new memories and sometimes uses confabulation to fill in the blanks. She asks the same questions repeatedly, sometimes struggling for the right word. She can no longer provide the correct names of items in her environment. She has no concept of time.

Joan visits Carmen daily, and Nancy visits weekly, each offering support to the other in person and by phone. Carmen always seems pleased to see them but can no longer call either of them by name. They are unsure if she knows who they are.

NURSING DIAGNOSES AND OUTCOME IDENTIFICATION

From the assessment data, the nurse develops the following nursing diagnoses for Carmen:

1. Risk for trauma related to impairments in cognitive and psychomotor functioning; wandering; falls
   a. Outcome criteria: Carmen will remain injury free during her nursing home stay.
   b. Short-term goals:
      • Carmen will not fall while wandering the halls.
      • Carmen will not fall out of bed.
2. Disturbed thought processes related to cerebral degeneration evidenced by disorientation, confusion, and memory deficits
   a. Outcome criteria: Carmen will maintain reality orientation to the best of her cognitive ability.
   b. Short-term goals:
      • Carmen will be able to find her room.
      • Carmen will be able to communicate her needs to staff.

CASE STUDY AND SAMPLE CARE PLAN—cont'd

3. Self-care deficit related to cognitive impairments, disorientation, confusion, and memory deficits
   a. Outcome criteria: Carmen will accomplish ADLs to the best of her ability.
   b. Short-term goals:
      • Carmen will assist with dressing herself.
      • Carmen will cooperate with trips to the bathroom.
      • Carmen will wash herself in the shower with help from the nurse.

PLANNING AND IMPLEMENTATION

RISK FOR TRAUMA

The following nursing interventions may be implemented *in an effort to ensure patient safety*:

1. Arrange the furniture in Carmen's room so that it will accommodate her moving around freely.
2. Store frequently used items within her easy reach.
3. Provide a "low bed," or possibly move her mattress from the bed to the floor, to prevent falls from the bed.
4. Attach a bed alarm to alert the nurse's station when Carmen has alighted from her bed.
5. Keep a dim light on in her room at night.
6. During the day and evening, provide a well-lighted area where Carmen can safely wander.
7. Ensure that all outside doors are electronically controlled.
8. Play soft music and maintain a low level of stimuli in the environment.

DISTURBED THOUGHT PROCESSES

The following nursing interventions may be implemented *to help maintain orientation and aid in memory and recognition*:

1. Use clocks and calendars with large numbers that are easy to read.
2. Put a sign on Carmen's door with her name on it and hang a personal item of hers on the door.
3. Ask Joan to bring some of Carmen's personal items for her room, even a favorite comfy chair, if possible. Ask also for some old photograph albums if they are available.
4. Keep staff and caregivers to a minimum to promote familiarity.
5. Speak slowly and clearly while looking into Carmen's face.
6. Use reminiscence therapy with Carmen. Ask her to share happy times from her life with you. This technique helps decrease depression and boost self-esteem.

7. Mention the date and time in casual conversation. Refer to "spring rain," "summer flowers," "fall leaves." Emphasize holidays.
8. Correct misperceptions gently and matter-of-factly and focus on real events and real people if false ideas should occur. Validate her feelings associated with current and past life situations.
9. Monitor for medication side effects because toxic effects from certain medications can intensify altered thought processes.

SELF-CARE DEFICIT

The following nursing interventions may be implemented *to ensure that all Carmen's needs are fulfilled*.

1. Assess what Carmen can do independently and with what she needs assistance.
2. Allow plenty of time for her to accomplish tasks that are within her ability. Clothing with easy removal or replacement, such as Velcro, facilitates independence.
3. Provide guidance and support for independent actions by talking her through tasks one step at a time.
4. Provide a structured schedule of activities that does not change from day to day.
5. Ensure that Carmen has snacks between meals.
6. Take Carmen to the bathroom regularly (according to her usual pattern, e.g., after meals, before bedtime, on arising).
7. To minimize nighttime wetness, offer fluid every 2 hours during the day and restrict fluid after 6:00 p.m.
8. To promote more restful nighttime sleep (and less wandering at night), reduce naps during late afternoon and encourage sitting exercises, walking, and ball toss. Carbohydrate snacks at bedtime may also be helpful.

EVALUATION

The outcome criteria identified for Carmen have been met. She has experienced no injury. She has not fallen out of bed. She continues to wander in a safe area. She can find her room by herself but occasionally requires some assistance when she is anxious and more confused. She has some difficulty communicating her needs to the staff, but those who work with her on a consistent basis are able to anticipate her needs. All ADLs are being fulfilled, and Carmen assists with dressing and grooming, accomplishing about half on her own. Nighttime wandering has been minimized. Soft bedtime music helps to relax her.

Summary and Key Points

■ NCDs constitute a large and growing public health concern.

■ Delirium is a disturbance of awareness and a change in cognition that develop rapidly over a short period. Level of consciousness is often affected, and psychomotor activity may fluctuate between agitated purposeless movements and a vegetative state resembling catatonic stupor.

■ The symptoms of delirium usually begin quite abruptly and often are reversible and brief.

■ Delirium may be caused by a general medical condition, substance intoxication or withdrawal, or ingestion of a medication or exposure to a toxin.

- NCD is a syndrome of acquired, persistent intellectual impairment with compromised function in multiple spheres of mental activity, such as memory, language, visuospatial skills, emotion or personality, and cognition.

- Dementia (also described as major NCD in the *DSM-5*) is a progressive decline of cognitive abilities in the presence of clear consciousness.

- Symptoms of NCD are insidious and develop slowly over time. In most patients, the disorder runs a progressive, irreversible course.

- NCD may be caused by genetics, cardiovascular disease, infections, neurophysiological disorders, and other general medical conditions.

- Nursing care of the patient with an NCD is presented around the six steps of the nursing process.

- Objectives of care for the patient experiencing an acute syndrome are aimed at eliminating the etiology, promoting patient safety, and a return to the highest possible level of functioning.

- Objectives of care for the patient experiencing a chronic, progressive disorder are aimed at preserving the dignity of the individual, promoting deceleration of the symptoms, and maximizing functional capabilities.

- WHELD is an evidence-based intervention for patients with dementia in long-term care settings that has demonstrated effectiveness in decreasing agitation, decreasing the need for antipsychotic medication, and improving the quality of life in this population.

- Nursing interventions are also directed toward helping the patient's family or primary caregivers learn about a chronic, progressive neurocognitive disorder.

- Education is provided about the disease process, expectations of patient behavioral changes, methods for facilitating care, and sources of assistance and support as they struggle, both physically and emotionally, with the demands brought on by a disease process that is slowly taking their loved one away from them.

Review Questions
Self-Examination/Learning Exercise

Select the answer that is most appropriate for each of the following questions:

1. An example of a treatable (reversible) form of NCD is one that is caused by which of the following? (Select all that apply.)
   a. Multiple sclerosis
   b. Multiple small brain infarcts
   c. Electrolyte imbalances
   d. HIV disease
   e. Folate deficiency

2. Mrs. G has been diagnosed with NCD due to Alzheimer's disease. This disorder is associated with the presence of which of the following?
   a. Multiple small brain infarcts
   b. Lewy bodies
   c. Cerebral abscess
   d. Amyloid beta plaques and neurofibrillary tangles

3. Mrs. G has been diagnosed with NCD due to Alzheimer's disease. The *primary* nursing intervention in working with Mrs. G is which of the following?
   a. Ensuring that she receives food she likes to prevent hunger
   b. Ensuring that the environment is safe to prevent injury
   c. Ensuring that she meets the other patients to prevent social isolation
   d. Ensuring that she takes care of her own ADLs to prevent dependence

4. Which of the following medications have been indicated for improvement in cognitive functioning in mild to moderate Alzheimer's disease? (Select all that apply.)
   a. Donepezil (Aricept)
   b. Rivastigmine (Exelon)
   c. Risperidone (Risperdal)
   d. Sertraline (Zoloft)
   e. Galantamine (Razadyne)

Review Questions—cont'd
Self-Examination/Learning Exercise

5. Mrs. G, who has NCD due to Alzheimer's disease, says to the nurse, "I have a date tonight. I always have a date on Christmas." Which of the following is the most appropriate response?
   a. "Don't be silly. It's not Christmas, Mrs. G."
   b. "Today is Tuesday, October 21, Mrs. G. We will have supper soon, and then your daughter will come to visit."
   c. "Who is your date with, Mrs. G?"
   d. "I think you need some more medication, Mrs. G. I'll bring it to you now."

6. In addition to disturbances in cognition and orientation, individuals with Alzheimer's disease may also show changes in which of the following? (Select all that apply.)
   a. Personality
   b. Vision
   c. Speech
   d. Hearing
   e. Mobility

7. Mrs. G, who has NCD due to Alzheimer's disease, has trouble sleeping and wanders around at night. Which of the following nursing actions would be *best* to promote sleep in Mrs. G?
   a. Ask the doctor to prescribe flurazepam (Dalmane).
   b. Ensure that Mrs. G gets an afternoon nap so she will not be overtired at bedtime.
   c. Make Mrs. G a cup of tea with honey before bedtime.
   d. Ensure that Mrs. G gets regular physical exercise during the day.

8. The night nurse finds Mrs. G, a client with Alzheimer's disease, wandering the hallway at 4 a.m. and trying to open the door to the side yard. Which statement by the nurse reflects the most patient-centered approach to the situation?
   a. "That door leads out to the patio, Mrs. G. It's nighttime. You don't want to go outside now."
   b. "You look confused, Mrs. G. What is bothering you?"
   c. "This is the patio door, Mrs. G. Are you looking for the bathroom?"
   d. "Are you lonely? Perhaps you'd like to go back to your room and talk for a while."

9. Which of the following factors is *not* associated with increased incidence of NCD due to Alzheimer's disease?
   a. Multiple small strokes
   b. Family history of Alzheimer's disease
   c. Head trauma
   d. Advanced age

10. Mr. Stone is a patient in the hospital with a diagnosis of vascular NCD. In explaining this disorder to Mr. Stone's family, which of the following statements by the nurse is correct?
    a. "He will probably live longer than if his disorder was of the Alzheimer's type."
    b. "Vascular NCD shows stepwise progression. This is why he sometimes seems okay."
    c. "Vascular NCD is caused by plaques and tangles that form in the brain."
    d. "The cause of vascular NCD is unknown."

11. Which of the following interventions is most appropriate in helping a patient with Alzheimer's disease with her ADLs? (Select all that apply.)
    a. Perform ADLs for her while she is in the hospital.
    b. Provide her with a written list of activities she is expected to perform.
    c. Assist her with step-by-step instructions.
    d. Tell her that if her morning care is not completed by 9:00 a.m., it will be performed for her by the nurse's aide so that she can attend group therapy.
    e. Encourage her and give her plenty of time to perform as many of her ADLs as possible independently.

TEST YOUR CRITICAL THINKING SKILLS

Joe, a 62-year-old accountant, began having difficulty remembering details necessary to perform his job. He was also having trouble at home, failing to keep his finances straight, and forgetting to pay bills. It became increasingly difficult for him to function properly at work, and eventually he was forced to retire. Cognitive deterioration continued, and behavioral problems soon began. He became stubborn, verbally and physically abusive, and suspicious of almost everyone in his environment. His wife and son convinced him to see a physician, who recommended hospitalization for testing.

At Joe's initial evaluation, he was fully alert and cooperative but obviously anxious and fidgety. He thought he was at his accounting office, and he could not state what year it was. He could not say the names of his parents or siblings, nor did he know who the current president of the United States was. He could not perform simple arithmetic calculations, write a proper sentence, or copy a drawing. He interpreted proverbs concretely and had difficulty stating similarities between related objects.

Laboratory serum studies revealed no abnormalities, but a CT scan showed marked cortical atrophy. The physician's diagnosis was Neurocognitive Disorder Due to Alzheimer's Disease.

Answer the following questions related to Joe:

1. What are the pertinent assessment data from which nursing care will be devised?
2. What is the primary nursing diagnosis for Joe?
3. How would outcomes be identified?

Communication Exercises

1. Mrs. B is a patient on the Alzheimer's unit. The nurse hears her yelling, "Waitress! Waitress! Why can't I get some service around here?!" How would the nurse respond appropriately to this statement by Mrs. B?

2. Mrs. B, who had breakfast an hour ago, says to the nurse, "I've been waiting and waiting for my breakfast. On the farm, we always had breakfast by six o'clock. Those were the good old days." How would the nurse respond appropriately to this statement by Mrs. B?

 MOVIE CONNECTIONS

The Notebook (Alzheimer's disease) • *Away From Her* (Alzheimer's disease) • *Iris* (Alzheimer's disease) • *Still Alice* (Early-onset Alzheimer's disease)

References

Alagiakrishnan, K. (2016). *Delirium medications.* Retrieved from http://emedicine.medscape.com/article/288890-medication

Allen, J. (2000). Using validation therapy to manage difficult behaviors. *Prism Innovations. ElderCare Online.* Retrieved from http://www.ec-online.net/community/Activists/difficultbehaviors.htm

Alzheimer's Association. (2018a). Alzheimer's disease facts and figures. *Alzheimer's Dementia, 14*(3), 367–429.

Alzheimer's Association. (2018b). *What is Alzheimer's?* Retrieved from https://www.alz.org/alzheimers_disease_what_is_alzheimers.asp

Alzheimer's Association. (2018c). *Depression and Alzheimer's.* Retrieved from http://www.alz.org/care/alzheimers-dementia-depression.asp

American Psychiatric Association (APA). (2000). *Diagnostic and statistical manual of mental disorders* (4th ed., text rev.). Washington, DC: Author.

American Psychiatric Association (APA). (2013). *Diagnostic and statistical manual of mental disorders* (5th ed.). Washington, DC: Author.

Ballard, C., Corbett, A., Orrell, M., Williams, G., Moniz-Cook, E., Romeo, R., . . . Fossey, J. (2018). Impact of person-centred care training and person-centred activities on quality of life, agitation, and antipsychotic use in people with dementia living in nursing homes: A cluster-randomised controlled trial. *PLoS Med, 15*(2), e1002500. https://doi.org/10.1371/journal.pmed.1002500

Ballard, C., Orrell, M., Yong Zhong, S., Moniz-Cook, E., Stafford, J., Whittaker, R., . . . Fossey, J. (2016). Impact of antipsychotic review and nonpharmacological intervention on antipsychotic use, neuropsychiatric symptoms, and mortality in people with dementia living in nursing homes: A factorial cluster-randomized controlled trial by the well-being and health for people with dementia (WHELD) program. *American Journal of Psychiatry, 173*(3), 252–262. doi:10.1176/appi.ajp.2015.15010130

Bateman, R. J., Xiong, C., Benzinger, T. L. S., Fagan, A. M., Goate, A., Fox, N. C., . . . Morris, J. C. (2012). Clinical and biomarker changes in dominantly inherited Alzheimer's disease. *New England Journal of Medicine, 367*(9), 795–804.

Birks, J., & Grimley, E. J. (2009). Ginkgo biloba for cognitive impairment and dementia. *Cochrane Database of Systematic Reviews, 21*(1), CD003120. doi:10.1002/14651858.CD003120

Crystal, H. A. (2017). Dementia with Lewy bodies: Treatment and management. *Medscape.* Retrieved from emedicine.medscape.com/article/1135041-treatment

Dancis, A., & Cotter, V. T. (2015). Diagnosis and management of cognitive impairment in Parkinson's disease. *Journal for Nurse Practitioner, 11*(30), 307–313.

Day, C. R. (2013). *Validation therapy: A review of the literature.* Retrieved from Validation Training Institute, Inc. website: http://www.vfvalidation.org/web.php?request=article1

Fabian, T. J., & Solai, L. K. (2017). Neurocognitive disorders. In B. J. Sadock, V. A. Sadock, & P. Ruiz (Eds.), *Comprehensive textbook of psychiatry* (pp. 1178–1191). Philadelphia, PA: Wolters Kluwer.

Feil, N. (2013). *It is never good to lie to a person who has dementia.* Retrieved from *Validation Training Institute, Inc. website:* http://www.vfvalidation.org//web.php?request=article5

Graff-Radford, J. (2017). *Can a head injury cause or hasten Alzheimer's disease or other types of dementia?* Retrieved from https://www.mayoclinic.org/diseases-conditions/alzheimers-disease/expert-answers/alzheimers-disease/faq-20057837

Graziane, J. A., & Sweet, R. A. (2017). Dementia. In B. J. Sadock, V. A. Sadock, & P. Ruiz (Eds.), *Comprehensive textbook of psychiatry* (pp. 1191–1221). Philadelphia, PA: Wolters Kluwer.

Herbert, J. (2016). Depression is a risk for Alzheimer's: We need to know why. *Psychology Today.* Retrieved from https://

www.psychologytoday.com/us/blog/hormones-and-the-brain/201604/depression-is-risk-alzheimer-s-we-need-know-why

Herbert, J., & Lucassen, P. J. (2016). Depression as a risk factor for Alzheimer's disease: Genes, steroids, cytokines and neurogenesis—What do we need to know? *Frontiers in Neuroendocrinology, 41,*153–171. doi:10.1016/j.yfrne.2015.12.001

Herdman, T. H., & Kamitsuru, S. (Eds.). (2018). *NANDA-I nursing diagnoses: Definitions and classification, 2018–2020.* New York, NY: Thieme.

Hung, S. Y., & Fu, W. M. (2017). Drug candidates in clinical trials for Alzheimer's disease. *Journal of Biomedical Medicine, 24,* 47. https://doi.org/10.1186/s12929-017-0355-7

Huntington's Disease Society of America (HDSA). (2018). *What is Huntington's disease?* Retrieved from http://hdsa.org/what-is-hd/

Institute of Medicine (IOM). (2003). *Health professions education: A bridge to quality.* Washington, DC: Author.

Johns Hopkins Medicine. (n.d.). Prion diseases. *Health Library.* Retrieved from https://www.hopkinsmedicine.org/healthlibrary/conditions/nervous_system_disorders/prion_diseases_134,56

Kishi, T., Hirota, T., Matsunaga, S., & Iwata, N. (2015). Antipsychotic medications for the treatment of delirium: A systematic review and meta-analysis of randomised controlled trials. *Journal of Neurology, Neurosurgery, and Psychiatry, 87*(7), 767–774. doi:10.1136/jnnp-2015-311049

Kou, X., & Chen, N. (2017). Resveratrol as a natural autophagy regulator for prevention and treatment of Alzheimer's disease. *Nutrients, 9*(9), 927. doi:10.3390/nu9090927

Langa, K. M., Larson, E. B., Crimmins, E. M., Faul, J. D., Levine, D. A., Kabeto, M. U., & Weir, D. R. (2017). A comparison of the prevalence of dementia in the United States in 2000 and 2012. *JAMA Internal Medicine, 177*(1), 51–58. doi:10.1001/jamainternmed.2016.6807

LaVigne, P. (2016). *Alzheimer's vaccine: Researchers target brain proteins in mouse study.* Retrieved from Vaccination Reaction website: http://www.thevaccinereaction.org/2016/08/alzheimers-vaccineresearchers-target-brain-proteins-in-mouse-study

Mayo Clinic. (2018a). *Dementia: Symptoms and causes.* Retrieved from https://www.mayoclinic.org/diseases-conditions/dementia/symptoms-causes/syc-20352013

Mayo Clinic. (2018b). *Alzheimer's disease: Diagnosis.* Retrieved from https://www.mayoclinic.org/diseases-conditions/alzheimers-disease/diagnosis-treatment/drc-20350453

McDonald, I. (2014). Could an Alzheimer's disease vaccine be a reality? *Dementia News.* Retrieved from http://dementiaresearchfoundation.org.au/blog/could-alzheimer%E2%80 %99s-disease-vaccine-be-reality

McShane, R. (2000). *Hallucinations and delusions.* London, UK: The Alzheimer's Society.

Mitchell, S. (2015). Advanced dementia. *New England Journal of Medicine, 372*(26), 2533–2540.

Moore, R. C., & Marquine, M. J. (2017). HIV and aging. In B. J. Sadock, V. A. Sadock, & P. Ruiz (Eds.), *Comprehensive textbook of psychiatry* (pp. 4268–4274). Philadelphia, PA: Wolters Kluwer.

Moussa, M. (2016). Alzheimer's disease. *Cardiology News.* Retrieved from http://www.mdedge.com/ecardiologynews/dsm/4936/hospital-medicine/alzheimers-disease

National Center for Advancing Translational Sciences. (2015). *Early-onset familial autosomal dominant Alzheimer disease.* Retrieved from https://rarediseases.info.nih.gov/diseases/12798/early-onset-autosomal-dominant-alzheimer-disease

National Institute of Neurological Disorders and Stroke (NINDS). (2017). *NINDS frontotemporal dementia information page.* Retrieved from https://www.ninds.nih.gov/Disorders/All-Disorders/Frontotemporal-Dementia-Information-Page

National Institute on Aging. (2011) Alzheimer's disease: Unraveling the mystery. NIH Publication No. 08-3782. Washington, DC: National Institutes of Health, U.S. Department of Health and Human Services.

National Institute on Aging (NIA). (2015). *Dietary treatments for cognitive impairment.* Retrieved from https://www.nia.nih.gov/alzheimers/clinical-trials/dietary-treatments-cognitive-impairment

National Institute on Aging (NIA). (2017). *Coping with late stage Alzheimer's disease.* Retrieved from https://www.nia.nih.gov/health/coping-late-stage-alzheimers-disease

Neufeld, K. J., Yue, J., Robinson, T. N., Inouye, S. K., & Needham, D. M. (2016). Antipsychotic medication for prevention and treatment of delirium in hospitalized adults: A systematic review and meta-analysis. *Journal of the American Geriatrics Society, 64*(4), 705–714. doi:10.1111/jgs.14076

Sadock, B. J., Sadock, V. A., & Ruiz, P. (2015). *Synopsis of psychiatry: Behavioral sciences/clinical psychiatry* (11th ed.). Philadelphia, PA: Wolters Kluwer.

Schwarz, S., Froelich, L., & Burns, A. (2012). Pharmacologic treatment of dementia. *Current Opinion in Psychiatry, 25*(6), 542–550. doi:10.1097/YCO.06013e328358e4f2

Sorrell, J. M. (2015). Meditation for older adults. *Journal of Psychosocial Nursing, 53*(5), 15–19.

Strub, R. L., & Black, F. W. (2000). *The mental status examination in neurology* (4th ed.). Philadelphia, PA: F.A. Davis.

Sullivan, M. (2018). Alzheimer's: Biomarkers, not cognition, will now define disorder. *Clinical Psychiatry News.* Retrieved from https://www.mdedge.com/clinicalpsychiatrynews/article/163073/alzheimers-cognition/alzheimers-biomarkers-not-cognition-will/page/0/6

Turner, R. S., Thomas, R. G., Craft, S., van Dyck, C. H., Mintzer, J., Reynolds, B. A., . . . Alzheimer's Disease Cooperative Study. (2015). A randomized, double-blind, placebo-controlled trial of resveratrol for Alzheimer disease. *Neurology, 85*(16), 1383–1391. doi:10.1212/WNL.0000000000002035

WebMD. (2017). *7 stages of Alzheimer's disease.* Retrieved from https://www.webmd.com/alzheimers/guide/alzheimers-disease-stages#2

Whitaker, R., Fossey, J., Ballard, C., Orrell, M., Moniz-Cook, E., Woods, R. T., . . . Khan, Z. (2014). Improving well-being and health for people with dementia (WHELD): Study protocol for a randomised controlled trial. *BioMed Central, 15*(284). doi:10.1186/1745-6215-15-284

Winblad, B., Andreasen, N., Minthon, L., Floesser, A., Imbert, G., Dumortier, T., . . . Graf, A. (2012). Safety, tolerability, and antibody response of active Aβ immunotherapy with CAD106 in patients with Alzheimer's disease: Randomized, double-blind, placebo-controlled, first-in-human study. *The Lancet Neurology, 11*(7), 597–604.Review Questions—cont'd

14 Substance Use and Addiction Disorders

OBJECTIVES

After reading this chapter, the student will be able to:

1. Define *addiction, intoxication,* and *withdrawal.*
2. Discuss predisposing factors implicated in the etiology of substance-related and addictive disorders.
3. Identify symptomatology and use the information in assessment of clients with various substance-related and addictive disorders.
4. Identify nursing diagnoses common to patients with substance-related and addictive disorders and select appropriate nursing interventions for each.
5. Identify topics for patient and family teaching relevant to substance-related and addictive disorders.
6. Describe relevant outcome criteria for evaluating nursing care of patients with substance-related and addictive disorders.
7. Discuss the issue of substance-related and addictive disorders within the profession of nursing.

8. Define *codependency* and identify behavioral characteristics associated with the disorder.
9. Discuss treatment of codependency.
10. Describe various modalities relevant to treatment of individuals with substance-related and addictive disorders.

HOMEWORK ASSIGNMENT
Please read the chapter and answer the following questions:

1. What are the physical consequences of thiamine deficiency in chronic alcohol use?
2. Define *tolerance* as it relates to physical addiction to a substance.
3. Describe two types of toxic reactions that can occur with the use of hallucinogens.
4. Describe current trends and national responses to the opiate use disorder epidemic in the United States.
5. What is medication-assisted treatment?

Introduction

Substance-related disorders comprise two groups: the substance use disorders (addiction) and the substance-induced disorders (intoxication, withdrawal, delirium, neurocognitive disorder, psychosis, bipolar disorder, depressive disorder, obsessive-compulsive disorder, anxiety disorder, sexual dysfunction, and sleep disorders). This chapter discusses addiction, intoxication, and withdrawal. The remainder of the substance-induced disorders are included in the chapters with which they share symptomatology (e.g., substance-induced depressive disorder is discussed in Chapter 16, Depressive Disorders; substance-induced anxiety disorder is discussed in Chapter 18, Anxiety, Obsessive-Compulsive, and Related Disorders). Also included in this chapter is a discussion of gambling disorder, a nonsubstance addiction disorder.

Drugs are a pervasive part of our society. Certain mood-altering substances are quite socially acceptable and are used moderately by many adult Americans. They include alcohol, caffeine, and nicotine. Society has even developed a relative indifference to an occasional abuse of these substances despite documentation of their negative impact on health.

A wide variety of substances are produced for medicinal purposes. These include central nervous system (CNS) stimulants (e.g., **amphetamines**), CNS depressants (e.g., sedatives, tranquilizers), as well as numerous over-the-counter preparations designed to relieve nearly every kind of human ailment, real or imagined.

Some illegal substances have achieved a degree of social acceptance by certain societal subcultures. These drugs, such as marijuana and hashish, are by no means harmless even though they are becoming legalized in some states. The long-term effects are still being studied, whereas the dangerous effects of other illegal substances (e.g., lysergic acid diethylamide [LSD], **phencyclidine,** cocaine, and heroin) have been well documented. Opiate use has increased dramatically in both prescriptions for medicinal purposes and those purchased illegally. Currently this substance use disorder has been identified as a national epidemic and is associated with an alarming number of deaths.

This chapter discusses the physical and behavioral manifestations and personal and social consequences related to the abuse of or addiction to alcohol, other CNS depressants, CNS stimulants, **opioids,** hallucinogens, cannabinols, and the nonsubstance addiction to gambling. Variations in attitudes regarding substance consumption and patterns of use are explored. For example, drinking alcohol is considered by many to be part of the culture of college life while, at the same time, substance *abuse* is especially prevalent among individuals between the ages of 18 and 24. Substance-related disorders are diagnosed more commonly in men than in women, but the gender ratios vary with the class of the substance.

Codependency is described in this chapter, as are aspects of treatment for the disorder. The issue of substance impairment within the profession of nursing is also explored. Nursing care for individuals with substance use and addictive disorders is presented in the context of the six steps of the nursing process. Various medical and other treatment modalities are also discussed.

Substance Use Disorder, Defined

CORE CONCEPT
Addiction
A compulsive or chronic requirement. The need is so strong as to generate distress (either physical or psychological) if left unfulfilled.

Substance Addiction

The *Diagnostic and Statistical Manual of Mental Disorders, Fifth Edition (DSM-5)* (American Psychiatric Association [APA], 2013) lists diagnostic criteria for addiction to specific substances, including alcohol, cannabis, hallucinogens, inhalants, opioids, sedative-hypnotics, stimulants, and tobacco. Individuals are considered to have a substance use disorder when use of the substance interferes with their ability to fulfill role obligations, such as at work, school, or home. Often the individual would like to cut down or control use of the substance, but attempts fail, and use of the substance continues to increase. There is an intense craving for the substance, and an excessive amount of time is spent trying to procure more of the substance or recover from the effects of its use. Use of the substance causes problems with interpersonal relationships, and the individual may become socially isolated. Individuals with substance use disorders often participate in hazardous activities when they are impaired by the substance and continue to use the substance despite knowing that its use is contributing to a physical or psychosocial problem. Addiction is evident when tolerance develops and the amount required to achieve the desired effect continues to increase. A syndrome of symptoms, characteristic of the specific substance, occurs when the individual with the addiction attempts to discontinue use of the substance.

Substance-Induced Disorders, Defined

CORE CONCEPT
Intoxication
A state of disturbance in cognition, perception, behavior, level of consciousness, judgment, and other functions that is directly attributable to the effects of a psychoactive drug. It may be marked by a physical and mental state of exhilaration and emotional frenzy or lethargy and stupor.

Substance Intoxication

Substance intoxication is defined as the development of a reversible syndrome of symptoms following excessive use of a substance. The symptoms are drug-specific and occur during or shortly after the ingestion of the substance. There is a direct effect on the CNS, and a disruption in physical and psychological functioning occurs. Judgment is disturbed, resulting in inappropriate and maladaptive behavior, and social and occupational functioning are impaired.

Substance Withdrawal

Substance withdrawal occurs upon abrupt reduction or discontinuation of a substance that has been used regularly over a prolonged period. The substance-specific syndrome includes clinically significant physical signs and symptoms as well as psychological changes such as disturbances in thinking, feeling, and behavior.

CORE CONCEPT
Withdrawal
The physiological and mental readjustment that accompanies the discontinuation of an addictive substance.

Classes of Psychoactive Substances

The following classes of psychoactive substances are associated with substance use and substance-induced disorders:

1. Alcohol
2. Caffeine
3. Cannabis
4. Hallucinogens
5. Inhalants
6. Opioids
7. Sedative-hypnotics
8. Stimulants
9. Tobacco (nicotine)

Predisposing Factors to Substance-Related Disorders

A number of factors have been implicated in the predisposition to abuse of substances. At present, there is no single theory that can adequately explain the etiology of this problem. No doubt the interaction between various elements forms a complex collection of determinants that influence a person's susceptibility to abuse substances.

Biological Factors

Genetics

Hereditary factors appear to be involved in the development of substance use disorders, especially alcoholism. Children of alcoholics are four times more likely than other children to become alcoholics (American Academy of Child and Adolescent Psychiatry, 2015). Studies of monozygotic and dizygotic twins have demonstrated that monozygotic (one egg, genetically identical) twins have a higher rate for concordance of alcoholism than dizygotic (two eggs, genetically nonidentical) twins (Schuckit, 2017). Furthermore, biological offspring of alcoholic parents have a significantly greater incidence of alcoholism than offspring of nonalcoholic parents whether the child was reared by the biological parents or by nonalcoholic adoptive parents (Schuckit, 2017). Although there is no single factor that determines whether someone will develop a substance use disorder, scientists estimate that genetics accounts for 40 to 60 percent of a person's vulnerability (National Institute on Drug Abuse [NIDA], 2018a). Some of this vulnerability may be related to heritable personality traits, such as high novelty seeking and low harm avoidance, both of which have been linked to substance use disorders (Iannucci & Weiss, 2017). Other variables include lifestyle influences such as diet, exercise, and types of social activities (e.g., frequency of engaging in social activities that include regular substance use).

Biochemical

There is good evidence that changes in brain structure and brain neurochemistry occur in the process of addiction, but whether these changes wholly explain etiology remains controversial. Alcohol has demonstrated effects on almost all neurotransmitters, but those most strongly linked to substance abuse include opioid, catecholamine (especially dopamine), glutamate (especially those binding to N-methyl-D-aspartate [NMDA]), and gamma-aminobutyric acid (GABA) systems (Sadock, Sadock, & Ruiz, 2015). Once activated, the neuronal pathways that are responsible for sensing pleasure and reward are believed to be responsible for pleasurable sensations associated with addictive substances as well as creating a "memory" that triggers desire for repeated use of the substance. These pathways are referred to as the *brain-reward circuitry*. Over time, the brain tries to compensate for this excessive activation by lowering levels of these neurotransmitters, and the result is that an individual begins to feel sick. At this point, the substance user may be drawn to continue use of the substance simply to feel less sick. Skeptics of the biochemical theories of addiction argue that because substance-dependent individuals have the capacity to change their behavior, addiction is more likely a complex interaction of several factors than strictly a single biochemical process. While ongoing research will continue to shed light on specific mechanisms in addiction, both the American Society of Addiction Medicine (ASAM, 2015) and the Surgeon General (U.S. Department of Health and Human Services [HHS], 2016) agree that addiction is a disease of the brain.

Psychological Factors

Developmental Influences

The psychodynamic approach to the etiology of substance abuse focuses on a punitive superego and fixation at the oral stage of psychosexual development (Sadock et al., 2015). Thus, individuals with punitive superegos turn to drugs to diminish unconscious anxiety and increase feelings of power and self-worth. Sadock and colleagues (2015) state, "As a form of self-medication, alcohol may be used to control panic, opioids to diminish anger, and amphetamines to alleviate depression" (pp. 619–620).

Personality Factors

Certain personality traits have been associated with an increased tendency toward addictive behavior. Some clinicians believe that low self-esteem, frequent depression, passivity, antisocial personality traits, high risk-taking traits, the inability to relax or to defer gratification, and the inability to communicate effectively are common in individuals who abuse substances. These personality characteristics cannot be called *predictive* of addictive behavior, yet for reasons not completely understood, they have been found to accompany addiction in many instances. In some cases, the substance user may be self-medicating to treat symptoms of depression or anxiety.

Cognitive Factors

Irrational thinking patterns have long been identified as a problem that is central in addictions. Whether these thought patterns contribute to the development or simply perpetuate an existing addiction is an unanswered question, but their influence is widely accepted. Twerski (1997) describes these thought patterns as "addictive thinking" and suggests that when these thought patterns are unchallenged, they may culminate in additional addictions (drugs, sex, gambling, etc.) even when a person stops using the substance to which he or she first became addicted. Some examples of irrational thinking patterns often associated with addiction include denial ("I'm not really addicted"), projection ("It's my wife's fault that I take drugs"), and rationalization ("I have to take drugs because I am in pain"). Exploring these thought patterns and their influence on problematic behavior, which is the basis of cognitive behavior therapy (CBT), has been identified as beneficial in addictions treatment (NIDA, 2018b).

Sociocultural Factors

Social Learning

The effects of modeling, imitation, and identification on behavior can be observed from early childhood onward. The family appears to be an important influence in individuals with substance use disorders. Various studies have shown that children and adolescents are more likely to use substances if they have parents who provide a model for substance use. Peers often exert a great deal of influence in the life of the child or adolescent who is being encouraged to use substances for the first time. Modeling may continue to be a factor in the use of substances once the individual enters the workforce, particularly if the work setting provides plenty of leisure time with coworkers and drinking is valued as a way to express group cohesiveness.

Conditioning

Conditioning is a learned response that occurs after repeated exposure to a stimulus. Substance abuse can become a learned response from the substance itself as well as from the environment where use occurs. Many substances create a pleasurable experience that encourages the user to repeat it; thus, it is the intrinsically reinforcing properties of addictive drugs that "condition" the individual to repeatedly seek out their use.

The environment in which the substance is taken also contributes to the reinforcement. If the environment is pleasurable, substance use is usually increased. In addition, as the substance induces a state of pleasure, the user may begin to associate that environment with these feelings and thus with drug use. Aversive stimuli within an environment are thought to be associated with a decrease in substance use within that environment.

Cultural and Ethnic Influences

Factors within an individual's culture may contribute to establishing patterns of substance use by molding attitudes, influencing patterns of consumption based on cultural acceptance, and determining the availability of the substance. However, it is important to remember that a person's risk for addiction is multifaceted and cannot be tied solely to ethnic or cultural factors. For centuries, the French and Italians have considered wine an essential part of the family meal, even for the children. The incidence of alcohol addiction is low, and acute intoxication from alcohol is not common. Conversely, alcohol problems in Ireland, where alcohol is a part of the social culture and pubs are considered a hub for social activity, are among the highest internationally; the National Alcohol Diary Survey (Alcohol Action Ireland, 2018) found that 54 percent of the population were classified as harmful drinkers.

Some races and ethnic groups (notably Asian or Native American individuals) have a higher risk for genetic variations that affect the activity of isoenzymes involved in alcohol metabolism. These changes cause alcohol to be converted quickly to acetaldehyde as well as a decrease in the rate at which acetaldehyde is oxidized. As a result of these changes, acetaldehyde rapidly accumulates in the body, producing unpleasant symptoms such as flushing, headaches, nausea, and palpitations when alcohol is consumed (Hanley, 2017). However, whether these genetic variations influence higher or lower prevalence of substance use disorders is unclear.

The Dynamics of Substance-Related Disorders

Alcohol Use Disorder

Profile of the Substance

Alcohol is a natural substance formed by the reaction of fermenting sugar with yeast spores. Although there are many alcohols, the type in alcoholic beverages is known scientifically as ethyl alcohol and chemically as C_2H_5OH. Its abbreviation, ETOH, is sometimes seen in medical records and in various other documents and publications.

By strict definition, alcohol is classified as a food because it contains calories; however, it has no nutritional value. Different alcoholic beverages are produced by using different sources of sugar for the fermentation process. For example, beer is made from malted barley, wine from grapes or berries, whiskey from malted grains, and rum from molasses. Distilled beverages (e.g., whiskey, scotch, gin, vodka, and other "hard" liquors) derive their name from further concentration of the alcohol through a process called *distillation.*

The alcohol content varies by type of beverage. For example, most American beers contain 3 to 6 percent alcohol, wines average 10 to 20 percent, and distilled beverages range from 40 to 50 percent alcohol. The average-sized drink, regardless of beverage, contains a similar amount of alcohol. That is, 12 ounces of beer, 3 to 5 ounces of wine, and a cocktail with 1 ounce of whiskey all contain approximately 0.5 ounce of alcohol. If consumed at the same rate, they all would have an equivalent effect on the body.

Alcohol exerts a depressant effect on the CNS, resulting in behavioral and mood changes. The effects of alcohol on the CNS are proportional to the alcoholic concentration in the blood. Most states consider that an individual is legally intoxicated with a blood alcohol level of 0.08 percent.

The body burns alcohol at the rate of about 0.5 ounce per hour, so behavioral changes would not be expected to occur in an individual who slowly consumed only one average-sized drink per hour. Other factors do influence these effects, however, such as individual size and whether or not the stomach contains food at the time the alcohol is consumed. Alcohol is also thought to have a more profound effect when an individual is emotionally stressed or fatigued.

Most alcohol is metabolized in the liver, and the outcome of this process is the production of acetaldehyde. Acetaldehyde is then broken down by aldehyde dehydrogenase. Increased exposure to acetaldehyde leads to CNS depression, and prolonged exposure is associated with many detrimental health effects. At high levels, acetaldehyde causes the release of histamines and catecholamines, which can affect blood pressure and produce flushing, nausea, and vomiting. Although acetaldehyde oxidation generally occurs rapidly, in individuals who have genetic variations that affect alcohol dehydrogenase and aldehyde dehydrogenase, the process occurs more slowly, which may result in negative physical reactions to alcohol. These genetic variations are more common in Asian (Japanese, Chinese, and Korean) individuals (Schuckit, 2017).

Historical Aspects

The use of alcohol can be traced back to the Neolithic age. Beer and wine are known to have been used around 6400 B.C. With the introduction of distillation by the Arabs in the Middle Ages, alchemists believed that alcohol was the answer to all of their ailments. The word *whiskey,* meaning "water of life," became widely known.

In America, American Indian and Alaska Native (AI/AN) peoples had been drinking beer and wine prior to the arrival of the first white immigrants. Refinement of the distillation process made beverages with high alcohol content readily available. By the early 1800s, one renowned physician of the time, Benjamin Rush, had begun to identify the widespread excessive, chronic alcohol consumption as a disease and an addiction. The strong religious mores on which the United States was founded soon led to the Temperance movement, which sought to prohibit the sale of alcoholic beverages. By the middle of the 19th century, 13 states had passed prohibition laws. The most widespread prohibition of alcohol in the United States was from 1920 to 1933. The mandatory restrictions on national social habits resulted in the creation of profitable underground markets, which in turn led to flourishing criminal enterprises. On the other hand, millions of dollars in federal, state, and local revenues from taxes and import duties on alcohol were lost when alcohol was illegal. Still, economic losses are difficult to justify when measured against the current prevalence of physical illness, injury, and loss of life secondary to alcohol abuse in the United States today.

Patterns of Use

About two-thirds (66.6%) of Americans aged 12 years and older report being current drinkers of alcohol and 6.4 percent meet criteria for alcohol use disorder (Substance Abuse and Mental Health Services Administration [SAMHSA], 2017). Studies of drinking patterns in the United States show that people use alcoholic beverages to enhance the flavor of food with meals; at social gatherings to encourage relaxation and conviviality among the guests; and to promote a feeling of celebration at special occasions such as weddings, birthdays, and anniversaries. An alcoholic beverage (wine) is also used as part of the sacred ritual in some religious ceremonies. Therapeutically, alcohol is the major ingredient in many over-the-counter and prescription medicines that are prepared in concentrated form. Therefore, alcohol can be harmless and enjoyable—sometimes even beneficial—if it is used responsibly and in moderation.

However, like any other mind-altering drug, alcohol has the potential for abuse. Alcohol is the third most commonly misused substance in the United States today, second only to prescription drugs followed by marijuana (SAMHSA, 2017). Annually, 88,000 deaths are related to excessive alcohol use, and it is the third-leading lifestyle-related cause of death in the United States (National Council on Alcoholism and Drug Dependence, 2015). In addition, it is a factor in more than one-half of all homicides, suicides, and traffic accidents. Incidents of domestic violence are commonly alcohol related. Heavy drinking contributes to illness in each of the top three causes of death: heart disease, cancer, and stroke. It is estimated that up to 40 percent of hospital beds in the United States are being used to treat health conditions related to alcohol consumption. Fetal alcohol syndrome, caused by prenatal exposure to alcohol, is the leading known cause of intellectual disability in the United States (Vaux, 2016).

Development of an Alcohol Use Disorder

Jellinek's classic work (1952) outlined four phases through which the pattern of drinking progresses to becoming an alcohol use disorder (commonly referred to as alcoholism). Some variability among individuals is to be expected within this model of progression.

Phase I. Prealcoholic Phase

This phase is characterized by the use of alcohol for its effects in relieving the everyday stress and tensions of life. As a child, the individual may have observed parents or other adults drinking alcohol and enjoying the effects; societally the individual learns that use of alcohol is an acceptable method of coping with stress. Tolerance develops, and the amount required to achieve the desired effect increases steadily.

Phase II. Early Alcoholic Phase

This phase begins with blackouts—brief periods of amnesia that occur during or immediately following a period of drinking. Now the alcohol is no longer a source of pleasure or relief for the individual but rather a drug that is *required* by the individual. Common behaviors include sneaking drinks or secret drinking, preoccupation with drinking and maintaining the supply of alcohol, rapid gulping of drinks, and further blackouts. The individual feels enormous guilt and becomes very defensive about his or her drinking. Excessive use of denial and rationalization is evident.

Phase III. Crucial Phase

In this phase, the individual has lost control, and physiological addiction is clearly evident. This loss of control has been described as the inability to choose whether or not to drink. Binge drinking, lasting from a few hours to several weeks, is common. These episodes are characterized by sickness, loss of consciousness, squalor, and degradation. In this phase, the individual is extremely ill. Anger and aggression are common manifestations. Drinking is the total focus, and he or she is willing to risk losing everything that was once important, in an effort to maintain the addiction. By this phase of the illness, it is not uncommon for the individual to have experienced the loss of job, marriage, family, friends, and most especially, self-respect.

Phase IV. Chronic Phase

This phase is characterized by emotional and physical disintegration. The individual is usually intoxicated more than he or she is sober. Emotional disintegration is evidenced by profound helplessness and self-pity. Impairment in reality testing may result in psychosis. Life-threatening physical manifestations may be evident in virtually every system of the body. Unmanaged withdrawal from alcohol results in a terrifying syndrome of symptoms that include hallucinations, tremors, convulsions, severe agitation, and panic. Depression and ideas of suicide are not uncommon. For long-term, heavy drinkers, abrupt withdrawal of alcohol can be fatal.

Effects on the Body

Alcohol can induce a general, nonselective, reversible depression of the CNS. About 20 percent of a single dose of alcohol is absorbed directly and immediately into the bloodstream through the stomach wall. Unlike other "foods," alcohol does not have to be digested. The blood carries alcohol directly to the brain where it acts on the brain's central control areas, slowing or depressing brain activity. The other 80 percent of the alcohol in one drink is processed only slightly more slowly through the upper intestinal tract and into the bloodstream. Only moments after alcohol is consumed, it can be found in all tissues, organs, and secretions of the body. Rapidity of absorption is influenced by various factors. For example, absorption is delayed when the drink is sipped rather than gulped, when the stomach contains food rather than being empty, and when the drink is wine or beer rather than distilled beverages.

At low doses, alcohol produces relaxation, loss of inhibitions, lack of concentration, drowsiness, slurred speech, and sleep. Chronic abuse results in multisystem physiological impairments. These complications include (but are not limited to) those outlined in the following sections.

Peripheral Neuropathy

Peripheral neuropathy, characterized by peripheral nerve damage, results in pain, burning, tingling, or prickly sensations of the extremities. Researchers believe that it is the direct result of deficiencies in the B vitamins, particularly thiamine. Nutritional deficiencies are common in chronic alcoholics because of insufficient intake of nutrients as well as the toxic effect of alcohol that results in malabsorption of nutrients. The process is often reversible with abstinence from alcohol and restoration of nutritional deficiencies, but for some individuals, pain and numbness may be permanent (Schuckit, 2017). With chronic alcohol use permanent muscle wasting and paralysis can occur.

Alcoholic Myopathy

Alcoholic myopathy may occur as an acute or chronic condition. In the acute condition, also called *alcoholic necrotizing myopathy* or *alcoholic rhabdomyolysis,* the individual experiences a sudden onset of muscle pain, swelling, and weakness along with myoglobinuria evidenced by a red tinge in the urine. Creatine kinase may be elevated before the appearance of symptoms. Experimental studies have suggested that alcohol use and malnourishment are necessary to produce this syndrome (Lanska, 2017). Muscle symptoms are usually generalized, but pain and swelling may selectively involve the calves or other muscle groups. Laboratory studies show elevations of the enzymes creatine phosphokinase (CPK), lactate dehydrogenase (LDH), aldolase, and aspartate aminotransferase (AST). The symptoms of chronic alcoholic myopathy include a gradual wasting and weakness in skeletal muscles. Neither the pain and tenderness nor the elevated muscle enzymes seen in acute myopathy are evident in the chronic condition.

Alcoholic myopathy is thought to be a result of the same B vitamin deficiency that contributes to peripheral neuropathy and to the general injurious effects of acetaldehyde. Improvement is observed with abstinence from alcohol and the return to a nutritious diet with vitamin supplements.

Wernicke's Encephalopathy

Wernicke's encephalopathy represents the most serious form of thiamine deficiency in alcoholics. Symptoms include paralysis of the ocular muscles, diplopia, ataxia, somnolence, and stupor. If thiamine replacement therapy is not undertaken quickly, death will ensue.

Korsakoff's Psychosis

Korsakoff's psychosis is identified by a syndrome of confusion, loss of recent memory, and confabulation in alcoholics. It is frequently encountered in clients recovering from Wernicke's encephalopathy. In the United States, the two disorders are usually considered together and are called *Wernicke-Korsakoff syndrome.* Treatment is with parenteral or oral thiamine replacement.

Alcoholic Cardiomyopathy

The effect of alcohol on the heart is an accumulation of lipids in the myocardial cells, resulting in enlargement and a weakened condition. The clinical findings of alcoholic cardiomyopathy generally relate to congestive heart failure or arrhythmia. Symptoms include decreased exercise tolerance, tachycardia, dyspnea, edema, palpitations, and nonproductive cough. Laboratory studies may show elevation of the enzymes CPK, AST, alanine aminotransferase (ALT), and LDH. Changes may be observed by electrocardiogram, and congestive heart failure may be evident on chest x-ray films.

Treatment involves total, permanent abstinence from alcohol. Specific treatment of the congestive heart failure may include rest, oxygen, digitalization, sodium restriction, and diuretics. Prognosis is encouraging if treated in the early stages. The death rate is high for individuals with advanced symptomatology.

Esophagitis

Esophagitis—inflammation and pain in the esophagus—occurs because of the toxic effects of alcohol on the esophageal mucosa. It also occurs because of frequent vomiting associated with alcohol abuse.

Gastritis

The effects of alcohol on the stomach include inflammation of the stomach lining characterized by epigastric distress, nausea, vomiting, and distention. Alcohol breaks down the stomach's protective mucosal barrier, allowing hydrochloric acid to erode the stomach wall. Damage to blood vessels may result in hemorrhage.

Pancreatitis

Pancreatitis may be categorized as *acute* or *chronic.* Acute pancreatitis usually occurs 1 or 2 days after a binge of excessive alcohol consumption. Symptoms include constant, severe epigastric pain; nausea and vomiting; and abdominal distention. Chronic pancreatitis leads to pancreatic insufficiency, resulting in steatorrhea, malnutrition, weight loss, and diabetes mellitus.

Alcoholic Hepatitis

Alcoholic hepatitis is inflammation of the liver caused by long-term heavy alcohol use. Clinical manifestations include an enlarged and tender liver, nausea and vomiting, lethargy, anorexia, elevated white blood cell count, fever, and jaundice. **Ascites** and weight loss may be evident in more severe cases. With treatment—which includes strict abstinence from alcohol, proper nutrition, and rest—the individual can experience complete recovery. Severe cases can lead to cirrhosis or **hepatic encephalopathy.**

Cirrhosis of the Liver

Cirrhosis of the liver may be caused by anything that results in chronic injury to the liver. It is the end-stage of alcoholic liver disease and results from long-term chronic alcohol abuse. There is widespread destruction of liver cells, which are replaced by fibrous (scar) tissue. Clinical manifestations include nausea and vomiting, anorexia, weight loss, abdominal pain, jaundice, edema, anemia, and blood coagulation abnormalities. Treatment includes abstention from alcohol, correction of malnutrition, and supportive care to prevent complications of the disease. Complications of cirrhosis include the following:

- **Portal hypertension:** Elevation of blood pressure through the portal circulation results from defective blood flow through the cirrhotic liver.
- **Ascites:** Ascites, a condition in which an excessive amount of serous fluid accumulates in the abdominal cavity, occurs in response to portal hypertension. The increased pressure results in the seepage of fluid from the surface of the liver into the abdominal cavity.
- **Esophageal varices: Esophageal varices** are veins in the esophagus that become distended because of excessive pressure from defective blood flow through the cirrhotic liver. As this pressure increases, these varicosities can rupture, resulting in hemorrhage and sometimes death.
- **Hepatic encephalopathy:** This serious complication occurs in response to the inability of the diseased liver to convert ammonia to urea for excretion. The continued rise in serum ammonia results in progressively impaired mental functioning, apathy, euphoria or depression, sleep disturbance, increasing confusion, and progression to coma and eventual death. Treatment includes complete abstention from alcohol; reduction of protein in the diet; reduction of intestinal ammonia using neomycin, rifaximin, or lactulose; and treatment of electrolyte imbalances (sodium and potassium), kidney failure, and infections (National Library of Medicine, 2017).

Leukopenia

The production, function, and movement of the white blood cells are impaired in chronic alcoholics. This condition, called *leukopenia*, places the individual at high risk for contracting infectious diseases and for complicated recovery.

Thrombocytopenia

Platelet production and survival are impaired as a result of the toxic effects of alcohol. Thrombocytopenia places the alcoholic at risk for hemorrhage. Abstinence from alcohol rapidly reverses this deficiency.

Sexual Dysfunction

Alcohol interferes with the normal production and maintenance of female and male hormones, and long-term alcohol use can interfere with the liver's ability to metabolize estrogenic compounds (Sadock et al., 2015). For women, this can mean changes in the menstrual cycle and a decreased or loss of ability to become pregnant. For men, the altered hormone levels result in a diminished libido, decreased sexual performance, and impaired fertility, and gynecomastia may develop secondary to testicular atrophy.

Use During Pregnancy

Fetal Alcohol Syndrome

Prenatal exposure to alcohol can result in a broad range of disorders to the fetus, known as fetal alcohol spectrum disorders (FASDs), the most common of which is fetal alcohol syndrome (FAS). Fetal alcohol syndrome includes physical, mental, behavioral, and/or learning disabilities with lifelong implications. There may be problems with learning, memory, attention span, communication, vision, hearing, or a combination of these (Centers for Disease Control and Prevention [CDC], 2018). Other FASDs include alcohol-related neurodevelopmental disorder (ARND) and alcohol-related birth defects (ARBD).

No amount of alcohol during pregnancy is considered safe, and alcohol can damage a fetus at any stage of pregnancy (CDC, 2018; Vaux, 2016). Therefore, drinking alcohol should be avoided by women who are pregnant and by women who could become pregnant. Estimates of the prevalence of FAS range from 0.2 to 1.5 per 1,000 live births, and studies of school-aged children estimate the prevalence to be as high as 5 percent of the population (CDC, 2018). Vaux (2016) adds that FAS crosses all races and ethnic groups. The common feature in the development

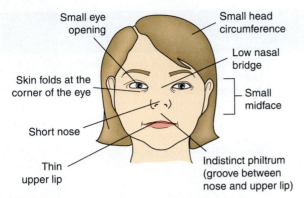

FIGURE 14–1 Facial features of fetal alcohol syndrome. (From the National Institute of Alcohol Abuse and Alcoholism of the National Institutes of Health, Washington, DC.)

Small eye opening

Small head circumference

Low nasal bridge

Skin folds at the corner of the eye

Small midface

Short nose

Thin upper lip

Indistinct philtrum (groove between nose and upper lip)

of FAS is women who drink heavily during pregnancy. Maier and West (2013) state:

> The number of women who engage in heavy alcohol consumption during pregnancy surpasses the total number of children diagnosed with either FAS or ARND, meaning that not every child whose mother drank alcohol during pregnancy develops FAS or ARND. Moreover, the degree to which people with FAS or ARND are impaired differs from person to person. Several factors may contribute to this variation in the consequences of maternal drinking.
>
> These factors include, but are not limited to, the following:
>
>   ▪ Maternal drinking pattern
>   ▪ Differences in maternal metabolism
>   ▪ Differences in genetic susceptibility
>   ▪ Timing of the alcohol consumption during pregnancy
>   ▪ Variation in the vulnerability of different brain regions

Sadock and colleagues (2015) report that women with alcohol-related disorders have a 35 percent risk of having a child with defects. Children with FAS may have the following characteristics or exhibit the following behaviors (CDC, 2018:

■ Abnormal facial features (Fig. 14–1)
■ Small head size
■ Shorter-than-average height
■ Low body weight
■ Poor coordination
■ Hyperactive behavior
■ Difficulty paying attention
■ Poor memory
■ Difficulty in school
■ Learning disabilities
■ Speech and language delays

■ Intellectual disability or low IQ
■ Poor reasoning and judgment skills
■ Sleep and sucking problems as a baby
■ Vision or hearing problems
■ Problems with the heart, kidneys, or bones

Neuroimaging of children with FAS shows abnormalities in the size and shape of their brains. The frontal lobes and cerebellum are often smaller than normal, and the corpus callosum and basal ganglia are commonly affected. Studies show that children with FAS are often at risk for psychiatric disorders, most commonly attention deficit-hyperactivity disorder (Vaux, 2016). FAS may also co-occur with mood disorders, anxiety disorders, eating disorders, reactive attachment disorder, and conduct disorder (Elias, 2013).

Children with FAS require lifelong care and treatment. There is no cure for FAS, but it can be prevented. The Collaborative for Alcohol-Free Pregnancy, a joint effort of the CDC along with FASD Practice and Implementation Centers and National Partners (CDC, 2018), stresses the importance of using evidence-based tools such as alcohol screening and brief intervention (SBI) to prevent alcohol-exposed pregnancy and risky alcohol use. Nurses who work with women of childbearing age or who are pregnant can play a vital role in ensuring that this type of screening is conducted. Online training and resources for nurses and other healthcare professionals are available at https://nccd.cdc.gov/FASD/

Alcohol Intoxication

Symptoms of alcohol intoxication include disinhibition of sexual or aggressive impulses, mood lability, impaired judgment, impaired social or occupational functioning, slurred speech, incoordination, unsteady gait, nystagmus, and flushed face. Intoxication usually occurs at blood alcohol levels between 100 and 200 mg/dL. Death has been reported at levels ranging from 400 to 700 mg/dL.

Alcohol Withdrawal

Within 4 to 12 hours of cessation of or reduction in heavy and prolonged (several days or longer) alcohol use, the following withdrawal symptoms may appear: coarse tremor of hands, tongue, or eyelids; nausea or vomiting; malaise or weakness; tachycardia; sweating; elevated blood pressure; anxiety; depressed mood or irritability; transient hallucinations or illusions; headache; and insomnia. In about 1 percent of alcoholic patients, complicated withdrawal syndrome may progress to *alcohol withdrawal delirium* (Sadock et al., 2015). Concomitant medical problems may increase the risk.

TABLE 14–1	Sedative, Hypnotic, and Anxiolytic Drugs	
CATEGORIES	**GENERIC (TRADE) NAMES**	**COMMON STREET NAMES**
Barbiturates	Amobarbital (Amytal) Pentobarbital (Nembutal) Secobarbital (Seconal) Butabarbital (Butisol) Phenobarbital Mephobarbital (Mebaral)	Bluebirds; blue angels (amobarbital); yellow jackets; yellow birds (pentobarbital); GBs; red birds; red devils (secobarbital)
Nonbarbiturate hypnotics	Chloral hydrate Diphenhydramine Estazolam Flurazepam Temazepam (Restoril) Triazolam (Halcion) Quazepam (Doral) Eszoplicone (Lunesta) Ramelteon (Rozerem) Zaleplon (Sonata) Zolpidem (Ambien)	Peter, Mickey (chloral hydrate); sleepers
Antianxiety agent	Alprazolam (Xanax) Chlordiazepoxide (Librium) Clonazepam (Klonopin) Clorazepate (Tranxene) Diazepam (Valium) Lorazepam (Ativan) Oxazepam (Serax) Meprobamate (Miltown)	Green and whites, roaches (Librium); candy, downers (benzodiazepines); Vs (Valium; color designates strength); dolls, dollies (meprobamate)
Club drugs	Flunitrazepam (Rohypnol) Gamma hydroxybutyric acid (gamma hydroxybutyrate; GHB)	Date-rape drug; roofies, R-2, rope (Rohypnol); G, liquid X, grievous bodily harm, easy lay (GHB)

Onset of delirium is usually on the second or third day following cessation of or reduction in prolonged, heavy alcohol use. Symptoms include those described under the syndrome of delirium (Chapter 13, Neurocognitive Disorders).

Sedative, Hypnotic, or Anxiolytic Use Disorder

Profile of the Substance

The sedative, hypnotic, and anxiolytic compounds are drugs of diverse chemical structures that are all capable of inducing varying degrees of CNS depression, from tranquilizing relief of anxiety to anesthesia, coma, and even death. They are generally categorized as (1) barbiturates, (2) nonbarbiturate hypnotics, and (3) antianxiety agents. Effects produced by these substances depend on size of dose and potency of drug administered.

Table 14–1 presents a selected list of drugs included in these categories. Generic names are followed in parentheses by the trade names. Common street names for each category are also included.

Several principles have been identified that apply fairly uniformly to all CNS depressants:

1. **The effects of CNS depressants are additive with one another and with the behavioral state of the user.** For example, when these drugs are used in combination with each other or in combination with alcohol, the depressive effects are compounded. These intense depressive effects are often unpredictable and can even be fatal. Similarly, a person who is mentally depressed or physically fatigued may have an exaggerated response to a dose of the drug that would only slightly affect a person in a normal or excited state. The U.S. Food and Drug Administration (FDA, 2016) began requiring black-box warnings, its strongest warning label, for opioid analgesics, opioid cough products, and benzodiazepines based on evidence that the combination of opioids and

benzodiazepines carries a particularly high risk for excessive sleepiness, respiratory depression, coma, and death.

2. **CNS depressants are capable of producing physiological addiction.** If large doses of CNS depressants are repeatedly administered over a prolonged duration, a period of CNS hyperexcitability occurs on withdrawal of the drug. The response can be quite severe, even leading to convulsions and death.

3. **CNS depressants are capable of producing psychological addiction.** CNS depressants have the potential to generate within the individual a psychic drive for periodic or continuous administration of the drug to achieve a maximum level of functioning or feeling of well-being.

4. **Cross-tolerance and cross-dependence may exist between various CNS depressants.** Cross-tolerance refers to a condition in which an individual becomes resistant to the effects of one drug because he or she has developed tolerance to another drug with similar pharmacological activity. Cross-dependence is a condition in which an individual can become dependent on more than one substance because of their similar activity and effects.

Historical Aspects

Anxiety and insomnia, two of the most common human afflictions, were treated during the 19th century with opiates, bromide salts, chloral hydrate, paraldehyde, and alcohol (Julien, 2014). Because the opiates were known to produce physical addiction, bromides carried the risk of chronic bromide poisoning, and chloral hydrate and paraldehyde had an objectionable taste and smell, alcohol became the prescribed depressant drug of choice. However, some people refused to use alcohol either because they did not like the taste or for moral reasons, and others tended to take more than was prescribed. Therefore, a search for a better sedative drug continued.

Although barbituric acid was first synthesized in 1864, it was not until 1912 that phenobarbital was introduced into medicine as a sedative drug, the first of the structurally classified group of drugs called barbiturates (Julien, 2014). Since that time, more than 2,500 barbiturate derivatives have been synthesized, but, currently, fewer than a dozen remain in medical use. Illicit use of the drugs for recreational purposes grew throughout the 1930s and 1940s.

Efforts to create depressant medications that were not barbiturate derivatives accelerated. By the mid-1950s, the market for depressants had been expanded by the appearance of the nonbarbiturates glutethimide, ethchlorvynol, methyprylon, and meprobamate. Benzodiazepines were introduced around 1960 with the marketing of chlordiazepoxide (Librium), followed shortly by its derivative diazepam (Valium). The use of these drugs, and others within their group, grew very rapidly, and they are prescribed widely in medical practice. Their margin of safety is greater than that of barbiturates and the other nonbarbiturates. However, prolonged use of even moderate doses is likely to result in physical and psychological addiction with a characteristic syndrome of withdrawal that can be severe.

Patterns of Use

Sadock and colleagues (2015) reported that about 15 percent of all persons in the United States have had a benzodiazepine prescribed by a physician. Of all the drugs used in clinical practice, the sedative, hypnotic, and anxiolytic drugs are among the most widely prescribed.

Two patterns of addiction are described. The first pattern is one of an individual whose physician originally prescribed the CNS depressant as treatment for anxiety or insomnia. Independently, the individual has increased the dosage or frequency from that which was prescribed. Use of the medication is justified on the basis of treating symptoms, but as tolerance grows, more and more of the medication is required to produce the desired effect. Substance-seeking behavior is evident as the individual seeks prescriptions from several physicians in order to maintain sufficient supplies.

The second pattern involves young people in their teens or early 20s who, in the company of their peers, use substances that are obtained illegally. The initial objective is to achieve a feeling of euphoria. The drug is usually used intermittently during recreational gatherings. This pattern of intermittent use leads to regular use and extreme levels of tolerance. Combining use with other substances is not uncommon. Physical and psychological addiction leads to intense substance-seeking behaviors, most often through illegal channels.

Effects on the Body

The sedative, hypnotic, and anxiolytic compounds induce a general depressant effect; that is, they depress the activity of the brain, nerves, muscles, and heart tissue. They reduce the rate of metabolism in a variety of tissues throughout the body, and in general,

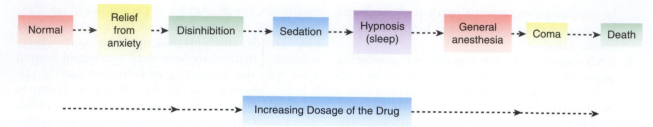

FIGURE 14–2 Continuum of CNS depression with increasing doses of sedative-hypnotic drugs.

they depress any system that uses energy. Large doses are required to produce these effects. In lower doses, these drugs appear to be more selective in their depressant actions by exerting their action on the centers within the brain that are concerned with arousal (e.g., the ascending reticular activating system, in the reticular formation, and the diffuse thalamic projection system).

As stated previously, these drugs are capable of producing all levels of CNS depression—from mild sedation to death. The level is determined by dosage and potency of the drug used. In Figure 14–2, a continuum demonstrates how increasing doses of the drugs affect the level of CNS depression.

Following is a discussion of the physiological effects of these medications.

Effects on Sleep and Dreaming

Barbiturate use decreases the amount of sleep time spent in dreaming. During drug withdrawal, dreaming becomes vivid and excessive. Rebound insomnia and increased dreaming (termed *REM rebound*) are not uncommon with abrupt withdrawal from long-term use of these drugs as sleeping aids.

Respiratory Depression

Barbiturates are capable of inhibiting the reticular activating system, resulting in respiratory depression, and can be lethal in overdose (Sadock et al., 2015). In addition, additive effects can occur with the concurrent use of other CNS depressants, also effecting a life-threatening situation.

Cardiovascular Effects

Hypotension may be a problem with large doses. Only a slight decrease in blood pressure is noted with normal oral dosage. High dosages of barbiturates also compromise cardiac contractility and vascular tone, which may result in cardiovascular collapse. Individuals with congestive heart failure are more susceptible to these effects (Lafferty, 2017).

Hepatic Effects

Barbiturates may produce jaundice with doses large enough to produce acute intoxication. Barbiturates stimulate the production of liver enzymes, resulting in a decrease in the plasma levels of both the barbiturates and other drugs metabolized in the liver. Preexisting liver disease may predispose an individual to additional liver damage with excessive barbiturate use.

Body Temperature

High doses of barbiturates can greatly decrease body temperature. Body temperature is not significantly altered with normal dosage levels.

Sexual Function

CNS depressants have a tendency to produce a biphasic response. There is an initial increase in libido, presumably from the primary disinhibitory effects of the drug. In men, this initial response is then followed by a decrease in the ability to maintain an erection.

Sedative, Hypnotic, or Anxiolytic Intoxication

The *DSM-5* (APA, 2013) describes sedative, hypnotic, or anxiolytic intoxication as the presence of clinically significant maladaptive behavioral or psychological changes that develop during or shortly after use of one of these substances. These maladaptive changes may include inappropriate sexual or aggressive behavior, mood lability, impaired judgment, or impaired social or occupational functioning. Other symptoms that may develop with excessive use of CNS depressants include slurred speech, incoordination, unsteady gait, nystagmus, impairment in attention or memory, and stupor or coma.

"Club drugs" in this category include gamma-hydroxybutyric acid (GHB) and flunitrazepam (Rohypnol). Like all of the depressants, they can produce a state of disinhibition, excitement, drunkenness, and amnesia. They have been widely implicated as "date rape" drugs, their presence being easily disguised in drinks. They produce anterograde amnesia, the inability to remember events experienced while under their influence.

Sedative, Hypnotic, or Anxiolytic Withdrawal

Withdrawal from sedatives, hypnotics, or anxiolytics produces a characteristic syndrome of symptoms that develops after a marked decrease in or cessation of heavy or prolonged intake (APA, 2013). Onset and duration of withdrawal symptoms depend on the half-life of the drug from which the individual is withdrawing. With short-acting sedative-hypnotics (e.g., alprazolam, lorazepam), symptoms may begin between 12 and 24 hours after the last dose, reach peak intensity between 24 and 72 hours, and subside in 5 to 10 days. Withdrawal symptoms from substances with longer half-lives (e.g., diazepam, phenobarbital, chlordiazepoxide) may begin within 2 to 7 days, peak on the fifth to eighth day, and subside in 10 to 16 days.

Severe withdrawal is most likely to occur when a substance has been used at high dosages for prolonged periods. However, withdrawal symptoms also have been reported with moderate dosages taken over a relatively short duration. Withdrawal symptoms associated with sedative-hypnotics include autonomic hyperactivity (e.g., sweating or pulse rate greater than 100), increased hand tremor, insomnia, nausea or vomiting, hallucinations, illusions, depersonalization, psychomotor agitation, anxiety, grand mal seizures, and delirium.

Stimulant Use Disorder

Profile of the Substance

The CNS stimulants are identified by the behavioral stimulation and psychomotor agitation that they induce. They differ widely in their molecular structures and in their mechanisms of action. The amount of CNS stimulation caused by a certain drug depends on both the area in the brain or spinal cord that is affected by the drug and the cellular mechanism fundamental to the increased excitability. The *DSM-5* (APA, 2013) categorizes caffeine-related disorders and tobacco-related disorders as separate and distinct diagnoses. For purposes of this text, these substances are discussed with the stimulant-related disorders.

Groups within this category are classified according to similarities in mechanism of action. The *psychomotor stimulants* induce stimulation by augmentation or potentiation of the neurotransmitters norepinephrine, epinephrine, or dopamine. The *general cellular stimulants* (caffeine and nicotine) exert their action directly on cellular activity. Caffeine inhibits the enzyme phosphodiesterase, allowing increased levels of 3', 5'-cyclic adenosine monophosphate (cAMP), a chemical substance that promotes increased rates of cellular metabolism. Nicotine stimulates ganglionic synapses. This results in increased acetylcholine, which stimulates nerve impulse transmission to the entire autonomic nervous system. A selected list of drugs included in these categories is presented in Table 14–2.

The two most prevalent and widely used stimulants are caffeine and nicotine. Caffeine is readily available in every supermarket and grocery store as a common ingredient in coffee, tea, colas, and chocolate. Nicotine is the primary psychoactive substance found in tobacco products. When used in moderation, these stimulants tend to relieve fatigue and increase alertness. They are a generally accepted part of our culture; however, with increased social awareness regarding the health risks associated with tobacco products, their use has become stigmatized in some circles.

The more potent stimulants, because of their potential for physiological addiction, are under regulation by the Controlled Substances Act. These controlled stimulants are available for therapeutic purposes by prescription only; however, they are also clandestinely manufactured and widely distributed on the illicit market. More recently, the synthetic stimulants mephedrone, 3,4 methylenedioxypyrovalerone (MDPV), methylone, and others have become available, and because their chemical structures had been altered, they were not initially identifiable as a controlled substance or regulated by the federal government. Known as "bath salts," their street names include, among others, blue silk, cloud 9, ivory wave, vanilla sky, white knight, white lightning stardust, and purple wave. In October 2011, the U.S. Drug Enforcement Administration (DEA) issued emergency scheduling of these substances to make their possession and sales illegal (except as authorized by law). They are currently designated as Schedule I substances, the most restrictive category under the Controlled Substances Act. This action was taken in response to reports of episodes of violent behavior associated with use of the substance. Since then, another synthetic cathinone, alpha-PVP (commonly known as flakka, gravel, $5 insanity, or the zombie drug), whose chemical structure is similar but not identical to bath salts, began to surface in the United States. This drug can be snorted, injected, eaten, and vaporized for inhalation in e-cigarettes, for example. Vaporization is a particularly dangerous route

CATEGORIES	GENERIC (TRADE) NAMES	COMMON STREET NAMES
Amphetamines	Dextroamphetamine (Dexedrine)	Dexies, uppers, truck drivers
	Methamphetamine (Desoxyn)	Meth, speed, crystal, ice, crank, chalk, fire, glass
	3,4-Methylenedioxyamphetamine (MDMA)*	Adam, ecstasy, EVE, XTC
	Amphetamine + dextroamphetamine (Adderall)	Beanies, pep pills, speed, uppers, study buddies, smart pills
Synthetic stimulants	3,4-Methylenedioxypyrovalerone* (MDPV)	Bath salts (also called blue silk, cloud 9, ivory wave, vanilla sky, white lightning, white knight, and others)
	4-Methylmethcathinone (mephedrone, 4-MMC)*	
	Methylone*	
	Ethylone	
	Dibutylone	flakka, gravel
	Alpha-PVP	
Nonamphetamine stimulants	Phendimetrazine (Bontril)	Diet pills
	Benzphetamine (Didrex)	
	Diethylpropion (Tenuate)	
	Phentermine (Adipex-P; Ionamin)	
	Sibutramine (Meridia)†	
	Methylphenidate (Ritalin, Concerta)	Speed, uppers
	Dexmethylphenidate (Focalin)	
	Modafinil (Provigil)	
Cocaine	Cocaine hydrochloride	Coke, blow, toot, snow, lady, flake, crack
Caffeine	Coffee, tea, colas, chocolate	Java, mud, brew, cocoa
Nicotine	Cigarettes, cigars, pipe tobacco, snuff	Weeds, fags, butts, chaw, cancer sticks

TABLE 14–2 Central Nervous System (CNS) Stimulants

*Cross-listed with the hallucinogens.
†No longer marketed in the United States.

because of its immediate absorption, and deaths have been reported secondary to overdose, suicide, and heart attack. Flakka has been considered a particularly dangerous drug because of reports of violent aggression, homicide, and suicide related to its use. Flakka was considered a significant threat in the United States in 2014 and 2015, but no deaths were reported in 2016 after China (the singular provider of the drug) banned the production and exportation of alpha-PVP (Storrs, 2016). Although flakka use has diminished, flakka-related erratic behavior and sometimes criminal activity continues to surface in some areas of the United States. Storrs (2016) additionally reports that when one synthetic substance is banned, it is often replaced by another. For example, when China banned methylone (a drug similar to flakka, in 2014), it was replaced by ethylone; after ethylone was banned, a similar drug called dibutylone surfaced. This pattern creates an ongoing challenge for the FDA and DEA to identify and take action on each new synthetic substance as it comes to public attention (usually through significant health consequences or

deaths). New synthetic drugs may also be difficult to identify because standard drug screens do not recognize these chemicals.

Historical Aspects

Cocaine is the most potent stimulant derived from nature. It is extracted from the leaves of the coca plant, which has been cultivated in the Andean highlands of South America since prehistoric times. Natives of the region chew the leaves of the plant for refreshment and relief from fatigue.

The coca leaves must be mixed with lime to release the cocaine alkaloid. The chemical formula for the pure form of the drug was developed in 1960. Physicians began using the drug as an anesthetic in eye, nose, and throat surgeries. It has also been used therapeutically in the United States in a morphine-cocaine elixir designed to relieve the suffering associated with terminal illness. These therapeutic uses are now obsolete.

Cocaine has achieved a degree of acceptability within some social circles. It is illicitly distributed as a white crystalline powder, often mixed with other ingredients to increase its volume and thereby create more profits. The drug is most commonly "snorted," and chronic users may manifest symptoms that resemble the congested nose of a common cold. The intensely pleasurable effects of the drug create the potential for extraordinary psychological addiction.

Another form of cocaine commonly used in the United States is made by processing powdered cocaine with ammonia or sodium bicarbonate and water and heating it to remove the hydrochloride (Publishers Group, 2017). The term "crack," which is the street name for this form of the drug, refers to the crackling sound heard when the mixture is smoked. Because this type of cocaine can be easily vaporized and inhaled, its effects have an extremely rapid onset. See "Real People, Real Stories" to learn more about Alan's experience with crack cocaine and alcohol addiction.

Amphetamine was first produced in 1887. Various derivatives of the drug soon followed, and clinical use of the drug began in 1927. Amphetamines were used extensively for medical purposes through the 1960s, but recognition of their abuse potential has sharply decreased clinical use. Today, they are prescribed only to treat narcolepsy (a rare disorder resulting in an uncontrollable desire for sleep), hyperactivity disorders in children, and in certain cases of obesity. Clandestine production of amphetamines for distribution on the illicit market has become a thriving business. Methamphetamine can be smoked, snorted, injected, or taken orally. The effects include an intense rush from smoking or IV injection to a slower onset of euphoria as a result of snorting or oral ingestion. Another form of the drug, crystal methamphetamine, is produced by slowly recrystallizing powder methamphetamine from a solvent such as methanol, ethanol, isopropanol, or acetone (Publishers Group, 2017). It is a colorless, odorless, large-crystal form of d-methamphetamine and is commonly called "glass" or "ice" because of its appearance. Crystal meth is usually smoked in a glass pipe like crack cocaine.

Although methamphetamine use is widespread, particularly on college campuses, its use has perhaps been overshadowed by the nationwide opiate epidemic with its associated deaths. An alarming recent trend has been the increasing use of methamphetamines in combination with opiates. Ellis and associates, as cited by Dotinga, (2018) report that the use of crystal meth increased by 82 percent in the last decade and combined use of opioids and methamphetamine almost doubled during the same time period.

Ellis notes that individuals with opiate-use disorder sometimes use amphetamines to create a state of arousal to counteract the sedative effects of opiates. The use of combinations of drugs increases the risk for adverse effects and overdose. It also underscores the importance of assessing for multisubstance use in any individual presenting with substance use issues.

The earliest history of caffeine is unknown and is shrouded by legend and myth. Caffeine was first discovered in coffee in 1820 and in tea 7 years later. Both beverages have been widely accepted and enjoyed as a "pick-me-up" by many cultures.

Tobacco was used by the aborigines from remote times. Introduced in Europe in the mid-16th century, its use grew rapidly and soon became prevalent in Asia. Tobacco came to America with the settlement of the earliest colonies. Today, it is grown in many countries of the world, and although smoking is decreasing in most industrialized nations, it continues to be a serious problem in developing areas.

Patterns of Use

Because of their pleasurable effects, CNS stimulants have a high abuse potential. In 2014, approximately 1.5 million Americans were current cocaine users (SAMHSA, 2016a). Use was highest among Americans ages 18 to 25.

Many individuals who abuse or are addicted to CNS stimulants began using the substance for the appetite-suppressant effect in an attempt at weight control. Increasingly higher doses are consumed in an effort to maintain the pleasurable effects. With continued use, these pleasurable effects diminish as dysphoric effects increase. A persistent craving for the substance remains even in the face of unpleasant adverse effects from continued use.

CNS stimulant use is usually characterized by either episodic or chronic daily, or almost daily, use. Individuals who use the substances on an episodic basis often "binge" on the drug with very high dosages followed by a day or two of recuperation. This recuperation period is characterized by extremely intense and unpleasant symptoms, often called a "crash."

The daily user may take large or small doses and may use the drug several times a day or only at a specific time during the day. The amount consumed usually increases over time as tolerance develops. Chronic users tend to rely on CNS stimulants to feel more powerful, more confident, and more decisive. They often fall into a pattern of taking "uppers" in the morning and "downers," such as alcohol or sleeping pills, at night.

Real People, Real Stories: Alan Brunner on Substance Use Disorder

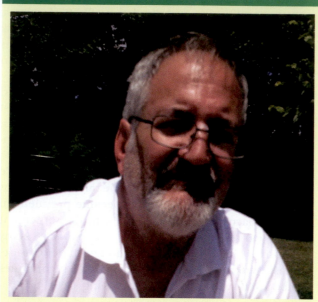

Substance use disorders often follow a progressive pattern that develops over a long period. Alan's story is an example of that process. See also Chapter 5, Relationship Development and Therapeutic Communication, for an interaction with Alan that incorporates motivational interviewing. Reflect on important issues for primary prevention education. Consider examples of interventions that are ineffective or unhealthy for the user and the care provider. Incorporate an understanding of codependency in this reflection.

Karyn: Tell me about when you first used drugs or alcohol.

Alan: I was 15 years old when I first started smoking pot and 16 when I had my first drink. The pot use went from occasional use to several times a week by the time I was a senior in high school. I knew that was a problem, but the drinking progressed much more gradually. For years, I only drank on weekends. For a while, my buddy and I would share a quart on the weekend. Eventually, we each had our own quart, then two quarts each. I only drank beer. Once when I was a teenager, I drank a fifth of vodka and I got extremely sick. My mom didn't try to rescue me or help me feel better or cover for me. I just had to live through the consequences, and that was probably a good thing; I never drank vodka again. But the beer drinking became more often and at higher amounts. Even so, it took another 35 years to recognize that it was a problem!

Karyn: Was there any history of alcoholism in your family?

Alan: Oh yeah . . . several relatives. My dad had a drinking problem, and that led to my parents divorcing when I was 14 years old. When I was 19, I moved in with my dad, and then I started drinking during the week, too—because

he did. My dad always worked and had a strong work ethic, even though he was a heavy drinker, so I thought, "As long as I'm able to drink and it's not interfering with work, then it's not a problem." I also remember thinking, "It's just beer, and I would never use the 'strong' or 'bad' drugs, like cocaine—I would NEVER do that."

Karyn: So your beer drinking increased while you were living with your father?

Alan: Initially, yes, but then I was surrounding myself with people and friends who liked to drink. I moved in with a friend, and we usually drank a case of beer each night. Then I started an auto repair business with a friend who was a heavy drinker, and we had beer at the shop. Pretty soon we weren't leaving the shop until all the beer was gone. Then I got involved with auto racing, and that was an environment with lots of alcohol and cocaine.

Karyn: I remember you said you were using cocaine. Is that when the use started?

Alan: No, actually I had become friends with a deacon at my church, probably because we both liked to drink. He was the one that introduced me to cocaine.

Karyn: So you started using cocaine along with drinking?

Alan: Yeah, even though I had said I would never do that. But I discovered that if I did cocaine, I had a lot more energy and I could stay awake longer, so I could be a much "better" drinker. (chuckles)

Karyn: Tell me about when you recognized that your use was a problem.

Alan: Well, eventually, I was drinking at home because it was a waste of "good drinking time" to get together with other people. So largely, I was sitting at home in the dark drinking by myself, and the beer never even made it into the fridge. The cocaine was putting me in the company of some very bad people. I knew I had to somehow get away from that . . . and when I started using cocaine, I said, "One thing I'll never do is crack," but then I started doing that, and that's when things completely fell apart.

Karyn: Fell apart?

Alan: I was racking up a lot of legal problems. I had some DUIs and reckless operation charges before that, but now I'm getting drug possession charges, paraphernalia charges, driving with a suspended license, driving with expired license plates, more DUIs, disorderly conduct charges. And the crack—that drug rips out your soul! You're always chasing the high that you got the first time you used it, and you never find that, so you keep using more. That's why one of my friends called crack "gotta" because you gotta have it. . . . And you don't care about ANYTHING else—you don't care if you die.

Karyn: You told me you've been clean and sober for seven years. How did you turn the corner?

Real People, Real Stories: Alan Brunner on Substance Use Disorder—cont'd

Alan: I had such a huge legal mess that my lawyer was recommending I just accept the jail time (3 to 10 days) and be done with it, but the judge offered treatment in lieu of jail, and I told him that's what I wanted because I knew I needed it. I was told, though, that if I violated the treatment program, I would spend a year in jail, so I knew I was taking a big risk by going into treatment. But I knew it was the only way out—and I knew I needed it.

Karyn: So what is your relapse prevention plan?

Alan: I have an AA sponsor, and I go to meetings sometimes, but not as often as I used to. I never allow myself to become too proud about my sobriety because I know all it would take is one drink. As long as I remember that, I'm vulnerable. . . . I don't get too cocky. I've also had a lot of support from family, especially my mom. She supported me every step of the way in treatment. Having supportive people around you is essential. The relationship I had been in for many years broke up largely because she was telling my counselors that she wanted me to cut down but she wasn't in favor of abstinence—she was quite a partier, too. Staying in that relationship, I believed (and my counselors believed), was putting my sobriety at risk.

Karyn: What do you think is important for healthcare providers to know or to do to help someone who has a substance use problem?

Alan: First of all, a person has to want help. You can't fix another person, and you can't help someone who doesn't want help.

Karyn: I agree, that is so important. I think healthcare providers (and family caregivers) are vulnerable sometimes to thinking they can fix any health problem, which can culminate in interventions that are ineffective and unhealthy for the user and for the care provider.

Alan: Yes, and I would also say that healthcare providers need to know how to recognize symptoms of problematic substance use.

Karyn: Like?

Alan: Like someone having "the shakes," someone not looking at you when they are answering questions, blaming other people for their circumstances and consequences, talking in circles. Don't ever ask someone, "Are you an alcoholic or a drug addict?" because we'll always say no unless we're in recovery—the denial is so strong. I also think not being too judgmental is important so you can find ways to open the door to discuss the issues. If someone is too "hard-nosed" and judgmental, I think it reinforces the denial. Asking a question like "Have you ever been drinking and couldn't remember events around that time?" is good because having blackouts is a good indication of an alcohol problem. You may not be able to "fix" someone but you can "plant seeds" and hope that the information and education will have an impact at some point. I think that's why people who are recovering themselves can be so effective as healthcare providers because they can share their own story of addiction and, since most people think they are completely unique, hearing someone else's story about having been in the same place you are now may turn on a light switch and help people recognize their own need for treatment.

The average American consumes two cups of coffee (about 200 mg of caffeine) per day. Caffeine is consumed in various amounts by about 90 percent of the population. At a level of 500 to 600 mg of daily caffeine consumption, symptoms of anxiety, insomnia, and depression are not uncommon. It is also at this level that caffeine dependence and withdrawal can occur. Caffeine consumption is prevalent among children as well as adults. Energy drinks have some of the highest caffeine contents of all beverages, and a Consumer Reports study (2012) found that several energy drinks had over 20 percent more caffeine than reported on the label. In addition, many beverages have multiple servings in one bottle and some beverages do not list the caffeine content on the label. Individuals may be at risk for consuming far more caffeine than they expected. Table 14–3 lists some common sources of caffeine.

Next to caffeine, nicotine, an active ingredient in tobacco, is the most widely used psychoactive substance in U.S. society. Currently more than 40 million Americans smoke (SAMHSA, 2017). Since 1964, when the results of the first public health report on smoking were issued, the percentage of total smokers has declined. However, the percentage of women and teenage smokers has declined more slowly than that of adult men. Even though tobacco use is on the decline, people with severe mental illness and those in addiction treatment continue to have higher rates than the general population; as many as 93 percent of people in addiction treatment and 40 percent of people with severe mental illness report using tobacco (SAMHSA, 2017). The dangers of secondhand smoke continue to be identified as a significant health hazard. The CDC (2017a) reports that, annually, secondhand smoke claims the lives of 41,000 nonsmokers from heart disease and lung cancer and 400 babies from sudden infant death syndrome.

Vaping, the use of a device to heat and release chemicals that can then be inhaled, is a current

TABLE 14–3 Common Sources of Caffeine

SOURCE	CAFFEINE CONTENT (MG)
FOOD AND BEVERAGES	
8 oz. brewed coffee	95–165
8 oz. instant coffee	63–110
8 oz. decaffeinated coffee	2–5
1 oz. espresso	47–64
8 oz. brewed tea	25–48
6 oz. instant tea	30
8 oz. green tea	25–29
8–12 oz. cola drinks	22–54
8–24 oz. energy drinks	142–375
2 oz. high energy drinks	215–240
1.93 oz. 10 hr energy shot	422
5–6 oz. cocoa	20
8 oz. chocolate milk	2–7
1 oz. chocolate bar	22
PRESCRIPTION MEDICATIONS	
APCs (aspirin, phenacetin, caffeine)	32
Cafergot	100
Fiorinal	40
Migralam	100
OVER-THE-COUNTER ANALGESICS	
Anacin, Empirin, Midol, Vanquish	32
Excedrin Migraine (aspirin, acetaminophen, caffeine)	65
OVER-THE-COUNTER STIMULANTS	
NoDoz	100
Vivarin	200
Caffedrine	250

Sources: Juliano, L. M. & Griffiths, R. R. (2017). Caffeine-related disorders. In B. J. Sadock, V. A. Sadock, & P. Ruiz (Eds.), *Comprehensive textbook of psychiatry* (10th ed., pp. 1291–1303). Philadelphia, PA: Wolters Kluwer; Mayo Clinic (2017). *Caffeine content for coffee, tea, soda, and more.* Retrieved from https://www.mayoclinic.org/healthy-lifestyle/nutrition-and-healthy-eating/in-depth/caffeine/art-20049372

trend. One such device is the e-cigarette, which typically contains nicotine. In addition to its addiction potential, nicotine is known to be harmful to developing brains and, therefore, particularly dangerous to teens and pregnant women. Its use has become common among youth, now surpassing conventional cigarette smoking (CDC, 2017a).

Effects on the Body

The CNS stimulants are a group of pharmacological agents that are capable of exciting the entire nervous system. This is accomplished by increasing the activity or augmenting the capability of the neurotransmitter agents known to be directly involved in physical and behavioral stimulation. Physiological responses vary markedly according to the potency and dosage of the drug.

Central Nervous System (CNS) Effects

Stimulation of the CNS results in tremor, restlessness, anorexia, insomnia, agitation, and increased motor activity. Amphetamines, nonamphetamine stimulants, and cocaine produce increased alertness, decrease in fatigue, elation and euphoria, and subjective feelings of greater mental agility and muscular power. Chronic use of these drugs may result in compulsive behavior, paranoia, hallucinations, and aggressive behavior (Publishers Group, 2017).

Cardiovascular and Pulmonary Effects

Amphetamines can induce increased systolic and diastolic blood pressure, increased heart rate, and cardiac arrhythmias (Publishers Group, 2017). These drugs also relax bronchial smooth muscle.

Cocaine intoxication typically produces an increase in myocardial demand for oxygen and an increased heart rate. Severe vasoconstriction may occur and can result in myocardial infarction, ventricular fibrillation, and sudden death. Inhaled cocaine can cause pulmonary hemorrhage, chronic bronchiolitis, and pneumonia. Nasal rhinitis is a result of chronic cocaine snorting.

Caffeine ingestion can result in increased heart rate, palpitations, extrasystoles, and cardiac arrhythmias. Caffeine induces dilation of pulmonary and general systemic blood vessels and constriction of cerebral blood vessels.

Nicotine stimulates the sympathetic nervous system, resulting in an increase in heart rate, blood pressure, and cardiac contractility, thereby increasing myocardial oxygen consumption and demand for blood flow. Contractions of gastric smooth muscle associated with hunger are inhibited, thereby producing a mild anorectic effect.

Gastrointestinal and Renal Effects

Gastrointestinal (GI) effects of amphetamines are somewhat unpredictable; however, a decrease in GI tract motility commonly results in constipation. Contraction of the bladder sphincter makes urination difficult. Caffeine exerts a diuretic effect on the kidneys. Nicotine stimulates the hypothalamus to release antidiuretic hormone, reducing the excretion of urine. Because nicotine increases the tone and activity of the bowel, it may occasionally cause diarrhea.

Most CNS stimulants induce a small increase in metabolic rate and various degrees of anorexia. Amphetamines and cocaine can cause a rise in body temperature.

Sexual Function

CNS stimulants appear to increase sexual urges in both men and women. Women, more than men, report that stimulants make them feel sexier and have more orgasms. Some men may experience sexual dysfunction with the use of stimulants. For the majority of individuals, however, these drugs exert a powerful aphrodisiac effect.

Stimulant Intoxication

Stimulant intoxication produces maladaptive behavioral and psychological changes that develop during or shortly after use of these drugs. Amphetamine and cocaine intoxication typically produces euphoria or affective blunting; changes in sociability; hypervigilance; interpersonal sensitivity; anxiety, tension, or anger; stereotyped behaviors; or impaired judgment. In severe amphetamine intoxication, symptoms may include memory loss, psychosis, and violent aggression. Physical effects include tachycardia or bradycardia, pupillary dilation, elevated or lowered blood pressure, perspiration or chills, nausea or vomiting, weight loss, psychomotor agitation or retardation, muscular weakness, respiratory depression, chest pain, cardiac arrhythmias, confusion, seizures, dyskinesias, dystonias, or coma (APA, 2013).

Intoxication from caffeine usually occurs following consumption in excess of 250 mg. Symptoms include restlessness, nervousness, excitement, insomnia, flushed face, diuresis, GI disturbance, muscle twitching, rambling flow of thought and speech, tachycardia or cardiac arrhythmia, periods of inexhaustibility, and psychomotor agitation (APA, 2013).

Stimulant Withdrawal

Stimulant withdrawal is the presence of a characteristic withdrawal syndrome that develops within a few hours to several days after cessation of or reduction in heavy and prolonged use (APA, 2013). This syndrome is often referred to as "crashing," which is an apt description because the symptoms include fatigue, cramps, depression, headaches, and nightmares. The dysphoria can be intense enough to result in increased risk for suicide. Peak withdrawal symptoms usually occur within 2 to 4 days of abstinence.

The *DSM-5* (APA, 2013) states that a withdrawal syndrome can occur with abrupt cessation of caffeine intake after a prolonged daily use of the substance. The symptoms begin within 24 hours after last consumption and may include the following symptoms: headache, fatigue, drowsiness, dysphoric mood, irritability, difficulty concentrating, flu-like symptoms, nausea, vomiting, and/or muscle pain and stiffness.

Withdrawal from nicotine results in dysphoric or depressed mood; insomnia; irritability, frustration, or anger; anxiety; difficulty concentrating; restlessness; decreased heart rate; and increased appetite or weight gain (APA, 2013). A mild syndrome of nicotine withdrawal can appear when a smoker switches from regular cigarettes to low-nicotine cigarettes (Sadock et al., 2015).

Inhalant Use Disorder

Profile of the Substance

Inhalant disorders are induced by inhaling the aliphatic and aromatic hydrocarbons found in substances such as fuels, solvents, adhesives, aerosol propellants, and paint thinners. Specific examples of these substances include gasoline, varnish remover, lighter fluid, airplane glue, rubber cement, cleaning fluid, spray paint, shoe conditioner, and typewriter correction fluid. Toluene (methylbenzene, toluol, phenylmethane) is a common ingredient in many of the substances that are inhaled, including paints, glues, and gasoline, and it is responsible for the mind-altering effects that occur after inhalation.

Patterns of Use

Inhalant substances are readily available, legal, and inexpensive—three factors that make them attractive to children, teens, and young adults. Younger teens more commonly inhale glue, gasoline, and spray paints. In older teens, nitrous oxide (also known as "whippets") use is more common, and in adults, nitrites, such as amyl nitrites (also called "poppers") are common inhalants used for mind-altering effects (NIDA, 2017a).

The National Survey of Drug Use and Health (NIDA, 2017a) reports that in 2016, 9.1 percent of people aged 12 and older reported using inhalants. Overall, use of illicit drugs among adolescents increased in 2017, with eighth graders showing the most significant increase for inhalant use. Because Johnston and associates (2018) note that inhalant use has been declining for over a decade, this trend reversal bears watching. Another finding in the national survey was a decline in the number of adolescents who believe that use of inhalants is harmful. Past education and advertising campaigns about the risks associated with inhalant use have contributed to the decline in use over the past decade (Johnston et al., 2018), and this education may need to be re-introduced and reinforced with today's adolescents. Nurses who work with children and adolescents can play a significant role in providing that education.

Methods of use include "huffing"—a procedure in which a rag soaked with the substance is applied to the mouth and nose and the vapors breathed in. Another common method is called "bagging," in which the substance is placed in a paper or plastic bag and inhaled from the bag by the user. The substance may also be inhaled directly from the container or sprayed in the mouth or nose.

Sadock and colleagues (2015) reported that

inhalant use among adolescents may be most common in those whose parents or older siblings use illegal substances. Inhalant use among adolescents is also associated with an increased likelihood of conduct disorder or antisocial personality disorder. (p. 657)

Tolerance to inhalants has been reported with heavy use. A mild withdrawal syndrome has been documented but does not appear to be clinically significant. Among children with inhalant disorder, the products may be used several times a week, often on weekends and after school. Adults with inhalant addiction may use the substance at varying times during each day, or they may binge on the substance during a period of several days.

Effects on the Body

Inhalants are absorbed through the lungs and reach the CNS very rapidly. Inhalants initially create rapid excitation followed by drowsiness, incoordination, and disinhibition. The effects are relatively brief, lasting from several minutes to a few hours, depending on the specific substance and amount consumed.

Central Nervous System

Inhalants can cause both central and peripheral nervous system damage. Neurological damage, such as ataxia, peripheral and sensorimotor neuropathy, speech problems, and tremor, can occur. Other CNS effects that have been reported with heavy inhalant use include ototoxicity, encephalopathy, parkinsonism, and damage to the protective sheath around certain nerve fibers in the brain and peripheral nervous system. These effects are particularly damaging to youth because their nervous systems are still developing. Chronic use has been associated with the development of several mental illnesses, including anxiety and psychotic disorders. Inhalant use in pregnant women has been linked to fetal development disorders, malformations, and death. Infants are at risk for *fetal solvent syndrome*, (similar to FAS) a syndrome of behavioral, language, and developmental impairments that may include hyperactivity and aggression (Howard, Bowen, & Garland, 2017).

Respiratory Effects

Respiratory effects of inhalant use range from coughing and wheezing to dyspnea, emphysema, and pneumonia. There is increased airway resistance due to inflammation of the passages. Death can occur from asphyxiation, suffocation when plastic bags are put over one's head to inhale substances, and from *sudden sniffing death,* a sudden fatal heart failure secondary to rapid and irregular heart rhythms.

Gastrointestinal Effects

Abdominal pain, nausea, and vomiting may occur. A rash may be present around the individual's nose and mouth. Unusual breath odors are common. Chronic inhalant use has been associated with liver failure (and renal failure) as well as liver tumors.

Renal System Effects

Acute and chronic renal failure and hepatorenal syndrome have occurred. Renal toxicity from toluene exposure has been reported, manifesting in renal tubular acidosis, hypokalemia, hypophosphatemia, hyperchloremia, azotemia, sterile pyuria, hematuria, and proteinuria (McKeown, 2015).

Inhalant Intoxication

The *DSM-5* defines *inhalant intoxication* as "clinically significant problematic behavioral or psychological changes that developed during or shortly after exposure to inhalants" (APA, 2013). Symptoms are similar to alcohol intoxication and may include the following (APA, 2013; Howard et al., 2017):

- Dizziness, ataxia
- Euphoria, excitation, disinhibition
- Nystagmus, blurred vision, double vision
- Slurred speech
- Hypoactive reflexes
- Psychomotor retardation, lethargy
- Generalized muscle weakness
- Stupor or coma (at higher doses)

Inhalant Withdrawal

Mild withdrawal symptoms may occur after chronic, long-term use. Reported symptoms include restlessness, nausea and vomiting, runny nose and watery eyes, poor attention and concentration, and mood changes. The *DSM-5,* however, does not include inhalant withdrawal as a diagnosis because the symptoms are either too mild or too inconsistent to be significant (American Addiction Centers, 2018).

Opioid Use Disorder

Profile of the Substance

The term *opioid* refers to a group of compounds that includes opium, opium derivatives, and synthetic substitutes. Opioids exert both sedative and analgesic effects, and their major medical uses are for the relief of pain, treatment of diarrhea, and relief of coughing. Under close supervision, opioids are indispensable in the practice of medicine. They are the most effective agents known for the relief of intense pain. However, they also induce a pleasurable effect that promotes misuse. And because opioids are capable of inducing tolerance, their use may lead to physiological and psychological addiction. The physiological and psychological addiction that occurs with opioids, as well as the development of profound tolerance, contribute to the addicted individual's ongoing quest for more of the substance, regardless of the means. The United States is currently facing an unprecedented opiate abuse epidemic and death toll.

Opioids are popular drugs of abuse because they desensitize an individual to both psychological and physiological pain and induce a sense of euphoria. Lethargy and indifference to the environment are common manifestations.

Opioid abusers usually spend much of their time acquiring opioids to sustain their addiction. Individuals who are addicted to opioids are seldom able to hold a steady job that will support their need. They must therefore secure funds from friends, relatives, or whomever they have not yet alienated with their addiction-related behavior. It is not uncommon for individuals who are addicted to opioids to resort to illegal means of obtaining funds, such as burglary, robbery, prostitution, or selling drugs.

Methods of administration of opioid drugs include oral, snorting, or smoking, and by subcutaneous, intramuscular, and intravenous injection. A selected list of opioid substances is presented in Table 14–4.

Historical Aspects

In its crude form, opium is a brownish-black, gummy substance obtained from the ripened pods of the opium poppy. References have been found to the use of opiates in the Egyptian, Greek, and Arabian cultures as early as 3000 B.C. The drug became widely used both medicinally and recreationally throughout Europe during the 16th and 17th centuries. Most of the opium supply came from China, where the drug was introduced by Arabic traders in the late 17th century. Morphine, the primary active ingredient of opium, was isolated in 1803 by the European chemist Friedrich Sertürner. Since that time, morphine, rather than crude opium, has been used throughout the world for the medical treatment of pain and

TABLE 14–4	Opioids and Related Substances	
CATEGORIES	**GENERIC (TRADE) NAMES**	**COMMON STREET NAMES**
Opioids of natural origin	Opium (ingredient in various antidiarrheal agents) Morphinan (Astramorph) Codeine (ingredient in various analgesics and cough suppressants) Kratom (opioid-like)	Black stuff, poppy, tar, big O M, white stuff, Miss Emma Terp, schoolboy, syrup, cody
Opioid derivatives	Heroin Hydromorphone (Dilaudid) Oxycodone (Percodan; OxyContin) Hydrocodone (Vicodin)	H, horse, junk, brown sugar, smack, skag, TNT, Harry DLs, 4s, lords, little D Perks, perkies, Oxy, O.C. Vike
Synthetic opiate-like drugs	Meperidine (Demerol) Methadone (Dolophine) Pentazocine (Talwin) Fentanyl (Fentora) Carfentanil Desomorphine U-47700 Sufentanil Tramadol	Doctors Dollies, done Ts Apache, China girl, China town, dance fever, goodfella, jackpot Krokodil Pink, pinky, U4

diarrhea. This process was facilitated in 1853 by the development of the hypodermic syringe, which made it possible to deliver the undiluted morphine quickly into the body for rapid relief from pain.

This development also created a new variety of opioid user in the United States: one who was able to self-administer the drug by injection. During this time, there was also a large influx into the United States of Chinese immigrants, who introduced opium smoking to this country. By the early part of the 20th century, opium addiction was widespread.

In response to the concerns over widespread addiction, in 1914 the U.S. government passed the Harrison Narcotic Act, which created strict controls on the accessibility of opiates. Until that time, these substances had been freely available to the public without a prescription. The Harrison Act banned the use of opiates for other than medicinal purposes and drove the use of heroin underground. To this day, the beneficial uses of these substances are widely acclaimed within the medical profession, but the illicit trafficking of the drugs for recreational purposes continues to resist most efforts aimed at control. Historically, the term "opiate" referred to naturally occurring (or slightly modified) components of opium and the term "opioid" described synthetic opiates. However, more recently, the term "opioid" has been used to describe the entire class of drugs. For the purposes of this discussion, these terms are used interchangeably.

Patterns of Use

The development of opioid addiction may follow one of two typical behavior patterns. The first occurs in the individual who has obtained the drug by prescription from a physician for the relief of a medical problem. Abuse and addiction occur when the individual increases the amount and frequency of use, justifying the behavior as symptom treatment. He or she becomes obsessed with obtaining more and more of the substance and may see several physicians in order to replenish and maintain supplies.

The second pattern of behavior associated with addiction to opioids occurs among individuals who use the drugs for recreational purposes and obtain them from illegal sources. Opioids may be used alone to induce the euphoric effects or in combination with stimulants or other drugs to enhance the euphoria or to counteract the depressant effects of the opioid. Tolerance develops and addiction occurs, leading the individual to procure the substance by whatever means is required to support the habit.

A recent government survey reported that there were 435,000 current heroin users aged 12 years and older in the United States in 2014 (SAMHSA, 2016b). The same survey revealed an estimated 4.3 million persons who used prescription psychotherapeutic drugs nonmedically. In 2016 deaths from prescription, illegal (like heroin), and illicitly manufactured fentanyl were five times higher than in 1999 (CDC, 2017b). Efforts have been made in some states to exert stricter controls on opiate prescription practices, and 2012 marked the first year of a trend toward a decline in prescription rates nationally. However, beginning in 2010, an increase in heroin use, and in 2013, an increase in the use of synthetic opioids (like illicitly manufactured fentanyl and carfentanil), are evidence that the opiate epidemic and associated deaths are ongoing problems. The CDC (2017b) reports that 66 percent of all drug overdose deaths in 2016 involved an opioid; on average, 115 deaths each day are related to opioid use. An alarming recent trend has been a significant increase in overdose deaths associated with fentanyl, which is being mixed with heroin and results in overdose because fentanyl is 30 to 50 times more potent than pure heroin and 50 to 100 times more potent than morphine (CDC, 2017b). Even more recently, carfentanil (carfentanyl), a potent drug used mainly in the capture of wild animals (100 times more potent than fentanyl and 10,000 times more potent than morphine), has been responsible for rapid overdose and often death when ingested along with heroin (National Institutes of Health [NIH], 2018). Late in 2018, the FDA approved a sublingual tablet form of sufentanil (five to ten times more potent than fentanyl) and although intended for the treatment of severe acute pain in certified, medically supervised healthcare settings, critics argue that it adds one more very potent opioid to the arsenal of those that may be diverted, easily administered, and potentially fatal (Brooks, 2018).

Similar to the trend in development of synthetic *amphetamines* discussed earlier in this chapter, a new synthetic *opioid,* U-47700, surfaced in 2015 and was responsible for 46 fatalities in 2016 before the substance underwent emergency classification as a Schedule I drug (Duffy, 2016). Kratom, a plant from Southeast Asia that triggers opiate-like effects, also surfaced in the United States and was subsequently banned; however, this decision was reversed when researchers argued that it may help in the development of treatments for opioid and alcohol addiction as well as chronic pain (MPR, 2016).

At present, the opioid epidemic remains out of control, but several national initiatives to address this public health crisis have been identified. A National Practice Guideline for use of medications to treat Opioid use disorder has been established (ASAM, 2015). For the first time in U.S. history, in 2016, the Surgeon General declared illicit drug use and misuse of prescription drugs a national healthcare priority and committed to the need for additional research and treatment options. In 2018, the Surgeon General advanced a public health advisory urging more Americans to carry naloxone kits to assist (along with rescue breathing) in preventing opiate overdose and death. Some state programs, like Project Dawn in Ohio, are providing naloxone education and distribution free of charge to individuals who are willing to carry naloxone kits for responding to opioid overdose victims. In 2018, the NIH launched the HEAL (Helping End Addiction Long-term) initiative, identifying 15 areas of critical focus for research and development to address the opiate epidemic. These areas include research on longer-acting naloxone-type drugs, better responses to chronic pain management, better management of neonatal opiate withdrawal, and better access to and efficacy of treatment options (Twachtman, 2018). All of these efforts underscore the gravity of this ongoing national public health issue.

Effects on the Body

Opiates are sometimes classified as *narcotic analgesics*. They exert their major effects primarily on the CNS, eyes, and GI tract. Chronic morphine use or acute morphine toxicity is manifested by a syndrome of sedation, chronic constipation, decreased respiratory rate, and pinpoint pupils. Intensity of symptoms is largely dose dependent. The following physiological effects are common with opioid use.

Central Nervous System

All opioids, opioid derivatives, and synthetic opioid-like drugs affect the CNS. Common manifestations include euphoria, mood changes, and mental clouding. Other common CNS effects include drowsiness and pain reduction. Pupillary constriction occurs in response to stimulation of the oculomotor nerve. CNS depression of the respiratory centers within the medulla results in respiratory depression. The antitussive response is due to suppression of the cough center within the medulla. The nausea and vomiting commonly associated with opiate ingestion is related to the stimulation of the centers within the medulla that trigger this response.

Gastrointestinal Effects

These drugs exert a profound effect on the GI tract. Both stomach and intestinal tone are increased, whereas peristaltic activity of the intestines is diminished. These effects lead to a marked decrease in the movement of food through the GI tract. This is a notable therapeutic effect in the treatment of severe diarrhea. In fact, no drugs have yet been developed that are more effective than the opioids for this purpose. However, constipation and even fecal impaction may be a serious problem for the chronic opioid user.

Cardiovascular Effects

In therapeutic doses, opioids have minimal effect on the action of the heart. Morphine is used extensively to relieve pulmonary edema and the pain of myocardial infarction in cardiac clients. At high doses, opioids induce hypotension, which may be caused by direct action on the heart or by opioid-induced histamine release. Although most opioids do not affect cardiac conductivity, "methadone and buprenorphine can prolong QTc, especially when used in patients at risk for QTc prolongation" (Chen & Ashburn, 2015). Abuse of loperamide, an over-the counter opiate-based antidiarrheal, is a growing problem that has been linked to cardiac dysrhythmias and death because at very high doses (needed to achieve other than antidiarrheal effects) this medication is highly cardiotoxic (Davenport, 2016).

Sexual Function

Opioid use causes decreased sexual function and diminished libido and long-term use has been associated with erectile dysfunction (Deyo et al., 2013). Delayed ejaculation, impotence, and orgasm failure (in both men and women) may occur.

Opioid Intoxication

Opioid intoxication constitutes clinically significant problematic behavioral or psychological changes that develop during or shortly after opioid use (APA, 2013). Symptoms include initial euphoria followed by apathy, dysphoria, psychomotor agitation or retardation, and impaired judgment. Physical symptoms include pupillary constriction (or dilation due to anoxia from severe overdose), drowsiness, slurred speech, and impairment in attention or memory (APA, 2013). Symptoms are consistent with the half-life of most opioid drugs and usually last for several hours. Severe opioid intoxication can lead to *respiratory depression*, coma, and death.

Opioid Withdrawal

Opioid withdrawal produces a syndrome of symptoms that develops after cessation of or reduction in heavy and prolonged use of an opiate or related substance. Symptoms include dysphoric mood, nausea or vomiting, muscle aches, lacrimation or rhinorrhea, pupillary dilation, piloerection, sweating, diarrhea, yawning, fever, and insomnia (APA, 2013). With short-acting drugs such as heroin, withdrawal symptoms occur within 6 to 8 hours after the last dose, peak within 1 to 3 days, and gradually subside over a period of 5 to 10 days. With longer-acting drugs such as methadone, withdrawal symptoms begin within 1 to 3 days after the last dose, peak between days 4 and 6, and are complete in 14 to 21 days. Withdrawal from the ultra-short-acting meperidine begins quickly, reaches a peak in 8 to 12 hours, and is complete in 4 to 5 days.

Hallucinogen Use Disorder

Profile of the Substance

Hallucinogenic substances are capable of distorting an individual's perception of reality. They have the ability to alter sensory perception and induce hallucinations. For this reason, they have sometimes been referred to as "mind-expanding drugs." Some of the manifestations have been likened to a psychotic break. The hallucinations experienced by an individual with schizophrenia, however, are most often auditory, whereas substance-induced hallucinations are usually visual. Perceptual distortions have been reported by some users as spiritual, as giving a sense of depersonalization (observing oneself having the experience), or as being at peace with self and the universe. Others, who describe their experiences as "bad trips," report feelings of panic and a fear of dying or going insane. A common danger reported with hallucinogenic drugs is that of "flashbacks," or a spontaneous reoccurrence of the hallucinogenic state without ingestion of the drug. These can occur months after the drug was last taken.

Recurrent use can produce tolerance, encouraging users to resort to higher and higher dosages. No evidence of physical addiction is detectable when the drug is withdrawn; however, recurrent use appears to induce a psychological addiction to the insight-inducing experiences that a user may associate with episodes of hallucinogen use (Sadock et al., 2015). This psychological addiction varies according to the drug, the dose, and the individual user. Hallucinogens are highly unpredictable in the effects they may induce each time they are used.

Many of the hallucinogenic substances have structural similarities. Some are produced synthetically; others are natural products of plants and fungi. A selected list of hallucinogens is presented in Table 14–5.

Historical Aspects

Hallucinogens have been used throughout history in many cultures for religious and mystical experiences, including in Aztec, Mexican Indian, and Hindu ceremonies (Parish, 2015). Use of the peyote cactus as

TABLE 14–5 **Hallucinogens**		
CATEGORIES	**GENERIC (TRADE) NAMES**	**COMMON STREET NAMES**
Naturally occurring hallucinogens	Mescaline (primary active ingredient of the peyote cactus) Psilocybin and psilocin (active ingredients of *Psilocybe* mushrooms) Ololiuqui (morning glory seeds) Salvia divinorum	Cactus, mesc, mescal, half moon, big chief, bad seed, peyote Magic mushroom, God's flesh, shrooms Heavenly blue, pearly gates, flying saucers Salvia
Synthetic compounds	Lysergic acid diethylamide (LSD)—synthetically produced from a fungal substance found on rye or a chemical substance found in morning glory seeds Dextromethorphan (DXM) Dimethyltryptamine (DMT) and diethyltryptamine (DET)—chemical analogues of tryptamine 2,5-Dimethoxy-4-methylamphetamine (DOM) Phencyclidine (PCP) Ketamine (Ketalar) 3,4-Methylene-dioxyamphetamine (MDMA)* Methoxy-amphetamine (MDA) 3,4-Methylenedioxypyrovalerone (MDPV)* 4-Methylmethcathinone (mephedrone, 4-MMC)* Methylone*	Acid, cube, big D, California sunshine, microdots, blue dots, sugar, orange wedges, peace tablets, purple haze, cupcakes Robo Businessman's trip STP (serenity, tranquility, peace) Angel dust, hog, peace pill, rocket fuel Special K, vitamin K, kit kat XTC, ecstasy, Adam, Eve Love drug, molly Bath salts (also called blue silk, cloud 9, ivory wave, vanilla sky, white knight, and others)

*Cross-listed with the CNS stimulants.

part of religious ceremonies in the southwestern part of the United States still occurs today, although this ritual use has greatly diminished.

LSD was first synthesized in 1943 by Dr. Albert Hoffman. It was used as a clinical research tool to investigate the biochemical etiology of schizophrenia. It soon reached the illicit market, however, and its abuse began to overshadow the research effort.

The abuse of hallucinogens reached a peak in the late 1960s, waned during the 1970s, and returned to favor in the 1980s with the so-called designer drugs (e.g., 3,4-methylene-dioxymethamphetamine [MDMA], also known as "Molly" or "ecstasy," and 3,4-methylene-dioxyamphetamine [MDA]). Another hallucinogen, PCP, originally was developed in the 1950s as an anesthetic but this use was discontinued because of serious adverse effects. It continues to be used illegally and is often combined with cannabis. A number of deaths have been directly attributed to the use of PCP, and numerous accidental deaths have occurred as a result of overdose and behavioral changes the drug precipitates. A derivative of PCP, ketamine, which is also used as a preoperative anesthetic, is abused for its psychedelic properties. It produces effects similar to, but somewhat less intense, than those of PCP. Ketamine is also currently being studied for potential benefits in the treatment of depression and post-traumatic stress disorder.

Several therapeutic uses of LSD have been proposed, including the treatment of chronic alcoholism and the reduction of intractable pain such as occurs in malignant disease. More research is required regarding the therapeutic uses of LSD. At this time, there is no real evidence of the safety and efficacy of this drug in humans.

Patterns of Use

Use of hallucinogens is usually episodic. Because cognitive and perceptual abilities are so markedly affected by these substances, the user must set aside time from normal daily activities for their use. According to a national study in 2014, 1.2 million people reported using hallucinogens in the prior month (SAMHSA, 2017).

LSD, like other hallucinogens, does not lead to the development of physical addiction or withdrawal symptoms (Sadock et al., 2015). However, tolerance for LSD and other hallucinogens develops quickly and to a high degree. In fact, tolerance is complete after 3 to 4 consecutive days of use. Recovery from the tolerance also occurs very rapidly (in 4 to 7 days), so that the individual is able to achieve the desired effect from the drug repeatedly and often.

PCP is usually taken episodically, in binges that can last for several days. However, some chronic users take the substance daily. Physical addiction does not occur with PCP; however, psychological addiction characterized by craving for the drug has been reported in chronic users, as has the development of tolerance. Tolerance apparently develops quickly with frequent use.

Psilocybin is an ingredient of the *Psilocybe* mushroom indigenous to the United States and Mexico. Ingestion of these mushrooms produces an effect similar to that of LSD but of a shorter duration. This hallucinogenic chemical can now be produced synthetically.

Mescaline is the only hallucinogenic compound used legally for religious purposes today by members of the Native American Church of the United States. It is the primary active ingredient of the peyote cactus. Neither physical nor psychological addiction occurs with the use of mescaline, although, as with other hallucinogens, tolerance can develop quickly with frequent use.

Salvia is an herb from the mint family that has hallucinogenic effects when dried leaves are chewed, extracted juices are consumed, or smoke from the leaves is inhaled. This particular hallucinogen is advertised and sold over the Internet because it is not currently regulated by the Controlled Substances Act, but some states have limited or banned its use. It is currently illegal in Delaware, Louisiana, Maine, Missouri, Oklahoma, and Tennessee (WebMD, 2018).

Among the very potent hallucinogens of the current drug culture are those that are categorized as amphetamine derivatives. These include 2, 5-dimethoxy-4-methylamphetamine (DOM [street name "STP"]), MDMA, and MDA. At lower doses, these drugs produce the "high" associated with CNS stimulants. At higher doses, hallucinogenic effects occur. These drugs have existed for many years but were "rediscovered" in the mid-1980s. Because of the rapid increase in recreational use, the DEA imposed an emergency classification of MDMA as a Schedule I drug in 1985. MDMA, or ecstasy, is a synthetic drug with both stimulant and hallucinogenic qualities. It has a chemical structure similar to methamphetamine and mescaline, and it has become widely available throughout the world. Because of its growing popularity, the demand for this drug has led to tablets and capsules being sold as "ecstasy" that are not pure MDMA. Many contain drugs such as methamphetamine, PCP, amphetamine, ketamine, and *p*-methoxyamphetamine (PMA, a stimulant with hallucinogenic properties; more toxic than MDMA). This practice has increased the dangers associated with MDMA use.

Effects on the Body

The effects produced by the various hallucinogens are highly unpredictable. The variety of effects may be related to dosage, the mental state of the individual, and the environment in which the substance is used. Some common effects have been reported (APA, 2013; Julien, 2014; Sadock et al., 2015) as discussed next.

Physiological Effects

- Nausea and vomiting
- Chills
- Pupil dilation
- Increased pulse, blood pressure, and temperature
- Mild dizziness
- Trembling
- Loss of appetite
- Insomnia
- Sweating
- Slowing of respirations
- Elevation in blood sugar

Psychological Effects

- Heightened response to color, texture, and sounds
- Heightened body awareness
- Distortion of vision
- Sense of slowing of time
- All feelings magnified: love, lust, hate, joy, anger, pain, terror, despair
- Fear of losing control
- Paranoia, panic
- Euphoria, bliss
- Projection of self into dreamlike images
- Serenity, peace
- Depersonalization
- Derealization
- Increased libido

The effects of hallucinogens are not always pleasurable for the user. Two types of toxic reactions are known to occur. The first is the *panic reaction*, or "bad trip." Symptoms include an intense anxiety, fear, and stimulation. The individual hallucinates and fears going insane. Paranoia and acute psychosis may be evident.

The second type of toxic reaction to hallucinogens is the *flashback*. This phenomenon refers to the transient, spontaneous repetition of a previous LSD-induced experience that occurs without taking the substance. The *DSM*-5 (APA, 2013) refers to this as *hallucinogen persisting perception disorder*. Various studies have reported that 15 to 80 percent of hallucinogen users report having experienced flashbacks (Sadock et al., 2015). These episodes typically last for a few minutes or less.

Hallucinogen Intoxication

Symptoms of hallucinogen intoxication develop during or shortly after hallucinogen use. Maladaptive behavioral or psychological changes include marked anxiety or depression, ideas of reference (a type of delusional thinking that all activity within one's environment is "referred to" [about] one's self), fear of losing one's mind, paranoid ideation, and impaired judgment. Perceptual changes occur while the individual is fully awake and alert and include intensification of perceptions, depersonalization, derealization, illusions, hallucinations, and synesthesias (APA, 2013). Because hallucinogens are sympathomimetics, they can cause tachycardia, hypertension, sweating, blurred vision, papillary (pupil) dilation, and tremors.

Symptoms of PCP intoxication are unpredictable. Specific symptoms are dose related and may be manifested by impulsiveness, impaired judgment, assaultiveness, and belligerence, or the individual may appear calm, stuporous, or comatose. Physical symptoms include vertical or horizontal nystagmus, hypertension, tachycardia, ataxia, diminished pain sensation, muscle rigidity, and seizures. Symptoms of ketamine intoxication appear similar to those of PCP.

General effects of MDMA (ecstasy) include increased heart rate, blood pressure, and body temperature; dehydration; confusion; insomnia; and paranoia. Overdose can result in panic attacks, hallucinations, severe hyperthermia, dehydration, and seizures. Death can occur from kidney or cardiovascular failure.

Cannabis Use Disorder

Profile of the Substance

Cannabis is the most commonly used illicit drug in the United States (NIDA, 2017a) and the fourth most commonly used psychoactive substance after caffeine, alcohol, and nicotine (Sadock et al., 2015). These trends may change because marijuana is becoming legalized in some states for recreational and/or medicinal use. The major psychoactive ingredient of this class of substances is delta-9-tetrahydrocannabinol (THC). It occurs naturally in the plant *Cannabis sativa*, which grows readily in warm climates. Marijuana, the most prevalent type of cannabis preparation, is composed of the dried leaves, stems, and flowers of the plant. Hashish is a more potent concentrate of the resin derived from the flowering tops of the plant. Hash oil is a very concentrated form of THC made by boiling hashish in a solvent and filtering out the solid matter (Publishers Group, 2017). Cannabis products are usually smoked in the form of loosely rolled cigarettes. Cannabis can also be taken orally when it is prepared in food, but about two to three times the amount of cannabis must be ingested orally to equal the potency of that obtained by the inhalation of its smoke (Sadock et al., 2015).

At moderate dosages, cannabis drugs produce effects resembling alcohol and other CNS depressants. By depressing higher brain centers, they release lower centers from inhibitory influences. There has been some controversy in the past over the classification of these substances. They are not narcotics, although they are legally classified as controlled substances. They are not hallucinogens, although in very high dosages they can induce hallucinations. They are not sedative-hypnotics, although they most closely resemble these substances. Like sedative-hypnotics, their action occurs in the ascending reticular activating system.

Psychological addiction has been shown to occur with cannabis, and tolerance can occur. Controversy has existed about whether physiological addiction occurs with cannabis. In the past, symptoms of cannabis withdrawal were considered less than clinically significant to include the diagnosis in the *DSM*. However, the *DSM-5* Substance-Related Work Group determined that subsequent research has provided significant data to support cannabis withdrawal as a valid and reliable syndrome that can negatively impact abstinence attempts of heavy cannabis users. The diagnosis of Cannabis Withdrawal is included in the *DSM-5*.

Synthetic cannabinoids, on the other hand, have been clearly identified as potentially addictive (NIDA, 2018c). Although some of these chemicals are illegal to buy, sell, or possess, manufacturers often sidestep the laws by altering their chemical formulas. Standard drug tests cannot easily detect many of these chemicals.

Common cannabis and synthetic cannabinoid preparations are presented in Table 14–6.

TABLE 14–6	**Cannabinoids**	
CATEGORY	**COMMON PREPARATIONS**	**STREET NAMES**
Cannabis	Marijuana	Joint, weed, pot, grass, Mary Jane, Texas tea, locoweed, MJ, hay, stick
	Hashish	Hash, bhang, ganja, charas
Synthetic cannabinoids	NPS (new psychoactive substances) powders or liquids to be inhaled	K2, Spice, Black Mamba, Joker, Kush, Kronic

Historical Aspects

Products of *Cannabis sativa* have been used therapeutically for nearly 5,000 years (Julien, 2014). Cannabis was first employed in China and India as an antiseptic and an analgesic. Its use later spread to the Middle East, Africa, and Eastern Europe.

In the United States, medical interest in the use of cannabis arose during the early part of the 19th century. Many articles were published espousing its use for varied reasons. The drug was almost as commonly used for medicinal purposes as aspirin is today, and it could be purchased without a prescription in any drug store. It was purported to have antibacterial and anticonvulsant capabilities, decrease intraocular pressure, decrease pain, help in the treatment of asthma, increase appetite, and generally raise one's morale.

The drug went out of favor primarily because of the large variation in potency across batches of medication caused by the variations in the THC content of different plants. Other medications were favored for their greater degree of solubility and faster onset of action than cannabis products. A federal law put an end to its legal use in 1937, after an association between marijuana and criminal activity became evident. In the 1960s, marijuana became the symbol of the "antiestablishment" generation, at which time it reached its peak as a drug of abuse.

Research continues in regard to the possible therapeutic uses of cannabis. It has been shown to be an effective agent for relieving the nausea and vomiting associated with cancer chemotherapy when other antinausea medications fail. It has also been used in the treatment of chronic pain, glaucoma, multiple sclerosis, AIDS, and epilepsy (Sadock et al., 2015).

Advocates who praise the therapeutic usefulness and support the legalization of the cannabinoids persist in the United States today. Groups such as the Alliance for Cannabis Therapeutics (ACT) and the National Organization for the Reform of Marijuana Laws (NORML) have lobbied extensively to allow disease sufferers easier access to the drug. The medical use of marijuana has been legalized in 30 states, and 8 states (and the District of Columbia) have legalized recreational use of marijuana (governing.com, 2018) nonetheless. The DEA (USDEA, 2013) has stated:

> The DEA supports ongoing research into potential medicinal uses of marijuana's active ingredients. At present, however, **the clear weight of the evidence is that smoked marijuana is harmful.** No matter what medical condition has been studied, other drugs already approved by the FDA have been proven to be safer and more effective than smoked marijuana. (p. 5)

In 2016, after several unsuccessful petitions to loosen restrictions on marijuana, the DEA maintained its stance that marijuana should continue to be in the most restrictive category for law enforcement purposes.

Several medications that have components of the marijuana plant or related synthetic compounds are currently approved by the FDA. Dronabinol, a synthetic compound in the medication Marinol, is approved for nausea and vomiting associated with cancer treatment and for severe weight loss associated with AIDS. Nabilone, a chemical similar to THC and found in the medication Cesamet, is a similar FDA-approved drug. A third medication, Sativex, which is an oromucosal spray containing THC and cannabidiol, can be prescribed in the United States only with a special exemption from the FDA for use in select patients (Sadock et al., 2015). In 2018, the first cannabis-based drug (Epidiolex) became FDA approved for the treatment of epilepsy.

Patterns of Use

In its 2016 National Survey on Drug Use and Health, SAMHSA (NIDA, 2017a) reported that 44 percent of Americans aged 12 years or older had used marijuana or hashish in their lifetime.

Many people incorrectly regard cannabis as a substance of low abuse potential. This lack of knowledge has promoted use of the substance by some individuals who believe it is harmless. Tolerance, although it tends to decline rapidly, does occur with chronic use. As tolerance develops, physical addiction also occurs, resulting in a withdrawal syndrome upon cessation of drug use.

One controversy that exists regarding marijuana (particularly because of several statewide efforts toward legalization) is whether its use leads to the use of other illicit drugs. Dupont (2016), the first director of NIDA, reports evidence that marijuana use is positively correlated with use of alcohol, tobacco, cocaine, and methamphetamine and that people addicted to marijuana are three times more likely to be addicted to heroin.

Effects on the Body

Following is a summary of some of the effects that have been attributed to marijuana in recent years. Undoubtedly, as research continues, evidence of additional physiological and psychological effects will be made available.

Cardiovascular Effects

Cannabis ingestion induces tachycardia and orthostatic hypotension (NIDA, 2018d). With the decrease in blood pressure, myocardial oxygen supply is decreased. Tachycardia in turn increases oxygen demand. Marijuana raises the heart rate for up to 3 hours after smoking.

Respiratory Effects

Marijuana produces a greater amount of "tar" than its equivalent weight in tobacco. Because of the method by which marijuana is smoked—that is, the smoke is held in the lungs for as long as possible to achieve the desired effect—larger amounts of tar are deposited in the lungs, promoting deleterious effects to the respiratory system.

Although the initial reaction to the marijuana is bronchodilation, thereby facilitating respiratory function, chronic use results in obstructive airway disorders. Frequent marijuana users often have laryngitis, bronchitis, cough, and hoarseness. Currently, researchers have not identified an increased risk for lung cancer among those who smoke marijuana (NIDA, 2018d).

Reproductive Effects

Some studies have shown that, with heavy marijuana use, men may have a decrease in sperm count, motility, and structure. In women, heavy marijuana use may result in a suppression of ovulation, disruption in menstrual cycles, and alteration of hormone levels. Marijuana use in pregnant women has been associated with low birth weight and increased risk of brain and behavioral problems in infants. Children exposed to marijuana during fetal development have a higher incidence of attention, problem-solving, and memory problems than unexposed children (NIDA, 2018d).

Central Nervous System Effects

Acute CNS effects of marijuana are dose related. Many people report a feeling of being high—the equivalent of being "drunk" on alcohol. Symptoms include feelings of euphoria, relaxed inhibitions, disorientation, depersonalization, and relaxation. At higher doses, sensory alterations may occur, including impairment in judgment of time and distance, recent memory, and learning ability. Physiological symptoms may include tremors, muscle rigidity, and conjunctival redness. Toxic effects are generally characterized by panic reactions. Very heavy usage has been shown to precipitate an acute psychosis that is self-limited and short-lived once the drug is removed from the body (Julien, 2014).

Heavy, long-term cannabis use is also associated with a condition called amotivational syndrome. *Amotivational syndrome* is defined as lack of motivation to persist in or complete a task that requires ongoing attention. Persons are described as "apathetic, anergic, usually gaining weight, and appearing slothful" (Sadock et al., 2015, p. 647). Evidence supports that long-term use also impairs cognitive functions of memory, attention, and organization, and these impairments may also contribute to some of the symptoms apparent in amotivational syndrome.

Sexual Function

Marijuana is reported to enhance the sexual experience in both men and women. The intensified sensory awareness and the subjective slowness of time perception are thought to increase sexual satisfaction. Marijuana also enhances sexual function by releasing inhibitions for certain activities that would normally be restrained.

Cannabis Intoxication

Cannabis intoxication is evidenced by the presence of clinically significant behavioral or psychological changes that develop during or shortly after cannabis use. Symptoms include impaired motor coordination, euphoria, anxiety, a sensation of slowed time, impaired judgment and memory, and social withdrawal. Physical symptoms include conjunctival injection (red eyes), increased appetite, dry mouth, and tachycardia (APA, 2013). The impairment of motor skills lasts for 8 to 12 hours and interferes with the operation of motor vehicles. These effects are additive to those of alcohol, which is commonly used in combination with cannabis (Sadock et al., 2015).

Cannabis intoxication delirium is marked by significant cognitive impairment and difficulty performing tasks. Higher doses also impair level of consciousness.

NIDA (2017b) reported a trend in overdoses associated with synthetic cannabinoids (such as K2, Spice, and others). There were over 177 different formulations of synthetic cannabinoids reported in 2014. Because the strengths are variable (up to 100 times more potent than THC), the risks of using these substances are unpredictable (NIDA, 2017b). Symptoms include agitation, high blood pressure, shaking and seizures, nausea and vomiting, hallucinations and paranoia, and violent behavior.

Cannabis Withdrawal

The *DSM-5* describes a syndrome of symptoms that occur upon cessation of cannabis use that has been heavy and prolonged. Symptoms occur within a week following cessation of use and may include any of the following:

- Irritability, anger, or aggression
- Nervousness, restlessness, or anxiety
- Sleep difficulty (e.g., insomnia, disturbing dreams)
- Decreased appetite or weight loss
- Depressed mood
- Physical symptoms, such as abdominal pain, tremors, sweating, fever, chills, or headache

Tables 14–7 and 14–8 include summaries of the psychoactive substances, including symptoms of intoxication, withdrawal, use, overdose, possible therapeutic uses, and trade and common names by which they may be referred.

Application of the Nursing Process

Assessment

In the pre-introductory phase of relationship development, the nurse must examine his or her feelings about working with a patient who abuses substances. If these behaviors are viewed as morally wrong and the nurse has internalized these attitudes from very early in life, it may be very difficult to suppress judgmental feelings. The role that alcohol or other substances has played (or plays) in the life of the nurse most certainly will affect the way in which he or she interacts with a patient who has a substance use disorder.

How are attitudes examined? Some individuals may have sufficient ability for introspection to be able to recognize on their own whether they have unresolved issues related to substance abuse. For others, it may be more helpful to discuss these issues in a group

TABLE 14–7 Psychoactive Substances: A Profile Summary

CLASS OF DRUGS	SYMPTOMS OF USE	THERAPEUTIC USES	SYMPTOMS OF OVERDOSE	TRADE NAMES	COMMON STREET NAMES
CNS DEPRESSANTS					
Alcohol	Relaxation, loss of inhibitions, lack of concentration, drowsiness, slurred speech, sleep	Antidote for methanol consumption; ingredient in many pharmacological concentrates	Nausea, vomiting; shallow respirations; cold, clammy skin; weak, rapid pulse; coma; possible death	Ethyl alcohol, beer, gin, rum, vodka, bourbon, whiskey, liqueurs, wine, brandy, sherry, champagne	Booze, alcohol, liquor, drinks, cocktails, highballs, nightcaps, moonshine, white lightening, firewater
Other (barbiturates and nonbarbiturates)	Same as alcohol	Relief from anxiety and insomnia; as anticonvulsants and anesthetics	Anxiety, fever, agitation, hallucinations, disorientation, tremors, delirium, convulsions, possible death	Seconal, amytal, Nembutal, Valium, Librium, Noctec, Miltown	Red birds, yellow birds, blue birds, blues, yellows, green & whites mickeys, downers
CNS STIMULANTS					
Amphetamines and related drugs	Hyperactivity, agitation, euphoria, insomnia, loss of appetite	Management of narcolepsy, hyperkinesia, and weight control	Cardiac arrhythmias, headache, convulsions, hypertension, rapid heart rate, coma, possible death	Dexedrine, Didrex, Tenuate, Bontril, Ritalin, Focalin, Meridia, Provigil	Uppers, pep pills, wakeups, bennies, eye-openers, speed, black beauties, sweet A's
Cocaine	Euphoria, hyperactivity, restlessness, talkativeness, increased pulse, dilated pupils, rhinitis		Hallucinations, convulsions, pulmonary edema, respiratory failure, coma, cardiac arrest, possible death	Cocaine hydrochloride	Coke, flake, snow, dust, happy dust, gold dust, girl, Cecil, C, toot, blow, crack
Synthetic stimulants	Agitation, insomnia, irritability, dizziness, decreased ability to think clearly, increased heart rate, chest pains	Depression, paranoia, delusions, suicidal thoughts, seizures, panic attacks, nausea, vomiting, heart attack, stroke	Increased heart rate, increased blood pressure, nosebleeds, hallucinations, aggressive behavior	Mephedrone, MDPV (3,4-methylene-dioxypyrovalerone), 4-Methylmethcathinone (mephedrone, 4-MMC),* Methylone,* Ethylone, Dibutylone, Alpha-PVP	Bath salts, bliss, vanilla sky, ivory wave, purple wave

Flakka |

CLASS OF DRUGS	SYMPTOMS OF USE	THERAPEUTIC USES	SYMPTOMS OF OVERDOSE	TRADE NAMES	COMMON STREET NAMES
OPIOIDS					
	Euphoria, lethargy, drowsiness, lack of motivation, constricted pupils	As analgesics; antidiarrheals, and antitussives; methadone in medication-assisted treatment; heroin has no therapeutic use	Shallow breathing, slowed pulse, clammy skin, pulmonary edema, respiratory arrest, convulsions, coma, possible death	Heroin	Snow, stuff, H, harry, horse
				Morphine	M, morph, Miss Emma
				Codeine	Schoolboy
				Dilaudid	Lords
				Demerol	Doctors
				Dolophine	Dollies
				Percodan	Perkies
				Talwin	Ts
				Opium	Big O, black stuff
HALLUCINOGENS					
	Visual hallucinations, disorientation, confusion, paranoid delusions, euphoria, anxiety, panic, increased pulse	LSD has been proposed in the treatment of chronic alcoholism and in the reduction of intractable pain	Agitation, extreme hyperactivity, violence, hallucinations, psychosis, convulsions, possible death	LSD	Acid, cube, big D
				PCP	Angel dust, hog, peace pill
				Mescaline	Mesc
				DMT	Businessman's trip
				STP, DOM	Serenity and peace
				MDMA	Ecstasy, XTC
				Ketamine	Special K, vitamin K, kit kat
				MDPV	Bath salts
CANNABINOLS					
	Relaxation, talkativeness, lowered inhibitions, euphoria, mood swings	Marijuana has been used for relief of nausea and vomiting associated with antineoplastic chemotherapy and to reduce eye pressure in glaucoma	Fatigue, paranoia, delusions, hallucinations, possible psychosis	Cannabis	Marijuana, pot, grass, joint, Mary Jane, MJ
				Hashish	Hash, rope, sweet Lucy
Synthetic cannabinoids	Highly variable from elevated mood and relaxation to extreme anxiety, confusion, paranoia, hallucinations	Pain management in multiple sclerosis, diabetic neuropathy, nausea and vomiting	Rapid heart rate, vomiting, violent behavior, suicidal thoughts	Many chemical names	Fake weed, K2, Spice (over 500 street names for various chemical formulas)

TABLE 14–8 Summary of Symptoms Associated With the Syndromes of Intoxication and Withdrawal

CLASS OF DRUGS	INTOXICATION	WITHDRAWAL	COMMENTS
Alcohol	Aggressiveness, impaired judgment, impaired attention, irritability, euphoria, depression, emotional lability, slurred speech, incoordination, unsteady gait, nystagmus, flushed face	Tremors, nausea/vomiting, malaise, weakness, tachycardia, sweating, elevated blood pressure, anxiety, depressed mood, irritability, hallucinations, headache, insomnia, seizures	Alcohol withdrawal begins within 4–6 hr after last drink. May progress to delirium tremens on 2nd or 3rd day. Use of Librium or Serax is common for medication-assisted treatment.
Amphetamines and related substances	Fighting, grandiosity, hypervigilance, psychomotor agitation, impaired judgment, tachycardia, pupillary dilation, elevated blood pressure, perspiration or chills, nausea and vomiting	Anxiety, depressed mood, irritability, craving for the substance, fatigue, insomnia or hypersomnia, psychomotor agitation, paranoid and suicidal ideation	Withdrawal symptoms usually peak within 2–4 days, although depression and irritability may persist for months. Antidepressants may be used.
Caffeine	Restlessness, nervousness, excitement, insomnia, flushed face, diuresis, gastrointestinal complaints, muscle twitching, rambling flow of thought and speech, cardiac arrhythmia, periods of inexhaustibility, psychomotor agitation	Headache	Caffeine is contained in coffee, tea, colas, cocoa, chocolate, some over-the-counter analgesics, "cold" preparations, and stimulants.
Cannabis	Euphoria, anxiety, suspiciousness, sensation of slowed time, impaired judgment, social withdrawal, tachycardia, conjunctival redness, increased appetite, hallucinations	Restlessness, irritability, insomnia, loss of appetite, depressed mood, tremors, fever, chills, headache, stomach pain	Intoxication occurs immediately and lasts about 3 hours. Oral ingestion is more slowly absorbed and has longer-lasting effects.
Cocaine	Euphoria, fighting, grandiosity, hypervigilance, psychomotor agitation, impaired judgment, tachycardia, elevated blood pressure, pupillary dilation, perspiration or chills, nausea/vomiting, hallucinations, delirium	Depression, anxiety, irritability, fatigue, insomnia or hypersomnia, psychomotor agitation, paranoid or suicidal ideation, apathy, social withdrawal	Large doses of the drug can result in convulsions or death from cardiac arrhythmias or respiratory paralysis.

CLASS OF DRUGS	INTOXICATION	WITHDRAWAL	COMMENTS
Inhalants	Belligerence, assaultiveness, apathy, impaired judgment, dizziness, nystagmus, slurred speech, unsteady gait, lethargy, depressed reflexes, tremor, blurred vision, stupor or coma, euphoria, irritation around eyes, throat, and nose		Intoxication occurs within 5 minutes of inhalation. Symptoms last 60–90 minutes. Large doses can result in death from CNS depression or cardiac arrhythmia.
Nicotine		Craving for the drug, irritability, anger, frustration, anxiety, difficulty concentrating, restlessness, decreased heart rate, increased appetite, weight gain, tremor, headaches, insomnia	Symptoms of withdrawal begin within 24 hr of last drug use and decrease in intensity over days, weeks, or sometimes longer.
Opioids	Euphoria, lethargy, somnolence, apathy, dysphoria, impaired judgment, pupillary constriction, drowsiness, slurred speech, constipation, nausea, decreased respiratory rate and blood pressure	Craving for the drug, nausea/vomiting, muscle aches, lacrimation or rhinorrhea, pupillary dilation, piloerection or sweating, diarrhea, yawning, fever, insomnia	Withdrawal symptoms appear within 6–8 hr after last dose, reach a peak in the 2nd or 3rd day, and subside in 5–10 days. Times are shorter with meperidine and longer with methadone.
Phencyclidine and related substances	Belligerence, assaultiveness, impulsiveness, psychomotor agitation, impaired judgment, nystagmus, increased heart rate and blood pressure, diminished pain response, ataxia, dysarthria, muscle rigidity, seizures, hyperacusis, delirium		Delirium can occur within 24 hr after use of phencyclidine or may occur up to a week following recovery from an overdose of the drug.
Sedatives, hypnotics, and anxiolytics	Disinhibition of sexual or aggressive impulses, mood lability, impaired judgment, slurred speech, incoordination, unsteady gait, impairment in attention or memory disorientation, confusion	Nausea/vomiting, malaise, weakness, tachycardia, sweating, anxiety, irritability, orthostatic hypotension, tremor, insomnia, seizures	Withdrawal may progress to delirium, usually within 1 week of last use. Long-acting barbiturates or benzodiazepines may be used in withdrawal medication-assisted treatment.

situation, where insight may be gained from feedback regarding the perceptions of others.

Whether alone or in a group, the nurse may gain a greater understanding about attitudes and feelings related to substance abuse by responding to the following types of questions. As written here, the questions are specific to alcohol, but they could be adapted for any substance:

■ What are my drinking patterns?
■ If I drink, why do I drink? When, where, and how much?
■ If I don't drink, why do I abstain?
■ Am I comfortable with my drinking patterns?
■ If I decided not to drink any more, would that be a problem for me?
■ What did I learn from my parents about drinking?
■ Have my attitudes changed as an adult?
■ What are my feelings about people who become intoxicated?
■ Does it seem more acceptable for some individuals than for others?
■ Do I ever use terms like "sot," "drunk," or "boozer," to describe some individuals who overindulge yet overlook it in others?
■ Do I ever overindulge?
■ Has the use of alcohol (by me or others) affected my life in any way?
■ Do I see alcohol/drug abuse as a sign of weakness? A moral problem? An illness?

Unless nurses fully understand and accept their own attitudes and feelings, they cannot be empathetic toward patients' problems. Clients in recovery need to know they are accepted for themselves, regardless of past behaviors. Nurses must be able to separate the patient from the behavior and to accept that individual with unconditional positive regard.

Motivational Interviewing

Motivational interviewing is an approach that can be used in the assessment and intervention process for clients with any disorder, although it first gained popularity in treatment of substance use disorders. Its focus is on using skills such as empathy and reflection to explore the client's motivation, strengths, and readiness for change. Some of the previously mentioned questions could easily be reframed to explore the client's attitudes and feelings. Through this process, the client is empowered to become an active partner in treatment goals while exploring reasons for any resistance to behavior change. For example, rather than telling a client that he or she must abstain from alcohol and must attend 12-step meetings, the healthcare

professional helps the client articulate what he or she wants to achieve and then facilitates the process of exploring advantages and disadvantages of desired behavior change. See Chapter 5, Relationship Development and Therapeutic Communication, for more discussion of this approach and a sample interview using motivational interviewing.

🔷 Because this is a patient-centered approach that encourages empowerment and active engagement, it articulates well with two current trends in psychiatric mental health nursing care: recognizing the importance of patient-centered care as an essential nursing competency (Institute of Medicine, 2003) and the recovery model (see Chapter 10, The Recovery Model, for more discussion of this model).

Assessment Tools

Nurses often perform the admission interview. A variety of assessment tools are appropriate for use in chemical dependency units. A nursing history and assessment tool is presented in Chapter 6, The Nursing Process in Psychiatric Mental Health Nursing. With some adaptation, it is an appropriate instrument for creating a database on clients who abuse substances. Box 14–1 presents a drug history and assessment that could be used in conjunction with the general biopsychosocial assessment.

The Clinical Institute Withdrawal Assessment of Alcohol Scale, Revised (CIWA-Ar) is an excellent tool that is used by many hospitals to assess risk and severity of withdrawal from alcohol. It may be used for initial assessment as well as ongoing monitoring of alcohol withdrawal symptoms. A copy of the CIWA-Ar is presented in Box 14–2.

Other screening tools exist for determining whether an individual has a problem with substances. Two such tools developed by the APA for the diagnosis of alcoholism include the Michigan Alcoholism Screening Test and the CAGE Questionnaire (Boxes 14–3 and 14–4). Some psychiatric units administer these surveys to all clients who are admitted to help determine if there is a secondary alcoholism problem in addition to the psychiatric problem for which the client is being admitted (sometimes called **dual diagnosis).** These tools can be adapted for use in diagnosing problems with other drugs as well.

Dual Diagnosis

If it is determined that the client has a coexisting substance disorder and mental illness, he or she may be assigned to a special program that targets both

BOX 14–1 Drug History and Assessment*

1. When you were growing up, did anyone in your family drink alcohol or take other kinds of drugs?
2. If so, how did the substance use affect the family situation?
3. When did you have your first drink/drugs?
4. How long have you been drinking/taking drugs on a regular basis?
5. What is your pattern of substance use?
   a. When do you use substances?
   b. What do you use?
   c. How much do you use?
   d. Where are you and with whom when you use substances?
6. When did you have your last drink/drug? What was it, and how much did you consume?
7. Does using the substance(s) cause problems for you? Describe. Include family, friends, job, school, other.
8. Have you ever experienced injury as a result of substance use?
9. Have you ever been arrested or incarcerated for drinking/using drugs?
10. Have you ever tried to stop drinking/using drugs? If so, what was the result? Did you experience any physical symptoms, such as tremors, headache, insomnia, sweating, or seizures?
11. Have you ever experienced loss of memory for times when you have been drinking/using drugs?
12. Describe a typical day in your life.
13. Are there any changes you would like to make in your life? If so, what are they?
14. What plans or ideas do you have for seeing that these changes occur?

*To be used in conjunction with general biopsychosocial nursing history and assessment tool.

BOX 14–2 Clinical Institute Withdrawal Assessment of Alcohol Scale, Revised (CIWA-Ar)

Patient: _____   Date: _____

Time: _____ (24-hour clock, midnight = 00:00)

Pulse or heart rate, taken for one minute: _____   Blood pressure: _____

NAUSEA AND VOMITING—Ask "Do you feel sick to your stomach? Have you vomited?" Observation. 0 no nausea and no vomiting 1 mild nausea with no vomiting 2 3 4 intermittent nausea with dry heaves 5 6 7 constant nausea, frequent dry heaves and vomiting	TACTILE DISTURBANCES—Ask "Have you any itching, pins and needles sensations, any burning, any numbness, or do you feel bugs crawling on or under your skin?" Observation. 0 none 1 very mild itching, pins and needles, burning or numbness 2 mild itching, pins and needles, burning or numbness 3 moderate itching, pins and needles, burning or numbness 4 moderately severe hallucinations 5 severe hallucinations 6 extremely severe hallucinations 7 continuous hallucinations
TREMOR—Arms extended and fingers spread apart. Observation. 0 no tremor 1 not visible, but can be felt fingertip to fingertip 2 3 4 moderate, with patient's arms extended 5 6 7 severe, even with arms not extended	AUDITORY DISTURBANCES—Ask "Are you more aware of sounds around you? Are they harsh? Do they frighten you? Are you hearing anything that is disturbing to you? Are you hearing things you know are not there?" Observation. 0 not present 1 very mild harshness or ability to frighten 2 mild harshness or ability to frighten 3 moderate harshness or ability to frighten 4 moderately severe hallucinations 5 severe hallucinations 6 extremely severe hallucinations 7 continuous hallucinations

Continued

BOX 14–2 Clinical Institute Withdrawal Assessment of Alcohol Scale, Revised (CIWA-Ar)—cont'd

PAROXYSMAL SWEATS—Observation. 0 no sweat visible 1 barely perceptible sweating, palms moist 2 3 4 beads of sweat obvious on forehead 5 6 7 drenching sweats	**VISUAL DISTURBANCES**—Ask "Does the light appear to be too bright? Is its color different? Does it hurt your eyes? Are you seeing anything that is disturbing to you? Are you seeing things you know are not there?" Observation. 0 not present 1 very mild sensitivity 2 mild sensitivity 3 moderate sensitivity 4 moderately severe hallucinations 5 severe hallucinations 6 extremely severe hallucinations 7 continuous hallucinations
ANXIETY—Ask "Do you feel nervous?" Observation. 0 no anxiety, at ease 1 mildly anxious 2 3 4 moderately anxious, or guarded, so anxiety is inferred 5 6 7 equivalent to acute panic states as seen in severe delirium or acute schizophrenic reactions	**HEADACHE, FULLNESS IN HEAD**—Ask "Does your head feel different? Does it feel like there is a band around your head?" Do not rate for dizziness or lightheadedness. Otherwise, rate severity. 0 not present 1 very mild 2 mild 3 moderate 4 moderately severe 5 severe 6 very severe 7 extremely severe
AGITATION—Observation. 0 normal activity 1 somewhat more than normal activity 2 3 4 moderately fidgety and restless 5 6 7 paces back and forth during most of the interview, or constantly thrashes about	**ORIENTATION AND CLOUDING OF SENSORIUM**—Ask "What day is this? Where are you? Who am I?" 0 oriented and can do serial additions 1 cannot do serial additions or is uncertain about date 2 disoriented for date by no more than 2 calendar days 3 disoriented for date by more than 2 calendar days 4 disoriented for place/or person
	Total CIWA-Ar Score _____ Rater's Initials _____ Maximum Possible Score 67

The CIWA-Ar is not copyrighted and may be reproduced freely. This assessment for monitoring withdrawal symptoms requires approximately 5 minutes to administer. The maximum score is 67 (see instrument). Patients scoring less than 10 do not usually need additional medication for withdrawal.

Source: From Sullivan, J. T., Sykora, K., Schneiderman, J., Naranjo, C A., & Sellers, E. M. (1989). Assessment of alcohol withdrawal: The revised Clinical Institute Withdrawal Assessment for Alcohol scale (CIWA-Ar). British Journal of Addiction, 84, 1353–1357.

problems. Traditional counseling approaches use more confrontation than that which is considered appropriate for clients with dual diagnoses. Most dual diagnosis programs take a more supportive and less confrontational approach.

Peer support groups are an important part of the treatment program. Group members offer encouragement and practical advice to each other. Psychodynamic therapy can be useful for some individuals with dual diagnoses by delving into the personal

BOX 14–3 Michigan Alcoholism Screening Test (MAST)

Answer the following questions by placing an X under yes or no.*	Yes	No
1. Do you enjoy a drink now and then?	0	0
2. Do you feel you are a normal drinker? (By *normal*, we mean you drink less than or as much as most people.)		2
3. Have you ever awakened the morning after some drinking the night before and found that you could not remember a part of the evening?	2	
4. Does your wife, husband, parent, or other near relative ever worry or complain about your drinking?	1	
5. Can you stop drinking without a struggle after one or two drinks?		2
6. Do you ever feel guilty about your drinking?	1	
7. Do friends or relatives think you are a normal drinker?		2
8. Are you able to stop drinking when you want to?		2
9. Have you ever attended a meeting of Alcoholics Anonymous (AA)?	5	
10. Have you gotten into physical fights when drinking?	1	
11. Has your drinking ever created problems between you and your wife, husband, a parent, or other relative?	2	
12. Has your wife, husband, or another family member ever gone to anyone for help about your drinking?	2	
13. Have you ever lost friends because of your drinking?	2	
14. Have you ever gotten into trouble at work or school because of drinking?	2	
15. Have you ever lost a job because of drinking?	2	
16. Have you ever neglected your obligations, your family, or your work for 2 or more days in a row because you were drinking?	2	
17. Do you drink before noon fairly often?	1	
18. Have you ever been told you have liver trouble? Cirrhosis?	2	
19. After heavy drinking, have you ever had delirium tremens (DTs) or severe shaking or heard voices or seen things that really were not there?	5	
20. Have you ever gone to anyone for help about your drinking?	5	
21. Have you ever been in a hospital because of drinking?	5	
22. Have you ever been a patient in a psychiatric hospital or on a psychiatric ward of a general hospital where drinking was part of the problem that resulted in hospitalization?	2	
23. Have you ever been seen at a psychiatric or mental health clinic or gone to any doctor, social worker, or clergyman for help with any emotional problem, where drinking was part of the problem?	2	
24. Have you ever been arrested for drunk driving, driving while intoxicated, or driving under the influence of alcoholic beverages? (If yes, how many times? _____)	2 ea	
25. Have you ever been arrested or taken into custody, even for a few hours, because of other drunk behavior? (If yes, how many times? _____)	2 ea	

*Items are scored under the response that would indicate a problem with alcohol.
Method of scoring:
   0–3 points = no problem with alcohol
   4 points = possible problem with alcohol
   5 or more = indicates problem with alcohol
Source: From Selzer, M. L. (1971). The Michigan alcohol screening test: The quest for a new diagnostic instrument. American Journal of Psychiatry, 127, 1653–1658, with permission.

history of how psychiatric disorders and substance abuse have reinforced one another and how the cycle can be broken. Cognitive and behavioral therapies are helpful in training clients to monitor moods and thought patterns that lead to substance abuse. Teaching patients about coping skills and stress management offers skills that promote abstinence and dealing with substance cravings. (See Chapter 21, Eating Disorders, for Vic's discussion of his dual diagnosis, alcohol use disorder and anorexia nervosa, in "Real People, Real Stories").

Individuals with dual diagnoses should be educated about 12-step recovery programs (e.g., Alcoholics Anonymous and Narcotics Anonymous). Some clients are resistant to attending 12-step programs, and they may do better in substance abuse support groups specifically designed for people with psychiatric disorders.

BOX 14–4 The CAGE Questionnaire

1. Have you ever felt you should **C**ut down on your drinking?
2. Have people **A**nnoyed you by criticizing your drinking?
3. Have you ever felt bad or **G**uilty about your drinking?
4. Have you ever had a drink first thing in the morning to steady your nerves or get rid of a hangover (**E**ye-opener)?

Scoring: 2 or 3 "yes" answers strongly suggest a problem with alcohol.
Source: From Mayfield, D., McLeod, G., & Hall, P. (1974). The CAGE questionnaire: Validation of a new alcoholism screening instrument. American Journal of Psychiatry, 131, 1121–1123, with permission.

Substance abuse groups are usually integrated into regular programming for the psychiatric patient with a dual diagnosis. An individual in a psychiatric facility or day treatment program may attend a substance abuse group periodically in lieu of another scheduled activity therapy. Topics are directed toward areas that are unique to clients with a mental illness, such as mixing medications with other substances, as well as topics that are common to primary substances abusers. Individuals are encouraged to discuss their personal problems.

Continued attendance at 12-step group meetings is encouraged on discharge from treatment. Family involvement is enlisted, and preventive strategies are outlined. Individual case management is common, and success is often promoted by this close supervision.

Diagnosis and Outcome Identification

The next step in the nursing process is to identify appropriate nursing diagnoses by analyzing the data collected during the assessment phase. The individual who abuses or is dependent on substances undoubtedly has many unmet physical and emotional needs. Table 14–9 presents a list of patient behaviors and the NANDA-I nursing diagnoses (Herdman & Kamitsuru, 2018) that correspond to those behaviors, which may be used in planning care for the patient with a substance use disorder.

Outcome Criteria

The following criteria may be used for measurement of outcomes in the care of the patient with substance-related disorders.

The patient:

■ Has not experienced physical injury.
■ Has not caused harm to self or others.

TABLE 14–9 Assigning Nursing Diagnoses to Behaviors Commonly Associated With Substance Use Disorders

BEHAVIORS	NURSING DIAGNOSES
Makes statements such as, "I don't have a problem with [substance]. I can quit any time I want to." Delays seeking assistance; does not perceive problems related to use of substances; minimizes use of substances; unable to admit impact of disease on life pattern	Denial
Abuse of chemical agents; destructive behavior toward others and self; inability to meet basic needs; inability to meet role expectations; risk taking	Ineffective coping
Loss of weight, pale conjunctiva and mucous membranes, decreased skin turgor, electrolyte imbalance, anemia, drinks alcohol or takes drugs instead of eating	Imbalanced nutrition: Less than body requirements Deficient fluid volume
Risk factors: malnutrition, altered immune system, failing to avoid exposure to pathogens	Risk for infection
Criticizes self and others, self-destructive behavior (abuse of substances as a coping mechanism), family conflicts	Chronic low self-esteem
Denies that substance is harmful; continues to use substance in light of obvious consequences	Deficient knowledge
FOR PATIENT WITHDRAWING FROM CNS DEPRESSANTS	
Risk factors: CNS agitation (tremors, elevated blood pressure, nausea and vomiting, hallucinations, illusions, tachycardia, anxiety, seizures)	Risk for injury
FOR PATIENT WITHDRAWING FROM CNS STIMULANTS	
Risk factors: intense feelings of lassitude and depression; "crashing," suicidal ideation	Risk for suicide

- Accepts responsibility for own behavior.
- Acknowledges association between personal problems and use of substance(s).
- Demonstrates adaptive coping mechanisms that can be used in stressful situations (instead of taking substances).
- Shows no signs or symptoms of infection or malnutrition.
- Exhibits evidence of increased self-worth by attempting new projects without fear of failure and by demonstrating less defensive behavior toward others.
- Verbalizes importance of abstaining from use of substances in order to maintain optimal wellness.

Planning and Implementation

Implementation of care with patients who abuse substances is a long-term process, often beginning with **detoxification** and progressing to total abstinence. The following are common major treatment objectives for each phase of this process.

Detoxification:

- Provide a safe and supportive environment for detoxification.

- Administer medication-assisted treatment (see section on "Treatment Modalities for Substance-Related Disorders" for definition and discussion) as ordered.

Intermediate Care:

- Provide explanations of physical symptoms.
- Promote understanding and identify the causes of substance dependency.
- Provide education and assistance in course of treatment to patient and family.

Rehabilitation

- Encourage continued participation in long-term treatment.
- Promote participation in outpatient support system (e.g., Alcoholics Anonymous [AA]).
- Assist patient to identify alternative sources of satisfaction.
- Provide support for health promotion and maintenance.

Table 14–10 provides a plan of care for the patient with substance-related disorders. Selected nursing diagnoses are presented, along with outcome criteria, appropriate nursing interventions, and rationales for each.

Table 14–10 | CARE PLAN FOR THE PATIENT WITH A SUBSTANCE-RELATED DISORDER

NURSING DIAGNOSIS: RISK FOR INJURY

RELATED TO: Central nervous system (CNS) agitation secondary to withdrawal from alcohol or other CNS depressant

OUTCOME CRITERIA	NURSING INTERVENTIONS	RATIONALE
Short-Term Goal ■ Patient's condition will stabilize within 72 hours. **Long-Term Goal** ■ Patient will not experience physical injury.	1. Assess patient's level of disorientation. 2. Obtain a drug history, if possible. It is important to determine the type of substance(s) used, the time and amount of last use, the length and frequency of use, and the amount used on a daily basis. 3. Obtain a urine sample for laboratory analysis of substance content. 4. Keep the patient in as quiet an environment as possible. A private room is ideal. 5. Observe the patient's behaviors frequently. If seriousness of the condition warrants, it may be necessary to assign a staff person on a one-to-one basis. 6. Accompany and assist the patient when ambulating and use a wheelchair for transporting the patient long distances.	1. Determination of specific requirements for safety must be made. 2. This information is essential to know what to expect during the withdrawal process and to establish an appropriate plan of care. 3. A subjective history is often not accurate. 4. Excessive stimuli may increase patient agitation. 5. Patient safety is a nursing priority. 6. In weakened condition, patient will require assistance to prevent falls.

Continued

Table 14–10	CARE PLAN FOR THE PATIENT WITH A SUBSTANCE-RELATED DISORDER—cont'd

OUTCOME CRITERIA	NURSING INTERVENTIONS	RATIONALE
	7. Pad the headboard and side rails of the bed with thick towels.	7. Individuals in withdrawal from CNS depressants are at risk for seizures. Padding will offer protection from injury should a seizure occur.
	8. Ensure that smoking materials and other potentially harmful objects are stored away from the patient's access. Institute suicide precautions, if necessary, for patients withdrawing from CNS stimulants.	8. A patient in withdrawal has impaired judgment. The environment must be made safe for him or her.
	9. Monitor the patient's vital signs every 15 minutes, and less frequently as acute symptoms subside.	9. Accurate assessment is vital for the provision of safe and effective nursing care.
	10. Follow the medication regimen as ordered by the physician.	10. Medication-assisted treatment will be prescribed to ease the symptoms of withdrawal from substances. (See section on " Medication-Assisted Treatment.")

NURSING DIAGNOSIS: **DENIAL**

RELATED TO: Weak, underdeveloped ego

EVIDENCED BY: Statements indicating no problem with substance use

OUTCOME CRITERIA	NURSING INTERVENTIONS	RATIONALE
Short-Term Goal ■ Patient will focus on behavioral outcomes associated with substance use rather than using deflection to focus on external issues. **Long-Term Goal** ■ Patient will verbalize acceptance of responsibility for own behavior and acknowledge association between substance use and personal problems.	1. Begin by working to develop a trusting nurse–patient relationship. Be honest. Keep all promises. 2. Convey an attitude of acceptance. Ensure that he or she understands "It is not *you* but your *behavior* that is unacceptable." 3. Provide information to correct misconceptions about substance abuse. 4. Identify recent maladaptive behaviors or situations that have occurred in the patient's life and discuss how use of substances may have been a contributing factor.	1. Trust is the basis of a therapeutic relationship. 2. An attitude of acceptance promotes feelings of dignity and self-worth. 3. Many myths abound regarding use of specific substances. In addition, the patient may rationalize his or her behavior with statements such as, "I'm not an alcoholic. I can stop drinking any time I want. Besides, I only drink beer." Or "I only smoke pot to relax before class. So what? I know lots of people who do. Besides, you can't get hooked on pot." Factual information presented in a matter-of-fact, nonjudgmental way explaining what behaviors constitute substance-related disorders may help the patient focus on his or her own behaviors as an illness that requires help. 4. The first step in decreasing use of denial is for the patient to see the relationship between substance use and personal problems.

Table 14–10 | CARE PLAN FOR THE PATIENT WITH A SUBSTANCE-RELATED DISORDER—cont'd

OUTCOME CRITERIA	NURSING INTERVENTIONS	RATIONALE
	5. 💬 Use confrontation with caring. Do not allow patient to fantasize about his or her lifestyle (e.g., "It is my understanding that the last time you drank alcohol, you . . ." or "The lab report shows that you were under the influence of alcohol when you had the accident that injured three people").	5. Confrontation interferes with patient's ability to use denial; a caring attitude preserves self-esteem and avoids putting the patient on the defensive.
	6. Do not accept rationalization or projection as patient attempts to make excuses for or blame his or her behavior on other people or situations.	6. Rationalization and projection prolong denial that problems exist in the patient's life because of substance use.
	7. Encourage participation in group activities.	7. Peer feedback is often more accepted than feedback from authority figures. Peer pressure can be a strong factor, as well as association with individuals who are experiencing or who have experienced similar problems.
	8. Offer immediate positive recognition of patient's expressions of insight gained regarding illness and acceptance of responsibility for his or her own behavior.	8. Positive reinforcement enhances self-esteem and encourages repetition of desirable behaviors.

NURSING DIAGNOSIS: INEFFECTIVE COPING

RELATED TO: Inadequate coping skills

EVIDENCED BY: Use of substances as coping mechanism; manipulative behavior

OUTCOME CRITERIA	NURSING INTERVENTIONS	RATIONALE
Short-Term Goal ■ Patient will express true feelings about using substances as a method of coping with stress. **Long-Term Goal** ■ Patient will be able to verbalize adaptive coping mechanisms to use, instead of substance abuse, in response to stress (and demonstrate, as applicable).	1. Spend time with the patient to establish a trusting relationship. 2. Set limits on manipulative behavior. Be sure that the patient knows what is acceptable, what is not, and the consequences for violating the limits set. Ensure that all staff maintains consistency with this intervention. 3. Encourage the patient to verbalize feelings, fears, and anxieties. Answer any questions he or she may have regarding the disorder. 4. Explain the effects of substance abuse on the body. Emphasize that the prognosis is closely related to abstinence. 5. Explore options available to assist with stressful situations rather than resorting to substance abuse (e.g., contacting various members of Alcoholics Anonymous or Narcotics Anonymous; physical exercise; relaxation techniques; meditation).	1. Establishing trust is the foundation for therapeutic intervention and relationship development. 2. The patient is unable to establish his or her own limits, so limits must be set for him or her. Unless administration of consequences for violation of limits is consistent, manipulative behavior will not be eliminated. 3. Verbalization of feelings in a nonthreatening environment may help the patient come to terms with long-unresolved issues. 4. Many patients lack knowledge regarding the deleterious effects of substance abuse on the body. 5. The patient may have persistently resorted to chemical abuse and thus may possess little or no knowledge of adaptive responses to stress.

Continued

Table 14–10 | **CARE PLAN FOR THE PATIENT WITH A SUBSTANCE-RELATED DISORDER—cont'd**

OUTCOME CRITERIA	NURSING INTERVENTIONS	RATIONALE
	6. Provide positive reinforcement for evidence of gratification delayed appropriately. Encourage the patient to be as independent as possible in performing his or her self-care. Provide positive feedback for independent decision making and effective use of problem-solving skills.	6. Positive reinforcement increases self-esteem and encourages repetition of adaptive behaviors.

NURSING DIAGNOSIS: IMBALANCED NUTRITION: LESS THAN BODY REQUIREMENTS/ DEFICIENT FLUID VOLUME

RELATED TO: Use of substances instead of eating

EVIDENCED BY: Loss of weight, pale conjunctiva and mucous membranes, poor skin turgor, electrolyte imbalance, anemias (and/or other signs and symptoms of malnutrition/dehydration)

OUTCOME CRITERIA	NURSING INTERVENTIONS	RATIONALE
Short-Term Goal ■ Abnormal lab values will be restored to normal. ■ Patient will gain weight on a regular, nutritious diet. **Long-Term Goal** ■ Patient will be free of signs/symptoms of malnutrition/ dehydration.	1. Parenteral support may be required initially. 2. Encourage cessation of smoking. 3. Consult dietitian. Determine the number of calories required based on body size and level of activity. Document intake and output and calorie count, and weigh patient daily. 4. Ensure that the amount of protein in the diet is correct for the individual patient's condition. Protein intake should be adequate to maintain nitrogen equilibrium but should be drastically decreased or eliminated if there is potential for hepatic coma. 5. Sodium may need to be restricted. 6. Provide foods that are nonirritating to patients with esophageal varices. 7. Provide small frequent feeding of patient's favorite foods. Supplement nutritious meals with multiple vitamin and mineral tablet.	1. To correct fluid and electrolyte imbalance, hypoglycemia, and some vitamin deficiencies. 2. To facilitate repair of damage to GI tract. 3. These interventions are necessary to maintain an ongoing nutritional assessment. 4. Diseased liver may be incapable of properly metabolizing proteins, resulting in an accumulation of ammonia in the blood that circulates to the brain and can result in altered consciousness. 5. To minimize fluid retention (e.g., ascites and edema). 6. To avoid irritation and bleeding of these swollen blood vessels. 7. To encourage intake and facilitate patient's achievement of adequate nutrition.

Concept Care Mapping

The concept map care plan (see Chapter 6) is a diagrammatic teaching and learning strategy that allows visualization of interrelationships between medical diagnoses, nursing diagnoses, assessment data, and treatments. An example of a concept map care plan for a patient with a substance use disorder is presented in Figure 14–3.

Patient and Family Education

The role of patient–teacher is important in the psychiatric area, as it is in all areas of nursing. A list of topics

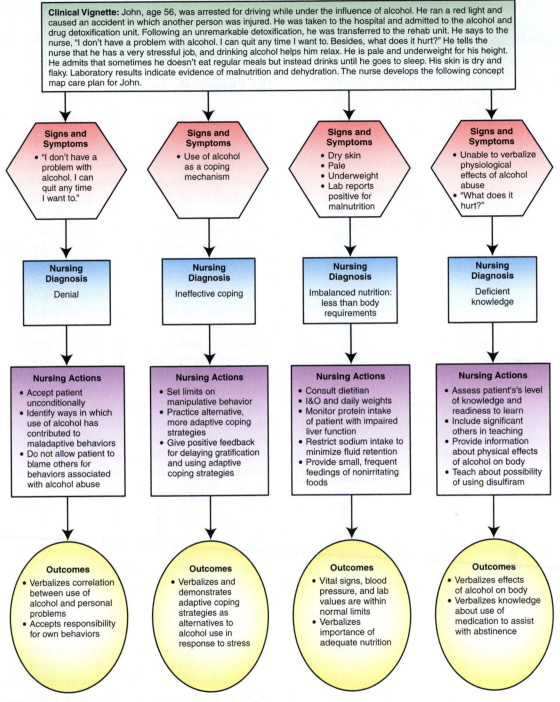

Clinical Vignette: John, age 56, was arrested for driving while under the influence of alcohol. He ran a red light and caused an accident in which another person was injured. He was taken to the hospital and admitted to the alcohol and drug detoxification unit. Following an unremarkable detoxification, he was transferred to the rehab unit. He says to the nurse, "I don't have a problem with alcohol. I can quit any time I want to. Besides, what does it hurt?" He tells the nurse that he has a very stressful job, and drinking alcohol helps him relax. He is pale and underweight for his height. He admits that sometimes he doesn't eat regular meals but instead drinks until he goes to sleep. His skin is dry and flaky. Laboratory results indicate evidence of malnutrition and dehydration. The nurse develops the following concept map care plan for John.

Signs and Symptoms
- "I don't have a problem with alcohol. I can quit any time I want to."

Signs and Symptoms
- Use of alcohol as a coping mechanism

Signs and Symptoms
- Dry skin
- Pale
- Underweight
- Lab reports positive for malnutrition

Signs and Symptoms
- Unable to verbalize physiological effects of alcohol abuse
- "What does it hurt?"

Nursing Diagnosis
Denial

Nursing Diagnosis
Ineffective coping

Nursing Diagnosis
Imbalanced nutrition: less than body requirements

Nursing Diagnosis
Deficient knowledge

Nursing Actions
- Accept patient unconditionally
- Identify ways in which use of alcohol has contributed to maladaptive behaviors
- Do not allow patient to blame others for behaviors associated with alcohol abuse

Nursing Actions
- Set limits on manipulative behavior
- Practice alternative, more adaptive coping strategies
- Give positive feedback for delaying gratification and using adaptive coping strategies

Nursing Actions
- Consult dietitian
- I&O and daily weights
- Monitor protein intake of patient with impaired liver function
- Restrict sodium intake to minimize fluid retention
- Provide small, frequent feedings of nonirritating foods

Nursing Actions
- Assess patient's's level of knowledge and readiness to learn
- Include significant others in teaching
- Provide information about physical effects of alcohol on body
- Teach about possibility of using disulfiram

Outcomes
- Verbalizes correlation between use of alcohol and personal problems
- Accepts responsibility for own behaviors

Outcomes
- Verbalizes and demonstrates adaptive coping strategies as alternatives to alcohol use in response to stress

Outcomes
- Vital signs, blood pressure, and lab values are within normal limits
- Verbalizes importance of adequate nutrition

Outcomes
- Verbalizes effects of alcohol on body
- Verbalizes knowledge about use of medication to assist with abstinence

FIGURE 14–3 Concept map care plan for patient with alcoholism.

for patient and family education relevant to substance-related disorders is presented in Box 14–5.

Evaluation

The final step of the nursing process involves reassessment to determine if the nursing interventions have

been effective in achieving the intended goals of care. Evaluation of the patient with a substance-related disorder may be accomplished by using information gathered from the following reassessment questions:

- Has detoxification occurred without complications?
- Is the patient no longer in denial?

BOX 14–5 Topics for Patient and Family Education Related to Substance Use Disorders

NATURE OF THE ILLNESS

1. Effects of (substance) on the body
   a. Alcohol
   b. Other CNS depressants
   c. CNS stimulants
   d. Hallucinogens
   e. Inhalants
   f. Opioids
   g. Cannabinols
2. Ways in which use of (substance) affects life.

MANAGEMENT OF THE ILLNESS

1. Activities to substitute for (substance) in times of stress
2. Relaxation techniques
   a. Progressive relaxation
   b. Tense and relax
   c. Deep breathing
   d. Autogenics
3. Problem-solving skills
4. The essentials of good nutrition
5. Medication-assisted treatment

SUPPORT SERVICES

1. Financial assistance
2. Legal assistance
3. Alcoholics Anonymous (or other support group specific to another substance)
4. One-to-one support person

■ Does the patient accept responsibility for his or her own behavior? Has he or she acknowledged a personal problem with substances?

■ Has a correlation been made between personal problems and the use of substances?

■ Has the patient remained substance free during treatment?

■ Does the patient cooperate with treatment?

■ Does the patient refrain from manipulative behavior and violation of limits?

■ Is the patient able to verbalize motivation toward alternative adaptive coping strategies to substitute for substance use? Has the use of these strategies been demonstrated? Does positive reinforcement encourage repetition of these adaptive behaviors?

■ Has nutritional status been restored? Does the patient consume diet adequate for his or her size and level of activity? Is the patient able to discuss the importance of adequate nutrition?

■ Has the patient remained free of infection during hospitalization?

■ Is the patient able to verbalize the effects of substance abuse on the body?

The Chemically Impaired Nurse

Substance abuse and addiction is a problem that has the potential for impairment in an individual's social, occupational, psychological, and physical functioning. This becomes an especially serious problem when the impaired person is responsible for the lives of others on a daily basis. It is estimated that 10 percent of nurses have substance use disorders which is the same as the prevalence in the general public (Worley, 2017). Alcohol is the most widely abused drug, followed closely by narcotics. Nurses who abuse substances have an added vulnerability because they often handle controlled substances when providing patient care.

For years, the impaired nurse was protected, promoted, transferred, ignored, or fired. These types of responses promoted the growth of the problem. Programs are needed that involve early reporting and treatment of chemical addiction as a disease with a focus on public safety and rehabilitation of the nurse.

How does one identify the impaired nurse? It is still easiest to overlook what *might* be a problem. Denial, on the part of the impaired nurse as well as nurse colleagues, is still the strongest reason for not dealing with substance abuse problems. Some states have mandatory reporting laws that require observers to report substance-abusing nurses to the state board of nursing. They are difficult laws to enforce, and hospitals are not always compliant with mandatory reporting. Some hospitals may choose not to report to the state board of nursing if the impaired nurse is actively seeking treatment and is not placing patients in danger.

A number of clues for recognizing substance impairment in nurses have been identified (Ellis & Hartley, 2012). Signs of substance impairment are not easy to detect, and they vary according to the substance being used. There may be high absenteeism if the person's source is outside the work area, or the individual may rarely miss work if the substance source is at work. There may be an increase in "wasting" of drugs, increased incidences of incorrect narcotic counts, and a higher record of signing out drugs than for other nurses.

Poor concentration, difficulty meeting deadlines, inappropriate responses, and poor memory or recall usually occur late in the disease process. The person may also have problems with relationships. Some other possible signs are irritability, mood swings, tendency to isolate, elaborate excuses for behavior, unkempt appearance, impaired motor coordination, slurred speech, flushed face, inconsistent job performance, and frequent use of the restroom. He or she may frequently medicate other nurses' patients, and there may be patient complaints of inadequate pain control. Discrepancies in documentation may occur. Ideally, suspicious behavior has been recognized by peers and intervention sought before the impaired nurse reaches late stages of the disease process. As uncomfortable as it may seem to tell a supervisor about suspected impairment in one of your peers, it is in the interest of the nurse's health and most critically important to ensuring patient safety.

If suspicious behavior occurs, it is important to keep careful, objective records. Confrontation with the impaired nurse will undoubtedly result in hostility and denial. Confrontation should occur in the presence of a supervisor or other nurse manager and should include the offer of assistance in seeking treatment. If a report is made to the state board of nursing, it should be a factual documentation of specific events and actions, not a diagnostic statement of impairment.

State boards generally decide each case on an individual basis. A state board may deny, suspend, or revoke a license based on a report of chemical abuse by a nurse. Several state boards of nursing have passed diversionary laws that allow impaired nurses to avoid disciplinary action by agreeing to seek treatment. Some of these state boards administer the treatment programs themselves, and others refer the nurse to community resources or state nurses' association assistance programs. Treatment may entail successful completion of inpatient, outpatient, group, or individual counseling treatment program(s); evidence of regular attendance at nurse support groups or 12-step program; random negative drug screens; and employment or volunteer activities during the suspension period. When a nurse is deemed safe to return to practice, he or she may be closely monitored for several years and required to undergo random drug screenings. The nurse also may be required to practice under specifically circumscribed conditions for a designated period.

In 1982, the American Nurses Association (ANA) House of Delegates adopted a national resolution to provide assistance to impaired nurses. Since that time, the majority of state nurses' associations have developed (or are developing) programs for nurses who are impaired by substances or psychiatric illness. The individuals who administer these efforts are nurse members of the state associations as well as nurses who are in recovery themselves. For this reason, they are called **peer assistance programs.**

The peer assistance programs strive to intervene early, reduce hazards to patients, and increase prospects for the nurse's recovery. Most states provide either a hot-line number that the impaired nurse or intervening colleague may call or phone numbers of peer assistance committee members, which are made available for the same purpose. Typically, a contract is drawn up detailing the method of treatment, which may be obtained from various sources, such as employee assistance programs, Alcoholics Anonymous, Narcotics Anonymous, private counseling, or outpatient clinics. Guidelines for monitoring the course of treatment are established. Peer support is provided through regular contact with the impaired nurse, usually for a period of 2 years. Peer assistance programs serve to assist impaired nurses to recognize their impairment, to obtain necessary treatment, and to regain accountability within their profession.

Codependency

The concept of **codependency** arose out of a need to define the dysfunctional behaviors that are evident among members of the family of a chemically addicted person. The term has been expanded to include all individuals from families who harbor secrets of physical or emotional abuse, other cruelties, or pathological conditions. Living under these conditions results in unmet needs for autonomy and self-esteem and a profound sense of powerlessness. The codependent person is able to achieve a sense of control only through fulfilling the needs of others. Personal identity is relinquished, and boundaries with the other person become blurred. The codependent person disowns his or her own needs and wants in order to respond to external demands and the demands of others. Codependence has been called "a dysfunctional relationship with oneself."

The traits associated with a codependent personality are varied. In a relationship, the codependent person derives self-worth from that of the partner, whose feelings and behaviors determine how the codependent should feel and behave. In order for the codependent to feel good, his or her partner must be happy and behave in appropriate ways. If the partner is not happy, the codependent feels responsible for *making* him or her happy. The codependent's home life is fraught with stress. Ego boundaries are weak, and behaviors are often enmeshed with those of the pathological partner. Denial that problems exist is common. Feelings are kept in control, and anxiety may be released in the form of stress-related illnesses or compulsive behaviors such as eating, spending, working, or use of substances.

Selected characteristics of the codependent individual (Beatty, 2011) include:

- Taking care of others at the expense of one's own needs
- Feeling responsible for fixing other people's problems
- Having low self-esteem; expecting to perform perfectly but never feeling "good enough"
- Desperately seeking approval from others; often identified as "people pleasers"
- Generally unhappy and seeking things outside oneself to attempt to fulfil unmet needs
- Tending to have come from dysfunctional families where there was abuse or neglect
- Having weak boundaries that lead to feelings of resentment, lack of trust, and anger toward others

The Codependent Nurse

Certain characteristics of codependence have been associated with the profession of nursing. A shortage of nurses combined with the increasing ranks of seriously ill patients may result in nurses providing care and fulfilling everyone's needs but their own. Many healthcare workers who are reared in homes with a chemically addicted person or otherwise dysfunctional family are at risk for having unresolved codependent tendencies activated. Nurses who, as children, assumed the "fixer" role in their dysfunctional families of origin may attempt to resume that role in their caregiving professions. They are attracted to a profession in which they are needed, but they nurture feelings of resentment for receiving so little in return. Their emotional needs go unmet; however, they continue to deny that these needs exist. Instead, these unmet emotional needs may be manifested through use of compulsive behaviors, such as work or spending excessively, or addictions, such as to food or substances.

Codependent nurses have a need to be in control. They often strive for an unrealistic level of achievement. Their self-worth comes from the feeling of being needed by others and of maintaining control over their environment. They nurture the dependence of others and accept the responsibility for the happiness and contentment of others. They rarely express their true feelings, and they do what is necessary to preserve harmony and maintain control. They are at high risk for physical and emotional burnout.

Treating Codependency

Cermak (1986) identified four stages in the recovery process for individuals with codependent personality:

Stage I: The Survival Stage. In this first stage, codependent persons must begin to let go of the denial that problems exist or that their personal capabilities are unlimited. This initiation of abstinence from blanket denial may be a very emotional and painful period.

Stage II: The Reidentification Stage. Reidentification occurs when the individuals are able to glimpse their true selves through a break in the denial system. They accept the label of codependent and take responsibility for their own dysfunctional behavior. Codependents tend to enter reidentification only after being convinced that it is more painful not to. They accept their limitations and are ready to face the issues of codependence.

Stage III: The Core Issues Stage. In this stage, the recovering codependent must face the fact that relationships cannot be managed by force of will. Each partner must be independent and autonomous. The goal of this stage is to detach from the struggles of life that exist because of prideful and willful efforts to control those things that are beyond the individual's power to control.

Stage IV: The Reintegration Stage. This is a stage of self-acceptance and willingness to change when codependents relinquish the power *over others* that was not rightfully theirs but reclaim the *personal* power that they do possess. Integrity is achieved out of awareness, honesty, and being in touch with one's spiritual consciousness. Control is achieved through self-discipline and self-confidence.

Self-help groups have been found to be helpful in the treatment of codependency. Groups developed for families of chemically addicted people, such as Al-Anon, may be of assistance. Groups specific to the problem of codependency also exist. One of these groups, which bases its philosophy on the Twelve Steps of Alcoholics Anonymous (see the section that follows) is:

Co-Dependents Anonymous (CoDA)
P.O. Box 33577
Phoenix, AZ 85067-3577P: (602) 277-7991
(888) 444-2359 (Toll free)
(888) 444-2379 (Spanish toll free)
www.coda.org

Treatment Modalities for Substance-Related Disorders

Self-Help Groups: Alcoholics Anonymous

Alcoholics Anonymous (AA) is a major self-help organization for the treatment of alcoholism. It was founded in 1935 by two alcoholics—a stockbroker, Bill Wilson, and a physician, Dr. Bob Smith—who discovered that they could remain sober through mutual support. They accomplished sobriety not as professionals but as peers who were able to share their common experiences. Soon they were working with other alcoholics, who in turn worked with others. The movement grew, and, remarkably, individuals who had been treated unsuccessfully by professionals were able to maintain sobriety through helping one another.

Today AA chapters exist in virtually every community in the United States. The self-help groups are based on the concept of peer support—acceptance and understanding from others who have experienced the same problems in their lives. The only requirement for membership is a desire on the part of the alcoholic person to stop drinking. Each new member is assigned a support person from whom he or she may seek assistance when the temptation to drink occurs.

A survey by the General Service Office of Alcoholics Anonymous in 2014 (Alcoholics Anonymous, 2015) revealed the following statistics: Members ages 30 and younger comprised 12 percent of the membership, and the average age of AA members was 50; women comprised 38 percent; 89 percent were white, 4 percent were African American, 3 percent were Hispanic, 1 percent were American Indian/Alaska Native, and 3 percent were Asian American and other minorities. Almost one-half (49%) of people involved in AA were referred by a healthcare professional or treatment facility. The sole purpose of AA is to help members stay sober. When sobriety has been achieved, members in turn are expected to help other alcoholic persons. The Twelve Steps that embody the philosophy of AA provide specific guidelines on how to attain and maintain sobriety (Box 14–6).

AA accepts alcoholism as an illness and promotes total abstinence as the only cure, emphasizing that the alcoholic person can never safely return to social drinking. They encourage the members to seek sobriety, taking one day at a time. The Twelve Traditions are the statements of principles that govern the organization.

AA has been the model for various other self-help groups associated with addiction problems. Some of these groups and the memberships for which they are organized are listed in Table 14–11. Nurses need to be fully and accurately informed about available self-help groups and their importance as a treatment resource on the healthcare continuum so they can use them as a referral source for patients with substance use disorders.

Pharmacotherapy

Disulfiram (Antabuse): Deterrent Therapy

Disulfiram (Antabuse) is a drug that can be administered as a deterrent to drinking to individuals who abuse alcohol. Ingestion of alcohol while disulfiram is in the body results in a syndrome of symptoms that can produce a great deal of discomfort for the individual. It can even result in death if the blood alcohol level is high. The reaction varies according to the sensitivity of the individual and how much alcohol was ingested.

Disulfiram works by inhibiting the enzyme aldehyde dehydrogenase, thereby blocking the oxidation of alcohol at the stage when acetaldehyde is converted to acetate. This results in an accumulation of acetaldehyde in the blood, which is thought to produce the symptoms associated with the disulfiram-alcohol reaction. These symptoms persist as long as alcohol is being metabolized. The rate of alcohol elimination does not appear to be affected.

Symptoms of disulfiram-alcohol reaction can occur within 5 to 10 minutes of ingestion of alcohol. Mild reactions can occur at blood alcohol levels as low as 5 to 10 mg/dL. Symptoms are fully developed at approximately 50 mg/dL and may include flushed skin, throbbing in the head and neck, respiratory difficulty, dizziness, nausea and vomiting, sweating, hyperventilation, tachycardia, hypotension, weakness, blurred vision, and confusion. With a blood alcohol level of approximately 125 to 150 mg/dL, severe reactions can occur, including respiratory depression, cardiovascular collapse, arrhythmias, myocardial infarction, acute congestive heart failure, unconsciousness, convulsions, and death.

Disulfiram should not be administered until it has been ascertained that the client has abstained from alcohol for at least 12 hours. If disulfiram is discontinued, it is important for the client to understand that the sensitivity to alcohol may last for as long as 2 weeks. Consuming alcohol or alcohol-containing substances during this 2-week period could result in the disulfiram- alcohol reaction.

BOX 14–6 Alcoholics Anonymous

The Twelve Steps

1. We admitted we were powerless over alcohol—that our lives have become unmanageable.
2. Came to believe that a Power greater than ourselves could restore us to sanity.
3. Made a decision to turn our will and our lives over to the care of God as we understood Him.
4. Made a searching and fearless moral inventory of ourselves.
5. Admitted to God, to ourselves, and to another human being the exact nature of our wrongs.
6. Were entirely ready to have God remove all these defects of character.
7. Humbly asked Him to remove our shortcomings.
8. Made a list of all persons we had harmed and became willing to make amends to them all.
9. Made direct amends to such people wherever possible except when to do so would injure them or others.
10. Continued to take personal inventory and when we were wrong promptly admitted it.
11. Sought through prayer and meditation to improve our conscious contact with God as we understood Him, praying only for knowledge of His will for us and the power to carry that out.
12. Having had a spiritual awakening as the result of these steps, we tried to carry this message to alcoholics and to practice these principles in all our affairs.

The Twelve Traditions

1. Our common welfare should come first; personal recovery depends upon AA unity.
2. For our group purpose there is but one ultimate authority—a loving God as He may express Himself in our group conscience. Our leaders are but trusted servants; they do not govern.
3. The one requirement for AA membership is a desire to stop drinking.
4. Each group should be autonomous except in matters affecting other groups or AA as a whole.
5. Each group has but one primary purpose—to carry its message to the alcoholic who still suffers.
6. An AA group ought never endorse, finance, or lend the AA name to any related facility or outside enterprise, lest problems of money, property, and prestige divert us from our primary purpose.
7. Every AA group ought to be fully self-supporting, declining outside contributions.
8. Alcoholics Anonymous should remain forever nonprofessional, but our service centers may employ special workers.
9. Alcoholics Anonymous, as such, ought never be organized; but we may create service boards of committees directly responsible to those they serve.
10. Alcoholics Anonymous has no opinion on outside issues; hence, the Alcoholics Anonymous name ought never be drawn into public controversy.
11. Our public relations policy is based on attraction rather than promotion; we need always maintain personal anonymity at the level of press, radio, and films.
12. Anonymity is the spiritual foundation of all our traditions, ever reminding us to place principles before personalities.

Source: The Twelve Steps and Twelve Traditions are reprinted with permission of Alcoholics Anonymous World Services, Inc. (AAWS). Permission to reprint the Twelve Steps and Twelve Traditions does not mean that AAWS has reviewed or approved the contents of this publication, or that AA necessarily agrees with the views expressed herein. AA is a program of recovery from alcoholism only. Use of the Twelve Steps and Twelve Traditions in connection with programs and activities which are patterned after AA, but which address other problems, or in any other non-AA context, does not imply otherwise.

The client receiving disulfiram therapy should be aware of the large number of alcohol-containing substances. These products, such as liquid cough and cold preparations, vanilla extract, aftershave lotions, colognes, mouthwash, nail polish removers, and isopropyl alcohol, if ingested or even rubbed on the skin, are capable of producing the symptoms described. The individual must read labels carefully and must inform any doctor, dentist, or other healthcare professional from whom assistance is sought that he or she is taking disulfiram. In addition, it is important that the client carry a card explaining participation in disulfiram therapy, possible consequences of the therapy, and symptoms that may indicate an emergency situation.

The client must be assessed carefully before beginning disulfiram therapy. A thorough medical screening is performed before starting therapy, and written informed consent is usually required. The drug is contraindicated for clients who are at high risk for alcohol ingestion. It is also contraindicated for psychotic clients and clients with severe cardiac, renal, or hepatic disease.

TABLE 14–11 **Addiction Self-Help Groups**	
GROUP	**MEMBERSHIP**
Adult Children of Alcoholics (ACOA)	Adults who grew up with an alcoholic in the home
Al-Anon	Families of alcoholics
Alateen	Adolescent children of alcoholics
Children Are People	School-age children with an alcoholic family member
Cocaine Anonymous	Individuals with cocaine addiction
Codependents Anonymous (CoDA)	Families of alcohol or other substance abusers
Families Anonymous	Parents of children who abuse substances
Fresh Start	Individuals with nicotine addiction
Gamblers Anonymous	Individuals with gambling addiction
Narcotics Anonymous	Individuals with narcotics addiction
Nar-Anon	Families of individuals with narcotics addiction
Overeaters Anonymous	Individuals with food addiction
Pills Anonymous	Individuals with polysubstance addictions
Pot Smokers Anonymous	Individuals with marijuana addiction
Smokers Anonymous	Individuals with nicotine addiction
Women for Sobriety	Women with alcohol addictions

Disulfiram therapy is not a cure for alcoholism. It provides a measure of control for the individual who desires to avoid impulse drinking. Clients receiving disulfiram therapy are encouraged to seek other assistance with their problem, such as AA or other support group, to aid in the recovery process.

Vitamin Replacement in Alcohol Use Disorder

Multivitamin therapy in combination with daily injections or oral administration of thiamine is common protocol. Thiamine is commonly deficient in chronic alcoholics. Replacement therapy is required to prevent neuropathy, confusion, and encephalopathy.

Medication-Assisted Treatment

Various medications have been used to decrease the intensity of symptoms in an individual who is withdrawing from, or who is experiencing the effects of excessive use of, alcohol and other drugs and to decrease cravings by administering a controlled dose of another medication. This is referred to as **medication-assisted treatment.**

Alcohol Withdrawal

Benzodiazepines are the most widely used group of drugs for medication-assisted treatment in alcohol

withdrawal. Benzodiazepines act similarly to alcohol in their effects but can be administered in controlled doses to prevent adverse effects of alcohol withdrawal. Chlordiazepoxide (Librium), oxazepam (Serax), lorazepam (Ativan), and diazepam (Valium) are the most commonly used agents. The approach to treatment with benzodiazepines for alcohol withdrawal is to start with relatively high doses and reduce the dosage by 20 to 25 percent each day until withdrawal is complete. Additional doses may be given for breakthrough signs or symptoms. In clients with liver disease, accumulation of the longer-acting agents (chlordiazepoxide and diazepam) may be problematic, and use of the shorter-acting benzodiazepines (lorazepam or oxazepam) is more appropriate.

Some physicians may order anticonvulsant medication (e.g., carbamazepine, valproic acid, phenobarbital, or gabapentin) for prevention of withdrawal seizures. These drugs are particularly useful in individuals who have had repeated episodes of alcohol withdrawal. Repeated episodes of withdrawal appear to "kindle" even more serious withdrawal episodes, including the production of withdrawal seizures that can result in brain damage (Julien, 2014). These anticonvulsants have been used successfully in both acute withdrawal and to reduce longer-term craving. Rosenson and associates (2013) found that a single IV dose of phenobarbital along with symptom-guided lorazepam for management of acute withdrawal reduced intensive care unit (ICU) admissions and did not have any adverse effects.

Alcohol Abstinence

The narcotic antagonist naltrexone (ReVia [oral], Vivitrol [injection]) was approved by the FDA in 1994 for the treatment of alcohol addiction. Naltrexone, which was approved in 1984 for the treatment of heroin abuse, works on the same receptors in the brain that produce the feelings of pleasure when heroin or other opiates bind to them, but it does not produce the "narcotic high" and is not habit forming. Although alcohol does not bind to these same brain receptors, studies have shown that naltrexone works equally well against it (O'Malley et al., 1992; Volpicelli et al., 1992). In comparison to the placebo-treated clients, participants on naltrexone therapy showed significantly lower overall relapse rates and fewer drinks per drinking day among those clients who did resume drinking.

In August 2004, the FDA approved acamprosate (Campral), which is indicated for the maintenance of abstinence from alcohol in patients with alcohol addiction who are abstinent at treatment initiation. The mechanism of action of acamprosate in maintenance of alcohol abstinence is not completely understood. It is thought to restore the normal balance between neuronal excitation and inhibition by interacting with glutamate and GABA neurotransmitter systems. Acamprosate is ineffective in clients who have not undergone detoxification and not achieved alcohol abstinence prior to beginning treatment. It is recommended for concomitant use with psychosocial therapy.

An over-the-counter antioxidant, n-acetylcysteine, has demonstrated in animal studies to be beneficial in reducing alcohol-seeking and withdrawal symptoms and preventing alcohol toxicity. However, only one study in humans has shown that it may decrease use in adolescents who are using alcohol and marijuana concurrently (Tomko et al., 2018). More research is needed, and currently n-acetylcysteine is not approved by the FDA for treatment of substance use disorders.

Opiate Intoxication

Examples of drugs in the opioid classification include opium, morphine, codeine, heroin, hydromorphone, oxycodone, and hydrocodone. Synthetic opiate-like narcotic analgesics include meperidine, methadone, pentazocine, tramadol, fentanyl, carfentanil, sufentanil, and U-47700.

Opiate intoxication is treated with narcotic antagonists such as naloxone (Narcan) or naltrexone (ReVia, Vivitrol). In 2015, the FDA approved an intranasal form of naloxone hydrochloride under a fast-track approval process in response to the continued increase in deaths associated with drug overdose, particularly from respiratory depression and arrest. It is reported to work within 2 minutes but must be given quickly to prevent death (Brown, 2015). Naloxone nasal spray can cause severe withdrawal in patients who are opioid dependent. A current concern identified by the recent NIH initiative, HEAL, is a need for stronger, more effective naloxone options, because overdoses secondary to fentanyl and carfentanil do not always respond to existing medications.

Opiate Withdrawal

Opiate withdrawal symptoms, as discussed previously, last for varying amounts of time depending on the type of opiate. Withdrawal therapy includes rest, adequate nutritional support, and medication-assisted treatment with drugs such as methadone or buprenorphine. Although not all patient treatment plans will include medication-assisted treatment (the administration of a controlled opiate agonist in substitution for the substance that was being abused), there is evidence that they are beneficial in reducing withdrawal symptoms, and recent studies have supported that addition of this treatment reduces overall mortality risks (Jancin, 2018). Methadone, if ordered, is given on the first day in a dose sufficient to suppress withdrawal symptoms. The dose is then gradually tapered over a specified time. As the dose of methadone diminishes, renewed abstinence symptoms may be ameliorated by the addition of clonidine. Some patients are maintained on medication-assisted treatment indefinitely, although this was not the original intent for these drugs. Grossman, as cited by Jancin (2018), reports that studies repeatedly demonstrate that when treatment stops, the risk of relapse increases. Methadone can only be administered in methadone clinics that are overseen at state and federal levels.

In October 2002, the FDA approved two forms of the drug buprenorphine for treating opiate addiction. Buprenorphine is an opioid partial agonist (where methadone is an opioid agonist, similar to morphine) and is considered to be somewhat safer and cause fewer side effects, making it especially attractive for clients who are mildly or moderately addicted. Individuals are able to access treatment with buprenorphine in office-based settings, providing an alternative to methadone clinics. Physicians are deemed qualified to prescribe buprenorphine if they hold an addiction certification from the American Society of Addiction Medicine, the American Academy of Addiction Psychiatry, the American Psychiatric Association, or other associations deemed appropriate. The number of patients to whom individual physicians may provide outpatient buprenorphine treatment was previously limited to 100 but in response to the growing opioid epidemic, a new federal rule became effective in August 2016 increasing the allowable number to 275 patients with stipulations about necessary credentialing in addictions medicine or addictions psychiatry and allowable practice settings. Currently, buprenorphine/naloxone combinations (in sublingual tablets or film, buccal film, extended release, and long-acting injectable forms) and injectable naltrexone are all options for medication-assisted treatment of opioid addiction.

Clonidine (Catapres) also has been used to suppress opiate withdrawal symptoms. As monotherapy, it is not as effective as substitution with methadone, but it is nonaddicting and serves effectively as a bridge to enable the client to stay opiate free long enough to facilitate termination of methadone maintenance.

Barbiturate Withdrawal

Medication-assisted treatment for CNS depressant withdrawal (particularly barbiturates) is most commonly used with the long-acting barbiturate phenobarbital (Luminal). The dosage required to suppress withdrawal symptoms is administered. When stabilization has been achieved, the dose is gradually decreased by 30 mg/day until withdrawal is complete. Long-acting benzodiazepines are commonly used for medication-assisted treatment when the abused substance is a nonbarbiturate CNS depressant.

Stimulant Intoxication

Treatment of stimulant intoxication usually begins with minor tranquilizers such as chlordiazepoxide and progresses to major tranquilizers such as haloperidol (Haldol). Antipsychotics should be administered with caution because of their propensity to lower seizure threshold. Repeated seizures are treated with IV diazepam.

Stimulant Withdrawal

Withdrawal from CNS stimulants does not constitute a medical emergency observed with CNS depressants.

Treatment is usually aimed at reducing drug craving and managing severe depression. The client is placed in a quiet atmosphere and allowed to sleep and eat as much as is needed or desired. Suicide precautions may need to be instituted. Antidepressant therapy may be helpful in treating symptoms of depression.

Hallucinogens and Cannabinols

Medication-assisted treatment is not required with these drugs and there are no FDA-approved medications for treatment of these substance use disorders. When adverse reactions such as anxiety or panic occur, benzodiazepines (e.g., diazepam or chlordiazepoxide) may be prescribed to prevent harm to the client or others. Psychotic reactions may be treated with antipsychotic medications.

Counseling

Counseling on a one-to-one basis is often used to help the client who abuses substances. The relationship is goal directed, and the length of the counseling may vary from weeks to years. The focus is on current reality, development of a working treatment relationship, and strengthening ego assets. The counselor must be warm, kind, and nonjudgmental yet able to set limits firmly. Research consistently demonstrates that personal characteristics of counselors are highly predictive of client outcome. In addition to technical counseling skills, many important therapeutic qualities affect the outcome of counseling, including insight, respect, genuineness, concreteness, and empathy (SAMHSA, 2014). Often counselors in substance use disorders treatment are themselves engaged in an ongoing recovery program from alcohol or drug addiction, or both. Having the shared experience of addiction is considered an opportunity to develop connection and compassion with the client and there is typically more self-disclosure about the counselor's own journey than is typical in psychiatric settings.

Counseling of the client who abuses substances passes through various phases, each of which is of indeterminate length. In the first phase, an assessment is conducted. Factual data are collected to determine whether the client does have a problem with substances; that is, that substances are regularly impairing effective functioning in a significant life area.

Following the assessment, in the working phase of the relationship, the counselor assists the individual to work on acceptance of the fact that the use of substances causes problems in significant life areas and that he or she cannot prevent it from occurring. The client states a desire to make changes. The strength of the denial system is determined by the duration and extent of substance-related adverse effects in the person's life. Thus, those individuals with rather minor substance-related problems of recent origin have less difficulty with this stage than those with long-term extensive impairment. The individual also works to gain self-control and abstain from substances.

Once the problem has been identified and sobriety is achieved, the client must have a concrete and workable plan for getting through the early weeks of abstinence. Anticipatory guidance through role-play helps the individual practice how he or she will respond when substances are readily obtainable and the impulse to partake is strong.

Counseling often includes the family or specific family members. In family counseling the therapist tries to help each member see how he or she has affected, and been affected by, the substance abuse behavior. Family strengths are mobilized, and family members are encouraged to move in a positive direction. Referrals are often made to self-help groups such as Al-Anon, Nar-Anon, Alateen, Families Anonymous, and Adult Children of Alcoholics.

Group Therapy

Group therapy with substance abusers has long been regarded as a powerful agent of change. In groups, individuals are able to share their experiences with others who are going through similar problems. They are able to "see themselves in others" and confront their defenses about giving up the substance. They may confront similar attitudes and defenses in others. Groups also give individuals the capacity for communicating needs and feelings directly.

Some groups may be task-oriented education groups in which the leader is charged with presenting material associated with substance abuse and its various effects on the person's life. Other educational groups that may be helpful with individuals who abuse substances include assertiveness techniques and relaxation training. Teaching groups differ from psychotherapy groups, whose focus is more on helping individuals understand and manage difficult feelings and situations, particularly as they relate to use of substances.

Therapy groups and self-help groups such as AA are complementary to each other. Whereas the self-help group focus is on achieving and maintaining sobriety, in the therapy group, the individual may learn more adaptive ways of coping, how to deal with problems that may have arisen or were exacerbated by the former substance use, and ways to improve quality of life and to function more effectively without substances.

Nonsubstance Addictions

Gambling Disorder

This disorder is defined by the *DSM-5* as persistent and recurrent problematic gambling behavior leading to clinically significant impairment or distress (APA, 2013). The preoccupation with and impulse to gamble often intensifies when the individual is under stress. Many impulsive gamblers describe a physical sensation of restlessness and anticipation that can only be relieved by placing a bet. Blume (2013) states:

> In some cases the initial change in gambling behavior leading to pathological gambling begins with a "big win," bringing a rapid development of preoccupation, tolerance, and loss of control. Winning brings feelings of special status, power, and omnipotence. The gambler increasingly depends on this activity to cope with disappointments, problems, and negative emotional states, pulling away from emotional attachment to family and friends.

As the need to gamble increases, the individual is forced to obtain money by any means available, which may include borrowing money from illegal sources or pawning personal items (or items that belong to others). As gambling debts accrue, or out of a need to continue gambling, the individual may desperately resort to forgery, theft, or even embezzlement. Family relationships are disrupted, and impairment in occupational functioning may occur because of absences from work in order to gamble.

Gambling behavior usually begins in adolescence; however, compulsive behaviors rarely occur before young adulthood. The disorder generally runs a chronic course, with periods of waxing and waning, largely dependent on periods of psychosocial stress. Prevalence estimates for problem gambling range from 3 to 5 percent, and about 1 percent meet the criteria for a gambling disorder (Sadock et al., 2015). It is more common among men than women.

Various personality traits have been attributed to pathological gambling. In a systematic review and meta-analysis (Dowling et al., 2015), the most prevalent included narcissistic, antisocial, avoidant, obsessive-compulsive, and borderline traits. The researchers concluded that in any treatment setting for gambling disorders, screening and treatment for these common comorbid conditions must be addressed.

Gambling problems may be episodic and increase during periods of stress or depression, or the behavior may be persistent (APA, 2013). Based on *DSM-5* diagnostic criteria, a gambling disorder is diagnosed when gambling leads to significant impairment, distress, or consequences evidenced by increases in money needed to gamble to achieve excitement; restlessness or irritation with attempts to reduce gambling; unsuccessful efforts to stop; and gambling when feeling guilty, helpless, anxious, or depressed, among others (APA, 2013).

Predisposing Factors to Gambling Disorder

Biological Influences

Genetic Familial and twin studies show an increased prevalence of pathological gambling in family members of individuals diagnosed with the disorder. Black and associates (2014) found that first-degree relatives of pathological gamblers were eight times more likely to develop the same condition, suggesting an underlying genetic predisposition.

Physiological Studies of dopamine receptor systems have implicated this neurotransmitter in the development of addictive personality traits, including pathological gambling (Weiss & Pontone, 2014). Support for this association comes from studies that demonstrated a correlation between the development of pathological gambling behaviors after individuals were treated with dopamine receptor agonist drugs (Moore, Glenmullen, & Mattison, 2014). Biochemical theories suggest that, ironically, both winning and losing (perhaps related to the excitement of taking a risk) stimulate the reward and pleasure centers in the brain. This could contribute to persistent and repeated desire to gamble even when one is not winning.

Psychosocial Influences

Sadock and colleagues (2015) report that the following may be predisposing factors to the development of pathological gambling: "loss of a parent by death, separation, divorce, or desertion before the child is 15 years of age; inappropriate parental discipline (absence, inconsistency, or harshness); exposure to and availability of gambling activities for the adolescent; a family emphasis on material and financial symbols; and a lack of family emphasis on saving, planning, and budgeting" (p. 691).

Treatment Modalities for Gambling Disorder

Because most pathological gamblers deny that they have a problem, treatment is difficult. In fact, most gamblers only seek treatment due to legal difficulties, family pressures, or other psychiatric complaints. Behavior therapy, cognitive therapy, motivational interviewing, 12-step programs (Gamblers Anonymous), and self-help strategies such as bibliotherapy have all been used with varying degrees of success. About one-third of individuals with gambling disorders recover without need for treatment (Rash, Weinstock, & Van Patten, 2016). Some medications have been used with effective results in the treatment of pathological gambling. SSRIs and clomipramine have been used to treat obsessive-compulsive disorders and may have benefits for those with gambling disorders who have comorbid obsessive-compulsive traits. Lithium and carbamazepine and naltrexone have also demonstrated some effectiveness.

Possibly the most effective treatment of pathological gambling is participation by the individual in **Gamblers Anonymous** (GA). This group therapy organization is modeled after Alcoholics Anonymous.

CASE STUDY AND SAMPLE CARE PLAN

NURSING HISTORY AND ASSESSMENT

The police bring Dan to the emergency department of the local hospital around 9:00 p.m. His wife, Carol, called 911 when Dan became violent and she began to fear for her safety. Dan was fired from his job as a foreman in a manufacturing plant for refusing to follow his supervisor's directions on a project. When cleaning up after his move, several partially used bottles of liquor were found in his work area.

Carol reports that Dan has been drinking since he came home shortly after noon today. He bloodied her nose and punched her in the stomach when she poured the contents of a bottle from which he was drinking down the kitchen sink. The police responded to her call and brought Dan to the hospital in handcuffs. By the time they arrive at the hospital, Dan has calmed down and appears drugged and drowsy. His blood alcohol level measures 247 mg/dL. He is admitted to the detoxification unit of the hospital with a diagnosis of Alcohol Intoxication.

Carol tells the admitting nurse that she and Dan have been married for 12 years. He was a social drinker before they were married, but his drinking has increased over the years. He has been under a lot of stress at work, hates his job, his boss, and his coworkers, and is depressed a lot of the time. He never had a loving relationship with his parents, who are now deceased. For the past few years, his pattern has been to come home, start drinking immediately, and drink until he passes out for the night. She states that she has tried to get him to go for help with his drinking, but he refuses and says that he doesn't have a problem. Carol begins to cry and says to the nurse, "We can't go on like this. I don't know what to do!"

Continued

CASE STUDY AND SAMPLE CARE PLAN—cont'd

NURSING DIAGNOSES AND OUTCOME IDENTIFICATION

From the assessment data, the nurse develops the following nursing diagnoses for Dan:

1. **Risk for injury** related to CNS agitation from alcohol withdrawal
   a. **Short-term goal:** Dan's condition will stabilize within 72 hours.
   b. **Long-term goal:** Dan will not experience physical injury.
2. **Denial** related to low self-esteem, weak ego development, and underlying fears and anxieties
   a. **Short-term goal:** Dan will focus immediate attention on behavioral changes required to achieve sobriety.
   b. **Long-term goal:** Dan will accept responsibility for his drinking behaviors and acknowledge the association between his drinking and personal problems.

PLANNING AND IMPLEMENTATION

RISK FOR INJURY

The following nursing interventions may be implemented *in an effort to ensure patient safety:*

1. Assess his level of disorientation; frequently orient him to reality and his surroundings.
2. Obtain a drug history.
3. Obtain a urine sample for analysis.
4. Place Dan in a quiet room (private, if possible).
5. Ensure that smoking materials and other potentially harmful objects are stored away.
6. Observe Dan frequently. Take vital signs every 15 to 30 minutes.
7. Monitor for signs of withdrawal within a few hours after admission. Watch for signs of
   a. Increased heart rate
   b. Tremors
   c. Headache
   d. Diaphoresis
   e. Agitation; restlessness
   f. Nausea
   g. Fever
   h. Convulsions
8. Follow medication regimen, as ordered by physician (commonly a benzodiazepine, thiamine, multivitamin).

DENIAL

The following nursing interventions may be implemented *in an effort to help Dan accept responsibility for the behavioral consequences associated with his drinking:*

1. Develop Dan's trust by spending time with him, being honest, and keeping all promises.
2. Ensure that Dan understands that it is not *him* but his *behavior* that is unacceptable.
3. Provide Dan with accurate information about the effects of alcohol. Do this in a matter-of-fact, nonjudgmental way.
4. Point out recent negative events that have occurred in Dan's life, and associate the use of alcohol with these events. Help him to see the association.
5. Use confrontation with caring: "Yes, your wife called the police. You were physically abusive. She was afraid. And your blood alcohol level was 247 when you were brought in. You were obviously not in control of your behavior at the time."
6. Don't accept excuses for his drinking. Point out rationalization and projection behaviors. These behaviors prolong denial that he has a problem. He must directly accept responsibility for his drinking (not make excuses and blame it on the behavior of others). He must come to understand that only *he* has control of his behavior.
7. Encourage Dan to attend group therapy during treatment and Alcoholics Anonymous following treatment. Peer feedback is a strong factor in helping individuals recognize their problems and to ultimately remain sober.
8. Encourage Carol to attend Al-Anon meetings. She can benefit from the experiences of others who have experienced and are experiencing the same types of problems as she.
9. Help Dan to identify ways that he can cope besides using alcohol, such as exercise, sports, and relaxation. He should choose what is most appropriate for him and should be given positive feedback for efforts made toward change.

EVALUATION

The outcome criteria identified for Dan have been met. He experienced an uncomplicated withdrawal from alcohol and exhibits no evidence of physical injury. He verbalizes understanding of the relationship between his personal problems and his drinking, and he accepts responsibility for his own behavior. He verbalizes understanding that alcohol addiction is an illness that requires ongoing support and treatment, and he regularly attends AA meetings. Carol regularly attends Al-Anon meetings.

Summary and Key Points

■ An individual is considered to be addicted to a substance when he or she is unable to control its use, even knowing that it interferes with normal functioning; when more and more of the substance is required to produce the desired effects; and when characteristic withdrawal symptoms develop upon cessation or drastic decrease in use of the substance.

■ *Substance intoxication* is defined as the development of a reversible syndrome of maladaptive cognitive, behavioral, or psychological changes that are due to the direct physiological effects of a substance on the CNS and develop during or shortly after ingestion of (or exposure to) a substance.

■ Substance withdrawal is the development of a substance-specific maladaptive behavioral change, with physiological and cognitive concomitants, that is due to the cessation of, or reduction in, heavy and prolonged substance use.

■ The etiology of substance use disorders is unknown. Various contributing factors have been implicated, such as genetics, biochemical changes, developmental influences, personality factors, social learning, conditioning, and cultural and ethnic influences.

■ Although multiple factors influence the development of a substance use disorder, it is clearly a disease of the brain.

■ Seven classes of substances are presented in this chapter in terms of a profile of the substance, historical aspects, patterns of use and abuse, and effects on the body. They include alcohol, other CNS depressants, CNS stimulants, opioids, hallucinogens, inhalants, and cannabinols.

■ The nurse uses the nursing process as the vehicle for delivery of care of the patient with a substance-related disorder.

■ The nurse must first examine his or her own feelings regarding personal substance use and substance use by others. Only the nurse who can be accepting and nonjudgmental of substance use behaviors will be effective in working with these clients.

■ Special care is given to patients with dual diagnoses of mental illness and substance use disorders.

■ Addiction to substances is a problem for many members of the nursing profession. Most state boards of nursing and state nurses' associations have established avenues for peer assistance to provide help to impaired members of the profession.

■ Individuals who are reared in families with chemically addicted persons learn patterns of dysfunctional behavior that carry over into adult life. These dysfunctional behavior patterns are termed *codependence.* Codependent persons sacrifice their own needs for the fulfillment of others in order to achieve a sense of control. Many nurses also have codependent traits.

■ Treatment modalities for substance-related disorders include self-help groups, deterrent therapy, individual counseling, and group therapy. Medication-assisted treatment is frequently implemented with clients experiencing substance withdrawal. Treatment modalities are implemented on an inpatient basis or in outpatient settings, depending on the severity of the impairment.

■ Gambling disorder is defined by the *DSM-5* as persistent and recurrent problematic gambling behavior leading to clinically significant impairment or distress.

■ Research indicates a possible genetic component in the etiology to gambling disorder. Abnormalities in the serotonergic, noradrenergic, and dopaminergic neurotransmitter systems have also been implicated.

■ A number of psychosocial influences have been implicated in the predisposition to gambling disorder, including dysfunctional family patterns.

Review Questions
Self-Examination/Learning Exercise

Select the answer that is most appropriate for each of the following questions:

1. Mr. White is admitted to the hospital after an extended period of binge alcohol drinking. His wife reports that he has been a heavy drinker for a number of years. Laboratory reports reveal that he has a blood alcohol level of 250 mg/dL. He is placed on the chemical addiction unit for detoxification. When would the first signs of alcohol withdrawal symptoms be expected to occur?
   a. Several hours after the last drink
   b. 2 to 3 days after the last drink
   c. 4 to 5 days after the last drink
   d. 6 to 7 days after the last drink

2. Symptoms of alcohol withdrawal include which of the following?
   a. Euphoria, hyperactivity, and insomnia
   b. Depression, suicidal ideation, and hypersomnia
   c. Diaphoresis, nausea and vomiting, and tremors
   d. Unsteady gait, nystagmus, and profound disorientation

Continued

Review Questions—cont'd
Self-Examination/Learning Exercise

3. Which of the following medications is the physician most likely to order for a patient experiencing alcohol withdrawal syndrome?
   a. Haloperidol (Haldol)
   b. Chlordiazepoxide (Librium)
   c. Methadone (Dolophine)
   d. Cannabidiol (Epidiolex)

4. Dan, who has been admitted to the alcohol rehabilitation unit after being fired for drinking on the job, states to the nurse, "I don't have a problem with alcohol. I can handle my booze better than anyone I know. My boss is a jerk! I haven't missed any more days than my coworkers." What is the nurse's best response?
   a. "Maybe your boss is mistaken, Dan."
   b. "You are here because your drinking was interfering with your work, Dan."
   c. "Get real, Dan! You're a boozer and you know it!"
   d. "Why do you think your boss is a jerk, Dan?"

5. Dan, who has been admitted to the alcohol rehabilitation unit after being fired for drinking on the job, states to the nurse, "I don't have a problem with alcohol. I can handle my booze better than anyone I know. My boss is a jerk! I haven't missed any more days than my coworkers." What defense mechanism is Dan using?
   a. Denial
   b. Projection
   c. Displacement
   d. Rationalization

6. Dan has been admitted to the alcohol rehabilitation unit after being fired for drinking on the job. Dan's drinking buddies come for a visit, and when they leave, the nurse smells alcohol on Dan's breath. Which of the following would be the best intervention with Dan at this time?
   a. Search his room for evidence.
   b. Ask, "Have you been drinking alcohol, Dan?"
   c. Send a urine specimen from Dan to the laboratory for drug screening.
   d. Tell Dan, "These guys cannot come to the unit to visit you again."

7. Dan begins to attend AA meetings. Which of the statements by Dan reflects the purpose of this organization?
   a. "They claim they will help me stay sober."
   b. "I'll dry out in AA, then I can have a social drink now and then."
   c. "AA is only for people who have reached the bottom."
   d. "If I lose my job, AA will help me find another."

8. From which of the following symptoms might the nurse identify a chronic cocaine user?
   a. Clear, constricted pupils
   b. Red, irritated nostrils
   c. Muscle aches
   d. Conjunctival redness

Review Questions—cont'd
Self-Examination/Learning Exercise

9. An individual who is addicted to heroin is likely to experience which of the following symptoms of withdrawal?
   a. Increased heart rate and blood pressure
   b. Tremors, insomnia, and seizures
   c. Incoordination and unsteady gait
   d. Nausea and vomiting, diarrhea, and diaphoresis

10. A polysubstance abuser makes the statement, "The green and whites do me good after speed." How might the nurse interpret the statement?
    a. The client abuses amphetamines and anxiolytics.
    b. The client abuses alcohol and cocaine.
    c. The client is psychotic.
    d. The client abuses narcotics and marijuana.

11. A client admitted to the emergency department smells strongly of alcohol, and his wife reports that he has been a heavy drinker for the last 25 years. Which of the following assessment findings are consistent with long-term chronic alcohol abuse? (Select all that apply.)
    a. The client reports weak leg muscles, and his gait is unsteady.
    b. The client's abdomen is distended.
    c. The client reports that he was coughing up some blood.
    d. The client reports that he has double vision.
    e. Blood tests reveal a low white blood cell count.

IMPLICATIONS OF RESEARCH FOR EVIDENCE-BASED PRACTICE

Majer, J. M., Payne, J. C., & Jason, L. A. (2015). Recovery resources and psychiatric severity among persons with substance use disorders. *Community Mental Health Journal, 51*(4), 437–444. doi:10.1007/s10597-014-9762-3

DESCRIPTION OF THE STUDY: This study examined social support and self-efficacy in maintaining abstinence among individuals discharged from inpatient treatment for substance use disorders. The participants (n = 270) were largely unemployed with an average of 6.3 prior convictions, and the majority (41.4%) reported using opiates/heroin, followed by cocaine (27.8%), alcohol (12.8%), polysubstance use (11.3%), and cannabis (6.4%). The researchers found that individuals with high psychiatric severity had lower levels of self-efficacy for abstinence even though there was not a significant difference in social support. The researchers suggest that usual social support resources such as 12-step programs may not be sufficient for individuals with comorbid psychiatric illness. Abstinence self-efficacy may be inhibited by cognitive dysfunction associated with the psychiatric illness, but whatever the contributing factors, abstinence self-efficacy is highly correlated with decreasing relapse.

IMPLICATIONS FOR NURSING PRACTICE: The researchers point out that interventions related to coping skills and stress management have been shown to increase abstinence self-efficacy. Nurses play an active role in this kind of education for clients in inpatient psychiatric units. Targeting these interventions for individuals with concurrent substance abuse disorders may provide a stronger foundation for relapse prevention in this group post-discharge.

TEST YOUR CRITICAL THINKING SKILLS

Kelly, age 23, is a first-year law student. She is engaged to a surgical resident at the local university hospital. She has been struggling to do well in law school because she wants to make her parents, two prominent local attorneys, proud of her. She had never aspired to do anything but go into law, and that is also what her parents expected her to do.

Kelly's mid-term grades were not as high as she had hoped, so she increased the number of hours of study time, staying awake all night several nights a week to study. She started drinking large amounts of coffee to stay awake but still found herself falling asleep as she tried to study at the library and in her apartment. As final exams approached, she began to panic that she would not be able to continue the pace of studying she felt she needed in order to make the grades she hoped for.

One of Kelly's classmates told her that she needed some "speed" to give her that extra energy to study. Her classmate said, "All the kids do it. Hardly anyone I know gets through law school without it." She gave Kelly the name of a source.

Kelly contacted the source, who supplied her with enough amphetamines to see her through final exams. Kelly was excited because she had so much energy, did not require sleep, and was able to study the additional hours she thought she needed for the exams.

However, when the results were posted, Kelly had failed two courses and would have to repeat them in summer school if she was to continue with her class in the fall. She continued to replenish her supply of amphetamines from her "contact" until he told her that he could not get her any more. She became frantic and stole a prescription blank from her fiancé and forged his name for more pills.

She started taking more and more of the medication in order to achieve the "high" she wanted to feel. Her behavior became erratic. Yesterday, her fiancé received a call from a pharmacy to clarify an order for amphetamines that Kelly had written. He insisted that she admit herself to the chemical addiction unit for detoxification.

On the unit, she appears tired, depressed, moves very slowly, and wants to sleep all the time. She keeps saying to the nurse, "I'm a real failure. I'll never be an attorney like my parents. I'm too dumb. I just wish I could die."

Answer the following questions related to Kelly:

1. What is the primary nursing diagnosis for Kelly?
2. Describe important nursing interventions to be implemented with Kelly.
3. In addition to physical safety, what are the primary short-term goals the nurses would strive to achieve with Kelly?

Communication Exercises

1. Tom is a patient on the alcohol treatment unit. He says to the nurse, "My boss and my wife ganged up on me. They think I have a drinking problem. I don't have a drinking problem! I can quit any time I want to!"
   How would the nurse respond appropriately to this statement by Tom?

2. Tom says to the nurse, "My head hurts. I didn't sleep very well last night. I'm getting shaky, and it's hot in here! I could sure use a cup of coffee and a cigarette."
   How would the nurse respond appropriately to this statement by Tom?

3. Tom says, "Sure, I missed a couple days of work. Everyone gets sick now and then. I don't think my wife cares about what happens to me. She and my boss got together and decided I needed to be here, or I lose my job!"
   How would the nurse respond appropriately to this statement by Tom?

🎦 MOVIE CONNECTIONS

Affliction (Alcoholism) • *Days of Wine and Roses* (Alcoholism) • *I'll Cry Tomorrow* (Alcoholism) • *When a Man Loves a Woman* (Alcoholism) • *Clean and Sober* (Cocaine addiction) • *28 Days* (Alcoholism) • *Lady Sings the Blues* (Heroin addiction) • *I'm Dancing as Fast as I Can* (Sedatives addiction) • *The Rose* (Polysubstance addiction)

References

Alcohol Action Ireland. (2018). *Alcohol facts: How much do we drink?* Retrieved from http://alcoholireland.ie/facts/how-much-do-we-drink/

Alcoholics Anonymous. (2015). *Alcoholics Anonymous 2014 membership survey.* Retrieved from http://www.aa.org/assets/en_US/p-48_membershipsurvey.pdf

American Academy of Child and Adolescent Psychiatry. (2015). *Children of alcoholics.* Retrieved from https://www.aacap.org/AACAP/Families_and_Youth/Facts_for_Families/FFF-Guide/Children-Of-Alcoholics-017.aspx

American Addiction Centers. (2018). *What is inhalant withdrawal and detoxification like?* Retrieved from https://www.withdrawal.net/learn/inhalant/

American Psychiatric Association. (2013). *Diagnostic and statistical manual of mental disorders* (5th ed.). Washington, DC: Author.

American Society of Addiction Medicine (ASAM). (2015). *The ASAM national practice guideline for the use of medications in the treatment of addiction involving opioid use.* Retrieved from http://www.asam.org/docs/default-source/practice-support/guidelines-and-consensus-docs/asam-national-practiceguideline-supplement.pdf

Beatty, M. (2011). *Codependent no more.* Center City, MN: Hazelden.

Black, D., Coryell, W., Crowe, R., McCormick, B., Shaw, M., & Allen, J. A. (2014). Direct, controlled, blind family study of DSM-IV pathological gambling. *Journal of Clinical Psychiatry, 75*(3), 215–221. doi:10.4088/JCP.13m08566

Blume, S. G. (2013). *Pathological gambling: Recognition and intervention.* Retrieved from http://education.iupui.edu/soe/programs/graduate/counselor/readings_n_docs/reading4.pdf

Brooks, M. (2018). *FDA goes ahead with approval of sufentanil despite controversy.* Retrieved from http: www.medscape.com Brown, T. (2015). *FDA approves Narcan nasal spray to treat opioid overdose.* Retrieved from http://www.medscape.com

Centers for Disease Control and Prevention (CDC). (2017a). *Smoking and tobacco use.* Retrieved from http://www.cdc.gov/tobacco/data_statistics/vital_signs/index.htm

Centers for Disease Control and Prevention (CDC). (2017b). *Opiate overdose: Understanding the epidemic.* Retrieved from https://www.cdc.gov/drugoverdose/epidemic/index.html

Centers for Disease Control and Prevention (CDC). (2018). *Facts about FASDs*. Retrieved from http://www.cdc.gov/ncbddd/fasd/facts.html

Chen, A. & Ashburn, M. A. (2015). Cardiac effects of opioid therapy. *Pain Medicine, 16*, S27–31. doi: 10.1111/pme.12915

Consumer Reports. (2012). *The buzz on energy-drink caffeine*. Retrieved from https://www.consumerreports.org/cro/magazine/2012/12/the-buzz-on-energy-drink-caffeine/index.htm

Davenport, L. (2016). Abuse of OTC antidiarrheal meds linked to cardiac deaths. *Medscape*. Retrieved from https://www.medscape.com/viewarticle/863232

Deyo, R.A., Smith, D.H., Johnson, E.S., Tillotson, C.J., Donovan, M.,Yang, X., & Dobscha, S.K. (2013). Prescription opioids for back pain and use of medications for erectile dysfunction. *Spine, 38*(11), 909-915. doi:10.1097/BRS.0b013e3182830482

Dotinga, R. (2018). Methamphetamine use climbing among opioid users. *Clinical Psychiatry News*. Retrieved from https://www.mdedge.com/psychiatry/article/169254/addiction-medicine/methamphetamine-use-climbing-among-opioid-users?utm_source=News_CPN_eNL_070418_F&utm_medium=email&utm_content=Opioid%20users%20turn%20to%20meth

Dowling, N.A., Cowlishaw, S., Jackson, A.C., Merkouris, S.S., Francis, K.L., & Christensen, D.R. (2015). The prevalence of comorbid personality disorders in treatment-seeking problemgamblers: A systematic review and meta-analysis. *Journal of Personality Disorders, 29*(6):735–754. doi:10.1521/pedi_2014_28_168

Duffy, S. (2016). *DEA classifies deadly synthetic opioid as schedule I*. Retrieved from http://www.empr.com/news/dea-classifies-deadly-syntheticopioid-as-schedule-i/article/572194

DuPont, R. L. (2016). *Marijuana has proven to be a gateway drug*. Retrieved from http://www.nytimes.com/roomfordebate/2016/04/26/is-marijuana-a-gateway-drug/marijuana-has-proven-to-be-a-gateway-drug

Elias, E. (2013). *Improving awareness and treatment of children with fetal alcohol spectrum disorders and co-occurring psychiatric disorders*. Retrieved from https://www.jbsinternational.com/sites/default/files/FASDpaperfinal_INT.pdf

Ellis, J. R., & Hartley, C. L. (2012). *Nursing in today's world: Trends, issues, and management* (10th ed.). Philadelphia, PA: Lippincott Williams & Wilkins.

Governing.com. (2018). *State marijuana laws in 2018 map*. Retrieved from http://www.governing.com/gov-data/state-marijuana-laws-map-medical-recreational.html

Hanley, C. E. (2017). Navajos. In J. N. Giger (Ed.), *Transcultural nursing: Assessment and intervention* (7th ed.). St. Louis, MO: Mosby.

Herdman, T. H., & Kamitsuru, S. (Eds.). (2018). *NANDA International nursing diagnoses: Definitions and classification: 2018–2020* (11th ed.). New York, NY: Thieme.

Howard, M. O., Bowen, S. E., & Garland, E. L. (2017). Inhalant-related disorders. In B. J. Sadock, V. A. Sadock, & P. Ruiz (Eds.), *Comprehensive textbook of psychiatry* (10th ed., pp. 1328–1342). Philadelphia, PA: Wolters Kluwer.

Iannucci, R. A., & Weiss, R. D. (2017). Stimulant-related disorders. In B. A. Sadock, V. A. Sadock, & P. Ruiz (Eds.), *Comprehensive textbook of psychiatry* (10th ed., pp. 1280–1290). Philadelphia, PA: Wolters Kluwer.

Institute of Medicine. (2003). *Health professions education: A bridge to quality*. Washington, DC: Author.

Jancin, B. (2018). How to prescribe effectively for opioid use disorder. *Family Practice News*. Retrieved from https://www.mdedge.com/familypracticenews/article/171003/addiction-medicine/how-prescribe-effectively-opioid-use-disorder

Johnston, L. D., Miech, R. A., O'Malley, P. M., Bachman, J. G., Schulenberg, J. E., & Patrick, M. E. (2018). Monitoring the future national survey results on drug use: 1975–2017: Overview, key findings on adolescent drug use. Ann Arbor: Institute for Social Research, The University of Michigan.

Juliano, L. M., & Griffiths, R. R. (2017). Caffeine-related disorders. In B. A. Sadock, V. A. Sadock, & P. Ruiz (Eds.), *Comprehensive textbook of psychiatry* (10th ed., pp. 1291–1303). Philadelphia, PA: Wolters Kluwer.

Julien, R. M. (2014). *A primer of drug action: A comprehensive guide to actions, uses and side effects of psychoactive drugs* (13th ed.). New York, NY: Worth.

Lafferty, K. A. (2017). *Barbiturate toxicity*. Retrieved from https://emedicine.medscape.com/article/813155-overview#a5

Lanska, D. (2017). Alcoholic myopathy. *Medlink Neurology*. Retrieved from http://www.medlink.com/article/alcoholic_myopathy

Maier, S. E., & West, J. R. (2013). *Drinking patterns and alcohol-related birth defects*. Retrieved from the National Institute on Alcohol Abuse and Alcohol, National Institutes of Health website: http://pubs.niaaa.nih.gov/publications/arh25-3/168-174.htm

Mayo Clinic. (2017). *Caffeine content for coffee, tea, soda, and more*. Retrieved from https://www.mayoclinic.org/healthy-lifestyle/nutrition-and-healthy-eating/in-depth/caffeine/art-20049372

McKeown, N. J. (2015). Toluene toxicity. *Medscape Reference: Drugs, diseases, and procedures*. Retrieved from http://emedicine.medscape.com/article/818939-overview

Moore, T. J., Glenmullen, J., & Mattison, D. R. (2014). Reports of pathological gambling, hypersexuality, and compulsive shopping associated with dopamine receptor agonist drugs. *JAMA Internal Medicine, 174*(12), 1930–1933. doi:10.1001/jamainternmed.2014.5262

MPR. (2016). *DEA reverses decision to ban kratom*. Retrieved from http://www.empr.com/news/dea-reverses-decision-to-ban-kratom/article/559547

National Council on Alcoholism and Drug Dependence. (2015). *Facts about alcohol*. Retrieved from http://www.ncadd.org

National Institute on Drug Abuse (NIDA). (2017a). *Trends and statistics*. National Institute of Health. Retrieved from https://www.drugabuse.gov/related-topics/trends-statistics

National Institute on Drug Abuse (NIDA). (2017b). *Synthetic cannabinoids (K2/Spice) unpredictable danger*. Retrieved from https://www.drugabuse.gov/related-topics/trends-statistics/infographics/synthetic-cannabinoids-k2spice-unpredictable-danger

National Institute on Drug Abuse (NIDA). (2018a). *Drugs, brains, and behavior: The science of addiction*. National Institute of Health. Retrieved from http://www.drugabuse.gov/publications/drugs-brains-behavior-science-addiction/drug-abuse-addiction

National Institute on Drug Abuse (NIDA). (2018b). *Principles of drug addiction treatment: A research-based guide (third edition)*. National Institute of Health. Retrieved from https://www.drugabuse.gov/publications/principles-drug-addiction-treatment-research-based-guide-third-edition/evidence-based-approaches-to-drug-addiction-treatment/behavioral

National Institute on Drug Abuse (NIDA). (2018c). *Synthetic cannabinoids*. Retrieved from https://www.drugabuse.gov/publications/drugfacts/synthetic-cannabinoids-k2spice

National Institute on Drug Abuse (NIDA). (2018d). *Marijuana: Drug facts*. Retrieved from https://www.drugabuse.gov/publications/drugfacts/marijuana

National Institutes of Health. (2018). *Carfentanil*. Retrieved from https://pubchem.ncbi.nlm.nih.gov/compound/carfentanil

National Library of Medicine. (2017). *Loss of brain function—Liver disease*. Retrieved from http://www.nlm.nih.gov/medlineplus/ency/article/000302.htm

Parish, B. S. (2015). *Hallucinogen use*. Retrieved from http://emedicine.medscape.com/article/293752-overview

Publishers Group. (2017). *Street drugs: A drug identification guide*. Lon Lake, MN: Author.

Rash, C. J., Weinstock, J., & Van Patten, R. (2016). A review of gambling disorder and substance use disorders. *Dovepress, 7*, 3–13. doi:https://doi.org/10.2147/SAR.S83460

Rosenson, J., Clements, C., Simon, B., Vieaux, J., Graffman, S., Vahidnia, F., . . . Alter, H. (2013). Phenobarbital for acute alcohol withdrawal: A prospective randomized double-blind placebo-controlled study. *The Journal of Emergency Medicine, 44*(3), 592–598.

Sadock, B. J., Sadock, V. A., & Ruiz, P. (2015). *Synopsis of psychiatry: Behavioral sciences/clinical psychiatry* (11th ed.). Philadelphia, PA: Wolters Kluwer.

Schuckit, M. A. (2017). Alcohol-related disorders. In B. A. Sadock, V. A. Sadock, & P. Ruiz (Eds.), *Comprehensive textbook of psychiatry* (10th ed., pp. 1264–1279). Philadelphia, PA: Wolters Kluwer.

Storrs, C. (2016). *Is street drug flakka gone for good?* Retrieved from http://www.cnn.com/2016/04/18/health/flakka-drugdisappearance/index.html

Substance Abuse and Mental Health Services Administration (SAMHSA). (2014). *Clinical supervision and professional development of the substance abuse counselor.* (Treatment Improvement Protocol (TIP) Series 52, DHHS Publication No. SMA 09-4435). Rockville, MD: Author.

Substance Abuse and Mental Health Services Administration (SAMHSA). (2016a). *Stimulants.* Retrieved from https://www.samhsa.gov/atod/stimulants

Substance Abuse and Mental Health Services Administration (SAMHSA) (2016b). *Opioids.* Retrieved from https://www.samhsa.gov/atod/opioids

Substance Abuse and Mental Health Services Administration (SAMHSA). (2017). Alcohol, tobacco, and other drugs. Retrieved from http://www.samhsa.gov/atod

Tomko, R. L., Jones, J. L., Gilmore, A. K., Brady, K. T., Back, S. E., & Gray, K. M. (2018). N-acetylcysteine: A potential treatment for substance use disorders. *Current Psychiatry, 17*(6), 31–41.

Twachtman, G. (2018). *NIH launches HEAL initiative to combat opioid crisis.* Retrieved from https://www.mdedge.com/psychiatry/article/167889

U.S. Department of Health and Human Services (HHS), Office of the Surgeon General. (2016). *Facing addiction in America: The surgeon general's report on alcohol, drugs, and health.* Washington, DC: Author.

U.S. Drug Enforcement Administration (USDEA). (2013). *The DEA position on marijuana.* Retrieved from http://www.justice.gov/dea/docs/marijuana_position_2011.pdf

U.S. Food and Drug Administration (FDA). (2016). *FDA requires strong warnings for opioid analgesics, prescription opioid cough products, and benzodiazepine labeling related to serious risks and death from combined use.* Retrieved from https://www.fda.gov/NewsEvents/Newsroom/PressAnnouncements/ucm518697.htm

Vaux, K. K. (2016). *Fetal alcohol syndrome.* Retrieved from http://emedicine.medscape.com/article/974016-overview

WebMD. (2018). *Salvia divinorum.* Retrieved from https://www.webmd.com/vitamins/ai/ingredientmono-1043/salvia-divinorum

Weiss, H. D., & Pontone, G. M. (2014). Dopamine receptor agonist drugs and impulse control disorders. *JAMA Internal Medicine, 174*(12), 1935–1937. doi:10.1001/jamainternmed.2014.4097

Worley, J. (2017). Nurses with substance use disorders: Where we are and what needs to be done. *Journal of Psychosocial Nursing and Mental Health Services. 55*(12):11-14. https://doi.org/10.3928/02793695-20171113-02

Classical References

Cermak, T. L. (1986). *Diagnosing and treating co-dependence.* Center City, MN: Hazelton.

Jellinek, E. M. (1952). Phases of alcohol addiction. *Quarterly Journal of Studies on Alcohol, 13,* 673–684.

Mayfield, D., McLeod, G., & Hall, P. (1974). The CAGE questionnaire: Validation of a new alcoholism screening instrument. *American Journal of Psychiatry, 131,* 1121–1123.

O'Malley, S. S., Jaffe, A. J., Chang, G., Schottenfeld, R. S., Meyer, R. E., & Rounsaville, B. (1992). Naltrexone and coping skills therapy for alcohol dependence: A controlled study. *Archives of General Psychiatry 49*(11), 881–887.

Selzer, M. L. (1971). The Michigan Alcoholism Screening Test: The quest for a new diagnostic instrument. *American Journal of Psychiatry, 127,* 1653–1658.

Sullivan, J. T., Sykora, K., Schneiderman, J., Naranjo, C. A., & Sellers, E. M. (1989). Assessment of alcohol withdrawal: The revised Clinical Institute Withdrawal Assessment for Alcohol scale (CIWA-Ar). *British Journal of Addiction, 84,* 1353–1357.

Twerski, A. (1997). *Addictive thinking: Understanding self-deception* (2nd ed.). Center City, MN: Hazeldon.

Volpicelli, J. R., Alterman, A. I., Hayashida, M., & O'Brien, C. P. (1992). Naltrexone in the treatment of alcohol dependence. *Archives of General Psychiatry 49*(11), 876–880.

Schizophrenia Spectrum and Other Psychotic Disorders

15

CORE CONCEPT

Psychosis

KEY TERMS

anhedonia	illusion
anosognosia	loose associations
catatonia	magical thinking
circumstantiality	neologism
clang association	neuroleptic malignant syndrome
delusions	paranoid delusions
echolalia	perseveration
echopraxia	social skills training
extrapyramidal symptoms	tangentiality
gynecomastia	waxy flexibility
hallucinations	word salad

OBJECTIVES
After reading this chapter, the student will be able to:

1. Discuss the concepts of schizophrenia and other psychotic disorders.
2. Identify predisposing factors in the development of these disorders.
3. Describe various types of schizophrenia and other psychotic disorders.
4. Identify symptomatology associated with these disorders and use this information in patient assessment.
5. Formulate nursing diagnoses and outcomes of care for patients with schizophrenia and other psychotic disorders.
6. Identify topics for patient and family teaching relevant to schizophrenia and other psychotic disorders.

7. Describe appropriate nursing interventions for behaviors associated with these disorders.
8. Describe relevant criteria for evaluating nursing care of patients with schizophrenia and other psychotic disorders.

9. Discuss various modalities relevant to treatment of schizophrenia and other psychotic disorders.

HOMEWORK ASSIGNMENT
Please read the chapter and answer the following questions:

1. An alteration in which of the neurotransmitters is most closely associated with the symptoms of schizophrenia?
2. What is schizoaffective disorder?

3. How do delusions differ from hallucinations?
4. What was the first atypical antipsychotic to be developed? Why is it not considered a first-line treatment for schizophrenia?

Introduction

The term *schizophrenia* was coined in 1908 by the Swiss psychiatrist Eugen Bleuler. The word was derived from the Greek "skhizo" (split) and "phren" (mind).

Over the years, much debate has surrounded the concept of schizophrenia. Various definitions of the disorder have evolved, and numerous treatment strategies have been proposed, but none have proven to be uniformly effective or sufficient.

Although the controversy lingers, two general factors appear to be gaining acceptance among clinicians. The first is that schizophrenia is probably not a homogeneous disease entity. The *Diagnostic and Statistical Manual of Mental Disorders, Fifth Edition (DSM-5)*, supports this concept by describing schizophrenia as one of the schizophrenia spectrum disorders (American Psychiatric Association [APA], 2013). Although current consensus points to schizophrenia as a neurodevelopmental disorder (Álvarez et al., 2015), schizophrenia spectrum disorders may have several etiological influences including genetic predisposition, biochemical dysfunction, physiological factors, and psychosocial stress.

The second agreed-upon factor among clinicians is that there may never be a single treatment that cures the disorder. Effective treatment requires a comprehensive, multidisciplinary effort, including pharmacotherapy and various forms of psychosocial care, such as living skills and **social skills training,** rehabilitation and recovery, and family therapy. Emerging evidence indicates that early intervention and a comprehensive, patient-centered approach offers hope for a recovery process and improved quality of life for this population.

Of all the mental illnesses that cause suffering in society, schizophrenia is likely responsible for longer hospitalizations, greater chaos in family life, more exorbitant costs to individuals and governments, and more fear than any other. In addition, studies have shown that people with a severe mental illness (SMI) like schizophrenia have, on average, a 25-year shorter life span than the general population (Chesney, Goodwin & Fazel, 2014; Druss et al., 2011; Roberts et al., 2017). Because it is such an enormous threat to life and happiness and because its causes are an unsolved puzzle, it has probably been studied more than any other mental disorder.

Risk for suicide is a significant concern among patients with schizophrenia. About 20 to 40 percent of people with schizophrenia attempt suicide, and current evidence suggests that about 5 percent die by suicide (Lewis, Escalona, & Keith, 2017). This chapter explores various theories of predisposing factors that have been implicated in the development of schizophrenia. Symptomatology associated with different diagnostic categories of the disorder is discussed. Nursing care is presented in the context of the six steps of the nursing process. Various dimensions of medical treatment are explored.

Nature of the Disorder

CORE CONCEPT
Psychosis
A severe mental condition in which there is disorganization of the personality, deterioration in social functioning, and loss of contact with or distortion of reality. There may be evidence of hallucinations (false sensory perceptions not associated with real external stimuli) and delusions (fixed, false beliefs). Psychosis can occur with or without the presence of organic impairment.

Perhaps no psychological disorder is more crippling than schizophrenia. Characteristically, disturbances in thought processes, perception, and affect invariably result in a severe deterioration of social and occupational functioning.

The lifetime prevalence of schizophrenia is about 1 percent in the general population (Sadock, Sadock, & Ruiz, 2015). Symptoms generally appear in late adolescence or early adulthood, although they may occur in middle or late adult life. Early-onset schizophrenia refers to symptoms that begin in childhood and adolescence before age 18 years. This condition, although rare, is recognized as a progressive neurodevelopmental disorder with a chronic and severely symptomatic course (Sadock et al., 2015). Some studies have indicated that symptoms occur earlier in men than in women.

Phases of Schizophrenia

The pattern of development of schizophrenia may be viewed in four phases: premorbid, prodromal, active psychotic (acute schizophrenic episode), and residual phases.

Phase I: The Premorbid Phase

Premorbid signs are those that occur before there is clear evidence of illness and may include distinctive personality traits or behaviors. Premorbid personality and behavioral measurements that have been noted include being very shy and withdrawn, having poor peer relationships, doing poorly in school, and demonstrating antisocial behavior. Sadock and associates (2015) stated:

> In the typical, but not invariable, premorbid history of schizophrenia, patients had schizoid or schizotypal personalities characterized as quiet, passive, and introverted; as children, they had few friends. Pre-schizophrenic adolescents may have no close friends and no dates and may avoid team sports. They may enjoy [solitary activities] to the exclusion of social activities. (p. 311)

Current research that focuses on the premorbid stage seeks to identify biomarkers and at-risk individuals with the hope of preventing transition to illness and providing greater opportunity for early intervention (Clark et al., 2016).

Phase II: The Prodromal Phase

Prodromal signs are differentiated from premorbid signs in that prodromal symptoms more clearly manifest as signs of the developing illness of schizophrenia. The prodromal phase of schizophrenia begins with a change from premorbid functioning and extends until the onset of frank psychotic symptoms. This phase can be as brief as a few weeks or months, but most studies indicate that the average length of the prodromal phase is between 2 and 5 years. During this phase, the individual begins to show signs of significant deterioration in function. Fifty percent complain of depressive symptoms (APA, 2013). Social withdrawal is not uncommon, and signs of cognitive impairment may begin to emerge. In addition, some adolescent patients develop sudden onset of obsessive-compulsive behavior as part of the prodromal picture (Sadock et al., 2015).

Recognition of the behaviors associated with the prodromal phase provides an opportunity for early intervention with a possibility for improvement in long-term outcomes. Current treatment guidelines suggest therapeutic interventions that offer support with identified problems, cognitive therapies to minimize functional impairment, family interventions to improve coping, and involvement with the schools to reduce the possibility of failure. Some controversy exists about the benefits of pharmaceutical therapy during the prodromal phase; however, evidence supports that comprehensive treatment begun at the time of the first psychotic episode is associated with better outcomes (Insel, 2015).

Phase III: Active Psychotic Phase (Acute Schizophrenic Episode)

Schizophrenia is a chronic illness but is characterized by acute episodes in which symptoms are more pronounced. During acute episodes, psychotic symptoms are typically prominent. Box 15–1 describes the *DSM-5* (APA, 2013) diagnostic criteria for schizophrenia.

Phase IV: Residual Phase

Schizophrenia is characterized by periods of remission and exacerbation. A residual phase usually follows an active phase of the illness (symptoms described in Phase III). During the residual phase, symptoms of the acute stage are either absent or no longer prominent. Positive symptoms (like delusions and hallucinations) are often ameliorated but negative symptoms may remain (see Box 15–2), and flat affect and impairment in role functioning are common. Residual impairment often increases with additional episodes of active psychosis.

Prognosis

Outcomes in schizophrenia are difficult to predict and are highly variable, but long-term follow-up studies indicate that significant clinical improvement occurs in about 44 percent of patients with schizophrenia (Os & Reininghaus, 2017). However, several factors have

BOX 15–1 *DSM-V* Criteria for Schizophrenia

A. Two (or more) of the following, each present for a significant portion of time during a 1-month period (or less if successfully treated). At least one of these must be (1), (2), or (3):

1. **Delusions**
2. **Hallucinations**
3. **Disorganized speech (e.g., frequent derailment or incoherence)**
4. Grossly disorganized or catatonic behavior
5. Negative symptoms (i.e., diminished emotional expression or avolition)

B. For a significant portion of the time since the onset of the disturbance, level of functioning in one or more major areas, such as work, interpersonal relations, or self-care, is markedly below the level achieved prior to the onset (or when the onset is in childhood or adolescence, there is failure to achieve expected level of interpersonal, academic, or occupational functioning).

C. Continuous signs of the disturbance persist for at least 6 months. This 6-month period must include at least 1 month of symptoms (or less if successfully treated) that meet Criterion A (i.e., active-phase symptoms) and may include periods of prodromal or residual symptoms. During these prodromal or residual periods, the signs of the disturbance may be manifested by only negative symptoms or by two or more symptoms listed in Criterion A present in an attenuated form (e.g., odd beliefs, unusual perceptual experiences).

D. Schizoaffective disorder and depressive or bipolar disorder with psychotic features have been ruled out because either (1) no major depressive or manic episodes have occurred concurrently with the active-phase symptoms; or (2) if mood episodes have occurred during active-phase symptoms, they have been present for a minority of the total duration of the active and residual periods of the illness.

E. The disturbance is not attributable to the physiological effects of a substance (e.g., a drug of abuse, a medication) or another medical condition.

F. If there is a history of autism spectrum disorder or a communication disorder of childhood onset, the additional diagnosis of schizophrenia is made only if prominent delusions or hallucinations, in addition to the other required symptoms of schizophrenia, are also present for at least 1 month (or less if successfully treated).

Specify if: First episode, currently in acute, partial, or full remission; Multiple episodes, currently in acute, partial or full remission; Continuous; Unspecified; With catatonia

Specify current severity.

Source: Reprinted with permission from the Diagnostic and Statistical Manual of Mental Disorders, Fifth Edition *(Copyright 2013). American Psychiatric Association.*

been associated with a more positive outcome. These factors include good premorbid functioning, later age at onset, female gender, abrupt onset of symptoms with obvious precipitating factor (as opposed to gradual, insidious onset of symptoms), associated mood disturbance, rapid resolution of active-phase symptoms, minimal residual symptoms, absence of structural brain abnormalities, normal neurological functioning, and no family history of schizophrenia (Black & Andreasen, 2016; Sadock et al., 2015).

Predisposing Factors

The cause of schizophrenia is still uncertain. Most likely, no single factor can be implicated in the etiology; rather, the disease probably results from a combination of influences, including biological, psychological, and environmental factors.

Biological Factors

Refer to Chapter 2, Biological Implications, for a more thorough review of the biological implications of psychiatric illness.

Genetics

The body of evidence for genetic vulnerability to schizophrenia is growing. Studies show that relatives of individuals with schizophrenia have a much higher probability of developing the disease than does the general population. Whereas the lifetime risk for developing schizophrenia is about 1 percent in most population studies, the siblings of an identified patient have a 10 percent risk of developing schizophrenia, and offspring with one parent who has schizophrenia have a 5 to 6 percent chance of developing the disorder (Black & Andreasen, 2016).

How schizophrenia is inherited is uncertain. Current research is focused on determining which gene or genes are important in the vulnerability to schizophrenia and what other biomarkers may predict risk for this illness. Okazaki and associates (2016) studied gene expression in peripheral blood samples of patients admitted with acute psychosis and found that a specific combination of genes (*CDK4, MCM7,* and *POLD 4*) differentiated these patients from controls. This finding suggests that the combination could be a genetic biomarker for schizophrenia and may also influence certain pathophysiological aspects of schizophrenia. The authors conclude that messenger ribonucleic acid (mRNA) expression changes occurring in *CDK4* are potentially biomarkers for both trait (stable features) and state (temporary changes) symptoms in schizophrenia. Research is ongoing to identify genetic influences in schizophrenia that will hone our understanding of the multivariate influences in the development of this disease and perhaps identify treatment implications.

In monozygotic (identical) twins, the rate of schizophrenia is four to five times greater than the rate in dizygotic (fraternal) twins and approximately 50 times that of the general population (Sadock et al., 2015). Identical twins reared apart have the same rate of development of the illness as do those reared together. Because in about one-half of the cases only one of a pair of identical twins develops schizophrenia, genetic makeup cannot be solely responsible for causing this disease. Os and Reininghaus (2017) suggest that additive and interacting combinations of genes, environmental factors, and the moderation of gene expression through interaction with environmental factors are probably all influential.

Biochemical Factors

The oldest and most thoroughly explored biological theory in the explanation of schizophrenia attributes a pathogenic role to abnormal brain biochemistry. Notions of a "chemical disturbance" as an explanation for insanity were suggested by some theorists as early as the mid-19th century.

The Dopamine Hypothesis

This theory suggests that schizophrenia (or schizophrenia-like symptoms) may be caused by an excess of dopamine-dependent neuronal activity in the brain (Fig. 15–1). This excess activity may be related to increased production or release of the substance at nerve terminals, increased receptor sensitivity, too many dopamine receptors, or a combination of these mechanisms (Sadock et al., 2015).

Pharmacological support for this hypothesis comes from the observation that amphetamines, which increase levels of dopamine, induce symptoms that mimic those of psychosis. Antipsychotics (e.g., chlorpromazine or haloperidol) lower brain levels of dopamine by blocking dopamine receptors, thus reducing psychotic symptoms, including those induced by amphetamines.

Postmortem brain studies of individuals with schizophrenia have revealed a significant increase in the average number of dopamine receptors in approximately two-thirds of cases. This finding suggests that an increased number of dopamine receptors may not be the central or sole issue in all individuals with schizophrenia. Clients with positive symptoms such as delusions and hallucinations (referred to as positive symptoms because they are "added" to the clinical picture) respond with greater efficacy to dopamine-reducing drugs than do clients with negative symptoms (deficits such as apathy, poverty of ideas, and loss of drive). Positive and negative symptoms are listed in Box 15–4.

Thus, the current position on the dopamine hypothesis is that positive symptoms of schizophrenia may be related to increased numbers of dopamine receptors in the brain, because these symptoms are ameliorated by antipsychotic drugs that block dopamine receptors.

Other Biochemical Hypotheses

Various other biochemicals have been implicated in the predisposition to schizophrenia. Abnormalities in the neurotransmitters norepinephrine, serotonin, acetylcholine, and gamma-aminobutyric acid and in the neuroregulators, such as prostaglandins and endorphins, have been suggested. Excess of serotonin has been hypothesized to be responsible for both positive and negative symptoms of schizophrenia, and the effectiveness of medications such as clozapine (a strong serotonin antagonist) lends support to this hypothesis (Sadock et al., 2015).

Recent research has implicated the neurotransmitter glutamate in the etiology of schizophrenia. The *N*-methyl-D-aspartate (NMDA) receptor is the receptor that is activated by the neurotransmitters glutamate and glycine. Psychopharmacological studies have shown that the drug class of glutamate antagonists (e.g., phencyclidine [PCP]; ketamine) can produce schizophrenic-like symptoms in individuals without the disorder (Hashimoto, 2006; Stahl, 2013). In one study, participants experiencing ketamine-induced schizophrenia-like psychotic symptoms were treated with a drug trial of a glycine transporter-1 inhibitor (D'Souza et al., 2012). Because this medication was shown to reduce the psychotic symptoms induced by the NMDA receptor antagonism of ketamine, it may also have benefits in schizophrenia treatment. Despite evidence of a glutamate link in schizophrenia (Hu et al., 2014) more research is needed on the implications for treatment. Previous studies have focused on reducing glutamate levels in patients who have advanced illness, but current research has identified that glutamate levels may be more important in the

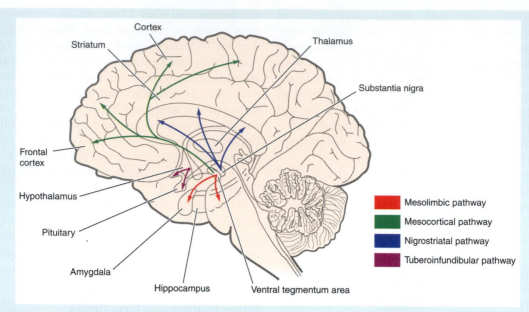

FIGURE 15-1   Neurobiology of schizophrenia.

NEUROTRANSMITTERS

A number of neurotransmitters have been implicated in the etiology of schizophrenia: dopamine, norepinephrine, serotonin, glutamate, and gamma-aminobutyric acid (GABA). The dopaminergic system has been most widely studied and closely linked to the symptoms associated with the disease.

AREAS OF THE BRAIN AFFECTED

Four major dopaminergic pathways (the pathways that transmit dopamine to different areas of the brain) have been identified:

- *Mesolimbic pathway:* Originates in the ventral tegmentum area (VTA) and projects to areas of the limbic system, including the nucleus accumbens, amygdala, and hippocampus. The mesolimbic pathway is associated with functions of memory, emotion, arousal, and pleasure. Excess activity in the mesolimbic tract has been implicated in the positive symptoms of schizophrenia (e.g., hallucinations, delusions). Dopamine blockade in this pathway is the target of antipsychotic medication to reduce hallucinations and delusions.
- *Mesocortical pathway:* Originates in the VTA and projects into the cortex. The mesocortical pathway is concerned with cognition, social behavior, planning, problem-solving, motivation, and reinforcement in learning. Negative symptoms of schizophrenia (e.g., flat affect, apathy, lack of motivation, and anhedonia) have been associated with diminished activity in the mesocortical tract.
- *Nigrostriatal pathway:* Originates in the substantia nigra and terminates in the striatum of the basal ganglia. This pathway is associated with the function of motor control. Degeneration in this pathway is associated with Parkinson's disease, and because typical antipsychotics may also block dopamine here, drug-induced Parkinson-like extrapyramidal side effects and tardive dyskinesia occur.
- *Tuberoinfundibular pathway:* Originates in the hypothalamus and projects to the pituitary gland. It is associated with endocrine function, digestion, metabolism, hunger, thirst, temperature control, and sexual arousal. Dopamine blockade in this pathway is associated with an increase in prolactin levels (hyperprolactinemia), which can result in galactorrhea (milk discharge from the nipples) in both men and women, erectile disorder, and anorgasmia.

ANTIPSYCHOTIC MEDICATIONS

Type	Receptor Affinity	Associated Side Effects
First generation (typical) antipsychotics		
Phenothiazines Haloperidol	Strong D_2 (dopamine)	Extrapyramidal symptoms (EPS), hyperprolactinemia, **neuroleptic malignant syndrome**
	Varying degrees of affinity for: ACh (acetylcholine) α_1 (norepinephrine)	Anticholinergic effects Tachycardia, tremors, insomnia, postural hypotension

ANTIPSYCHOTIC MEDICATIONS–cont'd		
Second generation (atypical) antipsychotics:		
Clozapine, olanzapine, quetiapine, aripiprazole, risperidone, iloperidone, ziprasidone, paliperidone, asenapine, lurasidone	H_1 (histamine) Weak 5-HT (serotonin) Strong 5-HT	Weight gain, sedation Low potential for ejaculatory difficulty Sexual dysfunction, GI disturbance, headache
	Low to moderate D_2 Varying degrees of affinity for: ACh α-adrenergic H_1	Low potential for EPS Anticholinergic effects Tachycardia, tremors, insomnia, postural hypotension

transition to psychosis. This theory is supported by the fact that first episodes of psychosis are often precipitated by stress, and glutamate increases under stress (Nauert, 2015). When glutamate levels are very high, the hippocampus becomes hypermetabolic and then begins to atrophy. Hippocampal atrophy has been identified as a significant finding in many individuals with schizophrenia. Future research may find that interventions targeting glutamate are beneficial in high-risk individuals or those in early stages of illness to prevent onset or slow the progression of the disease (Nauert, 2015).

Currently conventional antipsychotic medications largely target the dopamine receptors in the brain. Newer, second generation antipsychotics have strong affinity for serotonergic receptors. The glutamate model of schizophrenia suggests possibilities for new biomarkers signaling early illness and for new approaches to prevention and early treatment.

Physiological Factors

A number of physical factors of possible etiological significance have been identified in the medical literature. However, their specific mechanisms in the implication of schizophrenia are unclear.

Viral Infection

Sadock and colleagues (2015) report that epidemiological data indicate a high incidence of schizophrenia after prenatal exposure to influenza. They stated:

> Other data supporting a viral hypothesis are an increased number of physical anomalies at birth, an increased rate of pregnancy and birth complications, seasonality of birth consistent with viral infection, geographical clusters of adult cases, and seasonality of hospitalizations. (p. 305)

The effect of autoimmune antibodies in the brain is an area of ongoing study. Psychoneuroimmunological research suggests that such antibodies may be responsible for the development of at least some cases of schizophrenia following infection from a neurotoxic virus (particularly prenatal exposure to *Toxoplasma gondii*) (Matheson, Shepherd, & Carr, 2014). The role of cytokines in inflammation and the specific effects of these chemicals in the brain are still being explored through ongoing research.

Anatomical Abnormalities

With the use of neuroimaging technologies, structural brain abnormalities have been observed in individuals with schizophrenia. Ventricular enlargement is the most consistent finding; however, some reductions in gray matter are also reported.

Magnetic resonance imaging (MRI) has revealed reduced symmetry in several lobes of the brain and reductions in size of structures within the limbic system of individuals with schizophrenia. Considerable evidence from postmortem studies has shown abnormalities in the prefrontal cortex, and people who have had prefrontal lobotomies are reported to manifest many symptoms common to schizophrenia (Sadock et al., 2015).

Diffusion tensor imaging studies have identified widespread white matter abnormalities in schizophrenia (Viher et al., 2016). These abnormalities in white matter microstructure appear to be primarily associated with negative symptoms and psychomotor behavior abnormalities.

Long-term studies of patients with schizophrenia have noted brain volume reduction, particularly in the temporal and preventricular areas (Veijola et al., 2014). It has been postulated that long-term antipsychotic medication use may contribute to this reduction, but the implications are unclear. Veijola and associates found that symptom severity, level of functional ability, and decline in cognitive abilities were not correlated with this reduction in brain volume.

Electrophysiology

Several studies have evaluated 40 Hz auditory steady state response, a measure of electrical activity in the brain, and identified neural circuit dysfunctions in people with schizophrenia. A recent meta-analysis (Thunè, Recasens, & Uhlhaas, 2016) of these studies demonstrates robust evidence of such dysfunction in schizophrenia. The meaning of these circuit dysfunctions is not well understood but may indicate another biomarker for identifying risk or illness.

Physical Conditions

Several medical conditions are known to cause acute psychotic episodes, including Huntington's disease, hyperthyroidism or hypothyroidism, hypoglycemia, calcium imbalances, temporal lobe epilepsy, Wilson's disease, central nervous system (CNS) neoplasms, encephalitis, meningitis, neurosyphilis, and stroke (Mathews et al., 2013). See Box 15–2 for a list of many medical conditions associated with psychosis.

Psychological Factors

Early conceptualizations of schizophrenia focused on family relationship factors as major influences in the development of the illness, probably in light of the conspicuous absence of information related to a biological connection. These early theories implicated poor parent-child relationships, particularly condemning the mother as "schizophrenogenic" (inducing schizophrenia in her child) related to a troublesome communication style known as *double bind communication*. This theory is no longer credible. Researchers now focus on schizophrenia as a brain disorder. Although family relationships are not involved in the etiology of the illness, the symptoms in schizophrenia can contribute to significant disruption in communication and relationships among family members, so psychosocial factors should always be part of a comprehensive assessment. Furthermore, evidence suggests that childhood trauma, particularly multiple traumatizations, are associated (among many other influences) with the development of schizophrenia (Álvarez et al., 2015, Matheson et al., 2014). Trauma-informed care is an important part of comprehensive assessment and intervention for this client.

Environmental Influences

Sociocultural Factors

Many studies have attempted to link schizophrenia to social class. Epidemiological statistics have shown that greater numbers of individuals from the lower

---

BOX 15–2 General Medical Conditions That May Cause Psychotic Symptoms

Acute intermittent porphyria
Brain abscesses
Cerebrovascular disease
CNS infections
CNS trauma
Cushing's syndrome
Deafness
Encephalitis
Fluid or electrolyte imbalances
Hepatic disease
Herpes encephalitis
Huntington's disease
Hypoadrenocorticism
Hypo- or hyperparathyroidism
Hypo- or hyperthyroidism
Meningitis
Metabolic conditions (e.g., hypoxia; hypercarbia; hypoglycemia)
Migraine headache
Neoplasms
Neurosyphilis
Normal pressure hydrocephalus
Renal disease
Systemic lupus erythematosus
Temporal lobe epilepsy
Vitamin deficiency (e.g., B_{12})
Wilson's disease

Sources: Black, D. W., & Andreasen, N. C. (2016). Introductory textbook of psychiatry *(6th ed.). Washington, DC: American Psychiatric; Freudenreich, O. (2010). Differential diagnosis of psychotic symptoms: Medical "mimics."* Psychiatric Times, 27*(12), 52–61. Sadock, B. J., Sadock, V. A., & Ruiz, P. (2015).* Synopsis of psychiatry: Behavioral sciences/clinical psychiatry *(11th ed.). Philadelphia, PA: Lippincott Williams & Wilkins.*

---

socioeconomic classes (in urban neighborhoods) experience symptoms associated with schizophrenia than do those from higher socioeconomic groups (Os & Reininghaus, 2017). These studies consistently find that lack of material resources (including housing and access to healthcare) and fragmented social relationships increase the risk for schizophrenia, whereas social cohesion and ethnic density (the concentration of a given ethnic group in a particular area) are protective.

An alternative view is the *downward drift hypothesis*, which suggests that because of the characteristic symptoms of the disorder, individuals with schizophrenia have difficulty maintaining gainful employment and "drift down" to a lower socioeconomic level (or fail to rise out of a lower socioeconomic group). Proponents of this view consider poor social conditions to be a consequence rather than a cause of schizophrenia.

Stressful Life Events

Studies have been conducted in an effort to determine whether psychotic episodes may be precipitated by stressful life events. There is no scientific evidence to indicate that stress causes schizophrenia. It is probable, however, that stress may contribute to the severity and course of the illness. It is known that extreme stress can precipitate psychotic episodes. Stress may indeed precipitate symptoms in an individual who possesses a genetic vulnerability to schizophrenia. Stressful life events also may be associated with exacerbation of schizophrenic symptoms and increased rates of relapse.

Cannabis and Genetic Vulnerability

Studies of genetic vulnerability for schizophrenia have linked certain genes (*COMT* and *ATK1*) to increased risk for psychosis and particularly for adolescents with this genetic vulnerability who use cannabinoids (Radhakrishnan, Wilkinson, & D'Souza, 2014). Both cannabis and synthetic cannabinoids can induce many schizophrenia-like symptoms, and in individuals with a pre-existing psychosis, cannabinoids can exacerbate symptoms. More importantly, the increased risk for psychotic disorders such as schizophrenia with cannabis use suggests the influence of lifestyle factors in the expression of genes and points to the possibility of multiple factors playing a role in the causality of this illness.

Theoretical Integration

The etiology of schizophrenia remains unclear. No single theory or hypothesis has been postulated that substantiates a clear-cut explanation for the disease. Accumulating evidence supports the concept of multiple causation in the development of schizophrenia. In a systematic review of the literature on schizophrenia, Matheson and associates (2014) summarize that the most robust evidence suggests that schizophrenia is a widespread neural dysfunction accompanied by various psychological effects that respond moderately well to psychosocial and biomedical therapy:

> Patients have relatively poor cognitive functioning, and subtle, but diverse, structural brain alterations, altered electrophysiological functioning and

sleep patterns, minor physical anomalies, neurological soft signs, and sensory alterations. There are markers of infection, inflammation or altered immunological parameters; and there is increased mortality from a range of causes. Risk for schizophrenia is increased with cannabis use, pregnancy and birth complications, prenatal exposure to *T. gondii*, childhood central nervous system viral infections, childhood adversities, urbanicity, and immigration (first and second generation), particularly in certain ethnic groups. Developmental motor delays and lower intelligence quotient in childhood and adolescence are apparent. (p. 3387)

Despite the wealth of research and knowledge that we have about schizophrenia, much more investigation is needed before we will fully understand this illness.

Other Schizophrenia Spectrum and Psychotic Disorders

The *DSM-5* (APA, 2013) identifies a spectrum of psychotic disorders that are organized to reflect a gradient of psychopathology from least to most severe. Degree of severity is determined by the level, number, and duration of psychotic signs and symptoms.

Several of the disorders may *also have accompanying catatonic features.* **Catatonia** refers to a significant motor disturbance that may range from stupor (no motor activity) to excessive motor activity and agitation. The disorders in which catatonia may appear include brief psychotic disorder, schizophreniform disorder, schizophrenia, schizoaffective disorder, substance-induced psychotic disorder, neurodevelopmental disorder, major depressive disorder, and bipolar disorders I and II (APA, 2013).

The *DSM-5* initiates the spectrum of disorders with Schizotypal Personality Disorder. For purposes of this textbook, this disorder is presented in Chapter 22, Personality Disorders.

Delusional Disorder

Delusional disorder is characterized by the presence of delusions that have been experienced by the individual for at least 1 month. Although the individual with schizophrenia may experience similar delusions, this disorder does not meet the diagnostic criteria for schizophrenia (APA, 2013). If present at all, hallucinations are not prominent, and behavior is not bizarre. The subtype of delusional disorder is based on the predominant delusional theme. The *DSM-5* states that a specifier may be added to denote whether the delusions are considered *bizarre* (i.e., whether the thought is "clearly implausible, not understandable, and not derived from ordinary life experiences" (p. 91). Subtypes of delusional disorders include erotomanic, grandiose, jealous, persecutory, somatic, and mixed. These are discussed further in the section "Application of the Nursing Process."

Brief Psychotic Disorder

This disorder is identified by the sudden onset of psychotic symptoms that may or may not be preceded by a severe psychosocial stressor. These symptoms last at least 1 day but less than 1 month, and there is an eventual full return to the premorbid level of functioning (APA, 2013). The individual experiences emotional turmoil or overwhelming perplexity or confusion. Evidence of impaired reality testing may include incoherent speech, delusions, hallucinations, bizarre behavior, and disorientation. Individuals with pre-existing personality disorders (most commonly, histrionic, narcissistic, paranoid, schizotypal, and borderline personality disorders) appear to be susceptible to this disorder (Sadock et al., 2015). Catatonic features also may be associated with this disorder.

Substance- and Medication-Induced Psychotic Disorder

The prominent hallucinations and delusions associated with substance-induced or medication-induced disorder are found to be directly attributable to substance intoxication or withdrawal or after exposure to a medication or toxin. This diagnosis is made when the symptoms are more excessive and more severe than those usually associated with the intoxication or withdrawal syndrome (APA, 2013). The medical history, physical examination, and laboratory findings provide evidence that the appearance of the symptoms occurred in association with a substance intoxication or withdrawal or exposure to a medication or toxin. Substances that are believed to induce psychotic disorders are presented in Box 15–3. Catatonic features also may be associated with this disorder.

Psychotic Disorder Due to Another Medical Condition

The essential features of this disorder are prominent hallucinations and delusions that can be directly attributed to another medical condition (APA, 2013). The diagnosis is not made if the symptoms occur during the course of a delirium. A number of medical conditions that can cause psychotic symptoms are presented in Box 15–2.

BOX 15–3 Substances That May Cause Psychotic Disorders

DRUGS OF ABUSE
Alcohol
Amphetamines and related substances
Cannabis
Cocaine
Hallucinogens
Inhalants
Opioids
Phencyclidine and related substances
Sedatives, hypnotics, and anxiolytics

MEDICATIONS
Anesthetics and analgesics
Anticholinergic agents
Anticonvulsants
Antidepressant medication
Antihistamines
Antihypertensive agents
Antimicrobial medications
Antineoplastic medications
Antiparkinsonian agents
Cardiovascular medications
Corticosteroids
Disulfiram
Gastrointestinal medications
Muscle relaxants
Nonsteroidal Anti-Inflammatory Agents

TOXINS
Anticholinesterase
Organophosphate insecticides
Nerve gases
Carbon dioxide
Carbon monoxide
Volatile substances (e.g., fuel, paint, gasoline, toluene)

Sources: American Psychiatric Association. (2013). Diagnostic and statistical manual of mental disorders (5th ed.). Washington, DC: Author; Black, D. W., & Andreasen, N. C. (2016). Introductory textbook of psychiatry (6th ed.). Washington, DC: American Psychiatric; Freudenreich, O. (2010). Differential diagnosis of psychotic symptoms: Medical "mimics." Psychiatric Times, 27(12), 52–61.

Catatonic Disorder Due to Another Medical Condition

This diagnosis is made when catatonic features are evidenced from medical history, physical examination, or laboratory findings to be directly attributable to the physiological consequences of another medical condition (APA, 2013). Types of medical conditions that have been associated with catatonic disorder include metabolic disorders (e.g., hepatic encephalopathy, diabetic ketoacidosis, hypo- and hyperthyroidism, hypo- and hyperadrenalism, and vitamin B_{12} deficiency) and neurological conditions (e.g., epilepsy, tumors, cerebrovascular disease, head trauma, and encephalitis) (APA, 2013; Mathews et al., 2013).

Schizophreniform Disorder

The essential features of schizophreniform disorder are identical to those of schizophrenia with the exception that the duration, including prodromal, active, and residual phases, is at least 1 month but less than 6 months (APA, 2013). If the diagnosis is made while the individual is still symptomatic but has been so for less than 6 months, it is qualified as "provisional." The diagnosis is changed to schizophrenia if the clinical picture persists beyond 6 months. Schizophreniform disorder is thought to have a good prognosis if the individual's affect is not blunted or flat, if there is a rapid onset of psychotic symptoms from the time the unusual behavior is noticed, or if the premorbid social and occupational functioning was satisfactory (APA, 2013). Catatonic features also may be associated with this disorder.

Schizoaffective Disorder

This disorder is manifested by signs and symptoms of schizophrenia, along with a strong element of symptomatology associated with the mood disorders (depression or mania). The client may appear depressed with psychomotor retardation and suicidal ideation, or symptoms may include euphoria, grandiosity, and hyperactivity (see "Real People, Real Stories" interview with Josh, who describes his diagnosis and experience with schizoaffective disorder in Chapter 16, Depressive Disorders). The decisive factor in the diagnosis of schizoaffective disorder is the presence of hallucinations and/or delusions that occur for at least 2 weeks in the absence of a major mood episode (APA, 2013). However, prominent mood disorder symptoms must be evident for a majority of the time. The prognosis for schizoaffective disorder is generally better than that for other schizophrenic disorders but worse than that for mood disorders alone (Black & Andreasen, 2016). Catatonic features also may be associated with this disorder.

Application of the Nursing Process

Schizophrenia: Background Assessment Data

The diagnostic criteria for schizophrenia were presented earlier in this chapter. As previously stated, symptoms may present in phases with schizophrenia representing the active phase of the disorder. Symptoms associated with the active phase are discussed in this section.

In the first step of the nursing process, the nurse gathers a database from which nursing diagnoses are derived and a plan of care is formulated. This first step of the nursing process is extremely important because problem identification, objectives of care, and outcome criteria cannot be accurately determined without an accurate assessment.

Assessment of the client with schizophrenia may be a complex process based on information gathered from a number of sources. Clients in an acute episode of their illness may not be able to make accurate contributions to their history. Data may be obtained from family members if possible, from old medical records if available, or from other individuals who have been in a position to report on the progression of the client's behavior.

The nurse must be familiar with behaviors common to the disorder to be able to obtain an adequate assessment of the patient with schizophrenia. This includes positive and negative symptoms. Most but not all clients exhibit a mixture of both types of symptoms.

Cognitive deficits, including memory impairment, attention, language, and executive functioning deficits are often present and can be debilitating. Bora (2015) notes that in individuals who develop cognitive deficits, the age of onset is variable, and MacCabe and associates (2013) identify that a subgroup of individuals with schizophrenia have no cognitive impairment even in adulthood. Many factors contribute to functional impairment and decline beyond the symptoms themselves, including comorbid metabolic conditions, chronic substance use, stress, frequency and intensity of episodes, residual symptoms, and social defeat (Bora, 2015). A summary of positive and negative symptoms is presented in Box 15–4 and described in more detail in the following section.

Positive Symptoms

Disturbances in Thought Content

Delusions Delusions are fixed false beliefs that are irrational and that the individual maintains as true despite evidence to the contrary. These beliefs are

BOX 15–4 Positive and Negative Symptoms of Schizophrenia

POSITIVE SYMPTOMS

Delusions (Fixed, False Beliefs) (examples)

Persecutory—belief that one is going to be harmed by other(s)

Referential—belief that cues in the environment are specifically referring to them

Grandiose—belief that they have exceptional greatness

Somatic—beliefs that center on one's body functioning

Hallucinations (Sensory Perceptions Without External Stimuli)

Auditory (most common in schizophrenia)

Visual

Tactile

Olfactory

Gustatory

(NOTE: Hallucinations may be a normal part of religious experience in some cultural contexts.)

Disorganized Thinking (Manifested in Speech)

Loose association

Tangentiality

Circumstantiality

Incoherence (includes word salad)

Neologisms

Clang associations

Echolalia

Grossly Disorganized or Abnormal Motor Behavior (Including Catatonia)

Hyperactivity

Hypervigilance

Hostility

Agitation

Childlike silliness

Catatonia (ranging from rigid or bizarre posture and decreased responsivity to complete lack of verbal or behavioral response to the environment)

Catatonic excitement (excessive and purposeless motor activity)

Stereotyped, repetitive movements

Unusual mannerisms or postures

NEGATIVE SYMPTOMS

Lack of Emotional Expression

Blunted affect

Lack of movement in head and hands that adds expression in communication

Lack of intonation in speech

Decreased or Lack of Motivation to Complete Purposeful Activities (Avolition)

Neglect of activities of daily living

Decreased Verbal Communication (Alogia)

Decreased Interest in Social Interaction and Relationship (Asociality)

Withdrawal

Poor rapport

Diminished Ability for Abstract Thinking

Concrete interpretation of events and communication from others

Positive symptoms refer to symptoms that are present ("added") in people with schizophrenia and not typically present in people without the disease.
    Negative symptoms are referred to as deficits or impairments (things "taken away" by the illness) in individuals with schizophrenia.
Sources: American Psychiatric Association (APA). (2013). Diagnostic and statistical manual of mental disorders (5th ed.). Washington, DC: Author; Kay, S. R., Fiszbein, A., & Opler, L. A. (1987). The positive and negative syndrome scale (PANSS) for schizophrenia. Schizophrenia Bulletin, 13(2), 261–276.

not explainable as part of the person's usual religious or cultural precepts. Delusions are subdivided according to their content. Some of the more common ones are listed here.

Persecutory delusions: These are the most common type of delusion in which individuals believe they are being persecuted or malevolently treated in some way. Frequent themes include being plotted against, cheated or defrauded, followed and spied on, poisoned, or drugged. The individual may obsess about and exaggerate a slight rebuff (either real or imagined) until it becomes the focus of a delusional system. Repeated complaints may be directed at legal authorities. The individual feels threatened and believes that others intend harm or persecution toward him or her in some way (e.g., "The FBI has 'bugged' my room and intends to kill me"; "The government put a chip in my brain to erase my memories"). These may also be referred to as **paranoid delusions**, which describes the extreme suspiciousness of others and of their actions or perceived intentions (e.g., "I won't eat this food. I know it has been poisoned"). Aggression or violence may occur because the individual believes that he or she must defend him/herself against someone or something perceived to be a threat.

Grandiose delusions: The individual has an exaggerated feeling of importance, power, knowledge, or identity. The individual may believe that he or she has a special relationship with a famous person or even assume the identity of a famous person (believing that the actual person is an imposter). Grandiose delusions of a religious nature may lead to assumption of the identity of a deity or religious leader (e.g., "I am Jesus Christ").

Delusions of reference: Events within the environment are referred by the psychotic person to himself or herself (e.g., "Someone is trying to get a message to me through the articles in this magazine [or newspaper or TV program]; I must break the code so that I can receive the message") and these beliefs become fixed (as with other delusions) despite evidence to the contrary. *Ideas* of reference may have content similar to delusions of reference but they are less rigidly adhered to beliefs; when a person with ideas of reference is offered an alternative explanation, the person is more likely able to consider that he or she has misinterpreted the situation. For example, an individual with ideas of reference may think that other people in the room who are giggling must be laughing about him but with additional information can acknowledge that there could be other explanations for their laughter.

Delusions of control or influence: The individual believes that certain objects or persons have control over his or her behavior (e.g., "The dentist put a filling in my tooth; I now receive transmissions through the filling that control what I think and do") or the person believes that his or her thoughts or behaviors have control over specific situations or people (e.g., the mother who believed that if she scolded her son in any way, he would die). This is similar to **magical thinking**, which is common in children (e.g., "The sky is raining because I'm sad").

Somatic delusions: The individual has a false idea about the functioning of his or her body. This may be a false belief that the he or she has some type of general medical condition or that there has been an alteration in a body organ or its function (e.g., "The doctor says I'm not pregnant, but I know I am"; "There is an alien force that is eating my brain").

Nihilistic delusions: The individual has a false idea that the self, a part of the self, others, or the world is nonexistent (e.g., "The world no longer exists"; "I have no heart").

Erotomanic delusions: Individuals with erotomanic delusions falsely believe that someone, usually of a higher status, is in love with him or her. Famous persons are often the subjects of erotomanic delusions. Sometimes the delusion is kept secret, but some individuals may follow, contact, or otherwise try to pursue the object of their delusion.

Jealous delusions: The content of jealous delusions centers on the idea that the person's sexual partner is unfaithful. The idea is irrational and without cause, but the individual with the delusion searches for evidence to justify the belief. The sexual partner is confronted (and sometimes physically attacked) regarding the imagined infidelity. The imagined "lover" of the sexual partner also may be the object of the attack. Attempts to restrict the autonomy of the sexual partner in an effort to stop the imagined infidelity are common.

Disturbances in Thought Processes Manifested in Speech

Loose Associations Thinking is characterized by speech in which ideas shift from one unrelated subject to another. Typically, the individual with **loose associations** is unaware that the topics are not connected. When the condition is severe, speech may be incoherent (e.g., "We wanted to take the bus, but my lunch was cold. The FBI is watching me. No one needs to pay to get to heaven. We have it all in our pockets").

Neologisms The person invents new words, or **neologisms,** that are meaningless to others but have symbolic meaning to the individual (e.g., "She wanted to give me a ride in her new *uniphorum*").

Clang Associations Choice of words is governed by sounds. **Clang associations** often take the form of rhyming. For instance, "It is very cold. I am cold and bold. The gold has been sold."

Word Salad A **word salad** is a group of words that are put together randomly, without any logical connection (e.g., "Most forward action grows life double plays circle uniform").

Circumstantiality With **circumstantiality**, the individual delays in reaching the point of a communication because of unnecessary and tedious details. The point or goal is usually met but only with numerous interruptions by the interviewer to keep the person on track of the topic being discussed.

Tangentiality **Tangentiality** refers to a veering away from the topic of discussion and difficulty maintaining focus and attention.

Perseveration The individual who exhibits **perseveration** persistently repeats the same word or idea in response to different questions. It is a manifestation of a thought processing disturbance in which the person gets stuck on a particular thought.

Echolalia **Echolalia** refers to repeating words or phrases spoken by another. In toddlers this is a normal phase in development, but in children with autism, echolalia may persist beyond the toddler years. In adulthood, echolalia is a significant neurological symptom of thought disturbance that occurs in schizophrenia, strokes, and other neurological disorders.

Disturbances in Perception

Hallucinations **Hallucinations**, or false sensory perceptions not associated with real external stimuli, may involve any of the five senses. Types of hallucinations include the following:

- **Auditory:** Auditory hallucinations are false perceptions of sound. Most commonly they are of voices, but the individual may report clicks, rushing noises, music, and other noises. *Command hallucinations* are "voices" that issue commands to the individual. They are potentially dangerous when the commands are directing violence toward self or others. Auditory hallucinations are the most common type in schizophrenia.
- **Visual:** These hallucinations are false visual perceptions that may consist of formed images, such as of people, or of unformed images, such as flashes of light. Visual hallucinations occur about 27 percent of the time in individuals with schizophrenia (and 15 percent of the time in affective psychoses). They typically co-occur with auditory hallucinations and are associated with poorer outcomes (Waters et al., 2014).
- **Tactile:** Tactile hallucinations are false perceptions of the sense of touch, often of something on or under the skin. One specific tactile hallucination is formication, the sensation that something is crawling on or under the skin.
- **Gustatory:** This type of hallucination is a false perception of taste. Most commonly, gustatory hallucinations are described as unpleasant tastes.
- **Olfactory:** Olfactory hallucinations are false perceptions of the sense of smell.

Illusions **Illusions** are misperceptions or misinterpretations of real external stimuli. These may occur in the prodromal, active, and residual phases of schizophrenia and may co-occur with delusions.

Echopraxia The client who exhibits **echopraxia** imitates movements made by others. The mechanisms underlying echopraxia in schizophrenia are not well understood, but current evidence suggests that it may involve a disturbance in mirror neuron activity in the presence of social cognition impairments and self-monitoring deficits (Urvakhsh et al., 2014).

Negative Symptoms

Disturbances in Affect

Affect describes the behavior associated with an individual's feeling state or emotional tone.

Inappropriate Affect Affect is inappropriate when the individual's emotional tone is incongruent with the circumstances (e.g., a young woman who laughs when told of the death of her mother).

Bland or Flat Affect Affect is described as bland when the emotional tone is very weak. The individual with flat affect appears to be void of emotional tone (or overt expression of feelings).

Apathy

The client with schizophrenia often demonstrates an indifference to or disinterest in the environment. The bland or flat affect is a manifestation of the emotional apathy.

Avolition

Impaired volition has to do with the inability to initiate goal-directed activity. In the individual with schizophrenia, this may take the form of inadequate interest, lack of motivation, neglect of activities of daily living including personal hygiene and appearance, or inability to choose a logical course of action in a given situation.

Lack of Interest or Skills in Interpersonal Interaction

Impairment in social functioning may be reflected in social isolation, emotional detachment, and lack of regard for social convention. Some clients with acute schizophrenia cling to others and intrude on the personal space of others, exhibiting behaviors that are not socially and culturally acceptable. Others may exhibit ambivalence in social relationships. Still others may withdraw from relationships altogether (asociality).

Lack of Insight

Some individuals lack awareness of there being any illness or disorder even when symptoms appear obvious to others. The term for this is **anosognosia.** The *DSM-5* identifies this symptom as the "most common predictor of nonadherence to treatment, and it predicts higher relapse rates, increased number of involuntary treatments, poorer psychosocial functioning, aggression, and poorer course of illness" (APA, 2013, p. 101).

Anergia

Anergia is a deficiency of energy. The individual with schizophrenia may lack sufficient energy to carry out activities of daily living or to interact with others.

Anhedonia

Anhedonia is the inability to experience pleasure. This is a distressing symptom that may increase one's risk for suicide.

Lack of Abstract Thinking Ability

Concrete thinking, or literal interpretations of the environment, represents a regression to an earlier level of cognitive development. Abstract thinking becomes impaired in some individuals with schizophrenia. For example, the client with this deficit would have great difficulty describing the abstract meaning of sayings such as "I'm climbing the walls" or "It's raining cats and dogs."

Associated Features

Waxy Flexibility

Waxy flexibility describes a condition in which the client with schizophrenia allows body parts to be placed in bizarre or uncomfortable positions. This symptom is associated with catatonia. Once placed in position, the arm, leg, or head remains in that position for long periods, regardless of how uncomfortable it is for the client. For example, the nurse may position the client's arm in an outward position to take a blood pressure measurement. When the cuff is removed, the client may maintain the arm in the position in which it was placed to take the reading.

Posturing

This symptom is manifested by the voluntary assumption of inappropriate or bizarre postures.

Pacing and Rocking

Pacing back and forth and body rocking (a slow, rhythmic, backward-and-forward swaying of the trunk from the hips, usually while sitting) are common psychomotor behaviors of the client with schizophrenia.

Regression

Regression is the retreat to an earlier level of development. Regression, a primary defense mechanism of schizophrenia, is a dysfunctional attempt to reduce anxiety. It provides the basis for many of the behaviors associated with schizophrenia.

Eye Movement Abnormalities

Eye movement abnormalities may manifest in several ways including difficulty maintaining focus on a stationary object and difficulty with smooth pursuit of a moving object. Research (Benson et al., 2012) has found that simple eye movement tests can distinguish the abnormalities common in schizophrenia with exceptional accuracy.

Diagnosis and Outcome Identification

Using information collected during the assessment, the nurse completes the client database from which the selection of appropriate nursing diagnoses is determined. Table 15–1 presents a list of client behaviors and the NANDA International (NANDA-I) nursing diagnoses (Herdman & Kamitsuru, 2018) that correspond to those behaviors, which may be used in planning care for clients with psychotic disorders.

Outcome Criteria

The following criteria may be used for measurement of outcomes in the care of the patient with schizophrenia.

The patient:

■ Demonstrates an ability to relate satisfactorily with others.
■ Recognizes distortions of reality.
■ Has not harmed self or others.
■ Perceives self realistically.
■ Demonstrates the ability to perceive the environment correctly.
■ Maintains anxiety at a manageable level.
■ Relinquishes the need for delusions and hallucinations.
■ Demonstrates the ability to trust others.
■ Uses appropriate verbal communication in interactions with others.
■ Performs self-care activities independently.

Planning and Implementation

Table 15–2 provides a plan of care for the patient with schizophrenia. Selected nursing diagnoses are presented, along with outcome criteria, appropriate nursing interventions, and rationales for each. In general, nursing interventions should be geared toward establishing trust because suspiciousness is a common symptom in this disorder.

Use of a passive rather than a directive communication approach, which offers the client the opportunity to make his or her decisions about activities, treatment goals, and other aspects of care, is in the interest of establishing trust and incorporating a patient-centered approach.

TABLE 15–1 Assigning Nursing Diagnoses to Behaviors Commonly Associated With Psychotic Disorders	
BEHAVIORS	**NURSING DIAGNOSES**
Impaired communication (inappropriate responses), disordered thought sequencing, rapid mood swings, poor concentration, disorientation, stops talking in midsentence, tilts head to side as if to be listening	Disturbed sensory perception*
Delusional thinking; inability to concentrate; impaired volition; inability to problem solve, abstract, or conceptualize; extreme suspiciousness of others; inaccurate interpretation of the environment	Disturbed thought processes*
Withdrawal, sad dull affect, need-fear dilemma, preoccupation with own thoughts, expression of feelings of rejection or of aloneness imposed by others, uncommunicative, seeks to be alone	Social isolation
Risk factors: Aggressive body language (e.g., clenching fists and jaw, pacing, threatening stance); verbal aggression; catatonic excitement; command hallucinations; rage reactions; history of violence; overt aggressive acts; goal-directed destruction of objects in the environment; self-destructive behavior; active, aggressive suicidal acts	Risk for violence: Self-directed or other-directed
Loose association of ideas, neologisms, word salad, clang associations, echolalia, verbalizations that reflect concrete thinking, poor eye contact, difficulty expressing thoughts verbally, inappropriate verbalization	Impaired verbal communication
Difficulty carrying out tasks associated with hygiene, dressing, grooming, eating, and toileting	Self-care deficit
Neglectful care of client in regard to basic human needs or illness treatment, extreme denial or prolonged overconcern regarding client's illness, depression, hostility and aggression	Interrupted Family Processes
Inability to take responsibility for meeting basic health practices, history of lack of health-seeking behavior, lack of expressed interest in improving health behaviors, demonstrated lack of knowledge regarding basic health practices, anosognosia (lack of insight about illness)	Ineffective health maintenance
Unsafe, unclean, disorderly home environment; household members express difficulty in maintaining their home in a safe and comfortable condition	Impaired home maintenance

*These diagnoses have been resigned from the NANDA-I list of approved diagnoses. They are used in this instance because they are most compatible with the identified behaviors.
Source: Adapted from Herdman, T. H., & Kamitsuru, S. (Eds.). (2018). *NANDA International nursing diagnoses: Definitions and classifications, 2018–2020*. New York, NY: Thieme.

In addition, nurses must be aware of their own attitudes in order to avoid perpetuating stigmatization of this client because this concern has often been responsible for individuals avoiding treatment from healthcare professionals. One way to reduce stigma is to become familiar with real people who suffer from this disorder rather than relying on fictitious representations (and sometimes, misrepresentations) of this population in popular media. (See the "Real People, Real Stories" introduction to Dr. Fred Frese.)

Concept Care Mapping

The concept map care plan is a diagrammatic teaching and learning strategy that allows visualization of interrelationships between medical diagnoses,

nursing diagnoses, assessment data, and treatments (see Chapter 6, The Nursing Process in Psychiatric Mental Health Nursing). An example of a concept map care plan for a patient with schizophrenia is presented in Figure 15–2.

Patient and Family Education

The role of patient and family educator is important in the psychiatric area, as it is in all areas of nursing. A list of topics for patient and family education relevant to schizophrenia is presented in Box 15–5.

Evaluation

In the final step of the nursing process, a reassessment is conducted in order to determine if the nursing actions have been successful in achieving the

Table 15–2 | CARE PLAN FOR THE PATIENT WITH SCHIZOPHRENIA

NURSING DIAGNOSIS: DISTURBED SENSORY PERCEPTION: AUDITORY/VISUAL

RELATED TO: Panic anxiety, extreme loneliness and withdrawal into the self

EVIDENCED BY: Inappropriate responses, disordered thought sequencing, rapid mood swings, poor concentration, disorientation

OUTCOME CRITERIA	NURSING INTERVENTIONS	RATIONALE
Short-Term Goal ■ Patient will discuss content of hallucinations with nurse or therapist within 1 week. **Long-Term Goals** ■ Patient will be able to define and test reality, reducing or eliminating the occurrence of hallucinations. (This goal may not be realistic for the individual with severe and persistent illness who has experienced auditory hallucinations for many years.) A more realistic goal may be: ■ Patient will verbalize understanding that the voices are a result of his or her illness and demonstrate ways to interrupt the hallucination.	1. Observe for signs of hallucinations (listening pose, laughing or talking to self, stopping in midsentence). 2. Avoid touching the patient without warning him or her that you are about to do so. 3. An attitude of acceptance will encourage the patient to share the content of the hallucination with you. 4. 💬 Do not reinforce the hallucination. Use "the voices" instead of words like "they" that imply validation. Let patient know that you do not share the perception. Say, "Even though I realize the voices are real to you, I do not hear any voices speaking." 5. Help the patient understand the connection between increased anxiety and the presence of hallucinations. 6. Try to distract the patient from the hallucination. 7. For some patients, auditory hallucinations persist after the acute psychotic episode has subsided. Listening to the radio or watching television helps distract some patients from attention to the voices. Others have benefited from an intervention called *voice dismissal*. With this technique, the patient is taught to say loudly, "Go away!" or "Leave me alone!" in a conscious effort to dismiss the auditory perception.	1. Early intervention may prevent aggressive response to command hallucinations. 2. Patient may perceive touch as threatening and may respond in an aggressive manner. 3. This is important to prevent possible injury to the patient or others from command hallucinations. 4. It is important for the nurse to be honest, and the patient must accept the perception as unreal before hallucinations can be eliminated. 5. If the patient can learn to interrupt escalating anxiety, hallucinations may be prevented. 6. Involvement in interpersonal activities and explanation of the actual situation facilitates reality orientation. 7. These activities assist the patient to exert some conscious control over the hallucination.

Continued

Table 15–2 | CARE PLAN FOR THE PATIENT WITH SCHIZOPHRENIA–cont'd

NURSING DIAGNOSIS: DISTURBED THOUGHT PROCESSES

RELATED TO: Inability to trust, panic anxiety, possible hereditary or biochemical factors

EVIDENCED BY: Delusional thinking; inability to concentrate; impaired volition; inability to problem solve, abstract, or conceptualize; extreme suspiciousness of others

OUTCOME CRITERIA	NURSING INTERVENTIONS	RATIONALE

Short-Term Goal
■ By the end of 2 weeks, patient will recognize and verbalize that false ideas occur at times of increased anxiety.
 	
Long-Term Goals
■ By time of discharge from treatment, patient's verbalizations will reflect reality-based thinking with no evidence of delusional ideation.
■ By time of discharge from treatment, the patient will be able to differentiate between delusional thinking and reality.
	1. Convey acceptance of patient's need for the false belief but indicate that you do not share the belief.
	2. 💬 Do not argue or deny the belief. Use "reasonable doubt" as a therapeutic technique: "I understand that you believe this is true, but I personally find it hard to accept."
	3. Reinforce and focus on reality. Discourage long ruminations about the irrational thinking. Talk about real events and real people.
	4. If patient is highly suspicious, the following interventions may be helpful:
	  a. Use same staff as much as possible; be honest and keep all promises.
	  b. Avoid physical contact; ask the patient before touching to perform a procedure, such as taking a blood pressure.
	  c. Avoid laughing, whispering, or talking quietly where patient can see but cannot hear what is being said.
	  d. Provide canned food with can opener or serve food family style.
	  e. Mouth checks may be necessary following medication administration to verify whether the patient is actually swallowing the pills.
	  f. Provide activities that encourage a one-to-one relationship with the nurse or therapist.
	  g. Maintain an assertive, matter-of-fact, yet genuine approach.
		1. Patient must understand that you do not view the idea as real.
		2. Arguing with the patient or denying the belief serves no useful purpose, because delusional ideas are not eliminated by this approach, and the development of a trusting relationship may be impeded.
		3. Discussions that focus on the false ideas are purposeless and useless and may even aggravate the psychosis.
		4. To decrease patient's suspiciousness:
		
		  a. Familiar staff and honesty promotes trust.
		
		  b. Patients with suspicious ideation often perceive touch as threatening and may respond in an aggressive or defensive manner.
		  c. Patient may have ideas of reference and believe he or she is being talked about.
		
		  d. Suspicious patients may believe they are being poisoned and refuse to eat food from an individually prepared tray.
		  e. Suspicious patients may believe they are being poisoned with their medication and attempt to discard the tablets or capsules.
		  f. Competitive activities are very threatening to suspicious patients.
		
		  g. Patients with suspicious ideation are prone to distrust and are hypervigilant of people's behavior and communication. Approaches that are overly directive or cheerful may increase the patient's suspiciousness.

Table 15–2 | CARE PLAN FOR THE PATIENT WITH SCHIZOPHRENIA—cont'd

NURSING DIAGNOSIS: SOCIAL ISOLATION

RELATED TO: Inability to trust, panic anxiety, delusional thinking, regression, lack of interest or skills in interpersonal interaction

EVIDENCED BY: Withdrawal, sad, dull affect, preoccupation with own thoughts, expression of feelings of rejection or of aloneness imposed by others

OUTCOME CRITERIA	NURSING INTERVENTIONS	RATIONALE
Short-Term Goal ■ Patient will willingly attend therapy activities accompanied by trusted staff member within 1 week. **Long-Term Goal** ■ Patient will voluntarily spend time with other patients and staff members in group therapeutic activities.	1. Convey an accepting attitude by making brief, frequent contacts. 2. Show unconditional positive regard. 3. Offer to be with patient during group activities that he or she finds frightening or difficult. 4. Give recognition and positive reinforcement for patient's voluntary interactions with others.	1. An accepting attitude increases feelings of self-worth and facilitates trust. 2. This conveys a belief in the patient as a worthwhile human being. 3. The presence of a trusted individual provides emotional security for the patient. 4. Positive reinforcement enhances self-esteem and encourages repetition of acceptable behaviors.

NURSING DIAGNOSIS: RISK FOR VIOLENCE: SELF-DIRECTED OR OTHER-DIRECTED

RISK FACTORS: Extreme suspiciousness, panic anxiety, catatonic excitement, rage reactions, command hallucinations, overt and aggressive acts, goal-directed destruction of objects in the environment, self-destructive behavior or active aggressive suicidal acts

OUTCOME CRITERIA	NURSING INTERVENTIONS	RATIONALE
Short-Term Goals ■ Within [a specified time], patient will recognize signs of increasing anxiety and agitation and report to staff (or other care provider) for assistance with intervention. ■ Patient will not harm self or others. **Long-Term Goal** ■ Patient will not harm self or others.	1. Maintain low level of stimuli in patient's environment (low lighting, few people, simple decor, low noise level). 2. Observe behavior frequently. Do this while carrying out routine activities. 3. Remove all dangerous objects from patient's environment. 4. 💬 Intervene at the first sign of increased anxiety, agitation, or verbal or behavioral aggression. Offer empathetic response to the patient's feelings: "You seem anxious (or frustrated or angry) about this situation. How can I help?" 5. It is important to maintain a calm attitude toward the patient. As the patient's anxiety increases, offer some alternatives: participating in a physical activity (e.g., physical exercise), talking about the situation, taking some antianxiety medication.	1. Anxiety level rises in a stimulating environment. A suspicious, agitated patient may perceive individuals as threatening. 2. Observation during routine activities avoids creating suspiciousness on the part of the patient. Close observation is necessary so that intervention can occur if required to ensure patient (and others') safety. 3. Removal of dangerous objects prevents patient, in an agitated, confused state from using them to harm self or others. 4. Validation of the patient's feelings conveys a caring attitude and offering assistance reinforces trust. 5. Offering alternatives to the patient gives him or her a feeling of some control over the situation.

Continued

Table 15–2 | CARE PLAN FOR THE PATIENT WITH SCHIZOPHRENIA—cont'd

OUTCOME CRITERIA	NURSING INTERVENTIONS	RATIONALE
	6. Have sufficient staff available to indicate a show of strength to the patient if it becomes necessary.	6. This shows the patient evidence of control over the situation and provides some physical security for staff.
	7. If patient is not calmed by "talking down" or by medication, use of mechanical restraints may be necessary.	7. The avenue of the "least restrictive alternative" must be selected when planning interventions for a violent patient. Restraints should be used only as a last resort after all other interventions have been unsuccessful and the patient is clearly at risk of harm to self or others.
	8. If restraint is deemed necessary, ensure that sufficient staff is available to assist. Follow the protocol established by the institution.	8. These interventions are necessary for the protection of patient and staff.
	9. Ensure that the patient in restraints is assessed at least every 15 minutes to ensure that circulation to extremities is not compromised (check temperature, color, pulses); to assist the patient with needs related to nutrition, hydration, and elimination; and to position the patient so that comfort is facilitated, and aspiration is prevented. Maintain continuous one-to-one monitoring of restrained patients, to assess level of agitation and to prevent injury.	9. Patient safety is a nursing priority.
	10. As agitation decreases, assess the patient's readiness for restraint removal or reduction. Remove one restraint at a time while assessing the patient's response.	10. This minimizes the risk of injury to patient and staff.

NURSING DIAGNOSIS: IMPAIRED VERBAL COMMUNICATION

RELATED TO: Panic anxiety, regression, withdrawal, disordered and delusional thinking

EVIDENCED BY: Loose association of ideas, neologisms, word salad, clang association, echolalia, verbalizations that reflect concrete thinking, poor eye contact

Short-Term Goal		
■ Patient will demonstrate the ability to remain on one topic using appropriate, intermittent eye contact for 5 minutes with the nurse or therapist.	1. 💬 Attempt to decode incomprehensible communication patterns. Seek validation and clarification by stating, "Is it that you mean. . .?" or "I don't understand what you mean by that. Would you please explain it to me?"	1. These techniques reveal how the patient is being perceived by others and convey the nurse's desire to establish meaningful communication.
	2. Maintain staff assignments as consistently as possible.	2. This facilitates trust and understanding between patient and nurse.

Table 15–2 | CARE PLAN FOR THE PATIENT WITH SCHIZOPHRENIA—cont'd

Long-Term Goal
■ By time of discharge from treatment, the patient will demonstrate ability to carry on a verbal communication in a socially acceptable manner with healthcare providers and peers.

3. 💬 The technique of *verbalizing the implied* is used with the patient who is struggling to communicate thoughts and feelings. Example: "That must be frightening to worry that others are wiretapping your house."

4. Anticipate and fulfill patient's needs until functional communication pattern returns.

5. Orient patient to reality as needed. Call the patient by name. Validate those aspects of communication that help differentiate between what is real and not real.

6. 💬 Explanations must be provided at the patient's level of comprehension. Example: "Pick up the spoon, scoop some mashed potatoes into it, and put it in your mouth."

3. This approach conveys empathy and may encourage the patient to disclose thoughts and feelings.

4. Patient safety and comfort are nursing priorities.

5. These techniques may facilitate restoration of functional communication patterns in the patient.

6. Because concrete thinking prevails, abstract phrases and clichés must be avoided because they are likely to be misinterpreted.

NURSING DIAGNOSIS: SELF-CARE DEFICIT

RELATED TO: Withdrawal, regression, panic anxiety, perceptual or cognitive impairment, inability to trust

EVIDENCED BY: Difficulty carrying out tasks associated with hygiene, dressing, grooming, eating, toileting

OUTCOME CRITERIA	NURSING INTERVENTIONS	RATIONALE
Short-Term Goal ■ Patient will verbalize a desire to perform activities of daily living (ADLs) by end of 1 week. **Long-Term Goal** ■ Patient will perform ADLs in an independent manner and demonstrate a willingness to do so by time of discharge from treatment.	1. Provide assistance with self-care needs as required. Some patients who are severely withdrawn may require total care. 2. Encourage patient to perform as many activities as possible independently. Provide positive reinforcement for independent accomplishments. 3. 💬 Use concrete communication to show patient what is expected and to minimize misinterpretation by the patient. Provide step-by-step instructions for assistance in performing ADLs. Example: "Take your pajamas off and put them in the drawer. Take your shirt and pants from the closet and put them on. Comb your hair and brush your teeth." 4. Creative approaches may need to be taken with the patient who is not eating, such as allowing client to open own canned or packaged foods; family-style serving may also be an option. 5. If toileting needs are not being met, establish a structured schedule for the patient.	1. Patient safety and comfort are nursing priorities. 2. Independent accomplishment and positive reinforcement enhance self-esteem and promote repetition of desirable behaviors. 3. Because concrete thinking prevails, explanations must be provided at the patient's concrete level of comprehension. 4. These techniques may be helpful with the patient who is paranoid and may be suspicious that he or she is being poisoned with food or medication. 5. A structured schedule will help the patient establish a pattern so that he or she can develop a habit of toileting independently.

Real People, Real Stories: Dr. Fred Frese

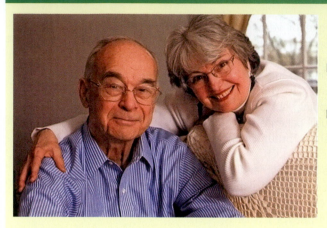

People with schizophrenia continue to be disenfranchised, misunderstood, and stigmatized. Even within healthcare, evidence has shown that some settings have been very hostile to people with severe mental illnesses. One way to begin combating stigmatization of people with mental illness is to get to know them personally. Dr. Fred Frese is a licensed psychologist and an internationally renowned speaker, writer, and advocate in the field of mental illness.

Karyn: Could you share a little bit about your history with the illness of schizophrenia?

Dr. Frese: I was 25 when I had my first episode. I was in the Marines and—I know I had seen the movie *The Manchurian Candidate* previously—and I began to think that the Vietnamese were using the same strategies from the movie to control us. When I let my commanding officer know my theories, I was hospitalized involuntarily, and for the next 10 years I was in and out of hospitals—mostly involuntarily—taking various medications, living many different places, and not employed.

Karyn: Were you getting any treatments or intervention that you thought were helpful to your recovery?

Dr. Frese: Well, at that time it was thought that schizophrenia was not an illness from which one could recover. Even recently, I've heard some folks who have a family member with schizophrenia say, "There's no way that anyone with this illness can get better." But that's starting to change, and now that the government, through SAMHSA (Substance Abuse and Mental Health Services Administration) is backing the recovery model approach, I think healthcare will improve. I remember being told that my brain was going to progressively deteriorate and that I would never be able to function on my own. All in all, I probably spent about a year of my life in hospitalizations. Once the laws changed and I knew you had to be of imminent harm to yourself or others in order to be hospitalized involuntarily, I talked some of the health professionals out of admitting

me. During the last attempt to hospitalize me, I actually escaped and ran away, even though I was in pretty bad shape.

Karyn: So since you were knowledgeable about the laws, you could essentially be your own self-advocate and argue your case, so to speak?

Dr. Frese: Yes, and by that time, I was in grad school and had secured a job at what is now the Department of Mental Health and Addiction Services. I remember I was living in the hallway of some university housing, and one of the students, who saw me day after day just hanging around and not really doing anything, suggested that I might be eligible for a government job because of my military background. When I applied, the receptionist saw my history of mental health commitments and said I would never get the job, but I did. The last time I went to the hospital, I went voluntarily because I knew I needed more medication, but they thought I needed to be hospitalized and I didn't; so I ran away.

Karyn: Sounds like you were managing a lot of stuff—grad school, working—and, at the same time, episodically struggling with symptoms of illness. You were working in the field of mental health, too. Was the work environment supportive?

Dr. Frese: Not always. It seemed like even among my coworkers, when something strange happened, they thought it was something wrong with me.

Karyn: What do you mean by "something strange"?

Dr. Frese: Like one time when they perceived I was spending too much time interacting with patients, they assumed I was "going off again," and next thing I knew, they called a "blue alert" and wanted to hospitalize me. But that time, the medical director just told me to take some time off. I never did find out why they called that blue alert.

Karyn: So you haven't been hospitalized for a very long time, and you are internationally renowned for all of your work and advocacy in the field of mental health. What do you think has contributed most to your recovery?

Dr. Frese: No, I haven't been hospitalized since I got married. I think that has been central in my recovery: having a person who you trust to give you feedback and let me know when I need more medication.

Karyn: What role do medications play in recovery?

Dr. Frese: It's very individual. We need more research to identify who, among people with schizophrenia, will benefit most by continuous medication versus episodic, reduced doses, or no medication. Genetic research is hopeful, but we're not there yet. It's hard to advise any individual what to do without knowing their individual circumstances, and even knowing, it can be very hard.

Real People, Real Stories: Dr. Fred Frese—cont'd

Karyn: What do you think is most important for future nurses to know about what they should do or say when they encounter someone with schizophrenia in a healthcare setting, such as ER, for example?

Dr. Frese: Even though Freud's theories about psychoanalysis and insight-oriented therapy have been shown in research to be not only *not* helpful in the treatment of people with schizophrenia but potentially harmful, these ideas continue to influence the thinking of healthcare professionals. I would tell nurses to wean themselves away from psychoanalytic concepts in treating people with schizophrenia. There continue to be assumptions that something bad must have happened in this patient's childhood, and the family is probably to blame. It's not a good way to forge relationships and may prejudge or isolate the people that can provide invaluable support.

So I would say to future nurses, don't make assumptions about me because you see a diagnosis or the kind of medication I'm on, and don't try to blame anyone for my symptoms. Treat me with civility and respect, don't respond to me with shock and disbelief, bullying, or laughing at me. Listening to the patient is the best way to establish and maintain a relationship. Even if the patient is saying something that doesn't make any sense to you, the best response is, "That's very interesting; tell me more."

To learn more about Dr. Frese, go to www.fredfrese.com.

---

objectives of care. Evaluation of the nursing actions for the patient with exacerbation of schizophrenic psychosis may be facilitated by gathering information utilizing the following types of questions:

- Has the patient established trust with at least one staff member?
- Is the anxiety level maintained at a manageable level?
- Is delusional thinking still prevalent?
- Is hallucinogenic activity evident? Does the patient share content of hallucinations, particularly if commands are heard?
- Is the patient able to manage escalating anxiety with adaptive coping mechanisms?
- Is the patient easily agitated?
- Is the patient able to interact with others appropriately?
- Does the patient voluntarily attend therapy activities?
- Is verbal communication comprehensible?
- Is the patient compliant with medication? Does the patient verbalize the importance of taking medication regularly and on a long-term basis? Does he or she verbalize understanding of possible side effects and when to seek assistance from the physician?
- Does the patient spend time with others rather than isolating self?
- Is the patient able to carry out all activities of daily living independently?
- Is the patient able to verbalize resources from which he or she may seek assistance outside the hospital?
- Does the family have information regarding support groups in which they may participate and from which they may seek assistance in dealing with their family member who is ill?
- If the patient lives alone, does he or she have a source for assistance with home maintenance and health management?

Quality and Safety Education for Nurses (QSEN)

The Institute of Medicine (IOM), in its 2003 report *Health Professions Education: A Bridge to Quality*, challenged faculties of medicine, nursing, and other health professions to ensure that their graduates have achieved a core set of competencies in order to meet the needs of the 21st-century healthcare system. These competencies include *providing patient-centered care, maintaining safety, working in interdisciplinary teams, employing evidence-based practice, incorporating quality improvement,* and *utilizing informatics.*

Patient-centered care is foundational to the recovery model (see Chapter 10, The Recovery Model), which has been advanced as an important framework for empowering clients with severe mental illnesses like schizophrenia. This model promotes active patient engagement in treatment with a focus on achieving their full recovery potential. However, in order to maintain *patient safety* and because some clients lack insight about their need for treatment, decisions may need to be made for these clients in their best interest. Supporting the client's recovery necessitates the use of several resources and disciplines, which may include housing and financial assistance, medication management, peer support, spiritual counsel, and case management services. It is essential that nurses working with this population have a good

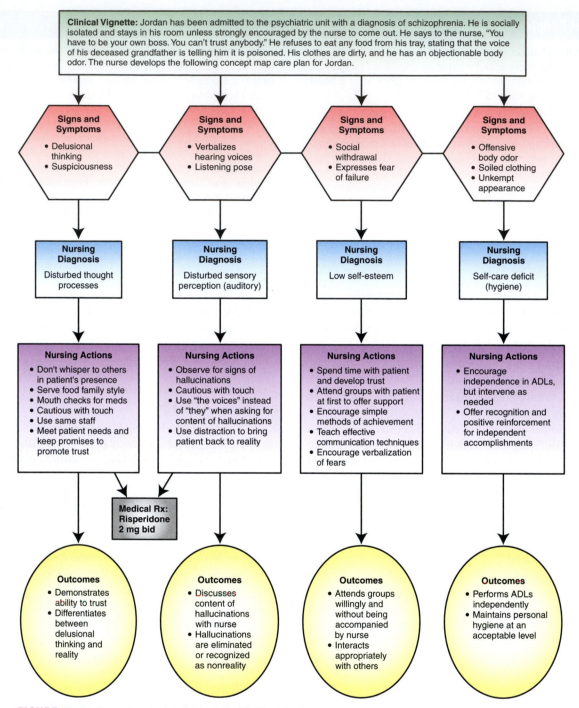

FIGURE 15–2 Concept map care plan for patient with schizophrenia.

understanding of the available support services for clients with schizophrenia and that they effectively work within *interdisciplinary teams* to meet this client's complex needs. A QSEN teaching strategy related to intervening with a combative patient is included in

Box 15–6. The use of this type of activity is intended to arm the instructor and the student with guidelines for attaining the knowledge, skills, and attitudes necessary for achievement of quality and safety competencies in nursing.

BOX 15–5 Topics for Patient and Family Education Related to Schizophrenia

NATURE OF THE ILLNESS
1. What to expect as the illness progresses
2. Symptoms associated with the illness
3. Ways for family to respond to behaviors associated with the illness

MANAGEMENT OF THE ILLNESS
1. Connection of exacerbation of symptoms to times of stress
2. Appropriate medication management
3. Side effects of medications
4. Importance of not stopping medications

5. When to contact healthcare provider
6. Relaxation techniques
7. Social skills training
8. Daily living skills training

SUPPORT SERVICES
1. Financial assistance
2. Housing
3. Legal assistance
4. Caregiver support groups
5. Respite care
6. Home healthcare

BOX 15–6 QSEN TEACHING STRATEGY

Assignment: Using Evidence to Address Clinical Problems
Intervention With a Combative Client

Competency Domain: Evidence-based practice

Learning Objectives: Student will:
- Differentiate clinical opinion from research and evidence summaries.
- Explain the role of evidence in determining the best clinical practice for intervening with combative clients.
- Identify gaps between what is observed in the treatment setting and what has been identified as best practice.
- Discriminate between valid and invalid reasons for modifying evidence-based clinical practice based on clinical expertise or other reasons.
- Participate effectively in appropriate data collection and other research activities.
- Acknowledge own limitations in knowledge and clinical expertise before determining when to deviate from evidence-based best practices.

Strategy Overview
1. Investigate the research related to intervening with a combative client.
2. Identify best practices described in the literature. How were these best practices determined?
3. Compare and contrast staff intervention with best practices described in the literature.
4. Investigate staff perceptions related to intervening with a combative client. How have they developed these perceptions?
5. Do staff members view any problems associated with their practice versus best practice described in the literature? If so, how would they like to see the problem addressed?
6. Describe ethical issues associated with intervening with a combative client.
7. What is your personal perception regarding the best evidence available to date related to intervening with a combative client? Are there situations that you can think of when you might deviate from the best practice model?
8. What questions do you have about intervening with a combative client that are not being addressed by current researchers?

Source: Adapted from teaching strategy submitted by Pamela M. Ironside, Associate Professor, Indiana University School of Nursing, Indianapolis, IN. © 2009 QSEN; http://qsen.org. With permission.

Treatment Modalities for Schizophrenia and Other Psychotic Disorders

Psychological Treatments

Individual Psychotherapy

Individual recovery-oriented psychotherapy and cognitive therapies are evidence-based interventions in the treatment of the client with schizophrenia, but these therapies should be adjunct to a multifaceted team approach. The primary focus in all cases must reflect efforts to decrease anxiety and increase trust.

Establishing a relationship is often particularly difficult because the individual with schizophrenia is desperately lonely yet defends against closeness and trust. He or she is likely to respond to attempts at closeness with suspiciousness, anxiety, aggression, or regression. Successful intervention may be achieved with honesty, simple directness, and a manner that respects the client's privacy and human dignity. Exaggerated warmth and professions of friendship are likely to be met with confusion and suspicion.

Once a therapeutic interpersonal relationship has been established, reality orientation is maintained through exploration of the client's behavior in relationships. Education is provided to help the client identify sources of real or perceived danger and ways of reacting appropriately. Methods for improving interpersonal communication, emotional expression, and frustration tolerance are attempted.

Group Therapy

Group therapy for individuals with schizophrenia has been shown to be effective, particularly with outpatients and when combined with drug treatment. Sadock and colleagues (2015) stated:

> Group therapy for persons with schizophrenia generally focuses on real-life plans, problems, and relationships. Some investigators doubt that dynamic interpretation and insight therapy are valuable for typical patients with schizophrenia. But group therapy is effective in reducing social isolation, increasing the sense of cohesiveness, and improving reality testing for patients with schizophrenia. (p. 322)

Group therapy in inpatient settings is less productive. Inpatient treatment usually occurs when symptomatology and social disorganization are at their most intense. At this time, the least amount of stimuli possible is most beneficial for the patient. Because group therapy can be intensive and highly stimulating, it may be counterproductive early in treatment.

Group therapy for schizophrenia has been most useful over the long-term course of the illness. The social interaction, sense of cohesiveness, identification, and reality testing achieved within the group setting have proven to be highly therapeutic processes for individuals with this illness. Groups that offer a supportive environment appear to be more helpful than those that follow a more confrontational approach.

Behavior Therapy

Behavior modification has a history of qualified success in reducing the frequency of bizarre, disturbing, and deviant behaviors and increasing appropriate behaviors. Features that have led to the most positive results include the following:

- Clearly defining goals and how they will be measured
- Attaching positive, negative, and aversive reinforcements to adaptive and maladaptive behavior
- Using simple, concrete instructions and prompts to elicit the desired behavior

In the treatment setting, the healthcare provider can use praise and other positive reinforcements to help the patient with schizophrenia reduce the frequency of maladaptive or deviant behaviors. A limitation of this type of therapy is the inability of some individuals with schizophrenia to generalize what they have learned from the treatment setting to the community setting.

Social Treatments

Social Skills Training

Social skills training is used to help clients manage struggles with interpersonal relationships and communication, which are often complicated by clients' inability to accurately perceive responses in others. Mueser, Bond, and Drake (2001) describe this training:

> The basic premise of social skills training is that complex interpersonal skills involve the smooth integration of a combination of simpler behaviors, including *nonverbal behaviors* (e.g., facial expression, eye contact); *paralinguistic features* (e.g., voice loudness and affect); *verbal content* (i.e., the appropriateness of what is said); and *interactive balance* (e.g., response latency, amount of time talking). These specific skills can be systematically taught, and, through the process of *shaping* (i.e., rewarding successive approximations toward the target behavior), complex behavioral repertoires can be acquired.

Social dysfunction is a hallmark of schizophrenia. Impairment in interpersonal relations is included as part of the defining diagnostic criteria for the condition in the *DSM-5* (APA, 2013). Considerable attention is now being given to enhancement of social skills for this population.

The educational procedure in social skills training focuses on role-play. A series of brief scenarios are selected. These should be typical of situations that clients experience in their daily lives and be graduated in terms of level of difficulty. The healthcare provider may serve as a role model for some behaviors. For example, "See how I sort of nod my head up and down and look at your face while you talk." This demonstration is followed by the client's role-playing. Immediate feedback is provided regarding the client's presentation. Only by countless repetitions does the response gradually become smooth and effortless.

Progress is geared toward the individual's needs and limitations. The focus is on small units of behavior, and the training proceeds very gradually. Highly threatening issues are avoided, and emphasis is placed on functional skills that are relevant to activities of daily living. Milieu therapy, which focuses on the client's interaction within a social environment, may provide opportunities for social skills training.

Family Therapy

Schizophrenia is an illness that can puzzle, disrupt, and sometimes tear apart families. Even when families appear to cope well, there is a notable impact on the mental and physical health of relatives when a family member has the illness.

The importance of the expanded role of family in the aftercare of relatives with schizophrenia has been recognized, thereby stimulating interest in family intervention programs designed to support the family system, prevent or delay relapse, and help the client to remain in the community. These psychoeducational programs treat the family as a resource rather than a stressor, with the focus on concrete problem-solving and specific helping behaviors for coping with stress. These programs recognize the biological basis for schizophrenia and the impact that stress has on the client's ability to function. By providing the family with information about the illness and suggestions for effective coping, psychoeducational programs reduce the likelihood of the client's relapse and the possible emergence of mental illness in previously nonaffected relatives.

Mueser and associates (2001) stated that although models of family intervention with schizophrenia differ in their characteristics and methods, effective treatment programs share a number of common features:

■ All programs are long term (usually 9 months to 2 years or more).
■ They all provide the client and family with information about the illness and its management.
■ They focus on improving adherence to prescribed medications.
■ They strive to decrease stress in the family and improve family functioning.

Asen (2002) suggested the following interventions with families of individuals with schizophrenia:

■ Forming a close alliance with the caregivers
■ Lowering the emotional intrafamily climate by reducing stress and burden on relatives
■ Increasing the ability of relatives to anticipate and solve problems
■ Reducing the expressions of anger and guilt by family members
■ Maintaining reasonable expectations for how the ill family member should perform
■ Encouraging relatives to set appropriate limits while maintaining some degree of separateness
■ Promoting desirable changes in the relatives' behaviors and belief systems

Family therapy typically consists of a brief program of family education about schizophrenia and a more extended program of family contact designed to reduce overt manifestations of conflict and to improve patterns of family communication and problem-solving. The response to this type of therapy has been very dramatic. Studies have clearly revealed that a more positive outcome in the treatment of the client with schizophrenia can be achieved by including the family system in the program of care (Caqueo-Urízar et al., 2015).

Assertive Community Treatment

Assertive community treatment (ACT) is an evidence-based program of case management that takes a team approach in providing comprehensive, community-based psychiatric treatment, rehabilitation, and support to persons with serious and persistent mental illness such as schizophrenia. Some states use other terms for this type of treatment, such as mobile treatment teams and community support programs. Assertive programs of treatment are individually tailored for each client, intended to be proactive, and include the teaching of basic living skills, helping clients work with community agencies, and assisting clients in developing a social support network. There is emphasis on vocational expectations, and supportive work settings (i.e., sheltered workshops) are an important part of the treatment program. Other services include substance abuse treatment, psychoeducational programs, family support and education, mobile crisis intervention, and attention to healthcare needs.

Responsibilities are shared by multiple team members, including psychiatrists, nurses, social workers, vocational rehabilitation therapists, and substance abuse counselors. Services are provided in the person's home; within the neighborhood; in local restaurants, parks, stores; or wherever assistance by the client is required. These services are available to the client 24 hours a day, 365 days a year, and ACT is considered a long-term intervention strategy. One recent study looked at the impact of a *Housing First* intervention (an intervention that prioritizes rapid re-housing for homeless individuals with schizophrenia) and found that when this type of intervention was combined with ACT, medication adherence improved from below 50 percent to 78 percent. Additionally, these combined interventions improved clients' integration into the community, increased residential stability, and decreased criminal convictions (Rezansoff et al., 2016).

ACT has been shown to reduce the number of hospitalizations and decrease costs of care. Although it has been called "paternalistic" and "coercive" by its critics, ACT has provided much-needed services and improved quality of life for many clients who are unable to manage in a less-structured environment. One limitation is that treatment programs of this kind are time and labor intensive.

The Recovery Model

Research provides support for recovery as an obtainable objective for individuals with schizophrenia. Lysaker, Roe, and Buck (2010) state,

> Recovery from schizophrenia, in the sense of a state in which persons experience no difficulties associated with the illness, can occur but the modal outcome seems to be one in which difficulties linked to symptoms, social function, and work appear periodically but can be successfully confronted. (p. 40)

Conceptual models of recovery from mental illness are presented in Chapter 10, The Recovery Model. The recovery model has been used primarily in caring for individuals with serious mental illness, such as schizophrenia and bipolar disorder. However, concepts of the model are amenable to use with all individuals experiencing emotional conditions with which they require assistance and who have a desire to take control and manage their lives more independently.

Weiden (2010) identifies two types of recovery with schizophrenia: functional and process. Functional recovery focuses on the individual's level of functioning in such areas as relationships, work, independent living, and other kinds of life functioning. He or she may or may not be experiencing active symptoms of schizophrenia.

Weiden (2010) suggests that recovery can also be considered as a process. With process recovery, there is no defined end point, but recovery is viewed as a process that continues throughout the individual's life and involves collaboration between the client and clinician. The individual identifies goals based on personal values or what he or she defines as giving meaning and purpose to life. The clinician and client work together to develop a treatment plan that is in alignment with the goals set forth by the client. In the process recovery model, the individual may still be experiencing symptoms. Weiden states:

> Patients do not have to be in remission, nor does remission automatically have to be a desired (or likely) goal when embarking on a recovery-oriented treatment plan. As long as the patient (and family) understands that a process recovery treatment plan is not to be confused with a promise of "cure" or even "remission," then one does not overpromise.

The concept of recovery in schizophrenia remains controversial among clinicians, and many challenges lie ahead for continued study. Recovery models have similarities with ACT in that they both necessarily engage the support of multiple resources, but recovery models also highlight the dimension of active engagement and empowerment of the client in decision making. Some argue that this approach is difficult to implement when the client lacks insight about his or her illness or the need for treatment. Furthermore, there is a lack of consistency in what constitutes "recovery," and many concepts exist.

Nevertheless, the potential and hope are that, as these models become better studied and more clearly defined, they will provide a treatment approach that is comprehensive, protective, and supportive of patient-centered care.

RAISE (Recovery After an Initial Schizophrenia Episode)

The RAISE approach to treatment for schizophrenia is based on a large National Institute of Mental Health (NIMH) initiative that began in 2008, and research findings published in 2015 demonstrated several benefits of this approach. Insel (2015) describes the RAISE approach as

> coordinated specialty care for first episode psychosis. With coordinated specialty care the young person experiencing first episode psychosis works with a team of specialists to create a personal treatment plan, combining recovery-oriented psychotherapy, low-dose medication management, family education and support, case management, and work or education support. Coordinated specialty care emphasizes shared decision making, including family members when possible.

The RAISE approach incorporates many elements from other treatment approaches, including community treatment, recovery model approaches, family approaches, and comprehensive care models. It adds the dimension of early intervention at the first episode of psychosis. The research findings after 5 years of studying this approach look very promising for improving care to this population when intervention begins at the earliest onset of psychotic symptoms. Findings have included greater adherence to treatment programs; greater improvement in symptoms, interpersonal relationships, and quality of life; more involvement in employment or educational pursuits; and less frequent hospitalizations for clients involved in RAISE than for clients involved in more traditional treatment approaches (Insel, 2015).

The hope for this approach to treatment is that, through early and comprehensive intervention, the long-term, debilitating consequences of schizophrenia can be averted or minimized.

Psychopharmacological Treatment

Chlorpromazine (Thorazine) was first introduced in the United States in 1952. At that time, it was used in conjunction with barbiturates in surgical anesthesia. With increased use, the drug's psychic properties were recognized, and by 1954 it was marketed as an antipsychotic medication in the United States. The manufacture and sale of other antipsychotic drugs followed in rapid succession.

Antipsychotic medications are also called *neuroleptics* and historically were referred to as *major tranquilizers*. They are effective in the treatment of acute and chronic manifestations of schizophrenia and in maintenance therapy to prevent exacerbation of schizophrenic symptoms. A meta-analysis of studies (Takeuchi et al., 2017) evaluating the benefits of maintenance antipsychotic medication found that there was a significant worsening of symptoms over the course of a year in patients who did not continue on medication.

The prognosis for schizophrenia has often been reported in a paradigm of thirds. About one-third of the people achieve significant and lasting improvement. They may never experience another episode of psychosis following the initial occurrence. One-third may achieve some improvement with intermittent relapses and residual disability. Their occupational level may have decreased because of their illness, or they may be socially isolated. Finally, one-third experience severe and permanent incapacity. They often do not respond to medication and remain severely ill for much of their lives. Men typically have poorer outcomes than women do; women respond better to treatment with antipsychotic medications. Although the paradigm of thirds provides a general guideline for understanding the variable course and prognosis in schizophrenia, Jablensky (2017) notes that with each successive decade there has been a trend toward a less deteriorating course in schizophrenia, which may be attributed to both treatment advances and changes in attitudes about this illness.

As mentioned earlier, the efficacy of antipsychotic medications is enhanced by adjunct psychosocial therapy. Because the psychotic manifestations of the illness subside with use of the drugs, clients are generally more cooperative with the psychosocial therapies. However, although the sedative effects are relatively immediate, it takes several weeks for the antipsychotics to effectively treat positive symptoms, a fact that often leads to discontinuation of the medication. Clients and families need to be educated about the importance of waiting, often for several weeks, to determine whether the drug will be effective.

These medications are classified as either "typical" (first generation, conventional antipsychotics) or "atypical" (the newer, novel antipsychotics). Examples of commonly used antipsychotic agents are presented in Table 15–3. A description of these medications follows. More detailed information is available in Chapter 4, Psychopharmacology, and online at FA Davis*Plus*.

Indications

Antipsychotic medications are used in the treatment of schizophrenia and other psychotic disorders. Selected agents are used in the treatment of bipolar

TABLE 15–3 Antipsychotic Agents

CATEGORY	GENERIC (TRADE NAME)	DAILY DOSAGE RANGE (MG)
Typical antipsychotic agents (first generation; conventional)	Chlorpromazine	40–400
	Fluphenazine	2.5–10
	Haloperidol (Haldol)	1–100
	Loxapine	20–250
	Perphenazine	12–64
	Pimozide (Orap)	1–10
	Prochlorperazine	15–150
	Thioridazine	150–800
	Thiothixene (Navane)	6–30
	Trifluoperazine	4–40
Atypical antipsychotic agents (second generation; novel)	Aripiprazole (Abilify)	10–30
	(Abilify MyCite; with tracking sensor)	2–30
	Aripiprazole lauroxil (Aristada)	441–662 (monthly), 882 q 6 weeks
	Asenapine (Saphris) (SL)	10–20
	Brexpiprazole (Rexulti)	2–4
	Cariprazine (Vraylor)	1.5–6
	Clozapine (Clozaril)	300–900
	Iloperidone (Fanapt)	12–24
	Lurasidone (Latuda)	40–80
	Olanzapine (Zyprexa)	5–20
	Paliperidone (Invega)	6–12
	Quetiapine (Seroquel)	300–400
	Risperidone (Risperdal)	4–8
	Long-acting risperidone (Perseris)	90 mg or 120 mg subcutaneously (once a month)
	Ziprasidone (Geodon)	40–160

mania (olanzapine, aripiprazole, chlorpromazine, quetiapine, risperidone, asenapine, ziprasidone).

Action

Typical antipsychotics work by blocking postsynaptic dopamine receptors in the basal ganglia, hypothalamus, limbic system, brainstem, and medulla. They also demonstrate varying affinity for cholinergic, alpha$_1$-adrenergic, and histaminic receptors. Antipsychotic effects may also be related to inhibition of dopamine-mediated transmission of neural impulses at the synapses.

Atypical antipsychotics are weaker dopamine receptor antagonists than the conventional antipsychotics but are more potent antagonists of the serotonin (5-hydroxytryptamine) type 2A (5-HT$_{2A}$) receptors. They also exhibit antagonism for cholinergic, histaminic, and adrenergic receptors.

Positive symptoms are associated with normal brain structures on computed tomography (CT) scan and respond relatively well to treatment with both typical (first generation) and atypical (second generation) antipsychotic medication. Sadock and associates (2015) identify that positive symptoms tend to become less severe over time, whereas the negative or "deficit" symptoms are socially debilitating and may increase in severity. Atypical antipsychotics have been advanced as being more effective than first generation antipsychotics in treating negative symptoms, but researchers continue to search for medications that will specifically treat the several cognitive deficits that are most problematic for patients with schizophrenia. These deficits include memory, attention, language, and executive functions, and they can dramatically impact an individual's overall functional ability (Fioravanti, Bianchi, & Cinti, 2012).

A detailed discussion of contraindications, precautions, side effects, and drug interactions associated with antipsychotic medications is available in Chapter 4, Psychopharmacology.

Side Effects

The effects of these medications are related to blockage of a number of receptors for which they exhibit various degrees of affinity. Blockage of the dopamine receptors is thought to be responsible for controlling positive symptoms of schizophrenia. Dopamine blockage also results in **extrapyramidal symptoms** (EPS) and prolactin elevation (galactorrhea; **gynecomastia**).

Cholinergic blockade causes anticholinergic side effects (dry mouth, blurred vision, constipation, urinary retention, and tachycardia). Blockage of the alpha$_1$-adrenergic receptors produces dizziness, orthostatic hypotension, tremors, and reflex tachycardia. Histamine blockade is associated with weight gain and sedation (Table 15–4).

The plan of care should include monitoring for the side effects from antipsychotic medications and educating the patient and family about safety precautions when taking antipsychotic medication. A list of side effects and relevant nursing interventions is included in Chapter 4.

There have been two recent and novel developments in psychopharmacological treatments for patients with schizophrenia. The first is a formulation of aripiprazole (AbilifyMyCite) with a tracking sensor that allows the client (and others) to monitor whether or not the medication was taken. Approved in late 2017, this formulation has spurred controversy and debate about the benefits versus the potential intrusiveness of such a monitoring device. The second novel treatment is valbenazine (Ingrezza), a drug for the treatment of tardive dyskinesia. Tardive dyskinesia, a movement disturbance that is more prevalent with first generation antipsychotics, is particularly troubling because it has been a permanent, incurable side effect. Valbenazine works by reducing dopamine release at the synaptic cleft and has demonstrated effectiveness in reducing abnormal involuntary movements such as tardive dyskinesia. Future research will determine its long-term effectiveness. Currently, the cost for this treatment is over $125,000 annually, which may limit its accessibility for many with chronic, severe mental illness.

Patient and Family Education Related to Antipsychotics

The patent receiving antipsychotic medication should:

- Use caution when driving or operating dangerous machinery. Drowsiness and dizziness can occur.
- Not stop taking the drug abruptly after long-term use. To do so might produce withdrawal symptoms, such as nausea, vomiting, dizziness, gastritis, headache, tachycardia, insomnia, tremulousness.
- Use sunblock lotion and wear protective clothing when spending time outdoors. Skin is more susceptible to sunburn, which can occur in as little as 30 minutes.
- Report weekly (if receiving clozapine therapy) to have blood levels drawn and to obtain a weekly supply of the drug.
- Immediately report to the physician the occurrence of any of the following symptoms: sore throat, fever, malaise, unusual bleeding, easy bruising, persistent nausea and vomiting, severe headache, rapid heart rate, difficulty urinating, muscle

TABLE 15–4	**Antiparkinsonian Agents Used to Treat Extrapyramidal Side Effects of Antipsychotic Drugs**
Indication	Used to treat parkinsonism of various causes and drug-induced extrapyramidal reactions.
Action	Restores the natural balance of acetylcholine and dopamine in the CNS. The imbalance is a deficiency in dopamine that results in excessive cholinergic activity.
Contraindications/Precautions	Antiparkinsonian agents are contraindicated in individuals with hypersensitivity. Anticholinergics should be avoided by individuals with angle-closure glaucoma; pyloric, duodenal, or bladder neck obstructions; prostatic hypertrophy; or myasthenia gravis. Caution should be used in administering these drugs to clients with hepatic, renal, or cardiac insufficiency; elderly and debilitated clients; those with a tendency toward urinary retention; and those exposed to high environmental temperatures.
Common Side Effects	Anticholinergic effects (dry mouth, blurred vision, constipation, paralytic ileus, urinary retention, tachycardia, elevated temperature, decreased sweating), nausea/GI upset, sedation, dizziness, orthostatic hypotension, exacerbation of psychoses.

CHEMICAL CLASS	GENERIC (TRADE) NAME	DAILY DOSAGE RANGE (MG)
Anticholinergics	Benztropine (Cogentin)	1–8
	Biperiden (Akineton)	2–6
	Trihexyphenidyl	1–15
Antihistamines	Diphenhydramine (Benadryl)	25–200
Dopaminergic Agonists	Amantadine	200–300

CNS, central nervous system; GI, gastrointestinal.

twitching, tremors, darkly colored urine, excessive urination, excessive thirst, excessive hunger, weakness, pale stools, yellow skin or eyes, muscular incoordination, or skin rash.

■ Rise slowly from a sitting or lying position to prevent a sudden drop in blood pressure.

■ Take frequent sips of water, chew sugarless gum, or suck on hard candy, if dry mouth is a problem. Good oral care (frequent brushing, flossing) is very important.

■ Consult the physician regarding smoking while on antipsychotic therapy. Smoking increases the metabolism of antipsychotics, requiring an adjustment in dosage to achieve a therapeutic effect.

■ Dress warmly in cold weather, and avoid extended exposure to very high or low temperatures. Body temperature is harder to maintain with this medication.

■ Avoid drinking alcohol while on antipsychotic therapy. These drugs potentiate each other's effects.

■ Avoid taking other medications (including over-the-counter products) without the physician's approval. Many medications contain substances that interact with antipsychotics in a way that may be harmful.

■ Be aware of possible risks of taking antipsychotics during pregnancy. Safe use during pregnancy has not been established. Antipsychotics are thought to readily cross the placental barrier; if so, a fetus could experience adverse effects of the drug. Inform the physician immediately if pregnancy occurs, is suspected, or is planned.

■ Be aware of side effects of antipsychotic drugs. Refer to written materials furnished by healthcare providers for safe self-administration.

■ Continue to take the medication even if feeling well and as though it is not needed. Symptoms may return if medication is discontinued.

■ Carry a card or other identification at all times describing medications being taken.

Smoking Cessation

Smoking cigarettes has long been identified as a particular health risk for clients with schizophrenia because the prevalence is three times that of the general population; it is estimated that as many as 88 percent of those with schizophrenia and 70 percent of those with bipolar disorder are smokers (Kranjac, 2016). Some clients report increased ability to concentrate when smoking tobacco, which has led to clinical trials of drugs that increase nicotine levels. However, to date, these drugs have not been proven to be effective. In addition to the obvious health risks of chronic lung diseases and cancers, smoking decreases the effectiveness of some psychotropic medications. Varenicline (Chantix), a nicotine agonist used as a smoking deterrent, was once thought to increase symptoms and even suicide risk in those with severe mental illness. However, a recent meta-analysis (Wu et al., 2016) concluded that varenicline is effective for assisting with smoking cessation in this population and that "there was no clear evidence of neuropsychiatric or other adverse events compared with placebo" (p. 1554). In any scenario, assessing the client's motivation to stop smoking and exploring viable treatment options, including psychological interventions, is an important component of treatment.

CASE STUDY AND SAMPLE CARE PLAN

NURSING HISTORY AND ASSESSMENT

Frank is 22 years old. He joined the Marines just out of high school at age 18 for a 3-year enlistment. His final year was spent in Afghanistan. When his 3-year enlistment was up, he returned to his hometown and married a young woman with whom he had been a high school classmate. Frank has always been quiet, somewhat withdrawn, and had very few friends. He was the only child of a single mom who never married, and he does not know his father. His mother was killed in an automobile accident the spring before he enlisted in the Marines.

During the past year, he has become increasingly isolated and withdrawn. He is without regular employment but finds work as a day laborer when he can. His wife, Suzanne, works as a secretary and is the primary wage earner. Lately, Frank

has become very suspicious of her and sometimes follows her to work. He also drops in on her at work and accuses her of having affairs with some of the men in the office.

Last evening, when Suzanne got home from work, Frank was hiding in the closet. She didn't know he was home. When she started to undress, he jumped out of the closet holding a large kitchen knife and threatened to kill her "for being unfaithful." Suzanne managed to flee their home and ran to the neighbor's house and called the police.

Frank told the police that he received a message over the radio from his Marine commanding officer telling him that he couldn't allow his wife to continue to commit adultery, and the only way he could stop it was to kill her. The police took Frank to the emergency department of the VA

CASE STUDY AND SAMPLE CARE PLAN—cont'd

Hospital, where he was admitted to the psychiatric unit. Suzanne is helping with the admission history.

Suzanne tells the nurse that she has never been unfaithful to Frank and she doesn't know why he believes that she has. Frank tells the nurse that he has been "taking orders from my commanding officer through my car radio ever since I got back from Afghanistan." He survived a helicopter crash in Afghanistan in which all were killed except Frank and one other man. Frank says, "I have to follow my CO's orders. God saved me to annihilate the impure."

Following an evaluation, the psychiatrist diagnoses Frank with Schizophrenia. He orders olanzapine 10 mg PO to be given daily and olanzapine 10 mg IM q6h prn for agitation.

NURSING DIAGNOSES AND OUTCOME IDENTIFICATION

From the assessment data, the nurse develops the following nursing diagnoses for Frank:

1. **Risk for self-directed or other-directed violence** related to unresolved grief over loss of mother; survivor's guilt associated with helicopter crash; command hallucinations; and history of violence
   a. **Short-Term Goals:**
      - Frank will seek out staff when anxiety and agitation start to increase.
      - Frank will not harm self or others.
   b. **Long-Term Goal:** Frank will not harm self or others.
2. **Disturbed sensory perception: Auditory** related to increased anxiety and agitation, withdrawal into self, and stress of sufficient intensity to threaten an already weak ego
   a. **Short-Term Goals:**
      - Frank will discuss the content of the hallucinations with the nurse.
      - Frank will maintain anxiety at a manageable level.
   b. **Long-Term Goal:** Frank will be able to define and test reality, reducing or eliminating the occurrence of hallucinations.

PLANNING AND IMPLEMENTATION

RISK FOR SELF-DIRECTED OR OTHER-DIRECTED VIOLENCE

1. Keep the stimuli as low as possible in Frank's environment.
2. Monitor Frank's behavior frequently but in a manner of carrying out routine activities so as not to create suspiciousness on his part.
3. Watch for the following signs (considered the prodrome to aggressive behavior): increased motor activity, pounding, slamming, tense posture, defiant affect, clenched teeth and fists, arguing, demanding, and challenging or threatening staff.

4. If Frank should become aggressive, maintain a calm attitude. Try talking. Offer medication. Provide physical activities.
5. If these interventions fail, indicate a show of strength with a team of staff members.
6. Utilize restraints only as a last resort and if Frank is clearly at risk of harm to himself or others.
7. Help Frank recognize unresolved grief and fixation in denial or anger stage of grief process.
8. Encourage him to talk about the loss of his mother and of fellow Marines in Afghanistan.
9. Encourage him to talk about guilt feelings associated with survival when others died.
10. Assess for presence of suicide risk and collaborate with the patient to develop a personal safety plan.

DISTURBED SENSORY PERCEPTION: AUDITORY

1. Monitor Frank's behavior for signs that he is hearing voices: listening pose, talking and laughing to self, stopping in midsentence.
2. If these behaviors are observed, ask Frank, "Are you hearing the voices again?"
3. Encourage Frank to share the content of the hallucinations. This information is important for early intervention in case the content contains commands to harm himself or others.
4. Say to Frank, "I understand that the voice is real to you, but I do not hear any voices speaking." It is important for him to learn the difference between what is real and what is not real.
5. Try to help Frank recognize that the voices often appear at times when he becomes anxious about something and his agitation increases.
6. Help him to recognize this increasing anxiety, and teach him methods to keep it from escalating.
7. Use distracting activities to bring him back to reality. Involvement with real people and real situations will help to distract him from the hallucination.
8. Teach him to use *voice dismissal*. When he hears the CO's (or others') voice, he should shout, "Go away!" or "Leave me alone!" These commands may help to diminish the sounds and give him a feeling of control over the situation.

EVALUATION

The outcome criteria identified for Frank have been met. When feeling especially anxious or becoming agitated, he seeks out staff for comfort and for assistance in maintaining his anxiety at a manageable level. He currently denies suicide ideation and has collaborated to develop a personal safety plan. He is experiencing fewer auditory hallucinations and has learned to use voice dismissal to interrupt the behavior. He is beginning to recognize his position in the grief process and is working toward resolution at his own pace.

Summary and Key Points

- Of all of the mental illnesses, schizophrenia undoubtedly results in the greatest amount of personal, emotional, and social costs. It presents an enormous threat to life and happiness.

- For many years, there was little agreement as to a definition of the concept of schizophrenia. The *DSM-5* (APA, 2013) identifies specific criteria for diagnosis of the disorder.

- The initial symptoms of schizophrenia most often occur in early adulthood. Development of the disorder can be viewed in four phases: (1) the premorbid phase, (2) the prodromal phase, (3) the active psychotic phase (schizophrenia), and (4) the residual phase.

- The cause of schizophrenia remains unclear. Most likely no single factor can be implicated; rather, the disease probably results from a complex interaction of genetic, biochemical, psychological, and environmental factors.

- A spectrum of schizophrenic and other psychotic disorders has been identified. These include (on a gradient of psychopathology from least to most severe): schizotypal personality disorder, delusional disorder, brief psychotic disorder, substance-induced psychotic disorder, psychotic disorder associated with another medical condition, catatonic disorder associated with another medical condition, schizophreniform disorder, schizoaffective disorder, and schizophrenia.

- Nursing care of the patient with schizophrenia is accomplished using the six steps of the nursing process.

- Nursing assessment is based on knowledge of symptomatology related to thought content and processes, perception, affect, volition, interpersonal functioning and relationship to the external world, and psychomotor behavior.

- Symptoms of schizophrenia are categorized as *positive* (an excess or distortion of normal functions) or *negative* (a diminution or loss of normal functions).

- Antipsychotic medications remain the mainstay of treatment for psychotic disorders. Atypical antipsychotics have become the first line of therapy and treat both positive and negative symptoms of schizophrenia. They have a more favorable side-effect profile than the conventional (typical) antipsychotics.

- Individuals with schizophrenia require long-term integrated treatment with pharmacological and other interventions. Some of these include individual psychotherapy, group therapy, behavior therapy, social skills training, milieu therapy, family therapy, and assertive community treatment. For the majority of clients, the most effective treatment appears to be a combination of psychotropic medication and psychosocial therapy.

- Some clinicians are choosing a course of therapy based on a model of recovery, somewhat like that which has been used for many years with problems of addiction. The basic premise of a recovery model is empowerment of the consumer. The recovery model is designed to allow consumers primary control over decisions about their own care and to enable persons with mental health problems to live a meaningful life in a community of their choice while striving to achieve their full potential.

- Families generally require support and education about psychotic illnesses. The focus is on coping with the diagnosis, understanding the illness and its course, teaching about medication, and learning ways to manage symptoms.

- The most current, evidence-based approach to treatment, RAISE, demonstrates that early intervention at the first episode of psychosis can significantly improve outcomes.

Review Questions
Self-Examination/Learning Exercise

Select the answer that is most appropriate for each of the following questions:

1. Josh, age 21, has been diagnosed with schizophrenia. He has been socially isolated and hearing voices telling him to kill his parents. He has been admitted to the psychiatric unit from the emergency department. The *initial* intervention for Josh is to:
   a. Give him an injection of haloperidol.
   b. Assess Josh to evaluate his safety toward himself and others.
   c. Place him in restraints.
   d. Order him a nutritious diet.

Review Questions—cont'd
Self-Examination/Learning Exercise

2. Which of the following is the primary goal in working with an actively psychotic, suspicious patient?
   a. Promote interaction with others.
   b. Decrease his anxiety and increase trust.
   c. Improve his relationship with his parents.
   d. Encourage participation in therapy activities.

3. The nurse is caring for a patient with schizophrenia. Orders from the physician include haloperidol (Haldol) 5 mg. IM STAT and then 3 mg PO tid, 2 mg benztropine PO bid prn. Why is haloperidol ordered?
   a. To reduce extrapyramidal symptoms
   b. To prevent neuroleptic malignant syndrome
   c. To decrease psychotic symptoms
   d. To induce sleep

4. The nurse is caring for a patient with schizophrenia. Orders from the physician include 5 mg haloperidol IM STAT and then 3 mg PO tid, 2 mg benztropine PO bid prn. Because benztropine was ordered on a prn basis, which of the following assessments by the nurse would convey a need for this medication?
   a. The patient's level of agitation increases.
   b. The patient complains of a sore throat.
   c. The patient's skin has a yellowish cast.
   d. The patient develops muscle spasms.

5. Brandon, a patient on the psychiatric unit, has been diagnosed with schizophrenia. He begins to tell the nurse about how the CIA is looking for him and will kill him if they find him. Which of the following is the most appropriate response by the nurse?
   a. "That's ridiculous, Brandon. No one is going to hurt you."
   b. "The CIA isn't interested in people like you, Brandon."
   c. "Why do you think the CIA wants to kill you?"
   d. "I know you believe that, Brandon, but it's really hard for me to believe."

6. Brandon, a patient on the psychiatric unit, has been diagnosed with schizophrenia. He begins to tell the nurse about how the CIA is looking for him and will kill him if they find him. Brandon's belief is an example of which of the following?
   a. Delusion of persecution
   b. Delusion of reference
   c. Delusion of control or influence
   d. Delusion of grandeur

7. The nurse is interviewing a patient on the psychiatric unit. The patient tilts his head to the side, stops talking in midsentence, and listens intently. The nurse recognizes from these signs that the patient is likely experiencing which of the following?
   a. Somatic delusions
   b. Catatonic stupor
   c. Auditory hallucinations
   d. Pseudoparkinsonism

Review Questions—cont'd
Self-Examination/Learning Exercise

8. The nurse is interviewing a patient on the psychiatric unit. The patient tilts his head to the side, stops talking in midsentence, and listens intently. The nurse recognizes these behaviors as a symptom of the patient's illness. What is the most appropriate nursing intervention for this symptom?
   a. Ask the patient to describe his physical symptoms.
   b. Ask the patient to describe what he is hearing.
   c. Administer a dose of benztropine.
   d. Call the physician for additional orders.

9. When a patient suddenly becomes aggressive and violent on the unit, which of the following approaches would be best for the nurse to use **first?**
   a. Provide large motor activities to relieve the patient's pent-up tension.
   b. Administer a dose of prn olanzapine to keep the patient calm.
   c. Call for sufficient help to control the situation safely.
   d. Convey to the patient that his behavior is unacceptable and will not be permitted.

10. Which of the following is the primary focus of family therapy for patients with schizophrenia and their families?
    a. To discuss concrete problem-solving and adaptive behaviors for coping with stress
    b. To introduce the family to others with the same problem
    c. To keep the patient and family in touch with the healthcare system
    d. To promote family interaction and increase understanding of the illness

11. A patient recently admitted to the hospital reports to the nurse, "I don't understand why I was brought here. I was simply hanging out in my apartment, and the police said I had to come with them." This is an example of what symptom of schizophrenia?
    a. Delusions of reference
    b. Loose association
    c. Anosognosia
    d. Auditory hallucinations

12. Recent research on the RAISE approach to treatment of schizophrenia incorporates which of the following elements as important to improving outcomes? (Select all that apply.)
    a. Early intervention at the first episode of psychosis
    b. Support for employment and/or educational pursuits
    c. Rapid, high-dose loading with antipsychotic medication
    d. Court-ordered sanctions for treatment
    e. Recovery-focused psychotherapy

IMPLICATIONS OF RESEARCH FOR EVIDENCE-BASED PRACTICE

Castillo, E. G., Rosati, J., Williams, C., Pessin, N., & Lindy, D. C. (2015). Metabolic syndrome screening and assertive community treatment: A quality improvement study. *Journal of the American Psychiatric Nurses Association, 21*(4), 233–243.

DESCRIPTION OF THE STUDY: As part of a quality improvement study, the authors sought to improve physical health screening for metabolic syndrome in clients with severe mental illness (SMI) who were being treated in an ACT program. An underlying assumption was that physical illnesses were not routinely being tracked and typically were not treated until after a medical event occurred. This was identified as a significant quality of care issue because studies have shown that people with SMI generally have a 25-year shorter life span than the general population, and one of the largest contributors (greater than suicide or injury) is metabolic syndrome and cardiometabolic sequelae such as hypertension, diabetes, and dyslipidemia. A large sample of clients (N = 199) agreed to participate in the study, and they were evaluated on five parameters that are diagnostic for metabolic syndrome: waist circumference, blood pressure, fasting blood glucose, triglycerides, and high-density lipoprotein cholesterol. ACT staff also provided additional support services to encourage adherence with laboratory test completion, such as reminders, assistance with overcoming transportation barriers, and even accompanying clients to appointments when requested.

RESULTS OF THE STUDY: Although some of the identified barriers to adherence necessitated time-consuming support from staff, 141 clients completed all five parameters of screening. Fifty-three percent of the clients met criteria for metabolic syndrome, and of those who did not meet criteria, only nine participants had *no* risk factors. As a result, the authors identified new preclinical or clinical diagnoses of hypertension for 68 percent of the clients, of diabetes for 15 percent of the clients, and of dyslipidemia for 53 percent of the clients. The authors concluded that the results justify routine screening for metabolic syndrome among those with SMI.

IMPLICATIONS FOR NURSING PRACTICE: The Institute of Medicine (2003) identified quality improvement as a core competency needed by nurses to improve safe, effective nursing care. This study is an example of healthcare professionals identifying a potential quality of care issue, studying the issue, and identifying outcomes needed to improve care based on the results of their study. Nurses, as they review current literature and think critically about the practice settings where they work, can take a leadership role in quality-improvement studies such as this one. This particular study highlighted the fact that significant healthcare risks for the SMI population can be missed unless screening for these risks is done routinely. The complex needs of the SMI client with regard to managing mental illness symptoms has, at times, taken precedence to the exclusion of attention to other health risks. Nurses need to be thoughtful about providing quality, holistic care to clients with SMI because some of these health risks contribute to a significantly shorter life span when they are not addressed.

TEST YOUR CRITICAL THINKING SKILLS

Sara, a 23-year-old single woman, has just been admitted to the psychiatric unit by her parents. They explain that over the past few months, she has become increasingly withdrawn. She stays in her room alone but lately has been heard talking and laughing to herself.

Sara left home for the first time at age 18 to attend college. She performed well during her first semester, but when she returned after Christmas, she began to accuse her roommate of stealing her possessions. She started writing to her parents that her roommate wanted to kill her and that her roommate was turning everyone against her. She said she feared for her life. She started missing classes and stayed in her bed most of the time. Sometimes she locked herself in her closet. Her parents took her home, and she was hospitalized and diagnosed with schizophrenia. Sara has since been maintained on antipsychotic medication while taking a few classes at the local community college.

Sara tells the admitting nurse that she quit taking her medication 4 weeks ago because the pharmacist who fills the prescriptions is plotting to have her killed. She believes he is trying to poison her. She says she got this information from a television message. As Sara speaks, the nurse notices that she sometimes stops in midsentence and listens; sometimes she cocks her head to the side and moves her lips as though she is talking.

Answer the following questions related to Sara:

1. From the assessment data, what would be the most immediate nursing concern in working with Sara?
2. What is the nursing diagnosis related to this concern?
3. What interventions must be accomplished before the nurse can be successful in working with Sara?

Communication Exercises

1. Hal, a patient on the psychiatric unit, has a diagnosis of schizophrenia. He lives in a halfway house, where last evening he began yelling that "aliens were on the way to take over our bodies! The message is coming through loud and clear!" The residence supervisor became frightened and called 911. As Hal was being admitted to the psychiatric unit, he told the nurse, "I'm special! I get messages from a higher being! We are in for big trouble!" How would the nurse respond appropriately to this statement by Hal?

2. The nurse notices that Hal is sitting off to himself in a corner of the dayroom. He appears to be talking to himself and tilts his head to the side as if listening to something. How would the nurse intervene with Hal in this situation?

3. Hal says to the nurse, "We must choose to take a ride. All alone we slip and slide. Now it's time to take a bride." How would the nurse respond appropriately to this statement by Hal?

 MOVIE CONNECTIONS

I Never Promised You a Rose Garden (Schizophrenia) • *A Beautiful Mind* (Schizophrenia) • *The Fisher King* (Schizophrenia) • *Bennie & Joon* (Schizophrenia) • *Out of Darkness* (Schizophrenia) • *Conspiracy Theory* (Paranoia) • *The Fan* (Delusional disorder) • *The Soloist* (Schizophrenia) • *Of Two Minds* (Schizophrenia)

References

Álvarez, M. J., Masramon, H., Peña, C., Pont, M., Gourdier, C., Roura-Poch, P., & Arrufat, F. (2015). Cumulative effects of childhood traumas: Polytraumatization, dissociation, and schizophrenia. *Community Mental Health Journal, 51*(1), 54–62. doi:10.1007/s10597-014-9755-2

American Psychiatric Association. (2013). *Diagnostic and statistical manual of mental disorders* (5th ed.) Washington, DC: Author.

Asen, E. (2002). Outcome research in family therapy: Family intervention for psychosis. *Advances in Psychiatric Treatment, 8,* 230–238.

Benson, P. J., Beedie, S. A., Shephard, E., Giegling, I., Rujescu, G., & St. Clair, D. (2012). Simple viewing tests can detect eye movement abnormalities that distinguish schizophrenia cases from controls with exceptional accuracy. *Biological Psychiatry, 72*(9), 716–724.

Black, D. W., & Andreasen, N. C. (2016). *Introductory textbook of psychiatry* (6th ed.). Washington, DC: American Psychiatric.

Bora, E. (2015). Neurodevelopmental origin of cognitive impairment in schizophrenia. *Psychological Medicine, 45*(1), 1–9. doi:10.1017/S0033291714001263

Caqueo-Urízar, A., Rus-Calafell, M., Urzúa, A., Escudero, J., & Gutiérrez-Maldonado, J. (2015). The role of family therapy in the management of schizophrenia: Challenges and solutions. *Neuropsychiatric Disease and Treatment, 11,* 145–151. doi:10.2147/NDT.S51331

Castillo, E. G., Rosati, J., Williams, C., Pessin, N., & Lindy, D. C. (2015). Metabolic syndrome screening and assertive community treatment: A quality improvement study. *Journal of the American Psychiatric Nurses Association, 21*(4), 233–243.

Chesney, E., Goodwin, G. M., & Fazel, S. (2014). Risks of all-cause and suicide mortality in mental disorders: A meta-review. *World Psychiatry.* https://doi.org/10.1002/wps.20128

Clark, S. R., Baune, B. T., Schubert, K. O., Lavoie, S., Smesny, S., Rice, S. M., & Amminger, G. P. (2016). Prediction of transition from ultra-high risk to first-episode psychosis using a probabilistic model combining history, clinical assessment and fatty-acid biomarkers. *Translational Psychiatry, 6*(9), e897. doi:10.1038/tp.2016.170

D'Souza, D. C., Singh, N., Elander, J., Carbuto, M., Pittman, B., Udo de Haes, J., . . . Schipper, J. (2012). Glycine transporter inhibitor attenuates the psychotomimetic effects of ketamine in healthy males: Preliminary evidence. *Neuropsychopharmacology, 37,* 1036–1046.

Druss, B. G., Zhao, L., Von Esenwein, S., Morrato, E. H., & Marcus, S. C. (2011). Understanding excess mortality in persons with mental illness: 17-year follow up of a nationally representative US survey. *Medical Care, 49*(6), 599–604.

Fioravanti, M., Bianchi, V., & Cinti, M. E. (2012). Cognitive deficits in schizophrenia: An updated meta-analysis of the scientific evidence. *BMJ Psychiatry, 12*(1), 1–20.

Freudenreich, O. (2010). Differential diagnosis of psychotic symptoms: Medical "mimics." *Psychiatric Times, 27*(12), 52–61.

Hashimoto, K. (2006). Glycine transporter inhibitors as therapeutic agents for schizophrenia. *Recent Patents on CNS Drug Discovery, 1,* 43–53.

Herdman, T. H., & Kamitsuru, S. (Eds.). (2018). *NANDA-I nursing diagnoses: Definitions and classification, 2018–2020.* New York, NY: Thieme.

Hu, W., MacDonald, M. L., Elswick, D. E., & Sweet, R. A. (2014). The glutamate hypothesis of schizophrenia: Evidence from human brain tissue studies [Abstract]. *Annals of the New York Academy of Sciences, 1338,* 38–57. doi:10.1111/nyas

Insel, T. (2015). *Director's blog: New hope for treating psychosis.* Retrieved from http://www.nimh.nih.gov/about/director/2015/new-hope-for-treating-psychosis.shtml

Institute of Medicine (IOM). (2003). *Health professions education: A bridge to quality.* Washington, DC: Author.

Jablensky, A. (2017). Worldwide burden of schizophrenia. In B. J. Sadock, V. A. Sadock, & P. Ruiz (Eds.), *Comprehensive textbook of psychiatry* (11th ed., pp. 1425–1437). Philadelphia, PA: Wolters Kluwer.

Kay, S. R., Fiszbein, A., & Opler, L. A. (1987). The positive and negative syndrome scale (PANSS) for schizophrenia. *Schizophrenia Bulletin, 13*(2), 261–276.

Kranjac, D. (2016). *Pharmacotherapy for smoking cessation in adults with neuropsychiatric illness.* Retrieved from http://www.psychiatryadvisor.com/addiction/smoking-cessation-inadults-with-neuropsychiatric-illness/article/518385

Lewis, S. F., Escalona, R., & Kieth, S. J. (2017). The phenomenology of schizophrenia. In B. J. Sadock, V. A. Sadock, & P. Ruiz (Eds.), *Comprehensive textbook of psychiatry* (11th ed., pp. 1406–1425). Philadelphia, PA: Wolters Kluwer.

Lysaker, P. H., Roe, D., & Buck, K. D. (2010). Recovery and wellness amidst schizophrenia: Definitions, evidence, and the implications for clinical practice. *Journal of the American Psychiatric Nurses Association, 16*(1), 36–42.

MacCabe, J. H., Wicks, S., Löfving, S., David, A. S., Berndtsson, Å., Gustafsson, . . . Dalman, C. (2013). Decline in cognitive performance between ages 13 and 18 years and the risk for psychosis in adulthood: A Swedish longitudinal cohort study in males. *JAMA Psychiatry 70*(3), 261–270. doi:10.1001/2013.jamapsychiatry.43

Matheson, S. L., Shepherd, A. M., & Carr, V. J. (2014). How much do we know about schizophrenia and how well do we know it? Evidence from the Schizophrenia Library. *Psychological Medicine—London, 44*(6), 3387–3405. doi:10.1017/S0033291714000166

Mathews, M., Tesar, G. E., Fattal, O., & Muzina, D. J. (2013). *Schizophrenia and acute psychosis*. Retrieved from http://www.clevelandclinicmeded.com/medicalpubs/diseasemanagement/psychiatry-psychology/schizophrenia-acute-psychosis

Mueser, K. T., Bond, G. R., & Drake, R. E. (2001). Community-based treatment of schizophrenia and other severe mental disorders: Treatment outcomes. *Medscape General Medicine 3*(1) [formerly published in Medscape Psychiatry & Mental Health eJournal 6(1), 2001]. Retrieved from http://www.medscape.com/viewarticle/430529

Nauert, R. (2015). Excess neurotransmitter in brain may trigger schizophrenia. *Psych Central*. Retrieved from http://psychcentral.com/news/2013/04/19/excess-neurotransmitterin-brain-may-trigger-schizophrenia/53880.html

Okazaki, S., Boku, S., Otsuka, I., Mouri, K., Aoyama, S., Shiroiwa, K., . . . Hishimoto, A. (2016). The cell cycle-related genes as biomarkers for schizophrenia. *Progress Neuropsychopharmacology and Biological Psychiatry, 70*(Suppl. 9), 85–91. doi:10.1016/j.pnpbp.2016.05.005

Os, J. V., & Reininghaus, U. (2017). The clinical epidemiology of schizophrenia. In B. J. Sadock, V. A. Sadock., & P. Ruiz (Eds.), *Comprehensive textbook of psychiatry* (10 ed., pp. 1445–1457). Philadelphia, PA: Wolters Kluwer.

Radhakrishnan, R., Wilkinson, S. T., & D'Souza, D. C. (2014). Gone to pot—A review of the association between cannabis and psychosis. *Frontiers in Psychiatry, 5*(54). doi:10.3389/fpsyt.2014.00054

Rezansoff, S., Moniruzzaman, A., Fazel, S., McCandless, L., Procyshyn, R., & Somers, J. M. (2016). Housing First improves adherence to antipsychotic medication among formerly homeless adults with schizophrenia: Results of a randomized controlled trial. *Schizophrenia Bulletin*. doi:10.1093/schbul/sbw136

Roberts, L. W., Louie, A. K., Guerrero, A., Balon, R., Beresin, E. V., Brenner, A., & Coverdale, J. (2017). Premature mortality among people with mental illness: Advocacy in academic psychiatry. *Academic Psychiatry, 41*, (4), 441–446.

Sadock, B. J., Sadock, V. A., & Ruiz, P. (2015). *Synopsis of psychiatry: Behavioral sciences/clinical psychiatry* (11th ed.). Philadelphia, PA: Wolters Kluwer.

Stahl, S. M. (2013). *Stahl's essential psychopharmacology: Neuroscientific basis and practical applications* (4th ed.). New York, NY: Cambridge University Press.

Takeuchi, H., Kantor, N., Sanches, M., Fervaha, G., Agid, O., & Remington, G. (2017). One-year symptom trajectories in patients with stable schizophrenia maintained on antipsychotics versus placebo: Meta-analysis. *British Journal of Psychiatry, 211*(3). doi:10.1192/bjp.bp.116.186007

Thunè, H., Recasens, M., & Uhlhaas, P. J. (2016). The 40-Hz auditory steady-state response in patients with schizophrenia: A meta-analysis. *JAMA Psychiatry*. Retrieved from http://jamanetwork.com/journals/jamapsychiatry/article-abstract/2566207

Urvakhsh, M. M., Thirthalli, J., Aneelraj, D., Jadhav, P., Gangadhar, B. N., & Keshavan, M. S. (2014). Mirror neuron dysfunction in schizophrenia and its functional implications: A systematic review. *Schizophrenia Research, 160*(1–3), 9–19. doi:http://dx.doi.org/10.1016/j.schres.2014.10.040

Veijola, J., Guo, J. Y., Moilanen, J. S., Jaaskelainen, E., Miettunen, J., Kyllonen, M., . . . Murray, G. (2014). Longitudinal changes in total brain volume in schizophrenia: Relation to symptom severity, cognition and antipsychotic medication. *PLoS ONE, 9*(7), e101689. doi:10.1371/journal.pone.0101689

Viher, P. V., Stegmayer, K., Giezendanner, S., Federspiel, A., Bohlhalter, S., Vanbellingen, T., . . . Walthera, S. (2016). Cerebral white matter structure is associated with DSM-5 schizophrenia symptom dimensions. *Neuroimage: Clinical, 12*(Suppl. 7), 93–99. doi:http://dx.doi.org/10.1016/j.nicl.2016.06.013

Waters, F., Collerton, D., Ffytche, D. H., Jardri, R., Pins, D., Dudley, R., . . . Laroi, F. (2014). Visual hallucinations in the psychosis spectrum and comparative information from neurodegenerative disorders and eye disease. *Schizophrenia Bulletin, 40*(Suppl. 4), 233–245. doi:10.1093/schbul/sbu036

Weiden, P. J. (2010). Is recovery attainable in schizophrenia? *Medscape Psychiatry & Mental Health*. Retrieved from http://www.medscape.com/viewarticle/729750

Wu, Q., Gilbody, S., Peckham, E., Brabyn, S., & Parrott, S. (2016). Varenicline for smoking cessation and reduction in people with severe mental illnesses: Systematic review and metaanalysis. *Addiction, 111*(9), 1554–1567. doi:10.1111/add.13415 [Epub 2016 Jun 9]

16

Depressive Disorders

CORE CONCEPTS

Depression

Mood

KEY TERMS

cognitive therapy

dysthymia

melancholia

postpartum depression

premenstrual dysphoric disorder

psychomotor retardation

OBJECTIVES

After reading this chapter, the student will be able to:

1. Recount historical perspectives of depression.
2. Discuss epidemiological statistics related to depression.
3. Describe various types of depressive disorders.
4. Identify predisposing factors in the development of depression.
5. Discuss implications of depression related to developmental stage.
6. Identify symptomatology associated with depression and use this information in patient assessment.
7. Formulate nursing diagnoses and goals of care for patients with depression.
8. Identify topics for patient and family teaching relevant to depression.
9. Describe appropriate nursing interventions for behaviors associated with depression.
10. Describe relevant criteria for evaluating nursing care of patients with depression.
11. Discuss various modalities relevant to treatment of depression.

HOMEWORK ASSIGNMENT

Please read the chapter and answer the following questions:

1. Alterations in which of the neurotransmitters are most closely associated with depression?
2. Depression in adolescence is very hard to differentiate from the normal stormy behavior associated with adolescence.

What is the best clue for determining a problem with depression in adolescence?

3. Behaviors of depression often change with the diurnal variation in the level of neurotransmitters. Describe the difference

in this phenomenon between moderate and severe depression.

4. All antidepressants carry a black-box warning. What is it?

Introduction

Depression is likely the oldest and still one of the most frequently diagnosed psychiatric illnesses. Symptoms of depression have been described almost as far back as there is evidence of written documentation.

An occasional bout with the "blues," a feeling of sadness or downheartedness, is common among healthy people and considered to be a normal response to everyday disappointments in life. These episodes are short-lived as the individual adapts to the loss, change, or failure (real or perceived) that has been experienced. Pathological depression occurs when adaptation is ineffective and the symptoms are significant enough to impair functioning.

CORE CONCEPT

Mood

Mood is a pervasive and sustained emotion that may have a major influence on a person's perception of the world. Examples of mood include depression, joy, elation, anger, and anxiety. *Affect* is described as the external, observable emotional reaction associated with an experience. A *flat affect* describes someone who lacks emotional expression and is often seen in severely depressed clients.

This chapter focuses on the different manifestations of depressive illness and implications for nursing intervention. A historical perspective and epidemiological statistics related to depression are presented. Predisposing factors that have been implicated in the etiology of depression provide a framework for studying the dynamics of the disorder. Similarities and differences between depressive disorders and grief are discussed.

Depressive illnesses specific to individuals at various developmental stages are reviewed. An explanation of the symptomatology is presented as background knowledge for assessing the client with depression. Nursing care is described in the context of the six steps of the nursing process. Various medical treatment modalities are explored.

CORE CONCEPT

Depression

An alteration in mood that is expressed by feelings of sadness, despair, and pessimism. There is a loss of interest in usual activities, and somatic symptoms may be evident. Changes in appetite, sleep patterns, and cognition are common.

Historical Perspective

Many ancient cultures (e.g., Babylonian, Egyptian, Hebrew) believed in the supernatural or divine origin of mood disorders. The Old Testament states in the Book of Samuel that King Saul's depression was inflicted by an "evil spirit" sent from God to "torment" him.

A clearly nondivine point of view regarding depression was held by the Greek medical community from the 5th century BC through the 3rd century AD and represented the thinking of Hippocrates, Celsus, and Galen, among others. They strongly rejected the idea of divine origin and considered the brain as the seat of all emotional states. Hippocrates believed that **melancholia** was caused by an excess of black bile, a heavily toxic substance produced in the spleen or intestine, which affected the brain. Melancholia is currently used to describe a severe form of major depressive disorder in which symptoms are exaggerated and interest or pleasure in virtually all activities is lost.

During the Renaissance, several new theories evolved. Depression was viewed by some as being the result of obstruction of vital air circulation, excessive brooding, or helpless situations beyond the client's control. Depression was reflected in major literary works of the time, including Shakespeare's *King Lear*, *Macbeth*, and *Hamlet*.

Contemporary thinking has been shaped a great deal by the works of Sigmund Freud, Emil Kraepelin, and Adolf Meyer. Having evolved from these early 20th-century models, current thinking about mood disorders generally encompasses the intrapsychic, behavioral, and biological perspectives. These various perspectives support the notion of multiple causation in the development of mood disorders.

Epidemiology

Major depressive disorder (MDD) is one of the leading causes of disability in the United States. In addition to the disability posed by the disorder itself, recent research links depression to an increased risk for several other medical conditions, including coronary artery disease (another leading cause of death), especially in women younger than age 65 (Jiang et al., 2016). Based on data collected in 2015 and 2016, 6.7 percent of persons aged 18 or older had at least one major depressive episode in the previous year (Substance Abuse and Mental Health Services Administration [SAMHSA], 2017). The lifetime prevalence of depression is about 17 percent, which makes it the most prevalent psychiatric disorder (Sadock, Sadock, & Ruiz, 2015). Akiskal (2017) reports that as diagnostic evaluation of bipolar disorders (alternating episodes of depression and manic or hypomanic symptoms) has improved, there is convincing data that up to 50 percent of all depressions may actually be bipolar illness.

There is evidence that the incidence of depression is increasing among American teens and young adults, particularly adolescent girls. From 2005 to 2014, the incidence rose from 4.5 to 5.7 percent for teenage boys and from 13.1 to 17.3 percent for teenage girls (Mojtabai, Olfson, & Han, 2016). The reasons for these increases are unclear but the overall preponderance of evidence has led some researchers to consider depression "the common cold of psychiatric disorders" and this generation as an "age of melancholia."

Age and Gender

Although the lifetime prevalence of depressive disorders is higher in those aged 45 years or younger (Merikangas & Rihmer, 2017), it is difficult to pinpoint a single age correlate because many factors influence age-related depressive symptoms. Research indicates that the incidence of depressive disorder is higher in women than it is in men by almost 2 to 1. Sadock and colleagues (2015) report that this is "an almost universal observation, independent of country or culture" (p. 349). Many biological explanations have been suggested, including that women have higher concentrations of monoamine oxidase (a neurotransmitter associated with depression); greater vulnerability to thyroid dysfunctions; and hormone changes that occur during the menstrual cycle, postpartum, and at menopause (Akiskal, 2017). Psychosocial factors contributing to depression in women may include increased sensitivity to stress (and higher prevalence of anxiety disorders), multiple social roles, and poorer coping mechanisms (Merikangas & Rihmer, 2017). In general, this gender-related increased risk for depression is influenced by many factors in complex interactions that are not yet clearly understood.

Socioeconomic Factors

Results of some studies have indicated an inverse relationship between social class and report of depressive symptoms. However, there has yet to be a definitive causal understanding in the socioeconomic status–mental illness relationship. A National Center for Health Statistics report identified that, for the 45 to 64 age group, depression was five times more prevalent among those below the poverty level (National Center for Health Statistics [NCHS], 2012) and a study of European countries (Freeman et al., 2016) reinforced that, internationally, lower socioeconomic status, including lower levels of education, are associated with increased prevalence of depression. Merikangas & Rihmer (2017) cite that depression is three times more prevalent among those without a workplace than those with one. Whether these findings are related to lack of access to resources and early treatment, difficulty managing multiple stressors associated with socioeconomic well-being, or a combination of many factors requires more research.

Race and Culture

Studies have shown no consistent relationship between race and affective disorders. One problem encountered in reviewing racial comparisons has to do with the socioeconomic class of the race being investigated. Sample populations of nonwhite clients are often predominantly lower socioeconomic class populations that are being compared with white populations from middle and upper social classes.

Other studies suggest a second problematic factor in the study of racial comparisons. Clinicians tend to underdiagnose mood disorders and to overdiagnose schizophrenia in clients who have racial or cultural backgrounds different from their own (Sadock et al., 2015). This misdiagnosis may result from language barriers between clients and physicians who are unfamiliar with cultural aspects of nonwhite clients' language and behavior.

Marital Status

A number of studies have suggested that marriage has a positive effect on the psychological well-being of an individual (as compared to those who are single or do not have a close relationship with another person). Other studies have suggested that marital status alone is not a valid indicator of risk for depression (Lapate et al., 2014; LaPierre, 2004). Some of those studies have identified that age is an important variable in risk for depression among married and single individuals. Lapate and colleagues (2014) report that marital *stress* was associated with increased risk for depression, suggesting that social stress may also be an important variable to consider.

In a broader context, it may be that lack of social connectedness rather than marital status is associated with higher incidence of depression. Holt-Lundstat, Robles, and Sbarra (2017) cite studies that associate lack of social connections (including high divorce rates, among others) with morbidity for many diseases (including cardiovascular disease, which has been associated with depression) and mortality. These authors suggest that there are so many factors that influence lack of social connectedness and illness that it is difficult to pinpoint one of those (such as marital status) as a singular cause.

Seasonality

Studies exploring whether seasonality is a cause of depression have yielded varying results. The *Diagnostic and Statistical Manual of Mental Disorders (DSM-5)* (American Psychiatric Association [APA], 2013) uses the term *seasonal pattern* to describe and specify any depressive disorder that occurs at "characteristic times of the year" (p. 187). The *DSM-5* notes that, most commonly, the episodes occur in fall or winter but in some cases clients have recurrent summer episodes. Authors of one large study report that prevalence rates of depression with seasonal patterns have varied from 1 to 12 percent, but in their study of 5,549 patients from primary care settings, there was no evidence of seasonal patterns for MDD (Winthorst et al., 2011). Another study (Cobb et al., 2014) found that a small but significant peak in depression symptoms occurred in winter months, but in over 20 years of following those clients, the winter seasonal pattern was not stable. Seasonal affective disorder continues to be popularly referred to as a separate condition, although the *DSM-5* does not list it as a distinct diagnosis. The reported benefits of light therapy seem to support a seasonal cause for depression during winter months when there may be less exposure to natural sunlight, but in a meta-analysis of the research on benefits of bright white light in treating depression the authors found that the evidence was not consistent or conclusive (Mårtensson et al., 2015).

Types of Depressive Disorders

Major Depressive Disorder

MDD is characterized by depressed mood or loss of interest or pleasure in usual activities. Evidence will show impaired social and occupational functioning that has existed for at least 2 weeks, no history of manic behavior, and symptoms that cannot be attributed to use of substances or a general medical condition. Additionally, the diagnosis of MDD is specified according to whether it is a *single episode* (the individual's first encounter with a major depressive episode) or *recurrent* (the individual has a history of previous major depressive episodes). The diagnosis will also identify the degree of severity of symptoms (mild, moderate, or severe) and whether there is evidence of psychotic, catatonic, or melancholic features. The presence of anxiety and severity of suicide risk may also be noted. MDD is differentiated from a schizoaffective disorder, a condition in which the individual expresses symptoms of a mood disorder as well as symptoms of schizophrenia. Read Josh's story on his experience with depression and an eventual diagnosis of schizoaffective disorder in "The Real People, Real Stories" feature that follows. The *DSM-5* (APA, 2013) diagnostic criteria for major depressive episode are presented in Box 16–1.

Persistent Depressive Disorder (Dysthymia)

Characteristics of **dysthymia** are similar to, if somewhat milder than, those ascribed to MDD. Individuals with this mood disturbance describe their mood as sad or "down in the dumps." There is no evidence of psychotic symptoms. The essential feature is a chronically depressed mood (or possibly an irritable mood in children or adolescents) for most of the day, more days than not, for at least 2 years (1 year for children and adolescents). The diagnosis is identified as *early onset* (occurring before age 21 years) or *late onset* (occurring at age 21 years or older). The *DSM-5* diagnostic criteria for dysthymia are presented in Box 16–2.

Premenstrual Dysphoric Disorder

The essential features of **premenstrual dysphoric disorder** include markedly depressed mood, excessive anxiety, mood swings, and decreased interest in activities during the week prior to menses, improving shortly after the onset of menstruation, and becoming minimal or absent in the week postmenses (APA, 2013). The major difference between the diagnosis of premenstrual dysphoric disorder and

Real People, Real Stories: Josh's Experience With Depression and the Eventual Diagnosis of Schizoaffective Disorder

(This individual preferred to remain anonymous so his name has been changed.)

Consider reflecting on factors that may contribute to Josh's perceptions about his illness and his perceptions about the contributions of healthcare providers in his recovery process.

Karyn: Tell me about the time when you first became aware that you had a mood disorder [Josh had told me he had depression. I was unaware when we began the interview that his actual diagnosis was schizoaffective disorder.]

Josh: I was in senior high school and was doing well. I was in advance placement (AP) courses, and suddenly I got an F in AP English. Nothing like that had ever happened before. I started becoming more withdrawn. I was smoking pot with my friends, and I wonder now if that had an impact. I graduated high school, then attended college for two years until the symptoms really surfaced. I was cut from the soccer team, so there were some disappointments, but I became very withdrawn and depressed. I had suicide ideas and a plan. I had to take a break from school, and I just wasn't doing anything; I was just very withdrawn. Four years later I was diagnosed with schizoaffective disorder.

Karyn: What did you think about that diagnosis?

Josh: I thought it was wrong. I did have some difficulty tracking objects with my eyes, and I still do when I don't get enough sleep [difficulty tracking objects with one's eyes is a common neurological symptom in schizophrenia]. I guess now that I think of it, there was a time in college when I thought my roommates were talking about me, and then I started thinking people in the next room were talking about me. I would read into things a lot. Sometimes I thought I saw something out of the corner of my eye, and sometimes I heard voices.

Karyn: It seems like that would be difficult, maybe even frightening, to have these symptoms and get this diagnosis. What was that like for you?

Josh: Yeah, it was, but I was glad to get a diagnosis because then I knew what I had to deal with. At the same time, though, I thought it was too quickly made and they were too quick to prescribe pills. If I had it to do over, I would have just trusted the doctors, but I rebelled against the drugs several times; sometimes because I was having side effects like tardive dyskinesia; one time because I was convinced the meds were holding me back and even hurting me; and one time because I just gave up, since I didn't have any of the things I wanted, like marriage, a college degree, or a career. Sometimes I thought, "I can just be smarter than this, and I'll get over it." But I was very disorganized and incoherent. Each time I didn't take the pills, I became withdrawn, depressed, and hearing voices,

and eventually I just couldn't find anything else to blame it on. I tried to hide the fact that I had stopped taking the pills, but it always became evident eventually. I stay on the medications now because I know I have to.

Karyn: You've come so far since then!

Josh: (smiles) Yeah, it took me eight years to finish my college degree, but now I have a good job in information technology at a large hospital system, and I live on my own. I was engaged, and although it didn't work out, I'm dating again and hopeful about pursuing a committed relationship.

Karyn: What do you think has been most important in supporting your recovery?

Josh: My parents supported me through all of it. They were my only support, and I didn't want other people to know my "stuff." I was able to stay with my parents until I got back on my feet, and that was really important. The last time I stopped taking my meds, I'd have to consult court records to remember everything that happened, but I know there were trespassing charges. I had run-ins with the police. I also had run-ins with my parents, who eventually called in a crisis team, and I was hospitalized against my will. I was in the hospital for around 30 days, and I saw people who were homeless and had no one supporting them, and they were really doing poorly. Knowing I had some place to live really helped me.

Also, I had a job and some successes at work, so that gave me focus. My job is largely mathematical and doesn't require a lot of social skills challenges. That was helpful for me because, while some people may be self-taught with social skills, I've always struggled with that. My job allows me to develop great insights, be quirky, and not have to try to figure people out.

Karyn: What are your thoughts about the impact of the healthcare providers with whom you've interacted?

Josh: I work in a hospital, so I have a great appreciation for their hard work. I saw an NP who gave me good advice and was very supportive. She asked some probing questions and confronted me at times, and that was challenging, but she was just doing her job and I was trying to hide from my illness. She told me the medications might end up being less effective if I didn't take them or stay on them early in my illness, so that may have encouraged me to keep taking them.

I had good community health services—a case worker, a psychiatrist, and a behavioral health specialist that I found to be particularly supportive because we talked about spiritual things, and that made it okay to explore other issues. In the hospital, the nurses mostly worked at the station, and that was probably better for their safety,

Real People, Real Stories: Josh's Experience With Depression and the Eventual Diagnosis of Schizoaffective Disorder—cont'd

but still I could talk to them and they made it seem like it was okay that I was there. That was important because I wasn't sure what was happening to me, and they just talked about normal, everyday stuff. They seemed more like warm people than cold or clinical.

I go to NAMI [National Alliance on Mental Illness] meetings now because I want to share the message with people who have a mental illness (and with their family members) that the professionals could see things I was unable to see at the time I was symptomatic, so it's important to trust the process. I also want families to know that having ongoing support from family members was a lifeline for me even when we were having run-ins and they were facilitating hospitalization against my will.

BOX 16-1 Diagnostic Criteria for Major Depressive Disorder

A. Five (or more) of the following symptoms have been present during the same 2-week period and represent a change from previous functioning; at least one of the symptoms is either (1) depressed mood or (2) loss of interest or pleasure. **Note:** Do not include symptoms that are clearly due to another medical condition.
1. Depressed mood most of the day, nearly every day, as indicated by either subjective report (e.g., feels sad, empty, or hopeless) or observation made by others (e.g., appears tearful) (**Note:** In children and adolescents, can be irritable mood.)
2. Markedly diminished interest or pleasure in all, or almost all, activities most of the day, nearly every day (as indicated by either subjective account or observation)
3. Significant weight loss when not dieting or weight gain (e.g., a change of more than 5% of body weight in a month), or decrease or increase in appetite nearly every day (**Note:** In children, consider failure to make expected weight gain.)
4. Insomnia or hypersomnia nearly every day
5. Psychomotor agitation or retardation nearly every day (observable by others, not merely subjective feelings of restlessness or being slowed down)
6. Fatigue or loss of energy nearly every day
7. Feelings of worthlessness or excessive or inappropriate guilt (which may be delusional) nearly every day (not merely self-reproach or guilt about being sick)
8. Diminished ability to think or concentrate, or indecisiveness, nearly every day (either by subjective account or as observed by others)
9. Recurrent thoughts of death (not just fear of dying), recurrent suicidal ideation without a specific plan, or a suicide attempt or a specific plan for committing suicide
B. The symptoms cause clinically significant distress or impairment in social, occupational, or other important areas of functioning.

C. The episode is not attributable to the physiological effects of a substance or another medical condition.

Note: Criteria A, B, and C represent a major depressive episode.

Note: Responses to a significant loss (e.g., bereavement, financial ruin, losses from a natural disaster, a serious medical illness or disability) may include feelings of intense sadness, rumination about the loss, insomnia, poor appetite, and weight loss noted in Criterion A, which may resemble a depressive episode. Although such symptoms may be understandable or considered appropriate to the loss, the presence of a major depressive episode in addition to the normal response to a significant loss should also be carefully considered. This decision inevitably requires the exercise of clinical judgment based on the individual's history and the cultural norms for the expression of distress in the context of loss.

D. The occurrence of the major depressive episode is not better explained by schizoaffective disorder, schizophrenia, schizophreniform disorder, delusional disorder, or other specified and unspecified schizophrenia spectrum and other psychotic disorders.
E. There has never been a manic episode or a hypomanic episode.

Specify:

With anxious distress
With mixed features
With melancholic features
With atypical features
With mood-congruent psychotic features
With mood-incongruent psychotic features
With catatonia
With peripartum onset
With seasonal pattern

Reprinted with permission from American Psychiatric Association. (2013). Diagnostic and statistical manual of mental disorders (5th ed.). Washington, DC: American Psychiatric Publishing.

BOX 16–2 Diagnostic Criteria for Persistent Depressive Disorder (Dysthymia)

A. Depressed mood for most of the day, for more days than not, as indicated by either subjective account or observation by others, for at least 2 years. **Note:** In children and adolescents, mood can be irritable and duration must be at least 1 year.

B. Presence, while depressed, of two (or more) of the following:
  1. Poor appetite or overeating
  2. Insomnia or hypersomnia
  3. Low energy or fatigue
  4. Low self-esteem
  5. Poor concentration or difficulty making decisions
  6. Feelings of hopelessness

C. During the 2-year period (1 year for children or adolescents) of the disturbance, the individual has never been without the symptoms in Criteria A and B for more than 2 months at a time.

D. Criteria for a major depressive disorder may be continuously present for 2 years.

E. There has never been a manic episode or a hypomanic episode, and criteria have never been met for cyclothymic disorder.

F. The disturbance is not better explained by a persistent schizoaffective disorder, schizophrenia, delusional disorder, or other specified or unspecified schizophrenia spectrum and other psychotic disorder.

G. The symptoms are not attributable to the physiological effects of a substance (e.g., a drug of abuse, a medication) or another medical condition (e.g., hypothyroidism).

H. The symptoms cause clinically significant distress or impairment in social, occupational, or other important areas of functioning.

Specify if:
With anxious distress
With mixed features
With melancholic features

With atypical features
With mood-congruent psychotic features
With mood-incongruent psychotic features
With peripartum onset

Specify if:
With pure dysthymic syndrome
With persistent major depressive episode
With intermittent major depressive episodes, with current episode
With intermittent major depressive episodes, without current episode

Specify if:
In partial remission
In full remission

Specify if:
Early onset (onset before age 21 years)
Late onset (onset at age 21 years or older)

Specify if:
Mild
Moderate
Severe

Reprinted with permission from American Psychiatric Association. (2013). Diagnostic and statistical manual of mental disorders (5th ed.). Washington, DC: American Psychiatric Publishing.

the premenstrual mood changes that many women experience is a matter of intensity and frequency of symptoms. The symptoms of premenstrual dysphoric disorder are severe enough to interfere with one's ability to function socially, at work, or at school and they are recurrent for the majority of menstrual cycles over the course of a year.

Substance/Medication-Induced Depressive Disorder

The symptoms associated with a substance/medication-induced depressive disorder are considered to be the direct result of physiological effects of a substance (e.g., a drug of abuse, a medication, or toxin exposure). This disorder causes clinically significant distress or impairment in social, occupational, or other important areas of functioning. The depressed mood is associated with *intoxication* or *withdrawal* from substances such as alcohol, amphetamines,

cocaine, hallucinogens, opioids, phencyclidine-like substances, sedatives, hypnotics, or anxiolytics. The symptoms meet the full criteria for a relevant depressive disorder (APA, 2013).

A number of medications have been known to evoke mood symptoms. Classifications include anesthetics, analgesics, anticholinergics, anticonvulsants, antihypertensives, antiparkinsonian agents, antiulcer agents, cardiac medications, oral contraceptives, psychotropic medications, muscle relaxants, steroids, and sulfonamides. Some specific examples are included in the discussion of predisposing factors to depressive disorders.

Depressive Disorder Due to Another Medical Condition

This disorder is characterized by symptoms associated with a major depressive episode that are the direct physiological consequence of another medical condition (APA, 2013). The depression causes clinically significant distress or impairment in social, occupational, or other important areas of functioning. Examples of medical conditions that influence depression include stroke, traumatic brain injuries, thyroid disorders, Cushing's disease, Huntington's disease, Parkinson's disease, and multiple sclerosis.

Predisposing Factors

The etiology of depression is unclear. No single theory or hypothesis has been postulated that substantiates a clear-cut explanation for the disease. Evidence continues to mount in support of multiple causations, recognizing the combined effects of genetic, biochemical, and psychosocial influences on an individual's susceptibility to depression. A number of theoretical postulates are presented here.

Biological Theories

Genetics

Affective illness has been the subject of considerable research on the relevance of hereditary factors. A genetic link has been suggested in numerous studies; however, a definitive mode of genetic transmission has yet to be demonstrated.

Twin Studies

Twin studies suggest a strong genetic factor in the etiology of affective illness, including depressive disorders and bipolar disorders. When compared to dizygotic twins, monozygotic twins have a two to four times greater incidence of depression but between monozygotic twins there is only a 70 to 80 percent chance of both twins having the illness (Kelsoe & Greenwood, 2017). These findings suggest that although twin studies do identify genetic risk, genetics does not explain all depressions. Environmental risks are not only an important variable but are uniquely individual.

Family Studies

Family studies have shown that major depression is seven times more common among first-degree biological relatives of people with the disorder than among the general population (Kelsoe & Greenwood, 2017). The evidence to support an increased risk of depressive disorder in individuals with positive family history is quite compelling. It is unlikely that random environmental factors could cause the concentration of illness that is seen within families.

Adoption Studies

Further support for heritability as an etiological influence in depression comes from studies of the adopted offspring of affectively ill biological parents. These studies have indicated that biological children of parents with mood disorders are at increased risk of developing a mood disorder, even when they are reared by adoptive parents who do not have the disorder (Kelsoe & Greenwood, 2017). Conversely, adoption studies have also been used to look at the effects of being reared by an adoptive parent (particularly the maternal parent) with depression and the risks for depression in nongenetically similar children. Interestingly, these studies have demonstrated an increased risk of depression (as well as oppositional defiant disorder and conduct disorder) in adopted children that cannot be explained by genetics (Natsuaki et al., 2014). Again, this finding suggests that environmental factors also play a role in the etiology of depressive illnesses.

Biochemical Influences

Biogenic Amines

It has been hypothesized that depressive illness may be related to a deficiency of the neurotransmitters norepinephrine, serotonin, and dopamine at functionally important receptor sites in the brain. Historically, the biogenic amine hypothesis of mood disorders grew out of the observation that reserpine, an antihypertensive, which depletes the brain of amines such as norepinephrine, was associated with the development of a depressive syndrome. The catecholamine norepinephrine has been identified as a key component in the mobilization of the body to deal with stressful situations. Neurons that contain serotonin are critically involved in the regulation of many psychobiological functions, such as mood, anxiety, arousal, vigilance, irritability, thinking, cognition, appetite, aggression, sleep–wake cycles, eating, and intestinal motility. Tryptophan, the amino acid precursor of serotonin, has been shown to enhance the efficacy of antidepressant medications and, on occasion, to be effective as an antidepressant itself. The level of dopamine in the mesolimbic system of the brain is thought to exert a strong influence over human mood and behavior. A diminished supply of these biogenic amines inhibits the transmission of impulses from one neuronal fiber to another, causing a failure of the cells to fire or become charged (Fig. 16–1).

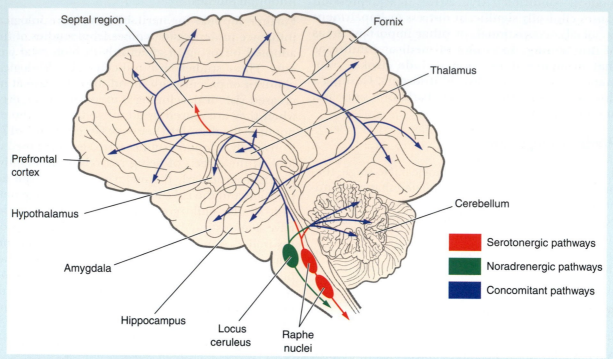

FIGURE 16–1 Neurobiology of depression.

NEUROTRANSMITTERS

Although other neurotransmitters have also been implicated in the pathophysiology of depression, disturbances in serotonin and norepinephrine have been the most extensively scrutinized.

Cell bodies of origin for the serotonin pathways lie within the raphe nuclei located in the brainstem. Those for norepinephrine originate in the locus ceruleus. Projections for both neurotransmitters extend throughout the forebrain, prefrontal cortex, cerebellum, and limbic system.

AREAS OF THE BRAIN AFFECTED

Areas of the brain affected by depression and the symptoms that they mediate include the following:

- Hippocampus: Memory impairments, feelings of worthlessness, hopelessness, and guilt
- Amygdala: Anhedonia, anxiety, reduced motivation
- Hypothalamus: Increased or decreased sleep and appetite; decreased energy and libido
- Other limbic structures: Emotional alterations
- Frontal cortex: Depressed mood; problems concentrating
- Cerebellum: Psychomotor retardation/agitation

MEDICATIONS AND THEIR EFFECTS ON THE BRAIN

All medications that increase serotonin or norepinephrine, or both, can improve the emotional and vegetative symptoms of depression. Medications that produce these effects include those that block the presynaptic reuptake of the neurotransmitters or block receptors at nerve endings (tricyclics, SSRIs, SNRIs) and those that inhibit monoamine oxidase, an enzyme that is involved in the metabolism of the monoamines serotonin, norepinephrine, and dopamine (MAOIs).

Side effects of these medications relate to their specific neurotransmitter receptor-blocking action. Tricyclic and tetracyclic drugs (e.g., imipramine, amitriptyline, mirtazapine) block reuptake and/or receptors for serotonin, norepinephrine, acetylcholine, and histamine. SSRIs are selective serotonin reuptake inhibitors. Others, such as bupropion, venlafaxine, and duloxetine block serotonin and norepinephrine reuptake and also are weak inhibitors of dopamine.

Blockade of norepinephrine reuptake results in side effects of tremors, cardiac arrhythmias, sexual dysfunction, and hypertension. Blockade of serotonin reuptake results in side effects of gastrointestinal disturbances, increased agitation, and sexual dysfunction. Blockade of dopamine reuptake results in side effects of psychomotor activation. Blockade of acetylcholine reuptake results in dry mouth, blurred vision, constipation, and urinary retention. Blockade of histamine reuptake results in sedation, weight gain, and hypotension.

More recently, the biogenic amine hypothesis has been expanded to include another neurotransmitter, acetylcholine. Because cholinergic agents have profound effects on mood, electroencephalograms, sleep, and neuroendocrine function, it has been suggested that the problem in depression and mania may be an imbalance between the biogenic amines and acetylcholine.

Cholinergic transmission is thought to be excessive in depression and inadequate in mania (Sadock et al., 2015). The precise role that any neurotransmitters play in the etiology of depression is unknown because these chemicals cannot be measured in the human brain. It has been theorized that because selective serotonin reuptake inhibitors (SSRIs) are drugs that elevate serotonin levels, low serotonin levels in the brain must be responsible for depression. However, SSRIs also seem to be beneficial in the treatment of anxiety, leading to the hypothesis that low serotonin levels are responsible for anxiety. Further, too much serotonin has also been implicated in anxiety states and in schizophrenia. All of this seemingly contradictory information has led many current researchers to believe that neurotransmitters such as serotonin might be better explained as modulators of intense emotional states rather than associated with any one particular emotion (Sadock et al., 2015). Newer antidepressants that act on both serotonergic and noradrenergic receptors suggest that the dysregulation of biogenic amines in depression is far more complex than can be explained by single neurotransmitter hypotheses (Akiskal, 2017). Ongoing research will hopefully clarify what are, at present, only hypotheses about the etiology of depression.

Neuroendocrine Disturbances

Neuroendocrine disturbances may play a role in the pathogenesis or persistence of depressive illness. This notion has arisen in view of the marked disturbances in mood observed with the administration of certain hormones or in the presence of spontaneously occurring endocrine disease.

Hypothalamic-Pituitary-Adrenocortical Axis

In clients who are depressed, the normal system of hormonal inhibition fails, resulting in a hypersecretion of cortisol. This elevated serum cortisol is the basis for the dexamethasone suppression test that is sometimes used to determine if an individual has somatically treatable depression.

Hypothalamic-Pituitary-Thyroid Axis

Thyrotropin-releasing factor (TRF) from the hypothalamus stimulates the release of thyroid-stimulating hormone (TSH) from the anterior pituitary gland. In turn, TSH stimulates the thyroid gland. Diminished TSH response to administered TRF is observed in approximately 25 percent of depressed persons and appears to be associated with increased risk for relapse despite treatment with antidepressants (Sadock et al., 2015). Individuals with hypothyroidism often manifest with signs of depression (in addition to a host of other symptoms), and nearly 20 million people in the United States (women are five to eight times more likely than men) suffer from thyroid conditions (American Thyroid Association, 2018). Laboratory testing to evaluate TSH is relevant to distinguish between depressive disorders and thyroid disorders because, in thyroid disorders, the symptoms of depression are treated with hormone replacement rather than antidepressants.

Although there is not a single diagnostic test for depression, several findings from tests that may indicate depression but are nonspecific, such as increased corticotropin releasing factor in cerebrospinal fluid, steroid overproduction (evidenced by the dexamethasone suppression test), and thyroid dysregulation (evidenced by thyrotropin challenge tests), lead Akiskal (2017) to conclude that there is clear evidence of midbrain disturbance (and thus, evidence of a legitimate disease process) in clinical depression.

Physiological Influences

Depressive symptoms that occur as a consequence of a non-mood disorder or as an adverse effect of certain medications are called *secondary* depression. Secondary depression may be related to medication side effects, neurological disorders, electrolyte or hormonal disturbances, nutritional deficiencies, and other physiological or psychological conditions.

Medication Side Effects

A number of drugs, either alone or in combination with other medications, can produce a depressive syndrome. Most common among these drugs are those that have a direct effect on the central nervous system. Examples of these include the anxiolytics, antipsychotics, sedative-hypnotics (including barbiturates and opioids), and anticonvulsant mood stabilizers. Many drugs that are used to treat general medical conditions have also been associated with inducing depression and several are listed here:

- Antibacterial, antifungal, and antiviral agents
- Antihypertensives (including beta blockers and calcium blockers)
- Antineoplastics (including vincristine and zidovudine)
- Dermatologics (including Accutane and finasteride)
- Hormones (including contraceptives)
- Respiratory agents (leukotriene inhibitors)
- Statins
- Steroids
- Smoking cessation agents (varenicline)
- Anticonvulsants

Neurological Disorders

An individual who has had a cardiovascular accident (CVA) may experience despondency unrelated to the severity of the CVA. These are true mood disorders, and antidepressant drug therapy may be indicated. Brain tumors, particularly in the area of the temporal lobe, often cause symptoms of depression. Agitated depression may be part of the clinical picture associated with Alzheimer's disease, Parkinson's disease, and Huntington's disease. Agitation and restlessness may also represent an underlying depression in the individual with multiple sclerosis.

Electrolyte Disturbances

Excessive levels of sodium bicarbonate or calcium can produce symptoms of depression, as can deficits in magnesium and sodium. Potassium is also implicated in the syndrome of depression. Symptoms have been observed with excesses of potassium in the body as well as in instances of potassium depletion. Interestingly, *hypo*natremia is a side effect of serotonergic antidepressants, especially in the elderly.

Hormonal Disturbances

Depression is associated with dysfunction of the adrenal cortex and is commonly observed in both Addison's disease and Cushing's syndrome. Other endocrine conditions that may result in symptoms of depression include hypoparathyroidism, hyperparathyroidism, hypothyroidism, and hyperthyroidism.

An imbalance of the hormones estrogen and progesterone has been implicated in the predisposition to premenstrual dysphoric disorder (PMDD), although the exact etiology is unknown. The interaction of these hormonal changes also has an impact on serotonin levels, which may contribute to the depression associated with this disorder. It is also noted that individuals with PMDD often have underlying depression and anxiety, so it is possible that the hormone changes are exacerbating an already existing condition (Thielen, 2015).

Nutritional Deficiencies

Deficiencies in proteins, carbohydrates, vitamin B_1 (thiamine), vitamin B_2 (riboflavin), vitamin B_6 (pyridoxine), vitamin B_9 (folate), vitamin B_{12}, iron, zinc, calcium, chromium, iodine, lithium, selenium, and potassium have all been associated with producing symptoms of depression (Holland, 2016; Sathyanarayana et al., 2008). It is not surprising that individuals with anorexia nervosa, who have significant nutritional deficiencies, commonly have comorbid depression.

Other Physiological Conditions

Other conditions that have been associated with secondary depression include collagen disorders, such as systemic lupus erythematosus (SLE) and polyarteritis nodosa; cardiovascular disease, such as cardiomyopathy, congestive heart failure, and myocardial infarction; infections, such as encephalitis, hepatitis, mononucleosis, pneumonia, and syphilis; and metabolic disorders, such as diabetes mellitus and porphyria.

The Role of Inflammation

The role of inflammation in the development of depression is an area of current research. The function of the immune system in the development of disease is being explored with regard to a host of illnesses including cancer, autoimmune disorders, and several psychiatric disorders. Not all patients with depression have signs of inflammation but individuals with treatment-resistant depression manifest with high C-reactive protein levels (CRP) and tumor necrosis factor (TNF), which are biomarkers of inflammation (Miller, 2018). Cytokines, part of the inflammatory response, have specific activities in the brain, including impacting neurotransmitters associated with depression (monoamines) and dopamine. Stress, another inflammatory process, has been shown to increase the permeability of the blood-brain barrier and consequently may have an impact on the development of depression when inflammatory responses in the brain trigger chemical changes. Does depression trigger inflammation or is inflammation one potential cause of depression? Much more research is needed but there is current evidence that elevated inflammation biomarkers can predict a patient's response to conventional antidepressants, psychotherapy, ketamine, and anti-cytokine immunotherapy (Miller, 2018). This research reinforces the complex interactions and dynamics associated with the disease of depression.

Psychosocial Theories

Psychoanalytical Theory

Freud (1957) presented his classic paper "Mourning and Melancholia" in 1917. He defined the distinguishing features of melancholia as

> a profoundly painful dejection, cessation of interest in the outside world, loss of the capacity to love, inhibition of all activity, and a lowering of the self-regarding feelings to a degree that finds utterances in self-reproaches and self-revilings, and culminates in a delusional expectation of punishment.

He observed that melancholia occurs after the loss of a loved object, either actually by death or emotionally by rejection, or the loss of some other abstraction of value to the individual. Freud indicated that in melancholia, the depressed patient's rage is internally directed because of identification with the lost object (Sadock et al., 2015).

Freud believed that the individual predisposed to melancholia experienced ambivalence in love relationships. He postulated, therefore, that once the loss had been incorporated into the self (ego), the hostile part of the ambivalence that had been felt for the lost object is then turned inward against the ego.

Learning Theory

The model of "learned helplessness" arises out of Seligman's (1973) experiments with dogs. The animals were exposed to electrical stimulation from which they could not escape. Later, when they were given the opportunity to avoid the traumatic experience, they reacted with helplessness and made no attempt to escape. A similar state of helplessness exists in humans who have experienced numerous failures (either real or perceived). The individual abandons any further attempt to succeed. Seligman theorized that learned helplessness predisposes individuals to depression by imposing a feeling of lack of control over their life situation. They become depressed because they feel helpless; they have learned that whatever they do is futile. This can be especially damaging very early in life because the sense of mastery over one's environment is an important foundation for future emotional development.

Object Loss Theory

The theory of object loss suggests that depressive illness occurs as a result of having been abandoned by or otherwise separated from a significant other during the first 6 months of life. Because during this period the mother represents the child's main source of security, she is considered to be the "object." This absence of attachment, which may be either physical or emotional, leads to feelings of helplessness and despair that contribute to lifelong patterns of depression in response to loss.

The concept of "anaclitic depression" was introduced in 1946 by psychiatrist René Spitz to refer to children who became depressed after being separated from their mothers for an extended period during the first year of life. The condition included behaviors such as excessive crying, anorexia, withdrawal, **psychomotor retardation,** stupor, and a generalized impairment in the normal process of growth and development. Object loss theory suggests that loss in adult life afflicts people much more severely in the form of depression if the individuals have suffered early childhood loss.

Cognitive Theory

Beck and colleagues (1979) proposed a theory suggesting that the primary disturbance in depression is cognitive rather than affective. The underlying cause of the depression is cognitive distortions that result in negative, defeated attitudes. Beck and colleagues identified three cognitive distortions that they believe serve as the basis for depression:

1. Negative expectations of the environment
2. Negative expectations of the self
3. Negative expectations of the future

These cognitive distortions arise out of a defect in cognitive development, and the individual feels inadequate, worthless, and rejected by others. Outlook for the future is one of pessimism and hopelessness.

Cognitive theorists believe that depression is the product of negative thinking. This is in contrast to the suggestions by other theorists that negative thinking occurs when an individual is depressed. **Cognitive therapy** focuses on helping the individual to alter mood by changing the way he or she thinks. The individual is taught to control negative thought distortions that lead to pessimism, lethargy, procrastination, indecisiveness, and low self-esteem.

The Transactional Model of Stress and Adaptation

As is clearly evident, no single theory or hypothesis exists to substantiate a clear-cut explanation for depressive disorder. Evidence continues to mount in support of multiple causation. The transactional model of stress and adaptation recognizes the combined effects of genetic, biochemical, and psychosocial influences on an individual's susceptibility to depression (for more information on the transactional model of stress and adaptation, see Chapter 19, Trauma- and Stressor-Related Disorders).

Developmental Implications

Childhood

Only in recent years has a consensus developed among investigators identifying MDD as an entity in children and adolescents that can be identified using criteria similar to those used for adults. It is not uncommon, however, for the symptoms of depression to be manifested differently in childhood, and the picture changes with age (Anxiety and Depression Association of America, 2016; Sadock et al., 2015):

1. **Up to age 3:** Signs may include feeding problems, tantrums, lack of playfulness and emotional expressiveness, failure to thrive, or delays in speech and gross motor development.
2. **From ages 3 to 5:** Common symptoms may include accident proneness, phobias, aggressiveness, and excessive self-reproach for minor infractions. The incidence among preschool children is estimated to be between 0.3 and 0.9 percent.
3. **From ages 6 to 8:** These children may have vague physical complaints and display aggressive behavior. They may cling to parents and avoid new people and challenges. They may lag behind their classmates in social skills and academic competence.
4. **From ages 9 to 12:** Common symptoms include morbid thoughts and excessive worrying. They may reason that they are depressed because they have disappointed their parents in some way. There may be lack of interest in playing with friends. The incidence of depression among school-age children is estimated to be around 2 to 3 percent.

Other symptoms of childhood and adolescent depression may include hyperactivity, delinquency, school problems, psychosomatic complaints, sleeping and eating disturbances, social isolation, delusional thinking, and suicidal thoughts or actions. Wagner and Brent (2017) note that youth with depression are more often irritable rather than dysphoric and consequently less likely to identify themselves as depressed. Additionally, they cite that anywhere from 40 to 90 percent of youth with depression have other comorbid psychiatric conditions so comprehensive assessment is essential.

The APA (2013) has included a new diagnostic category in the Depressive Disorders chapter of the *DSM-5*. This childhood disorder is called *Disruptive Mood Dysregulation Disorder*. The diagnostic criteria for disruptive mood dysregulation disorder are presented in Box 16–3.

Children may become depressed for various reasons. In many depressed children, there is a genetic predisposition toward the condition, which is then precipitated by a stressful situation. Common precipitating factors include physical or emotional detachment by the primary caregiver, parental separation or divorce, death of a loved one (person or pet), a move, academic failure, or physical illness. In any event, the common denominator is loss.

The focus of therapy for depressed children is to alleviate the child's symptoms and strengthen the child's coping and adaptive skills with the hope of possibly preventing future psychological problems. Some studies have shown that untreated childhood depression may lead to subsequent problems in adolescence and adult life. Most children are treated on an outpatient basis. Hospitalization of the depressed child usually occurs only if he or she is actively suicidal, when the home environment precludes adherence to a treatment regimen, or if the child needs to be separated from the home because of psychosocial deprivation.

Parental and family therapy are commonly used to help the younger depressed child. Recovery is facilitated by emotional support and guidance to family members. Children older than age 8 years usually participate in family therapy. In some situations, individual treatment may be appropriate for older children. Medications, such as antidepressants, can be important in the treatment of children, especially for the more serious and recurrent forms of depression. The SSRIs have been used with success, particularly in combination with psychosocial therapies. However, because there has been some concern that the use of antidepressant medications may cause suicidal behavior in young people, the U.S. Food and Drug Administration (FDA) has applied a black-box label warning (described in the next section) to all

BOX 16–3 Diagnostic Criteria for Disruptive Mood Dysregulation Disorder

A. Severe recurrent temper outbursts manifested verbally (e.g., verbal rages) and/or behaviorally (e.g., physical aggression toward people or property) that are grossly out of proportion in intensity or duration to the situation or provocation.

B. The temper outbursts are inconsistent with developmental level.

C. The temper outbursts occur, on average, three or more times per week.

D. The mood between temper outbursts is persistently irritable or angry most of the day, nearly every day, and is observable by others (e.g., parents, teachers, peers).

E. Criteria A–D have been present for 12 or more months. Throughout that time, the individual has not had a period lasting 3 or more consecutive months without all of the symptoms of Criteria A–D.

F. Criteria A and D are present in at least two of three settings (i.e., at home, at school, with peers) and are severe in at least one of these.

G. The diagnosis should not be made for the first time before age 6 or after age 18 years.

H. By history or observation, the age at onset of Criteria A–E is before 10 years.

I. There has never been a distinct period lasting more than 1 day during which the full symptom criteria, except duration, for a manic or hypomanic episode have been met. *Note:* Developmentally appropriate mood elevation, such as occurs in the context of a highly positive event or its anticipation, should not be considered as a symptom of mania or hypomania.

J. The behaviors do not occur exclusively during an episode of major depressive disorder and are not better explained by another mental disorder (e.g., autism spectrum disorder, post-traumatic stress disorder, separation anxiety disorder, persistent depressive disorder [dysthymia]).

Note: This diagnosis cannot coexist with oppositional defiant disorder, intermittent explosive disorder, or bipolar disorder, though it can coexist with others, including major depressive disorder, attention-deficit/ hyperactivity disorder, conduct disorder, and substance use disorders. Individuals whose symptoms meet criteria for both disruptive mood dysregulation disorder and oppositional defiant disorder should only be given the diagnosis of disruptive mood dysregulation disorder. If an individual has ever experienced a manic or hypomanic episode, the diagnosis of disruptive mood dysregulation disorder should not be assigned.

K. The symptoms are not attributable to the physiological effects of a substance or to another medical or neurological condition.

Reprinted with permission from American Psychiatric Association. (2013). Diagnostic and statistical manual of mental disorders (5th ed.). Washington, DC: American Psychiatric Publishing.

---

antidepressant medications. The National Institute of Mental Health (NIMH, 2018) stated:

> In some cases, children, teenagers, and young adults under 25 may experience an increase in suicidal thoughts or behavior when taking antidepressants, especially in the first few weeks after starting or when the dose is changed. This warning from the U.S. Food and Drug Administration (FDA) also says that patients of all ages taking antidepressants should be watched closely, especially during the first few weeks of treatment.

Adolescence

Depression may be even harder to recognize in an adolescent than in a younger child. Feelings of sadness, loneliness, anxiety, and hopelessness associated with depression may be perceived as the normal emotional stresses of growing up. Therefore, many young people whose symptoms are attributed to the "normal adjustments" of adolescence do not get the help they need. Depression is a major cause of suicide among teens, and suicide is the second-leading cause of death in the 15- to 24-year-old age group (NCHS, 2018).

Common symptoms of depression in the adolescent are inappropriately expressed anger, aggressiveness, running away, delinquency, social withdrawal, sexual acting out, substance abuse, restlessness, and apathy. Loss of self-esteem, sleeping and eating disturbances, and psychosomatic complaints are also common.

What, then, is the indicator that differentiates mood disorder from the typical turbulent behavior of adolescence? A visible manifestation of *behavioral change that lasts for several weeks* is the best clue for a mood disorder. Examples include the normally outgoing and extroverted adolescent who becomes withdrawn and isolates herself, the good student who previously received consistently high marks but is now failing and skipping classes, and the usually self-confident teenager who is now inappropriately irritable and defensive with others.

Adolescents become depressed for the same reasons that were discussed under childhood depression. In adolescence, however, depression is a common manifestation of the stress and independence conflicts associated with the normal maturation process. Depression may also be the response to death of a parent, other relative, or friend or to a breakup with a boyfriend or girlfriend. This perception of abandonment by parents or closest peer relationship is thought to be the most frequent immediate precipitant to adolescent suicide.

Treatment of the depressed adolescent is often conducted on an outpatient basis. Hospitalization may be required in cases of severe depression or threat of imminent suicide, when a family situation is such that treatment cannot be carried out in the home, when the physical condition precludes self-care of biological needs, or when the adolescent has indicated possible harm to self or others in the family.

In addition to supportive psychosocial intervention, antidepressant therapy may be part of the treatment of adolescent mood disorders. However, as mentioned previously, the FDA has issued a public health advisory warning the public about the increased risk of suicidal thoughts and behavior in children and adolescents being treated with antidepressant medications. The black-box warning label on all antidepressant medications describes this risk and emphasizes the need for close monitoring of clients started on these medications. The advisory language does not prohibit the use of antidepressants in children and adolescents. Rather, it warns of the risk of suicidality and encourages prescribers to balance this risk with clinical need.

Fluoxetine (Prozac) has been approved by the FDA to treat depression in children and adolescents, and escitalopram (Lexapro) was approved in 2009 for treatment of MDD in adolescents aged 12 to 17 years. The other SSRI medications, such as sertraline, citalopram, and paroxetine, and the serotonin-norepinephrine reuptake inhibitor (SNRI) antidepressants duloxetine, venlafaxine, and desvenlafaxine have not been approved for treatment of depression in children or adolescents, although they have been prescribed to children by physicians in "off-label use"—a use other than the FDA-approved use. In June 2003, the FDA recommended that paroxetine not be used in children and adolescents for the treatment of MDD. The FDA analysis of antidepressant medications, as reported by the Mayo Clinic (2016), identified that a small percentage of those taking antidepressants had an increase in suicidal thoughts and that none of the children in the study actually took their own life. Nonetheless, the potential risk is considered significant enough to carefully evaluate risks versus benefits before prescribing antidepressants to children and adolescents.

Senescence

The elderly make up 14.5 percent of the general population of the United States (United States Census Bureau, 2017) and depression (along with dementia) is one of the most common psychiatric disorders in this group. Estimates are that about 1 to 5 percent of older adults living in the community have depression but that incidence increases to 13.5 percent for those requiring home healthcare. Depression is also more common in older adults with other medical conditions, such as heart disease and limited functioning (Centers for Disease Control [CDC], 2017).

Depression among the elderly may be influenced by the value our society places on youth, vigor, and uninterrupted productivity. These societal attitudes reinforce feelings of low self-esteem, helplessness, and hopelessness that become more pervasive and intensive with advanced age. Further, the aging individual's adaptive coping strategies may be seriously challenged by major stressors, such as financial problems, physical illness, changes in bodily functioning, and an increasing awareness of approaching death. The problem is often intensified by the numerous losses that individuals experience during this period in life, such as spouse, friends, children, home, and independence. A phenomenon called *bereavement overload* occurs when individuals experience so many losses in their lives that they are not able to resolve one grief response before another one begins. Bereavement overload predisposes elderly individuals to depressive illness. Evidence-based treatments for depression will continue to be a focal point of care for this population.

Although they make up only about 14.5 percent of the population, the elderly account for a proportionately larger percentage of the suicides in the United States. The rate of suicide in those aged 65 to 74 is 15.38 percent; in those aged 75 to 84 the rate increases to 18.3 percent; and for those 85 years of age and older the rate jumps to 18.98 percent (American Foundation for Suicide Prevention, 2018). For all ages and races, including the elderly, the highest number of these suicides is among white men at almost four times the national rate.

Symptoms of depression in the elderly are not very different from those in younger adults. However, depressive syndromes may be confused with those of other illnesses associated with the aging process. Symptoms of depression are often misdiagnosed as neurocognitive disorder (NCD) when, in fact, the memory loss, confused thinking, or apathy symptomatic of NCD may be the result of depression. The early awakening and reduced appetite typical of depression are common among many older people who are not depressed. Compounding this situation is that many medical conditions, including endocrinological, neurological, nutritional, and metabolic disorders, often present with classic symptoms of depression. Many medications commonly used by the elderly, such as antihypertensives, corticosteroids, and analgesics, can also produce a depressant effect.

Depression accompanies many of the illnesses that affect older people, such as Parkinson's disease, cancer, arthritis, and the early stages of Alzheimer's disease. Treating depression in these situations can reduce unnecessary suffering and help individuals cope with their medical problems.

The most effective treatment for depression in the elderly individual is thought to be a combination of psychosocial and biological approaches. Antidepressant medications are administered with consideration for age-related physiological changes in absorption, distribution, elimination, and brain receptor sensitivity. Because of these changes, plasma concentrations of these medications can reach very high levels despite moderate oral doses. Anticholinergic side effects associated with tricyclic antidepressants can be problematic for the elderly, and SSRIs have been associated with inducing significant hyponatremia in this population, so careful evaluation and monitoring are essential.

In the elderly, especially considering the problematic side effects of antidepressants in this population, the response to electroconvulsive therapy (ECT) may be slower with advancing age, and the therapeutic effects are of limited duration. In a systematic review, researchers concluded that use of ECT in the elderly is "highly effective, safe, and well tolerated" in the geriatric population (Geduldig & Kellner, 2016). It may be considered the treatment of choice for the elderly individual who is an acute suicidal risk or is unable to tolerate antidepressant medications. Confusion, a side effect of ECT that typically lasts a few minutes to several hours, is generally more pronounced in the elderly (Mayo Clinic, 2018).

Other therapeutic approaches include interpersonal, behavioral, cognitive, group, and family psychotherapies. Appropriate treatment of the depressed elderly individual can bring relief from suffering and offer a new lease on life with a feeling of renewed productivity.

Postpartum Depression

The severity of depression in the postpartum period varies from a feeling of the blues to moderate depression to severe depression with psychotic features. About 50 percent of these episodes actually begin prior to delivery (APA, 2013) and the onset of symptoms during pregnancy increases risk for major depression in the postpartum period. Major depression with psychotic features occurs in about 1 or 2 out of 1,000 postpartum women.

Symptoms of the "baby blues" include worry, sadness, and fatigue after having a baby. These symptoms affect about 80 percent of mothers and usually subside within a week or two (National Institute of Mental Health, n.d.).

Symptoms of moderate **postpartum depression** have been described as depressed mood varying from day to day, with more bad days than good, tending to be worse toward evening and associated with fatigue, irritability, loss of appetite, sleep disturbances, and loss of libido. In addition, the new mother expresses a great deal of concern about her inability to care for her baby. These symptoms begin somewhat later than those described in the maternity blues and take from a few weeks to several months to abate.

Postpartum depression with psychotic features is characterized by depressed mood, agitation, indecision, lack of concentration, guilt, and an abnormal attitude toward bodily functions. The symptoms can be severe and incapacitating. There may be lack of interest in or rejection of the baby or a morbid fear that the baby may be harmed, accompanied by delusions and hallucinations. Risks of suicide and infanticide should not be overlooked. There is a 30 to 50 percent likelihood of postpartum psychosis recurring with subsequent pregnancies (APA, 2013).

The etiology of postpartum depression remains unclear. Maternity blues may be associated with hormonal changes, tryptophan metabolism, or alterations in membrane transport during the early postpartum period. Besides being exposed to these same somatic changes, the woman who experiences moderate to severe symptoms probably possesses a vulnerability to depression related to heredity, upbringing, early life experiences, personality, or social circumstances. A history of depression appears to be a risk factor for postpartum depression (NIMH, 2018) and family history of psychiatric disorders, including schizophrenia, bipolar, depression, and other psychiatric disorders, also increases risk (Bauer et al., 2018). The etiology of postpartum depression may very likely be a combination of hormonal, metabolic, and psychosocial influences.

Treatment of postpartum depression varies with the severity of the illness. Psychotic depression may be treated with antidepressant medication, along with supportive psychotherapy, group therapy, and possibly family therapy. Moderate depression may be relieved with supportive psychotherapy and continuing assistance with home management until the symptoms subside. Maternity blues usually needs no treatment beyond reassurance from the physician or nurse that these feelings are common and will soon pass. Extra support and comfort from significant others also is important.

Application of the Nursing Process

Background Assessment Data

Symptomatology of depression can be viewed on a continuum from transient symptoms to severe depression according to severity of the illness. All individuals become depressed from time to time in response to life's disappointments, and these symptoms tend to be transient. Severe depression, however, is marked by significant distress that interferes with social, occupational, cognitive, and emotional functioning.

The individual who is severely depressed may also demonstrate a loss of contact with reality. This level is associated with a complete lack of pleasure in all activities, and ruminations about suicide are common. MDD is an example of severe depression. A continuum of depression is presented in Figure 16–2.

A number of assessment rating scales are available for measuring severity of depressive symptoms. Some are meant to be clinician administered, whereas others may be self-administered. Examples of self-rating scales include the Zung Self-Rating Depression Scale and the Beck Depression Inventory. One of the most widely used clinician-administered scales is the Hamilton Depression Rating Scale (HDRS) (Box 16–4). It has been reviewed and revised over the years and exists today in several versions. The original version contains seventeen items and is designed to measure mood, guilty feelings, suicidal ideation, sleep disturbances, anxiety levels, and weight loss.

Symptoms of depression can be described as alterations in four spheres of human functioning: (1) affective, (2) behavioral, (3) cognitive, and (4) physiological. Alterations within these spheres differ according to degree of severity of symptomatology.

Transient Depression

Symptoms at this level of the continuum are not necessarily dysfunctional; in fact, they may be considered part of the broad range of typical human emotional responses that accompany everyday disappointments in life. Transient depression subsides quickly, and the individual is able to refocus on other goals and achievements. Alterations include the following:

- **Affective:** Sadness, dejection, feeling downhearted, having the blues
- **Behavioral:** Some crying
- **Cognitive:** Some difficulty getting mind off one's disappointment
- **Physiological:** Feeling tired and listless

Mild Depression

Symptoms at the mild level of depression are like those associated with uncomplicated grieving. Alterations at the mild level include the following:

- **Affective:** Denial of feelings, anger, anxiety, guilt, helplessness, hopelessness, sadness, despondency
- **Behavioral:** Tearfulness, regression, restlessness, agitation, withdrawal
- **Cognitive:** Preoccupation with the loss, self-blame, ambivalence, blaming others
- **Physiological:** Anorexia or overeating, insomnia or hypersomnia, headache, backache, chest pain, or other symptoms associated with the loss of a significant other

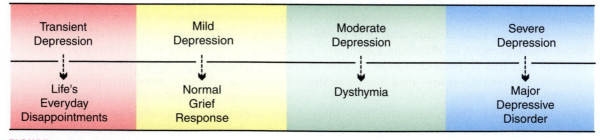

FIGURE 16–2 A continuum of depression.

BOX 16–4 Hamilton Depression Rating Scale (HDRS)

Instructions: For each item, circle the number to select the one "cue" that best characterizes the patient.

1. Depressed Mood (sadness, hopeless, helpless, worthless)
- 0 = Absent
- 1 = These feeling states indicated only on questioning
- 2 = These feeling states spontaneously reported verbally
- 3 = Communicates feeling states nonverbally (e.g., through facial expression, posture, voice, tendency to weep)
- 4 = Patient reports virtually only these feeling states in spontaneous verbal and nonverbal communication

2. Feelings of Guilt
- 0 = Absent
- 1 = Self-reproach; feels he/she has let people down
- 2 = Ideas of guilt or rumination over past errors or sinful deeds
- 3 = Present illness is a punishment; delusions of guilt
- 4 = Hears accusatory or denunciatory voices and/or experiences threatening visual hallucinations

3. Suicide
- 0 = Absent
- 1 = Feels life is not worth living
- 2 = Wishes he/she were dead or any thoughts of possible death to self
- 3 = Suicidal ideas or gesture
- 4 = Attempts at suicide (any serious attempt rates 4)

4. Insomnia: Early in the Night
- 0 = No difficulty falling asleep
- 1 = Complains of occasional difficulty falling asleep (i.e., more than ½ hour)
- 2 = Complains of nightly difficulty falling asleep

5. Insomnia: Middle of the Night
- 0 = No difficulty
- 1 = Complains of being restless and disturbed during the night
- 2 = Waking during the night—any getting out of bed rates 2 (except for purposes of voiding)

6. Insomnia: Early Hours of the Morning
- 0 = No difficulty
- 1 = Wakes in early hours of the morning but goes back to sleep
- 2 = Unable to fall asleep again if he/she gets out of bed

7. Work and Activities
- 0 = No difficulty
- 1 = Thoughts and feelings of incapacity, fatigue, or weakness related to activities, work, or hobbies
- 2 = Loss of interest in activity, hobbies, or work—either directly reported by patient or indirectly in listlessness, indecision, and vacillation (feels he/she has to push self to work or do activities)
- 3 = Decrease in actual time spent in activities or decrease in productivity. Rate 3 if patient does not spend at least 3 hours a day in activities (job or hobbies), excluding routine chores
- 4 = Stopped working because of present illness. Rate 4 if patient engages in no activities except routine chores or does not perform routine chores unassisted

8. Psychomotor Retardation (slowness of thought and speech, impaired ability to concentrate, decreased motor activity)
- 0 = Normal speech and thought
- 1 = Slight retardation during the interview
- 2 = Obvious retardation during the interview
- 3 = Interview difficult
- 4 = Complete stupor

9. Agitation
- 0 = None
- 1 = Fidgetiness
- 2 = Playing with hands, hair, etc.
- 3 = Moving about, can't sit still
- 4 = Hand wringing, nail biting, hair pulling, biting of lips

10. Anxiety (Psychic)
- 0 = No difficulty
- 1 = Subjective tension and irritability
- 2 = Worrying about minor matters
- 3 = Apprehensive attitude apparent in face or speech
- 4 = Fears expressed without questioning

11. Anxiety (Somatic): Physiological concomitants of anxiety (e.g., dry mouth, indigestion, diarrhea, cramps, belching, palpitations, headache, tremor, hyperventilation, sighing, urinary frequency, sweating, flushing)
- 0 = Absent
- 1 = Mild
- 2 = Moderate
- 3 = Severe
- 4 = Incapacitating

12. Somatic Symptoms (Gastrointestinal)
- 0 = None
- 1 = Loss of appetite, but eating without encouragement; heavy feelings in abdomen
- 2 = Difficulty eating without urging from others; requests or requires medication for constipation or gastrointestinal symptoms

13. Somatic Symptoms (General)
- 0 = None
- 1 = Heaviness in limbs, back or head; backaches, headache, muscle aches; loss of energy and fatigability
- 2 = Any clear-cut symptom rates 2

Continued

BOX 16-4 Hamilton Depression Rating Scale (HDRS)—cont'd

14. **Genital Symptoms** (e.g., loss of libido, impaired sexual performance, menstrual disturbances)
   - 0 = Absent
   - 1 = Mild
   - 2 = Severe
15. **Hypochondriasis**
   - 0 = Not present
   - 1 = Self-absorption (bodily)
   - 2 = Preoccupation with health
   - 3 = Frequent complaints, requests for help, etc.
   - 4 = Hypochondriacal delusions
16. **Loss of Weight** (rate *either* A *or* B)
   - **A. According to subjective patient history:**
     - 0 = No weight loss
     - 1 = Probably weight loss associated with present illness
     - 2 = Definite weight loss associated with present illness
   - **B. According to objective weekly measurements:**
     - 0 = Less than 1 lb. weight loss in week

   - 1 = Greater than 1 lb. weight loss in week
   - 2 = Greater than 2 lb. weight loss in week
17. **Insight**
   - 0 = Acknowledges being depressed and ill
   - 1 = Acknowledges illness but attributes cause to bad food, climate, overwork, virus, need for rest, etc.
   - 2 = Denies being ill at all

SCORING:
   - 0–6 = No evidence of depressive illness
   - 7–17 = Mild depression
   - 18–24 = Moderate depression
   - >24 = Severe depression

TOTAL SCORE_____

Source: Hamilton, M. (1960). *A rating scale for depression.* Journal of Neurology, Neurosurgery, & Psychiatry, 23, 56–62. The HDRS is in the public domain.

Moderate Depression

Dysthymia (also called *persistent depressive disorder*) is an example of moderate depression and represents a more problematic disturbance that, according to the *DSM-5,* is characterized by symptoms that are enduring for at least 2 years (APA, 2013). Symptoms associated with this disorder include the following:

■ **Affective:** Feelings of sadness, dejection, helplessness, powerlessness, hopelessness; gloomy and pessimistic outlook; low self-esteem; difficulty experiencing pleasure in activities
■ **Behavioral:** Sluggish physical movements (i.e., psychomotor retardation); slumped posture; slowed speech; limited verbalizations, possibly consisting of ruminations about life's failures or regrets; social isolation with a focus on the self; increased use of substances possible; self-destructive behavior possible; decreased interest in personal hygiene and grooming
■ **Cognitive:** Slowed thinking processes; difficulty concentrating and directing attention; obsessive and repetitive thoughts, generally portraying pessimism and negativism; verbalizations and behavior reflecting suicidal ideation
■ **Physiological:** Anorexia or overeating; insomnia or hypersomnia; sleep disturbances; amenorrhea; decreased libido; headaches; backaches; chest pain; abdominal pain; low energy level; fatigue

and listlessness; feeling best early in the morning and continually worse as the day progresses (this may be related to the diurnal variation in the level of neurotransmitters that affect mood and level of activity)

Severe Depression

Severe depression (also called *major depressive disorder*) is characterized by an intensification of the symptoms described for moderate depression (see Box 16–1). Symptoms at the severe level of depression include the following:

■ **Affective:** Feelings of total despair, hopelessness, and worthlessness; flat (unchanging) affect, appearing devoid of emotional tone; prevalent feelings of nothingness and emptiness; apathy; loneliness; sadness; inability to feel pleasure
■ **Behavioral:** Psychomotor retardation so severe that physical movement may literally come to a standstill, or psychomotor behavior manifested by rapid, agitated, purposeless movements; slumped posture; sitting in a curled-up position; walking slowly and rigidly; virtually nonexistent communication (when verbalizations do occur, they may reflect delusional thinking); no personal hygiene and grooming; social isolation is common, with virtually no inclination toward interaction with others

■ **Cognitive:** Prevalent delusional thinking with delusions of persecution and somatic delusions being most common; confusion, indecisiveness, and an inability to concentrate; hallucinations reflecting misinterpretations of the environment; excessive self-deprecation, self-blame, and thoughts of suicide

NOTE: Because of the low energy level and slow thought processes, the individual may be unable to follow through on suicidal ideas. However, the desire is strong at this level.

■ **Physiological:** A general slowdown of the entire body, reflected in sluggish digestion, constipation, and urinary retention; amenorrhea; impotence; diminished libido; anorexia; weight loss; difficulty falling asleep and awakening very early in the morning; feeling worse early in the morning and somewhat better as the day progresses (as with moderate depression, this may reflect the diurnal variation in the level of neurotransmitters that affect mood and activity)

Diagnosis and Outcome Identification

Using information collected during the assessment, the nurse completes the patient database from which the selection of appropriate nursing diagnoses is determined. Table 16–1 presents a list of behaviors and the NANDA International nursing diagnoses (Herdman & Kamitsuru, 2018) that correspond to those behaviors, which may be used in planning care for the depressed patient.

Outcome Criteria

The following criteria may be used for measurement of outcomes in the care of the depressed patient.

The patient:

■ Has experienced no physical harm to self.
■ Discusses feelings with staff and family members.
■ Expresses hopefulness.
■ Sets realistic goals for self.
■ Is no longer afraid to attempt new activities.
■ Is able to identify aspects of self-control over life situation.

TABLE 16–1 Assigning Nursing Diagnoses to Behaviors Commonly Associated With Depression

BEHAVIORS	NURSING DIAGNOSES
Depressed mood; feelings of hopelessness and worthlessness; anger turned inward in the self; misinterpretations of reality; suicidal ideation, plan, and available means	Risk for suicide
Depression, preoccupation with thoughts of loss, self-blame, grief avoidance, inappropriate expression of anger, decreased functioning in life roles	Complicated grieving
Expressions of helplessness, uselessness, guilt, and shame; hypersensitivity to slight or criticism; negative, pessimistic outlook; lack of eye contact; self-negating verbalizations	Low self-esteem
Apathy, verbal expressions of having no control, dependence on others to fulfill needs	Powerlessness
Expresses anger toward God, expresses lack of meaning in life, sudden changes in spiritual practices, refuses interactions with significant others or with spiritual leaders	Spiritual distress
Withdrawn, uncommunicative, seeks to be alone, dysfunctional interaction with others, discomfort in social situations	Social isolation/Impaired social interaction
Inappropriate thinking, confusion, difficulty concentrating, impaired problem-solving ability, inaccurate interpretation of environment, memory deficit	Disturbed thought processes*
Weight loss, poor muscle tone, pale conjunctiva and mucous membranes, poor skin turgor, weakness	Imbalanced nutrition: Less than body requirements
Difficulty falling asleep, difficulty staying asleep, lack of energy, difficulty concentrating, verbal reports of not feeling well rested	Insomnia
Uncombed hair, disheveled clothing, offensive body odor	Self-care deficit (hygiene, grooming)

*This diagnosis has been resigned from the NANDA-I list of approved diagnoses. It is used in this instance because it is most compatible with the identified behaviors.

- Expresses personal satisfaction and support from spiritual practices.
- Interacts willingly and appropriately with others.
- Is able to maintain reality orientation.
- Is able to concentrate, reason, solve problems, and make decisions.
- Eats a well-balanced diet with snacks to prevent weight loss and maintain nutritional status.
- Sleeps 6 to 8 hours per night and reports feeling well rested.
- Bathes, washes and combs hair, and dresses in clean clothing without assistance.

Planning and Implementation

Table 16–2 presents a plan of care for the depressed patient. Selected nursing diagnoses are presented, along with outcome criteria, appropriate nursing interventions, and rationales for each.

Some institutions use a case management model to coordinate care (see Chapter 6 for more detailed explanation). In case management models, the plan of care may take the form of a critical pathway.

Concept Care Mapping

The concept map care plan is an approach to planning and organizing nursing care (see Chapter 6). It is a diagrammatic teaching and learning strategy that allows visualization of interrelationships between medical diagnoses, nursing diagnoses, assessment data, and treatments. An example of a concept map care plan for a patient with depression is presented in Figure 16–3.

Patient and Family Education

The role of patient teacher is important in the psychiatric area, as it is in all areas of nursing. A list of topics for patient and family education relevant to depression is presented in Box 16–5.

Evaluation of Care for the Depressed Patient

In the final step of the nursing process, a reassessment is conducted to determine if the nursing actions have been successful in achieving the objectives of care. Evaluation of the nursing actions for the depressed patient may be facilitated by gathering information using the following types of questions:

- Has self-harm to the individual been avoided?
- Have suicidal ideations subsided?
- Does the individual know where to seek assistance outside the hospital when suicidal thoughts occur?

- Has the patient discussed the recent loss with staff and family members?
- Is he or she able to verbalize feelings and behaviors associated with each stage of the grieving process and recognize own position in the process?
- Have obsession with and idealization of the lost object subsided?
- Is anger toward the lost object expressed appropriately?
- Does the patient set realistic goals for self?
- Is he or she able to verbalize positive aspects about self, past accomplishments, and future prospects, including a desire to live?
- Can the patient identify areas of life situation over which he or she has control?
- Is the patient able to participate in usual religious practices and feel satisfaction and support from them?
- Is the patient seeking interaction with others in an appropriate manner?
- Does the patient maintain reality orientation with no evidence of delusional thinking?
- Is he or she able to concentrate and make decisions concerning own self-care?
- Is the patient selecting and consuming foods sufficiently high in nutrients and calories to maintain weight and nutritional status?
- Does the patient sleep without difficulty and wake feeling rested?
- Does the patient attend to personal hygiene and grooming?
- Have somatic complaints subsided?

Quality and Safety Education for Nurses (QSEN)

The 2003 report *Health Professions Education: A Bridge to Quality* (Greiner, Knebel, & Institute of Medicine, 2003) challenged faculties of medicine, nursing, and other health professions to ensure that their graduates have achieved a core set of competencies to meet the needs of the 21st-century healthcare system. These competencies include *providing patient-centered care, maintaining safety, working in interdisciplinary teams, employing evidence-based practice, incorporating quality improvement,* and *utilizing informatics.* A QSEN teaching strategy is included in Box 16–6. The use of this type of activity is intended to arm the instructor and the student with guidelines for attaining the knowledge, skills, and attitudes necessary for achievement of quality and safety competencies in nursing.

Table 16–2 | CARE PLAN FOR THE DEPRESSED PATIENT

NURSING DIAGNOSIS: RISK FOR SUICIDE

RELATED TO: Depressed mood, feelings of hopelessness and worthlessness, anger turned inward on the self, misinterpretations of reality

OUTCOME CRITERIA	NURSING INTERVENTIONS	RATIONALE
Short-Term Goals ■ Patient will seek out staff when feeling urge to harm self. ■ Patient will not harm self. **Long-Term Goal:** ■ Patient will not harm self.	1. 💬 Ask patient directly: "Have you thought about killing yourself?" or "Have you thought about harming yourself in any way? If so, what do you plan to do? Do you have the means to carry out this plan? How strong are your intentions to die?" 2. Create a safe environment for the patient. Remove all potentially harmful objects from patient's access (sharp objects, straps, belts, ties, glass items, alcohol). Supervise closely during meals and medication administration. Perform room searches as deemed necessary. 3. Convey an attitude of unconditional acceptance of the patient as a worthwhile individual. Encourage the patient to actively participate in establishing a safety plan. 4. Maintain close observation of the patient. Depending on level of suicide precaution, provide one-to-one contact, constant visual observation, or every-15-minute checks. Place in room close to nurse's station; do not assign to private room. Accompany to off-unit activities if attendance is indicated and, if necessary, to the bathroom. 5. Maintain special care in administration of medications. 6. Make rounds at frequent, *irregular* intervals (especially at night, toward early morning, at change of shift, or other predictably busy times for staff). 7. Encourage patient to express honest feelings, including anger. Provide hostility release if needed. Help the patient to identify the true source of anger and to work on adaptive coping skills for use outside the treatment setting. 8. Identify community resources that the patient can access for support and assistance as needed post-discharge.	1. The risk of suicide is greatly increased if the patient has developed a plan, has strong intentions to die, and particularly if means exist for the patient to execute the plan. 2. Patient safety is a nursing priority. 3. A relationship founded on trust and acceptance is essential for collaboration with the patient in developing a plan for his or her ongoing safety. Suicidal clients are often ambivalent about their feelings related to suicide and discussion (and "buy in") about strategies for maintaining safety. Empower the patient to collaborate in preventing a crisis situation. 4. Close observation is necessary to ensure that patient does not harm self in any way. Being alert for suicidal and escape attempts facilitates being able to prevent or interrupt harmful behavior. 5. Prevents saving up to overdose or discarding and not taking. 6. Prevents staff surveillance from becoming predictable. To be aware of patient's location is important, especially when staff is busy, unavailable, or less observable. 7. Depression and suicidal behaviors may be viewed as anger turned inward on the self. If this anger can be verbalized in a non-threatening environment, the client may eventually be able to resolve these feelings. 8. Having a concrete plan for seeking assistance should suicidal ideation recur or intensify post-discharge assists the client to manage symptoms and prevent self-destructive behaviors.

Continued

Table 16–2 | CARE PLAN FOR THE DEPRESSED PATIENT–cont'd

NURSING DIAGNOSIS: COMPLICATED GRIEVING

RELATED TO: Real or perceived loss, bereavement overload

EVIDENCED BY: Denial of loss, inappropriate expression of anger, idealization of or obsession with lost object, inability to carry out activities of daily living

OUTCOME CRITERIA	NURSING INTERVENTIONS	RATIONALE
Short-Term Goals ■ Patient will express anger about the loss. ■ Patient will verbalize behaviors associated with normal grieving. **Long-Term Goal** ■ Patient will be able to recognize his or her own position in the grief process, while progressing at own pace toward resolution.	1. Determine the stage of grief in which the patient is fixed. Identify behaviors associated with this stage. 2. Develop a trusting relationship with the patient. Show empathy, concern, and unconditional positive regard. Be honest and keep all promises. 3. Convey an accepting attitude and enable the patient to express feelings openly. 4. Encourage the patient to express anger. Do not become defensive if the initial expression of anger is displaced on the nurse or therapist. Help the patient explore angry feelings so that they may be directed toward the actual intended person or situation. 5. Help the patient to discharge pent-up anger through participation in large motor activities (e.g., brisk walks, jogging, physical exercises, volleyball, exercise bike). 6. Teach the normal stages of grief and behaviors associated with each stage. Help the patient to understand that feelings such as guilt and anger toward the lost concept are appropriate and acceptable during the grief process and should be expressed rather than held inside. 7. Encourage the patient to review the relationship with the lost entity. With support and sensitivity, point out the reality of the situation in areas where misrepresentations are expressed. 8. Communicate to the patient that crying is acceptable. Use of touch may also be therapeutic. 9. Encourage the patient to reach out for spiritual support during this time in whatever form is desirable to him or her. Assess spiritual needs of the patient (see online Chapter 31) and assist as necessary in the fulfillment of those needs.	1. Accurate baseline assessment data are necessary to effectively plan care for the grieving patient. 2. Trust is the basis for a therapeutic relationship. 3. An accepting attitude conveys to the patient that you believe he or she is a worthwhile person. Trust is enhanced. 4. Verbalization of feelings in a nonthreatening environment may help the client come to terms with unresolved issues. 5. Physical exercise provides a safe and effective method for discharging pent-up tension. 6. Knowledge of acceptability of the feelings associated with normal grieving may help to relieve some of the guilt that these responses generate. 7. The patient must give up an idealized perception and be able to accept both positive and negative aspects about the lost entity before the grief process is complete. 8. Some individuals believe it is important to remain stoic and refrain from crying openly and some are uncomfortable with touch. It is important to be aware of individual preferences before employing these interventions. 9. Patient may find comfort in religious rituals with which he or she is familiar.

Table 16–2 | CARE PLAN FOR THE DEPRESSED PATIENT—cont'd

NURSING DIAGNOSIS: LOW SELF-ESTEEM

RELATED TO: Learned helplessness, feelings of abandonment by significant other, impaired cognition fostering negative view of self

EVIDENCED BY: Expressions of worthlessness, hypersensitivity to slights or criticism, negative and pessimistic outlook

OUTCOME CRITERIA	NURSING INTERVENTIONS	RATIONALE
Short-Term Goals: ■ Patient will verbalize areas he or she likes about self. ■ Patient will attempt new activities without fear of failure. **Long-Term Goal** ■ By time of discharge from treatment, client will exhibit increased feelings of self-worth as evidenced by verbal expression of positive aspects of self, past accomplishments, and future prospects.	1. Be accepting of patient and spend time with him or her even though pessimism and negativism may seem objectionable. Focus on strengths and accomplishments and minimize limitations and failures. 2. Promote attendance in therapy groups that offer patient simple methods of accomplishment. Encourage patient to be as independent as possible. 3. Encourage patient to recognize areas of change and provide assistance toward this effort. 4. Teach assertiveness techniques: the ability to recognize the differences among passive, assertive, and aggressive behaviors; and the importance of respecting the human rights of others while protecting one's own basic human rights. 5. 💬 Teach effective communication techniques, such as the use of "I" messages (e.g., "I feel hurt when you say those things").	1. Interventions that focus on the positive contribute toward feelings of self-worth. 2. Success and independence promote feelings of self-worth. 3. Patient will need assistance with problem-solving. 4. Self-esteem is enhanced by the ability to interact with others in an assertive manner. 5. "I" statements help to avoid making judgmental statements.

NURSING DIAGNOSIS: POWERLESSNESS

RELATED TO: Dysfunctional grieving process, lifestyle of helplessness

EVIDENCED BY: Feelings of lack of control over life situation, overdependence on others to fulfill needs

OUTCOME CRITERIA	NURSING INTERVENTIONS	RATIONALE
Short-Term Goal ■ Patient will participate in decision making regarding own care within 5 days.	1. Encourage patient to take as much responsibility as possible for own self-care practices. In the most acute stage of severe depression, patients may have extreme difficulty making decisions. 💬 It may be more helpful to use active communication to help the client accomplish even basic ADLs. For example, "It's time to eat lunch," rather than, "Would you like to eat lunch now?" Ongoing assessment is important so that the client can be encouraged to make choices as soon as possible. Examples: a. Include patient in setting the goals of care he or she wishes to achieve. b. Allow patient to establish own schedule for self-care activities.	1. Providing patient with choices will increase his or her feelings of control.

Continued

Table 16–2 | CARE PLAN FOR THE DEPRESSED PATIENT–cont'd

OUTCOME CRITERIA	NURSING INTERVENTIONS	RATIONALE
Long-Term Goal ■ Patient will be able to effectively problem solve ways to take control of his or her life situation by time of discharge from treatment, thereby decreasing feelings of powerlessness.	c. Provide privacy as need is determined. d. Provide positive feedback for decisions made. Respect patient's right to make those decisions independently, and refrain from attempting to influence him or her toward those that may seem more logical. 2. Help patient set realistic goals. 3. Help patient identify areas of life situation that he or she can control. 4. Help patient identify areas of life situation that are not within his or her ability to control. Encourage verbalization of feelings related to this inability.	2. Realistic goals will avoid setting patient up for failure and reinforcing feelings of powerlessness. 3. Patient's emotional condition interferes with his or her ability to solve problems. Assistance is required to perceive the benefits and consequences of available alternatives accurately. 4. Verbalization of unresolved issues may help patient accept what cannot be changed.

NURSING DIAGNOSIS: SPIRITUAL DISTRESS

RELATED TO: Dysfunctional grieving over loss of valued object

EVIDENCED BY: Anger toward God, questioning meaning of own existence, inability to participate in usual religious practices

OUTCOME CRITERIA	NURSING INTERVENTIONS	RATIONALE
Short-Term Goal ■ Patient will identify meaning and purpose in life, moving forward with hope for the future. **Long-Term Goal** ■ Patient will express achievement of support and personal satisfaction from spiritual practices.	1. Be accepting and nonjudgmental when patient expresses anger and bitterness toward God. Stay with patient. 2. Encourage patient to express feelings related to meaning of own existence in the face of current loss. 3. Encourage patient as part of grief work to reach out to previous religious practices for support. Encourage patient to discuss these practices and how they provided support in the past. 4. Reassure patient that he or she is not alone when feeling inadequate in the search for life's answers. 5. Contact spiritual leader of patient's choice, if he or she requests.	1. The nurse's presence and nonjudgmental attitude increase the patient's feelings of self-worth and promote trust in the relationship. 2. Patient may believe he or she cannot go on living without the lost entity. Catharsis can provide relief and put life back into realistic perspective. 3. Patient may find comfort in religious rituals with which he or she is familiar. 4. Validation of patient's feelings and the assurance that others share them offers reassurance and an affirmation of acceptability. 5. These individuals serve to provide relief from spiritual distress and often can do so when other support persons cannot.

Table 16–2 | CARE PLAN FOR THE DEPRESSED PATIENT—cont'd

NURSING DIAGNOSIS: HOPELESSNESS

RELATED TO: Absence of support systems and perception of worthlessness

EVIDENCED BY: Verbal cues (despondent content, "I can't"); decreased affect; lack of initiative; suicidal ideas or attempts

OUTCOME CRITERIA	NURSING INTERVENTIONS	RATIONALE
Short-Term Goal ■ Patient will express acceptance of life and situations over which he or she has no control. **Long-Term Goal** ■ Patient will verbalize a measure of hope for the future by identifying reachable goals. and ways to achieve them.	1. Identify stressors in patient's life that precipitated current crisis. 2. Determine coping behaviors previously used and patient's perception of effectiveness then and now. 3. Encourage patient to explore and verbalize feelings and perceptions. 4. 💬 Provide expressions of hope to patient in positive, low-key manner (e.g., "I know you feel you cannot go on, but I believe that things can get better for you. What you are feeling is temporary. It is okay if you don't see it just now. You are very important to the people who care about you"). 5. Help patient identify areas of life situation that are under own control. 6. Identify sources that patient may use after discharge when crises occur or feelings of hopelessness and possible suicidal ideation prevail.	1. Important to identify causative or contributing factors in order to plan appropriate assistance. 2. Reviewing coping behaviors assists the patient to recognize personal strengths that have been helpful in the past. 3. Identification of feelings underlying behaviors helps patient to begin process of taking control of own life. 4. Even though the patient feels hopeless, it is helpful to hear positive expressions from others. The patient's current state of mind may prevent him or her from identifying anything positive in life. It is important to accept the patient's feelings nonjudgmentally and to affirm the individual's personal worth and value. 5. The patient's emotional condition may interfere with ability to problem solve. Assistance may be required to perceive the benefits and consequences of available alternatives accurately. 6. Providing information about local suicide hotlines or other local support services from which he or she may seek assistance following discharge from the hospital promotes follow-through with an ongoing safety plan

Treatment Modalities for Depression

Individual Psychotherapy

Research has documented both the importance of close, satisfactory attachments in the prevention of depression and the role of disrupted attachments in the development of depression. With this concept in mind, interpersonal psychotherapy focuses on the client's current interpersonal relations. Interpersonal psychotherapy with the depressed person proceeds through three phases.

Phase I

During the first phase, the client is assessed to determine the extent of the illness. Complete information is then given to the individual regarding the nature of depression, symptom pattern, frequency, clinical course, and alternative treatments. If the level of depression is severe, interpersonal psychotherapy has been shown to be more effective if conducted in combination with antidepressant medication. The client is encouraged to continue working and participating in regular activities

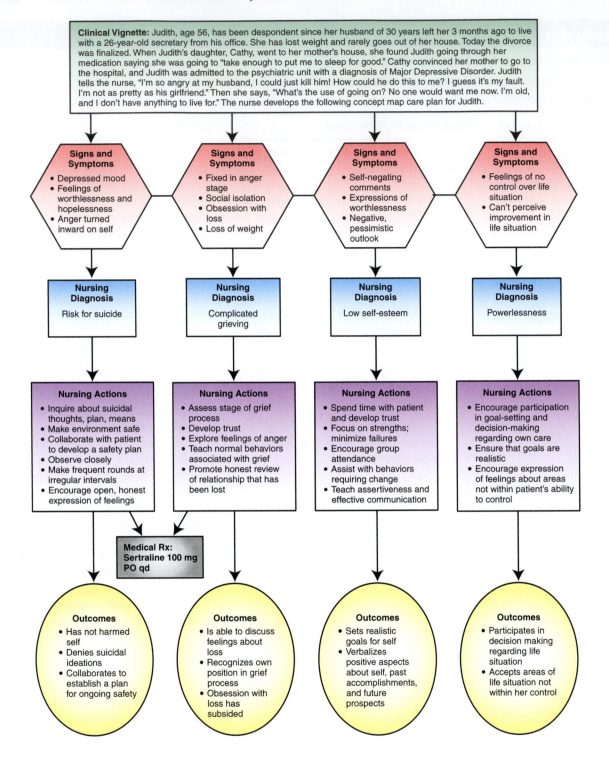

Clinical Vignette: Judith, age 56, has been despondent since her husband of 30 years left her 3 months ago to live with a 26-year-old secretary from his office. She has lost weight and rarely goes out of her house. Today the divorce was finalized. When Judith's daughter, Cathy, went to her mother's house, she found Judith going through her medication saying she was going to "take enough to put me to sleep for good." Cathy convinced her mother to go to the hospital, and Judith was admitted to the psychiatric unit with a diagnosis of Major Depressive Disorder. Judith tells the nurse, "I'm so angry at my husband, I could just kill him! How could he do this to me? I guess it's my fault. I'm not as pretty as his girlfriend." Then she says, "What's the use of going on? No one would want me now. I'm old, and I don't have anything to live for." The nurse develops the following concept map care plan for Judith.

Signs and Symptoms
- Depressed mood
- Feelings of worthlessness and hopelessness
- Anger turned inward on self

Signs and Symptoms
- Fixed in anger stage
- Social isolation
- Obsession with loss
- Loss of weight

Signs and Symptoms
- Self-negating comments
- Expressions of worthlessness
- Negative, pessimistic outlook

Signs and Symptoms
- Feelings of no control over life situation
- Can't perceive improvement in life situation

Nursing Diagnosis
Risk for suicide

Nursing Diagnosis
Complicated grieving

Nursing Diagnosis
Low self-esteem

Nursing Diagnosis
Powerlessness

Nursing Actions
- Inquire about suicidal thoughts, plan, means
- Make environment safe
- Collaborate with patient to develop a safety plan
- Observe closely
- Make frequent rounds at irregular intervals
- Encourage open, honest expression of feelings

Nursing Actions
- Assess stage of grief process
- Develop trust
- Explore feelings of anger
- Teach normal behaviors associated with grief
- Promote honest review of relationship that has been lost

Nursing Actions
- Spend time with patient and develop trust
- Focus on strengths; minimize failures
- Encourage group attendance
- Assist with behaviors requiring change
- Teach assertiveness and effective communication

Nursing Actions
- Encourage participation in goal-setting and decision-making regarding own care
- Ensure that goals are realistic
- Encourage expression of feelings about areas not within patient's ability to control

Medical Rx: Sertraline 100 mg PO qd

Outcomes
- Has not harmed self
- Denies suicidal ideations
- Collaborates to establish a plan for ongoing safety

Outcomes
- Is able to discuss feelings about loss
- Recognizes own position in grief process
- Obsession with loss has subsided

Outcomes
- Sets realistic goals for self
- Verbalizes positive aspects about self, past accomplishments, and future prospects

Outcomes
- Participates in decision making regarding life situation
- Accepts areas of life situation not within her control

FIGURE 16–3   Concept map care plan for a patient with depression.

BOX 16–5 Topics for Patient and Family Education Related to Depression

NATURE OF THE ILLNESS
1. Stages of grief and symptoms associated with each stage
2. What is depression?
3. Why do people get depressed?
4. What are the symptoms of depression?

MANAGEMENT OF THE ILLNESS
1. Medication management
   a. Nuisance side effects
   b. Side effects to report to physician
   c. Importance of taking regularly
   d. Length of time to take effect
   e. Diet (related to MAOIs)
2. Assertiveness techniques
3. Stress-management techniques
4. Ways to increase self-esteem
5. Electroconvulsive therapy

Support Services
1. Suicide hotline
2. Support groups
3. Legal/financial assistance

during therapy. A mutually agreeable therapeutic contract is negotiated.

Phase II

Treatment at this phase focuses on helping the client resolve complicated grief reactions, which may include resolving the ambivalence with a lost relationship and assistance with establishing new relationships. Other areas of treatment focus may include interpersonal disputes between the client and a significant other, difficult role transitions at various developmental life cycles, and correction of interpersonal deficits that may interfere with the client's ability to initiate or sustain interpersonal relationships.

Phase III

During the final phase of interpersonal psychotherapy, the therapeutic alliance is terminated. With emphasis on reassurance, clarification of emotional states, improvement of interpersonal communication, testing of perceptions, and performance in interpersonal settings, interpersonal psychotherapy has been successful in helping depressed persons recover enhanced social functioning.

Group Therapy

Group therapy forms an important dimension of multimodal treatment for the depressed client. Once an acute phase of the illness is passed, groups can provide an atmosphere in which individuals may discuss issues in their lives that cause, maintain, or arise out of having a serious affective disorder. The element of peer support provides a feeling of security, because troublesome or embarrassing issues are discussed and resolved. Some groups have other specific purposes, such as helping to monitor medication-related issues or serving as an avenue for promoting education related to the affective disorder and its treatment. Therapy groups help members gain a sense of perspective on their condition and tangibly encourage them to link up with others who have common problems. A sense of hope is conveyed when the individual is able to see that he or she is not alone or unique in experiencing affective illness.

Self-help groups offer another avenue of support for the depressed client. These groups are usually peer led and are not meant to substitute for or compete with professional therapy. They offer supplementary support that frequently enhances compliance with the medical regimen. Examples of self-help groups are the Depression and Bipolar Support Alliance (DBSA), Depressives Anonymous, Recovery International, and GriefShare (grief recovery support group). Although self-help groups are not psychotherapy groups, they do provide important adjunctive support experiences, which often have therapeutic benefit for participants.

Family Therapy

The ultimate objectives in working with families of clients with mood disorders are to resolve the symptoms and initiate or restore adaptive family functioning. Similar to group therapy, the most effective approach appears to be a combination of psychotherapeutic and pharmacotherapeutic treatments. Sadock and colleagues (2015) stated:

> Family therapy is indicated if the disorder jeopardizes the patient's marriage or family functioning or if the mood disorder is promoted or maintained by the family situation. Family therapy examines the role of the mood-disordered member in the overall psychological well-being of the whole family; it also examines the role of the entire family in the maintenance of the patient's symptoms. (p. 373)

Cognitive Therapy

In cognitive therapy, the individual is taught to control thought distortions that are considered to be a factor in the development and maintenance of mood disorders. In the cognitive model, depression is characterized by a triad of negative distortions related to expectations of the environment, self, and future.

BOX 16–6 QSEN TEACHING STRATEGY

Assignment: Staff Workarounds
Placing a Patient on Suicide Precautions

Competency Domains: Evidence-Based Practice; Patient-Centered Care; Quality Improvement; Safety; Teamwork and Collaboration

Learning Objectives: Student will:
- Demonstrate skills in identifying gaps between practice on the unit and what has been identified as best practice.
- Demonstrate skills at finding professional practice standards and research literature related to placing a patient on suicide precautions.
- Demonstrate skills in accounting for patient preferences within the boundaries of safe and therapeutic practice.
- Demonstrate attitudes and behaviors that show that student values teamwork and wants to contribute to maintaining standards of safe and effective care.

Strategy Overview

This assignment is meant to familiarize the student with standardized nursing policies, procedures, standards of care, and other evidence-based nursing practice guidelines and to encourage students to observe actual nursing practice on the units to note compliance with, deviations from, or workarounds by registered nurses (RNs) when implementing nursing procedures. The following aspects of the assignment can guide students in preparation for clinical conference discussion, in writing a paper, or in putting together a poster presentation.

1. Identify a need to place a patient on suicide precautions.
2. Find the current written nursing policy or procedure in place for your institution and/or unit and answer these questions:
   a. How easy or difficult was it to find the policy or procedure?
   b. Did the RNs know where to find the written policy or procedure?
   c. How was the policy or procedure originally disseminated to the staff?
   d. Is the policy or procedure evidence-based? (Review the current practice standards from professional organizations and/or oversight and accreditation groups [e.g., The Joint Commission, Centers for Disease Control and Prevention], and/or review the research literature.)
3. Observe RNs on the unit putting a patient on suicide precautions and describe:
   a. Steps taken by the RN
   b. In what ways the RN deviated from the written policy or procedure
   c. What prompted the RN to make the deviations she or he made
   d. As many details as you can recollect
4. Discuss why RNs may or may not follow the institution's written policies and/or procedures. Reflect on the opportunities and challenges of evidence-based practice and its implementation into actual bedside nursing practice.
5. Discuss what the proper response should be when you, as an RN, discover an unsafe practice that deviates from standards, policies, or procedures.

Source: Adapted from Day, L., & Smith, E. L. (2007). Integrating quality and safety content into clinical teaching in the acute care setting. Nursing Outlook, 55(3), 138–143. With permission.

The environment and activities within it are viewed as unsatisfying, the self is unrealistically devalued, and the future is perceived as hopeless.

The general goals in cognitive therapy are to obtain symptom relief as quickly as possible, to assist the client in identifying dysfunctional patterns of thinking and behaving, and to guide the client to evidence and logic that effectively test the validity of the dysfunctional thinking. Therapy focuses on changing "automatic thoughts" that occur spontaneously and contribute to the distorted affect. Following are examples of automatic thoughts that may be common cognitive distortions in depression:

- **Personalizing:** "I'm the only one who failed."
- **All or nothing:** A person who had a failure or disappointment thinks I can't do anything right, I'm a complete failure."

- **Mind reading:** "He thinks I'm foolish."
- **Discounting positives:** "The other questions were so easy. Any dummy could have gotten them right."

The client is asked to describe evidence that both supports and disputes the automatic thought. The logic underlying the inferences is then reviewed with the client. Another technique involves evaluating what would most likely happen if the client's automatic thoughts were true. Implications of the consequences are then discussed.

Clients should not become discouraged if one technique seems not to be working. No single technique works with all clients. He or she should be reassured that any of a number of techniques may be used, and both the therapist and client may explore these possibilities.

Cognitive therapy has offered encouraging results in the treatment of depression. In fact, the results of several studies with depressed clients show that in some cases cognitive therapy may be equally or even more effective than antidepressant medication (Amick et al., 2015; Page & Hooke, 2012; Siddique et al., 2012).

Electroconvulsive Therapy

Electroconvulsive therapy (ECT) is the induction of a grand mal (generalized) seizure through the application of electrical current to the brain. ECT is effective with clients who are acutely suicidal and in the treatment of severe depression, particularly in those clients who are also experiencing psychotic symptoms and those with psychomotor retardation and neurovegetative changes, such as disturbances in sleep, appetite, and energy. It is often considered for treatment only after a trial of therapy with antidepressant medication has proved ineffective.

Mechanism of Action

The exact mechanism by which ECT effects a therapeutic response is unknown. In a longitudinal study of imaging research, the preponderance of evidence supported that ECT response is associated with several effects on the brain, including decreased frontal perfusion, changes in metabolism, functional connectivity, volume, and neuronal chemical metabolites all of which support anticonvulsant and neurotrophic effects of ECT (Abbott et al., 2014). Other studies have demonstrated increased gamma-aminobutyric acid (GABA) levels, increased sensitization of 5-HT1A serotonin receptors, increased dopamine binding, and normalized dexamethasone suppression tests in patients who received ECT (Sharma et al., 2018).

The results of studies relating to the mechanism underlying the effectiveness of ECT continue to be controversial.

Side Effects

The most common side effects of ECT are temporary memory loss (retrograde and anterograde amnesia) and confusion. Critics of the therapy argue that these changes represent irreversible brain damage. Proponents insist that they are temporary and reversible. Other cognitive deficits in the immediate post-ECT period include processing speed, attention, verbal and visual memory, spatial problem-solving, and executive functioning deficits, but Semovska and Mcloughlin's meta-analysis demonstrated that most of those resolve within 3 days after treatment and some improve beyond baseline after 15 days (Sharma et al., 2018). It has been argued that bilateral electrode placement may be more effective than right unilateral (RUL) placement but is associated with more cognitive side effects. However, evidence supports that a more aggressive stimulus in RUL placement improves its efficacy (Pulia et al., 2013).

Risks Associated With ECT

Mortality

In 2011, the American Psychiatric Nurses Association (APNA) advanced a position statement in support of ECT for "severe depression that has been shown to be refractory to medication administration" (APNA, 2011). The APNA cites a mortality rate less than that of childbirth. Studies indicate that the mortality rate from ECT is about 0.002 percent per treatment and 0.01 percent for each patient (Sadock et al., 2015). Although the occurrence is rare, the major cause of death with ECT is from cardiovascular complications (e.g., acute myocardial infarction or CVA), usually in individuals with previously compromised cardiac status. Assessment and management of cardiovascular disease prior to treatment is vital in the reduction of morbidity and mortality rates associated with ECT.

Memory Loss

Memory impairment almost always occurs to some degree during the course of ECT treatments, but follow-up studies indicate that most patients return to their cognitive baselines after 6 months (Sadock et al., 2015). Some clients do report persistent memory impairment, and, in most cases, this impairment occurs among patients who showed little improvement with ECT (Sadock et al., 2015). Nonetheless, this issue should be reviewed with the patient when the physician obtains informed consent for the procedure.

Brain Damage

The question of brain damage secondary to ECT treatments has been advanced as a concern by critics of the procedure. The subject has been studied using a variety of brain imaging modalities, and virtually all conclude that there is no evidence of brain damage caused by ECT treatments (McClintock & Husain, 2011; Sadock et al., 2015). Previously cited studies on the *neurorestorative* effects of ECT have argued that this, too, is evidence in contradiction to ideas about brain-damaging effects of ECT.

Medications Used With ECT

Several medications are associated with ECT. A pre-treatment medication, such as atropine sulfate or glycopyrrolate (Robinul), is administered intramuscularly approximately 30 minutes before the treatment. Either of these medications may be ordered to decrease secretions (to prevent aspiration) and counteract the effects of vagal stimulation (bradycardia) induced by the ECT.

In the treatment room, the anesthesiologist administers intravenously a short-acting anesthetic, such as propofol (Diprivan) or etomidate (Amidate). A muscle relaxant, usually succinylcholine chloride (Anectine), is given intravenously to prevent severe muscle contractions during the seizure, thereby reducing the possibility of fractured or dislocated bones. Because succinylcholine paralyzes respiratory muscles as well, the client is oxygenated with pure oxygen during and after the treatment, except for the brief interval of electrical stimulation, until spontaneous respirations return.

Clients and families must also understand that ECT is voluntary and that consent may be withdrawn at any time (APA, 2001; Fetterman & Ying, 2011; Vera, 2012). This kind of education supports patient-centered care.

Repetitive Transcranial Magnetic Stimulation (rTMS)

Repetitive transcranial magnetic stimulation (rTMS) is a noninvasive procedure that is used to treat depression by stimulating nerve cells in the brain. rTMS involves the use of very short pulses of magnetic energy to stimulate nerve cells at localized areas in the cerebral cortex, similar to the electrical activity observed with ECT. However, unlike ECT, the electrical waves generated by rTMS do not result in generalized seizure activity (George, Taylor, & Short, 2013). The waves are passed through a coil placed on the scalp to areas of the brain involved in mood regulation. It is noninvasive and considered generally safe. High-frequency waves are used to stimulate the left prefrontal cortex and low-frequency waves are used to stimulate the right prefrontal cortex. This combination has been shown most effective in treating depression (Sharma et al., 2018). A typical course of treatment is 40-minute sessions, three to five times a week for 4 to 6 weeks (Raposelli, 2015). In rare instances, seizures have been triggered with the use of TMS therapy, particularly with high-frequency rTMS, but more common adverse effects include tinnitus, headache, or facial twitching (Sharma et al., 2018). Gaynes and associates (2014) conducted a meta-analysis demonstrating that rTMS had a remission rate of 30 percent. Effectiveness ratings for ECT have varied from 17 to 70 percent. Although the effectiveness ratings may seem small or highly variable, both treatments provide an option for patients who are otherwise treatment resistant. Magnezi and associates (2016) compared ECT to rTMS and found that although ECT was more effective than rTMS and additionally relieved anxiety symptoms, ECT had a much higher incidence (60 percent) of adverse effects, mostly related to memory loss. From the client's perspective, rTMS was still deemed preferable to ECT (if it was covered by insurance), which may be related to the stigma associated with ECT.

George and associates (2013) stated:

> Since FDA approval, TMS has been generally safe and well tolerated with a low incidence of treatment discontinuation, and the therapeutic effects once obtained appear at least as durable as other antidepressant treatments. TMS also shows promise in several other psychiatric disorders, particularly treating acute and chronic pain. (p. 17)

More recently, researchers compared rTMS to pharmacotherapy and found them both effective but identified rTMS as more cost effective (Raposelli, 2015). Currently, not all insurance companies cover this treatment, so from the client's standpoint, this may be a more expensive alternative. Raposelli reports that up to 40 percent of patients with MDD do not respond to pharmacotherapy, so alternatives such as ECT and rTMS may offer some hope of recovery for treatment-resistant conditions.

Vagal Nerve Stimulation and Deep Brain Stimulation

During studies for the treatment of epilepsy, researchers found that vagal nerve stimulation (VNS) improved mood. This treatment involves implanting an electronic device in the skin to stimulate the vagus nerve. The mechanism of action is not known, but preliminary studies have shown that many patients with chronic recurrent depression improved when treated with VNS (Sadock et al., 2015). Positive emission tomography studies performed during treatment demonstrate metabolic changes in areas of the brain associated with mood disorders (Sharma et al., 2018), including the amygdala, hippocampus, and cingulate gyrus. Response rates vary from 13 to 40 percent and remission rates are around 13 percent. Trials are ongoing to determine its effectiveness.

A novel approach is deep brain stimulation (DBS), which is a form of psychosurgery. In this procedure, as in VNS, an electrode is implanted with the intent of stimulating brain function. The implant is deeper than that used in VNS and requires craniotomy. DBS has been well studied to determine its safety and effectiveness for other conditions, and controlled trials are ongoing. The procedure is reversible and stimulation levels can easily be adjusted (Sharma et al., 2018). There is no consensus on the best area of the brain for implantation but studies have reported improvement regardless of the site of electrode placement (Sharma et al., 2018). Berlim and associates (2014) conducted a systematic review of several studies using DBS and determined a response rate of approximately 40 percent and a remission rate of approximately 26 percent. Currently, DBS is reserved for patients with severe, incapacitating depression or obsessive-compulsive disorder who have not responded to any other more conservative treatments (Sadock et al., 2015).

Light Therapy

The prevalence of depression with a seasonal pattern is reported to be up to 10 percent but varies on the basis of geographic location (Kurlansik & Ibay, 2013). The *DSM-5* identifies this disorder as Major Depressive Disorder, Recurrent, With Seasonal Pattern. It is commonly known as seasonal affect disorder (SAD). One theory suggests that SAD is related to the presence of the hormone melatonin (Cotterell, 2010), which is produced by the pineal gland. Melatonin plays a role in the regulation of biological rhythms for sleep and activation. It is produced during the cycle of darkness and shuts off in the light of day. During the months of longer hours of darkness, there is increased production of melatonin, which seems to trigger the symptoms of SAD in susceptible people. Other research has pointed to seasonal serotonin transporter fluctuations associated with variation in exposure to daylight (McMahon et al., 2016).

Light therapy, or exposure to light, has been shown, in several studies, to be an effective short-term treatment for SAD. The light therapy is administered by a 10,000-lux light box, which contains white fluorescent light tubes covered with a plastic screen that blocks ultraviolet rays. The individual sits in front of the box with the eyes open (although the client should not look directly into the light). Therapy usually begins with 10- to 15-minute sessions and gradually progresses to 30 to 45 minutes. The mechanism of action is believed to be related to retinal stimulation, which triggers a reduction of melatonin and an increase in serotonin in the brain (Rodriguez, 2015). A recent study demonstrated benefits of bright light therapy in non-SADs as well (Lam et al., 2015). Some people notice improvement rapidly, within a few days, whereas others may take several weeks to feel better. Side effects appear to be dosage related and include headache, eyestrain, nausea, irritability, photophobia (eye sensitivity to light), insomnia (when light therapy is used late in the day), and (rarely) hypomania (Kurlansik & Ibay, 2013). Light therapy and antidepressants have shown comparable efficacy in studies of SAD treatment. One study compared the efficacy of light therapy for SAD to daily treatment with 20 mg of fluoxetine (Lam et al., 2015). The authors concluded that "light treatment showed earlier response onset and lower rate of some adverse events relative to fluoxetine, but there were no other significant differences in outcome between light therapy and antidepressant medication" (p. 805). Although improvement is often noted within 2 weeks, most clients relapse in the short term. Treatment should therefore be continued until an expected time of spontaneous remission, such as the change in season to spring or summer (Kurlansik & Ibay, 2013). More recent studies have demonstrated that cognitive behavior therapy (CBT) is as effective as light therapy with the added benefit of preventing recurrences over time (Rohan et al., 2016).

Psychopharmacology

Antidepressant medication is generally considered first-line treatment for severe clinical depression, but antidepressants are also used in the treatment of other depressive disorders. These include tricyclic, tetracyclic, and heterocyclic antidepressants; monoamine oxidase inhibitors (MAOIs); SSRIs; SNRIs; and SSRI/SNRI combination drugs. Examples of commonly used antidepressant medications are presented in Table 16–3. A detailed description of these medications can be found in Chapter 4, Psychopharmacology. In addition to the side effects and safety issues addressed in Chapter 4, it is important to highlight that antidepressant medication can be lethal in overdose. Depressed, suicidal patients must be observed closely and suicide risk assessed frequently in the use of this treatment modality.

Ketamine is increasingly being used off-label for the treatment of depression. Although not yet FDA approved for the treatment of depression, early clinical trials of an intranasal application of esketamine are reportedly improving depression and suicide symptoms within 4 hours; a revolutionary claim (Canuso et al., 2018). Concerns that will need to be addressed in ongoing research and use of ketamine preparations include the fact that there is addiction potential. But there is hope that its use will provide an option for individuals with treatment-resistant depression and recurrent suicide risk.

> **CLINICAL PEARL** All antidepressants carry an FDA black-box warning for increased risk of suicidality in children and adolescents.

> **CLINICAL PEARL** As antidepressant drugs take effect and mood begins to lift, the individual may have increased energy with which to implement a suicide plan. Suicide potential often increases as level of depression decreases. The nurse should be particularly alert to sudden lifts in mood.

Patient and Family Education Related to Antidepressants

The patient should:

■ Continue to take the medication even though the symptoms have not subsided. The therapeutic effect may not be seen for as long as 4 weeks. If after this length of time no improvement is noted, the physician may prescribe a different medication.

■ Use caution when driving or operating dangerous machinery. Drowsiness and dizziness can occur. If these side effects become persistent or interfere with activities of daily living (ADLs), the patient should report them to the physician. Dosage adjustment may be necessary.

■ Not discontinue use of the drug abruptly. To do so might produce withdrawal symptoms, such as nausea, vertigo, insomnia, headache, malaise, nightmares, and return of symptoms for which the medication was prescribed.

■ Use sunblock lotion and wear protective clothing when spending time outdoors. The skin may be sensitive to sunburn.

■ Immediately report occurrence of any of the following symptoms to the physician: sore throat, fever, malaise, yellowish skin, unusual bleeding, easy bruising, persistent nausea/vomiting, severe headache, rapid heart rate, difficulty urinating, anorexia/weight loss, seizure activity, stiff or sore neck, and chest pain.

■ Rise slowly from a sitting or lying position to prevent a sudden drop in blood pressure.

■ Take frequent sips of water, chew sugarless gum, or suck on hard candy if dry mouth is a problem. Good oral care (frequent brushing, flossing) is very important.

■ Not consume the following foods or medications while taking MAOIs: aged cheese, wine (especially Chianti), beer, chocolate, colas, coffee, tea, sour cream, smoked and processed meats, beef or chicken liver, canned figs, soy sauce, overripe and fermented foods, pickled herring, raisins, caviar, yogurt, yeast products, broad beans, cold remedies, diet pills. To do so could cause a life-threatening hypertensive crisis.

■ Avoid smoking while receiving tricyclic therapy. Smoking increases the metabolism of tricyclics, requiring an adjustment in dosage to achieve the therapeutic effect.

■ Avoid drinking alcohol while taking antidepressant therapy. These drugs potentiate the effects of each other.

■ Avoid use of other medications (including over-the-counter medications) without the physician's approval while receiving antidepressant therapy. Many medications contain substances that, in combination with antidepressant medication, could precipitate a life-threatening hypertensive crisis.

■ Notify the physician immediately if inappropriate or prolonged penile erections occur while taking trazodone. If the erection persists longer than 1 hour, seek emergency department treatment. This condition is rare but has occurred in some men who have taken trazodone. If measures are not instituted immediately, impotence can result.

■ Not "double up" on medication if a dose of bupropion (Wellbutrin) is missed, unless advised to do so by the physician. Taking bupropion in divided doses will decrease the risk of seizures and other adverse effects.

■ Follow the correct procedure for applying the selegiline transdermal patch:
   ■ Apply to dry, intact skin on upper torso, upper thigh, or outer surface of upper arm.

TABLE 16–3 Medications Used in the Treatment of Depression

CHEMICAL CLASS	GENERIC (TRADE) NAME*	DAILY ADULT DOSAGE RANGE (MG)†	THERAPEUTIC PLASMA RANGES
TRICYCLICS	Amitriptyline	50–300	110–250 (including metabolite)
	Amoxapine	50–300	200–500
	Clomipramine (Anafranil)	25–250	80–100
	Desipramine (Norpramin)	25–300	125–300
	Doxepin	25–300	100–200 (including metabolite)
	Imipramine (Tofranil)	30–300	200–350 (including metabolite)
	Nortriptyline (Aventyl; Pamelor)	30–100	50–150
	Protriptyline (Vivactil)	15–60	100–200
	Trimipramine (Surmontil)	50–300	180 (including metabolite)
SELECTIVE SEROTONIN REUPTAKE INHIBITORS (SSRIS)	Citalopram (Celexa)	20–40	Not well established
	Escitalopram (Lexapro)	10–20	Not well established
	Fluoxetine (Prozac; Serafem)	20–80	Not well established
	Fluvoxamine (Luvox)	50–300	Not well established
	Paroxetine (Paxil)	10–50 (CR: 12.5–75)	Not well established
	Sertraline (Zoloft)	25–200	Not well established
	Vilazodone (Viibryd) (also acts as a partial serotonergic agonist)	40	Not well established
	Vortioxetine (Brintellix)	10–20	Not well established
MONOAMINE OXIDASE INHIBITORS	Isocarboxazid (Marplan)	20–60	Not well established
	Phenelzine (Nardil)	45–90	Not well established
	Tranylcypromine (Parnate)	30–60	Not well established
	Selegiline Transdermal System (Emsam)	6/24 hr–12/24 hr patch	Not well established
ATYPICAL ANTIDEPRESSANTS	Bupropion (Wellbutrin)	200–450	Not well established
	Maprotiline	25–225	200–300 (including metabolite)
	Mirtazapine (Remeron)	15–45	Not well established
	Nefazodone	200–600	Not well established
	Trazodone	150–600	800–1600
SEROTONIN-NOREPINEPHRINE REUPTAKE INHIBITORS (SNRIS)	Desvenlafaxine (Pristiq)	50–400	Not well established
	Duloxetine (Cymbalta)	40–60	Not well established
	Venlafaxine (Effexor)	75–375	Not well established
PSYCHOTHERAPEUTIC COMBINATIONS	Olanzapine and fluoxetine (Symbyax)	6/25–12/50	Not well established
	Chlordiazepoxide and fluoxetine (Limbitrol)	20/50–40/100	Not well established
	Perphenazine and amitriptyline (Etrafon)	6/30–16/200	Not well established

- Apply approximately same time each day to new spot on skin after removing and discarding old patch.
- Wash hands thoroughly after applying the patch.
- Avoid exposing application site to direct heat (e.g., heating pads, electric blankets, heat lamps, hot tub, or prolonged direct sunlight).
- If patch falls off, apply new patch to a new site and resume previous schedule.

■ Be aware of possible risks of taking antidepressants during pregnancy. Safe use during pregnancy and lactation has not been fully established. These drugs are believed to readily cross the placental barrier; if so, the fetus could experience adverse effects of the drug. Inform the physician immediately if pregnancy occurs, is suspected, or is planned.

■ Be aware of the side effects of antidepressants. Refer to written materials furnished by healthcare providers for safe self-administration.

■ Carry a card or other identification at all times describing the medications being taken.

Pharmacogenomics

Recent genetic studies have demonstrated that variations in genes can predict whether someone will respond to SSRIs (Lee, 2015), which may offer clinicians important guidance in prescribing antidepressants according to a client's genetic makeup. As Lee reports, between 30 and 50 percent of people don't respond to the first antidepressant they are prescribed. Patients and family members often express frustration as prescriptions are changed in an effort to find the right antidepressant and dose that are most effective for each individual. Genotyping has also demonstrated benefits in identifying which individuals may be more prone to certain side effects. One study cited by Lee demonstrated that Asian populations with a specific genotype were at increased risk for sexual dysfunction side effects associated with SSRIs. This information could be useful because sexual dysfunction is a primary reason that many people choose to stop taking these medications. Currently, this area of study is in its infancy, and further study is needed to identify benefits of routine genotyping, its cost-effectiveness, and the ability to provide timely results so that therapy can be initiated promptly.

CASE STUDY AND SAMPLE CARE PLAN

NURSING HISTORY AND ASSESSMENT

Seth is a 45-year-old white male admitted to the psychiatric unit of a general medical center by his family physician, Dr. Jones, who reported that Seth had become increasingly despondent over the past month. His wife reported that he had made statements such as "Life is not worth living" and "I think I could just take all those pills Dr. Jones prescribed at one time; then it would all be over." Seth says he loves his wife and children and does not want to hurt them, but he feels they no longer need him. He states, "They would probably be better off without me." His wife appears to be very concerned about his condition, although in his despondency, he seems oblivious to her feelings. His mother (a widow) lives in a neighboring state, and he sees her infrequently. His father was an alcoholic and physically abused Seth and his siblings. He admits that he is somewhat bitter toward his mother for allowing him and his siblings to "suffer from the physical and emotional brutality of their father." His siblings and their families live in distant states, and he sees them rarely, during holiday gatherings.

Seth earned a college degree working full time at night to pay his way. He is employed in the administration department of a large corporation. Over the past 12 years, Seth has watched while a number of his peers were promoted to management positions. Seth has been considered for several of these positions but has never been selected. Last month, a management position became available for which Seth felt he was qualified. He applied for this position, believing he had a good chance of being promoted. However, when the

announcement was made, the position had been given to a younger man who had been with the company for only 5 years. Seth seemed to accept the decision, but over the past few weeks, he has become increasingly withdrawn. He speaks to very few people at the office and is falling behind in his work. At home, he eats very little, talks to family members only when they ask a direct question, withdraws to his bedroom early in the evenings, and does not come out until it is time to leave for work the next morning. Today, he refused to get out of bed or to go to work. His wife convinced him to talk to their family doctor, who admitted him to the hospital. The referring psychiatrist diagnosed Seth with Major Depressive Disorder.

NURSING DIAGNOSES AND OUTCOME IDENTIFICATION

From the assessment data, the nurse develops the following nursing diagnoses for Seth:

1. **Risk for suicide** related to depressed mood and expressions of having nothing to live for
   a. **Short-Term Goals:**
      • Seth will discuss suicide ideation and intentions with staff.
      • Seth will collaborate with the nurse to identify a plan for maintaining safety.
   b. **Long-Term Goal:** Seth will not harm himself during his hospitalization.

CASE STUDY AND SAMPLE CARE PLAN—cont'd

2. **Complicated grieving** related to unresolved losses (job promotion and unsatisfactory parent/child relationships) evidenced by anger turned inward on self and desire to end his life
   a. **Short-Term Goal:** Seth will discuss anger toward boss and parents within 1 week.
   b. **Long-Term Goal:** Seth will verbalize his position in the grief process and begin movement in the progression toward resolution by time of discharge from treatment.

PLANNING AND IMPLEMENTATION

RISK FOR SUICIDE

The following nursing interventions have been identified for Seth:

1. Develop a trusting relationship with Seth that facilitates open, nonjudgmental discussion of suicide ideation and related thoughts and feelings.
2. Ask Seth directly, "Have you thought about killing yourself? If so, what do you plan to do? Do you have the means to carry out this plan?"
3. Create a safe environment. Remove all potentially harmful objects from immediate access (sharp objects, straps, belts, ties, glass items).
4. Assess suicide risk each shift and identify any changes in level of hopelessness. Encourage honest verbalization of feelings. Through discussion and exploration, assist Seth to identify symbols of hope in his life (reasons for wanting to live).
5. Allow Seth to express angry feelings within appropriate limits. Encourage use of the exercise room and other activities for releasing energy appropriately. Help him to identify the true source of his anger, and work on adaptive coping skills for use outside the hospital (e.g., jogging, exercise club available to employees of his company).
6. Identify community resources that he may use as a support system and from whom he may request help if feeling suicidal (e.g., suicidal or crisis hotline, psychiatrist or social worker at community mental health center, hospital "HELP" line).
7. Introduce Seth to support and education groups for adult children of alcoholics (ACoA).
8. Spend time with Seth. Doing so will help him to feel safe and secure while conveying the message that he is a worthwhile person.

COMPLICATED GRIEVING

The following nursing interventions have been identified for Seth:

1. Discuss with Seth the stages in the grief process and encourage him to explore his feelings so that he may come to realize the connection between grief and his anger.
2. Develop a trusting relationship with Seth. Show empathy and caring. Be honest and keep all promises.
3. Convey an accepting attitude—one in which Seth is not afraid to express feelings openly.

4. Facilitate Seth's verbalization of feelings of anger. The initial expression of anger may be displaced onto the healthcare provider. Do not become defensive if this should occur. Assist him to explore these angry feelings so that they may be directed toward the intended persons (boss, parents). Help Seth write letters *(not to be mailed)* expressing his feelings toward his boss and his parents. Discuss the "letters" and then destroy them.
5. Assist Seth to discharge pent-up anger through participation in large motor activities (brisk walks, jogging, physical exercises, volleyball, exercise bike, or other equipment).
6. Help Seth to understand that feelings such as guilt and anger toward his boss and parents are appropriate and acceptable during this stage of the grieving process. Help him also to understand that he must work through these feelings and move past this stage in order to eventually feel better. Knowledge of acceptability of the feelings associated with normal grieving may help to relieve some of the guilt that these responses generate. Knowing why he is experiencing these feelings may also help to resolve them.
7. Encourage Seth to review the relationship with his parents. Educate Seth about the common roles and behaviors of members in families with alcoholic parents. Encourage Seth to explore his roles and behavior within his family of origin.
8. Assist Seth in problem-solving as he attempts to determine methods for more adaptive coping. Suggest alternatives to automatic negative thinking patterns (e.g., thought-stopping techniques). Provide positive feedback for strategies identified and decisions made.
9. Encourage Seth to reach out for spiritual support during this time in whatever form is desirable to him. Assess spiritual needs (see online Chapter 31, Cultural and Spiritual Concepts Relevant to Psychiatric Mental Health Nursing, for an assessment tool), and assist as necessary in the fulfillment of those needs. Seth may find comfort in religious rituals with which he is familiar.

EVALUATION

The outcome criteria identified for Seth have been met. He sought out staff when feelings of suicide surfaced and identified a safety plan for which he reports willingness to engage. He has not harmed himself in any way. He verbalizes no further thought of suicide and expresses hope for the future. He is able to verbalize names of resources outside the hospital from whom he may request help if thoughts of suicide return. He is able to verbalize normal stages of the grief process and behaviors associated with each stage. He is able to identify his own position in the grief process and express honest feelings related to the loss of the job promotion and satisfactory parent/child relationships. He expresses willingness to continue exploring behaviors and coping mechanisms through a local ACoA meeting.

Summary and Key Points

- Depression is one of the oldest recognized psychiatric illnesses that is still prevalent today. It is so common that it has been referred to as the "common cold of psychiatric disorders."

- The cause of depressive disorders is not entirely known. A number of factors, including genetics, biochemical influences, and psychosocial experiences, likely enter into the development of the disorder.

- Secondary depression occurs in response to other physiological disorders and may be induced by a variety of substances or medications.

- Symptoms of depression occur along a continuum according to the degree of severity from transient to severe.

- The disorder occurs at all developmental levels, including childhood, adolescence, senescence, and during the puerperium.

- Treatment of depression may include individual therapy, group and family therapy, cognitive therapy, electroconvulsive therapy, light therapy, repetitive transcranial magnetic stimulation, vagal nerve or deep brain stimulation, and psychopharmacology.

- Nursing care of the depressed patient is provided using the six steps of the nursing process.

Review Questions
Self-Examination/Learning Exercise

Select the answer that is most appropriate for each of the following questions:

1. Margaret, age 68, is a widow of 6 months. Since her husband died, her sister reports that Margaret has become socially withdrawn, has lost weight, and does little more each day than visit the cemetery where her husband was buried. She told her sister today that "she doesn't have anything more to live for." She has been hospitalized with a diagnosis of Major Depressive Disorder. The *priority* nursing diagnosis for Margaret is:
   a. Imbalanced nutrition: Less than body requirements
   b. Complicated grieving
   c. Risk for suicide
   d. Social isolation

2. The physician orders sertraline (Zoloft) 50 mg PO bid for Margaret, a 68-year-old woman with major depressive disorder. After 3 days of taking the medication, Margaret says to the nurse, "I don't think this medicine is doing any good. I don't feel a bit better." What is the most appropriate response by the nurse?
   a. "Cheer up, Margaret. You have so much to be happy about."
   b. "Sometimes it takes a few weeks for the medicine to bring about an improvement in symptoms."
   c. "I'll report that to the physician, Margaret. Maybe he will order something different."
   d. "Try not to dwell on your symptoms, Margaret. Why don't you join the others down in the dayroom?"

3. The goal of cognitive therapy with depressed clients is to:
   a. Identify and change dysfunctional patterns of thinking.
   b. Resolve the symptoms and initiate or restore adaptive family functioning.
   c. Alter the neurotransmitters that are creating the depressed mood.
   d. Provide feedback from peers who are having similar experiences.

Review Questions—cont'd
Self-Examination/Learning Exercise

4. Education for the patient who is taking MAOIs should include which of the following?
   a. Fluid and sodium replacement when appropriate, frequent drug blood levels, signs and symptoms of toxicity
   b. Lifetime of continuous use, possible tardive dyskinesia, advantages of an injection every 2 to 4 weeks
   c. Short-term use, possible tolerance to beneficial effects, careful tapering of the drug at end of treatment
   d. Tyramine-restricted diet, prohibitive concurrent use of over-the-counter medications without physician notification

5. A patient expresses interest in alternative treatments for depression with seasonal variations and asks the nurse about light therapy. Which of the following are evidence-based teaching points that the nurse may share with the patient? (Select all that apply.)
   a. Light therapy has demonstrated effectiveness that is comparable to antidepressants.
   b. Light therapy should be used regularly until the season changes.
   c. Light therapy should only be used when ECT has proven to be ineffective.
   d. Side effects such as headache, nausea, or agitation, when they occur, are usually mild and transient.
   e. Light therapy can cause sedation so the best time to use it is before bedtime.

6. A patient has just been admitted to the psychiatric unit with a diagnosis of Major Depressive Disorder. Which of the following manifestations may be apparent in a patient with this diagnosis? (Select all that apply.)
   a. Slumped posture
   b. Delusional thinking
   c. Feelings of despair
   d. Feels best early in the morning and worse as the day progresses
   e. Anorexia

7. A patient with depression asks the nurse, "Why would they be checking my thyroid function when I clearly have depression and I'm not overweight?" Which of these is an accurate response?
   a. An underactive thyroid gland can manifest as depression.
   b. Depression has been proven to be a hormonal illness.
   c. Thyroid hormone replacement is a first-line treatment for most people with depression.
   d. Abnormal thyroid function predicts positive response to antidepressant medication.

8. A patient whose husband died 6 months ago is diagnosed with major depressive disorder. She says to the nurse, "I start feeling angry that Harold died and left me all alone; he should have stopped smoking years ago! But then I start feeling guilty for feeling that way." What is an appropriate response by the nurse?
   a. "Yes, he should have stopped smoking. Then he probably wouldn't have gotten lung cancer."
   b. "I can understand how you must feel."
   c. "Those feelings are a normal part of the grief response."
   d. "Just think about the good times that you had while he was alive."

9. An acutely depressed patient isolates herself in her room and just sits and stares into space. Which of these is the best example of an active communication approach with this patient?
   a. "Do you like exercise?"
   b. "Come with me. I will go with you to group therapy."
   c. "Would you like to go to group therapy, stay in bed, or come out to the day lounge for some activities?"
   d. "Why do you stay in your room all the time?"

Continued

Review Questions—cont'd
Self-Examination/Learning Exercise

10. Shondra is admitted to the hospital with major depressive disorder and repeatedly makes negative statements about herself. Which of the following interventions is identified as an approach that promotes positive self-esteem in the patient? (Select all that apply.)
    a. Teach assertive communication skills.
    b. Make observations to Shondra when she completes a goal or task.
    c. Instruct Shondra that you will not talk with her unless she stops talking negatively about herself.
    d. Offer to spend time with Shondra using a nonjudgmental, accepting approach.

11. Demitrius informs the nurse that his doctor is considering ECT and asks for some information about the procedure. Which of the following are accurate statements that the nurse can share with this patient? (Select all that apply.)
    a. ECT is typically used to treat patients who have not responded to antidepressant therapy.
    b. A long-acting anesthetic agent is given to the patient the morning of the treatment.
    c. One treatment is usually all that is needed to relieve depression.
    d. Side effects may include headache and some confusion or memory loss.

IMPLICATIONS OF RESEARCH FOR EVIDENCE-BASED PRACTICE

Schomerus, G., Matschinger, H., & Angermeyer, M. C. (2014). Causal beliefs of the public and social acceptance of persons with mental illness: A comparative analysis of schizophrenia, depression, and alcohol dependence. *Psychological Medicine, 44,* 303–314.

DESCRIPTION OF THE STUDY: The aim of the study was to identify whether biological explanations for mental illness (including schizophrenia, depression, and alcohol dependence) improved people's perceptions about and tolerance of people with these conditions. This study was conducted in Germany with a large sample (N = 3,642). The researchers used path models to compare different variables such as beliefs that these illnesses are caused by biogenetic factors, current stress, and/or childhood adversity. Then the researchers identified the participants' attitudes and social acceptance of patients with a mental illness based on those beliefs.

RESULTS OF THE STUDY: Biogenetic beliefs as a cause for mental illness were associated with lower acceptance of people with schizophrenia and depression but higher acceptance of individuals with alcohol dependence. Lower social acceptance was related to the perceptions of differentness and dangerousness that were believed to be "etched in stone" if the illness is genetic in origin (an oversimplification of the influence of genetic factors). Current stress as a cause for mental illness was associated with higher acceptance of people with schizophrenia, whereas belief in childhood adversity as a cause was associated with lower acceptance of people with depression.

IMPLICATIONS FOR NURSING PRACTICE: Stigmatization (a devaluing attitude about people's ability to function in society based on an illness or disability) has been identified as a major barrier to recovery for people with mental illnesses. This study provides evidence that we need to be thoughtful as we educate patients and families. In reality, mental illnesses, based on current evidence, are probably caused by many factors including genetic vulnerability, current stress, and past trauma. Oftentimes mental illnesses are explained strictly as biogenetic diseases of the brain and, at times, this is misrepresented as completely known when, in fact, much of our current knowledge about causality in mental illness is theoretical. The researchers conclude that we may not be helping our patients or combating stigma when we try to oversimplify causality explanations.

When interpreting findings from a study such as this, it is important to consider what variables might influence the findings. For example, might cultural beliefs about mental illness and biogenetics in Germany differ from those in other parts of the world? These questions become the foundation for additional research. Interestingly, the researchers cite a study by Hansell and colleagues in 2011* that reviewed Web sites in the United States and found that information supplied by universities and government agencies more often provided a balanced view of potential causative factors where nongovernment agencies

IMPLICATIONS OF RESEARCH FOR EVIDENCE-BASED PRACTICE—cont'd

and pharmaceutical Web sites tended to overemphasize biological causes. Nurses need to be cautious about the reliability of their sources for information to maintain the public trust in the information that is shared. The bottom line is, as nurses, we need to ensure that we are providing balanced information, based on current evidence when we provide patient education. This is critical to providing accurate information to patients and families and, as the study suggests, may help in the battle against stigmatization of people with mental illness.

*Hansell, J., Bailin, A. P., Franke, K. A., Kraft, J. M., Wu, H. Y., Dolsen, M. R., . . . Kazi, N. F. (2011). Conceptually sound thinking about depression: An Internet survey and its implications. *Professional Psychology: Research and Practice, 42*(5), 382–390. doi:10.1037/a0025608

TEST YOUR CRITICAL THINKING SKILLS

Carol is a 17-year-old high school senior. She will graduate in 1 month and has plans to attend the state university a few hours from her home. Carol has always made good grades in school, has participated in many activities, and has been a pep squad cheerleader. She had been dating the star quarterback, Alan, since last summer, and they had spoken a number of times about going to the senior prom together. About a month before the prom, Alan broke up with Carol and began dating Salima, whom he subsequently took to the prom. Since that time, Carol has become despondent. She does not go out with her friends, she dropped out of the pep squad, her grades have fallen, and she has lost 10 pounds. She attends classes most of the time, but she spends evenings and weekends in her room alone listening to her music, crying, and sleeping. Her parents are very concerned and contacted the family physician, who has admitted Carol to the psychiatric unit of the local hospital. The admitting psychiatrist has made the diagnosis of Major Depressive Disorder. Carol tells the nurse, "Sometimes I drive around and try to find Alan and Salima. I don't know why he broke up with me. I hate myself! I just want to die!"

Answer the following questions related to Carol:

1. What is the primary nursing diagnosis that is identified for Carol?
2. To determine the seriousness of this problem, what are important nursing assessments that must be made?
3. What medication might the physician order for Carol?
4. What concern has the FDA identified that is associated with this medication?

Communication Exercises

1. Carrie, age 75, is a patient on the psychiatric unit with a diagnosis of Major Depressive Disorder. She says to the nurse, "I never knew my life would end up like this. I've lost my husband, all my friends, and my home."
   What would be an appropriate response by the nurse to this statement by Carrie?

2. "I have spent my whole life taking care of others. Now someone else has to take care of me. I feel so useless."
   What would be an appropriate response by the nurse to this statement by Carrie?

3. "I don't know why anyone would want to bother taking care of me. I really have nothing left to live for."
   What would be an appropriate response by the nurse to this statement by Carrie?

🎬 MOVIE CONNECTIONS

Prozac Nation (Depression) • *The Butcher Boy* (Depression) • *Night, Mother* (Depression) • *The Prince of Tides* (Depression/suicide)

References

Abbott, C. C., Gallegos, P., Rediske, N., Lemke, N. T., & Quinn, D. K. (2014). A review of longitudinal electroconvulsive therapy: Neuroimaging investigations. *Journal of Geriatric Psychiatry and Neurology, 27*(1), 33–46. doi:10.1177/0891988713516542. PMID 24381234

Akiskal, H. S. (2017). Mood disorders: Historical introduction and conceptual overview. In B. J. Sadock, V. A. Sadock, & P. Ruiz (Eds.), *Comprehensive textbook of psychiatry* (10th ed., pp. 1599–1603). Philadelphia, PA: Wolters Kluwer.

American Foundation for Suicide Prevention. (2018). *Suicide statistics.* Retrieved from https://afsp.org/about-suicide/suicide-statistics/

American Psychiatric Association (APA). (2001). The practice of electroconvulsive therapy: Recommendations for treatment, training, and privileging (2nd ed.). Washington, DC: Author.

American Psychiatric Association (APA). (2013). *Diagnostic and statistical manual of mental disorders* (5th ed.). Washington, DC: Author.

American Psychiatric Nurses Association. (2011). Position statement: Electroconvulsive therapy. Retrieved from https://www.apna.org/files/public/ECT_POSITION_STATEMENT.pdf

American Thyroid Association. (2018). *Prevalence and impact of thyroid disease.* Retrieved from https://www.thyroid.org/media-main/about-hypothyroidism/

Amick, H. R., Gartlehner, G., Gaynes, B. N., Forneris, C., Asher, G. N., Morgan, L. C., . . . Lohr, K. N. (2015). Comparative benefits and harms of second generation antidepressants and cognitive behavioral therapies in initial treatment of major depressive disorder: Systematic review and meta-analysis. *British Medical Journal, 351*, h6019. doi:http://dx.doi.org/10.1136/bmj.h6019

Anxiety and Depression Association of America. (2016). *Anxiety and depression in children*. Retrieved from https://www.adaa.org/living-with-anxiety/children/anxiety-and-depression

Bauer, A. E., Maegbaek, M. L., Liu, X., Wray, N. R., Sullivan, P. F., Miller, W. C., . . . Munk-Olsen, T. (2018). Familiality of psychiatric disorders and risk of postpartum psychiatric episodes: A population-based cohort study. *American Journal of Psychiatry*. doi:10.1176/appi.ajp.2018.17111184

Berlim, M. T., McGirr, A., Van den Eynde, F., Fleck, M. P., & Giacobbe P. (2014). Effectiveness and acceptability of deep brain stimulation (DBS) of the subgenual cingulate cortex for treatment-resistant depression: A systematic review and exploratory meta-analysis. *Journal of Affective Disorders, 159*, 31–38. doi:10.1016/j.jad.2014.02.016

Canuso, C. M., Singh, J. B., Fedgchin, M., Alphs, L., Lane, R., Lim, P., . . . Drevets, W. C. (2018). Efficacy and safety of intranasal esketamine for the rapid reduction of symptoms of depression and suicidality in patients at imminent risk for suicide: Results of a double-blind, randomized, placebo-controlled study. *The American Journal of Psychiatry*. doi.org/10.1176/appi.ajp.2018.17060720

Centers for Disease Control and Prevention (CDC). (2017). *Depression is not a normal part of growing older*. Retrieved from https://www.cdc.gov/aging/mentalhealth/depression.htm

Cobb, B. S., Coryell, W. H., Cavanough, J., Keller, M., Solomon, D., Endicott, J., & Fiedorowicz, J. G. (2014). Seasonal variation of depressive symptoms in unipolar major depressive disorder. *Comprehensive Psychiatry, 55*(8), 1891–1899. doi:10.1016/j.comppsych.2014.07.021

Cotterell, D. (2010). Pathogenesis and management of seasonal affective disorder. *Progress in Neurology and Psychiatry, 14*(5), 18–25. doi:10.1002/pnp.173

Day, L., & Smith, E. L. (2007). Integrating quality and safety content into clinical teaching in the acute care setting. *Nursing Outlook, 55*(3), 138–143.

Fetterman, T. C., & Ying, P. (2011). Informed consent and electroconvulsive therapy. *Journal of the American Psychiatric Nurses Association, 17*(3), 219–222. doi:10.1177/1078390311408604

Freeman, A., Tyrovolas, S., Koyanagi, A., Chatterji, S., Leonardi, M., Ayuso-Mateos, J. L., . . . Josep Maria Haro, J. M. (2016). The role of socio-economic status in depression: Results from the COURAGE (aging survey in Europe). *BMC Public Health, 16*, 1098. doi: 10.1186/s12889-016-3638-0

Gaynes, B. N., Lloyd, S. W., Lux, L., Gartlehner, G., Hansen, R. A., Brode, S., . . . Lohr, K. N. (2014). Repetitive transcranial magnetic stimulation for treatment-resistant depression. *Journal of Clinical Psychiatry, 75*(5), 477–489.

Geduldig, E. T., & Kellner, C. H. (2016). Electroconvulsive therapy in the elderly: New findings in geriatric depression. *Current Psychiatry Reports, 18*, 40. https://doi.org/10.1007/s11920-016-0674-5

George, M. S., Taylor, J. J., & Short, E. B. (2013). The expanding evidence base for rTMS treatment of depression. *Current Opinion in Psychiatry, 26*(1), 13–18.

Greiner, A., Knebel, E., & Institute of Medicine Board on Health Care Services and Committee on the Health Professions Education Summit. (2003). *Health professions education: A bridge to quality*. Washington, DC: National Academies Press.

Hansell, J., Bailin, A. P., Franke, K. A., Kraft, J. M., Wu, H. Y., Dolsen, M. R., . . . Kazi, N. F. (2011). Conceptually sound thinking about depression: An Internet survey and its implications. *Professional Psychology: Research and Practice, 42*, 382–390.

Herdman, T. H., & Kamitsuru, S. (Eds.). (2018). *NANDA-I nursing diagnoses: Definitions and classification, 2018–2020*.

Holland, K. (2016). *Herbs, vitamins, and supplements for depression*. Retrieved from https://www.healthline.com/health/depression/herbs-vitamins-supplements

Holt-Lundstat, J., Robles, T. F., & Sbarra, D. A. (2017). Advancing social connection as a public health priority in the United States. *American Psychologist, 72*(6), 517–530. doi.org/10.1037/amp0000103

Jiang, X., Asmaro, R., O'Sullivan, D. O., Budnik, E., & Schnatz, P. F. (2016). Depression may be one of the strongest risk factors for coronary artery disease in women aged <65 years: A 10-year prospective longitudinal study [Abstract S-17]. Presented at the NAMS 2016 Annual Meeting, October 5–8, 2016, Orlando, FL.

Kelsoe, J. R., & Greenwood, T. A. (2017). Mood disorders: Genetics. In B. J. Sadock, V. A. Sadock, & P. Ruiz (Eds.), *Comprehensive textbook of psychiatry* (10 ed., pp. 1619–1630). Philadelphia, PA: Wolters Kluwer.

Kurlansik, S. L., & Ibay, A. D. (2013). Seasonal affective disorder. *Indian Journal of Clinical Practice, 24*(7), 607–610.

Lam, R. W., Levitt, A. J., Levitan, R. D., Michelak, E., Morehouse, R., Rammasubbu, R., & Tam, E. M. (2015). Efficacy of bright light treatment, fluoxetine, and the combination in patients with non-seasonal major depressive disorder: A randomized clinical trial. *JAMA Psychiatry*. doi:10.1001/jamapsychiatry.2015.2235

Lapate, R. C., Van Reekum, C. M., Schaefer, S. M., Greischar, L. L., Norris, C. J., Bachhuber, D., & Davidson, R. J. (2014). Prolonged marital stress is associated with short-lived responses to positive stimuli. *Psychophysiology, 51*(6), 499–509. doi:10.1111/psyp.12203

LaPierre, T. A. (2004). *An investigation of the role of age and life stage in the moderation and mediation of the effect of marital status on depression*. Paper presented at the annual meeting of the American Sociological Association, Hilton San Francisco & Renaissance Parc 55 Hotel, San Francisco, CA, August 14, 2004. Retrieved from http://www.allacademic.com/meta/p109917_index.html

Lee, K. C. (2015). Using pharmacogenomics to aid antidepressant prescribing. *Psychiatry Advisor*. Retrieved from http://www.psychiatryadvisor.com/mood-disorders/using-pharmacogenomics-to-aid-antidepressant-prescribing/article/394244/2

Magnezi, R., Aminov, E., Shmuel, D., Dreifuss, M., & Dannon, P. (2016). Comparison between neurostimulation techniques repetitive transcranial magnetic stimulation vs electroconvulsive therapy for the treatment of resistant depression: Patient preference and cost-effectiveness. *Patient Preference and Adherence, 10*, 1481–1487. doi:10.2147/PPA.S105654

Mårtensson, B., Pettersson, A., Berglund, L., & Ekselius, L. (2015). Bright white light therapy in depression: A critical review of the evidence. *Journal of Affective Disorders, 182*, 1–7. doi: 10.1016/j.jad.2015.04.013.

Mayo Clinic. (2016). *Antidepressants for children and teens*. Retrieved from http://www.mayoclinic.org/diseases-conditions/teen-depression/in-depth/antidepressants/art-20047502

Mayo Clinic. (2018). *Electroconvulsive therapy*. Retrieved from https://www.mayoclinic.org/tests-procedures/electroconvulsive-therapy/about/pac-20393894

McClintock, S.M., & Husain, M.M. (2011). Electroconvulsive therapy does not damage the brain. *Journal of the American Psychiatric Nurses Association, 17*(3), 212–213. doi:10.1177/1078390311407667

McMahon, B., Andersen, S. B., Madsen, M. K., Hjordt, L. V., Hageman, I., Dam, H., . . . Knudsen, G. M. (2016). Seasonal difference in brain serotonin transporter binding predicts symptom severity in patients with seasonal affective disorder. *Brain, 139*(Pt. 5), 1605–1614. doi:10.1093/brain/aww043

Merikangas, K. R., & Rihmer, Z. (2017). Mood disorders: Epidemiology. In B. J. Sadock, V. A. Sadock, & P. Ruiz (Eds.), *Comprehensive textbook of psychiatry* (10th ed., pp. 1614–1619). Philadelphia, PA: Wolters Kluwer.

Miller, A. H. (2018). *Five things to know about inflammation and depression*. Retrieved from http://www.psychiatrictimes.com/special-reports/five-things-know-about-inflammation-and-depression/page/0/1

Mojtabai, R., Olfson, M., & Han, B. (2016). National trends in the prevalence and treatment of depression in adolescents and young adults. *Pediatrics, 138*(6), 9. doi:10.1542/peds.2016-1878

National Center for Health Statistics (NCHS). (2012). *Health, United States, 2011* (DHS Publication No. 2012-1232). Hyattsville, MD: Author.

National Center for Health Statistics (NCHS). (2018). *Faststats: Adolescent health.* Retrieved from https://www.cdc.gov/nchs/fastats/adolescent-health.htm

National Institute of Mental Health (NIMH). (n.d.). *Postpartum depression facts.* Retrieved from https://www.nimh.nih.gov/health/publications/postpartum-depression-facts/index.shtml

National Institute of Mental Health (NIMH). (2018). *Depression.* Retrieved from https://www.nimh.nih.gov/health/topics/depression/index.shtml

Natsuaki, M. N., Shaw, D. S., Neiderhiser, J. M., Ganiban, J., Gordon, H. T., Reiss, D., & Leve, L. D. (2014). Raised by depressed parents: Is it an environmental risk? *Clinical Child and Family Psychology Review, 17*(4), 357–367. doi:10.1007/s10567-014-0169-z

Page, A. C., & Hooke, G. R. (2012). Effectiveness of cognitive behavioral therapy modified for inpatients with depression. *International Scholarly Research Notices, 2012*(4). doi:http://dx.doi.org/10.5402/2012/461265

Pulia, K., Vaidya, P., Jayaram, G., Hayat, M. J., & Reti, I. M. (2013). ECT treatment outcomes following performance improvement changes. *Journal of Psychosocial Nursing and Mental Health Services, 51*(11), 20–25. doi:10.3928/02793695-20130628-02

Raposelli, D. (2015). Is TMS cost effective? *Psychiatric Times.* Retrieved from http://www.psychiatrictimes.com/major-depressive-disorder/tms-cost-effective

Rodriguez, T. (2015). Using bright light therapy beyond seasonal affective disorder. *Psychiatry Advisor.* Retrieved from http://www.psychiatryadvisor.com/mood-disorders/depression-mood-winter-season-light-sad-antidepressant/article/457643

Rohan, K. J., Mahon, J. N., Evans, M., Ho, S-Y., Meyerhoff, J., Postolache, T. T., & Vacek, P. M. (2016). Outcomes one and two winters following cognitive-behavioral therapy or light therapy for seasonal affective disorder. *American Journal of Psychiatry, 173,* 244–251.

Sadock, B. J., Sadock, V. A., & Ruiz, P. (2015). *Synopsis of psychiatry: Behavioral sciences/clinical psychiatry* (11th ed.). Philadelphia, PA: Wolters Kluwer.

Sathyanarayana, T. S., Asha, M. R., Ramsh, B. M., & Rao, K. S. (2008). Understanding nutrition, depression, and mental illness. *Indian Journal of Psychiatry, 50*(2), 77–82. doi:10.4103/0019-5545.42391

Schomerus, G., Matschinger, H., & Angermeyer, M. C. (2014). Causal beliefs of the public and social acceptance of persons with mental illness: A comparative analysis of schizophrenia, depression, and alcohol dependence. *Psychological Medicine, 44,* 303–314. doi:10.1017/S003321971300072X

Sharma, M. S., Ang-Rabeanes, M., Selek, S., Gajwani, P., & Soares, J. C. (2018). Neuromodulatory options for treatment-resistant depression. *Current Psychiatry, 17*(3), 26–37.

Siddique, J., Chung, J. Y., Brown, C. H., & Miranda, J. (2012). Comparative effectiveness of medication versus cognitive-behavioral therapy in a randomized controlled trial of low income young minority women with depression. *Journal of Consulting and Clinical Psychology, 80*(6), 995–1006. doi:10.1037/a0030452

Substance Abuse and Mental Health Services Administration (SAMHSA). (2017). 2015–2016 National survey on drug use and health: Model-based prevalence estimates (50 states and the District of Columbia). Retrieved from https://www.samhsa.gov/data/sites/default/files/NSDUHsaePercents2016/NSDUHsaePercents2016.pdf

Thielen, J. (2015). Premenstrual syndrome. *Mayo Clinic.* Retrieved from http://www.mayoclinic.org/diseases-conditions/premenstrual-syndrome/expert-answers/pmdd/faq-20058315

United States Census Bureau. (2017). *American fact finder: 2016 American Community Survey.* Retrieved from https://factfinder.census.gov/faces/nav/jsf/pages/community_facts.xhtml

Vera, M. (2012). *Nursing notes: Electroconvulsive therapy.* Retrieved from http://nurseslabs.com/electroconvulsivetherapy-nursing-care

Wagner, K. D., & Brent, D. A. (2017). Mood disorders in children and adolescents: Depressive disorders and suicide. In B. J. Sadock, V. A. Sadock, & P. Ruiz (Eds.), *Comprehensive textbook of psychiatry* (10th ed., pp. 3674–3685). Philadelphia, PA: Wolters Kluwer.

Winthorst, W., Post, W., Meesters, Y., Penninx, B., & Nolen, W. A. (2011). Seasonality in depressive and anxiety symptoms among primary care patients and in patients with depressive and anxiety disorders; results from the Netherlands Study of Depression and Anxiety. *BMC Psychiatry, 11*(1), 1–18. doi:10.1186/1471-244X-11-198

Classical References

Beck, A. T., Rush, A. J., Shaw, B. F., & Emery, G. (1979). *Cognitive theory of depression.* New York, NY: Guilford Press.

Freud, S. (1957). *Mourning and melancholia, Vol. 14* (Standard ed.). London, England: Hogarth Press. (Original work published 1917)

Hamilton, M. (1960). A rating scale for depression. *Journal of Neurology, Neurosurgery, & Psychiatry, 23,* 56–62.

Seligman, M. E. P. (1973). Fall into helplessness. *Psychology Today, 7,* 43–48.

17

Bipolar and Related Disorders

CORE CONCEPT

Mania

KEY TERMS

bipolar disorder

cyclothymic disorder

delirious mania

flight of ideas

hypomania

OBJECTIVES

After reading this chapter, the student will be able to:

1. Recount historical perspectives of bipolar disorder.
2. Discuss epidemiological statistics related to bipolar disorder.
3. Describe various types of bipolar disorders.
4. Identify predisposing factors in the development of bipolar disorder.
5. Discuss implications of bipolar disorder related to developmental stage.
6. Identify symptomatology associated with bipolar disorder and use this information in client assessment.
7. Formulate nursing diagnoses and goals of care for clients experiencing a manic episode.
8. Identify topics for patient and family teaching relevant to bipolar disorder.
9. Describe appropriate nursing interventions for patients experiencing a manic episode.
10. Describe relevant criteria for evaluating nursing care of patients experiencing a manic episode.
11. Discuss various modalities relevant to treatment of bipolar disorder.

HOMEWORK ASSIGNMENT

Please read the chapter and answer the following questions:

1. What is the most common medication that has been known to trigger manic episodes?
2. What is the speech pattern of a person experiencing a manic episode?
3. What is the difference between cyclothymic disorder and bipolar disorder?
4. Why should a person on lithium therapy have blood levels drawn regularly?

Introduction

Mood is defined in Chapter 16, Depressive Disorders, as a pervasive and sustained emotion that may have a major influence on a person's perception of the world. Examples of mood include depression, joy, elation, anger, and anxiety. *Affect* is described as the external, observable emotional reaction associated with an experience.

Chapter 16 focuses on the consequences of complicated grieving as it is manifested by depressive disorders. This chapter addresses mood disorders as they are manifested by cycles of mania and depression—called **bipolar disorder.** A historical perspective and epidemiological statistics related to bipolar disorder are presented. Predisposing factors that have been implicated in the etiology of bipolar disorder provide a framework for studying the dynamics of the disorder.

The implications of bipolar disorder relevant to children and adolescents are discussed. An explanation of the symptomatology is presented as background knowledge for assessing the client with bipolar disorder. Nursing care is described in the context of the six steps of the nursing process. Various medical treatment modalities are explored.

CORE CONCEPT

Mania

An alteration in mood that may be expressed by feelings of elation, inflated self-esteem, grandiosity, hyperactivity, agitation, racing thoughts, and accelerated speech. Mania can occur as part of the psychiatric disorder bipolar disorder, as part of some other medical conditions, or in response to some substances.

Historical Perspective

Documentation of the symptoms associated with bipolar disorder dates back to about the second century in ancient Greece. Aretaeus of Cappadocia, a Greek physician, is credited with associating these extremes of mood as part of the same illness. He described patients who could at times laugh and play all night and day but at other times appeared "torpid, dull, and sorrowful (Burton, 2012). His view that these mood swings were part of the same illness did not gain acceptance until much later.

In early writings, mania was categorized with all forms of "severe madness." In 1025, the Persian physician Avicenna wrote *The Canon of Medicine* in which he described mania as "bestial madness characterized by rapid onset and remission, with agitation and irritability." The modern concept of manic-depressive illness began to emerge in the 19th century. In 1854, Jules Baillarger presented information to the French Imperial Academy of Medicine in which he used the term *dual-form insanity* to describe the illness. In the same year, Jean-Pierre Falret described the same disorder, which he termed *circular insanity* (Burton, 2012). Falret also noted that this disorder appeared to have genetic underpinnings, a belief that is adhered to today (Krans & Cherney, 2018).

Contemporary thinking has been shaped a great deal by the works of Emil Kraepelin, who first coined the term *manic-depressive* in 1913. He added that this disorder was characterized by acute episodes followed by relatively symptom-free periods. In 1980, the American Psychiatric Association (APA) adopted the term *bipolar disorder* as the diagnostic category for manic-depressive illness in the third edition of the *Diagnostic and Statistical Manual of Mental Disorders (DSM-III)*. This term identified a period of mood elevation and excitation as a defining characteristic that distinguishes it from other mood and psychotic disorders. The term *mania* was replaced in the diagnostic label because the description of people as "maniacs" was considered stigmatizing (Krans & Cherney, 2018). The term itself, however, is still currently used to describe an abnormal mood state of elation with symptoms that include agitation, insomnia, grandiose delusions, racing thoughts, boundless energy, and increased libido among others.

Epidemiology

Bipolar disorder affects approximately 4.4 percent of American adults and 82.9 percent of these cases are considered severe (National Institute of Mental Health [NIMH], 2017). In terms of gender, bipolar disorder occurs roughly the same between men and women. The average age of onset for bipolar disorder is 25 years, and following the first manic episode, the disorder tends to be recurrent. Bipolar disorder is associated with increased mortality in general and particularly with death by suicide (Merikangas & Rihmer, 2017).

Unlike depressive disorders, bipolar disorder appears to occur more frequently among the higher socioeconomic classes with an overrepresentation among socially active, creative individuals (Merikangas & Rihmer, 2017). Bipolar disorder is the sixth leading cause of disability in the middle-age group, but for those who respond to lithium treatment (about 33 percent of those treated with lithium), bipolar disorder may be completely treatable with no further episodes. Unfortunately, many individuals go for years without an accurate diagnosis or treatment, and for some the consequences can be devastating.

Types of Bipolar Disorders

A bipolar disorder is characterized by mood swings from profound depression to extreme euphoria (mania) with intervening periods of normalcy. Delusions or hallucinations may or may not be a part of the clinical picture, and onset of symptoms may reflect a seasonal pattern.

During a manic episode, the mood is elevated, expansive, or irritable. The disturbance is sufficiently severe to cause marked impairment in occupational functioning or in usual social activities or relationships with others or to require hospitalization to prevent harm to self or others. Motor activity is excessive and frenzied. Psychotic features may be present. The *Diagnostic and Statistical Manual of Mental Disorders, Fifth Edition (DSM-5)* (APA, 2013) diagnostic criteria for a manic episode are presented in Box 17–1.

A somewhat milder degree of this clinical symptom picture is called **hypomania.** Hypomania is not severe enough to cause marked impairment in social or occupational functioning or to require hospitalization, and it does not include psychotic features. The *DSM-5* diagnostic criteria for a hypomanic episode are presented in Box 17–2.

The diagnostic picture for depression associated with bipolar disorder is similar to that described for major depressive disorder, with one major distinction: the client must have a history of one or more manic episodes. When the presentation includes symptoms associated with both depression and mania, the diagnosis is further specified as *with mixed features.*

Bipolar I Disorder

Bipolar I disorder is the diagnosis given to an individual who is experiencing a manic episode or has a history of one or more manic episodes. The client may also have experienced episodes of depression. This diagnosis is further specified by the current or most recent behavioral episode experienced. For example, the specifier might be *single manic episode* (to describe individuals having a first episode of mania) or *current* (or most recent) *episode manic, hypomanic, mixed,* or *depressed* (to describe individuals who have had recurrent mood episodes). Psychotic or catatonic features may also be noted. Although the length of manic episodes (and depressive episodes) is variable when an

---

BOX 17–1 Diagnostic Criteria for a Manic Episode

A. A distinct period of abnormally and persistently elevated, expansive, or irritable mood and abnormally and persistently increased goal-directed activity or energy, lasting at least 1 week and present most of the day, nearly every day (or of any duration if hospitalization is necessary).

B. During the period of mood disturbance and increased energy or activity, three (or more) of the following symptoms (four if the mood is only irritable) are present to a significant degree and represent a noticeable change from usual behavior:
  1. Inflated self-esteem or grandiosity
  2. Decreased need for sleep (e.g., feels rested after only 3 hours of sleep)
  3. More talkative than usual or pressure to keep talking
  4. Flight of ideas or subjective experience that thoughts are racing
  5. Distractibility (i.e., attention too easily drawn to unimportant or irrelevant external stimuli), as reported or observed

  6. Increase in goal-directed activity (either socially, at work or school, or sexually) or psychomotor agitation (i.e., purposeless non-goal-directed activity)
  7. Excessive involvement in activities that have a high potential for painful consequences (e.g., engaging in unrestrained buying sprees, sexual indiscretions, or foolish business investments)

C. The mood disturbance is sufficiently severe to cause marked impairment in social or occupational functioning or to necessitate hospitalization to prevent harm to self or others, or there are psychotic features.

D. The episode is not attributable to the physiological effects of a substance (e.g., a drug of abuse, a medication, or other treatment) or to another medical condition.

Note: A full manic episode that emerges during antidepressant treatment (e.g., medication, electroconvulsive therapy) but persists at a fully syndromal level beyond the physiological effect of that treatment is sufficient evidence for a manic episode and, therefore, a bipolar I diagnosis.

BOX 17–2 Diagnostic Criteria for a Hypomanic Episode

A. A distinct period of abnormally and persistently elevated, expansive, or irritable mood and abnormally and persistently increased activity or energy, lasting at least 4 consecutive days and present most of the day, nearly every day.

B. During the period of mood disturbance and increased energy and activity, three (or more) of the following symptoms (four if the mood is only irritable) have persisted, represent a noticeable change from usual behavior, and have been present to a significant degree:
1. Inflated self-esteem or grandiosity
2. Decreased need for sleep (e.g., feels rested after only 3 hours of sleep)
3. More talkative than usual or pressure to keep talking
4. Flight of ideas or subjective experience that thoughts are racing
5. Distractibility (i.e., attention too easily drawn to unimportant or irrelevant external stimuli), as reported or observed
6. Increase in goal-directed activity (either socially, at work or school, or sexually) or psychomotor agitation
7. Excessive involvement in pleasurable activities that have a high potential for painful consequences (e.g., engaging in unrestrained buying sprees, sexual indiscretions, or foolish business investments)

C. The episode is associated with an unequivocal change in functioning that is uncharacteristic of the individual when not symptomatic.

D. The disturbance in mood and the change in functioning are observable by others.

E. The episode is not severe enough to cause marked impairment in social or occupational functioning or to necessitate hospitalization. If there are psychotic features, the episode is, by definition, manic.

F. The episode is not attributable to the physiological effects of a substance (e.g., a drug of abuse, a medication, or other treatment).

Note: A full hypomanic episode that emerges during antidepressant treatment (medication, electroconvulsive therapy) but persists at a fully syndromal level beyond the physiological effect of that treatment is sufficient evidence for a hypomanic episode diagnosis. However, caution is indicated so that one or two symptoms (particularly increased irritability, edginess or agitation following antidepressant use) are not taken as sufficient for diagnosis of a hypomanic episode, nor necessarily indicative of a bipolar diathesis.

Reprinted with permission from American Psychiatric Association. (2013). Diagnostic and statistical manual of mental disorders (5th ed.). Washington, DC: American Psychiatric Publishing.

individual has more than four manic and depressive episodes in a year, he or she is referred to as having *rapid cycling* bipolar disorder.

Bipolar II Disorder

The bipolar II disorder diagnostic category is characterized by recurrent bouts of major depression with episodic occurrence of hypomania. The individual who is assigned this diagnosis may present with symptoms (or history) of depression or hypomania. The client has never experienced a full manic episode, and the symptoms are "not severe enough to cause marked impairment in social or occupational functioning or to necessitate hospitalization" (APA, 2013, p. 133). The diagnosis may specify whether the current or most recent episode is hypomanic, depressed, or with mixed features. If the current syndrome is a major depressive episode, psychotic or catatonic features may be noted.

Cyclothymic Disorder

The essential feature of **cyclothymic disorder** is a chronic mood disturbance of at least 2 years' duration, involving numerous periods of elevated mood

that do not meet the criteria for a hypomanic episode and numerous periods of depressed mood of insufficient severity or duration to meet the criteria for major depressive episode. The individual is never without the symptoms for more than 2 months. The *DSM-5* criteria for cyclothymic disorder are presented in Box 17–3.

Substance/Medication-Induced Bipolar Disorder

The disturbance of mood associated with this disorder is considered to be the direct result of physiological effects of a substance (e.g., ingestion of or withdrawal from a drug of abuse or a medication). The mood disturbance may involve elevated, expansive, or irritable mood with inflated self-esteem, decreased need for sleep, and distractibility. The disorder causes clinically significant distress or impairment in social, occupational, or other important areas of functioning.

Mood disturbances are associated with *intoxication* from substances such as alcohol, amphetamines, cocaine, hallucinogens, inhalants, opioids,

---

BOX 17-3 Diagnostic Criteria for Cyclothymic Disorder

A. For at least 2 years (at least 1 year in children and adolescents) there have been numerous periods with hypomanic symptoms that do not meet criteria for hypomanic episode and numerous periods with depressive symptoms that do not meet the criteria for a major depressive episode.

B. During the above 2-year period (1 year in children and adolescents), the hypomanic and depressive periods have been present for at least half the time, and the individual has not been without the symptoms for more than 2 months at a time.

C. Criteria for a major depressive, manic, or hypomanic episode have never been met.

D. The symptoms in Criterion A are not better explained by schizoaffective disorder, schizophrenia, schizophreniform disorder, delusional disorder, or other specified or unspecified schizophrenia spectrum and other psychotic disorder.

E. The symptoms are not attributable to the physiological effects of a substance (e.g., a drug of abuse, a medication) or another medical condition (e.g., hyperthyroidism).

F. The symptoms cause clinically significant distress or impairment in social, occupational, or other important areas of functioning.

Specify if:
With anxious distress

Reprinted with permission from American Psychiatric Association. (2013). Diagnostic and statistical manual of mental disorders (5th ed.). Washington, DC: American Psychiatric Publishing.

---

phencyclidine, sedatives, hypnotics, and anxiolytics. Symptoms can also occur during *withdrawal* from substances such as alcohol, amphetamines, cocaine, sedatives, hypnotics, and anxiolytics.

A number of medications have been known to evoke mood symptoms. Classifications include anesthetics, analgesics, anticholinergics, anticonvulsants, antihypertensives, antiparkinsonian agents, antiulcer agents, cardiac medications, oral contraceptives, psychotropic medications, muscle relaxants, steroids, and sulfonamides. Some specific examples are included in the discussion of predisposing factors associated with bipolar disorders.

Bipolar Disorder Due to Another Medical Condition

This disorder is characterized by an abnormally and persistently elevated, expansive, or irritable mood and excessive activity or energy that is judged to be the result of direct physiological consequence of another medical condition (APA, 2013). The mood disturbance causes clinically significant distress or impairment in social, occupational, or other important areas of functioning. Types of physiological influences are included in the discussion of predisposing factors associated with bipolar disorders.

Predisposing Factors

The exact etiology of bipolar disorder has yet to be determined. Scientific evidence supports a chemical imbalance in the brain, although the cause of the imbalance remains unclear. Theories that consider a combination of hereditary factors and environmental triggers (stressful life events) appear to hold the most credibility.

Biological Theories

Genetics

Research suggests that bipolar disorder strongly reflects an underlying genetic vulnerability. Evidence from family, twin, and adoption studies exists to support this observation. In a large study that looked at genetic variations associated with five major mental illnesses, the researchers found that schizophrenia and bipolar disorders had about 15 percent of genetic variations in common (NIMH, 2013).

Twin Studies

Twin studies have indicated a concordance rate for bipolar disorder among monozygotic twins at 60 to 80 percent compared to 10 to 20 percent in dizygotic twins. Because monozygotic twins have identical genes and dizygotic twins share only approximately half their genes, this is strong evidence that genes play a major role in the etiology. However, because identical twins do not always develop the illness, other factors must also be involved. It is likely that many different genes as well as environmental factors are involved, although researchers do not yet know how these factors interact to cause bipolar disorder.

Family Studies

In general, family studies have shown that if one parent has a mood disorder, the risk that a child will have a mood disorder is between 10 and 25 percent (Sadock, Sadock, & Ruiz, 2015). Sadock and associates report that "a family history of bipolar disorder conveys a greater risk for mood disorders in general and, specifically, a much greater risk for bipolar disorder" (p. 352). If both parents have the disorder, the risk is two to three times as great. This has also been shown to be the case in studies of children born to parents with bipolar disorder who were adopted at birth and reared by adoptive parents without evidence of the disorder.

Other Genetic Studies

Soreff and McInnes (2018) state:

> The first series of genome-wide association studies . . . gave combined support for two particular genes, *ANK3* (ankyrin G) and *CACNA1C* (alpha 1C subunit of the L-type voltage-gated calcium channel) in a sample of 4,387 cases and 6,209 controls.

The *ANK3* protein is located on the first part of the axon and is involved in making the determination of whether a neuron will fire. Studies have shown that lithium carbonate, the most common medication used to prevent manic episodes, reduces expression of *ANK3* (Leussis et al., 2013). The *CACNA1C* protein regulates the influx and outflow of calcium from the cells and is the site of action of the calcium channel blockers sometimes used in the treatment in bipolar disorder.

Recent research looking specifically at factors associated with lithium's effectiveness identified "a number of candidate genes related to neurotransmitters, intracellular signaling, neuroprotection, circadian rhythms, and other pathogenic mechanisms of bipolar disorder [that] were found to be associated with lithium's prophylactic response" (Rybakowski, 2014, p. 353). Evidence from another recent study identified that common gene sets demonstrated altered expression in patients with schizophrenia, bipolar disorder, and depression (Darby, Yolken, & Sabunciyan, 2016). Specifically, ribosomal genes were overexpressed, and those involved with neuronal connections such as gamma aminobutyric acid (GABA) signaling were underexpressed.

The researchers suggest that this finding may lead the way to RNA processing and protein synthesis as targets for therapeutic intervention. Ongoing genetic research will continue to shed light on the genetic influences in the development of bipolar disorder and the genetic factors that influence treatment response.

Biochemical Influences

Biogenic Amines

Early studies have associated symptoms of mania with a functional excess of norepinephrine and dopamine. The neurotransmitter serotonin is believed to remain low in both depression and mania. However, the exact mechanisms and biochemical influences are complex and not yet completely understood. For example, even though serotonin is believed to be low in both depression and manic states, selective serotonin reuptake inhibitors (SSRIs) have been shown to sometimes trigger manic episodes and rapid cycling of mood swings in clients with bipolar disorders. Likely, multiple factors influence serotonin's role in this illness. Acetylcholine is another neurotransmitter believed to be related to symptoms in bipolar disorder. Medications that have an effect on cholinergic transmission, particularly cholinergic agonists, can reduce symptoms in mania (Sadock et al., 2015). Excessive levels of glutamate, an excitatory neurotransmitter have been associated with bipolar disorder. Many of the mood stabilizers used to treat bipolar disorder inhibit the actions of glutamate. The primary support for neurotransmitter hypotheses has been the effects that neuroleptic drugs have on the levels of these biogenic amines and the resulting reduction in symptoms of the disorder. Although several neurotransmitters have been implicated in influencing symptoms, the cause of bipolar disorder remains unknown.

Physiological Influences

Neuroanatomical Factors

Neuroanatomical changes have been correlated with dysfunction in the prefrontal cortex, basal ganglia, temporal and frontal lobes of the forebrain, and parts of the limbic system, including the amygdala, thalamus, and striatum. The different symptoms in bipolar disorder may be correlated to those specific areas of dysfunction (Semeniken & Dudás, 2012). Sadock and associates (2015) report that widely replicated positive emission tomography (PET) demonstrates decreased anterior brain function on the left side in depression and, in mania, greater right-side reductions in brain activity. Akiskal (2017) adds that circadian disturbances seen in both depression and manic episodes can be conceptualized as dysfunction in the limbic system. Although causality of bipolar disorder cannot yet be defined as solely a neuroanatomical disorder, it is clear that mood disorders, including bipolar disorder, involve pathology in the brain.

Medication Side Effects

Certain medications used to treat somatic illnesses have been known to trigger a manic response. The most common of these are the steroids frequently used to treat chronic illnesses such as multiple sclerosis and systemic lupus erythematosus (SLE). Some clients whose first episode of mania occurred during steroid therapy have reported spontaneous recurrence of manic symptoms years later. Amphetamines, antidepressants, and high doses of anticonvulsants and narcotics also have the potential for initiating a manic episode.

Psychosocial Theories

Interest in psychosocial theories has declined in recent years with the focus of research on genetic and biochemical predisposing factors. Consequently, conditions such as schizophrenia and bipolar disorder are more often viewed as diseases of the brain with biological etiologies. However, several studies have confirmed a link between childhood trauma (emotional, physical, and sexual abuse) and the development of bipolar disorder (Aas et al., 2016; Etain et al., 2013; Janiri et al., 2015; Watson et al., 2013). Aas and associates (2016) identify that childhood trauma interacts with genes along several pathways, which influences not only an increased risk for bipolar disorder but also earlier onset, more severe symptoms, substance abuse, and suicide risk. As research continues, the interaction of genetics and psychosocial stressors will become more apparent. More research is needed to translate these connections into practical applications for treatment or prevention.

The Transactional Model of Stress and Adaptation

Bipolar disorder most likely results from an interaction among genetic, biological, and psychosocial determinants. The transactional model takes into consideration these various etiological influences as well as those associated with past experiences, existing conditions, and the individual's perception of the event.

Developmental Implications

The lifetime prevalence of adolescent bipolar disorders is estimated to be about 1 percent and in younger children the incidence is very rare, but children and adolescents are often difficult to diagnose (Sadock et al., 2015). In the past decade, diagnosis of bipolar I disorder in youth has rapidly increased, prompting researchers to look more closely at factors contributing to this trend. It was thought that there was a connection between attention deficit-hyperactivity disorder (ADHD) and the development of bipolar disorder in youth, but research has not supported this hypothesis (Hassan et al., 2011; Sadock et al., 2015). Studies also found that youth who were given this diagnosis more often manifested with a host of atypical symptoms, including nondiscrete mood episodes, chronic irritability, and temper tantrums. The *DSM-5* incorporated a new diagnosis, *disruptive mood dysregulation disorder,* that more aptly describes the symptom profile. Since then, a longitudinal study of children with nonepisodic irritability found that although these children had higher risk for anxiety and depression, they were not typically at higher risk for developing bipolar disorder (Sadock et al., 2015). In addition, Sadock and associates report that when true mania associated with bipolar disorder does occur in adolescents, it is frequently accompanied by flight of ideas, grandiose or persecutory delusions, and hallucinations. Because family studies show a familial risk for bipolar disorder, whenever a child is exhibiting mood-related symptoms (including depression) and there is a family history of bipolar disorders, the possibility for a developing bipolar disorder should be carefully evaluated. True bipolar disorder in adolescents, as with adults, is considered a chronic illness (much like diabetes) and medication treatment is typically lifelong.

Treatment Strategies

Psychopharmacology

Monotherapy with the traditional mood stabilizers (e.g., lithium, divalproex, carbamazepine) or atypical antipsychotics (e.g., olanzapine, quetiapine, risperidone, aripiprazole) has historically been the first-line treatment. In the event of inadequate response to initial monotherapy, an alternate monotherapeutic agent is suggested. Augmentation with a second medication is indicated when monotherapy fails.

In an analysis to examine the preponderance of research data on medications for treating acute mania in children and adolescents with bipolar disorder, Hazell and Jairam (2012) reported "evidence favoring the use of second- generation antipsychotics (SGAs), limited evidence favoring the use of combinations of SGA with a mood stabilizer, and no evidence supporting the use of mood stabilizer monotherapy" (p. 264). From their study, they suggest that the first-line treatment for mania in children and adolescents is an SGA with combination therapies offering no clear advantage.

ADHD has been identified as the most common comorbid condition in children and adolescents with bipolar disorder. Because stimulants can exacerbate mania, it is suggested that medication for ADHD be initiated only after bipolar symptoms have been controlled with a mood-stabilizing agent (Jain & Jain, 2014). Nonstimulant medications indicated for ADHD (e.g., atomoxetine, bupropion, the tricyclic antidepressants) may also induce switches to mania or hypomania.

Bipolar disorder in children and adolescents appears to be a chronic condition with a high risk of relapse. Maintenance therapy incorporates the same medications used to treat acute symptoms, although few research studies exist that deal with long-term maintenance of bipolar disorder in children.

Family Interventions

Although pharmacological treatment is acknowledged as the primary method of stabilizing acute symptoms, a combination of medications with psychosocial interventions has been recognized as serving an important role in preventing relapses and improving adjustment. Treatment adherence must be emphasized as an essential component of relapse prevention.

Family dynamics and attitudes can play a crucial role in the outcome of a client's recovery. Interventions with family members must include education that promotes understanding that at least part of the client's negative behaviors are attributable to an illness that must be managed.

Family-focused treatment (FFT) is an evidence-based intervention for reducing relapses and increasing medication adherence in bipolar clients (Miklowitz, 2016). This treatment may be useful with adult clients as well as children and adolescents with bipolar disorder. FFT includes sessions that deal with psychoeducation about bipolar disorder (i.e., symptoms, early recognition, etiology, treatment, self-management), communication training, and problem-solving skills training. Teaching the client and family about early warning signs and management strategies provides the client with a needed support system and the family with tools and resources to provide that support.

Application of the Nursing Process to Bipolar Disorder (Mania)

Background Assessment Data

Symptoms of manias can be described according to three levels of severity: hypomania, acute mania, and **delirious mania.** Symptoms of mood, cognition and perception, and activity and behavior are presented for each stage.

Hypomania

At this stage, the disturbance is not sufficiently severe to cause marked impairment in social or occupational functioning or to require hospitalization (APA, 2013).

Mood

The mood of a hypomanic person is cheerful and expansive. There is an underlying irritability that surfaces rapidly when the person's wishes and desires go unfilled, however. The nature of the hypomanic person is very volatile and fluctuating (after See Box 17-2: diagnostic criteria for a hypomanic episode).

Cognition and Perception

Perceptions of the self are exalted—the individual has ideas of great worth and ability. Thinking is flighty with a rapid flow of ideas. Perception of the environment is heightened, but the individual is so easily distracted by irrelevant stimuli that goal-directed activities are difficult.

Activity and Behavior

Hypomanic individuals exhibit increased motor activity. They are perceived as being very extroverted and sociable, and, consequently, they attract numerous acquaintances. However, they lack the depth of personality and warmth to formulate close friendships. They talk and laugh a great deal, usually very loudly and often inappropriately. Increased libido is common. Some individuals experience anorexia and weight loss. The exalted self-perception leads some hypomanic individuals to engage in inappropriate behaviors, such as phoning the president of the United States or buying huge amounts of merchandise on a credit card without having the resources to pay.

Acute Mania

Symptoms of acute mania may be a progression in intensification of those experienced in hypomania, or they may be manifested directly. Most individuals experience marked impairment in functioning and require hospitalization (see Box 17–1 diagnostic criteria for a manic episode).

Mood

Acute mania is characterized by euphoria and elation. The person appears to be on a continuous "high." However, the mood is always subject to frequent variation, easily changing to irritability and anger or even to sadness and crying.

Cognition and Perception

Cognition and perception become fragmented and often psychotic in acute mania. Accelerated thinking proceeds to racing thoughts; overconnection of ideas; and rapid, abrupt movement from one thought to another (**flight of ideas**) and may be manifested by a continuous flow of accelerated, pressured speech (loquaciousness) to the point where trying to converse with this individual may be extremely difficult. When flight of ideas is severe, speech may be disorganized and incoherent. Distractibility becomes all-pervasive. Attention can be diverted by even the smallest of stimuli. Hallucinations and delusions (usually paranoid and grandiose) are common.

Activity and Behavior

Psychomotor activity is excessive. Sexual interest is increased. There is poor impulse control, low frustration tolerance, and the individual who is normally discreet may become socially and sexually uninhibited. Excessive spending is common. In acute mania, individuals typically have little insight with regard to their behavior and communication. This manifests, at times, as unreliable reporting of events and denial of problems when confronted by friends or family, both of which may be interpreted as lying. Energy seems inexhaustible, and the need for sleep is diminished. Individuals may go for many days without sleep and still not feel tired. Hygiene and grooming may be neglected. Dress may be disorganized, flamboyant, or bizarre, and the use of excessive makeup or jewelry is common.

Delirious Mania

Delirious mania is a grave form of the disorder characterized by severe clouding of consciousness and an intensification of the symptoms associated with acute mania. This condition has become relatively rare since the availability of antipsychotic medication.

Mood

The mood of the delirious person is very labile. He or she may exhibit feelings of despair, quickly converting to unrestrained merriment and ecstasy or becoming irritable or totally indifferent to the environment. Panic anxiety may be evident.

Cognition and Perception

Cognition and perception are characterized by a clouding of consciousness with accompanying confusion, disorientation, and sometimes stupor. Other common manifestations include religiosity, delusions of grandeur or persecution, and auditory or visual hallucinations. The individual is extremely distractible and incoherent.

Activity and Behavior

Psychomotor activity is frenzied and characterized by agitated, purposeless movements. The safety of these individuals is at stake unless this activity is curtailed. Exhaustion, injury to self or others, and eventually death could occur without intervention.

Diagnosis and Outcome Identification

Using information collected during the assessment, the nurse completes the patient database from which the selection of appropriate nursing diagnoses is determined. Table 17–1 presents a list of patient behaviors and the NANDA-I nursing diagnoses (Herdman & Kamitsuru, 2018) that correspond to those behaviors, which may be used in planning care for the patient experiencing a manic episode.

Outcome Criteria

The following criteria may be used for measuring outcomes in the care of the patient experiencing a manic episode.

The patient:

- Exhibits no evidence of physical injury.
- Has not harmed self or others.
- Is no longer exhibiting signs of physical agitation.
- Eats a well-balanced diet with snacks to prevent weight loss and maintain nutritional status.
- Verbalizes an accurate interpretation of the environment.
- Verbalizes that hallucinatory activity has ceased and demonstrates no outward behavior indicating hallucinations.
- Accepts responsibility for own behaviors.
- Does not manipulate others for gratification of own needs.
- Interacts appropriately with others.
- Is able to fall asleep within 30 minutes of retiring.
- Is able to sleep 6 to 8 hours per night without medication.

Planning and Implementation

Table 17–2 provides a plan of care for the patient experiencing a manic episode. Selected nursing diagnoses are presented, along with outcome criteria, appropriate nursing interventions, and rationales for each.

TABLE 17–1 Assigning Nursing Diagnoses to Behaviors Commonly Exhibited by Individuals Experiencing a Manic Episode

BEHAVIORS	NURSING DIAGNOSES
Extreme hyperactivity; increased agitation and lack of control over purposeless and potentially injurious movements	Risk for injury
Manic excitement, delusional thinking, hallucinations, impulsivity	Risk for violence: Self-directed or other-directed
Loss of weight, amenorrhea, refusal or inability to sit still long enough to eat	Imbalanced nutrition: Less than body requirements
Delusions of grandeur and persecution; inaccurate interpretation of the environment	Disturbed thought processes*
Auditory and visual hallucinations; disorientation	Disturbed sensory-perception*
Inability to develop satisfying relationships, manipulation of others for own desires, use of unsuccessful social interaction behaviors	Impaired social interaction
Difficulty falling asleep, sleeping only short periods	Insomnia

*These diagnoses have been resigned from the NANDA-I list of approved diagnoses. They are used in this instance because they are most compatible with the identified behaviors.

Table 17–2 | CARE PLAN FOR THE PATIENT EXPERIENCING A MANIC EPISODE

NURSING DIAGNOSIS: RISK FOR INJURY

RELATED TO: Extreme hyperactivity

EVIDENCED BY: Increased agitation and lack of control over purposeless and potentially injurious movements

OUTCOME CRITERIA	NURSING INTERVENTIONS	RATIONALE
Short-Term Goal ■ Patient will no longer exhibit potentially injurious movements after 24 hours, with administration of tranquilizing medication. **Long-Term Goal** ■ Patient will not experience injury.	1. Reduce environmental stimuli. Assign private room with simple decor on quiet unit if possible. Keep lighting and noise level low. 2. Remove hazardous objects and substances (including smoking materials). 3. Stay with the patient who is hyperactive and agitated. 4. Provide structured schedule of activities that includes established rest periods throughout the day. Limit group activities. 5. Provide physical activities. 6. Administer tranquilizing medication as ordered by physician.	1. Patient is extremely distractible and responses to even the slightest stimuli are exaggerated. A milieu unit may be too stimulating. 2. Rationality is impaired, and patient may harm self inadvertently. 3. Nurse's presence may offer support and provide feeling of security for the patient. 4. A structured schedule and one-to-one activities provide a feeling of security for the client. 5. Physical activities help relieve pent-up tension. 6. Antipsychotics are common and are very effective for providing rapid relief from symptoms of hyperactivity.

Continued

Table 17–2 | CARE PLAN FOR THE PATIENT EXPERIENCING A MANIC EPISODE–cont'd

NURSING DIAGNOSIS: RISK FOR VIOLENCE: SELF-DIRECTED OR OTHER-DIRECTED

RELATED TO: Manic excitement, delusional thinking, hallucinations

OUTCOME CRITERIA	NURSING INTERVENTIONS	RATIONALE
Short-Term Goal ■ Patient's agitation will be maintained at a manageable level with the administration of tranquilizing medication during the first week of treatment (decreasing risk of violence to self or others). **Long-Term Goal** ■ Patient will not harm self or others.	1. Maintain low level of stimuli in patient's environment (low lighting, few people, simple décor, low noise level). 2. Assess for concurrent substance use issues. 3. Observe patient's behavior frequently. Do this while carrying out routine activities so as to avoid creating suspiciousness in the individual. 4. Remove all sharp objects, glass or mirrored items, belts, ties, and smoking materials from patient's environment. 5. 💬 Intervene at the first signs of increased anxiety, agitation, or verbal or behavioral aggression using empathic responses such as "You seem anxious" or "How can I help?" 6. Maintain and convey a calm attitude. Respond matter-of-factly to verbal hostility. 7. As anxiety increases, offer some alternatives: to participate in a physical activity (e.g., walking or other physical exercise), talking about the situation, taking some antianxiety medication. 8. Have sufficient staff available to indicate a show of strength to patient if it becomes necessary. 9. If patient is not calmed by "talking down" or by medication, use of mechanical restraints may be necessary. 10. If restraint is deemed necessary, ensure that sufficient staff is available to assist. Follow protocol established by the institution.	1. This intervention minimizes anxiety, agitation, and suspiciousness. 2. There is a high incidence of comorbid substance use disorders in clients with bipolar disorder and these can increase risk for harm to self or others. Also, the use of other mood-altering chemicals makes evaluation of pharmacotherapy more difficult. 3. Close observation is important to identify the need for redirection or limit setting and to protect patient safety. 4. Dangerous objects are removed to minimize risks that patient (in an agitated, hyperactive state) harms self or others. 5. Validation of the patient's feelings conveys an attitude of caring and collaboration and facilitates establishing trust. Because the patient is highly distractible, providing a distraction can also aid in diffusing anxiety and agitation. 6. Maintaining a calm attitude facilitates de-escalation of patient's anxiety and agitation. 7. Offering alternatives to the patient empowers him or her to have a sense of control over the situation. 8. This intervention ensures staff and patient safety and shows the patient evidence of control over the situation, which can be comforting to a patient when he or she is feeling fearful of losing control of self. 9. Patient should be offered the "least restrictive alternative" to maintain safety. Restraints should be used only as a last resort, after all other interventions have been unsuccessful, and the patient is imminently at risk of harm to self or others. 10. Patient safety is a nursing priority.

Table 17–2 | CARE PLAN FOR THE PATIENT EXPERIENCING A MANIC EPISODE—cont'd

OUTCOME CRITERIA	NURSING INTERVENTIONS	RATIONALE
	11. Observe the patient in restraints continuously and assess patient at least every 15 minutes to ensure that circulation to extremities is not compromised (check temperature, color, pulses); to assist the patient with needs related to nutrition, hydration, and elimination; and to position the patient so that comfort is facilitated and aspiration can be prevented.	11. This intervention ensures that needs for circulation, nutrition, hydration, and elimination are met. Patient safety is a nursing priority.
	12. As agitation decreases, assess the patient's readiness for restraint removal or reduction. Remove restraints gradually, one at a time while assessing the patient's response.	12. Gradual removal of restraints minimizes potential for injury to patient and staff.

NURSING DIAGNOSIS: IMBALANCED NUTRITION: LESS THAN BODY REQUIREMENTS

RELATED TO: Refusal or inability to sit still long enough to eat

EVIDENCED BY: Weight loss, amenorrhea

OUTCOME CRITERIA	NURSING INTERVENTIONS	RATIONALE
Short-Term Goal ■ Patient will consume sufficient finger foods and between-meal snacks to meet recommended daily allowances of nutrients. **Long-Term Goal** ■ Patient will exhibit no signs or symptoms of malnutrition.	1. Provide high-protein, high-calorie, nutritious finger foods and drinks that can be consumed "on the run." 2. Have juice and snacks available on the unit at all times. 3. Maintain accurate record of intake, output, calorie count, and weight. Monitor daily laboratory values. 4. Determine patient's likes and dislikes and collaborate with dietitian to provide favorite foods. 5. Supplement diet with vitamins and minerals. 6. Walk or sit with patient while he or she eats.	1. Because the patient has difficulty sitting still long enough to eat a meal, the likelihood is greater that he or she will consume food and drinks that can be carried around and eaten with little effort. 2. Nutritious intake is required on a regular basis to compensate for increased caloric requirement due to hyperactivity. 3. These are important nutritional assessment data. 4. Patient is more likely to eat foods that he or she particularly enjoys. 5. Improvement of nutritional status. 6. The nurse's presence offers support and encouragement to patient to eat food that will maintain physical wellness.

Continued

Table 17–2 | CARE PLAN FOR THE PATIENT EXPERIENCING A MANIC EPISODE–cont'd

NURSING DIAGNOSIS: IMPAIRED SOCIAL INTERACTION

RELATED TO: Delusional thought processes (grandeur and/or persecution); underdeveloped ego and low self-esteem

EVIDENCED BY: Inability to develop satisfying relationships and manipulation of others for own desires

OUTCOME CRITERIA	NURSING INTERVENTIONS	RATIONALE
Short-Term Goal ■ Patient will verbalize which of his or her interaction behaviors are appropriate and which are inappropriate within 1 week. **Long-Term Goal** ■ Patient will demonstrate use of appropriate interaction skills as evidenced by lack of, or marked decrease in, manipulation of others to fulfill own desires.	1. Recognize the purpose manipulative behaviors serve for the patient: to reduce feelings of insecurity by increasing feelings of power and control. 2. Set limits on manipulative behaviors. Explain to the patient what is expected and what the consequences are if the limits are violated. Terms of the limitations must be agreed on by all staff who will be working with the patient. 3. Do not argue, bargain, or try to reason with the patient. Merely state the limits and expectations. Confront the patient as soon as possible when interactions with others are manipulative or exploitative. Follow through with established consequences for unacceptable behavior. 4. Provide positive reinforcement for nonmanipulative behaviors. Explore feelings and help the patient seek more appropriate ways of dealing with them. 5. Help the patient recognize that he or she must accept the consequences of own behaviors and refrain from attributing them to others. 6. Help the patient identify positive aspects about self, recognize accomplishments, and feel good about them.	1. Understanding the motivation behind the manipulation may facilitate acceptance of the individual and his or her behavior. 2. When the patient is unable to establish own limits this must be done for him or her. Unless administration of consequences for violation of limits is consistent, manipulative behavior will not be eliminated. 3. Because the patient may be vulnerable to impulsive, reckless, or pleasure-seeking behavior without considering consequences, he or she should receive immediate feedback when behavior is unacceptable. Consistency in enforcing the consequences is essential if positive outcomes are to be achieved. Inconsistency creates confusion and encourages testing of limits. 4. Positive reinforcement enhances self-esteem and promotes repetition of desirable behaviors. 5. The patient must accept responsibility for own behaviors before adaptive change can occur. 6. As self-esteem is increased, patient will feel less need to manipulate others for own gratification.

Concept Care Mapping

The concept map care plan (see Chapter 6, The Nursing Process in Psychiatric Mental Health Nursing) is a diagrammatic teaching and learning strategy that allows visualization of interrelationships between medical diagnoses, nursing diagnoses, assessment data, and treatments. An example of a concept map care plan for a patient experiencing a manic episode is presented in Figure 17–1.

Patient and Family Education

The role of patient teacher is important in the psychiatric area, as it is in all areas of nursing. A list of topics for patient and family education relevant to bipolar disorder is presented in Box 17–4.

Evaluation of Care for the Patient Experiencing a Manic Episode

In the final step of the nursing process, a reassessment is conducted to determine if the nursing actions have been successful in achieving the objectives of care. Evaluation of the nursing actions for the patient experiencing a manic episode may be facilitated by gathering information using the following types of questions:

■ Has the individual avoided personal injury?
■ Has violence to the patient and others been prevented?
■ Has agitation subsided?
■ Have nutritional status and weight been stabilized? Is the patient able to select foods to maintain adequate nutrition?

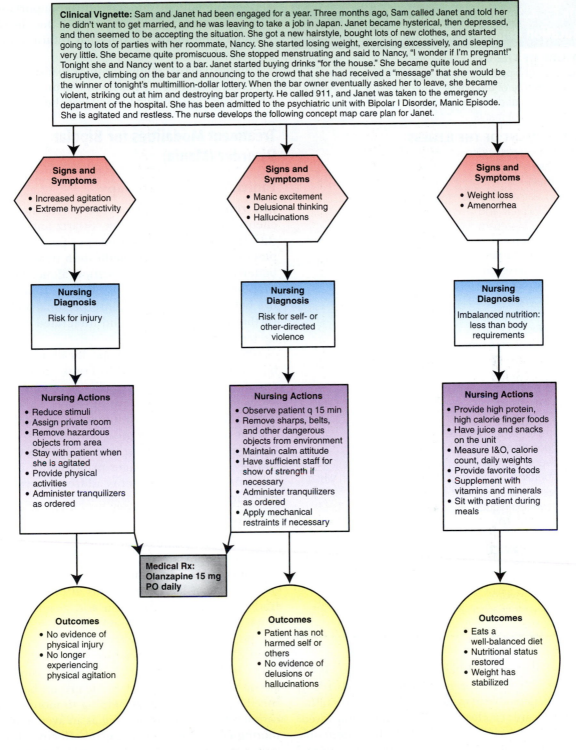

Clinical Vignette: Sam and Janet had been engaged for a year. Three months ago, Sam called Janet and told her he didn't want to get married, and he was leaving to take a job in Japan. Janet became hysterical, then depressed, and then seemed to be accepting the situation. She got a new hairstyle, bought lots of new clothes, and started going to lots of parties with her roommate, Nancy. She started losing weight, exercising excessively, and sleeping very little. She became quite promiscuous. She stopped menstruating and said to Nancy, "I wonder if I'm pregnant!" Tonight she and Nancy went to a bar. Janet started buying drinks "for the house." She became quite loud and disruptive, climbing on the bar and announcing to the crowd that she had received a "message" that she would be the winner of tonight's multimillion-dollar lottery. When the bar owner eventually asked her to leave, she became violent, striking out at him and destroying bar property. He called 911, and Janet was taken to the emergency department of the hospital. She has been admitted to the psychiatric unit with Bipolar I Disorder, Manic Episode. She is agitated and restless. The nurse develops the following concept map care plan for Janet.

Signs and Symptoms
- Increased agitation
- Extreme hyperactivity

Signs and Symptoms
- Manic excitement
- Delusional thinking
- Hallucinations

Signs and Symptoms
- Weight loss
- Amenorrhea

Nursing Diagnosis
Risk for injury

Nursing Diagnosis
Risk for self- or other-directed violence

Nursing Diagnosis
Imbalanced nutrition: less than body requirements

Nursing Actions
- Reduce stimuli
- Assign private room
- Remove hazardous objects from area
- Stay with patient when she is agitated
- Provide physical activities
- Administer tranquilizers as ordered

Nursing Actions
- Observe patient q 15 min
- Remove sharps, belts, and other dangerous objects from environment
- Maintain calm attitude
- Have sufficient staff for show of strength if necessary
- Administer tranquilizers as ordered
- Apply mechanical restraints if necessary

Nursing Actions
- Provide high protein, high calorie finger foods
- Have juice and snacks on the unit
- Measure I&O, calorie count, daily weights
- Provide favorite foods
- Supplement with vitamins and minerals
- Sit with patient during meals

Medical Rx:
Olanzapine 15 mg PO daily

Outcomes
- No evidence of physical injury
- No longer experiencing physical agitation

Outcomes
- Patient has not harmed self or others
- No evidence of delusions or hallucinations

Outcomes
- Eats a well-balanced diet
- Nutritional status restored
- Weight has stabilized

FIGURE 17–1   Concept map care plan for a patient with bipolar mania.

BOX 17–4 Topics for Patient and Family Education Related to Bipolar Disorder

NATURE OF THE ILLNESS
1. Causes of bipolar disorder
2. Cyclic nature of the illness
3. Symptoms of depression
4. Symptoms of mania

MANAGEMENT OF THE ILLNESS
1. Medication management
   a. Lithium
   b. Others
      1) Carbamazepine
      2) Valproic acid
      3) Clonazepam
      4) Verapamil
      5) Lamotrigine
      6) Gabapentin
      7) Topiramate
      8) Oxcarbazepine
      9) Olanzapine
      10) Risperidone
      11) Chlorpromazine
      12) Aripiprazole
      13) Quetiapine
      14) Ziprasidone
      15) Asenapine
   c. Side effects
   d. Symptoms of lithium toxicity
   e. Importance of regular blood tests
   f. Adverse effects
   g. Importance of not stopping medication, even when feeling well
2. Assertive techniques
3. Anger management

SUPPORT SERVICES
1. Crisis hotline
2. Support groups
3. Individual psychotherapy
4. Legal and/or financial assistance

■ Have delusions and hallucinations ceased? Is the patient able to interpret the environment correctly?

■ Is the patient able to make decisions about his or her own self-care? Has hygiene and grooming improved?

■ Is behavior socially acceptable? Is the patient able to interact with others in a satisfactory manner? Has the patient stopped manipulating others to fulfill own desires?

■ Is the patient able to sleep 6 to 8 hours per night and awaken feeling rested?

■ Does the patient understand the importance of maintenance medication therapy? Does he or she understand that symptoms may return if medication is discontinued?

■ Can the patient taking lithium verbalize early signs of lithium toxicity? Does he or she understand the necessity for monthly blood level checks?

Treatment Modalities for Bipolar Disorder (Mania)

Individual Psychotherapy

In a review of the evidence on psychotherapy for clients with bipolar disorder, Swartz and Swanson (2014) conclude that bipolar-specific psychotherapies in conjunction with medication treatment have better outcomes than medication alone. Evidence supports the benefits of psychoeducation, cognitive behavior therapy, FFT, interpersonal and social rhythm therapy (IPSRT), and integrated care management (Strakowski, 2016).

IPSRT is a type of therapy specifically designed for bipolar patients. Developed by Frank (2005), the focus of this therapy is helping clients to regulate their social rhythms, or daily activities such as the sleep–wake cycle and exercise routines, that may otherwise disrupt underlying biological rhythms and contribute to mood disturbances. In combination with this strategy, IPSRT also engages principles of interpersonal therapy to help clients address interpersonal problems.

Group Therapy

Once an acute phase of the illness is passed, groups can provide an atmosphere in which individuals may discuss issues in their lives that cause, maintain, or arise out of having a serious affective disorder. Both group psychoeducation and group cognitive behavior therapy have demonstrated benefits for this population (Swartz & Swanson, 2014). The element of peer support may provide a feeling of security because troublesome or embarrassing issues are discussed and resolved. Some groups have other specific purposes, such as helping to monitor medication-related issues or serving as an avenue for promoting education related to the affective disorder and its treatment.

Support groups help members gain a sense of perspective on their condition and tangibly encourage them to link up with others who have common problems. A sense of hope is conveyed when the individual is able to see that he or she is not alone or unique in experiencing affective illness.

Self-help groups offer another avenue of support for the individual with bipolar disorder. These groups are usually peer led and are not meant to substitute for or compete with professional therapy. They offer supplementary support that frequently enhances compliance with the medical regimen. Examples of self-help groups are the Depression and Bipolar Support Alliance (DBSA) and the Child and Adolescent Bipolar Foundation; these organizations put individuals in touch with their local support groups. Although self-help groups are not psychotherapy groups, they do provide important adjunctive support experiences, which often have therapeutic benefit for participants.

Family Therapy

The ultimate objectives in working with families of clients with mood disorders are to resolve the symptoms and initiate or restore adaptive family functioning. Some studies with bipolar disorder have shown that behavioral family treatment combined with medication substantially reduces relapse rate compared with medication therapy alone.

Sadock and associates (2015) state:

> Family therapy is indicated if the disorder jeopardizes the patient's marriage or family functioning or if the mood disorder is promoted or maintained by the family situation. Family therapy examines the role of the mood-disordered member in the overall psychological well-being of the whole family; it also examines the role of the entire family in the maintenance of the patient's symptoms. (p. 373)

Family functioning and marital relationships are often disrupted in clients with bipolar disorder, especially when symptoms are contributing to disloyalty in the marriage and to financial problems related to the client's excessive spending behaviors. Whether intervention occurs in the form of family education, support, formal therapy, or a combination of these approaches, it is clear that families need to be involved in treatment whenever possible.

Cognitive Therapy

In cognitive therapy, the individual is taught to control thought distortions that are considered to be a factor in the development and maintenance of mood disorders. In the cognitive model, depression is characterized by a triad of negative distortions related to expectations of the environment, self, and future. The environment and activities within it are viewed as unsatisfying, the self is unrealistically devalued, and the future is perceived as hopeless. In the same model, mania is characterized by exaggeratedly positive cognitions and perceptions. The individual perceives the self as highly valued and powerful. Life is experienced with overstated self-assurance and the future is viewed with unrealistic optimism.

The general goals in cognitive therapy are to obtain symptom relief as quickly as possible, assist the client in identifying dysfunctional patterns of thinking and behaving, and guide the client to evidence and logic that effectively test the validity of the dysfunctional thinking. Therapy focuses on changing "automatic thoughts" that occur spontaneously and contribute to the distorted affect. Examples of automatic thoughts in bipolar mania include the following:

- **Personalizing:** "I'm the only reason my husband is a successful businessman."
- **All or nothing:** "Everything I do is great."
- **Mind reading:** "She thinks I'm wonderful."
- **Discounting negatives:** "None of those mistakes are really important."

The client is asked to describe evidence that both supports and disputes the automatic thought. The logic underlying the inferences is then reviewed with the client. Another technique involves evaluating what would most likely happen if the client's automatic thoughts were true. Implications of the consequences are then discussed.

Clients should not become discouraged if one technique seems not to be working. No single technique works with all clients. Clients should be reassured that any of a number of techniques may be used, and both the therapist and client may explore these possibilities.

The Recovery Model

Research provides support for recovery as an obtainable objective for individuals with bipolar disorder. See "Real, People, Real Stories" to learn more about Bridget's recovery journey. Conceptual models of recovery from mental illness are presented in Chapter 10, The Recovery Model. The recovery model has been used primarily in caring for individuals with serious mental illness, such as schizophrenia and bipolar disorder. However, concepts of the model are amenable to use with all individuals experiencing emotional conditions with which they require assistance and who have a desire to take control and manage their lives more independently.

Real People, Real Stories

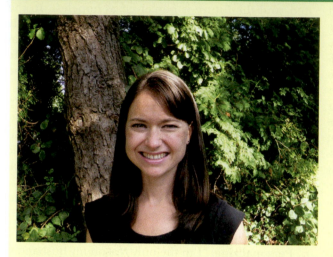

BRIDGET'S STORY

Bridget is an advanced practice registered nurse and doctoral student with bipolar disorder. Her story highlights the progression of her illness, her insights about illness management, and her courageous efforts to advocate for herself and others.

Karyn: I really appreciate you sharing your insights with other healthcare professionals. So tell me about your history with bipolar disorder.

Bridget: I was diagnosed with depression at the age of 13, was on medication for that, and was stable until about 24 years of age. At that time I was working on night shift as a labor and delivery nurse. I remember having a very stressful night and some ethical disagreements with some others and I couldn't sleep for a couple of nights. It threw me into a manic episode. I took melatonin and Nyquil and had a bad reaction. I was having visual hallucinations of interconnecting lights. I have heard other people say that Nyquil can trigger that.

Karyn: I have also read of accounts of people having hallucinations in reaction to dextromethorphan. What happened next?

Bridget: I didn't sleep for days. It was acute and recognizable; very uncomfortable and very scary. I was too sick to return to work and still very upset about ongoing disagreements about patient care issues so when I returned to work it was at a different hospital that rotated shifts. Rotating working the night and day shift worked better for my health. I would work 2 weeks of the night shift and then rotate to working 4 weeks of the day shift. Although not as ideal as working straight day shifts, this month of day shifts allowed me to catch up and stabilize my sleep.

I got accepted into a midwifery program and between the stresses of work, moving, and school, I had a second episode; first manic then depressive. I was concerned that I would have to drop out of school because I couldn't manage graduate school classes along with my recovery. In addition, I read about the importance of regulating sleep patterns in managing this illness and a midwife's schedule requires very irregular sleep patterns. Babies are not born nine to five. However, I couldn't drop out or even go part-time or else I would lose my health insurance. My professors really helped me work out arrangements and accommodations so I could remain a student and keep my insurance and continue working on my degree in midwifery.

The next couple years I was stable but it was frightening; I never knew how well I would recover from episodes. I had a counselor tell me I might have to cut back my expectations for my life. I went to support groups and felt like they brought me down more; there was a lot of complaining and one person told me I would probably only be able to work part-time. I had different expectations for what I wanted to do.

Karyn: How long does an acute episode typically last?

Bridget: The manic episodes seem to be sudden in onset then it "gets dark" and then it's a slow return. The worst episode has been for 2 months but I would say full recovery takes around nine months to one year. After that I'm able to get back into the swing of things.

Karyn: What do you mean when you say it "gets dark"?

Bridget: It's very frightening. There is a sense of loss of control. I lose weight quickly and people think I'm anorexic but it's just that my metabolism gets really fast. Not being able to sleep adds to the traumatization. Then there's the depression and suicidal thoughts. That's when it gets really dark. But I was stable for a 2–3 year period before I had a third episode. That was the worst one. I was going through another stressful period but some of it was positive stress; graduating from school, in a new relationship, accepted to a prestigious program for doctoral nursing study, and I was going through some medication changes. It seemed like any treatment was just "putting a bottle cap on a tidal wave." I was hospitalized three times, was having symptoms of psychosis, and it took about a year to get back on track. It's been six years since that last episode.

Karyn: What do you think has been most helpful in moving toward this recovery?

Bridget: Having a supportive family. My family has knowledge and history with mental illnesses and that has been a blessing. In my family, recovery is the expectation and chronic illness is the exception. Also, I have long-term friends that stuck with me and never gave up on me; even my doctor said I have amazing friends.

The medications are important even though I have a love-hate relationship with them. The only time I refused medication it was because I thought I was having a bad reaction, but people thought I was just not recognizing

Real People, Real Stories—cont'd

I was sick. It's still a blurry line . . . the judgments were snap . . . in fairness, I was a lot to handle . . . but it was scary. I was being told I had to take something I felt was hurting me so I was uncooperative. Now I recognize they were well-intentioned people doing the best they could.

Also I found work I love; as a childbirth educator. I got married and that has been a stabilizing factor. The medications seem to be working. I had been taking Trileptal but I stopped taking that so I wouldn't have to worry about its effects when I got pregnant, and my workplace has been accommodating.

Karyn: Accommodating?

Bridget: Well, I had been in circumstances prior to my current job; like once I was shoved by a coworker and I threw milk at her. The coworker maintained they were justified. In another circumstance when a coworker found out I had bipolar disorder she told my supervisor I should not be able to work there. I was very scared and felt like I had to become a strong advocate for myself. The truth is my illness requires little accommodation most of the time. When I am well, I am very well and a fairly high functioning person. I get sick fairly infrequently and when I do, I just need some time to recover, just like any other illness. It does help to have understanding and compassion from my superiors. When I've been able to garner support from them I've been able to pursue recovery and my life goals.

There was a journal editor and a mentor I connected with after grad school that was so encouraging in terms of me pursuing my PhD. At the time, I had so much shame and guilt about having bipolar disorder, but she extended compassion to me that I wasn't even able to extend to myself. She saw and encouraged me to work to my full potential.

Karyn: What are the most important things that you want nurses to know about providing care for patients with bipolar disorder, particularly in an acute manic episode?

Bridget: Number One: Better listening is key. Even if the patient does not seem to be making sense, there most likely is a kernel of truth in what they are saying. Be patient. Listen and look for that kernel of truth. I remember trying to talk to my psychiatrist about wanting lithium but we never got to discuss that because he was yelling at me that I was being uncooperative with the hospital treatment plan. I signed out AMA because . . . it felt safer. That's a whole other story.

Number two: A little compassion goes a long way. Patients can tell right away who is there to help them and who is just there for the paycheck.

Number three: Look patients in the eye and call them by their name. Many people, when they are in an acute episode of illness, feel very lost and confused; talking to them directly and personally is really grounding. It helps people reclaim their dignity.

Remember, being sick is hard: whether it's cancer or diabetes or bipolar disorder. It takes a lot to manage. Trust that people are truly doing the best that they can with the resources they are given. The mental health system can be very difficult to navigate, especially when someone is acutely ill. It makes it hard to get stabilized and get better. The more you can treat people with dignity, respect their requests when possible, listen, and offer compassion, the better they will do.

In bipolar disorder, recovery is a continuous process. The individual identifies goals based on personal values or what he or she defines as giving meaning and purpose to life. The clinician and client work together to develop a treatment plan that is in alignment with the goals set forth by the client. In the recovery process, the individual may still be experiencing symptoms. Weiden (2010) states:

> Patients do not have to be in remission, nor does remission automatically have to be a desired (or likely) goal when embarking on a recovery-oriented treatment plan. As long as the patient (and family) understands that a process recovery treatment plan is not to be confused with a promise of "cure" or even "remission," then one does not overpromise.

In the process of recovery, the client and clinician work on strategies to help the individual with bipolar disorder take control of and manage his or her illness. Some of these strategies include the following:

■ Become an expert on the disorder.
■ Take medications regularly.
■ Become aware of earliest symptoms.
■ Develop a plan for emergencies.
■ Identify and reduce sources of stress: Know when to seek help.
■ Develop a personal support system.
■ Develop a plan for emergencies.

During the process of recovery, individuals actively work on the strategies they have identified to keep themselves well. The clinician serves as a support person to help the individual take the necessary steps to achieve the goals previously set forth by the client.

Although there is no cure for bipolar disorder, there are effective treatments and interventions. Recovery is possible when the client is empowered and actively engaged in a multifaceted illness management approach.

Electroconvulsive Therapy

Episodes of acute mania are occasionally treated with electroconvulsive therapy (ECT), particularly when the client does not tolerate or fails to respond to lithium or other drug treatment, or when life is threatened by dangerous behavior or exhaustion (see Chapter 16, Depressive Disorders, for more information on ECT).

Psychopharmacology With Mood-Stabilizing Agents

For many years, the drug of choice for treatment and management of bipolar mania was lithium carbonate. However, in recent years, a number of investigators and clinicians in practice have achieved satisfactory results with several other medications, including anticonvulsant drugs, which have a mood-stabilizing effect either alone or in combination with lithium. (See Chapter 4, Psychopharmacology, for a detailed discussion of indications, actions, contraindications, and other safety issues related to mood-stabilizing agents.)

Both lithium and mood stabilizers demonstrate effectiveness in managing bipolar depression. Three mood stabilizer products are currently approved by the U.S. Food and Drug Administration (FDA) for that purpose: the combination of olanzapine and fluoxetine, quetiapine, and lurasidone (Strakowski, 2016). Antidepressants have shown little evidence of effectiveness in treating bipolar depression as an adjunct to mood stabilizers. Additionally, Strakowski identifies that antidepressants carry as high as a 40 percent risk of potentially triggering a switch from depression to mania in individuals with bipolar disorder.

Clients who respond to lithium can virtually be symptom free over the long term. About 33 percent of people treated with lithium respond positively (Rybakowski, 2014), so having other pharmacological treatments available is important in the treatment of this illness. Because bipolar disorder is a chronic, episodic illness, most people will remain on medication throughout their lives. See Table 17–3 for a list of commonly used medications in the treatment of bipolar disorder. Lithium, like other medications, has side effects. Most notably its therapeutic range (0.6–1.2 mEq/L) can have toxic side effects and is potentially fatal when exceeded.

Patient and Family Education for Lithium

The patient should:

- Take medication on a regular basis, even when feeling well. Discontinuation can result in return of symptoms.

- Not drive or operate dangerous machinery until lithium levels are stabilized. Drowsiness and dizziness can occur.

- Not skimp on dietary sodium intake. He or she should eat a variety of healthy foods and avoid junk foods. The patient should drink six to eight large glasses of water each day and avoid excessive use of beverages containing caffeine (coffee, tea, colas), which promote increased urine output.

- Notify the physician if vomiting or diarrhea occurs. These symptoms can result in sodium loss and an increased risk of lithium toxicity.

- Carry a card or other identification noting that he or she is taking lithium.

- Be aware of appropriate diet should weight gain become a problem. Include adequate sodium and other nutrients while decreasing number of calories.

- Be aware of risks of becoming pregnant while receiving lithium therapy. Use information furnished by healthcare providers regarding methods of contraception. Notify the physician as soon as possible if pregnancy is suspected or planned.

- Be aware of side effects and symptoms associated with toxicity. Notify the physician if any of the following symptoms occur: persistent nausea and vomiting, severe diarrhea, ataxia, blurred vision, tinnitus, excessive output of urine, increasing tremors, or mental confusion.

- Refer to written materials furnished by healthcare providers while receiving self-administered maintenance therapy. Keep appointments for outpatient follow-up; have serum lithium level checked every 1 to 2 months or as advised by physician.

Patient and Family Education for Anticonvulsant Mood Stabilizers

The patient should:

- Refrain from discontinuing the drug abruptly. Physician will administer orders for tapering the drug when therapy is to be discontinued.

- Report the following symptoms to the physician immediately: skin rash, unusual bleeding, spontaneous bruising, sore throat, fever, malaise, dark urine, and yellow skin or eyes.

- Not drive or operate dangerous machinery until reaction to the medication has been established.

- Avoid consuming alcoholic beverages and nonprescription medications without approval from physician.

- Carry a card at all times identifying the name of medications being taken.

TABLE 17–3 Mood-Stabilizing Agents

CLASSIFICATION: GENERIC (TRADE)	HALF-LIFE/INDICATIONS	MECHANISM OF ACTION	CONTRAINDICATIONS/ PRECAUTIONS	DAILY ADULT DOSAGE RANGE/ THERAPEUTIC PLASMA RANGE
ANTIMANIC				
Lithium carbonate (Eskalith, Lithobid)	24 hr/ ■ Prevention and treatment of manic episodes of bipolar disorder. *Unlabeled uses:* ■ Neutropenia ■ Cluster headaches (prophylaxis) ■ Alcohol dependence ■ Bulimia ■ Postpartum affective psychosis ■ Corticosteroid–induced psychosis	Not fully understood but may modulate the effects of various neurotransmitters, such as norepinephrine, serotonin, dopamine, glutamate, and GABA, that are thought to play a role in the symptomatology of bipolar disorder (may take 1–3 weeks for symptoms to subside).	Hypersensitivity. Cardiac or renal disease, dehydration; sodium depletion; brain damage; pregnancy and lactation. Caution with thyroid disorders, diabetes, urinary retention, history of seizures, and with elderly.	Acute mania: 1,800–2,400 mg Maintenance: 900–1,200 mg/ Acute mania: 0.5–1.5 mEq/L Maintenance: 0.6–1.2 mEq/L
ANTICONVULSANTS				
Carbamazepine (Tegretol)	25–65 hr (initial); 12–17 hr (repeated doses) ■ Epilepsy ■ Trigeminal neuralgia *Unlabeled uses:* ■ Bipolar disorder ■ Resistant schizophrenia ■ Management of alcohol withdrawal ■ Restless legs syndrome ■ Postherpetic neuralgia	Action in the treatment of bipolar disorder is unclear.	Hypersensitivity. With MAOIs, lactation. Caution with elderly; liver, renal, cardiac disease; pregnancy.	200–1,600 mg/ 4–12 mcg/mL
Clonazepam (Klonopin)	18–60 hr/ ■ Petit mal, akinetic, and myoclonic seizures ■ Panic disorder *Unlabeled uses:* ■ Acute manic episodes ■ Uncontrolled leg movements during sleep ■ Neuralgias	Action in the treatment of bipolar disorder is unclear.	Hypersensitivity, glaucoma, liver disease, lactation. Caution in elderly, liver and renal disease, pregnancy.	0.5–20 mg/ 20–80 mg/mL
Valproic acid (Depakene; Depakote)	5–20 hr/ ■ Epilepsy ■ Manic episodes ■ Migraine prophylaxis ■ Adjunct therapy in schizophrenia	Action in the treatment of bipolar disorder is unclear.	Hypersensitivity; liver disease. Caution in elderly, renal and cardiac diseases, pregnancy and lactation.	5–60 mg/kg/ 50–150 mcg/mL

Continued

TABLE 17–3 Mood-Stabilizing Agents—cont'd

CLASSIFICATION: GENERIC (TRADE)	HALF-LIFE/INDICATIONS	MECHANISM OF ACTION	CONTRAINDICATIONS/ PRECAUTIONS	DAILY ADULT DOSAGE RANGE/ THERAPEUTIC PLASMA RANGE
Lamotrigine (Lamictal)	~33 hr/ ■ Epilepsy *Unlabeled use:* ■ Bipolar disorder	Action in the treatment of bipolar disorder is unclear.	Hypersensitivity. Caution in renal and hepatic insufficiency, pregnancy, lactation, and children <16 years old.	100–200 mg/ Not established
Gabapentin (Neurontin)	5–7 hr/ ■ Epilepsy ■ Postherpetic neuralgia *Unlabeled uses:* ■ Bipolar disorder ■ Migraine prophylaxis ■ Neuropathic pain ■ Tremors associated with multiple sclerosis	Action in the treatment of bipolar disorder is unclear.	Hypersensitivity and children <3 years. Caution in renal insufficiency, pregnancy, lactation, children, and the elderly.	900–1,800 mg/ Not established
Topiramate (Topamax)	21 hr/ ■ Epilepsy ■ Migraine prophylaxis *Unlabeled uses:* ■ Bipolar disorder ■ Cluster headaches ■ Bulimia ■ Binge eating disorder ■ Weight loss in obesity	Action in the treatment of bipolar disorder is unclear.	Hypersensitivity. Caution in renal and hepatic impairment, pregnancy, lactation, children, and the elderly.	50–400 mg/ Not established
Oxcarbazepine (Trileptal)	2–9 hr/ ■ Epilepsy *Unlabeled uses:* ■ Bipolar disorder ■ Diabetic neuropathy ■ Neuralgia	Action in the treatment of bipolar disorder is unclear.	Hypersensitivity. Caution in renal and hepatic impairment, pregnancy, lactation, children, and the elderly.	600–2,400 mg/ Not established
CALCIUM CHANNEL BLOCKER				
Verapamil (Calan; Isoptin) Diltiazem (Cardizem, Tiazac) Isradipine (DynaCirc) Nimodipine (Nymalize)		Action in the treatment of bipolar disorder is unclear.	Hypersensitivity; severe left ventricular dysfunction, heart block, hypotension, cardiogenic shock, congestive heart failure. Caution in liver or renal disease, cardiomyopathy, intracranial pressure, elderly patients, pregnancy, and lactation.	80–320 mg/ Not established

TABLE 17–3 Mood-Stabilizing Agents—cont'd

CLASSIFICATION: GENERIC (TRADE)	HALF-LIFE/INDICATIONS	MECHANISM OF ACTION	CONTRAINDICATIONS/PRECAUTIONS	DAILY ADULT DOSAGE RANGE/THERAPEUTIC PLASMA RANGE
ANTIPSYCHOTICS		**ALL ANTIPSYCHOTICS**	**ALL ANTIPSYCHOTICS**	
Olanzapine (Zyprexa)	21–54 hr/ ■ Schizophrenia ■ Acute manic episodes ■ Management of bipolar disorder ■ Agitation associated with schizophrenia or mania *Unlabeled uses:* ■ Obsessive-compulsive disorder	Efficacy in schizophrenia is achieved through a combination of dopamine and serotonin type 2 (5-HT$_2$) antagonism. Mechanism of action in the treatment of mania is unknown.	Hypersensitivity, children, lactation. Caution with hepatic or cardiovascular disease, history of seizures, comatose or other CNS depression, prostatic hypertrophy, narrow-angle glaucoma, diabetes or risk factors for diabetes, pregnancy, elderly and debilitated patients, history of suicide attempts.	10–20 mg/ Not established
Olanzapine and fluoxetine (Symbyax)	(see individual drugs) ■ For the treatment of depressive episodes associated with bipolar disorder			6/25–12/50 mg/ Not established
Aripiprazole (Abilify)	50–80 hr/ ■ Bipolar mania ■ Schizophrenia	Action may be mediated via effects on dopamine and serotonin (5-HT$_{2A}$) receptor antagonism.		10–30 mg/ Not established
Lurasidone (Latuda)	18 hr/ ■ Depressive episodes in bipolar I disorder ■ Schizophrenia			20–120 mg/ Not established
Chlorpromazine	24 hr/ ■ Bipolar mania ■ Schizophrenia ■ Emesis/hiccoughs ■ Acute intermittent porphyria ■ Preoperative apprehension *Unlabeled uses:* ■ Migraine headaches			75–400 mg/ Not established
Quetiapine (Seroquel)	6 hr/ ■ Schizophrenia ■ Acute manic episodes			100–800 mg/ Not established

Continued

TABLE 17–3   **Mood-Stabilizing Agents—cont'd**

CLASSIFICATION: GENERIC (TRADE)	HALF-LIFE/INDICATIONS	MECHANISM OF ACTION	CONTRAINDICATIONS/ PRECAUTIONS	DAILY ADULT DOSAGE RANGE/ THERAPEUTIC PLASMA RANGE
Risperidone (Risperdal)	3–20 hr/ ■ Bipolar mania ■ Schizophrenia *Unlabeled uses:* ■ Severe behavioral problems in children ■ Behavioral problems associated with autism ■ Obsessive–compulsive disorder			1–6 mg/ Not established
Ziprasidone (Geodon)	7 hr (oral)/ ■ Bipolar mania ■ Schizophrenia ■ Acute agitation in schizophrenia			40–160 mg/ Not established
Asenapine (Saphris)	24 hr/ ■ Schizophrenia ■ Bipolar mania			10–20 mg/ Not established

CLINICAL PEARL The U.S. Food and Drug Administration requires that all antiepileptic (anticonvulsant) drugs carry a warning label indicating that use of the drugs increases risk for suicidal thoughts and behaviors. Patients being treated with these medications should be monitored for the emergence or worsening of depression, suicidal thoughts or behavior, or any unusual changes in mood or behavior.

Patient and Family Education for Calcium Channel Blocker

The patient should:

■ Take medication with meals if gastrointestinal upset occurs.

■ Use caution when driving or when operating dangerous machinery. Dizziness, drowsiness, and blurred vision can occur.

■ Refrain from discontinuing the drug abruptly. To do so may precipitate cardiovascular problems. Physician will administer orders for tapering the drug when therapy is to be discontinued.

■ Report occurrence of any of the following symptoms to physician immediately: irregular heartbeat, shortness of breath, swelling of the hands and feet, pronounced dizziness, chest pain, profound mood swings, severe and persistent headache.

■ Rise slowly from a sitting or lying position to prevent a sudden drop in blood pressure.

■ Avoid taking other medications (including over-the-counter medications) without physician's approval.

■ Carry a card at all times describing medications being taken.

Patient and Family Education for Antipsychotics

The patient should:

■ Use caution when driving or operating dangerous machinery. Drowsiness and dizziness can occur.

■ Refrain from discontinuing the drug abruptly after long-term use. To do so might produce withdrawal symptoms, such as nausea, vomiting, dizziness, gastritis, headache, tachycardia, insomnia, and tremulousness. Physician will administer orders for tapering the drug when therapy is to be discontinued.

■ Use sunblock lotion and wear protective clothing when spending time outdoors. Skin is more sus-

ceptible to sunburn, which can occur in as little as 30 minutes.

■ Report the occurrence of any of the following symptoms to the physician immediately: sore throat, fever, malaise, unusual bleeding, easy bruising, persistent nausea and vomiting, severe headache, rapid heart rate, difficulty urinating, muscle twitching, tremors, darkly colored urine, excessive urination, excessive thirst, excessive hunger, weakness, pale stools, yellow skin or eyes, muscular incoordination, or skin rash.

■ Rise slowly from a sitting or lying position to prevent a sudden drop in blood pressure.

■ Take frequent sips of water, chew sugarless gum, or suck on hard candy, if dry mouth is a problem. Good oral care (frequent brushing, flossing) is very important.

■ Consult the physician regarding smoking while on antipsychotic therapy. Smoking increases the metabolism of these drugs, requiring an adjustment in dosage to achieve a therapeutic effect.

■ Dress warmly in cold weather and avoid extended exposure to very high or low temperatures. Body temperature is harder to maintain with this medication.

■ Avoid drinking alcohol while on antipsychotic therapy. These drugs potentiate each other's effects.

■ Avoid taking other medications (including over-the-counter products) without the physician's approval. Many medications contain substances that interact with antipsychotic medications in a way that may be harmful.

■ Be aware of possible risks of taking antipsychotics during pregnancy. Safe use during pregnancy has not been established. Antipsychotics are thought to readily cross the placental barrier; if so, a fetus could experience adverse effects of the drug. Inform the physician immediately if pregnancy occurs, is suspected, or is planned.

■ Be aware of side effects of antipsychotic medications. Refer to written materials furnished by healthcare providers for safe self-administration.

■ Continue to take the medication, even if feeling well and feeling as though it is not needed. Symptoms may return if medication is discontinued.

■ Carry a card or other identification at all times describing medications being taken.

CASE STUDY AND SAMPLE CARE PLAN

NURSING HISTORY AND ASSESSMENT

Candace, age 32, recently moved to New York City from Omaha, Nebraska, where she had been working as a television reporter. She felt that Omaha had become "too boring" and wanted to experience the big city life. Candace has a history of bipolar I disorder and has been maintained on lithium since she was 23 years old. Since she arrived in New York, she has run out of her medication and has not found a doctor to have her prescription renewed. She has been staying in an inexpensive apartment, using her savings to live on. She has been seeking employment in her chosen line of work, but it has been 2 months now, and she has been unable to find a job. Candace is becoming anxious because her savings are becoming depleted. She has lost weight and has trouble sleeping.

Today, after two failed interviews, Candace went to a bar and began drinking. She ordered several rounds of drinks for everyone in the bar and told the bartender to "put it on my tab." The bartender called the police when Candace refused to pay her tab and became loud and belligerent. He said she began shouting that she knew the mayor, and he was going to help her find a job, and if they didn't leave her alone, she would tell the mayor how they were treating her. She took out her cell phone and said she was calling the mayor. When others in the room began laughing at her, she began cursing and saying that they would be sorry one day that they laughed at her. When the police arrived, Candace was resistant and had to be physically restrained. The police took Candace to the emergency department of the community hospital, where she was admitted with a diagnosis of Bipolar I Disorder, current episode manic. The psychiatrist ordered olanzapine 10 mg IM STAT, olanzapine 10 mg PO qd, lithium carbonate 600 mg PO bid, and vitamin supplement daily. He ordered a lithium level to be drawn prior to first dose of lithium.

NURSING DIAGNOSES AND OUTCOME IDENTIFICATION

From the assessment data, the admitting nurse develops the following nursing diagnoses for Candace:

1. **Risk for self- or other-directed violence** related to manic hyperactivity, delusional thinking, impulsivity
   a. **Short-Term Goal:** Agitation and hyperactivity will be maintained at manageable level with the administration of tranquilizing medication.
   b. **Long-Term Goal:** Candace will not harm self or others during hospitalization.
2. **Imbalanced nutrition: Less than body requirements** related to lack of appetite and excessive physical agitation, evidenced by loss of weight
   a. **Short-Term Goal:** Candace will consume sufficient finger foods and between-meal snacks to meet recommended daily allowances of nutrients.

b. **Long-Term Goal:** Candace will begin to regain weight and exhibit no signs or symptoms of malnutrition.

PLANNING AND IMPLEMENTATION

RISK FOR SELF- OR OTHER-DIRECTED VIOLENCE

The following nursing interventions have been identified for Candace:

1. Place Candace in a private room near the nurse's station. Observe her behavior frequently.
2. Remove all dangerous objects from her environment.
3. Plan some physical activities for Candace (e.g., treadmill, punching bag) and regular rest periods during the day.
4. Administer tranquilizing medication as ordered by physician.
5. Monitor lithium levels three times during first week of therapy. Monitor for signs and symptoms of toxicity (e.g., ataxia, blurred vision, severe diarrhea, persistent nausea and vomiting, tinnitus).
6. Ensure that sufficient staff is available to intervene should Candace become agitated and aggressive.

IMBALANCED NUTRITION: LESS THAN BODY REQUIREMENTS

The following nursing interventions have been identified for Candace:

1. Consult dietitian to determine appropriate diet for Candace to restore nutrition and increase weight. Ensure that her diet includes foods that she particularly likes.
2. Ensure that Candace has access to finger foods and between-meal snacks if she cannot or will not sit still to eat from a meal tray.
3. Maintain an accurate record of intake, output, and calorie count.
4. Obtain daily weights.
5. Administer vitamin supplement, as ordered by physician.
6. Sit with Candace during mealtime.

EVALUATION

The outcome criteria identified for Candace have been met. She has not harmed herself or others in any way. She is able to verbalize names of resources outside the hospital from whom she may request help if needed. With help from the social worker, she has applied for unemployment assistance and will begin receiving help within 2 weeks. She has gained 3 pounds in the hospital, and she verbalizes understanding of the importance of maintaining good nutrition. She is taking her medication regularly and has a follow-up appointment with the psychiatric nurse practitioner who will see Candace biweekly and ensure that Candace is adherent with medication and laboratory requirements. Candace verbalizes understanding of the importance of taking her medication on a continuous basis. She has a hopeful but realistic attitude about finding work in New York City and states that she will give herself a deadline, after which she plans to return to her home in Omaha, where she may be near family and friends.

Summary and Key Points

- Bipolar disorder is manifested by mood swings from profound depression to extreme elation and euphoria.
- Genetic influences have been strongly implicated in the development of bipolar disorder. Various other physiological factors, such as biochemical and electrolyte alterations, as well as cerebral structural changes, have been implicated. Side effects of certain medications may also induce symptoms of mania. No single theory can explain the etiology of bipolar disorder, and it is likely that the illness is caused by a combination of factors.
- Symptoms of mania may be observed on a continuum of three phases, each identified by the degree of severity: phase I, hypomania; phase II, acute mania; and phase III, delirious mania.
- The symptoms of bipolar disorder may occur in children and adolescents as well as in adults.
- Treatment of bipolar disorders includes individual therapy, group and family therapy, cognitive therapy, electroconvulsive therapy, and psychopharmacology. For the majority of clients, the most effective treatment appears to be a combination of psychotropic medication and psychosocial therapy.
- Some clinicians choose a course of therapy based on a model of recovery similar to that used for many years to treat addiction. The basic premise of a recovery model is empowerment; it allows clients primary control over decisions about their own care and enables a person with a mental health problem to live a meaningful life in a community of choice while striving to achieve his or her full potential.
- For many years, the pharmacological treatment of choice for bipolar mania was lithium carbonate. A number of other medications are now being used with satisfactory results, including anticonvulsants and antipsychotics.
- There is a narrow margin between the therapeutic and toxic levels of lithium. Serum lithium levels must be monitored regularly while the client is on maintenance therapy.

Review Questions
Self-Examination/Learning Exercise

Select the answer that is most appropriate for each of the following questions:

1. Margaret, a 68-year-old widow, is brought to the emergency department by her sister-in-law. Margaret has a history of bipolar disorder and has been maintained on medication for many years. Her sister-in-law reports that Margaret quit taking her medication a few months ago, thinking she didn't need it anymore. Margaret is agitated, pacing, demanding, and speaking very loudly. Her sister-in-law reports that Margaret eats very little, is losing weight, and almost never sleeps. "I'm afraid she's going to just collapse!" Margaret is admitted to the psychiatric unit. What is the *priority* nursing diagnosis for Margaret?
   a. Imbalanced nutrition: Less than body requirements related to not eating
   b. Risk for injury related to hyperactivity
   c. Disturbed sleep pattern related to agitation
   d. Ineffective coping related to denial of depression

2. Margaret, age 68, is diagnosed with bipolar I disorder, current episode manic. She is extremely hyperactive and has lost weight. What is one way to promote adequate nutritional intake for Margaret?
   a. Sit with her during meals to ensure that she eats everything on her tray.
   b. Have her sister-in-law bring all her food from home because she knows Margaret's likes and dislikes.
   c. Provide high-calorie, nutritious finger foods and snacks that Margaret can eat "on the run."
   d. Tell Margaret that she will be on room restriction until she starts gaining weight.

Continued

Review Questions—cont'd
Self-Examination/Learning Exercise

3. The physician orders lithium carbonate 600 mg tid for a client newly diagnosed with Bipolar I Disorder. There is a narrow margin between the therapeutic and toxic levels of lithium. What is the therapeutic range for *acute* mania?
   a. 0.5 to 1.5 mEq/L
   b. 10 to 15 mEq/L
   c. 0.5 to 1 mEq/L
   d. 5 to 10 mEq/L

4. Although historically lithium has been the medication of choice for mania, several others have been used with good results. Which of the following are used in the treatment of bipolar disorder? (Select all that apply.)
   a. Olanzapine (Zyprexa)
   b. Oxycodone (Oxycontin)
   c. Carbamazepine (Tegretol)
   d. Gabapentin (Neurontin)
   e. Tranylcypromine (Parnate)

5. Margaret, a 68-year-old widow experiencing a manic episode, is admitted to the psychiatric unit after being brought to the emergency department by her sister-in-law. Margaret yells, "My sister-in-law is just jealous of me! She's trying to make it look like I'm insane!" This behavior is an example of which of the following?
   a. A delusion of grandeur
   b. A delusion of persecution
   c. A delusion of reference
   d. A delusion of control or influence

6. Which of the following is the most common comorbid condition in children with bipolar disorder?
   a. Schizophrenia
   b. Substance disorders
   c. Oppositional defiant disorder
   d. Attention deficit-hyperactivity disorder

7. A nurse is educating a patient about his lithium therapy. She is explaining signs and symptoms of lithium toxicity. Which of the following would she instruct the patient to be on the alert for?
   a. Fever, sore throat, malaise
   b. Tinnitus, severe diarrhea, ataxia
   c. Occipital headache, palpitations, chest pain
   d. Skin rash, marked rise in blood pressure, bradycardia

8. Katerina, who is experiencing a manic episode, enters the milieu area dressed in a provocative and physically revealing outfit. Which of the following is the most appropriate intervention by the nurse?
   a. Tell her, in front of the other patients, that she cannot dress like a whore while she is in the hospital.
   b. Do nothing and allow her to learn from the responses of her peers.
   c. Quietly walk with her back to her room and help her change into something more appropriate.
   d. Explain to her that if she wears this outfit, she must remain in her room.

Review Questions—cont'd
Self-Examination/Learning Exercise

9. The nurse is prioritizing nursing diagnoses in the plan of care for a patient experiencing a manic episode. Number the diagnoses in order of the appropriate priority.
   a. Disturbed sleep pattern evidenced by sleeping only 4 to 5 hours per night
   b. Risk for injury related to manic hyperactivity
   c. Impaired social interaction evidenced by manipulation of others
   d. Imbalanced nutrition: Less than body requirements evidenced by loss of weight and poor skin turgor

10. A child with bipolar disorder also has attention deficit-hyperactivity disorder (ADHD). How would these comorbid conditions most likely be treated?
   a. No medication would be given for either condition.
   b. Medication would be given for both conditions simultaneously.
   c. The bipolar condition would be stabilized first before medication for the ADHD would be given.
   d. The ADHD would be treated before consideration of the bipolar disorder.

IMPLICATIONS OF RESEARCH FOR EVIDENCE-BASED PRACTICE

Morriss, R., Lobban, F., Riste, L., Davies, L., Holland, F., Long, R., . . . Jones, S. (2016). Clinical effectiveness and acceptability of structured group psychoeducation versus optimised unstructured peer support for patients with remitted bipolar disorder (Parades): A pragmatic, multicentre, observer-blind, randomised controlled superioritytrial. *The Lancet Psychiatry, 3*(11), 1029–1038. doi:10.1016/S2215-0366(16)30302-9

DESCRIPTION OF THE STUDY: This study sought evidence for efficacy of group psychoeducation versus peer support for patients with bipolar disorder in remission. The participants (n = 304) were randomly assigned to one of the two intervention strategies, and efficacy was measured by time from randomization to the next bipolar episode.

RESULTS OF THE STUDY: The researchers found that there was no significant difference in effectiveness between the two interventions. However, in the subset of participants with fewer than eight previous bipolar episodes, psychoeducation did improve outcomes.

IMPLICATIONS FOR NURSING PRACTICE: Both peer support and group psychoeducation demonstrated good outcomes, but as the researchers note, findings suggest that early intervention with group psychoeducation may have important benefits for patients with bipolar disorder. Nurses play an important role both in providing psychoeducation and referring clients for group treatment. Assessing the patient's history of bipolar episodes and providing psychoeducation early in the illness process may improve outcomes. Nurses can also play an active role in conducting and participating in similar research to identify which interventions demonstrate the best evidence of positive outcomes. This forms the foundation for evidence-based practice.

TEST YOUR CRITICAL THINKING SKILLS

Allie, age 29, had been working in the typing pool of a large corporation for 6 years. Her immediate supervisor recently retired, and Alice was promoted to supervisor in charge of 20 people in the department. Allie was flattered by the promotion but anxious about the additional responsibility of the position. Shortly after the promotion, she overheard two of her former coworkers saying, "Why in the world did they choose her? She's not the best one for the job. I know *I* certainly won't be able to respect her as a boss!" Hearing these comments added to Allie's anxiety and self-doubt.

Shortly after Allie began her new duties, her friends and coworkers noticed a change. She had a great deal of energy and worked long hours on her job. She began to speak very loudly and rapidly. Her roommate noticed that Allie slept very little yet seldom appeared tired. Every night, she would go out to bars and dances. Sometimes she brought men she had just met home to the apartment, something she had never done before. She bought lots of clothes and makeup and had her hair restyled in a more youthful look. She failed to pay her share of the rent and bills but came home with a brand new convertible. She lost her temper and screamed at her roommate, "Mind your own business!" when asked to pay her share.

Allie became irritable at work, and several of her subordinates reported her behavior to the corporate manager. When the manager confronted Allie about her behavior, she lost control, shouting, cursing, and striking out at anyone and anything that happened to be within her reach. The security officers restrained her and took her to the emergency department of the hospital, where she was admitted to the psychiatric unit. She had no previous history of psychiatric illness.

The psychiatrist assigned a diagnosis of Bipolar I Disorder and wrote orders for olanzapine (Zyprexa) 10 mg IM STAT, olanzapine 15 mg PO daily, and lithium carbonate 600 mg qid.

Answer the following questions related to Allie:

1. What are the most important considerations with which the nurse who is taking care of Allie should be concerned?
2. Why was Allie given the diagnosis of Bipolar I Disorder?
3. The doctor should order a lithium level drawn after 4 to 6 days. For what symptoms should the nurse be on the alert?
4. Why did the physician order olanzapine in addition to the lithium carbonate?

Communication Exercises

1. Bob, a newly admitted patient, diagnosed with bipolar disorder states to the nurse, "I was looking at the sky, blue is the color of my eyes, too. I went to Florida on a plane."
   How might the nurse respond to this patient's statement?

2. John, who is in a manic phase of bipolar disorder is jumping from chair to chair in the patient lounge during visiting hours, loudly proclaiming to the visitors that he is a famous gymnast. He begins doing somersaults, nearly tripping a visitor.
   How might the nurse respond to the patient at this point?

 MOVIE CONNECTIONS

Lust for Life • *Call Me Anna* • *Blue Sky* • *A Woman Under the Influence* • *Silver Linings Playbook* • *No Letting Go* • *A Light Beneath Their Feet*

References

Aas, M., Henry, C., Andreassen, O. A. Bellivier, F., Melle, I., & Etain, B. (2016). The role of childhood trauma in bipolar disorders. *International Journal of Bipolar Disorders, 4*(2), 1–10. doi:10.1186/s40345-015-0042-0

Akiskal, H. S. (2017). Mood disorders: Historical introduction and conceptual overview. In B. J. Sadock, V. A. Sadock, & P. Ruiz (Eds.), *Comprehensive textbook of psychiatry* (10th ed., pp. 1599–1603). Philadelphia, PA: Wolters Kluwer.

American Psychiatric Association. (2013). *Diagnostic and statistical manual of mental disorders* (5th ed.). Washington, DC: Author.

Burton, N. (2012). *A short history of bipolar disorder.* Retrieved from https://www.psychologytoday.com/blog/hide-and-seek/201206/short-history-bipolar-disorder

Darby, M. M., Yolken, R. H., & Sabunciyan, S. (2016). Consistently altered expression of gene sets in postmortem brains of individuals with major psychiatric disorders. *Translational Psychiatry, 6*(9), e890. doi:10.1038/tp.2016.173

Etain, B., Aas, M., Andreassen, O. A., Lorentzen, S., Dieset, I., Gard, S., . . . Henry, C. (2013). Childhood trauma is associated with severe clinical characteristics of bipolar disorders. *Journal of Clinical Psychiatry, 74*(10), 991–998.

Frank, E. (2005). *Treating bipolar disorder: A clinician's guide to interpersonal and social rhythm therapy.* New York, NY: Guilford Press.

Hassan, A., Agha, S. S., Langley, K., & Thapar, A. (2011). Prevalence of bipolar disorder in children and adolescents with attention-deficit hyperactivity disorder. *British Journal of Psychiatry, 198* (3), 195–198. doi:10.1192/bjp.bp.110.078741

Hazell, P., & Jairam, R. (2012). Acute treatment of mania in children and adolescents. *Current Opinion in Psychiatry, 25*(4), 264–270.

Herdman, T. H., & Kamitsuru, S. (Eds.). (2018). *NANDA-I nursing diagnoses: Definitions and classification, 2018–2020.* New York, NY: Thieme.

Jain, R., & Jain, S. (2014). *Facing the diagnostic challenge of comorbid bipolar disorder and ADHD.* Retrieved from http://www.psychiatryadvisor.com/adhd/facing-the-diagnosticchallenge-of-comorbid-bipolar-disorder-and-adhd/article/370068

Janiri, D., Sani, G., Danese, E., Simonetti, A., Ambrosi, E., Angeletti, G., . . . Girardi, P. (2015). Childhood traumatic experiences of patients with bipolar disorder type I and type II. *Journal of Affective Disorders, 175*(8), 92–97. doi:http://dx.doi.org/10.1016/j.jad.2014.12.055

Krans, B., & Cherney, K. (2018). *The history of bipolar disorder.* Retrieved from http://www.healthline.com/health/bipolar-disorder/history-bipolar#1

Leussis, M. P., Berry-Scott, E. M., Saito, M., Jhuang, H., Haan, G., Alkan, O., . . . Petryshen, T. L. (2013). The ANK3 bipolar disorder gene regulates psychiatric-related behaviors that are modulated by lithium and stress. *Biological Psychiatry, 73*(7), 683–696. doi:10.1016/j.biopsych.2012.10.016

Merikangas, K. R., & Rihmer, Z. (2017). Mood disorders: Epidemiology. In B. J. Sadock, V. A. Sadock, & P. Ruiz (Eds.), *Comprehensive textbook of psychiatry* (10th ed., pp.1614–1619). Philadelphia, PA: Wolters Kluwer.

Miklowitz, D. J. (2016). Evidence-based psychotherapies for adolescents and young adults with bipolar disorder. *Journal of Clinical Psychiatry, 77*(Suppl. E1), e5, 1–8.

Morriss, R., Lobban, F., Riste, L., Davies, L., Holland, F., Long, R., . . . Jones, S. (2016). Clinical effectiveness and acceptability of structured group psychoeducation versus optimized unstructured peer support for patients with re-mitted bipolar disorder (PARADES): A pragmatic, multicen-tre, observer-blind, randomised controlled superiority trial. *The Lancet Psychiatry, 3*(11), 1029–1038. doi:10.1016/S2215-0366(16)30302-9

National Institute of Mental Health (NIMH). (2013). *New data reveal the extent of genetic overlap between major mental disorders: Schizophrenia, bipolar disorder share the most common genetic varia-tion* [Press release]. Retrieved from http://www.nimh.nih.gov/news/science-news/2013/new-data-reveal-extent-of-genetic-overlap-between-major-mental-disorders.shtml

National Institute of Mental Health (NIMH). (2017). *Bipolar disorder.* Retrieved from https://www.nimh.nih.gov/health/statistics/bipolar-disorder.shtml

Rybakowski, J. (2014). Factors associated with lithium efficacy in bipolar disorder. *Harvard Review of Psychiatry, 22*(6), 353–357. doi:10.1097/HRP.0000000000000006

Sadock, B. J., Sadock, V. A., & Ruiz, P. (2015). *Synopsis of psychiatry: Behavioral sciences/clinical psychiatry* (11th ed.). Philadelphia, PA: Wolters Kluwer.

Semeniken, K. R., and Dudás, B. (2012). Bipolar disorder: Diagnosis, neuroanatomical and biochemical background. In M. Juruena (Ed.), *Clinical, research and treatment approaches to affective disorders* (chap. 8). Rijeka, Croatia: InTech. Retrieved from http://www.intechopen.com/books/clinical-research-and-treatment-approaches-to-affective-disorders/bipolar-dis order-diagnosis-neuroanatomical-and-biochemical-background

Soreff, S., & McInnes, L. A. (2018). Bipolar affective disorder. *E-medicine: Psychiatry.* Retrieved from http://emedicine.med-scape.com/article/286342-overview

Strakowski, S. (2016). *A guide to treating unipolar and bipolar depression.* Retrieved from http://www.medscape.com/viewarticle/871539#vp_6

Swartz, H., & Swanson, J. (2014). Psychotherapy for bipolar dis-order in adults: A review of the evidence. *American Psychiatric Publishing, 12*(3), 251–266. doi:10.1176/appi.focus.12.3.251

Watson, S., Gallagher, P., Dougall, D., Porter, R., Moncrieff, J., Ferrier, I. N., & Young, A. H. (2013). Childhood trauma in bipolar disorder. *Australian and New Zealand Journal of Psychia-try, 48*(6), 564–570. doi:10.1177/0004867413516681

Weiden, P. J. (2010). Is recovery attainable in schizophrenia? *Med-scape Psychiatry & Mental Health.* Retrieved from http://www.medscape.com/viewarticle/729750

18

Anxiety, Obsessive-Compulsive, and Related Disorders

CORE CONCEPTS

Anxiety

Compulsions

Obsessions

Panic

Phobia

KEY TERMS

agoraphobia

body dysmorphic disorder

generalized anxiety disorder

habit reversal training

hoarding disorder

implosion therapy (flooding)

obsessive-compulsive disorder

panic disorder

social anxiety disorder

specific phobia

systematic desensitization

trichotillomania (hair-pulling disorder)

OBJECTIVES
After reading this chapter, the student will be able to:

1. Differentiate among the terms *stress, anxiety,* and *fear.*
2. Discuss historical aspects and epidemiological statistics related to anxiety, obsessive-compulsive, and related disorders.
3. Differentiate between normal anxiety and clinically significant anxiety.
4. Describe various types of anxiety, obsessive-compulsive, and related disorders and identify symptomatology associated with each. Incorporate this information in patient assessment.
5. Identify predisposing factors in the development of anxiety, obsessive-compulsive, and related disorders.
6. Formulate nursing diagnoses and outcome criteria for patients with anxiety, obsessive-compulsive, and related disorders.
7. Describe appropriate nursing interventions for behaviors associated with anxiety, obsessive-compulsive, and related disorders.
8. Identify topics for patient and family teaching relevant to anxiety, obsessive-compulsive, and related disorders.
9. Evaluate nursing care of patients with anxiety, obsessive-compulsive, and related disorders.
10. Discuss various modalities relevant to treatment of anxiety, obsessive-compulsive, and related disorders.

Introduction

Singer, actor, and producer Barbra Streisand relates her experience of dealing with an anxiety disorder following a performance in which she forgot the lyrics to a song:

> I couldn't come out of it. . . . It was shocking to me to forget the words. So I didn't have any sense of humor about it. Some performers do really well when they forget the words. They forget the words all the time, but they somehow have humor about it. I remember I didn't have a sense of humor about it. I was quite shocked. I didn't sing and charge people for 27 years because of that night. . . . I was like, "God, I don't know. What if I forget the words again?" (ABC News, 2005)

Streisand's story is like that of many others who experience anxiety disorders (she was diagnosed specifically with social anxiety disorder); the interference with occupational, social, and other areas of functioning can be profound. She has sought therapy and medication and has since returned to performing on stage. Her story highlights not only the impact that anxiety disorders can have on one's functioning but also that treatment can be successful and improve one's quality of life.

CORE CONCEPT

Anxiety
A feeling of discomfort, apprehension, or dread related to anticipation of danger, the source of which is often nonspecific or unknown. Anxiety is considered a disorder (or pathology) when fears and anxieties are excessive (in a cultural context) and there are associated behavioral disturbances such as interference with social and occupational functioning (APA, 2013).

Individuals face anxiety on a daily basis. Anxiety, which provides the motivation for achievement, is a necessary force for survival. The term *anxiety* is often used interchangeably with the word *stress;* however, they are not the same. Stress, or more properly, a

stressor, is an external pressure that is brought to bear on the individual. Anxiety is the subjective emotional response to that stressor. (See Chapter 1, Mental Health and Mental Illness, for an overview of anxiety as a psychological response to stress.)

Anxiety may be distinguished from *fear* in that the former is an emotional process, whereas fear is a cognitive one. Fear involves the intellectual appraisal of a threatening stimulus; anxiety involves the emotional response to that appraisal.

This chapter focuses on disorders that are characterized by exaggerated and often disabling anxiety reactions. Historical aspects and epidemiological statistics are presented. Predisposing factors that have been implicated in the etiology of the disorders provide a framework for studying the dynamics of phobias, obsessive-compulsive disorders, generalized anxiety disorder, panic disorder, and other anxiety disorders. Various theories of causation are presented, although it is most likely that a combination of factors contribute to the etiology of these disorders. The neurobiology of anxiety disorders is presented in Figure 18–1.

An explanation of the symptomatology is presented as background knowledge for assessing the client with an anxiety or obsessive-compulsive disorder. Nursing care is described in the context of the nursing process. Various treatment modalities are explored.

Historical Aspects

Individuals have experienced anxiety throughout the ages. Yet anxiety, like fear, was not clearly defined or isolated as a separate entity by psychiatrists or psychologists until the 19th and 20th centuries. In fact, what we now know as anxiety was once solely identified by its physiological symptoms, focusing largely on the cardiovascular system. Clinicians used a myriad of diagnostic terms in attempting to identify these symptoms. For example, cardiac neurosis, DaCosta's syndrome, irritable heart, nervous

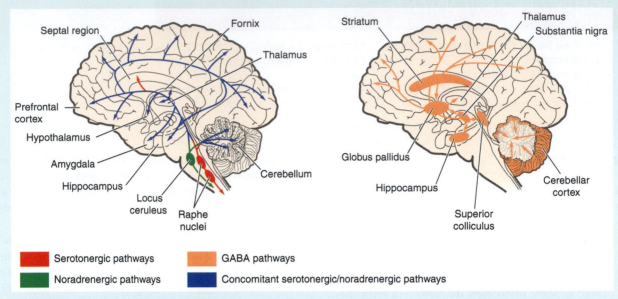

FIGURE 18–1 Neurobiology of anxiety disorders.

NEUROTRANSMITTERS

Although other neurotransmitters have also been implicated in the pathophysiology of anxiety disorders, disturbances in serotonin, norepinephrine, and gamma-aminobutyric acid (GABA) appear to be most significant.

Cell bodies of origin for the serotonin pathways lie within the raphe nuclei located in the brainstem. Serotonin is thought to be decreased in anxiety disorders (based on the efficacy of SSRIs in the treatment of anxiety disorders), but some studies suggest that serotonin may have a modulating effect in response to intense emotions in general. Cell bodies for norepinephrine originate in the locus ceruleus. Norepinephrine is thought to be increased in anxiety disorders. GABA is the major inhibitory neurotransmitter in the brain. It is involved in the reduction and slowing of cellular activity. It is synthesized from glutamic acid, with vitamin B_6 as a cofactor. It is found in almost every region of the brain. GABA is thought to be decreased in anxiety disorders (allowing for increased cellular excitability).

AREAS OF THE BRAIN AFFECTED

Areas of the brain affected by anxiety disorders and the symptoms that they mediate include the following:

- Amygdala: Fear, which is particularly important in panic and phobic disorders
- Hippocampus: Associated with memory related to fear responses
- Locus ceruleus: Arousal
- Brainstem: Respiratory activation, heart rate
- Hypothalamus: Activation of stress response
- Frontal cortex: Cognitive interpretations
- Thalamus: Integration of sensory stimuli
- Basal ganglia: Tremor

Anxiolytic Agents	Action	Side Effects
Benzodiazepines	Increases the affinity of the GABA_A receptor for GABA	Sedation, dizziness, weakness, ataxia, decreased motor performance, dependence, withdrawal
SSRIs	Block reuptake of serotonin into the presynaptic nerve terminal, increasing synaptic concentration of serotonin	Nausea, diarrhea, headache, insomnia, somnolence, sexual dysfunction
SNRIs	Inhibit reuptake of neuronal serotonin and norepinephrine; mild reuptake of dopamine	Headache, dry mouth, nausea, somnolence, dizziness, insomnia, asthenia, constipation, diarrhea

Anxiolytic Agents	Action	Side Effects
Noradrenergic agents (e.g., propranolol, clonidine)	Propranolol: blocks beta adrenergic receptor activity Clonidine: stimulates alpha-adrenergic receptors	Propranolol: Bradycardia, hypotension, weakness, fatigue, impotence, gastrointestinal upset, bronchospasm Clonidine: Dry mouth, sedation, fatigue, hypotension
Barbiturates	CNS depression; also produces effects in the hepatic and cardiovascular systems	Somnolence, agitation, confusion, ataxia, dizziness, bradycardia, hypotension, constipation
Buspirone	Partial agonist of 5-HT$_{1A}$ receptor	Dizziness, drowsiness, dry mouth, headache, nervousness, nausea, insomnia

tachycardia, neurocirculatory asthenia, soldier's heart, vasomotor neurosis, and vasoregulatory asthenia are just a few of the names under which anxiety has been concealed over the years (Sadock, Sadock, & Ruiz, 2015).

Freud first introduced the term *anxiety neurosis* in 1895. Freud wrote, "I call this syndrome 'anxiety neurosis' because all its components can be grouped round the chief symptom of anxiety" (Freud, 1959). This notion attempted to negate the previous concept of the problem as strictly physical, although it was some time before physicians of internal medicine were ready to accept the psychological implications for the symptoms. In fact, it was not until the years during World War II that the psychological dimensions of these various functional heart conditions were recognized.

For many years, anxiety disorders were viewed as purely psychological or purely biological in nature. Researchers have begun to focus on the interrelatedness of mind and body, and anxiety disorders provide an excellent example of this complex relationship. It is likely that various factors, including genetic, developmental, environmental, and psychological, play a role in the etiology of anxiety disorders.

Epidemiological Statistics

Anxiety disorders are the most common of all mental illnesses in the United States, affecting 18.1 percent of the population each year (American Depression Association of America [ADAA], 2018) and result in considerable functional impairment and distress. Statistics vary widely, but most agree that anxiety disorders are more common in women than in men by at least two to one. Prevalence rates (ADAA, 2018) for

anxiety disorders within the general population are identified as follows:

Specific phobias: 8.7 percent
Social anxiety disorder: 6.8 percent
Post-traumatic stress disorder: 3.5 percent
Generalized anxiety disorder: 3.1 percent
Panic disorder: 2.7 percent
Obsessive-compulsive disorder: 1 percent

The lifetime prevalence for any anxiety disorder is estimated at 31.1 percent for adults and 31.9 percent for children aged 13 to 18 years of age (National Institute of Mental Health [NIMH], 2017). Common comorbidities include another anxiety disorder, depression, and substance abuse. Vulnerability to comorbidities includes parental psychiatric history, childhood trauma, and negative life events (Hofmeijer-Sevink et al., 2012), but regardless of the contributing factors, comorbidities are associated with poorer outcomes, higher healthcare utilization, and greater impairment in functioning. Studies suggest that a familial predisposition to anxiety disorders probably exists.

How Much Is Too Much?

Anxiety is usually considered a normal reaction to a realistic danger or threat to biological integrity or self-concept. Normal anxiety dissipates when the danger or threat is no longer present.

It is difficult to draw a precise line between normal and abnormal anxiety. Normalcy is determined by societal standards; what is considered normal in Chicago, Illinois, may not be considered as such in Cairo, Egypt. There may even be regional differences within a country or cultural differences within a region. So what criteria can be used to determine if an individual's anxious response is normal? Anxiety can be considered abnormal or pathological if:

1. *It is out of proportion to the situation that is creating it.*

EXAMPLE

Mrs. K witnessed a serious automobile accident 4 weeks ago when she was out driving in her car, and since that time refuses to drive even to the grocery store a few miles from her house. When he is available, her husband must take her wherever she needs to go.

2. *The anxiety interferes with social, occupational, or other important areas of functioning.*

EXAMPLE

Because of the anxiety associated with driving her car, Mrs. K has been forced to quit her job in a downtown bank for lack of transportation.

It is clear that when anxiety becomes excessive and persistent, humans respond in a variety of ways that are likely a complex interaction of genetic vulnerability, biochemical influences, and environmental factors. Various manifestations of pathological anxiety are discussed in the following section.

Application of the Nursing Process–Assessment

CORE CONCEPT

Panic
A sudden, overwhelming feeling of terror or impending doom. This most severe form of emotional anxiety is usually accompanied by behavioral, cognitive, and physiological signs and symptoms considered to be outside the expected range of normalcy.

Panic Disorder

Background Assessment Data

Panic disorder is characterized by recurrent *panic attacks,* the onseta of which are unpredictable. Panic attacks are manifested by intense apprehension, fear, or terror, often associated with feelings of impending doom (clients often fear they are dying) and accompanied by intense physical discomfort. The physical sensations can be so intense that the individual believes he or she is having a heart attack or other critical illness. The symptoms come on suddenly and unexpectedly; that is, they do not occur immediately before or on exposure to a situation that usually causes anxiety

(as in specific phobia). They are not triggered by situations in which the person is the focus of others' attention (as in social anxiety disorder). The role of organic factors in the etiology has been ruled out.

The *Diagnostic and Statistical Manual of Mental Disorders, Fifth Edition (DSM-5)* (American Psychiatric Association [APA], 2013) states that at least four of the following symptoms must be present to identify the presence of a panic attack:

- Palpitations, pounding heart, or accelerated heart rate
- Sweating
- Trembling or shaking
- Sensations of shortness of breath or smothering
- Feelings of choking
- Chest pain or discomfort
- Nausea or abdominal distress
- Feeling dizzy, unsteady, lightheaded, or faint
- Chills or heat sensations
- Paresthesias (numbness or tingling sensations)
- Derealization (feelings of unreality) or depersonalization (feelings of being detached from oneself)
- Fear of losing control or going crazy
- Fear of dying

Attacks usually last minutes, or more rarely, hours. The individual often experiences varying degrees of nervousness and apprehension between attacks. Symptoms of depression are common.

The average age of onset of panic disorder is the late 20s. Frequency and severity of the panic attacks vary widely. Some individuals may have attacks of moderate severity weekly; others may have less severe or limited-symptom attacks several times a week. Still others may experience panic attacks that are separated by weeks or months. The disorder may last for a few weeks or months or for a number of years. Sometimes the individual experiences periods of remission and exacerbation. Limited-symptom attacks ("fearful spells" that do not meet criteria for panic attacks) may be a risk factor for later panic attacks and panic disorder. Genetic vulnerability, tendency toward negative emotions, history of childhood physical and sexual abuse, and smoking have also been identified as risk factors (APA, 2013).

Generalized Anxiety Disorder

Background Assessment Data

Generalized anxiety disorder (GAD) is characterized by persistent, unrealistic, and excessive anxiety and worry, which have occurred more days than not for at least 6 months and cannot be attributed to specific organic factors, such as caffeine intoxication or hyperthyroidism. The anxiety and worry are associated with muscle tension, restlessness, or feeling keyed up or on edge (APA, 2013).

These symptoms are like those often associated with anxiety in the general population but, unlike the typical experience of anxiety, the symptoms in GAD are intense enough to cause clinically significant impairment in social, occupational, or other important areas of functioning. The individual often avoids activities or events that may result in negative outcomes or spends considerable time and effort preparing for such activities. Anxiety and worry often result in procrastination in behavior or decision making, and the individual repeatedly seeks reassurance from others.

The disorder may begin in childhood or adolescence, but onset is not uncommon after age 20. Depressive symptoms are common, and numerous somatic complaints may also be a part of the clinical picture. GAD tends to be chronic, with frequent stress-related exacerbations and fluctuations in the course of the illness.

Theories of Etiology Related to Panic and Generalized Anxiety Disorders

Psychodynamic Theory

The psychodynamic view focuses on the inability of the ego to intervene when conflict occurs between the id and the superego, producing anxiety. For various reasons (unsatisfactory parent-child relationship, conditional love, or provisional gratification), ego development is delayed. When developmental defects in ego functions compromise the capacity to modulate anxiety, the individual resorts to unconscious mechanisms to resolve the conflict. Use of defense mechanisms rather than coping and management skills results in maladaptive responses to anxiety.

Cognitive Theory

The main thesis of the cognitive view is that faulty, distorted, or counterproductive thinking patterns accompany or precede maladaptive behaviors and emotional disorders (Sadock et al., 2015). A disturbance in this central mechanism of cognition causes a consequent disturbance in feeling and behavior. Because of distorted thinking, anxiety is maintained by erroneous or dysfunctional appraisal of a situation. There is a loss of ability to reason regarding the problem, whether it is physical or interpersonal. The individual feels vulnerable in a given situation, and the distorted thinking results in an irrational appraisal, fostering a negative outcome.

Biological Aspects

Research investigations into the psychobiological correlation of panic and generalized anxiety disorders (GAD) have implicated a number of possibilities.

Genetics Genetic studies have identified variations in specific genes that may be associated with anxiety disorders (including panic disorder and obsessive-compulsive disorder), and some studies suggest that genetic variations may affect the sensitivity of emotional processing centers in the brain (Ressler & Smoller, 2016). Twin studies identify a 30 to 40 percent risk of heritability. But as Ressler and Smoller point out, genetic findings are indicative of risk rather than determinants of illness, and, in fact, many current genetic studies reveal that environmental factors in interaction with genes have more of an impact on risk than genetic influences alone.

Neuroanatomical Structural brain imaging studies in patients with panic disorder have implicated pathological involvement in the temporal lobes, particularly the hippocampus and the amygdala (Sadock et al., 2015). Dysfunctions in the limbic system (often referred to as "the emotional brain") and the frontal cerebral cortex have also been noted in clients with anxiety disorders.

Biochemical Abnormal elevations of blood lactate have been noted in clients with panic disorder. Likewise, infusion of sodium lactate in clients with anxiety neuroses produces symptoms of panic disorder. Studies have suggested that people with panic disorders may be more sensitive to hypercapnia (which increases lactate levels), and carbon dioxide (CO_2) challenge tests have supported this sensitivity (Amaral et al., 2013). Additionally, studies of various medications and treatments such as cognitive behavior therapy have demonstrated decreased sensitivity to CO_2 inhalation after treatment, suggesting a relationship between lactate levels and anxiety reduction.

Neurochemical Strong evidence exists for the involvement of the neurotransmitter norepinephrine in the etiology of panic disorder. Norepinephrine is known to mediate arousal, and it causes hyperarousal and anxiety. This fact has been demonstrated by a notable increase in anxiety following the administration of drugs that increase the synaptic availability of norepinephrine, such as yohimbine. The neurotransmitters serotonin and gamma aminobutyric acid (GABA) are thought to be decreased in anxiety disorders. These hypotheses are related to the efficacy of benzodiazepines, which enhance the activity of GABA and the efficacy of selective serotonin reuptake inhibitors (SSRIs), which enhance the activity of serotonin. Similarly, deep-breathing exercises have been shown to elevate thalamic GABA levels through stimulation of vagal nerve pathways with a subsequent reduction in heart rate and improvement in emotional regulation and stress responses (Gerbard & Brown, 2016). Studies of serotonin's function in anxiety disorders have had mixed results (Sadock et al., 2015).

CORE CONCEPT

Phobia

A persistent, intensely felt, and irrational fear of a specific object, activity, or situation that results in a compelling desire to avoid the feared stimulus (Venes, 2017). Responses typically include intense anxiety or panic attacks.

Phobias

Two common phobia disorders include agoraphobia and social anxiety disorder (social phobia). The estimated lifetime prevalence of agoraphobia among U.S. adults is 1.3 percent, and approximately 40 percent of those cases are considered severe (NIMH, 2017). Social anxiety disorder (formerly called social phobia) is more common, with an estimated lifetime prevalence of 7 percent (APA, 2013). A specific phobia, in which a person has an exaggerated fear response to a specific object or situation, is estimated to affect 7 to 9 percent of the population in the United States (APA, 2013).

Agoraphobia

Background Assessment Data

The Greek translation of the word **agoraphobia** is "fear of the marketplace." Agoraphobia is the fear of being in open shops and markets, but more specifically, it is the fear of being vulnerable and unable to get help or escape the setting (Kimmel & Roy-Burn, 2017), should panic symptoms occur. It is possible that the individual may have experienced symptoms in the past and is preoccupied with fears of their recurrence. The *DSM-5* diagnostic criteria for agoraphobia are presented in Box 18–1.

Onset of symptoms most commonly occurs in the 20s and 30s and persists for many years. It is diagnosed more commonly in women than in men. Impairment can be severe. In extreme cases, the individual is unable to leave his or her home without being accompanied by a friend or relative. If this is not possible, the person may become totally confined to his or her home.

BOX 18–1 Diagnostic Criteria for Agoraphobia

A. Marked fear or anxiety about two (or more) of the following five situations:
 1. Using public transportation (e.g., automobiles, buses, trains, ships, planes)
 2. Being in open spaces (e.g., parking lots, marketplaces, bridges)
 3. Being in enclosed places (e.g., shops, theaters, cinemas)
 4. Standing in line or being in a crowd
 5. Being outside of the home alone
B. The individual fears these situations because of thoughts that escape might be difficult or help might not be available in the event of panic-like symptoms or other incapacitating or embarrassing symptoms (e.g., fear of falling in the elderly, fear of incontinence).
C. The agoraphobic situations almost always provoke fear or anxiety.
D. The agoraphobic situations are actively avoided, require the presence of a companion, or are endured with intense fear or anxiety.
E. The fear or anxiety is out of proportion to the actual danger posed by the agoraphobic situations and to the sociocultural context.
F. The fear, anxiety, or avoidance is persistent, typically lasting 6 months or more.
G. The fear, anxiety, or avoidance causes clinically significant distress or impairment in social, occupational, or other important areas of functioning.
H. If another medical condition (e.g., inflammatory bowel disease, Parkinson's disease) is present, the fear, anxiety, or avoidance is clearly excessive.
I. The fear, anxiety, or avoidance is not better explained by the symptoms of another mental disorder—for example, the symptoms are not confined to specific phobia, situational type; do not involve only social situations (as in social anxiety disorder); and are not related exclusively to obsessions (as in obsessive-compulsive disorder), perceived defects or flaws in physical appearance (as in body dysmorphic disorder), reminders of traumatic events (as in posttraumatic stress disorder), or fear of separation (as in separation anxiety disorder).

Reprinted with permission from American Psychiatric Association. (2013). Diagnostic and Statistical Manual of Mental Disorders (5th ed.). Washington, DC: American Psychiatric Publishing.

Social Anxiety Disorder (Social Phobia)

Background Assessment Data

Social anxiety disorder is an excessive fear of situations in which a person might do something embarrassing or be evaluated negatively by others. The individual has extreme concerns about being exposed to possible scrutiny by others and fears social or performance situations in which embarrassment may occur (APA, 2013). In some instances, the fear may be quite defined, such as the fear of speaking or eating in a public place, fear of using a public restroom, or fear of writing in the presence of others. In other cases, the social phobia may involve general social situations, such as making comments or answering questions in a manner that would provoke laughter on the part of others. Exposure to the phobic situation usually results in feelings of panic anxiety with sweating, tachycardia, and dyspnea.

Onset of symptoms of this disorder often begins in late childhood or early adolescence and runs a chronic, sometimes lifelong, course. It appears to be more common in women than in men (Kimmel & Roy-Burn, 2017). Impairment interferes with social or occupational functioning and causes marked distress. The *DSM-5* diagnostic criteria for social anxiety disorder are presented in Box 18–2.

Specific Phobia

Background Assessment Data

Specific phobia is identified by fear of specific objects or situations that could conceivably cause harm (e.g., snakes, heights), but the person's reaction to them is excessive, unreasonable, and inappropriate.

Specific phobias are often identified when other anxiety disorders have become a focus of clinical attention. Treatment is generally aimed at the primary diagnosis because it usually produces the greatest distress and interferes with functioning more so than does a specific phobia. A diagnosis of specific phobia is made only when the irrational fear restricts the individual's activities and interferes with his or her daily living.

The phobic person may be no more (or less) anxious than anyone else until exposed to the phobic object or situation. Exposure to the phobic stimulus produces overwhelming symptoms of panic, including palpitations, sweating, dizziness, and difficulty breathing. These symptoms may occur in response to the individual's merely *thinking* about the phobic stimulus. Invariably, the person recognizes that his or her fear is excessive or unreasonable but is powerless to change, even though the individual may occasionally endure the phobic stimulus when experiencing intense anxiety.

Phobias may begin at almost any age. Those that begin in childhood often disappear without treatment, but those that begin or persist into adulthood usually require assistance with therapy. The disorder is diagnosed more often in women than in men.

BOX 18–2 Diagnostic Criteria for Social Anxiety Disorder (Social Phobia)

A. Marked fear or anxiety about one or more social situations in which the individual is exposed to possible scrutiny by others. Examples include social interactions (e.g., having a conversation, meeting unfamiliar people), being observed (e.g., eating or drinking), and performing in front of others (e.g., giving a speech). *Note:* In children, the anxiety must occur in peer settings and not just during interactions with adults.

B. The individual fears that he or she will act in a way or show anxiety symptoms that will be negatively evaluated (i.e., will be humiliating or embarrassing; will lead to rejection or offend others).

C. The social situations almost always provoke fear or anxiety. **Note:** In children, the fear or anxiety may be expressed by crying, tantrums, freezing, clinging, shrinking, or failing to speak in social situations.

D. The social situations are avoided or are endured with intense fear or anxiety.

E. The fear or anxiety is out of proportion to the actual threat posed by the social situation and to the sociocultural context.

F. The fear, anxiety, or avoidance is persistent, typically lasting 6 months or more.

G. The fear, anxiety, or avoidance causes clinically significant distress or impairment in social, occupation, or other important areas of functioning.

H. The fear, anxiety, or avoidance is not attributable to the physiological effects of a substance (e.g., a drug of abuse, a medication) or another medical condition.

I. The fear, anxiety, or avoidance is not better explained by the symptoms of another mental disorder, such as panic disorder, body dysmorphic disorder, or autism spectrum disorder.

J. If another medical condition (e.g., Parkinson's disease, obesity, disfigurement from burns or injury) is present, the fear, anxiety, or avoidance is clearly unrelated or is excessive.

Specify if:

Performance only: If the fear is restricted to speaking or performing in public

Reprinted with permission from American Psychiatric Association. (2013). Diagnostic and Statistical Manual of Mental Disorders (5th ed.). Washington, DC: American Psychiatric Publishing.

Even though the disorder is relatively common among the general population, people seldom seek treatment unless the phobia interferes with ability to function. Obviously, the individual who has a fear of snakes but who lives on the 23rd floor of an urban, high-rise apartment building is not likely to be bothered by the phobia unless he or she decides to move to an area where snakes are prevalent. On the other hand, a fear of elevators may very well interfere with this individual's daily functioning.

Specific phobias have been classified according to the phobic stimulus. A list of some of the identified phobias appears in Table 18–1. This list is by no means all-inclusive. People can become phobic about almost any object or situation, and anyone with a little knowledge of Greek or Latin can produce a phobia classification, thereby making possibilities for the list almost infinite.

Theories of Etiology Related to Phobias

The cause of phobias is unknown. However, various theories exist that may offer insight into the etiology.

Psychoanalytic Theory Modern-day psychoanalysts believe that unconscious fears may be expressed in a symbolic manner as phobias. For example, a female child who was sexually abused by an adult male family friend when he was taking her for a ride in his boat grew up with an intense, irrational fear of all water vessels. Psychoanalytic theory postulates that fear of the man was repressed and displaced onto boats. Boats became an unconscious symbol for the feared person but one that the young girl viewed as safer because her fear of boats prevented her from having to confront the real fear.

Learning Theory Classic conditioning in the case of phobias may be explained as follows: a stressful stimulus produces an "unconditioned" response of fear. When the stressful stimulus is repeatedly paired with a harmless object, eventually the harmless object alone produces a "conditioned" response: fear. This conditioning becomes a phobia when the individual consciously avoids the harmless object to escape fear.

Some learning theorists hold that fears are conditioned responses and thus are learned by imposing rewards for certain behaviors. In the instance of phobias, when the individual avoids the phobic object, he or she escapes fear, which is indeed a powerful reward.

Phobias also may be acquired by direct learning or imitation (modeling; e.g., a mother who exhibits fear toward an object will provide a model for the child, who may also develop a phobia of the same object).

Cognitive Theory Cognitive theorists espouse that anxiety is the product of faulty cognitions or anxiety-inducing self-instructions. Two types of faulty thinking have been investigated: negative self-statements and irrational beliefs. Cognitive theorists believe that some individuals engage in negative and irrational

TABLE 18–1	**Classifications of Specific Phobias**
CLASSIFICATION	**FEAR**
Acrophobia	Height
Ailurophobia	Cats
Algophobia	Pain
Anthophobia	Flowers
Anthropophobia	People
Aquaphobia	Water
Arachnophobia	Spiders
Astraphobia	Lightning
Belonephobia	Needles
Brontophobia	Thunder
Claustrophobia	Closed spaces
Cynophobia	Dogs
Dementophobia	Insanity
Equinophobia	Horses
Gamophobia	Marriage
Herpetophobia	Lizards, reptiles
Homophobia	Homosexuality
Murophobia	Mice
Mysophobia	Dirt, germs, contamination
Numerophobia	Numbers
Nyctophobia	Darkness
Ochophobia	Riding in a car
Ophidiophobia	Snakes
Pyrophobia	Fire
Scoleciphobia	Worms
Siderodromophobia	Railroads or train travel
Taphophobia	Being buried alive
Thanatophobia	Death
Trichophobia	Hair
Triskaidekaphobia	The number 13
Xenophobia	Strangers
Zoophobia	Animals

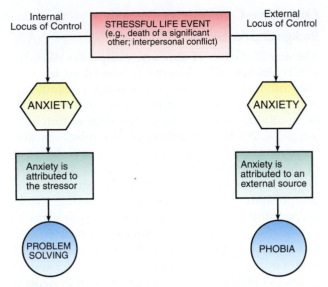

FIGURE 18–2 Locus of control as a variable in the etiology of phobias.

thinking that produces anxiety reactions. The individual begins to seek out avoidance behaviors to prevent the anxiety reactions, and phobias result.

Somewhat related to the cognitive theory is the involvement of locus of control. Johnson and Sarason (1978) suggested that individuals with internal locus of control and those with external locus of control might respond differently to life change. These researchers proposed that locus of control orientation may be an important variable in the development of phobias. Individuals with an external control orientation experiencing anxiety attacks in a stressful period are likely to mislabel the anxiety and attribute it to external sources (e.g., crowded areas) or to a disease (e.g., heart attack). They may perceive the experienced anxiety as being outside of their control. Figure 18–2 depicts a graphic model of the relationship between locus of control and the development of phobias.

Biological Aspects

■ Neuroanatomical: Specific areas in the prefrontal cortex and the amygdala play a role in storing and recalling information about threatening or potentially deadly events. Similar future events can trigger those memories, after which the amygdala triggers release of fight-or-flight hormones and the individual experiences heightened stress and fear as though the original threat was happening again (Nordqvist, 2017). Other researchers (Dias & Ressler, 2014) have found that parental traumatic exposure creates genetic "memories" that are passed down to subsequent generations via parental gametes, which are then expressed as phobias in their offspring. Kimmel & Roy-Burn (2017) note that although there may be a genetic vulnerability to phobias, environmental factors such as trauma play a more central role.

■ Temperament: Children experience fears as a part of normal development. Most infants are afraid of loud noises. Common fears of toddlers and preschoolers include strangers, animals, darkness, and fears of being separated from parents or attachment figures. During the school-age years, there is fear of death and anxiety about school achievement. Fears of social rejection and sexual anxieties are common among adolescents. Innate fears represent a part of the overall characteristics or tendencies with which one is born that influence how he or she responds throughout life to specific situations. Innate fears usually do not reach phobic intensity but may have the capacity for such development if reinforced by events in later life. For example, a 4-year-old girl is afraid of dogs. By age 5, however, she has overcome her fear and plays with her own dog and the neighbors' dogs without fear. Then, when she is 19, she is bitten by a stray dog and develops a phobia of dogs.

Life Experiences Certain early experiences may set the stage for phobic reactions later in life. Some researchers believe that phobias, particularly specific phobias, are symbolic of original anxiety-producing objects or situations that have been repressed. Examples include the following:

■ A child who is punished by being locked in a closet develops a phobia of elevators or other closed places.
■ A child who falls down a flight of stairs develops a phobia of high places.
■ A young woman who, as a child, survived a plane crash in which both her parents were killed has a phobia of airplanes.

Anxiety Disorder Due to Another Medical Condition and Substance/Medication-Induced Anxiety Disorder

Background Assessment Data

The symptoms associated with these disorders are judged to be the direct physiological consequence of another medical condition or due to the direct physiological effects of substance intoxication or withdrawal or exposure to a medication. A number of medical conditions have been associated with the development of anxiety symptoms. Some of these include cardiac conditions, such as myocardial infarction, congestive heart failure, and mitral valve prolapse; endocrine conditions, such as hypoglycemia, hypo- or hyperthyroidism, and pheochromocytoma; respiratory conditions, such as chronic obstructive pulmonary disease and hyperventilation; and neurological conditions, such as complex partial seizures, neoplasms, and encephalitis.

Nursing care of patients with this disorder must take into consideration the underlying cause of the anxiety. Holistic nursing care is essential to ensure that the patient's physiological and psychosocial needs are met. Nursing actions appropriate for the specific medical condition must be considered.

The diagnosis of substance-induced anxiety disorder is made only if the anxiety symptoms are in excess of those usually associated with the intoxication or withdrawal syndrome and warrant independent clinical attention. Evidence of intoxication or withdrawal must be available from history, physical examination, or laboratory findings to substantiate the diagnosis. Substance-induced anxiety disorder may be associated with use of the following substances: alcohol, amphetamines, cocaine, hallucinogen, sedatives, hypnotics, anxiolytics, caffeine, cannabis, or other substances (APA, 2013). Nursing care of the patient with substance-induced anxiety disorder must take into consideration the nature of the substance and the context in which the symptoms occur—that is, intoxication or withdrawal.

CORE CONCEPT

Obsessions

Intrusive thoughts that are recurrent and stressful. Although they are recognized by the individual as irrational, they continue to be repetitive and cannot be ignored.

CORE CONCEPT

Compulsions

Repetitive ritualistic behaviors or mental acts that the individual feels driven to perform, which are intended to reduce the anxiety associated with obsessive thoughts (APA, 2013).

Obsessive-Compulsive Disorder
Background Assessment Data

The manifestations of **obsessive-compulsive disorder** (OCD) include the presence of obsessions or compulsions, or both, the severity of which is significant enough to cause distress or impairment in social, occupational, or other important areas of functioning (APA, 2013). The individual recognizes that the behavior is excessive or unreasonable but, because of the feeling of relief from discomfort that it promotes, is compelled to continue the act. Common compulsions include hand washing, ordering, checking, praying, counting, and repeating words silently.

The disorder is equally common among men and women. It may begin in childhood but more often begins in adolescence or early adulthood. The course is usually chronic and may be complicated by depression or substance abuse. OCD is identified more frequently in single people than in married people, but this finding probably reflects the difficulty that individuals with this disorder have with maintaining interpersonal relationships (Sadock et al., 2015). The *DSM-5* diagnostic criteria for OCD are presented in Box 18–3.

Body Dysmorphic Disorder
Background Assessment Data

Body dysmorphic disorder is characterized by the exaggerated belief that the body is deformed or defective in some specific way. The most common complaints involve flaws of the face or head, such as wrinkles or scars, the shape of the nose, excessive facial hair, and facial asymmetry that are slight or not observable by others (Stein & Lochner, 2017). Other complaints involve the ears, eyes, mouth, lips, or teeth. Some clients may present with complaints involving other parts of the body, and in some instances a true defect is present. The significance of the defect is unrealistically exaggerated, however, and the person's concern is grossly excessive. These beliefs are differentiated from delusions in that the individual with body dysmorphic disorder is aware that his or her beliefs are exaggerated. In some cases, though, people with body dysmorphic disorder also develop psychotic disorders.

People with body dysmorphic disorder often have other comorbid mental disorders. One study found that 90 percent of people with body dysmorphic disorder had major depressive disorder, about 70 percent had an anxiety disorder (often OCD), and 30 percent had

BOX 18–3 Diagnostic Criteria for Obsessive-Compulsive Disorder

A. Presence of obsessions, compulsions, or both:

Obsessions are defined by (1) and (2)

1. Recurrent and persistent thoughts, urges, or images that are experienced, at some time during the disturbance, as intrusive and unwanted, and that in most individuals cause marked anxiety or distress.
2. The individual attempts to ignore or suppress such thoughts, urges, or images, or to neutralize them with some other thought or action (i.e., by performing a compulsion).

Compulsions are defined by (1) and (2):

1. Repetitive behaviors (e.g., hand washing, ordering, checking) or mental acts (e.g., praying, counting, repeating words silently) that the person feels driven to perform in response to an obsession or according to rules that must be applied rigidly.
2. The behaviors or mental acts are aimed at preventing or reducing anxiety or distress, or preventing some dreaded event or situation; however, these behaviors or mental acts either are not connected in a realistic way with what they are designed to neutralize or prevent or are clearly excessive. *Note:* Young children may not be able to articulate the aims of these behaviors or mental acts.

B. The obsessions or compulsions are time consuming (e.g., take more than 1 hour a day) or cause clinically significant distress or impairment in social, occupational, or other important areas of functioning.

C. The obsessive-compulsive symptoms are not attributable to the direct physiological effects of a substance (e.g., a drug of abuse, a medication) or another medical condition.

D. The disturbance is not better explained by the symptoms of another mental disorder (e.g., excessive worries, as in generalized anxiety disorder; preoccupation with appearance, as in body dysmorphic disorder; difficulty discarding or parting with possessions, as in hoarding disorder; hair pulling, as in trichotillomania [hair-pulling disorder]; skin picking, as in excoriation [skin-picking] disorder; stereotypies, as in stereotypic movement disorder; ritualized eating behavior, as in eating disorders; preoccupation with substances or gambling, as in substance-related and addictive disorders; preoccupation with having an illness, as in illness anxiety disorder; sexual urges or fantasies, as in paraphilic disorders; impulses, as in disruptive, impulse-control, and conduct disorders; guilty ruminations, as in major depressive disorder; thought insertion or delusional preoccupations, as in schizophrenia spectrum and other psychotic disorders; or repetitive patterns of behavior, as in autism spectrum disorder).

Specify if:

With good or fair insight

With poor insight

With absent insight/delusional beliefs

Specify if:

Tic-related

Reprinted with permission from American Psychiatric Association. (2013). Diagnostic and Statistical Manual of Mental Disorders *(5th ed.). Washington, DC: American Psychiatric Publishing.*

experienced a psychotic disorder (Sadock et al., 2015). Social and occupational impairment may occur because of the excessive anxiety experienced by the individual in relation to the imagined defect. The person's medical history may reflect numerous visits to plastic surgeons and dermatologists in an unrelenting drive to correct the imagined defect. He or she may undergo unnecessary surgical procedures toward this effort.

The *DSM-5* diagnostic criteria for body dysmorphic disorder are presented in Box 18–4.

Trichotillomania (Hair-Pulling Disorder)

Background Assessment Data

The *DSM-5* defines **trichotillomania (hair-pulling disorder)** as the recurrent pulling out of one's hair that results in hair loss (APA, 2013). The impulse is preceded by an increasing sense of tension and results in a sense of release or gratification from pulling out

the hair. The most common sites for hair pulling are the scalp, eyebrows, and eyelashes but may occur in any area of the body on which hair grows. These areas of hair loss are often found on the opposite side of the body from the dominant hand. Pain is seldom reported to accompany the hair pulling, although tingling and pruritus in the area are not uncommon.

Comorbid psychiatric disorders are common with hair-pulling disorder. The most common are mood and other anxiety disorders (Stein & Lochner, 2017).

The disorder usually begins in childhood and is seven times more prevalent in children (between the ages of 4 and 17) than adults (Yasgur, 2015). It may be accompanied by nail biting, head banging, scratching, biting, or other acts of self-mutilation. This phenomenon occurs more often in women than in men. Studies indicate that it affects about 4 percent of the population (Yasgur, 2015).

BOX 18–4 **Diagnostic Criteria for Body Dysmorphic Disorder**

A. Preoccupation with one or more perceived defects or flaws in physical appearance that are not observable or appear slight to others.

B. At some point during the course of the disorder, the individual has performed repetitive behaviors (e.g., mirror checking, excessive grooming, skin picking, reassurance seeking) or mental acts (e.g., comparing his or her appearance with that of others) in response to the appearance concerns.

C. The preoccupation causes clinically significant distress or impairment in social, occupational, or other important areas of functioning.

D. The appearance preoccupation is not better explained by concerns with body fat or weight in an individual whose symptoms meet diagnostic criteria for an eating disorder.

Specify if:

With muscle dysmorphia

Specify if:

With good or fair insight

With poor insight

With absent insight/delusional beliefs

Reprinted with permission from American Psychiatric Association. (2013). Diagnostic and Statistical Manual of Mental Disorders (5th ed.). Washington, DC: American Psychiatric Publishing.

Hoarding Disorder

Background Assessment Data

The *DSM-5* defines the essential feature of **hoarding disorder** as "persistent difficulties discarding or parting with possessions, regardless of their actual value" (APA, 2013, p. 248). Additionally, the diagnosis may be specified as "with excessive acquisition," which identifies the excessive need for continual acquiring of items (either by buying them or by other means). In previous editions of the *DSM*, hoarding was considered a symptom of OCD. However, in the *DSM-5*, it has been reclassified as a diagnostic disorder.

Individuals with this disorder collect items until virtually all surfaces within the home are covered. There may be only narrow pathways, winding through stacks of clutter, in which to walk. Some individuals also hoard food and animals, keeping dozens or hundreds of pets, often in unsanitary conditions (Mayo Clinic, 2018).

Hoarding disorder affects an estimated 700,000 to 1.4 million Americans, but few receive adequate treatment (Symonds & Janney, 2013). More men than women are diagnosed with the disorder, and it is almost three times more prevalent in older adults (ages 55–94) than in younger adults (ages 34–44) (APA, 2013). The symptoms, regardless of when they begin, appear to become more severe with each decade of life. Associated symptoms include perfectionism, indecisiveness, anxiety, depression, distractibility, and difficulty planning and organizing tasks (APA, 2013; Symonds & Janney, 2013). In addition to OCD, hoarding is associated with high comorbidity for dependent, avoidant, schizotypal, and paranoid personality disorders (Sadock et al., 2015). Research has shown that hoarding disorder runs in families, and there may be a genetic vulnerability.

Treatment of hoarding disorder has been met with mixed results. It is often difficult to convince individuals with the disorder that they are actually ill. Change is slow, and the relapse rate is high; when possessions are taken away, they are often quickly replaced to provide emotional comfort (Mayo Clinic, 2018). Psychoeducation about the disorder is almost always the initial intervention, and treatment is most commonly a combination of cognitive behavioral therapy and psychopharmacology with SSRIs. Family and friends may misinterpret hoarding behavior as laziness or uncleanliness. Psychoeducation that includes the client's identified support system assists the client in a recovery plan. Some experts have identified unresolved grief issues associated with hoarding behavior, which may provide another avenue for psychological intervention.

Theories of Etiology in Obsessive-Compulsive and Related Disorders

Psychoanalytic Theory

Psychoanalytic theorists propose that individuals with OCD have weak, underdeveloped egos (for any of a variety of reasons: unsatisfactory parent-child relationship, conditional love, or provisional gratification). The psychoanalytical concept views clients with OCD as having regressed to earlier developmental stages of the infantile superego—the harsh, exacting, punitive characteristics that now reappear as part of the psychopathology. Regression and use of defense mechanisms (isolation, undoing, displacement, reaction formation) produce the clinical symptoms of obsessions and compulsions (Sadock et al., 2015).

Learning Theory

Learning theorists explain obsessive-compulsive behavior as a conditioned response to a traumatic event. The traumatic event produces anxiety and discomfort, and the individual learns to prevent the anxiety and discomfort by avoiding the situation with which they are associated. This type of learning is called *passive avoidance* (staying away from the source). When passive avoidance is not possible, the individual learns to engage in behaviors that provide relief from the anxiety and discomfort associated with the traumatic situation. This type of learning is called *active avoidance* and describes the behavior pattern of the individual with OCD (Sadock et al., 2015).

According to this classic conditioning interpretation, a traumatic event should mark the beginning of the obsessive-compulsive behaviors. However, in a significant number of cases, the onset of the behavior is gradual, and the clients relate the onset of their problems to life stress in general rather than to one or more traumatic events.

Psychosocial Influences

In general, OCDs have more often been described in the context of neuropsychiatric influences, but some specific disorders have been connected to psychosocial influences. The onset of trichotillomania can be related to stressful situations in more than one quarter of cases. Additional factors that have been implicated include disturbances in mother-child relationship, fear of abandonment, and recent object loss. Trichotillomania has at times been connected to childhood trauma, but Woods (as cited by Kaplan, 2012) indicates that only 5 percent of patients with trichotillomania also meet diagnostic criteria for post-traumatic stress disorder. Hoarding disorder has been associated with unmanaged stress following the sudden loss of a loved one, divorce, or other significant life stressors (Mayo Clinic, 2018).

Biological Aspects

Genetics Twin studies and family studies support a genetic susceptibility for OCD, especially in childhood onset OCD (Stein & Lochner, 2017). Trichotillomania has commonly been associated with OCDs among first-degree relatives, leading researchers to conclude that the disorder has a possible hereditary or familial predisposition. Structural abnormalities in various areas

of the brain, as well as alterations in the serotonin and endogenous opioid systems, have also been noted.

Genetics also may play a role in the development of hoarding disorder. Family and twin studies indicate that approximately 50 percent of individuals who hoard report having a relative who also hoards (APA, 2013).

Neuroanatomy Recent findings suggest that neurobiological disturbances may play a role in the pathogenesis and maintenance of OCD. Abnormalities in various regions of the brain have been implicated in the neurobiology of OCD. Neuroimaging and neurocognitive assessment have identified impairment in motor inhibition responses (the ability to stop an action once initiated) in patients with OCD and trichotillomania (Kaplan, 2012). In individuals with hoarding disorder, neuroimaging studies have indicated less activity in the cingulate cortex, the area of the brain that connects the emotional part of the brain with the parts that control higher-level thinking (Saxena, 2013).

Yasgur (2015) reports that "animal models and brain imaging studies of patients with trichotillomania suggest abnormalities in neural regions involved in cognition (frontal cortex), affect regulation (amygdala-hippocampal formation), and habit learning (putamen). One study suggests that [trichotillomania] may be associated with altered reward processing within the central nervous system."

Physiology Electrophysiological studies, sleep electroencephalogram studies, and neuroendocrine studies have suggested that there are commonalities between depressive disorders and OCD (Sadock et al., 2015). Neuroendocrine commonalities were suggested in studies in which about one-third of OCD clients show nonsuppression on the dexamethasone-suppression test and decreased growth hormone secretion with clonidine infusions.

Biochemical Factors A number of studies have implicated the neurotransmitter serotonin as influential in the etiology of obsessive-compulsive behaviors. Drugs that have been used successfully in alleviating the symptoms of OCD include clomipramine (a tricyclic antidepressant) and SSRIs, which are believed to block the neuronal reuptake of serotonin, thereby potentiating serotonergic activity in the central nervous system (see Figure 18–1). The serotonergic system may also be a factor in the etiology of body dysmorphic disorder. This can be reflected in a high incidence of comorbidity with major mood disorder and anxiety disorder and the positive responsiveness of the condition to the serotonin-specific drugs.

Genome studies have implicated glutamatergic function in OCD but more research is needed (Stein & Lochner, 2017).

Assessment Scales

A number of assessment rating scales are available for measuring severity of anxiety symptoms. Some are meant to be clinician administered, whereas others may be self-administered. Examples of self-rating scales include the Beck Anxiety Inventory and the Zung Self-Rated Anxiety Scale. One of the most widely used clinician-administered scales is the Hamilton Anxiety Rating Scale (HAM-A), which is used in both clinical and research settings. The scale consists of 14 items and measures both psychic and somatic anxiety symptoms (psychological distress and physical complaints associated with anxiety). The HAM-A scale is presented in Box 18–5.

BOX 18–5 Hamilton Anxiety Rating Scale (HAM-A)

Below are descriptions of symptoms commonly associated with anxiety. Assign the client the rating between 0 and 4 (for each of the 14 items) that best describes the extent to which he/she has these symptoms.

0 = Not present, 1 = Mild, 2 = Moderate, 3 = Severe, 4 = Very severe

1. **Anxious mood** _____ Worries, anticipation of the worst, fearful anticipation, irritability	8. **Somatic (sensory)** _____ Tinnitus, blurred vision, hot/cold flushes, feelings of weakness, tingling sensation
2. **Tension** _____ Feelings of tension, fatigability, startle response, moved to tears easily, trembling, feelings of restlessness, inability to relax	9. **Cardiovascular symptoms** _____ Tachycardia, palpitations, pain in chest, throbbing of vessels, feeling faint
3. **Fears** _____ Of dark, of strangers, of being left alone, of animals, of traffic, of crowds	10. **Respiratory symptoms** _____ Pressure or constriction in chest, choking feelings, sighing, dyspnea
4. **Insomnia** _____ Difficulty in falling asleep, broken sleep, unsatisfying sleep and fatigue on waking, dreams, nightmares, night terrors	11. **Gastrointestinal symptoms** _____ Difficulty swallowing, flatulence, abdominal pain and fullness, burning sensations, nausea/vomiting, borborygmi, diarrhea, constipation, weight loss
5. **Intellectual** _____ Difficulty in concentration, poor memory	12. **Genitourinary symptoms** _____ Urinary frequency, urinary urgency, amenorrhea, menorrhagia, loss of libido, premature ejaculation, impotence
6. **Depressed mood** _____ Loss of interest, lack of pleasure in hobbies, depression, early waking, diurnal swing	13. **Autonomic symptoms** _____ Dry mouth, flushing, pallor, tendency to sweat, giddiness, tension headache
7. **Somatic (muscular)** _____ Pains and aches, twitching, stiffness, myoclonic jerks, grinding of teeth, unsteady voice, increased muscular tone	14. **Behavior at interview** _____ Fidgeting, restlessness or pacing, tremor of hands, furrowed brow, strained face, sighing or rapid respiration, facial pallor, swallowing, clearing throat

Client's Total Score _____

SCORING
14 – 17 = Mild Anxiety
18 – 24 = Moderate Anxiety
25 – 30 = Severe Anxiety

Source: Hamilton, M. (1959). The assessment of anxiety states by rating. British Journal of Medical Psychology, 32, 50–55. The HAM-A is in the public domain.

TABLE 18–2	**Assigning Nursing Diagnoses to Behaviors Commonly Associated With Anxiety, Obsessive-Compulsive, and Related Disorders**
BEHAVIORS	**NURSING DIAGNOSES**
Palpitations, trembling, sweating, chest pain, shortness of breath, fear of going crazy, fear of dying (panic disorder); excessive worry, difficulty concentrating, sleep disturbance (generalized anxiety disorder)	**Anxiety (severe/panic)**
Verbal expressions of having no control over life situation; nonparticipation in decision making related to own care or life situation; expressions of doubt regarding role performance (panic and generalized anxiety disorders)	**Powerlessness**
Behavior directed toward avoidance of a feared object or situation (phobic disorder)	**Fear**
Stays at home alone, afraid to venture out alone (agoraphobia)	**Social isolation**
Ritualistic behavior; obsessive thoughts, inability to meet basic needs; severe level of anxiety (OCD)	**Ineffective coping**
Inability to fulfill usual patterns of responsibility because of need to perform rituals (OCD)	**Ineffective role performance**
Preoccupation with imagined defect; verbalizations that are out of proportion to any actual physical abnormality that may exist; numerous visits to plastic surgeons or dermatologists seeking relief (body dysmorphic disorder)	**Disturbed body image**
Repetitive and impulsive pulling out of one's hair (trichotillomania)	**Ineffective impulse control**

Diagnosis and Outcome Identification

Nursing diagnoses are formulated from the data gathered during the assessment phase and with background knowledge regarding predisposing factors to the disorder. Table 18–2 presents a list of patient behaviors and the NANDA International (NANDA-I) nursing diagnoses (Herdman & Kamitsuru, 2018) that correspond to those behaviors, which may be used in planning care for patients with anxiety, obsessive-compulsive, and related disorders.

Outcome Criteria

The following criteria may be used for measurement of outcomes in the care of the patient with anxiety disorders.

The patient:

■ Is able to recognize signs of escalating anxiety and intervene before reaching panic level (*panic and generalized anxiety disorders*).
■ Is able to maintain anxiety at manageable level and make independent decisions about life situation (*panic and generalized anxiety disorders*).

■ Functions adaptively in the presence of the phobic object or situation without experiencing panic anxiety (*phobic disorder*).
■ Verbalizes a future plan of action for responding in the presence of the phobic object or situation without developing panic anxiety (*phobic disorder*).
■ Is able to maintain anxiety at a manageable level without resorting to the use of ritualistic behavior (*OCD*).
■ Demonstrates adaptive coping strategies for dealing with anxiety instead of ritualistic behaviors (*OCD*).
■ Verbalizes a realistic perception of his or her appearance and expresses feelings that reflect a positive body image (*body dysmorphic disorder*).
■ Verbalizes and demonstrates more adaptive strategies for coping with stressful situations (*trichotillomania*).

Planning and Implementation

Table 18–3 provides a plan of care for the patient with anxiety, obsessive-compulsive, and related disorders. Nursing diagnoses are presented, along with outcome criteria, appropriate nursing interventions, and rationales for each.

Table 18–3 | CARE PLAN FOR THE PATIENT WITH ANXIETY, OBSESSIVE-COMPULSIVE, AND RELATED DISORDERS

NURSING DIAGNOSIS: PANIC ANXIETY

RELATED TO: Real or perceived threat to biological integrity or self-concept

EVIDENCED BY: Any or all of the physical symptoms identified by the *DSM-5*

OUTCOME CRITERIA	NURSING INTERVENTIONS	RATIONALE
Short-Term Goal ■ The patient will verbalize ways to intervene in escalating anxiety within 1 week. **Long-Term Goal** ■ By time of discharge from treatment, the patient will be able to recognize symptoms of onset of anxiety and intervene before reaching panic level.	1. Stay with the patient and offer reassurance of safety and security. Do not leave the patient in panic anxiety alone. 2. Maintain a calm, nonthreatening, matter-of-fact approach. 3. Use simple words and brief messages, spoken calmly and clearly, to explain hospital experiences. 4. Hyperventilation may occur during periods of extreme anxiety. Hyperventilation causes the amount of carbon dioxide (CO_2) in the blood to decrease, possibly resulting in lightheadedness, rapid heart rate, shortness of breath, numbness or tingling in the hands or feet, and syncope. If hyperventilation occurs, assist the patient to breathe into a small paper bag held over the mouth and nose. Six to 12 natural breaths should be taken, alternating with short periods of diaphragmatic breathing. 5. Keep immediate surroundings low in stimuli (dim lighting, few people, simple decor). 6. Administer tranquilizing medication, as ordered by physician. Assess for effectiveness and for side effects. 7. When level of anxiety has been reduced, explore possible reasons for occurrence. 8. Teach signs and symptoms of escalating anxiety, and ways to interrupt its progression (relaxation techniques, such as deep-breathing exercises and meditation, or physical exercise, such as brisk walks and jogging).	1. The patient may fear for his or her life. Presence of a trusted individual provides a feeling of security and assurance of personal safety. 2. Anxiety is contagious and may be transferred from staff to patient or vice versa. Patient develops a feeling of security in the presence of a calm staff person. 3. In an intensely anxious situation, the patient is unable to comprehend anything but the most elemental communication. 4. Hyperventilation may result in injury to the patient, and patient safety is a nursing priority. The technique here should not be used with patients who have coronary or respiratory disorders, such as coronary artery disease, asthma, or chronic obstructive pulmonary disease. 5. A stimulating environment may increase level of anxiety. 6. Antianxiety medication provides relief from the immobilizing effects of anxiety. 7. Recognition of precipitating factor(s) is the first step in teaching client to interrupt escalation of anxiety. 8. Relaxation techniques result in a physiological response opposite that of the anxiety response. Physical activities discharge excess energy in a healthful manner.

Table 18–3 | CARE PLAN FOR THE PATIENT WITH ANXIETY, OBSESSIVE-COMPULSIVE, AND RELATED DISORDERS—cont'd

NURSING DIAGNOSIS: FEAR

RELATED TO: Causing embarrassment to self in front of others, being in a place from which one is unable to escape, or a specific stimulus

EVIDENCED BY: Behavior directed toward avoidance of the feared object or situation

OUTCOME CRITERIA	NURSING INTERVENTIONS	RATIONALE
Short-Term Goal ■ Patient will discuss the phobic object or situation with the healthcare provider within (time specified). **Long-Term Goal** ■ By time of discharge from treatment, patient will be able to function in presence of phobic object or situation without experiencing panic anxiety.	1. Reassure patient that he or she is safe. 2. Explore patient's perception of the threat to physical integrity or threat to self-concept. 3. Discuss reality of the situation with patient to recognize aspects that can be changed and those that cannot. 4. Include patient in making decisions related to selection of alternative coping strategies. (e.g., client may choose either to avoid the phobic stimulus or to attempt to eliminate the fear associated with it). 5. If patient elects to work on elimination of the fear, techniques of desensitization or implosion therapy may be employed. (See explanation of these techniques under "Treatment Modalities" at the end of this chapter.) 6. Encourage patient to explore underlying feelings that may be contributing to irrational fears and to face them rather than suppress them.	1. At the panic level of anxiety, patient may fear for his or her own life. 2. It is important to understand patient's perception of the phobic object or situation to assist with the desensitization process. 3. Patient must accept the reality of the situation (aspects that cannot change) before the work of reducing the fear can progress. 4. Allowing the patient choices provides a measure of control and serves to increase feelings of self-worth. 5. Fear is decreased as the physical and psychological sensations diminish in response to repeated exposure to the phobic stimulus under nonthreatening conditions. 6. Exploring underlying feelings may help the patient to confront unresolved conflicts and develop more adaptive coping abilities.

NURSING DIAGNOSIS: INEFFECTIVE COPING

RELATED TO: Underdeveloped ego, punitive superego; avoidance learning; possible biochemical changes

EVIDENCED BY: Ritualistic behavior or obsessive thoughts

OUTCOME CRITERIA	NURSING INTERVENTIONS	RATIONALE
Short-Term Goal ■ Within 1 week, the patient will decrease participation in ritualistic behavior by half. **Long-Term Goal** ■ By time of discharge from treatment, patient will demonstrate ability to cope effectively without resorting to obsessive-compulsive behaviors.	1. Work with patient to determine types of situations that increase anxiety and result in ritualistic behaviors. 2. In the beginning of treatment, allow plenty of time for rituals. Do not be judgmental or verbalize disapproval of the behavior.	1. Recognition of precipitating factors is the first step in teaching the patient to interrupt the escalating anxiety. 2. To deny patient this activity may precipitate panic anxiety. Conversely, indulging the patient's need for ritualistic behavior initially decreases anxiety and promotes the ability to learn alternative coping strategies. Learning is best accomplished when the patient's anxiety is at a mild level.

continued

Table 18–3 | CARE PLAN FOR THE PATIENT WITH ANXIETY, OBSESSIVE-COMPULSIVE, AND RELATED DISORDERS—cont'd

OUTCOME CRITERIA	NURSING INTERVENTIONS	RATIONALE
	3. Support patient's efforts to explore the meaning and purpose of the behavior.	3. Patient may be unaware of the relationship between emotional problems and compulsive behaviors. Recognition is important before change can occur.
	4. Provide structured schedule of activities for patient, including adequate time for completion of rituals.	4. Structure provides a feeling of security for the anxious patient.
	5. Gradually begin to limit amount of time allotted for ritualistic behavior as patient becomes more involved in other activities.	5. Anxiety is minimized when patient is able to replace ritualistic behaviors with more adaptive ones.
	6. Give positive reinforcement for nonritualistic behaviors.	6. Positive reinforcement enhances self-esteem and encourages repetition of desired behaviors.
	7. Help patient learn ways of interrupting obsessive thoughts and ritualistic behavior with techniques such as thought stopping, relaxation, and physical exercise.	7. Knowledge and practice of coping techniques that are more adaptive will help patient change and let go of maladaptive responses to anxiety.

NURSING DIAGNOSIS: DISTURBED BODY IMAGE

RELATED TO: Repressed severe anxiety

EVIDENCED BY: Preoccupation with imagined defect; verbalizations that are out of proportion to any actual physical abnormality that may exist; and numerous visits to plastic surgeons or dermatologists seeking relief

OUTCOME CRITERIA	NURSING INTERVENTIONS	RATIONALE
Short-Term Goal ■ Patient will verbalize understanding that changes in bodily structure or function are exaggerated out of proportion to the change that actually exists. (Time frame for this goal must be determined according to individual patient's situation.) **Long-Term Goal** ■ Patient will verbalize perception of own body that is realistic to actual structure or function by time of discharge from treatment.	1. Assess patient's perception of his or her body image. Keep in mind that this image is real to the patient. 2. Help patient to see that his or her body image is distorted or that it is out of proportion in relation to the significance of an actual physical anomaly. 3. Encourage verbalization of fears and anxieties associated with identified stressful life situations. Discuss alternative adaptive coping strategies.	1. Assessment information is necessary in developing an accurate plan of care. Denial of the patient's feelings impedes the development of a trusting, therapeutic relationship. 2. Recognition that a misperception exists is necessary before the patient can accept reality and reduce the significance of the imagined defect. 3. Verbalization of feelings with a trusted individual may help the patient come to terms with unresolved issues. Knowledge of alternative coping strategies may help the patient respond to stress more adaptively in the future.

Table 18–3 | CARE PLAN FOR THE PATIENT WITH ANXIETY, OBSESSIVE-COMPULSIVE, AND RELATED DISORDERS–cont'd

4. Involve patient in activities that reinforce a positive sense of self not based on appearance.

4. When the patient is able to develop self-satisfaction based on accomplishments and unconditional acceptance, significance of the imagined defect or minor physical anomaly will diminish.

5. Make referrals to support groups of individuals with similar histories (e.g., Adult Children of Alcoholics [ACOA], Victims of Incest, Survivors of Suicide [SOS], Adults Abused as Children).

5. Having a support group of understanding, empathic peers can help the patient accept the reality of the situation, correct distorted perceptions, and make adaptive life changes.

NURSING DIAGNOSIS: INEFFECTIVE IMPULSE CONTROL

RELATED TO: Possible genetic or biochemical factors; poor parent-child relationship; history of child abuse or neglect

EVIDENCED BY: Recurrent pulling out of the hair in response to stressful situations

OUTCOME CRITERIA	NURSING INTERVENTIONS	RATIONALE
Short-Term Goal ■ Patient will verbalize adaptive ways to cope with stress by means other than pulling out own hair (time dimension to be individually determined). **Long-Term Goal** ■ Patient will be able to demonstrate adaptive coping strategies in response to stress and a discontinuation of pulling out own hair (time dimension to be individually determined).	1. Support patient in his or her effort to stop hair pulling. Help patient understand that it is possible to discontinue the behavior. 2. Ensure that a nonjudgmental attitude is conveyed, and criticism of the behavior is avoided. 3. Assist patient with habit reversal training (HRT). Three components of HRT include the following: a. Awareness training. Help the patient become aware of times when the hair pulling most often occurs (e.g., client learns to recognize urges, thoughts, or sensations that precede the behavior; the therapist points out to the patient each time the behavior occurs). b. Competing response training. In this step, the patient learns to substitute another response to the urge to pull his or her hair. For example, when a patient experiences a hair-pulling urge, suggest that the individual ball up his/her hands into fists, tightening arm muscles, and "locking" his/her arms so as to make hair pulling impossible at that moment. c. Social support. Encourage family members to participate in the therapy process and to offer positive feedback for attempts at habit reversal.	1. Patient realizes that the behavior is maladaptive but feels helpless to stop. Support from the nurse builds trust. 2. An attitude of acceptance promotes feelings of dignity and self-worth. 3. HRT has been shown to be an effective tool in treatment of hair-pulling disorder. a. This helps the patient identify situations in which the behavior occurs or is most likely to occur. Awareness gives the patient a feeling of increased self-control. b. Substituting an incompatible behavior may help to extinguish the undesirable behavior. c. Positive feedback enhances self-esteem and increases patient's desire to continue with the therapy. It also provides cues for family members to use in their attempts to help the patient in treatment.

Continued

Table 18–3 | CARE PLAN FOR THE PATIENT WITH ANXIETY, OBSESSIVE-COMPULSIVE, AND RELATED DISORDERS–cont'd

OUTCOME CRITERIA	NURSING INTERVENTIONS	RATIONALE
	4. Once patient has become aware of hair-pulling times, suggest that patient hold something (a ball, paperweight, or other item) in his or her hand at times when hair pulling is anticipated.	4. This would help to prevent behaviors occurring without patient being aware that they are happening.
	5. Practice stress management techniques: deep breathing, meditation, stretching, physical exercise, listening to soft music.	5. Hair pulling is thought to occur at times of increased anxiety.
	6. Offer support and encouragement when setbacks occur. Help patient to understand the importance of not quitting when it seems that change is not happening as quickly as he or she would like.	6. Although some people see a decrease in the behavior within a few days, most will take several months to notice the greatest change.

Concept Care Mapping

The concept map care plan (see Chapter 6) is a diagrammatic teaching and learning strategy that allows visualization of interrelationships between medical diagnoses, nursing diagnoses, assessment data, and treatments. An example of a concept map care plan for the client with an anxiety disorder is presented in Figure 18–3.

Patient and Family Education

The role of patient teacher is important in the psychiatric area, as it is in all areas of nursing. A list of topics for patient and family education relevant to anxiety disorders is presented in Box 18–6.

Evaluation

In the final step of the nursing process, a reassessment is conducted in order to determine if the nursing actions have been successful in achieving the objectives of care. Evaluation of the nursing actions for the patient with an anxiety, OCD, or related disorder may be facilitated by asking whether the patient can:

■ Recognize signs and symptoms of escalating anxiety?
■ Use skills learned to interrupt the escalating anxiety before it reaches the panic level?
■ Demonstrate the activities most appropriate for him or her that can be used to maintain anxiety at a manageable level (e.g., relaxation techniques, physical exercise)?

■ Maintain anxiety at a manageable level without medication?
■ Verbalize a long-term plan for preventing panic anxiety in the face of a stressful situation?
■ Discuss the phobic object or situation without becoming anxious?
■ Function in the presence of the phobic object or situation without experiencing panic anxiety?
■ Refrain from performing rituals when anxiety level rises?
■ Demonstrate substitute behaviors to maintain anxiety at a manageable level?
■ Recognize the relationship between escalating anxiety and the dependence on ritualistic behaviors for relief?
■ Refrain from hair pulling (for patients with trichotillomania)?
■ Successfully substitute a more adaptive behavior when urges to pull hair occur (for patients with trichotillomania)?
■ Verbalize a realistic perception and satisfactory acceptance of personal appearance (for patients with body dysmorphic disorder)?

Treatment Modalities

Individual Psychotherapy

Most clients experience a marked decrease in anxiety when given the opportunity to discuss their difficulties with a concerned and sympathetic therapist. Supportive psychotherapy is designed to help clients

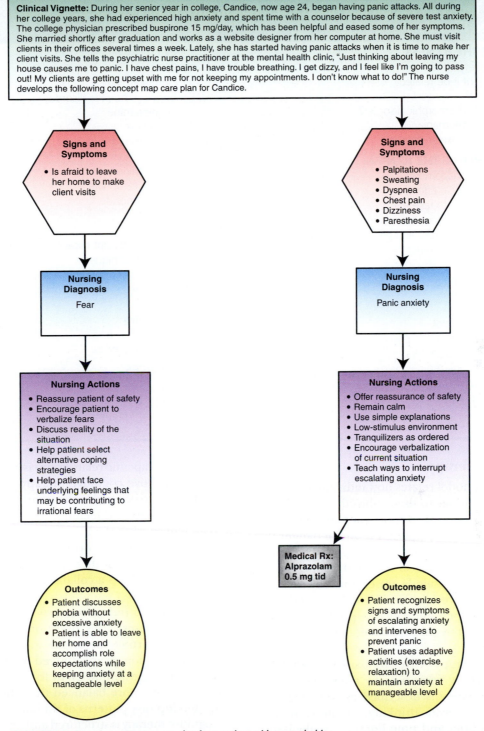

Clinical Vignette: During her senior year in college, Candice, now age 24, began having panic attacks. All during her college years, she had experienced high anxiety and spent time with a counselor because of severe test anxiety. The college physician prescribed buspirone 15 mg/day, which has been helpful and eased some of her symptoms. She married shortly after graduation and works as a website designer from her computer at home. She must visit clients in their offices several times a week. Lately, she has started having panic attacks when it is time to make her client visits. She tells the psychiatric nurse practitioner at the mental health clinic, "Just thinking about leaving my house causes me to panic. I have chest pains, I have trouble breathing. I get dizzy, and I feel like I'm going to pass out! My clients are getting upset with me for not keeping my appointments. I don't know what to do!" The nurse develops the following concept map care plan for Candice.

Signs and Symptoms

- Is afraid to leave her home to make client visits

Signs and Symptoms

- Palpitations
- Sweating
- Dyspnea
- Chest pain
- Dizziness
- Paresthesia

Nursing Diagnosis

Fear

Nursing Diagnosis

Panic anxiety

Nursing Actions

- Reassure patient of safety
- Encourage patient to verbalize fears
- Discuss reality of the situation
- Help patient select alternative coping strategies
- Help patient face underlying feelings that may be contributing to irrational fears

Nursing Actions

- Offer reassurance of safety
- Remain calm
- Use simple explanations
- Low-stimulus environment
- Tranquilizers as ordered
- Encourage verbalization of current situation
- Teach ways to interrupt escalating anxiety

Medical Rx:
Alprazolam 0.5 mg tid

Outcomes

- Patient discusses phobia without excessive anxiety
- Patient is able to leave her home and accomplish role expectations while keeping anxiety at a manageable level

Outcomes

- Patient recognizes signs and symptoms of escalating anxiety and intervenes to prevent panic
- Patient uses adaptive activities (exercise, relaxation) to maintain anxiety at manageable level

FIGURE 18–3   Concept map care plan for a patient with agoraphobia.

identify their personal strengths and explore adaptive coping mechanisms. Insight-oriented psychotherapy, which is rooted in Freudian psychology, is designed to help clients identify, explore, and resolve internal psychological conflicts that are contributing to anxiety.

The psychotherapist also can use logical and rational explanations to increase the client's understanding about various situations that create anxiety in his or her life. Psychoeducational information may also be presented in individual psychotherapy.

BOX 18–6 Topics for Patient and Family Education Related to Anxiety, OCD, and Related Disorders

NATURE OF THE ILLNESS
1. What is anxiety?
2. To what might it be related?
3. What is OCD?
4. What is body dysmorphic disorder?
5. What is trichotillomania?
6. Symptoms of anxiety disorders.

MANAGEMENT OF THE ILLNESS
1. Medication Management:
   • Possible adverse effects
   • Length of time to take effect
   • What to expect from the medication
     a. For panic disorder and generalized anxiety disorder
        1) Benzodiazepines
        2) Buspirone (BuSpar)
        3) Tricyclics
        4) SSRIs
        5) SNRIs
        6) Propranolol
        7) Clonidine
     b. For phobic disorders
        1) Benzodiazepines
        2) Tricyclics
        3) Propranolol
        4) SSRIs

   c. For OCD
      1) SSRIs
      2) Clomipramine
   d. For body dysmorphic disorder
      1) Clomipramine
      2) Fluoxetine
   e. For hair-pulling disorder (trichotillomania)
      1) Chlorpromazine
      2) Amitriptyline
      3) Lithium carbonate
      4) SSRIs/pimozide
      5) Olanzapine
2. Stress management:
   a. Teach ways to interrupt escalating anxiety
      1) Relaxation techniques
         (a) Progressive muscle relaxation
         (b) Imagery
         (c) Music
         (d) Meditation
         (e) Yoga
         (f) Physical exercise

SUPPORT SERVICES
1. Crisis hotline
2. Support groups
3. Individual psychotherapy

Cognitive Therapy

The cognitive model relates how individuals respond in stressful situations to their subjective cognitive appraisal of the event. Anxiety is experienced when an individual's cognitive appraisal is one of danger that he or she is unable to cope with. Impaired cognition can contribute to anxiety and related disorders when the individual's appraisals are chronically negative. Automatic negative appraisals provoke self-doubts, negative evaluations, and negative predictions. Anxiety is maintained by this dysfunctional appraisal of a situation.

Cognitive therapy strives to assist the individual to reduce anxiety responses by altering cognitive distortions. Anxiety is described as resulting from exaggerated, *automatic* thinking. Cognitive therapy for anxiety is brief and time limited, usually lasting from 5 to 20 sessions. Brief therapy discourages the client's dependency on the therapist, which is prevalent in anxiety disorders, and encourages the client's self-sufficiency.

A sound therapeutic relationship is a necessary condition for effective cognitive therapy. For the therapeutic process to occur, the client must be able to talk openly about fears and feelings. A major component of treatment consists of encouraging the client to face frightening situations in order to view them realistically, and talking about them is one way of achieving this goal. Treatment is a collaborative effort between client and therapist.

Rather than offering suggestions and explanations, the therapist uses questions to encourage the client to correct his or her anxiety-producing thoughts. The client is encouraged to become aware of the thoughts, examine them for cognitive distortions, substitute more balanced thoughts, and eventually develop new patterns of thinking.

Cognitive therapy is structured and orderly, which is important for the client with an anxiety or related disorder who is often confused and lacks self-assurance. The focus is on solving current problems. Together, the client and therapist work to identify and correct maladaptive thoughts and behaviors that maintain a problem and block its solution.

Cognitive therapy is based on education. The premise is that anxiety develops because of learned, inappropriate ways of thinking about and responding to life experiences. The belief is that with practice, individuals can learn more effective ways of responding to these experiences through cognitive reframing. Homework assignments, a central feature of cognitive therapy, provide an experimental, problem-solving approach to overcoming long-held anxieties. Through fulfillment of these personal "experiments," the effectiveness of specific strategies and techniques is determined.

Behavior Therapy

Behavior modification has been used to treat trichotillomania. Various techniques have been used, including covert desensitization and **habit reversal training** (HRT). These may include a system of positive and negative reinforcements in an effort to modify the hair-pulling behaviors. With HRT, in an attempt to extinguish the unwanted behavior, the individual learns to become more aware of the hair pulling, identifies times of occurrence, and substitutes a more adaptive coping strategy. (See interventions listed under the nursing diagnosis "Ineffective Impulse Control.")

Other forms of behavior therapy include **systematic desensitization** and **implosion therapy (flooding).** They are commonly used to treat clients with phobic disorders and to modify the stereotyped behavior of clients with OCD. They have also been shown to be effective in a variety of other anxiety-producing situations.

Systematic Desensitization

In systematic desensitization, the client is gradually exposed to the phobic stimulus, in either a real or an imagined situation. The concept was introduced by Joseph Wolpe in 1958 and is based on behavioral conditioning principles. Emphasis is placed on reciprocal inhibition or counterconditioning.

Reciprocal inhibition is described as the restriction of anxiety prior to the effort of reducing avoidance behavior. The rationale behind this concept is that because relaxation is antagonistic to anxiety, individuals cannot be anxious and relaxed at the same time.

Systematic desensitization with reciprocal inhibition involves two main elements:

1. Training in relaxation techniques
2. Progressive exposure to a hierarchy of fear stimuli while in the relaxed state

The individual is taught several relaxation techniques and is encouraged to use the one that is most effective for him or her (e.g., progressive relaxation, mental imagery, tense and relax, meditation). When the individual has mastered the relaxation technique, exposure to the phobic stimulus is initiated. The client is asked to present a hierarchal list of situations involving the phobic stimulus in order from most disturbing to least disturbing. While in a state of maximum relaxation, the client may be asked to imagine the phobic stimulus. Initial exposure is focused on a concept of the phobic stimulus that produces the least amount of fear or anxiety. In subsequent sessions, the individual is gradually exposed to stimuli that are more fearful. Sessions may be executed in fantasy, in real-life *(in vivo)* situations, or sometimes in a combination of both. Following is a case study describing systematic desensitization.

CASE STUDY: SYSTEMATIC DESENSITIZATION

Carlos was afraid to ride on elevators. He had been known to climb 24 flights of stairs in an office building to avoid riding the elevator. Carlos's office had plans for moving the company to a high-rise building soon with offices on the 32nd floor. Carlos sought assistance from a therapist for help to treat this fear. He was taught to achieve a sense of calmness and well-being by using a combination of mental imagery and progressive relaxation techniques. In the relaxed state, Carlos was initially instructed to imagine the entry level of his office building with a clear image of the bank of elevators. In subsequent sessions, and always in the relaxed state, Carlos progressed to images of walking onto an elevator, having the elevator door close after he had entered, riding the elevator to the 32nd floor, and emerging from the elevator once the doors were opened. The progression included being accompanied in the activities by the therapist and eventually accomplishing them alone.

Therapy for Carlos also included in vivo sessions in which he was exposed to the phobic stimulus in real-life situations (always after achieving a state of relaxation). This technique, combining imagined and in vivo procedures, proved successful for Carlos, and his employment in the high-rise complex was no longer in jeopardy because of his fear of elevators.

Implosion Therapy (Flooding)

Implosion therapy, or flooding, is a therapeutic process in which the client, for a prolonged period, must imagine situations or participate in real-life situations that he or she finds extremely frightening.

In implosion therapy, the therapist "floods" the client with information concerning situations that trigger the client's anxiety by describing anxiety-provoking situations in vivid detail. The more anxiety is provoked, the more expedient the therapeutic endeavor. This tactic is continued for as long as it arouses anxiety in the client. The therapy concludes when a topic no longer elicits inappropriate anxiety on the part of the client.

Relaxation training is not a part of this technique. Plenty of time must be allowed for these sessions because brief periods may be ineffective or even harmful. A session is terminated when the client responds with considerably less anxiety than at the beginning of the session. Sadock and colleagues (2015) state:

> Many patients refuse flooding because of the psychological discomfort involved. It is also contraindicated when intense anxiety would be hazardous to a patient (e.g., those with heart disease or fragile psychological adaptation). The technique works best with specific phobias. (p. 879)

Other Nonpharmacological Treatments for Anxiety

Many treatment modalities are available that may be used alone or in combination with medication to treat anxiety. Examples include deep breathing exercises, progressive muscle relaxation, imagery, mindfulness meditation, and exercise. (See online Chapter 30, Complementary and Psychosocial Therapies, for further discussion of these topics.)

Psychopharmacology

Antianxiety Agents

Antianxiety drugs are also called *anxiolytics* and historically were referred to as *minor tranquilizers*. Antianxiety agents are used in the treatment of anxiety disorders, anxiety symptoms, acute alcohol withdrawal, skeletal muscle spasms, convulsive disorders, status epilepticus, and preoperative sedation. Their use and efficacy for periods greater than 4 months have not been evaluated.

Benzodiazepines have been the traditional medication used for the treatment of acute anxiety states. By reducing anxiety, they allow learning and adaptation to take place. However, because they also have the potential for dependence, they are typically a short-term intervention. In addition, they pose certain risks for some patients, including those who are pregnant; the elderly; those who have current or past substance use disorders; current users of prescribed opioids (risk of respiratory depression and death); and patients with chronic obstructive pulmonary disease (Weber & Duchemin, 2018). Buspirone and SSRIs have demonstrated efficacy in treating anxiety disorders as well and have the added benefit of not being addictive chemicals. (See Chapter 4, Psychopharmacology, for a detailed description of contraindications, precautions, and other safety issues for these medications.)

Several drugs can be used off-label to treat anxiety, including atypical antipsychotics; mirtazapine (a tetracyclic antidepressant); gabapentin or pregabalin (analgesic and mood stabilizer that also carries a risk for dependence); antihistamines such as diphenhydramine; and other anticonvulsants such as lamotrigine and topiramate (Weber & Duchemin, 2018). Examples of antianxiety agents are presented in Table 18–4.

Medications for Specific Disorders

For Panic and Generalized Anxiety Disorders

Anxiolytics Benzodiazepines have been used with success in the treatment of GAD. They can be prescribed on an as-needed basis when the client is feeling particularly anxious. Alprazolam, lorazepam, and clonazepam have been particularly effective in the treatment of panic disorder. The major risks with benzodiazepine therapy are physical dependence and tolerance, which may encourage abuse. Because withdrawal symptoms can be life threatening, clients must be warned against abrupt discontinuation of the drug and should be tapered off the medication at the end of therapy. Because of this addiction potential, benzodiazepines have been surpassed as first-line choice of treatment by SSRIs, serotonin and norepinephrine reuptake inhibitors (SNRIs), and buspirone.

The antianxiety agent buspirone is effective in about 60 to 80 percent of clients with GAD (Sadock et al., 2015). One disadvantage of buspirone is its 10- to 14-day delay in alleviating symptoms. However, the benefit of lack of physical dependence and tolerance with buspirone may make it the drug of choice in the treatment of GAD.

Antidepressants Several antidepressants are effective as major antianxiety agents. The tricyclics clomipramine and imipramine have been used with success

TABLE 18–4 Antianxiety Agents

CHEMICAL CLASS	GENERIC (TRADE) NAME	CONTROLLED CATEGORIES	HALF-LIFE (HR)	DAILY ADULT DOSAGE RANGE (MG)	COMMON SIDE EFFECTS OF ANTIANXIETY AGENTS
Antihistamines	Hydroxyzine (Vistaril)		(3)	100–400	■ Drowsiness, confusion, lethargy.
Benzodiazepines	Alprazolam (Xanax, Niravam)	CIV	(6.3–26.9)	0.75–4	■ Tolerance; physical and psychological dependence (does not apply to buspirone or hydroxyzine). Client should be tapered off long-term use.
	Chlordiazepoxide (Librium)	CIV	(5–30)	15–100	■ Potentiates the effects of other CNS depressants. Client should not take alcohol or other CNS depressants with the medication.
	Clonazepam (Klonopin)	CIV	(18–50)	1.5–20	
	Clorazepate (Tranxene)	CIV	(40–50)	15–60	
	Diazepam (Valium, Diastat)	CIV	(20–80)	4–40	■ May aggravate symptoms of depression.
	Lorazepam (Ativan)	CIV	(10–20)	2–6	■ Orthostatic hypotension. Client should rise slowly from lying or sitting position.
	Oxazepam (Serax)	CIV	5–20 (5–20)	30–120	■ Paradoxical excitement. If symptoms opposite of desired effect occur, notify physician immediately.
	Oxazepam (Serax)	CIV	(2–6)	30–120	
	Midazolam (Versed)*	CIV	Adults	5	
Carbamate derivative	Meprobamate (Miltown, Equanil)	CIV	(6–17)	400–1,600	■ Dry mouth. ■ Nausea and vomiting. May be taken with food or milk. ■ Blood dyscrasias. Symptoms of sore throat, fever, malaise, easy bruising, or unusual bleeding should be reported to the physician immediately.
Azaspirodecanedione	Buspirone (BuSpar)		(14)	15–60	■ Delayed onset (with buspirone). Lag time of 10 to 14 days for anxiety symptoms to diminish with buspirone. Buspirone is not recommended for prn administration.

*Primarily used for preoperative sedation, antianxiety, and conscious sedation.

in clients experiencing panic disorder. However, since the advent of SSRIs, the tricyclics are less widely used because of their tendency to produce severe side effects at the high doses required to relieve symptoms of panic disorder.

SSRIs have been effective in the treatment of panic disorder. Paroxetine, fluoxetine (Prozac), and sertraline have been approved by the U.S. Food and Drug Administration (FDA) for this purpose. Venlafaxine, an SNRI, is also FDA approved for the treatment of panic disorder. Clients with panic disorder are often sensitive to treatment with antidepressants so doses are typically lower initially and titrated slowly.

SSRIs and SNRIs are considered first-line treatments for GAD. The FDA has approved paroxetine (Paxil), escitalopram (Lexapro), duloxetine (Cymbalta), and extended-release venlafaxine (Effexor XR) in the treatment of GAD. Atypical antidepressants such as nefazodone (Serzone) and mirtazapine (Remeron), although not FDA approved for anxiety disorder treatment, have also been identified as beneficial (Bhatt, 2018).

Antihypertensive Agents Several studies have noted the effectiveness of beta blockers (e.g., propranolol) and alpha$_2$-receptor agonists (e.g., clonidine) in the amelioration of anxiety symptoms (Bhatt, 2018). Propranolol has potent effects on the somatic manifestations of anxiety (e.g., palpitations, tremors) with less dramatic effects on the psychic component of anxiety. It appears to be most effective in the treatment of acute situational anxiety (e.g., performance anxiety, test anxiety), but it is not the first-line drug of choice in the treatment of panic disorder and GAD.

Clonidine is effective in blocking the acute anxiety effects in conditions such as opioid and nicotine withdrawal. However, it has had limited usefulness in the long-term treatment of panic and generalized anxiety disorders, particularly because of the development of tolerance to its antianxiety effects.

For Phobic Disorders

Anxiolytics Benzodiazepines have been successful in the treatment of social anxiety disorder (social phobia). Controlled studies have shown the efficacy of alprazolam and clonazepam in reducing symptoms of social anxiety. Both are well tolerated and have a rapid onset of action. However, because of their potential for abuse and dependence, they are not considered first-line choice of treatment.

Antidepressants The tricyclic imipramine and the monoamine oxidase inhibitors (MAOIs) such as phenelzine, selegiline, isocarboxazid, and tranylcypromine have been effective in diminishing symptoms of agoraphobia and social anxiety disorder. MAOIs are typically reserved for patients who don't respond to SSRIs. In recent years, SSRIs have become the first-line treatment of choice for social anxiety disorder, and paroxetine and sertraline have been approved for this purpose. Additional clinical trials have also indicated efficacy with other antidepressants, including nefazodone, venlafaxine, and bupropion. Specific phobias are generally not treated with medication unless panic attacks accompany the phobia.

Antihypertensive Agents The beta blockers propranolol and atenolol have been tried with success in clients experiencing anticipatory performance anxiety or "stage fright." This type of phobic response produces symptoms such as sweaty palms, racing pulse, trembling hands, dry mouth, labored breathing, nausea, and memory loss. The beta blockers appear to be quite effective in reducing these symptoms in some individuals.

For Obsessive-Compulsive Disorder

Antidepressants The SSRIs fluoxetine, paroxetine, sertraline, and fluvoxamine have been approved by the FDA for the treatment of OCD. Doses in excess of what is effective for treating depression may be required for OCD. Common side effects include sleep disturbances, headache, and restlessness. These effects are often transient and are less troublesome than those of the tricyclics.

The tricyclic antidepressant clomipramine was the first drug approved by the FDA in the treatment of OCD. Clomipramine is more selective for serotonin reuptake than any of the other tricyclics. Its efficacy in the treatment of OCD is well established, although adverse effects, such as those associated with all the tricyclics, may make it less desirable than the SSRIs.

For Body Dysmorphic Disorder

Antidepressants The most positive results of pharmacological therapy for body dysmorphic disorder have been with clomipramine and fluoxetine. These medications have been shown to reduce symptoms in more than 50 percent of clients with the disorder (Sadock et al., 2015).

For Trichotillomania

No medications have demonstrated consistent benefits for clients with trichotillomania but SSRIs have yielded moderate results for some clients with this condition (Elston, 2016).

CASE STUDY AND SAMPLE CARE PLAN

NURSING HISTORY AND ASSESSMENT

Stephanie is a 34-year-old mother of a 7-year-old girl named April. Stephanie's husband, Chris, brought her to the emergency department when she began complaining of chest pain and shortness of breath. Diagnostic testing ruled out cardiac problems, and Stephanie was referred for psychiatric evaluation.

Chris was present at the admission interview. He explained to the nurse that Stephanie has become increasingly "nervous and high-strung" over the past few years. Four years ago, April, then 3 years old, was attending nursery school 2 days a week. April came down with a severe case of influenza that developed into pneumonia. She was hospitalized, and her prognosis was questionable for a short while, although she eventually made a complete recovery. Since that time, however, Stephanie has been extremely anxious about her family's health. She is fastidious about housekeeping and scrubs her floors three times a week. She launders the bedclothes daily and uses bleach on all the countertops and door handles several times a day. She washes the woodwork twice a week. She washes her hands incessantly, and they are red and noticeably chapped. Chris explained that Stephanie becomes very upset if she is not able to perform all of her cleaning "chores" according to her self-assigned schedule. This afternoon, April came home from school with a note from the teacher saying that a child in April's class had been diagnosed with a case of meningitis. Chris told the nurse, "Stephanie just lost it. She got all upset and started crying and had trouble breathing. Then she got those pains in her chest. That's when I brought her to the hospital." Stephanie is admitted to the psychiatric unit with a diagnosis of obsessive-compulsive disorder. The physician orders alprazolam 0.5 mg tid and paroxetine 20 mg every morning.

The night nurse finds her up at 2 a.m. scrubbing the shower with a hand towel. She refuses to sleep in the bed, stating that it must certainly be contaminated. When the day nurse makes morning rounds, she finds Stephanie in the bathroom washing her hands.

NURSING DIAGNOSES AND OUTCOME IDENTIFICATION

From the assessment data, the nurse develops the following nursing diagnoses for Stephanie:

1. **Panic anxiety** related to perceived threat to biological integrity evidenced by chest pain and shortness of breath
   a. **Short-Term Goal:** Stephanie will be able to relax with effects of medication.
   b. **Long-Term Goal:** Stephanie will be able to maintain anxiety at manageable level.
2. **Ineffective coping** related to panic anxiety and weak ego strength evidenced by compulsive cleaning and washing hands
   a. **Short-Term Goal:** Stephanie will reduce amount of time performing rituals within 3 days.
   b. **Long-Term Goal:** Stephanie will demonstrate ability to cope effectively without resorting to ritualistic behavior.

PLANNING AND IMPLEMENTATION

PANIC ANXIETY

The following nursing interventions have been identified for Stephanie:

1. Stay with Stephanie and reassure her that she is safe and that she is not going to die.
2. Maintain a calm, nonthreatening manner.
3. Speak very clearly, calmly, and use simple words and messages to communicate with Stephanie.
4. Keep the lights low, the noise level down as much as possible, and as few people in her environment as is necessary.
5. Administer the alprazolam and paroxetine as ordered by the physician. Monitor for effectiveness and side effects.
6. After several days, when the anxiety has subsided, discuss with her the reasons that precipitated this attack.
7. Teach her the signs that indicate her anxiety level is rising.
8. Teach strategies that Stephanie may employ to interrupt the escalation of the anxiety. She could choose which is best for her: relaxation exercises, physical exercise, meditation.

INEFFECTIVE COPING

The following nursing interventions have been identified for Stephanie:

1. Initially, allow Stephanie all the time she needs to wash her hands, straighten up her room, change her own sheets, and so on. To deny her these rituals would result in panic anxiety.
2. Initiate discussions with Stephanie about her behavior. She ultimately must come to understand that these rituals are her way of keeping her anxiety under control.
3. Within a couple of days, begin to limit the amount of time Stephanie may spend on her rituals. Assign her to groups and activities that take up her time and distract her from her obsessions.
4. Explore with Stephanie the types of situations that cause her anxiety to rise. Help her to correlate these times of increased anxiety to initiation of the ritualistic behavior.

Continued

CASE STUDY AND SAMPLE CARE PLAN—cont'd

5. Help her with problem-solving and with making decisions about more adaptive ways to respond to situations that cause her anxiety to rise.

6. Explore her fears surrounding the health of her daughter. Help her to recognize which fears are legitimate and which are irrational.

7. Discuss possible activities in which she may participate that may distract from obsessions about contamination. Make suggestions and encourage her to follow through. Examples may include enrollment in classes at the local community college, volunteer work at the local hospital, or part-time employment.

8. Explain to her that she will likely be discharged from the hospital with a prescription for paroxetine. Teach her about the medication, how it should be taken, possible side effects, and what to report to the physician.

9. Suggest that she may benefit from attendance in an anxiety disorder support group. If she is interested, help locate one that would be convenient and appropriate for her.

EVALUATION

The outcome criteria for Stephanie have been met. She has remained calm during her hospital stay with the use of the medication. The use of ritualistic behavior in the hospital setting diminished rapidly. She has discussed situations that she knows cause her anxiety to rise. She has learned relaxation exercises and practices them daily. Stephanie plans to start jogging and has the phone number for an anxiety support group that she plans to call. She says that she hopes the support group will help her maintain rationality about her daughter's health. She knows about paroxetine and plans to take it every morning.

Summary and Key Points

- Anxiety is a necessary force for survival and has been experienced by humanity throughout the ages.

- Anxiety was first described as a physiological disorder and identified by its physical symptoms, particularly cardiac symptoms. The psychological implications for the symptoms were not recognized until the early 1900s.

- Anxiety is considered a normal reaction to a realistic danger or threat to biological integrity or self-concept.

- Normality of the anxiety experienced in response to a stressor is defined by societal and cultural standards.

- Anxiety disorders are more common in women than in men by at least two to one.

- Studies of familial patterns suggest that a familial predisposition to anxiety disorders probably exists.

- The *DSM-5* identifies several broad categories of anxiety and related disorders. They include panic and generalized anxiety disorders, phobic disorders, and obsessive-compulsive (OCD) and related disorders, such as body dysmorphic disorder and trichotillomania. Anxiety disorders may also be the result of other medical conditions and intoxication or withdrawal from substances.

- Panic disorder is characterized by recurrent panic attacks, manifested by intense apprehension, fear, and physical discomfort and the onset of which is unpredictable.

- Generalized anxiety disorder is characterized by chronic, unrealistic, and excessive anxiety and worry.

- Social anxiety disorder is an excessive fear of situations in which a person might do something embarrassing or be evaluated negatively by others.

- Specific phobia is a marked, persistent, and excessive or unreasonable fear when in the presence of, or when anticipating an encounter with, a specific object or situation.

- Agoraphobia is a fear of being in places or situations from which escape might be difficult or in which help might not be available in the event that the person becomes anxious.

- OCD involves recurrent obsessions or compulsions that are severe enough to interfere with social and occupational functioning.

- Body dysmorphic disorder is an exaggerated belief that the body is deformed or defective in some specific way.

- Trichotillomania (also known as hair-pulling disorder) is a disorder of impulse characterized by the recurrent pulling out of one's own hair that results in noticeable hair loss.

- Hoarding disorder is defined by the persistent difficulty of discarding or parting with possessions, regardless of their actual value.

- A number of elements, including psychosocial factors, biological influences, and learning experiences most likely contribute to the development of these disorders.

- Treatment of anxiety and related disorders includes individual psychotherapy, cognitive therapy, behavior therapy (including implosion therapy, systematic desensitization, and HRT), and psychopharmacology.

■ Nurses can help patients with anxiety and related disorders gain insight and increase self-awareness in relation to their illness.

■ Intervention focuses on assisting patients to learn techniques with which they may interrupt the escalation of anxiety before it reaches unmanageable proportions and to replace maladaptive behavior patterns with new, more adaptive coping skills.

Review Questions
Self-Examination/Learning Exercise

Select the answer that is most appropriate for each of the following questions:

1. Ms. T has been diagnosed with agoraphobia. Which behavior would be most characteristic of this disorder?
   a. Ms. T experiences panic anxiety when she encounters snakes.
   b. Ms. T refuses to fly in an airplane.
   c. Ms. T will not eat in a public place.
   d. Ms. T stays in her home for fear of being in a place from which she cannot escape.

2. Which of the following is the most appropriate therapy for a client with agoraphobia?
   a. 10 mg Valium qid
   b. Group therapy with other people with agoraphobia
   c. Facing her fear in gradual step progression
   d. Hypnosis

3. With implosion therapy, a client with phobic anxiety would be:
   a. Taught relaxation exercises.
   b. Subjected to graded intensities of the fear.
   c. Instructed to stop the therapeutic session as soon as anxiety is experienced.
   d. Presented with massive exposure to a variety of stimuli associated with the phobic object or situation.

4. A patient with OCD spends many hours each day washing her hands. What is the most likely reason she washes her hands so much?
   a. To relieve her anxiety
   b. To reduce the probability of infection
   c. To gain a feeling of control over her life
   d. To increase her self-concept

5. The *initial* care plan for a patient with OCD who washes her hands obsessively would include which of the following nursing interventions?
   a. Keep the patient's bathroom locked so she cannot wash her hands all the time.
   b. Structure the patient's schedule so that she has plenty of time for washing her hands.
   c. Place the patient in isolation until she promises to stop washing her hands so much.
   d. Explain the patient's behavior to her because she is probably unaware that it is maladaptive.

6. Sandy, a patient with OCD says to the nurse, "I've been here four days now, and I'm feeling better. I feel comfortable on this unit, and I'm not ill-at-ease with the staff or other patients anymore." In light of this change, which nursing intervention is most appropriate?
   a. Give attention to the ritualistic behaviors each time they occur and point out their inappropriateness.
   b. Ignore the ritualistic behaviors, and they will be eliminated for lack of reinforcement.
   c. Set limits on the amount of time Sandy may engage in the ritualistic behavior.
   d. Continue to allow Sandy all the time she wants to carry out the ritualistic behavior.

Continued

Review Questions—cont'd
Self-Examination/Learning Exercise

7. Annie has hair-pulling disorder. She is receiving treatment at the mental health clinic with HRT. Which of the following elements would be included in this therapy? (Select all that apply.)
   a. Awareness training
   b. Competing response training
   c. Social support
   d. Hypnotherapy
   e. Aversive therapy

8. Joselyn is a new patient at the mental health clinic. She has been diagnosed with Body Dysmorphic Disorder. Which of the following medications is the psychiatric nurse practitioner most likely to prescribe for Joanie?
   a. Alprazolam (Xanax)
   b. Diazepam (Valium)
   c. Fluoxetine (Prozac)
   d. Olanzapine (Zyprexa)

9. Tina, who is experiencing a panic attack, has just arrived at the emergency department. Which is the *priority* nursing intervention for this patient?
   a. Stay with Tina and reassure her of her safety.
   b. Administer a dose of diazepam.
   c. Leave Tina alone in a quiet room so that she can calm down.
   d. Encourage Tina to talk about what triggered the attack.

10. Jareth has a diagnosis of generalized anxiety disorder. His physician has prescribed buspirone 15 mg daily. Jareth says to the nurse, "Why do I have to take this every day? My friend's doctor ordered Xanax for her, and she only takes it when she is feeling anxious." Which of the following would be an appropriate response by the nurse?
   a. "Xanax is not effective for generalized anxiety disorder."
   b. "Buspirone must be taken daily in order to be effective."
   c. "I will ask the doctor if he will change your dose of buspirone to prn so that you don't have to take it every day."
   d. "Your friend really should be taking the Xanax every day."

IMPLICATIONS OF RESEARCH FOR EVIDENCE-BASED PRACTICE

Uebelacker, L. A., Weisberg, R., Millman, M., Yen, S., & Keller, M. (2013). Prospective study of risk factors for suicidal behavior in individuals with anxiety disorders. *Psychological Medicine, 43,* 1465–1474.

DESCRIPTION OF THE STUDY: Recognizing that there is an increased risk of suicide among people with anxiety disorders, the researchers initiated a prospective study of 676 individuals with a diagnosed anxiety disorder to identify associated factors that might predict an increased incidence of suicide attempts in this population. They studied the sample population for 12 years in an attempt to identify whether specific types of anxiety disorders, comorbid psychiatric disorders, physical health, or social/occupational functioning were associated with future risk of suicide attempts in people with anxiety disorders.

RESULTS OF THE STUDY: As the researchers hypothesized, comorbid post-traumatic stress disorder, major depressive disorder (MDD), intermittent depressive disorder (IDD), epilepsy, pain, and poor social/occupational functioning all predicted a shorter time to a suicide attempt. MDD and IDD were independent predictors of time to a suicide attempt even when they controlled for a past history of suicide attempts. No specific type of anxiety disorder predicted a shorter time to suicide attempts. The researchers conclude that the most powerful predictors

IMPLICATIONS OF RESEARCH FOR EVIDENCE-BASED PRACTICE–cont'd

of future suicide attempts in this sample of people with anxiety disorders are previous history of suicide attempts and comorbid mood disorders.

IMPLICATIONS FOR NURSING PRACTICE: Suicide is a major health problem in the United States, and the increase in incidence has prompted researchers to explore variables that are most associated with suicide risk. The findings in this study highlight the importance of assessing for

symptoms of depression and suicidal ideation in individuals with anxiety disorders. (See Chapter 11, Suicide Prevention, for a more thorough discussion of current assessment tools and interventions associated with risks for suicide.) Current research on the topic of suicide is rapidly expanding the evidence base related to this health concern, and nurses in any practice setting need to remain informed of the latest research to improve safety and quality care for this population.

TEST YOUR CRITICAL THINKING SKILLS

Sarah, age 25, was taken to the emergency department by her friends. They were at a dinner party when Sarah suddenly clasped her chest and started having difficulty breathing. She complained of nausea and was perspiring profusely. She had calmed down some by the time they reached the hospital. She denied any pain, and electrocardiogram and laboratory results were unremarkable.

Sarah told the admitting nurse that she had a history of these "attacks." She began having them in her sophomore year of college. She knew her parents had expectations that she should follow in their footsteps and become an attorney. They also expected her to earn grades that would promote acceptance by an Ivy League university. Sarah experienced her first attack when she made a B in English during her third semester of college. Since that time, she has experienced these symptoms sporadically, often in conjunction

with her perception of the need to excel. She graduated with top honors from Harvard.

Last week, Sarah was promoted within her law firm. She was assigned her first solo case of representing a couple whose baby had died at birth and who were suing the physician for malpractice. She has experienced these panic symptoms daily for the past week, stating, "I feel like I'm going crazy!"

Sarah is transferred to the psychiatric unit. The psychiatrist diagnoses Panic Disorder.

Answer the following questions related to Sarah:

1. What would be the priority nursing diagnosis for Sarah?
2. What is the priority nursing intervention with Sarah?
3. What medical treatment might you expect the physician to prescribe?

COMMUNICATION EXERCISES

1. John, who was just admitted to the psychiatric unit with panic disorder, approaches the nurse with complaints of numbness in his fingers and shortness of breath.
   What would be some appropriate responses by the nurse?
2. After attending a group that discussed irrational thinking patterns, John asks the nurse, "How does this cognitive behavior therapy work?"
   What would be some appropriate responses to John's question?

🎬 MOVIE CONNECTIONS

As Good As It Gets (OCD) • *The Aviator* (OCD) • *What About Bob?* (Phobias) • *Copycat* (Agoraphobia) • *Analyze This* (Panic disorder) • *Vertigo* (Specific phobia) • *Dirty, Filthy Love* (Trichotillomania and other anxiety disorders)

References

ABC News (2005). *Barbra Streisand looks back on twenty-five years.* Retrieved from http://abcnews.go.com/Primetime/Entertainment/story?id=1147020&page=1

Amaral, J. M., Spadaro, P. T., Pereira, V. M., Oliveira e Silva, A. C., & Nardi, A. E. (2013). The carbon dioxide challenge test in panic disorder: A systematic review of preclinical and clinical research. *Revista Brasileira de Psiquiatria, 35*(3), 318–331. doi:http://dx.doi.org/10.1590/1516-4446-2012-1045

American Psychiatric Association. (2013). *Diagnostic and statistical manual of mental disorders* (5th ed.). Washington, DC: Author.

Anxiety and Depression Association of America (ADAA). (2018). *Facts and statistics.* Retrieved from https://www.adaa.org/about-adaa/press-room/facts-statistics

Bhatt, N. (2018). *Anxiety disorders.* Retrieved from http://emedicine.medscape.com/article/286227-overview#a2

Dias, B. G., & Ressler, K. J. (2014). Parental olfactory experience influences behavior and neural structure in subsequent generations. *Nature Neuroscience, 17,* 86–96. doi:10.1038/nn.3594

Elston, D. M. (2016). *Trichotillomania.* Retrieved from http://emedicine.medscape.com/article/1071854-overview#a3

Gerbard, P. L., & Brown, R. P. (2016). Neurobiology and neurophysiology of breath practices in psychiatric care. *Psychiatric Times.* Retrieved from http://www.psychiatrictimes.com/specialreports/neurobiology-and-neurophysiology-breath-practicespsychiatric-care

Herdman, T. H., & Kamitsuru, S. (Eds.). (2018). *NANDA-I nursing diagnoses: Definitions and classification, 2018–2020.* New York, NY: Thieme.

Hofmeijer-Sevink, M. K., Batelaan, N. M., van Megen, H. J., Penninx, B. W., Cath, D. C., van den Hout, M. A., & van Balkom, A. J. (2012). Clinical relevance of comorbidity in anxiety disorders: A report from the Netherlands Study of Depression and Anxiety (NESDA). *Journal of Affective Disorders, 137*(1–3), 106–112. doi:http://dx.doi.org/10.1016/j.jad.2011.12.008

Kaplan, K. (2012). Update on trichotillomania. *Psychiatric Times.* Retrieved from http://www.psychiatrictimes.com/apa2012/updatetrichotillomania

Kimmel, R. J., & Roy-Burn, P. (2017). Clinical features of the anxiety disorders. In B. J. Sadock, V. A. Sadock, & P. Ruiz (Eds.), *Comprehensive textbook of psychiatry* (10th ed., pp. 1723–1730). Philadelphia, PA: Wolters Kluwer.

Mayo Clinic. (2018). *Hoarding.* Retrieved from http://www.mayoclinic.com/health/hoarding/DS00966

National Institute of Mental Health (NIMH). (2017). *Statistics.* Retrieved from https://www.nimh.nih.gov/health/statistics/index.shtml

Nordqvist, C. (2017). *Phobias: Causes, symptoms, and diagnosis.* Retrieved from http://www.medicalnewstoday.com/articles/249347.php

Ressler, K., & Smoller, J. (2016). *The genetics of anxiety disorders.* Retrieved from https://www.adaa.org/resources-professionals/podcasts/genetics-anxiety-disorders

Sadock, B. J., Sadock, V. A., & Ruiz, P. (2015). *Synopsis of psychiatry: Behavioral sciences/clinical psychiatry* (11th ed.). Philadelphia, PA: Wolters Kluwer.

Saxena, S. (2013). Medicines for the treatment of hoarding. *International OCD Foundation.* Retrieved from http://www.ocfoundation.org/hoarding/medication.aspx

Stein, D. J., & Lochner, C. (2017). Obsessive-compulsive and related disorders. In B. J. Sadock, V. A. Sadock, & P. Ruiz (Eds.), *Comprehensive textbook of psychiatry* (10th ed., pp. 1785–1798). Philadelphia, PA: Wolters Kluwer.

Symonds, A., & Janney, R. (2013). Shining a light on hoarding disorder. *Nursing2013, 43*(10), 22–28.

Uebelacker, L. A., Weisberg, R., Millman, M., Yen, S., & Keller, M. (2013). Prospective study of risk factors for suicidal behavior in individuals with anxiety disorders. *Psychological Medicine, 43,* 1465–1474. doi:10.1017/50033291712002504

Venes, D. (Ed.). (2017). *Taber's medical dictionary* (23rd ed.). Philadelphia, PA: F.A. Davis.

Weber, S. R., & Duchemin, A. M. (2018). Benzodiazepines: Sensible prescribing in light of the risks. *Current Psychiatry, 17*(2), 23–27.

Yasgur, B. S. (2015). Managing trichotillomania: A coordinated approach to compulsive hair pulling. *Psychiatry Advisor.* Retrieved from http://www.psychiatryadvisor.com/obsessive-compulsive-disorders/managing-trichotillomania-compulsive-hair-pulling/article/432260/?

Classical References

Freud, S. (1959). On the grounds for detaching a particular syndrome from neurasthenia under the description "anxiety neurosis." In *The standard edition of the complete psychological works of Sigmund Freud* (Vol. 3). London, England: Hogarth Press.

Hamilton, M. (1959). The assessment of anxiety states by rating. *British Journal of Medical Psychology, 32,* 50–55.

Johnson, J. H., & Sarason, I. B. (1978). Life stress, depression and anxiety: Internal-external control as moderator variable. *Journal of Psychosomatic Research, 22*(3), 205–208.

Trauma- and Stressor-Related Disorders

19

CORE CONCEPTS

Stress

Trauma

KEY TERMS

acute stress disorder
adjustment disorder

post-traumatic stress disorder
trauma-informed care

OBJECTIVES
After reading this chapter, the student will be able to:

1. Discuss historical aspects and epidemiological statistics related to trauma- and stressor-related disorders.
2. Describe various types of trauma- and stressor-related disorders and identify symptomatology associated with each; use this information in client assessment.
3. Identify predisposing factors in the development of trauma- and stressor-related disorders.
4. Formulate nursing diagnoses and goals of care for patients with trauma- and stressor-related disorders.

5. Describe the concepts and principles associated with trauma-informed care.
6. Describe appropriate nursing interventions for behaviors associated with trauma- and stressor-related disorders.
7. Evaluate the nursing care of patients with trauma- and stressor-related disorders.
8. Discuss various modalities relevant to treatment of trauma- and stressor-related disorders.

HOMEWORK ASSIGNMENT
Please read the chapter and answer the following questions:

1. What two variables are considered to be the best predictors of post-traumatic stress disorder (PTSD) according to the psychosocial theory?
2. What is associated with the onset of an adjustment disorder?
3. What are the elements that determine one's response (and subsequent adjustment) to a stressful situation?

4. What are four principles advanced by the Substance Abuse and Mental Health Services Administration (SAMHSA) as foundational to providing trauma-informed care?
5. What agents are considered first-line psychopharmacological treatment for PTSD?

Introduction

In 2011, a massive earthquake and tsunami claimed the lives of thousands and destroyed communities in eastern Japan. Yuri Sato, a public health nurse charged with helping survivors, shares her courageous experience (Frances, 2015):

> As public health nurses, our immediate task was to treat the injured and sick; collect and dispense medicines; and respond to the desperate conditions of the townspeople. We launched and managed an aid station and a welfare evacuation site for those in need of urgent nursing care; established countermeasures against infectious disorders; and arranged for emergency food supplies and sanitation. . . . With the entire town disaster-stricken, I was overcome with a sense of doubt and anxiety. Questions continually spun around in my mind: "What is mental health care when all of us have suffered so greatly?" But with everyone in mourning, we were single-mindedly focused on not losing any more lives to suicide or accident. . . . People continued to be unable to accept the deaths of family members, relatives and friends—and the fact that so many were still missing. I often heard "I should have died," "Why did I survive?" or "I want my time to come soon." I also felt this way, but had too much work to do to linger on my own losses and feelings about them.

Disasters such as the Japan earthquake and tsunami of 2011 test the very fiber of our human spirit and sense of emotional well-being. The events recounted by Yuri Sato were painfully traumatic. For some, the stress associated with such traumas continues to cause enduring, significant distress and interference with their ability to function. Such conditions are called *trauma- and stressor-related disorders.*

The *Diagnostic and Statistical Manual of Mental Disorders, Fourth Edition, Text Revision (DSM-IV-TR)* (American Psychiatric Association [APA], 2000) classified **post-traumatic stress disorder** (PTSD) and **acute stress disorder** with the anxiety disorders. **Adjustment disorder** carried its own classification and was identified as "a psychological response to an identifiable stressor or stressors" (p. 679). Clearly, however, anxiety is a component in each of these disorders. In the *DSM-5* (APA, 2013) these disorders have been combined into a single chapter, "Trauma- and Stressor-Related Disorders." The classification of these disorders in this manner "reflects increased recognition of trauma as a precipitant, emphasizing common etiology over common phenomenology" (Friedman et al., 2011, p. 737).

This chapter focuses on disorders that occur following exposure to an identifiable stressor or to an extreme traumatic event. Epidemiological statistics are presented, and predisposing factors associated with the etiology of these disorders are discussed. Concepts and principles of trauma-informed care are discussed. An explanation of the symptomatology is presented as background knowledge for assessing clients with trauma- and stressor-related disorders. Nursing care is described in the context of the nursing process. Various treatment modalities are explored.

Historical and Epidemiological Data

The concept of a post-trauma response has been referred to as *shell shock, battle fatigue, accident neurosis,* and *post-traumatic neurosis.* Reports of symptoms and syndromes with features resembling post-traumatic stress disorder (PTSD) have existed in writing throughout the centuries. In the early part of the 20th century, traumatic neurosis was viewed as the ego's inability to master the degree of disorganization brought about by a traumatic experience. Very little was written about "post-traumatic neurosis" during the years between 1950 and 1970. This absence was followed in the 1970s and 1980s with expansive research and writing on the subject. Many of the papers written during this time were about Vietnam War veterans. Although the renewed interest in PTSD was linked to the psychological casualties of war, it is well recognized that any experience of significant trauma may be associated with the development of this disorder.

The diagnostic category of PTSD did not appear until the third edition of the *Diagnostic and Statistical Manual of Mental Disorders (DSM-III)* in 1980, after a need was indicated by increasing numbers of problems identified in Vietnam veterans and victims of multiple disasters. The *DSM-5* (2013) describes the trauma that precedes PTSD as an event that is either directly experienced, witnessed, occurring in a close family member or close friend, or involving repeated exposure to aversive details about a traumatic event. Examples of such events include (but are not limited to) threatened or actual sexual violence, exposure to war, threatened or actual physical attack, torture, natural or man-made disasters, and severe motor vehicle accidents.

About 60 percent of men and 50 percent of women are exposed to a traumatic event in their lifetime (Department of Veterans Affairs, 2016). Women are more likely to experience sexual assault and childhood sexual abuse, whereas men are more likely to experience accidents, physical assaults, combat, or proximity to death or injury. Although the exposure to trauma is high, the National Center for PTSD reports that less than 10 percent of trauma victims develop PTSD (Department of Veterans Affairs, 2016). The disorder appears to be more common in women than in men.

Historically, as previously stated, individuals who experienced stress reactions that followed exposure to an extreme traumatic event were given the diagnosis of PTSD. Accordingly, stress reactions from "less extreme" events (e.g., divorce, failure, rejection) were characterized as adjustment disorders rather than PTSD (Friedman, 1996). Currently, the definition of an adjustment disorder is broader in spectrum and may involve single, multiple, recurrent, or continuous stressors. It is primarily differentiated from PTSD and acute stress disorders by the time of onset and duration of symptoms (APA, 2013).

A number of studies have indicated that adjustment disorders are probably quite common. Sadock, Sadock, and Ruiz (2015) report:

> Adjustment disorders are one of the most common psychiatric diagnoses for disorders of patients hospitalized for medical and surgical problems. In one study, 5 percent of people admitted to a hospital over a 3-year period were classified as having an adjustment disorder. Up to 50 percent of people with specific medical problems or stressors have been diagnosed with adjustment disorders. (p. 446)

Various studies have found that adjustment disorders are more common in women than in men. Examples of situations that result in adjustment disorders include giving birth to a stillborn child, enduring a stressful experience such as a major life change, being a victim of bullying or harassment, or being incarcerated (Katzman & Geppert, 2017).

Application of the Nursing Process— Trauma-Related Disorders

CORE CONCEPT

Trauma

An extremely distressing experience that causes severe emotional shock and may have long-lasting psychological effects.

Post-Traumatic Stress Disorder and Acute Stress Disorder

Background Assessment Data

PTSD is described as a multisymptom response triggered by an extremely traumatic event. These symptoms are not related to common experiences such as uncomplicated bereavement, marital conflict, or chronic illness but are associated with events that would be markedly distressing to almost anyone. The individual may experience or witness the trauma alone or in the presence of others.

Characteristic symptoms include reexperiencing the traumatic event, a sustained high level of anxiety or arousal, or a general numbing of responsiveness. Intrusive recollections or nightmares of the event are common. Some individuals may be unable to remember certain aspects of the trauma.

Symptoms of depression are common with this disorder and may be severe enough to warrant a diagnosis of a depressive disorder in addition to PTSD. In the case of a life-threatening trauma shared with others, survivors often describe painful guilt feelings about surviving when others lost their lives. They may also express trauma and guilt feelings about the things they had to do to survive. Substance abuse, anger and aggressive behavior, and relationship problems are common. The full symptom picture must be present for more than 1 month and cause significant interference with social, occupational, and other areas of functioning. The disorder can occur at any age. Symptoms may begin within the first 3 months after the trauma, or there may be a delay of several months or even years. The *DSM-5* diagnostic criteria for PTSD are presented in Box 19–1.

The *DSM-5* describes another disorder that is similar to PTSD called *acute stress disorder* (ASD). There are similarities between the two disorders in terms of precipitating traumatic events and symptomatology, but in ASD, the symptoms are time limited, up to 1 month following the trauma. By definition, if the symptoms last longer than 1 month, the diagnosis is PTSD. The *DSM-5* diagnostic criteria for ASD are presented in Box 19–2.

Predisposing Factors Related to Trauma-Related Disorders

Psychosocial Aspects

The widely accepted psychosocial model seeks to explain why certain persons exposed to massive trauma develop trauma-related disorders and others do not.

BOX 19–1 Diagnostic Criteria for Post-traumatic Stress Disorder

Note: The following criteria apply to adults, adolescents, and children older than 6 years.

A. Exposure to actual or threatened death, serious injury, or sexual violence, in one (or more) of the following ways:
   1. Directly experiencing the traumatic event(s).
   2. Witnessing, in person, the event(s) as it occurred to others.
   3. Learning that the traumatic event(s) occurred to a close family member or close friend. In cases of actual or threatened death of a family member or friend, the event(s) must have been violent or accidental.
   4. Experiencing repeated or extreme exposure to aversive details of the traumatic event(s) (e.g., first responders collecting human remains; police officers repeatedly exposed to details of child abuse). *Note:* Criterion A4 does not apply to exposure through electronic media, television, movies, or pictures unless this exposure is work related.

B. Presence of one (or more) of the following intrusion symptoms associated with the traumatic event(s), beginning after the traumatic event(s) occurred:
   1. Recurrent, involuntary, and intrusive distressing memories of the traumatic event(s). **Note:** In children older than 6 years, repetitive play may occur in which themes or aspects of the traumatic event(s) are expressed.
   2. Recurrent distressing dreams in which the content and/or effect of the dream is related to the traumatic event(s). **Note:** In children, there may be frightening dreams without recognizable content.
   3. Dissociative reactions (e.g., flashbacks) in which the individual feels or acts as if the traumatic event(s) were recurring. (Such reactions may occur on a continuum, with the most extreme expression being a complete loss of awareness of present surroundings.) **Note:** In children, trauma-specific reenactment may occur in play.
   4. Intense or prolonged psychological distress at exposure to internal or external cues that symbolize or resemble an aspect of the traumatic event(s).
   5. Marked physiological reactions to internal or external cues that symbolize or resemble an aspect of the traumatic event(s).

C. Persistent avoidance of stimuli associated with the traumatic event(s) beginning after the traumatic event(s) occurred, as evidenced by one or both of the following:
   1. Avoidance of or efforts to avoid distressing memories, thoughts, or feelings about or closely associated with the traumatic event(s).
   2. Avoidance of or efforts to avoid external reminders (people, places, conversations, activities, objects, situations) that arouse distressing memories, thoughts, or feelings about or closely associated with the traumatic event(s).

D. Negative alterations in cognitions and mood associated with the traumatic event(s), beginning or worsening after the traumatic event(s) occurred, as evidenced by two or more of the following:
   1. Inability to remember an important aspect of the traumatic event(s) (typically due to dissociative amnesia and not to other factors such as head injury, alcohol, or drugs).
   2. Persistent and exaggerated negative beliefs or expectations about oneself, others, or the world (e.g., "I am bad," "No one can be trusted," "The world is completely dangerous," "My whole nervous system is permanently ruined").
   3. Persistent, distorted cognitions about the cause or consequences of the traumatic event(s) that lead the individual to blame himself/herself or others.
   4. Persistent negative emotional state (e.g., fear, horror, anger, guilt, or shame).
   5. Markedly diminished interest or participation in significant activities.
   6. Feelings of detachment or estrangement from others.
   7. Persistent inability to experience positive emotions (e.g., inability to experience happiness, satisfaction, or loving feelings).

E. Marked alterations in arousal and reactivity associated with the traumatic event(s), beginning or worsening after the traumatic event(s) occurred, as evidenced by two or more of the following:
   1. Irritable behavior and angry outbursts (with little or no provocation) typically expressed as verbal or physical aggression toward people or objects.
   2. Reckless or self-destructive behavior.
   3. Hypervigilance.
   4. Exaggerated startle response.
   5. Problems with concentration.
   6. Sleep disturbance (e.g., difficulty falling or staying asleep or restless sleep).

F. Duration of the disturbance (Criteria B, C, D, and E) is more than 1 month.

G. The disturbance causes clinically significant distress or impairment in social, occupation, or other important areas of functioning.

H. The disturbance is not attributable to the physiological effects of a substance (e.g., medication, alcohol) or another medical condition.

Specify whether:
With dissociative symptoms (depersonalization or derealization)
With delayed expression (full diagnostic criteria not met until at least 6 months after the event)

BOX 19–2 Diagnostic Criteria for Acute Stress Disorder

A. Exposure to actual or threatened death, serious injury, or sexual violation, in one (or more) of the following ways:
  1. Directly experiencing the traumatic event(s).
  2. Witnessing, in person, the event(s) as it occurred to others.
  3. Learning that the event(s) occurred to a close family member or close friend. Note: In cases of actual or threatened death of a family member or friend, the event(s) must have been violent or accidental.
  4. Experiencing repeated or extreme exposure to aversive details of the traumatic event(s) (e.g., first responders collecting human remains, police officers repeatedly exposed to details of child abuse). Note: This does not apply to exposure through electronic media, television, movies, or pictures, unless this exposure is work related.
B. Presence of nine (or more) of the following symptoms from any of the five categories of intrusion, negative mood, dissociation, avoidance, and arousal, beginning or worsening after the traumatic event(s) occurred:

INTRUSION SYMPTOMS

  1. Recurrent, involuntary, and intrusive distressing memories of the traumatic event(s). Note: In children, repetitive play may occur in which themes or aspects of the traumatic event(s) are expressed.
  2. Recurrent distressing dreams in which the content and/or affect of the dream are related to the event(s). Note: In children, there may be frightening dreams without recognizable content.
  3. Dissociative reactions (e.g., flashbacks) in which the individual feels or acts as if the traumatic event(s) were recurring. (Such reactions may occur on a continuum, with the most extreme expression being a complete loss of awareness of present surroundings.) Note: In children, trauma-specific reenactment may occur in play.
  4. Intense or prolonged psychological distress or marked physiological reactions in response to internal or external cues that symbolize or resemble an aspect of the traumatic event(s).

NEGATIVE MOOD

  5. Persistent inability to experience positive emotions (e.g., inability to experience happiness, satisfaction, or loving feelings).

DISSOCIATIVE SYMPTOMS

  6. An altered sense of the reality of one's surroundings or oneself (e.g., seeing oneself from another's perspective, being in a daze, time slowing).
  7. Inability to remember an important aspect of the traumatic event(s) (typically due to dissociative amnesia and not to other factors such as head injury, alcohol, or drugs).

AVOIDANCE SYMPTOMS

  8. Efforts to avoid distressing memories, thoughts, or feelings about or closely associated with the traumatic event(s).
  9. Efforts to avoid external reminders (people, places, conversations, activities, objects, situations) that arouse distressing memories, thoughts, or feelings about or closely associated with the traumatic event(s).

AROUSAL SYMPTOMS

  10. Sleep disturbance (e.g., difficulty falling or staying asleep, or restless sleep).
  11. Irritable behavior and angry outbursts (with little or no provocation), typically expressed as verbal or physical aggression toward people or objects.
  12. Hypervigilance.
  13. Problems with concentration.
  14. Exaggerated startle response.
C. Duration of the disturbance (symptoms in Criteria B) is 3 days to 1 month after trauma exposure. Note: Symptoms typically begin immediately after the trauma, but persistence for at least 3 days and up to a month is needed to meet disorder criteria.
D. The disturbance causes clinically significant distress or impairment in social, occupational, or other important areas of functioning.
E. The disturbance is not attributable to the direct physiological effects of a substance (e.g., medication or alcohol) or another medical condition (e.g., mild traumatic brain injury), and is not better explained by brief psychotic disorder.

Variables include characteristics that relate to (1) the traumatic experience, (2) the individual, and (3) the recovery environment.

The Traumatic Experience

Specific characteristics relating to the trauma have been identified as crucial elements in the determination of an individual's long-term response to stress. They include the following:

- Severity and duration of the stressor
- Extent of anticipatory preparation for the event
- Exposure to death
- Numbers affected by life threat
- Amount of control over recurrence

■ Location where the trauma was experienced (e.g., familiar surroundings, at home, in a foreign country)

The Individual

The variables that follow are considered important in determining an individual's response to trauma:

■ Degree of ego strength
■ Effectiveness of coping resources
■ Presence of pre-existing psychopathology
■ Outcomes of previous experiences with stress or trauma
■ Behavioral tendencies (temperament)
■ Current psychosocial developmental stage
■ Demographic factors (e.g., age, socioeconomic status, education)

The Recovery Environment

It has been suggested that the quality of the environment in which the individual attempts to work through the traumatic experience is correlated with the outcome. Environmental variables include the following:

■ Availability of social supports
■ The cohesiveness and protectiveness of family and friends
■ The attitudes of society regarding the experience
■ Cultural and subcultural influences

In research with Vietnam veterans, it was shown that the best predictors of PTSD were the severity of the stressor and the degree of psychosocial isolation in the recovery environment.

Learning Theory

Learning theorists view negative reinforcement as behavior that leads to a reduction in an aversive experience, thereby reinforcing and resulting in repetition of the behavior. The avoidance behaviors and psychic numbing in response to a trauma are mediated by negative reinforcement (behaviors that decrease the emotional pain of the trauma). Behavioral disturbances, such as anger and aggression and drug and alcohol abuse, are the behavioral patterns that are reinforced by their capacity to reduce objectionable feelings.

Cognitive Theory

These models take into consideration the cognitive appraisal of an event and focus on assumptions that an individual makes about the world. Epstein (1991) outlines three fundamental beliefs that most people construct within a personal theory of reality:

1. The world is benevolent and a source of joy.
2. The world is meaningful and controllable.
3. The self is worthy (e.g., lovable, good, and competent).

As life situations occur, some disequilibrium is to be expected until accommodation for the change has been made and it has become assimilated into one's personal theory of reality. An individual is vulnerable to trauma-related disorders when fundamental beliefs are invalidated by a trauma that cannot be comprehended and a sense of helplessness and hopelessness prevails. One's appraisal of the environment can be drastically altered.

Biological Aspects

Exposure to trauma has been associated with hyperarousal of the sympathetic nervous system, excessive amygdala activity, and decreased hippocampus volume, all of which are neurobiological reactions to heightened stress. Dysfunctions in the hypothalamic-pituitary-adrenal (HPA) axis, either from chronic stress or exposure to an extreme stressor, have been linked to many psychiatric illnesses including PTSD, depression, Alzheimer's disease, and substance abuse and to medical conditions such as inflammatory disorders and cardiovascular disease (Valentino & Van Bockstaele, 2015). In addition, neuroendocrine abnormalities, including serotonin, glutamate, thyroid, and endogenous opioids (among others), have been associated with stress responses and PTSD. Valentino and Van Bockstaele (2015) identify that the activation of endogenous opioids both reduces stress and mimics the stress response depending on which opioid receptors are activated. Studies have shown that opioids administered shortly after exposure to a trauma reduced the incidence of PTSD, suggesting a protective effect. Chronic activation, however, may sensitize neurons in a way that increases vulnerability to stress-induced relapse. Lanius (2013) discusses the effects of repeated activation of opioid receptors, including the effect of increasing one's addiction potential to other drugs or even to the learned experience of relief when traumatic stress is reexperienced. He identifies that opiate antagonists such as naltrexone have demonstrated effectiveness in treatment.

Other biological systems have also been implicated in the symptomatology of PTSD. Norepinephrine, dopamine, and benzodiazepine receptors (on GABA receptors) are some of the neurotransmitters believed to be dysregulated in individuals with PTSD. Whether these factors are suggestive of vulnerability to PTSD or are changes that result from the brain's efforts to process trauma remains unclear. As with other disorders, it is likely that a complex dynamic of biological, social, and psychological factors is involved.

Trauma-Informed Care

Experts highlight the importance of trauma-informed care as essential to improving the quality of care for clients both in and outside of behavioral healthcare settings (Hopper, Bassuk, & Olivet, 2010; Substance Abuse and Mental Health Service Administration, 2018). **Trauma-informed care** generally describes a philosophical approach that values awareness and understanding of trauma when assessing, planning, and implementing care. SAMHSA advances the following principles in defining this approach. Trauma-informed care

- *Realizes* the widespread impact of trauma and various paths for recovery.
- *Recognizes* the signs and symptoms of trauma in clients, families, staff, and all those involved with the system.
- *Responds* by fully integrating knowledge about trauma in policies, procedures, and practices.
- Seeks to actively resist *retraumatization*.

Hopper and associates (2010) discuss applying this approach with the homeless population (many of whom are people with severe mental illness). The authors describe the many traumatic experiences that culminate in homelessness and the often co-occurring illnesses such as depression, substance abuse, and severe mental illness. To ignore the significance of trauma or to provide uninformed care leaves this population vulnerable to revictimization and "further complicates their service needs" (p. 81).

These authors advance the following definition of trauma-informed care:

> Trauma-informed care is a strength-based framework that is grounded in understanding of and responsiveness to the impact of trauma that emphasizes physical, psychological, and emotional safety for both providers and survivors to rebuild a sense of control and empowerment. (p. 82)

Inherent in this definition is the importance of *healthcare providers* also being aware of the impact of trauma on themselves because it may impact their effectiveness in providing care to clients.

Interventions that are considered trauma informed highlight the importance of respect for the client, collaboration and connection, providing information about the links between trauma and other health concerns, instilling hope, and empowering the trauma survivor to guide and direct his or her recovery plan (the essence of patient-centered care).

Childhood trauma, including physical, emotional, and sexual abuse, is identified as significant in the development of behavioral problems, eating disorders, some personality disorders, depression, and substance abuse. Healthcare providers, if they do not fully understand the impact of previous trauma on the client's current health concerns, may unwittingly retraumatize clients. This includes interventions such as seclusion and restraint, which are designed to protect the client's safety when they are at imminent risk of harm to themselves or others, but these actions may be retraumatizing to a client with a history of trauma. Much attention has been given to the importance of trauma-informed care in behavioral healthcare settings because of the recognition that trauma history may be associated with other mental illnesses. However, nurses in every practice setting must incorporate this approach in assessment and care provision because trauma history can impact any patient's response to care. See Chapter 25, Survivors of Abuse or Neglect, "Real People, Real Stories" feature for Diana's perspective on how previous traumas impact her response in general healthcare settings.

Diagnosis and Outcome Identification

Nursing diagnoses are formulated from the data gathered during the assessment phase and with background knowledge regarding predisposing factors to the disorder. Following are some common nursing diagnoses for patients with trauma-related disorders:

- Post-trauma syndrome related to distressing event considered to be outside the range of usual human experience evidenced by flashbacks, intrusive recollections, nightmares, psychological numbness related to the event, dissociation, or amnesia
- Complicated grieving related to loss of self as perceived before the trauma or other actual or perceived losses incurred during or after the event evidenced by irritability and explosiveness, self-destructiveness, substance abuse, verbalization of survival guilt, or guilt about behavior required for survival

The following criteria may be used for measurement of outcomes in the care of the patient with a trauma-related disorder.

The patient:

- Can acknowledge the traumatic event and the impact it has had on his or her life.
- Is experiencing fewer flashbacks, intrusive recollections, and nightmares than he or she was on admission (or at the beginning of therapy).
- Can demonstrate adaptive coping strategies (e.g., relaxation techniques, mental imagery, music, art).
- Can concentrate and has made realistic goals for the future.

- Includes significant others in the recovery process and willingly accepts their support.
- Verbalizes no ideas or intent of self-harm.
- Has worked through feelings of survivor's guilt.
- Gets enough sleep to avoid risk of injury.
- Verbalizes community resources from which he or she may seek assistance in times of stress.
- Attends support group of individuals who have recovered or are recovering from similar traumatic experiences.
- Verbalizes desire to put the trauma in the past and progress with his or her life.

Planning and Implementation

Tables 19–1 and 19–2 provide care plans for patients with trauma-related disorders. Nursing diagnoses are presented, along with outcome criteria, appropriate nursing interventions, and rationales for each.

See Chapter 28, Military Families, "Real People, Real Stories" feature to learn more about Sean's post-military experience with PTSD and the importance of compassionate nursing care in his recovery.

Concept Care Mapping

The concept map care plan (see Chapter 6, The Nursing Process in Psychiatric Mental Health Nursing) is a diagrammatic teaching and learning strategy that allows visualization of interrelationships between medical diagnoses, nursing diagnoses, assessment data, and treatments. An example of a concept map care plan for a patient with a trauma-related disorder is presented in Figure 19–1.

Table 19–1 | CARE PLAN FOR THE PATIENT WITH A TRAUMA-RELATED DISORDER

NURSING DIAGNOSIS: POST-TRAUMA SYNDROME

RELATED TO: Distressing event considered to be outside the range of usual human experience

EVIDENCED BY: Flashbacks, intrusive recollections, nightmares, psychological numbness related to the event, dissociation, or amnesia

OUTCOME CRITERIA	NURSING INTERVENTIONS	RATIONALE
Short-Term Goals ■ Patient will begin a healthy grief resolution, initiating the process of psychological healing (within time frame specific to individual).Patient will demonstrate ability to deal with emotional reactions in an individually appropriate manner.	1. a. Assign the same staff as often as possible. b. Use a nonthreatening, matter-of-fact but friendly approach. c. Respect patient's wishes regarding interaction with individuals of opposite gender at this time (especially important if the trauma was rape). d. Be consistent; keep all promises; convey acceptance; spend time with patient.	1. A post-trauma patient may be suspicious of others in his or her environment. All of these interventions serve to facilitate a trusting relationship.
Long-Term Goal ■ The patient will integrate the traumatic experience into his or her persona, renew significant relationships, and establish meaningful goals for the future.	2. Stay with patient during periods of flashbacks and nightmares. Offer reassurance of safety and security and that these symptoms are not uncommon following a trauma of the magnitude he or she has experienced. 3. Obtain accurate history from significant others about the trauma and the patient's specific response.	2. Presence of a trusted individual may calm fears for personal safety and reassure patient that he or she is not "in danger." 3. Various types of traumas elicit different responses (e.g., human-engendered traumas often generate a greater degree of humiliation and guilt in victims than trauma associated with natural disasters).

Table 19–1 | CARE PLAN FOR THE PATIENT WITH A TRAUMA-RELATED DISORDER—cont'd

OUTCOME CRITERIA	NURSING INTERVENTIONS	RATIONALE
	4. Encourage the patient to talk about the trauma at his or her own pace. Provide a nonthreatening, private environment, and include a significant other if the patient wishes. Acknowledge and validate patient's feelings as they are expressed.	4. This debriefing process is the first step in the progression toward resolution.
	5. Discuss coping strategies used in response to the trauma as well as those used during stressful situations in the past. Determine those that have been most helpful and discuss alternative strategies for the future. Include available support systems, including religious and cultural influences. Identify maladaptive coping strategies (e.g., substance use, psychosomatic responses) and practice more adaptive coping strategies for possible future post-trauma responses.	5. Resolution of the post-trauma response is largely dependent on the effectiveness of the coping strategies employed.
	6. Assist the individual to comprehend the trauma if possible. Discuss feelings of vulnerability and the individual's "place" in the world following the trauma.	6. Post-trauma response is largely a function of the shattering of basic beliefs the survivor holds about self and world. Assimilation of the event into one's persona requires that some degree of meaning associated with the event be incorporated into the basic beliefs, which will affect how the individual eventually comes to reappraise self and world (Epstein, 1991).

NURSING DIAGNOSIS: COMPLICATED GRIEVING

RELATED TO: Loss of self as perceived prior to the trauma or other actual/perceived losses incurred during/following the event

EVIDENCED BY: Irritability and explosiveness, self-destructiveness, substance abuse, verbalization of survival guilt or guilt about behavior required for survival

OUTCOME CRITERIA	NURSING INTERVENTIONS	RATIONALE
Short-Term Goal ■ Patient will verbalize feelings (guilt, anger, self-blame, hopelessness) associated with the trauma.	1. Acknowledge feelings of guilt or self-blame that patient may express.	1. Guilt at having survived a trauma in which others died is common. The patient needs to discuss these feelings and recognize that he or she is not responsible for what happened but must take responsibility for own recovery.
	2. Assess stage of grief in which the patient is fixed. Discuss normalcy of feelings and behaviors related to stages of grief.	2. Knowledge of grief stages is necessary for accurate intervention. Guilt may be generated if patient believes it is unacceptable to have these feelings. Knowing these are part of the normal grief response can provide a sense of relief.

Continued

Table 19–1 | CARE PLAN FOR THE PATIENT WITH A TRAUMA-RELATED DISORDER—cont'd

OUTCOME CRITERIA	NURSING INTERVENTIONS	RATIONALE
Long-Term Goal ■ Patient will demonstrate progress in dealing with stages of grief and will verbalize a sense of optimism and hope for the future.	3. Assess impact of the trauma on patient's ability to resume regular activities of daily living (ADLs). Consider employment, marital relationship, and sleep patterns. 4. Assess for self-destructive ideas and behavior. 5. Assess for maladaptive coping strategies, such as substance abuse. 6. Identify available community resources from which the individual may seek assistance if problems with complicated grieving persist.	3. Following a trauma, individuals are at high risk for physical injury because of disrupted concentration and problem-solving abilities and lack of sufficient sleep. Isolation and avoidance behaviors may interfere with interpersonal relatedness. 4. The trauma may result in feelings of hopelessness and worthlessness, leading to high risk for suicide. 5. These behaviors interfere with and delay the recovery process. 6. Support groups for victims of various types of traumas exist within most communities. The presence of support systems in the recovery environment has been identified as a major predictor in the successful recovery from trauma.

Table 19–2 | CARE PLAN FOR THE PATIENT WITH AN ADJUSTMENT DISORDER

NURSING DIAGNOSIS: COMPLICATED GRIEVING

RELATED TO: Death of a significant other; lack of social support; emotional instability

EVIDENCED BY: Decreased ability to function in life roles; inappropriate anger; persistent emotional distress; self-blame

OUTCOME CRITERIA	NURSING INTERVENTIONS	RATIONALE
Short-Term Goal ■ By end of 1 week, patient will express anger toward lost entity. **Long-Term Goal** ■ The patient will be able to verbalize behaviors associated with the normal stages of grief and identify own position in grief process, while progressing at own pace toward resolution.	1. Determine the stage of grief in which patient is fixed. Identify behaviors associated with this stage. 2. Develop a trusting relationship with the patient. Show empathy and caring. Be honest and keep all promises. 3. Convey an accepting attitude so that the patient is not afraid to express feelings openly. 4. Allow the patient to express anger. Do not become defensive if the initial expression of anger is displaced on the nurse or therapist. Help the patient explore angry feelings so that they may be directed toward the intended object or person. 5. Assist the patient to discharge pent-up anger through participation in large motor activities (e.g., brisk walks, jogging, physical exercises, volleyball, exercise bike).	1. Accurate baseline assessment data are necessary to plan effective care for the grieving patient. 2. Trust is the basis for a therapeutic relationship. 3. An accepting attitude conveys to the patient that you believe he or she is a worthwhile person. Trust is enhanced. 4. Verbalization of feelings in a nonthreatening environment may help the patient come to terms with unresolved issues. 5. Physical exercise provides a safe and effective method for discharging pent-up tension.

Table 19–2 | CARE PLAN FOR THE PATIENT WITH AN ADJUSTMENT DISORDER–cont'd

OUTCOME CRITERIA	NURSING INTERVENTIONS	RATIONALE
	6. Explain to the patient the normal stages of grief and the behaviors associated with each stage. Help the patient to understand that feelings such as guilt and anger toward the lost entity/concept are natural and acceptable during the grief process.	6. Knowledge of the acceptability of the feelings associated with normal grieving may help to relieve some of the guilt that these responses generate.
	7. Encourage the patient to review his or her perception of the loss or change. With support and sensitivity, point out the reality of the situation in areas where misrepresentations are expressed.	7. The patient must give up an idealized perception and be able to accept both positive and negative aspects about the painful life change before the grief process is complete.
	8. Communicate to the patient that crying is acceptable. The use of touch is therapeutic and appropriate with most patients.	8. Knowledge of cultural influences specific to the patient is important before employing this technique. Touch is considered inappropriate in some cultures.
	9. Help the patient to solve problems as he or she attempts to determine methods for more adaptive coping with the stressor. Provide positive feedback for strategies identified and decisions made.	9. Positive reinforcement enhances self-esteem and encourages repetition of desirable behaviors.
	10. Encourage the patient to reach out for spiritual support during this time in whatever form is desirable. Assess the patient's spiritual needs and assist as necessary in the fulfillment of those needs.	10. For some individuals, spiritual support can enhance successful adaptation to painful life experiences.

NURSING DIAGNOSIS: RISK-PRONE HEALTH BEHAVIOR

RELATED TO: Inadequate coping strategies; inadequate social support; low self-efficacy

EVIDENCED BY: Demonstrates nonacceptance of health status change

OUTCOME CRITERIA	NURSING INTERVENTIONS	RATIONALE
Short-Term Goals ■ The patient and primary nurse will discuss the kinds of lifestyle changes that will occur because of the change in health status. With the help of the primary nurse, the patient will formulate a plan of action for incorporating those changes into his or her lifestyle.	1. Encourage the patient to talk about his or her lifestyle prior to the change in health status. Discuss coping mechanisms that were used at stressful times in the past. 2. Encourage the patient to discuss the change or loss and particularly to express anger associated with it.	1. It is important to identify the patient's strengths so that they may be used to facilitate adaptation to the change or loss that has occurred. 2. Anger is a normal stage in the grieving process and, if not released in an appropriate manner, may be turned inward on the self, leading to pathological depression.

Continued

Table 19–2 | CARE PLAN FOR THE PATIENT WITH AN ADJUSTMENT DISORDER—cont'd

OUTCOME CRITERIA	NURSING INTERVENTIONS	RATIONALE
■ The patient will demonstrate movement toward independence, considering the change in health status. **Long-Term Goal** ■ The patient will demonstrate competence to function independently to his or her optimal ability, considering the change in health status, by the time of discharge from treatment.	3. Encourage the patient to express fears associated with the change or loss or alteration in lifestyle that it has created.	3. Change often creates a feeling of disequilibrium, and the individual may respond with fears that are irrational or unfounded. The patient may benefit from feedback that corrects misperceptions about how life will be with the change in health status.
	4. Provide assistance with activities of daily living as required but encourage independence to the limit that the patient's ability will allow. Give positive feedback for activities accomplished independently.	4. Independent accomplishments and positive feedback enhance self-esteem and encourage repetition of desired behaviors. Successes also provide hope that adaptive functioning is possible and decrease feelings of powerlessness.
	5. Help the patient with decision making regarding incorporation of the change or loss into his or her lifestyle. Identify problems the change or loss is likely to create. Discuss alternative solutions, weighing potential benefits and consequences of each alternative. Support the patient's decision in the selection of an alternative.	5. The great amount of anxiety that usually accompanies a major life change often interferes with an individual's ability to solve problems and to make appropriate decisions. The patient may need assistance with this process in an effort to progress toward successful adaptation.
	6. Use role-play to practice stressful situations that might occur in relation to the health status change.	6. Role-playing decreases anxiety and provides a feeling of security by providing the patient with a plan of action for responding in an appropriate manner when a stressful situation occurs.
	7. Ensure that the patient and family are fully knowledgeable regarding the physiology of the change in health status and understand the necessity of such knowledge for optimal wellness. Encourage them to ask questions, and provide printed material explaining the change to which they may refer.	7. Having knowledge about the health status and knowing what to expect regarding the change or loss decreases anxiety and enhances the capacity for wellness.
	8. Ensure that the patient can identify resources within the community from which he or she may seek assistance in adapting to the change in health status. Examples include self-help and support groups and public health nurses, counselors, or social worker. Encourage the patient to keep follow-up appointments with his or her physician or to call the physician's office prior to the follow-up date if problems or concerns arise.	8. Support services provide a feeling of security that one is not alone and provide a means to prevent decompensation when stress becomes intolerable

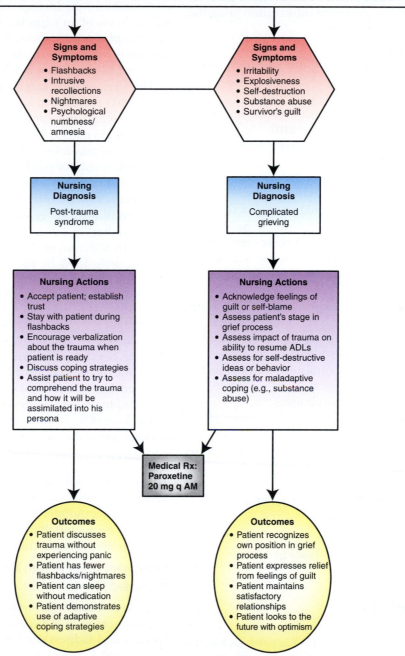

Clinical Vignette: Charles is a 29-year-old veteran of two deployments to Afghanistan. He was honorably discharged from the army 2 years ago and has resumed his position as an assemblyman with a large automobile manufacturing company. His wife reports that he has begun having nightmares, seems angry and bitter, and feels guilty that he survived while many of his friends had not. Recently, while working in their backyard, he threw himself on the ground at the sound of a helicopter flying overhead. Lately, at work, he becomes very agitated and irritable at the sounds of loud noises in the factory, a behavior that is interfering with his productivity. Charles has been diagnosed with Post-traumatic Stress Disorder. The mental health nurse develops the following concept map care plan for Charles.

Signs and Symptoms
- Flashbacks
- Intrusive recollections
- Nightmares
- Psychological numbness/amnesia

Signs and Symptoms
- Irritability
- Explosiveness
- Self-destruction
- Substance abuse
- Survivor's guilt

Nursing Diagnosis
Post-trauma syndrome

Nursing Diagnosis
Complicated grieving

Nursing Actions
- Accept patient; establish trust
- Stay with patient during flashbacks
- Encourage verbalization about the trauma when patient is ready
- Discuss coping strategies
- Assist patient to try to comprehend the trauma and how it will be assimilated into his persona

Nursing Actions
- Acknowledge feelings of guilt or self-blame
- Assess patient's stage in grief process
- Assess impact of trauma on ability to resume ADLs
- Assess for self-destructive ideas or behavior
- Assess for maladaptive coping (e.g., substance abuse)

Medical Rx: Paroxetine 20 mg q AM

Outcomes
- Patient discusses trauma without experiencing panic
- Patient has fewer flashbacks/nightmares
- Patient can sleep without medication
- Patient demonstrates use of adaptive coping strategies

Outcomes
- Patient recognizes own position in grief process
- Patient expresses relief from feelings of guilt
- Patient maintains satisfactory relationships
- Patient looks to the future with optimism

FIGURE 19–1 Concept map care plan for a patient with post-traumatic stress disorder.

Evaluation

Reassessment is conducted in order to determine if the nursing actions have been successful in achieving the objectives of care. Evaluation of the nursing actions for the patient with a trauma-related disorder may be facilitated by gathering information using the following types of questions:

Can the patient:

■ Discuss the traumatic event without experiencing panic anxiety?
■ Voluntarily discuss the traumatic event?
■ Discuss changes that have occurred in his or her life because of the traumatic event?
■ Verbalize that flashbacks have decreased in intensity or frequency?
■ Sleep without medication?
■ Verbalize that nightmares have subsided?
■ Identify new, adaptive coping strategies for assistance with recovery?
■ Demonstrate successful use of these new coping strategies in times of stress?
■ Verbalize stages of grief and the normal behaviors associated with each?
■ Recognize his or her own position in the grieving process?
■ Verbalize that feelings of guilt have decreased in intensity or subsided?
■ Maintain satisfactory relationships with significant others?
■ Look to the future with optimism?
■ Verbalize intent to attend a regular support group for victims of similar traumatic experiences?
■ Identify a plan of action for dealing with symptoms if they return?

Application of the Nursing Process—Stressor-Related Disorders

Adjustment Disorders—Background Assessment Data

> ### CORE CONCEPT
> **Stress**
> Perceptions, emotions, anxieties, interpersonal, social, or economic events that are considered threatening to one's physical health, personal safety, or well-being (Venes, 2017).

An adjustment disorder is characterized by a maladaptive reaction to an identifiable stressor or stressors that results in the development of clinically significant emotional or behavioral symptoms (APA, 2013). The response occurs within 3 months after onset of the stressor and has persisted for no longer than 6 months after the stressor or its consequences have ended.

The individual shows impairment in social and occupational functioning or exhibits symptoms that are in excess of an expected reaction to the stressor. The symptoms are expected to remit soon after the stressor is relieved, or if the stressor persists, when a new level of adaptation is achieved.

The stressor itself can be almost anything, but an individual's response to any particular stressor cannot be predicted. If an individual is highly predisposed or vulnerable to maladaptive response, a severe form of the disorder may follow what most people would consider only a mild or moderate stressor. On the other hand, a less vulnerable individual may develop only a mild form of the disorder in response to what others might consider a severe stressor.

A number of clinical presentations are associated with adjustment disorders. The following categories, identified by the *DSM-5* (APA, 2013), are distinguished by the predominant features of the maladaptive response.

Adjustment Disorder With Depressed Mood

This category is the most commonly diagnosed adjustment disorder. The clinical presentation is one of predominant mood disturbance, although it is less pronounced than that of major depressive disorder (MDD). The symptoms, such as depressed mood, tearfulness, and feelings of hopelessness, exceed what is an expected or normative response to an identified stressor.

Adjustment Disorder With Anxiety

This category denotes a maladaptive response to a stressor in which the predominant manifestation is anxiety. For example, the symptoms may reveal nervousness, worry, and jitteriness. The clinician must differentiate this diagnosis from those of anxiety disorders.

Adjustment Disorder With Mixed Anxiety and Depressed Mood

The predominant features of this category include disturbances in mood (depression, feelings of hopelessness and sadness) and manifestations of anxiety (nervousness, worry, jitteriness) that are more intense than what would be expected or considered to be a normative response to an identified stressor.

Adjustment Disorder With Disturbance of Conduct

This category is characterized by conduct in which there is violation of the rights of others or of major age-appropriate societal norms and rules. Examples include truancy, vandalism, reckless driving, fighting, and defaulting on legal responsibilities. Differential diagnosis must be made from conduct disorder or antisocial personality disorder.

Adjustment Disorder With Mixed Disturbance of Emotions and Conduct

The predominant features of this category include emotional disturbances (e.g., anxiety or depression) as well as disturbances of conduct in which there is violation of the rights of others or of major age-appropriate societal norms and rules (e.g., truancy, vandalism, fighting).

Adjustment Disorder Unspecified

This subtype is used when the maladaptive reaction is not consistent with any of the other categories. The individual may have physical complaints, withdraw from relationships, or exhibit impaired work or academic performance but without significant disturbance in emotions or conduct.

Predisposing Factors to Adjustment Disorders

Biological Aspects

Chronic disorders, such as neurocognitive or intellectual developmental disorders, are thought to impair the ability of an individual to adapt to stress, causing increased vulnerability to adjustment disorder. Genetic factors also may influence individual risks for maladaptive response to stress (Sadock et al., 2015).

Psychosocial Theories

Some proponents of psychoanalytic theory view adjustment disorder as a maladaptive response to stress that is caused by early childhood trauma, increased dependency, and retarded ego development. Other psychoanalysts give considerable weight to the constitutional factors or birth characteristics that contribute to the manner in which individuals respond to stress. In many instances, adjustment disorder is precipitated by a specific meaningful stressor having found a point of vulnerability in an individual of otherwise adequate ego strength.

Some studies relate a predisposition to adjustment disorder to factors such as developmental stage, timing of the stressor, and available support systems. When a stressor occurs, and the individual does not have the developmental maturity, available support systems, or adequate coping strategies to adapt, normal functioning is disrupted, resulting in psychological or somatic symptoms. The disorder also may be related to a dysfunctional grieving process. The individual may remain in the denial or anger stage with inadequate defense mechanisms to complete the grieving process.

Transactional Model of Stress and Adaptation

Why are some individuals able to confront stressful situations adaptively and even gain strength from the experience, whereas others not only fail to cope adaptively but may even encounter psychopathological dysfunction? The transactional model of stress and adaptation takes into consideration the interaction between the individual and the environment.

The type of stressor that one experiences may influence one's adaptation. Sudden-shock stressors occur without warning, and continuous stressors are those that an individual is exposed to over an extended period. Although many studies have been directed to individuals' responses to sudden-shock stressors, it has been found that continuous stressors are more commonly cited than sudden-shock stressors as precipitants to maladaptive functioning.

Both situational and intrapersonal factors most likely contribute to an individual's stress response. Situational factors include personal and general economic conditions; occupational and recreational opportunities; and the availability of social supports such as family, friends, neighbors, and cultural or religious support groups.

Intrapersonal factors such as constitutional vulnerability have also been implicated in the predisposition to adjustment disorder. Some studies have indicated that a child with a difficult temperament (defined as one who cries loudly and often; adapts to changes slowly; and has irregular patterns of hunger, sleep, and elimination) is at greater risk of developing a behavior disorder. Other intrapersonal factors that might influence one's ability to adjust to a painful life change include social skills, coping strategies, the presence of psychiatric illness, degree of flexibility, and level of intelligence.

Diagnosis and Outcome Identification

Nursing diagnoses are formulated from the data gathered during the assessment phase and with background knowledge regarding predisposing factors to the disorder. Nursing diagnoses that may be used for the patient with an adjustment disorder include the following:

■ Complicated grieving related to real or perceived loss of any concept of value to the individual, evidenced by interference with life functioning, developmental regression, or somatic complaints

- Risk-prone health behavior related to change in health status requiring modification in lifestyle (e.g., chronic illness, physical disability), as evidenced by inability to problem solve or set realistic goals for the future (appropriate diagnosis for the person with adjustment disorder if the precipitating stressor was a change in health status)
- Anxiety (moderate to severe) related to situational and/or maturational crisis as evidenced by restlessness, increased helplessness, and diminished productivity

Outcome Criteria

The following criteria may be used for measurement of outcomes in the care of the patient with an adjustment disorder.

The patient:

- Verbalizes acceptable behaviors associated with each stage of the grief process.
- Demonstrates a reinvestment in the environment.
- Accomplishes activities of daily living independently.
- Demonstrates ability for adequate occupational and social functioning.
- Verbalizes awareness of change in health status and the effect it will have on lifestyle.
- Solves problems and sets realistic goals for the future.
- Demonstrates ability to cope effectively with change in lifestyle.

Planning and Implementation

The following section presents a group of selected nursing diagnoses, with short- and long-term goals and nursing interventions for each.

Complicated Grieving

Complicated grieving is defined as "a disorder that occurs after the death of a significant other [or any other loss of significance to the individual], in which the experience of distress accompanying bereavement fails to follow normative expectations and manifests in functional impairment" (Herdman & Kamitsuru, 2018, p. 340).

Patient Goals

Outcome criteria include short- and long-term goals. Timelines are individually determined.
Short-Term Goal
  - By end of 1 week, patient will express anger toward lost entity.

Long-Term Goal
  - Patient will be able to verbalize behaviors associated with the normal stages of grief and identify own position in grief process, while progressing at own pace toward resolution.

Interventions

- Determine the stage of grief in which the patient is fixed. Identify behaviors associated with this stage. Accurate baseline assessment data are necessary to plan effective care.
- Develop a trusting relationship. Show empathy and caring. Be honest and keep all promises. Trust is the basis for a therapeutic relationship.
- Convey an accepting attitude so that the patient is not afraid to express feelings openly. An accepting attitude enhances trust.
- Allow the patient to express anger. Do not become defensive if the initial expression of anger is displaced on the nurse or therapist. Help the patient explore angry feelings so that they may be directed toward the intended object or person. Verbalization of feelings in a nonthreatening environment may help the patient come to terms with unresolved issues.
- Assist the patient to discharge pent-up anger through participation in large motor activities (e.g., brisk walks, jogging, physical exercises, volleyball, exercise bike). Physical exercise provides a safe and effective method for discharging pent-up tension.
- Explain the normal stages of grief and the behaviors associated with each stage. Educate the patient that feelings such as guilt and anger toward the lost entity/concept are natural and acceptable during the grief process. Knowledge of the acceptability of the feelings associated with normal grieving may help to relieve some of the guilt that these responses generate.
- Encourage the patient to review his or her perception of the loss or change. With support and sensitivity, point out the reality of the situation in areas where misrepresentations are expressed. The patient must give up an idealized perception and be able to accept both positive and negative aspects about the painful life change before the grief process is complete.
- Communicate to the patient that crying is acceptable. The use of touch is therapeutic and appropriate with most patients. Knowledge of cultural influences specific to the patient is important before employing this technique. Touch is considered inappropriate in some cultures.

■ Assist the patient to explore alternatives as he or she attempts to determine methods for more adaptive coping with the stressor. Provide positive feedback for strategies identified and decisions made. Positive reinforcement enhances self-esteem and encourages repetition of desirable behaviors.

■ Assess the patient's spiritual needs and assist as necessary in the fulfillment of those needs. Encourage the patient to reach out for spiritual support during this time in whatever form is desirable. For some individuals, spiritual support can enhance successful adaptation to painful life experiences.

Risk-Prone Health Behavior

Risk-prone health behavior is defined as "impaired ability to modify lifestyle/behaviors in a manner that improves health status" (Herdman & Kamitsuru, 2018, p. 149).

Patient Goals

Short-Term Goals
■ Patient and primary nurse will discuss the kinds of lifestyle changes that will occur because of the change in health status.
■ With the help of the primary nurse, the patient will formulate a plan of action for incorporating those changes into his or her lifestyle.
■ Patient will demonstrate movement toward independence, considering the change in health status.

Long-Term Goal
■ Patient will demonstrate competence to function independently to his or her optimal ability, considering the change in health status, by the time of discharge from treatment.

Interventions

■ Encourage the patient to talk about his or her lifestyle prior to the change in health status. Discuss coping mechanisms that were used at stressful times in the past. It is important to identify the patient's strengths so that they may be used to facilitate adaptation to the change or loss that has occurred.

■ Encourage the patient to discuss the change or loss and particularly to express anger associated with it. Anger is a normal stage in the grieving process and, if not released in an appropriate manner, may be turned inward on the self, leading to depression.

■ Encourage the patient to express fears associated with the change or loss or alteration in lifestyle that it has created. Change often creates a feeling of disequilibrium, and the individual may respond with fears that are irrational or unfounded. The patient may benefit from feedback that corrects misperceptions about how life will be with the change in health status.

■ Provide assistance with activities of daily living as required but encourage independence to the limit that the patient's ability will allow. Give positive feedback for activities accomplished independently. Independent accomplishments and positive feedback enhance self-esteem and encourage repetition of desired behaviors. Successes also provide hope that adaptive functioning is possible and decrease feelings of powerlessness.

■ Explore with the patient ways to incorporate the change or loss into his or her lifestyle. Identify problems the change or loss is likely to create. Discuss alternative solutions, weighing potential benefits and consequences of each alternative. Support the patient's decision in the selection of an alternative. The great amount of anxiety that usually accompanies a major lifestyle change often interferes with an individual's ability to solve problems and to make appropriate decisions. The patient may need assistance with this process in an effort to progress toward successful adaptation.

■ Use role-play to practice stressful situations that might occur in relation to the health status change. Role-playing decreases anxiety and provides a feeling of security by providing the patient with a plan of action for responding in an appropriate manner when a stressful situation occurs.

■ Ensure that the patient and family are fully knowledgeable regarding the physiology of the change in health status and understand the necessity of such knowledge for optimal wellness. Encourage them to ask questions, and provide printed material explaining the change to which they may refer. Having knowledge about the health status and knowing what to expect regarding the change or loss decreases anxiety and enhances the capacity for wellness.

■ Ensure that the patient can identify resources within the community from which he or she may seek assistance in adapting to the change in health status. Examples include self-help or support groups and public health nurse, counselor, or social worker. Encourage the patient to keep follow-up appointments with his or her physician or to call the physician's office prior to the follow-up date if problems or concerns arise. Support services provide a feeling of security that one is not alone and provide a means to prevent decompensation when stress becomes intolerable.

Concept Care Mapping

The concept map care plan is a diagrammatic teaching and learning strategy that allows visualization of interrelationships between medical diagnoses, nursing diagnoses, assessment data, and treatments. An example of a concept map care plan for a patient with an adjustment disorder is presented in Figure 19–2.

Evaluation

Reassessment is conducted to determine if the nursing actions have been successful in achieving the objectives of care. Evaluation of the nursing actions for the patient with an adjustment disorder may be facilitated by gathering information using the following types of questions:

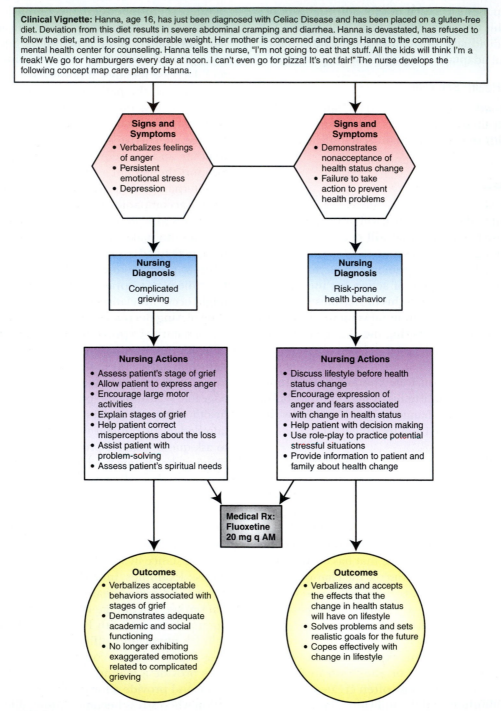

Clinical Vignette: Hanna, age 16, has just been diagnosed with Celiac Disease and has been placed on a gluten-free diet. Deviation from this diet results in severe abdominal cramping and diarrhea. Hanna is devastated, has refused to follow the diet, and is losing considerable weight. Her mother is concerned and brings Hanna to the community mental health center for counseling. Hanna tells the nurse, "I'm not going to eat that stuff. All the kids will think I'm a freak! We go for hamburgers every day at noon. I can't even go for pizza! It's not fair!" The nurse develops the following concept map care plan for Hanna.

Signs and Symptoms
- Verbalizes feelings of anger
- Persistent emotional stress
- Depression

Signs and Symptoms
- Demonstrates nonacceptance of health status change
- Failure to take action to prevent health problems

Nursing Diagnosis

Complicated grieving

Nursing Diagnosis

Risk-prone health behavior

Nursing Actions
- Assess patient's stage of grief
- Allow patient to express anger
- Encourage large motor activities
- Explain stages of grief
- Help patient correct misperceptions about the loss
- Assist patient with problem-solving
- Assess patient's spiritual needs

Nursing Actions
- Discuss lifestyle before health status change
- Encourage expression of anger and fears associated with change in health status
- Help patient with decision making
- Use role-play to practice potential stressful situations
- Provide information to patient and family about health change

Medical Rx: Fluoxetine 20 mg q AM

Outcomes
- Verbalizes acceptable behaviors associated with stages of grief
- Demonstrates adequate academic and social functioning
- No longer exhibiting exaggerated emotions related to complicated grieving

Outcomes
- Verbalizes and accepts the effects that the change in health status will have on lifestyle
- Solves problems and sets realistic goals for the future
- Copes effectively with change in lifestyle

FIGURE 19–2 Concept map care plan for a patient with an adjustment disorder.

Does the patient:

- Verbalize understanding of the grief process and his or her position in the process?
- Recognize his or her adaptive and maladaptive behaviors associated with the grief response?
- Demonstrate evidence of progression along the grief response?
- Accomplish activities of daily living independently?
- Demonstrate the ability to perform occupational and social activities adequately?
- Discuss the change in health status and modification of lifestyle it will affect?
- Demonstrate acceptance of the modification?
- Participate in decision making and problem-solving for his or her future?
- Set realistic goals for the future?
- Demonstrate new adaptive coping strategies for dealing with the change in lifestyle?
- Verbalize available resources to whom he or she may go for support or assistance should it be necessary?

Treatment Modalities

Trauma-Related Disorders

Cognitive Therapy

Cognitive therapy for PTSD and ASD strives to help the individual recognize and modify trauma-related thoughts and beliefs. The individual learns to modify the relationships between thoughts and feelings and to identify and challenge inaccurate or extreme automatic negative thoughts. The goal is to replace these negative thoughts with more accurate and less distressing thoughts and to cope more effectively with feelings such as anger, guilt, and fear. The individual is assisted to modify the appraisal of self and the world as it has been affected by the trauma and to regain hope and optimism about safety, trust, power and control, esteem, and intimacy. Stress inoculation therapy (SIT) is a type of cognitive behavior therapy (CBT) that focuses on learning new ways of coping with stressful events through education and practicing alternative responses like meditation, deep breathing, and other relaxation exercises.

Prolonged Exposure Therapy

Prolonged exposure therapy is a type of behavioral therapy somewhat similar to implosion therapy or flooding. It can be conducted in an imagined or real (in vivo) situation. In the imagined situation, the individual is exposed to repeated and prolonged mental recounting of the traumatic experience. In vivo exposure involves systematic confrontation, within safe limits, of trauma-related situations that are feared and avoided. This intense emotional processing of the traumatic event serves to neutralize the memories so that they no longer result in anxious arousal or escape and avoidance behaviors. Prolonged exposure therapy has four main parts: (1) education about the treatment, (2) breathing retraining for relaxation, (3) imagined exposure through repeated discussion about the trauma with a therapist, and (4) exposure to real-world situations related to the trauma.

Group and Family Therapy

Group therapy has been strongly advocated for clients with PTSD. It has proved especially effective with military veterans (Sadock et al., 2015). The importance of being able to share their experiences with empathetic fellow veterans, to talk about problems in social adaptation, and to discuss options for managing their aggression toward others has been emphasized. Some PTSD groups are informal and leaderless, such as self-help or support groups, and some are led by experienced group therapists who may have had some first-hand experience with the trauma. Some groups involve family members, thereby recognizing that the symptoms of PTSD may also severely affect them. For example, family members of military veterans sometimes develop PTSD as a result of exposure to their loved one's symptoms of PTSD (see Chapter 28, Military Families, for further discussion of this topic).

Eye Movement Desensitization and Reprocessing

Eye movement desensitization and reprocessing (EMDR) is a type of psychotherapy that was developed in 1989 by psychologist Francine Shapiro. It "has evolved from a simple technique into an integrative psychotherapy approach with a theoretical model that emphasizes the brain's information processing system and memories of disturbing experiences as the basis of pathology" (Shapiro, 2007, p. 3). EMDR has been shown to be an effective therapy for PTSD and other trauma-related disorders. It has been used experimentally in the treatment of other disorders, including depression, adjustment disorder, phobias, addictions, generalized anxiety disorder, and panic disorder. However, Aetna Healthcare (2017) concludes that EMDR has only been empirically validated for PTSD. Clinical practice guidelines from both the American Psychiatric Association and the Department of Veterans Affairs support the effectiveness of EMDR for PTSD (WebMD, 2017), yet it remains a controversial treatment among some healthcare professionals. Special precautions may be needed when using EMDR in clients with neurological impairments (e.g., seizure disorders), severe dissociative disorders, or unstable substance abuse and those who are suicidal or experiencing psychosis (UPMC, Center for Integrative Medicine, 2018).

The exact biological mechanisms by which EMDR achieves its therapeutic effects are unknown. Some studies have indicated that eye movements cause a decrease in imagery vividness and distress as well as an increase in memory access. The process involves rapid eye movements while processing painful emotions. The EMDR International Association (2018) stresses that "processing" information does not mean "talking about it" but rather "setting up a learning state that will allow experiences that are causing problems to be 'digested' and stored appropriately in your brain." While concentrating on a particular emotion or physical sensation surrounding the traumatic event, the client is asked to focus his or her eye movements on the therapist's fingers as the therapist moves them from left to right and back again. Although some individuals report rapid results with this therapy, research has indicated that from 5 to 12 sessions are required to achieve lasting treatment effects. The treatment encompasses an eight-phase process:

Phase 1: History and treatment planning. The therapist takes a thorough history and develops a treatment plan. The problem for which the client is seeking treatment and current symptoms are discussed. However, the client is not required to discuss the traumatic event in detail, unless he or she chooses to do so. Instead, emphasis is placed on the emotions and physical sensations surrounding the traumatic event.

Phase 2: Preparation. The therapist teaches the client certain self-care techniques (e.g., relaxation techniques) for dealing with emotional disturbances that may arise during or between sessions. Self-care is an important component of EMDR. It is important for the client to develop a sense of trust in the therapist during this phase.

Phase 3: Assessment. The therapist asks the client to identify a specific scene or picture from the target event identified in phase 1 that best represents the memory. The client is then directed to express a negative self-belief associated with the memory (e.g., "I am bad" or "I'm in danger"). The next step is to identify a self-statement that he or she would *rather* believe (e.g., "I am good" or "I'm safe now"). When the self-statements

have been identified, the client is asked to rate the validity of each of the statements on the Validity of Cognition (VOC) scale from "completely false" (a score of 1) to "completely true" (a score of 7). In this phase, the client is also asked to rank the disturbing emotions on the 0 to 10 Subjective Units of Disturbance (SUD) scale (with 0 meaning the disturbance is not disturbing at all and 10 meaning it is the worst feeling he or she has ever had).

Phase 4: Desensitization. The client gives attention to the negative beliefs and disturbing emotions associated with the traumatic event while focusing his or her vision on the back-and-forth motion of the therapist's fingers. All personal feelings and physical reactions experienced during this time are noted. Following each set of rapid eye movements, the therapist reassesses the level of disturbance associated with the feelings, images, and beliefs. This desensitization process continues until the distress level (as measured by the SUD scale) is reduced to 0 or 1.

Phase 5: Installation. The client gives attention to the positive belief that he or she has identified to replace the negative belief associated with the trauma. This is accomplished while simultaneously visually tracking the therapist's fingers. Following each set of rapid eye movements, the client is asked to rate the positive belief on the VOC scale. The goal is to strengthen the positive belief or self-statement until it is accepted as completely true (a score of 7 on the VOC scale).

Phase 6: Body scan. When the positive cognition has been strengthened, the therapist asks the client to concentrate on any lingering physical sensations. While focusing on the traumatic event, the client is asked to identify any areas of the body where residual tension is experienced. Because positive self-beliefs must be believed on more than just an intellectual level, phase 6 is not complete until the client is able to think about or discuss the traumatic event (or the feelings associated with it) without experiencing bodily tension.

Phase 7: Closure. Closure ensures that the client leaves each session feeling better than he or she felt at the beginning. If the processing that took place during the session is not complete, the therapist will direct the client through a variety of self-calming relaxation techniques to help him or her regain emotional equilibrium. The client is briefed about what to expect between sessions. Until processing of the trauma is complete, disturbing images, thoughts, and emotions may arise between therapy sessions. The therapist instructs the client to record these experiences in a journal so that they may be used as targets for processing in future therapy sessions.

Phase 8: Reevaluation. Reevaluation begins each new therapy session. The therapist assesses whether the positive changes have been maintained, determines if previous target areas need reprocessing, and identifies any new target areas that need attention.

Clients often feel relief quite rapidly with EMDR. However, to achieve lasting results, it is important that each of the eight phases be completed. Treatment is not complete until "EMDR therapy has focused on the past memories that are contributing to the problem, the present situations that are disturbing, and what skills the client may need for the future" (EMDR International Association, 2018).

Psychopharmacology

Trauma-focused psychotherapy is considered the first-line treatment for PTSD (Jeffreys, 2018); however, many medications have demonstrated benefits as well.

Antidepressants Specific selective serotonin reuptake inhibitors (SSRIs) are considered the first-line pharmacological choice for PTSD because of their efficacy, tolerability, and safety ratings (Sadock et al., 2015). Paroxetine and sertraline have been approved by the FDA for this purpose. Additionally, fluoxetine and the SNRI venlafaxine (although not FDA-approved for PTSD) have demonstrated effectiveness (Jeffreys, 2018). The tricyclic antidepressants amitriptyline (Elavil) and imipramine (Tofranil) have been supported by several well-controlled studies and may be an alternative if the client is not responding to an SSRI. The monoamine oxidase inhibitor phenelzine has also demonstrated efficacy in the treatment of PTSD.

Anxiolytics Alprazolam (a benzodiazepine) has been prescribed for PTSD clients for its antidepressant and antipanic effects despite the absence of controlled studies demonstrating their efficacy for this condition. Jeffreys (2018) recommends against using benzodiazepines in PTSD based on a meta-analysis finding that they worsened patients' PTSD symptoms. In addition, their addictive properties make them less desirable than some of the other medications in the treatment of post-trauma patients.

Buspirone, which has serotonergic properties similar to those of SSRIs, may be useful for treating anxiety in PTSD, and these drugs also have less addiction potential than benzodiazepines. More controlled trials with this drug are needed to validate its efficacy in treating PTSD.

Antihypertensives The beta-blocker propranolol and alpha$_2$-receptor agonist clonidine have been success-

ful in alleviating some of the symptoms associated with PTSD. Some clinical trials have reported reduction in symptoms, such as nightmares and angry outbursts. Although beta blockers are known to reduce hyperarousal states and may decrease aggression, Jeffreys (2018) reports that current evidence is insufficient to support their use in PTSD treatment.

Other Medications Sadock and colleagues (2015) report that little positive evidence exists concerning the use of antipsychotics in PTSD. They suggest that these drugs "should be reserved for the short-term control of severe aggression and agitation" (p. 621).

Ketamine, an anesthetic agent that has demonstrated benefits in treatment of depression and obsessive-compulsive disorder was found in clinical trials (Feder et al., 2014) to benefit some patients with PTSD. It modulates glutaminergic activity at N-methyl-D-aspartate receptors and serotonergic activity at 5HT1 receptors and is thought to disrupt the fear associated with trauma. Currently, ketamine is not FDA approved for this use but is prescribed as an off-label use. It is administered intravenously at subanesthetic doses and usually involves a series of treatments. Jeffreys (2018) cautions that its effects are short term and there is potential for addiction.

The endocannabinoid system may be another avenue for treatment, since decreased levels of endogenous cannabinoids have been found in PTSD patients (Jeffreys, 2018). Although direct stimulation of this pathway has demonstrated negative effects on PTSD and potential for addiction, indirect stimulation of this pathway might provide some additional treatment options. More research is needed to confirm its benefits.

The alpha$_1$ antagonist prazosin (Minipress) has been studied for its potential benefit in reducing nightmares and enhancing normal dreaming patterns in clients with PTSD. However, Veterans Health Administration clinical practice guidelines now recommend against its use in PTSD based on a large trial that found no difference between prazosin and placebo (Jeffreys, 2018). Low-dose glucocorticoids have been studied for possible benefit in decreasing recall of traumatic memories; other actions of glucocorticoids that may affect response to PTSD symptoms include potentiating glutamate at NMDA receptors and interactions with noradrenergic systems (Jeffreys, 2018), but more research is needed.

Adjustment Disorders

Various treatments are used for clients with adjustment disorder. The primary focus of intervention is to maximize the potential for adaptation.

Individual Psychotherapy

Individual psychotherapy is the most common treatment for adjustment disorder. Individual psychotherapy allows the client to examine the stressor that is causing the problem, possibly assign personal meaning to the stressor, and confront unresolved issues that may be exacerbating this crisis. Treatment works to remove these blocks to adaptation so that normal developmental progression can resume. Techniques are used to clarify links between the current stressor and past experiences and to assist with the development of more adaptive coping strategies.

Family Therapy

The focus of treatment is shifted from the individual to the system of relationships in which the individual is involved. The maladaptive response of the identified client is viewed as symptomatic of a dysfunctional family system. All family members are included in the therapy, and treatment serves to improve the functioning within the family network. Emphasis is placed on communication, family rules, and interaction patterns among the family members.

Behavior Therapy

The goal of behavior therapy is to replace ineffective response patterns with more adaptive ones. The situations that promote ineffective responses are identified, and carefully designed reinforcement schedules, along with role modeling and coaching, are used to alter the maladaptive response patterns. This type of treatment is very effective when implemented in an inpatient setting where the client's behavior and its consequences may be more readily controlled.

Self-Help Groups

Group experiences, with or without a professional facilitator, provide an arena in which members may consider and compare their responses with those of individuals with similar life experiences. Members benefit from learning that they are not alone in their painful experiences. Hope is derived from knowing that others have survived and even grown from similar experiences. Members of the group exchange advice, share coping strategies, and provide support and encouragement for each other.

Crisis Intervention

In crisis intervention, the therapist or other intervener becomes a part of the individual's life situation. Because of increased anxiety, the individual with adjustment disorder is unable to problem solve, so he or she requires guidance and support from another to help mobilize the resources needed to resolve the crisis. Crisis intervention is short term and relies heavily on orderly problem-solving techniques and structured activities that are focused on change. The ultimate goal of crisis intervention in the treatment of adjustment disorder is to resolve the immediate crisis, restore adaptive functioning, and promote personal growth.

Psychopharmacology

Adjustment disorder is not commonly treated with medications because (1) their effect may be temporary and only mask the real problem, interfering with the possibility of finding a more permanent solution, and (2) psychoactive drugs carry the potential for physiological and psychological dependence.

When the client with adjustment disorder has symptoms of anxiety or depression, the physician may prescribe antianxiety or antidepressant medication. These medications are considered only adjuncts to psychotherapy and should not be given as the primary therapy. In these instances, they are given to alleviate symptoms so that the individual may more effectively cope while attempting to adapt to the stressful situation.

CASE STUDY AND SAMPLE CARE PLAN

NURSING HISTORY AND ASSESSMENT

Marissa, age 22, was born in a small town in Oklahoma. She has lived there her whole life, even living at home while she attended a nearby college to earn a Baccalaureate degree in education. She is an only child, and her parents were in their 40s when she was born. She was engaged throughout her college years to her high school sweetheart, Dave, who graduated 6 months ago from the state university with a degree in aeronautical engineering. Upon his graduation, he accepted a position with NASA at Kennedy Space Center in Florida. Marissa and Dave were married 5 months ago and moved to a small apartment in Cape Canaveral, where Dave began his work with NASA. The plan was for Marissa to seek employment upon their arrival, but she has been unable to move ahead with those plans. She stays in their apartment most days, talking on the phone to her parents and crying about how much she misses them and her home in Oklahoma. Marissa has met very few people and has no desire to do so. She sleeps a lot and has lost weight. She has been having severe

CASE STUDY AND SAMPLE CARE PLAN—cont'd

headaches. Her husband is very concerned about her and made an appointment for her with a private physician. Following a complete and unremarkable physical examination, the physician referred Marissa to the mental health clinic where she was admitted to the day treatment center with a diagnosis of adjustment disorder with depressed mood.

NURSING DIAGNOSES AND OUTCOME IDENTIFICATION

From the assessment data, the nurse develops the following nursing diagnoses for Marissa:

1. **Complicated grieving** related to feelings of loss associated with leaving her parents and her lifetime home
   a. **Short-Term Goal:** Within 1 week, Marissa will express anger about the loss associated with her move.
   b. **Long-Term Goal:** Marissa will be able to verbalize behaviors associated with the normal stages of grief and identify her own position in the grief process, while progressing at her own pace toward resolution.
2. **Relocation stress syndrome** related to moving away from parents and familiar environment in which she had spent her whole life
   a. **Short-Term Goal:** Within 1 week, Marissa will verbalize at least one positive aspect regarding relocation to her new environment.
   b. **Long-Term Goal:** Within 1 month, Marissa will demonstrate positive adaptation to her new environment as evidenced by involvement in activities, expression of satisfaction with new acquaintances, and elimination of previously evident physical and psychological symptoms associated with the relocation.

PLANNING AND IMPLEMENTATION

COMPLICATED GRIEVING
The following nursing interventions have been identified for Marissa:

1. Determine the stage of grief in which Marissa is fixed. Identify behaviors associated with this stage.
2. Develop a trusting relationship with Marissa. Show empathy and caring. Be honest and keep all promises.
3. Convey an accepting attitude so that Marissa is not afraid to express her feelings openly.
4. Allow Marissa to express her anger. Do not become defensive if the initial expression of anger is displaced on nurse or therapist. Help Marissa explore angry feelings so that they may be directed toward the intended object or situation.
5. Help Marissa discharge pent-up anger through participation in large motor activities (e.g., brisk walks, jogging, physical exercises, or activity of her choice).
6. Explain to Marissa the normal stages of grief and the behaviors associated with each stage. Help her to

understand that these feelings are normal and acceptable during a grief process.
7. Encourage Marissa to review her personal perception of the move. With support and sensitivity, point out the reality of the situation in areas where misrepresentations are expressed.
8. Help Marissa solve problems as she attempts to determine methods for more adaptive coping with the life change. Provide positive feedback for strategies identified and decisions made.
9. Encourage Marissa to reach out for spiritual support during this time in whatever form is desirable to her. Assess her spiritual needs and assist as necessary in the fulfillment of those needs.

RELOCATION STRESS SYNDROME
The following nursing interventions have been identified for Marissa:

1. Encourage Marissa to discuss feelings (concerns, fears, anger) regarding this relocation.
2. Encourage Marissa to discuss how the change will affect her life. Ensure that Marissa is involved in decision making and problem-solving regarding the move.
3. Help Marissa identify positive aspects about the move.
4. Help Marissa identify resources within the new community from which assistance with various types of services may be obtained.
5. Identify groups within the community that specialize in helping individuals adapt to relocation. Examples include Newcomers' Club, Welcome Wagon International, and school and church organizations.
6. Refer Marissa to a support group (e.g., Depression and Bipolar Support Alliance [DBSA]).

EVALUATION

The outcome criteria for Marissa have been met. She is no longer having headaches, and she has regained some of her weight. She has joined a chapter of DBSA and has made some new acquaintances. She has applied to become a substitute teacher in the local school district, and she and Dave have joined the local Methodist church, where they have started to socialize with several couples their age. They have also adopted Molly, a 2-year-old mutt from the local shelter, who showers Marissa with love and keeps her company when no one else is around. They take daily walks together. Marissa still talks to her parents on the phone daily, but she no longer has feelings of despair about living so far away from them. Her parents provide encouragement and give her positive feedback for achieving a satisfactory adaptation to her new environment. They are planning a visit to see Marissa and Dave in the near future.

Summary and Key Points

- Post-traumatic stress disorder (PTSD) is the development of characteristic symptoms following exposure to an extreme traumatic stressor involving a personal threat to physical integrity or to the integrity of others. Symptoms may begin within the first 3 months after the trauma, or there may be a delay of several months or even years.

- The symptoms of PTSD are associated with events that would be markedly distressing to almost anyone and include reexperiencing the trauma, a sustained high level of anxiety or arousal, or a general numbing of responsiveness.

- A disorder that is similar in terms of precipitating traumatic events and symptomatology to PTSD is called acute stress disorder (ASD). In ASD, the symptoms are time limited, up to 1 month following the trauma. If the symptoms last longer than 1 month, the diagnosis would be PTSD.

- Predisposing factors to trauma-related disorders include psychosocial, learning, cognitive, and biological influences.

- Adjustment disorders are relatively common. Some studies indicate that they are the most commonly ascribed psychiatric diagnoses.

- Clinical symptoms associated with adjustment disorders include inability to function socially or occupationally in response to an identifiable stressor.

- Adjustment disorder is distinguished by the predominant features of the maladaptive response. These include depression, anxiety, mixed anxiety and depression, disturbance of conduct, and mixed disturbance of emotions and conduct.

- Of the two types of stressors discussed (sudden-shock and continuous), more individuals respond with maladaptive behaviors to long-term, continuous stressors.

- Treatment modalities for PTSD include cognitive therapy, prolonged exposure therapy, group and family therapy, EMDR, and psychopharmacology.

- Treatment modalities for adjustment disorders include individual psychotherapy, family therapy, behavior therapy, self-help groups, crisis intervention, and medications to treat anxiety or depression.

- Nursing care of individuals with trauma- and stressor-related disorders is accomplished using the steps of the nursing process.

- Trauma-informed care identifies and considers the impact of previous trauma when developing a care plan for clients in any setting because this client is vulnerable to retraumatization.

Review Questions
Self-Examination/Learning Exercise

Select the answer that is most appropriate for each of the following questions:

1. John, a veteran of the war in Iraq, is diagnosed with PTSD. He says to the nurse, "I can't figure out why God took my buddy instead of me." From this statement, the nurse assesses which of the following in John?
   a. Repressed anger
   b. Survivor's guilt
   c. Intrusive thoughts
   d. Spiritual distress

2. John, a veteran of the war in Iraq, is diagnosed with PTSD. He experiences a nightmare during his first night in the hospital. He explains to the nurse that he was dreaming about gunfire all around and people being killed. Which of the following is the nurse's most appropriate *initial* intervention?
   a. Administer alprazolam as ordered prn for anxiety.
   b. Call the physician and report the incident.
   c. Stay with John and reassure him of his safety.
   d. Have John listen to a tape of relaxation exercises.

Review Questions—cont'd
Self-Examination/Learning Exercise

3. John, a veteran of the war in Iraq, is diagnosed with PTSD. Which of the following therapy regimens would most appropriately be ordered for John?
   a. Paroxetine and group therapy
   b. Diazepam and implosion therapy
   c. Alprazolam and behavior therapy
   d. Carbamazepine and cognitive therapy

4. Which of the following may be influential in the predisposition to PTSD?
   a. Unsatisfactory parent-child relationship
   b. Excess of the neurotransmitter serotonin
   c. Distorted, negative cognitions
   d. Severity of the stressor and availability of support systems

5. Nina recently left her husband of 10 years. She was very dependent on her husband and is having difficulty adjusting to an independent lifestyle. She has been hospitalized with a diagnosis of adjustment disorder with depressed mood. Which of the following is the *priority* nursing diagnosis for Nina?
   a. Risk-prone health behavior related to loss of dependency
   b. Complicated grieving related to breakup of marriage
   c. Ineffective communication related to problems with dependency
   d. Social isolation related to depressed mood

6. Nina, who is depressed following the breakup of a very stormy marriage, says to the nurse, "I feel so bad. I thought I would feel better once I left, but I feel worse!" Which is the *best* response by the nurse?
   a. "Cheer up, Nina. You have a lot to be happy about."
   b. "You are grieving the loss of your marriage. It's natural for you to feel bad."
   c. "Try not to dwell on how you feel. If you don't think about it, you'll feel better."
   d. "You did the right thing, Nina. Knowing that should make you feel better."

7. Nina has been hospitalized with adjustment disorder with depressed mood following the breakup of her marriage. Which of the following is true regarding the diagnosis of adjustment disorder?
   a. Nina will require long-term psychotherapy to achieve relief.
   b. Nina likely inherited a genetic tendency for the disorder.
   c. Nina's symptoms will likely remit once she has accepted the change in her life.
   d. Nina probably would not have experienced adjustment disorder if she had a higher level of intelligence.

8. The physician orders sertraline (Zoloft) for a client who is hospitalized with adjustment disorder with depressed mood. What is this medication intended to do?
   a. Increase energy and elevate mood
   b. Stimulate the central nervous system
   c. Prevent psychotic symptoms
   d. Produce a calming effect

Continued

Review Questions—cont'd
Self-Examination/Learning Exercise

9. Shane, a patient diagnosed with PTSD tells the nurse that his social worker is recommending EMDR and asks the nurse to describe this treatment. Which of these is the most accurate response?
   a. EMDR is a therapy designed to help you process thoughts and emotions related to the trauma you've experienced.
   b. EMDR is a treatment to cure insomnia using hypnosis.
   c. EMDR is a treatment that uses electrical stimulation to induce a seizure and is beneficial in relieving depression associated with PTSD.
   d. EMDR is an acronym that stands for Emotional Motivation to Decrease Responsiveness and it will help you forget the trauma.

10. Emma, age 16, has recently been diagnosed with diabetes mellitus. She must watch her diet and take an oral hypoglycemic medication daily. She has become very depressed, and her mother reports that Emma refuses to change her diet and often skips her medication. Emma has been hospitalized for stabilization of her blood sugar. The psychiatric nurse practitioner has been called in as a consultant. Which of the following nursing diagnoses by the psychiatric nurse would be a priority for Emma at this time?
    a. Anxiety related to hospitalization evidenced by noncompliance
    b. Low self-esteem related to feeling different from her peers evidenced by social isolation
    c. Risk for suicide related to new diagnosis of diabetes mellitus
    d. Risk-prone health behavior related to denial of seriousness of her illness evidenced by refusal to follow diet and take medication

11. Trauma-informed care is a philosophical approach that includes which of the following principles? (Select all that apply.)
    a. Nurses need to be aware of the potential for trauma in any patient and provide care that minimizes the risk of revictimization or retraumatization.
    b. Medications need to be given before any other interventions are considered.
    c. Trauma-informed care highlights the importance of providing care that protects the physical, psychological, and emotional safety of the patient.
    d. Trauma-informed care is based on the principle that traumas are not correlated with depression or increased risk for suicide.

TEST YOUR CRITICAL THINKING SKILLS

Alice, age 48, underwent a mastectomy of the right breast after her mammogram revealed a lump that proved to be malignant when biopsied. Since her surgery 6 weeks ago, Alice has refused to see any of her friends. She stays in her bedroom, speaks to her husband only when he speaks first, is having difficulty sleeping, and eats very little. She refuses to look at the mastectomy scar and has refused to see the Reach to Recovery representative who has tried several times to help fit her with a prosthesis. Her husband is very worried about her and spoke to the family doctor, who recommended a psychiatrist. Alice has been admitted to the psychiatric unit with a diagnosis of adjustment disorder with depressed mood.

Answer the following questions about Alice:

1. What would be the primary nursing diagnosis for Alice?
2. Describe a short-term goal and a long-term goal for Alice.
3. Discuss a priority nursing intervention in working with Alice.

References

Aetna Healthcare. (2017). *Clinical policy bulletin: Eye movement desensitization and Reprocessing (EMDR) therapy.* Retrieved from http://www.aetna.com/cpb/medical/data/500_599/0583.html

American Psychiatric Association (APA). (2000). *Diagnostic and statistical manual of mental disorders, Fourth Edition, Text Revision (DSM-IV-TR).* Washington, DC: Author.

American Psychiatric Association (APA). (2013). *Diagnostic and statistical manual of mental disorders* (5th ed.). Washington, DC: Author.

Department of Veterans Affairs. (2016). *How common is PTSD?* Retrieved from https://www.ptsd.va.gov/public/PTSD-overview/basics/how-common-is-ptsd.asp

EMDR International Association. (2018). *What is the actual EMDR session like?* Retrieved from https://emdria.site-ym.com/?120

Feder, A., Parides, M. K., Murrough, J. W., Perez, A. M., Morgan, J. E., Saxena, S., . . . Charney, D. S. (2014). Efficacy of intravenous ketamine for treatment of chronic posttraumatic stress disorder: A randomized clinical trial. *JAMA Psychiatry, 71*(6), 681–688. doi:10.1001/jamapsychiatry.2014.62

Frances, A. (2015). "We should live"—Surviving after catastrophic death. *Psychiatric Times.* Retrieved from http://www.psychi

atrictimes.com/major-depressive-disorder/we-should-live-surviving-after-catastrophic-death

Friedman, M. J. (1996). PTSD diagnosis and treatment for mental health clinicians. *Community Mental Health Journal, 32*(2), 173–189.

Friedman, M. J., Resick, P. A., Bryant, R. A., Strain, J., Horowitz, M., & Spiegel, D. (2011). Classification of trauma and stressor-related disorders in DSM-5. *Depression and Anxiety, 28*(9), 737–749.

Herdman, T. H., & Kamitsuru, S. (Eds.). (2018). *NANDA-I nursing diagnoses: Definitions and classification, 2018–2020.* New York, NY: Thieme.

Hopper, E. K., Bassuk, E. L., & Olivet, J. (2010). Shelter from the storm: Trauma-informed care in homelessness services settings. *Open Health Services and Policy Journal, 3,* 80–100.

Jeffreys, M. (2018). *Clinician's guide to medications for PTSD.* Retrieved from http://www.ptsd.va.gov/professional/treatment/overview/clinicians-guide-to-medications-for-ptsd.asp

Katzman, J. W., & Geppert, C. M. (2017). Adjustment disorders. In B. J. Sadock, V. A. Sadock, & P. Ruiz (Eds.), *Comprehensive textbook of psychiatry* (10th ed., pp. 2116–2125). New York, NY: Wolters Kluwer.

Lanius, U. (2013). *Neurobiology and treatment of traumatic dissociation.* Retrieved from http://www.isst-d.org/downloads/AnnualConference/2013/Baltimore2013handout.pdf

Sadock, B. J., Sadock, V. A., & Ruiz, P. (2015). *Synopsis of psychiatry: Behavioral sciences/clinical psychiatry* (11th ed.). Philadelphia, PA: Wolters Kluwer.

Shapiro, F. (2007). EMDR and case conceptualization from an adaptive information processing perspective. In F. Shapiro, F. W. Kaslow, & L. Maxfield (Eds.), *Handbook of EMDR and family therapy processes* (pp. 3–34). Hoboken, NJ: John Wiley & Sons.

Substance Abuse and Mental Health Services Administration (SAMHSA) (2018). *Trauma-informed care and alternatives to seclusion and restraint.* Retrieved from https://www.samhsa.gov/nctic/trauma-interventions

UPMC, Center for Integrative Medicine. (2018). *Eye movement desensitization and reprocessing.* Retrieved from http://www.upmc.com/Services/integrative-medicine/services/Pages/eye-movement.aspx

Valentino, R. J., & Van Bockstaele, E. (2015). Endogenous opioids: The downside to opposing stress. *Neurobiology of Stress, 1,* 23–32. doi:http://dx.doi.org/10.1016/j.ynstr.2014.09.006

Venes, D. (Ed.). (2017). *Taber's medical dictionary* (23rd ed.). Philadelphia, PA: F.A. Davis.

WebMD. (2017). *EMDR: Eye movement desensitization and reprocessing.* Retrieved from https://www.webmd.com/mental-health/emdr-what-is-it#1

Classical Reference

Epstein, S. (1991). Beliefs and symptoms in maladaptive resolutions of the traumatic neurosis. In D. Ozer, J. M. Healy, Jr., & A. J. Stewart (Eds.), *Perspectives on personality* (Vol. 3). London, England: Jessica Kingsley.

20

Somatic Symptom and Dissociative Disorders

CORE CONCEPTS

Amnesia

Dissociation

CHAPTER OUTLINE

Objectives

Homework Assignment

Introduction

Historical Aspects

Epidemiological Statistics

Application of the Nursing Process

Treatment Modalities

Summary and Key Points

Review Questions

Implications of Research for
   Evidence-Based Practice

Test Your Critical Thinking Skills

Movie Connections

KEY TERMS

abreaction

amnesia, generalized

amnesia, localized

amnesia, selective

anosmia

aphonia

depersonalization

derealization

factitious disorder

fugue

integration

Munchausen syndrome

primary gain

pseudocyesis

secondary gain

somatization

tertiary gain

OBJECTIVES

After reading this chapter, the student will be able to:

1. Discuss historical aspects and epidemiological statistics related to somatic symptom and dissociative disorders.
2. Describe various types of somatic symptom and dissociative disorders and identify symptomatology associated with each; use this information in patient assessment.
3. Identify predisposing factors in the development of somatic symptom and dissociative disorders.

4. Formulate nursing diagnoses and goals of care for patients with somatic symptom and dissociative disorders.
5. Describe appropriate nursing interventions for behaviors associated with somatic symptom and dissociative disorders.
6. Evaluate the nursing care of patients with somatic symptom and dissociative disorders.
7. Discuss various modalities relevant to treatment of somatic symptom and dissociative disorders.

Introduction

Disorders with primarily somatic symptoms are characterized by physical symptoms, suggesting medical disease, but without demonstrable organic pathology. For this reason, most clients with a somatic symptom or related disorder are seen in primary care and hospital settings rather than in mental healthcare settings. It is important to note that in cases in which modern medicine cannot determine the existence of pathophysiology to explain a client's symptoms, the lack of pathophysiology is not sufficient to diagnose the client with a mental illness. Somatic symptoms and related disorders are classified as mental disorders, according to the *Diagnostic and Statistical Manual of Mental Disorders, Fifth Edition (DSM-5),* because the excessive focus on somatic symptoms is beyond any medical explanation *and* because somatic symptoms cause significant distress and impairment in one's functioning (American Psychiatric Association [APA], 2013).

The *DSM-5* identifies a specific disorder called *somatic symptom disorder* and several related disorders, including *illness anxiety disorder, conversion disorder, factitious disorders, psychological factors affecting other medical conditions, and others* (APA, 2013). Their common focus is distress and impairment secondary to somatic symptoms, as described previously. The prevalence of somatic symptom disorder in primary care settings is estimated to be as high as 11 percent, and prevalence of hypochondriasis (no longer a diagnostic category in the *DSM-5* but similar to *illness anxiety disorder)* is estimated to be 4 to 6 percent (Yates, 2014). The prevalence of conversion disorders, based on studies of hospital psychiatric consults, is estimated to be as high as 15 percent. But estimates vary widely, which highlights the difficulties associated with consensus about diagnosing and reporting of these conditions.

Dissociative disorders are defined by a disruption in psychobiological functions that would otherwise be integrated aspects of experience and cognition including memory, identity, consciousness, perception, behavior, emotion, body representation, and motor control (Lowenstein, Frewen, & Lewis-Fernandez, 2017). Dissociative responses occur when anxiety becomes overwhelming and the personality becomes disorganized. Defense mechanisms that normally govern consciousness, identity, and memory break down, and behavior occurs with little or no participation on the part of the conscious personality. Types of dissociative disorders described by the *DSM-5* include *depersonalization-derealization disorder, dissociative amnesia, dissociative identity disorder, and others.*

This chapter focuses on disorders characterized by severe anxiety that has been repressed and is being expressed in the form of physical symptoms, fear of illness, and dissociative behaviors. Historical and epidemiological statistics are presented. Predisposing factors that have been implicated in the etiology of these responses provide a framework for studying the dynamics of somatic symptom and dissociative disorders. An explanation of the symptomatology of these disorders is presented as background knowledge for assessing the patient, and nursing care is described in the context of the nursing process. Additional treatment modalities are explored.

Historical Aspects

Historically, somatic symptom disorders were identified as *hysterical neuroses.* The concept of hysteria is at least 4,000 years old and probably originated in Egypt. The name has been in use since the time of Hippocrates.

Over the years, symptoms of hysterical neuroses have been associated with witchcraft, demonology, and sorcery; dysfunction of the nervous system; and unexpressed emotion. They have also historically been viewed as primarily an affliction of women. Critics have argued that the depiction of women as prone to hysteria is not only sexist but has interfered, at times, with women receiving adequate medical evaluation for symptoms. Somatic symptom disorders are thought to occur in response to repressed severe anxiety. Freud observed that, under hypnosis, clients with hysterical neurosis could recall past memories and emotional experiences that would relieve their symptoms. This observation led to his proposal that unexpressed emotion can be "converted" into physical symptoms.

CORE CONCEPT

Dissociation

An unconscious defense mechanism in which there is separation of identity, memory, and cognition from affect; the segregation of ideas and memories about oneself from their emotional and historical underpinnings (Sadock, Sadock, & Ruiz, 2015; Venes, 2017).

Freud (1962) viewed dissociation as a type of repression, an active defense mechanism used to remove threatening or unacceptable mental contents from conscious awareness. He also described the defense of splitting of the ego in the management of incompatible mental contents. Despite that the study of dissociative processes dates back to the 19th century, scientists know remarkably little about the phenomena. Questions still remain unanswered: Are dissociative disorders psychopathological processes or ego-protective devices? Are dissociative processes under voluntary control, or are they a totally unconscious effort? In either case, they may serve to reduce a person's awareness and anxiety associated with events that are perceived as extremely stressful.

Whereas symptoms such as dissociation are an unconscious defense mechanism, some individuals consciously fabricate symptoms. The syndrome of fabricating symptoms for emotional gain was first described by Richard Asher in 1951. He described a pattern of behavior in which individuals fabricated or embellished their histories and signs and symptoms of illness. He termed this condition **Munchausen syndrome** after Baron Friedrich Hieronymus Freiherr von Munchhausen, a German cavalry officer and nobleman who was known for his fabricated stories and fanciful exaggerations about himself (Asher, 1951). Currently, the *DSM-5* describes these syndromes as **factitious disorders.** These include *factitious disorders imposed on self,* or when someone deceptively induces injury or illness in another person, *factitious disorder imposed on another.*

Epidemiological Statistics

The prevalence of somatic symptom disorder is estimated to be from 0.1 to 11.6 percent (Yates, 2014). Although historically this disorder was thought to be more prevalent in women, Sadock et al. (2015) identify it as a disorder that affects men and women equally. The *DSM-5* (APA, 2013) suggests that the higher reported prevalence of this disorder in women may be related to the fact that females tend to report somatic symptoms more often than males.

Lifetime prevalence rates of conversion disorder vary widely. Statistics within the general population range from 5 to 30 percent. The disorder occurs more frequently in women than in men and more frequently in adolescents and young adults than in other age groups. A higher prevalence exists in lower socioeconomic groups, rural populations, among those with less education, and among military personnel who have been exposed to combat situations (Sadock et al., 2015).

The prevalence of illness anxiety disorder, which along with somatic symptom disorder replaces hypochondriasis in the *DSM-5*, is especially difficult to establish because this disorder is new in the *DSM-5*. The best estimate is based on data about the prevalence of hypochondriasis, which is identified at between 3 and 8 percent (APA, 2013). Some people who were previously diagnosed with hypochondriasis might better meet diagnostic criteria for somatic symptom disorder under this new classification. There are similarities in these two disorders, but the distinguishing feature between illness anxiety disorder and somatic symptom disorder is that in somatic symptom disorder the primary symptom is significant somatic sensations, and in illness anxiety disorder there are few to no somatic symptoms but anxiety or fear about having or acquiring an illness is a primary concern. More research is needed to better understand the epidemiological statistics for each of these disorders. Hypochondriasis was relabeled as illness anxiety disorder, at least in part, to eliminate myths and stigmas associated with the former diagnosis (Dimsdale, 2015). Illness anxiety disorder is equally common among men and women, and onset most commonly occurs in early adulthood. Data on the prevalence of factitious disorder are limited, so the frequency of the disorder is unknown. Estimates based on samples of hospital patients identify that about 1 percent meet criteria for factitious disorder (APA, 2013). Factitious disorder imposed on another is most often perpetrated by mothers against infants, and it accounts for less than 0.04 percent of reported cases of child abuse in the United States (Sadock et al., 2015).

Dissociative syndromes, although often portrayed in fictional media, are statistically quite rare. However, when they do occur, they may present very dramatic clinical pictures of severe disturbance in normal personality functioning. Dissociative amnesia occurs most frequently under conditions of war or during natural disasters. In recent years, there has been an increase in the number of reported cases, possibly attributed to increased awareness of the phenomenon and identification of cases that were previously undiagnosed. It appears to be equally common in men and women. Dissociative amnesia can occur at any age but is difficult to diagnose in children because it is easily confused with inattention or oppositional behavior.

Estimates of the prevalence of dissociative identity disorder (DID), previously called *multiple personality disorder,* also vary. The disorder occurs from five to nine times more frequently in women than in men (Sadock et al., 2015). Onset likely occurs in childhood, although manifestations of the disorder may not be recognized until late adolescence or early adulthood. The prevalence of severe episodes of depersonalization-derealization disorder is unknown. Transient symptoms or brief episodes are not uncommon in the general population and may occur at some time in as many as one-half of all adults, particularly when under severe psychosocial stress; when sleep deprived; during travel to unfamiliar places; or when intoxicated with hallucinogens, marijuana, or alcohol. Symptoms usually begin in adolescence or early adulthood. The disorder is chronic with periods of remission and exacerbation. The incidence of depersonalization-derealization disorder is high under conditions of sustained traumatization, such as in military combat or prisoner-of-war camps. It has also been reported in many individuals who endure near-death experiences.

Application of the Nursing Process

Background Assessment Data: Types of Somatic Symptom Disorders

Somatic Symptom Disorder

Somatic symptom disorder is a syndrome of multiple somatic symptoms that cannot be explained medically and are associated with psychosocial distress and long-term seeking of assistance from healthcare professionals. Symptoms may be vague, dramatized, or exaggerated in their presentation, and an excessive amount of time and energy is devoted to worry and concern about the symptoms. Individuals with somatic symptom disorder are so convinced that their symptoms are related to organic pathology that they adamantly reject, and are often irritated by, any implication that stress or psychosocial factors play any role in their condition. The disorder is chronic, with symptoms beginning before age 30. Anxiety and depression are frequent comorbidities, and, consequently, the disorder is associated with an increased risk for suicide attempts (Yates, 2014).

Somatic symptom disorder usually runs a fluctuating course with periods of remission and exacerbation. Clients often receive medical care from several physicians, sometimes concurrently, leading to the possibility of dangerous combinations of treatments. They tend to seek relief through overmedicating with prescribed analgesics or antianxiety agents. Drug abuse and dependence are common complications of somatic symptom disorder. The *DSM-5* diagnostic criteria for somatic symptom disorder are presented in Box 20–1.

Illness Anxiety Disorder

Illness anxiety disorder may be defined as an unrealistic or inaccurate interpretation of physical symptoms or sensations, leading to preoccupation and fear of having a serious disease. The fear becomes disabling and persists despite appropriate reassurance that no organic pathology can be detected. Symptoms may be minimal or absent, but the individual is highly anxious about and suspicious of the presence of an undiagnosed, serious medical illness (APA, 2013).

Individuals with illness anxiety disorder are extremely conscious of bodily sensations and changes and may become convinced that a rapid heart rate indicates they have heart disease or that a small sore is skin cancer. They are profoundly preoccupied with their bodies and are totally aware of even the slightest change in feeling or sensation. Their response to these small changes, however, is usually unrealistic and exaggerated.

Some individuals with illness anxiety disorder have a long history of "doctor shopping" and are convinced that they are not receiving the proper care. Others avoid seeking medical assistance because to do so would increase their anxiety to intolerable levels. Psychiatric comorbidities are common, including generalized anxiety disorder, depression,

---

BOX 20–1 **Diagnostic Criteria for Somatic Symptom Disorder**

A. One or more somatic symptoms that are distressing or result in significant disruption in daily life.
B. Excessive thoughts, feelings, or behaviors related to the somatic symptoms or associated health concerns as manifested by at least one of the following:
   1. Disproportionate and persistent thoughts about the seriousness of one's symptoms.
   2. Persistently high level of anxiety about health or symptoms.
   3. Excessive time and energy devoted to these symptoms or health concerns.
C. Although any one symptom may not be continuously present, the state of being symptomatic is persistent (typically more than 6 months).

Specify if:

With predominant pain (the somatic symptoms predominantly involve pain)

Persistent (a persistent course is characterized by severe symptoms, marked impairment, and long duration [more than 6 months])

Specify current severity:

Mild (only one of the symptoms specified in Criterion B is fulfilled)

Moderate (two or more of the symptoms specified in Criterion B are fulfilled)

Severe (two or more of the symptoms specified in Criterion B are fulfilled, plus there are multiple somatic complaints [or one very severe somatic symptom])

Reprinted with permission from American Psychiatric Association. (2013). Diagnostic and statistical manual of mental disorders (5th ed.). Washington, DC: American Psychiatric Publishing.

BOX 20–2 **Diagnostic Criteria for Illness Anxiety Disorder**

A. Preoccupation with having or acquiring a serious illness.
B. Somatic symptoms are not present or, if present, are only mild in intensity. If another medical condition is present or there is a high risk for developing a medical condition (e.g., strong family history is present), the preoccupation is clearly excessive or disproportionate.
C. There is a high level of anxiety about health, and the individual is easily alarmed about personal health status.
D. The individual performs excessive health-related behaviors (e.g., repeatedly checks his or her body for signs of illness) or exhibits maladaptive avoidance (e.g., avoids doctors' appointments and hospitals).
E. Illness preoccupation has been present for at least 6 months, but the specific illness that is feared may change over that period of time.
F. The illness-related preoccupation is not better explained by another mental disorder, such as somatic symptom disorder, panic disorder, generalized anxiety disorder, body dysmorphic disorder, obsessive-compulsive disorder, or delusional disorder, somatic type.

Specify whether:

Care-seeking type: Medical care, including physician visits or undergoing tests and procedures, is frequently used.

Care-avoidant type: Medical care is rarely used.

Reprinted with permission from American Psychiatric Association. (2013). Diagnostic and statistical manual of mental disorders (5th ed.). Washington, DC: American Psychiatric Publishing.

---

somatization disorder, and panic disorder; in addition, patients with illness anxiety disorder are three times more likely to have a concurrent personality disorder (Soreff, 2018). Preoccupation with the fear of serious disease may interfere with social or occupational functioning. Some individuals are able to function appropriately on the job, however, while limiting their physical complaints to nonwork time.

Individuals with illness anxiety disorder are so apprehensive and fearful that they become alarmed at the slightest intimation of serious illness. Even reading about a disease or hearing that someone they know has been diagnosed with an illness precipitates alarm on their part. Both somatic symptom disorder and illness anxiety disorder have features similar to the now removed hypochondriasis, but the

DSM-5 identifies two separate disorders to distinguish between individuals who are primarily preoccupied with perceived physical symptoms (somatic symptom disorder) and those who are primarily focused on fear of illness in general (illness anxiety disorder). The *DSM-5* diagnostic criteria for illness anxiety disorder are presented in Box 20–2.

Conversion Disorder (Functional Neurological Symptom Disorder)

Conversion disorder is a loss of or change in body function that cannot be explained by any known medical disorder or pathophysiological mechanism. Although there is a psychological component involved in the initiation, exacerbation, or perpetuation of the symptom, it may or may not be obvious or easily identifiable.

Conversion symptoms affect voluntary motor or sensory functioning suggestive of neurological disease. Examples include paralysis, **aphonia** (inability to produce voice), seizures, coordination disturbance, difficulty swallowing, urinary retention, akinesia, blindness, deafness, double vision, **anosmia** (inability to perceive smell), loss of pain sensation, and hallucinations. Abnormal limb shaking with impaired or loss of consciousness that resembles epileptic seizures is another type of conversion disorder symptom that is referred to as *psychogenic* or *nonepileptic seizures*. **Pseudocyesis** (false pregnancy) is a conversion symptom and may represent a strong desire to be pregnant.

The *DSM-5* clarifies that "although the diagnosis [of conversion disorder] requires that the symptom is not explained by neurological disease, it should not be made simply because results from investigations are normal or because the symptom is 'bizarre.' There must be clear evidence of incompatibility with neurological disease" (APA, 2013, p. 319). For example, a client who appears to be having a seizure but has a normal electroencephalogram, whose eyes are closed and resist opening, and who has no urinary incontinence may be diagnosed with conversion disorder. It is likely that multiple factors play a role in the etiology.

Although not diagnostic of a conversion disorder, an associated symptom is the client's apparent indifference to symptoms that seem very serious to others. This feature is termed *la belle indifference*. Most symptoms of conversion disorder resolve within a few weeks. About 20 percent of individuals with the diagnosis have a relapse within 1 year. The *DSM-5* states that the prognosis is better when the symptoms are of short duration, when the client accepts the diagnosis, when there is absence of comorbid physical disease, and when the client has no identified maladaptive personality traits (APA, 2013). The *DSM-5* diagnostic criteria for conversion disorder are presented in Box 20–3.

Psychological Factors Affecting Other Medical Conditions

Psychological factors play a role in virtually any medical condition. However, in this disorder, it is evident that psychological or behavioral factors are clearly implicated in the development, exacerbation, or delayed recovery from a medical condition.

Factitious Disorder

Factitious disorders involve conscious, intentional feigning of physical or psychological symptoms. Individuals with factitious disorder pretend to be ill in order to receive emotional care and support

---

> ## BOX 20–3 Diagnostic Criteria for Conversion Disorder (Functional Neurological Symptom Disorder)
>
> A. One or more symptoms of altered voluntary motor or sensory function.
> B. Clinical findings provide evidence of incompatibility between the symptom and recognized neurological or medical conditions.
> C. The symptom or deficit is not better explained by another medical or mental disorder.
> D. The symptom or deficit causes clinically significant distress or impairment in social, occupational, or other important areas of functioning or warrants medical evaluation.
>
> *Specify symptom type:*
> **With weakness or paralysis**
> **With abnormal movement**
> **With swallowing symptoms**
> **With speech symptom**
> **With attacks or seizures**
> **With anesthesia or sensory loss**
> **With special sensory symptom**
> **With mixed symptoms**
>
> *Specify if:*
> **Acute episode**
> **Persistent**
>
> *Specify if:*
> **With psychological stressor**
> **Without psychological stressor**

Reprinted with permission from American Psychiatric Association. (2013). Diagnostic and statistical manual of mental disorders (5th ed.). Washington, DC: American Psychiatric Publishing.

---

commonly associated with the role of patient. Even though the behaviors are deliberate and intentional, there may be an associated compulsive element that diminishes personal control. Individuals with this disorder characteristically become skilled at presenting their "symptoms" so well that they successfully gain admission to hospitals and treatment centers. To accomplish this, they may aggravate existing symptoms, induce new ones, or even inflict painful injuries on themselves (Sadock et al., 2015). The disorder has also been identified as Munchausen syndrome, and symptoms may be psychological or physical, or a combination of both.

The disorder may be imposed on oneself or on another person (previously called *factitious disorder by proxy*). In the latter case, physical symptoms are intentionally imposed on a person who is under the care of the perpetrator. Diagnosis of factitious disorder can be very difficult because individuals become very inventive in their quest to produce symptoms. "The most common case of factitious disorder by proxy involves a mother who deceives medical personnel into believing her child is ill" (Sadock et al., 2015, p. 492). This deception may be accomplished by lying about the child's medical history, manipulating data such as by contaminating laboratory samples, and inducing illness or injury in the child through use of substances or other physical assaults.

Predisposing Factors Associated With Somatic Symptom and Related Disorders

Genetic

Escobar and Dimsdale (2017) report that somatic symptom and related disorders should be conceptualized as a complex interaction of genetic vulnerabilities; history of trauma; learning; environmental, psychological, and behavioral influences. Although the specific genetic vulnerabilities are not well understood the authors report that there is no evidence of familial aggregation in somatic symptom disorder.

Biochemical

Studies have indicated that tryptophan catabolism may be abnormal in clients with somatic symptom disorders (Yates, 2014). Decreased levels of serotonin and endorphins may play a role in the sensation of pain.

Neuroanatomical

Brain dysfunction has been proposed by some researchers as a factor in factitious disorders (Sadock et al., 2015). The hypothesis is that impairment in information processing contributes to the aberrant behaviors associated with the disorder. Sadock and associates (2015) report that brain imaging studies have found hypometabolism in the dominant hemisphere, hypermetabolism in the nondominant hemisphere, and impaired hemispheric communication in conversion disorders (p. 474).

Psychodynamic

Some psychodynamicists view illness anxiety disorder as an ego defense mechanism. Physical complaints are the expression of low self-esteem and feelings of worthlessness because it is easier to feel that something is wrong with the body than to feel that something is wrong with the self. Another psychodynamic view of illness anxiety disorder (as well as somatic

symptom disorder, predominantly pain) is related to a defense against guilt. The individual views the self as "bad" because of real or imagined past misconduct and views physical suffering as the deserved punishment required for atonement. This view has also been related to individuals with factitious disorders.

The psychodynamic theory of conversion disorder proposes that emotions associated with a traumatic event that the individual cannot express because of moral or ethical unacceptability are "converted" into physical symptoms. The unacceptable emotions are repressed and converted to a somatic symptom that is symbolic in some way of the original emotional trauma.

Another view suggests that individuals with factitious disorders were victims of child abuse or neglect. Frequent childhood hospitalizations provided a supportive caring that was absent in the child's family; in adulthood, the individual attempts to recapture the only positive support he or she may have known by seeking out the environment in which it was received as a child. Regarding factitious disorder imposed on another, Sadock and associates (2015) have stated, "One apparent purpose of the behavior is for the caretaker to indirectly assume the sick role; another is to be relieved of the caretaking role by having the child hospitalized" (p. 492).

Escobar and Dimsdale (2017) report that up to two-thirds of patients in primary care settings complain of symptoms for which no disease entity can be identified and up to two-thirds of those patients meet criteria for a major psychiatric disorder. The authors suggest that this reinforces the belief that individuals with psychiatric disorders more typically present with physical rather than psychological complaints in primary care settings.

Family Dynamics

Another view suggests that in families who have difficulty resolving conflicts, a child's illness creates a shift in focus from the unresolved conflicts to the child's illness. This provides a reprieve from the instability posed by issues that the family cannot confront openly, and the child in turn receives positive reinforcement for the illness. **Somatization** becomes reinforced as a way to shift the focus away from family issues and discord. The stabilization of the family achieved by somatizing is referred to as a **tertiary gain.**

Learning Theory

Somatic complaints are often reinforced when the sick role relieves the individual from the need to deal with a stressful situation, whether it be within society or within the family. The sick person learns that he or she may avoid stressful obligations; may postpone unwelcome challenges; is excused from troublesome duties (**primary gain**); becomes the prominent focus of attention because of the illness (**secondary gain**); or relieves conflict within the family as concern is shifted to the ill person and away from the real issue (tertiary gain). These types of positive reinforcement virtually guarantee repetition of the response.

Past experience with serious or life-threatening physical illness, either personal or that of close family members, can predispose an individual to illness anxiety disorder. Once an individual has experienced a threat to biological integrity, he or she may develop a fear of recurrence. The fear of recurring illness generates an exaggerated response to minor physical changes, leading to excessive anxiety and health concerns.

Background Assessment Data: Types of Dissociative Disorders

Dissociative Amnesia

CORE CONCEPT

Amnesia

Partial or total, permanent or transient loss of memory. The term is often applied to episodes during which patients forget recent events, although they may conduct themselves appropriately and after which no memory of the period persists. Such episodes may be caused by strokes, seizures, trauma, senility, alcoholism, or intoxication (Venes, 2017).

Dissociative amnesia is an inability to recall important personal information, usually of a traumatic or stressful nature, that is too extensive to be explained by ordinary forgetfulness and is not due to the direct effects of substance use or a neurological or other medical condition (APA, 2013). The *DSM-5* states that the most common types of dissociative amnesia are localized, selective, or generalized. Localized and selective amnesia are related to a specific stressful event that has occurred. For example, the individual with **localized amnesia** is unable to recall all incidents associated with a stressful event. It may be broader than just a single event, however, such as being unable to remember months or years of child abuse (APA, 2013). In **selective amnesia**, the individual can recall only certain incidents associated with a stressful event for a specific period after the event. In the **generalized** type, the individual has amnesia for his or her identity and total life history.

The individual with amnesia usually appears alert and may give no indication to observers that anything is wrong, although some clients may present with alterations in consciousness, with conversion symptoms, or in trance states. Clients suffering from amnesia are often brought to general hospital emergency departments by police who have found them wandering confusedly around the streets.

Onset of an amnestic episode usually follows severe psychosocial stress. Termination is typically abrupt and followed by complete recovery. Recurrences are unusual. A specific subtype of dissociative amnesia is *dissociative fugue*. Dissociative **fugue** is characterized by a sudden, unexpected travel away from the customary place of daily activities or by bewildered wandering with the inability to recall some or all of one's past. An individual in a fugue state may not be able to recall personal identity and sometimes assumes a new identity. The *DSM-5* diagnostic criteria for dissociative amnesia are presented in Box 20–4.

BOX 20–4 Diagnostic Criteria for Dissociative Amnesia

A. An inability to recall important autobiographical information, usually of a traumatic or stressful nature, that is inconsistent with ordinary forgetting. *Note*: Dissociative amnesia most often consists of localized or selective amnesia for a specific event or events; or generalized amnesia for identity and life history.

B. The symptoms cause clinically significant distress or impairment in social, occupational, or other important areas of functioning.

C. The disturbance is not attributable to the physiological effects of a substance (e.g., alcohol or other drug of abuse, a medication) or a neurological or other medical condition (e.g., partial complex seizures, transient global amnesia, sequelae of a closed head injury/traumatic brain injury, other neurological condition).

D. The disturbance is not better explained by dissociative identity disorder, posttraumatic stress disorder, acute stress disorder, somatic symptom disorder, or major or mild neurocognitive disorder.

Specify if:

With dissociative fugue (Apparently purposeful travel or bewildered wandering that is associated with amnesia for identity or for other important **autobiographical** information.)

Reprinted with permission from American Psychiatric Association. (2013). Diagnostic and statistical manual of mental disorders (5th ed.). Washington, DC: American Psychiatric Publishing.

Dissociative Identity Disorder

DID was formerly called *multiple personality disorder.* This disorder is characterized by the existence of two or more personality states in a single individual. These different personality states are sometimes referred to as *alter identities* or just *alters.* Only one of the personalities is evident at any given moment, and one of them is dominant most of the time over the course of the disorder. Each personality is unique and composed of a complex set of memories, behavior patterns, and social relationships that surface at different times. Transition from one personality state to another may be sudden or gradual and is sometimes quite dramatic. Sadock and associates (2015) state, "Patients often describe a profound sense of concretized internal division or personified internal conflicts between parts of themselves. . . . These parts may have proper names or be designated by their predominant affect or function, for example, 'the angry one' or 'the wife'" (p. 460).

DID has been a controversial disorder that gained attention after the 1976 movie *Sybil* portrayed the presumed true story of a woman who reported having 16 different personalities. Diagnosis of this disorder increased significantly in the years following the movie, and in 1980, the APA formally recognized the disorder as a psychiatric illness (Haberman, 2014). Since then, critics have reported that both patient "Sybil" and her psychiatrist acknowledged her case as much fabrication. Dr. David Speigel, a psychiatrist who was involved in promoting the APA's adoption of DID as the preferred term for this condition, is quoted in Haberman's review (2014) as saying "[the term] multiple personality carries with it the implication that they really have more than one personality. The problem is fragmentation of identity, not that you really are 12 people . . . that you have not more than one but less than one personality."

Although questions persist about whether this disorder has been overdiagnosed, there are certainly individuals who present with this condition of fragmented identity, and most have been victims of severe childhood physical and sexual abuse. It is not uncommon for clients with DID to also manifest with symptoms of other dissociative disorders, such as amnesia, fugue states, depersonalization, and derealization (Sadock et al., 2015). Generally, there is amnesia for the events that took place when another personality was being manifested, and clients report "gaps" in autobiographical histories, "lost time" or "blackouts." They may "wake up" in unfamiliar situations with no idea of where they are, how they got there, or the identities of the people around them. They may be accused of lying when they deny remembering or being responsible for events or actions.

DID is not always incapacitating. Some individuals with DID maintain responsible positions, complete graduate degrees, and are successful spouses and parents before diagnosis and while in treatment. Before they are diagnosed with DID, many individuals are misdiagnosed with depression, borderline and antisocial personality disorders, schizophrenia, epilepsy, or bipolar disorder. The *DSM-5* diagnostic criteria for DID are presented in Box 20–5.

Depersonalization-Derealization Disorder

Depersonalization-derealization disorder is characterized by a temporary change in the quality of self-awareness, which often takes the form of feelings of unreality, changes in body image, feelings of detachment from the environment, or a sense of observing oneself from outside the body. For example, a soldier in recalling an experience in combat describes that he saw himself observing himself

---

BOX 20–5 Diagnostic Criteria for Dissociative Identity Disorder

A. Disruption of identity characterized by two or more distinct personality states, which may be described in some cultures as an experience of possession. The disruption in identity involves marked discontinuity in sense of self and sense of agency, accompanied by related alterations in affect, behavior, consciousness, memory, perception, cognition, and/or sensory-motor functioning. These signs and symptoms may be observed by others or reported by the individual.

B. Recurrent gaps in the recall of everyday events, important personal information, and/or traumatic events that are inconsistent with ordinary forgetting.

C. The symptoms cause clinically significant distress or impairment in social, occupational, or other important areas of functioning.

D. The disturbance is not a normal part of a broadly accepted cultural or religious practice. *Note:* In children, the symptoms are not better explained by imaginary playmates or other fantasy play.

E. The symptoms are not attributable to the physiological effects of a substance (e.g., blackouts or chaotic behavior during alcohol intoxication) or another medical condition (e.g., complex partial seizures).

Reprinted with permission from American Psychiatric Association. (2013). Diagnostic and statistical manual of mental disorders (5th ed.). Washington, DC: American Psychiatric Publishing.

from a distance and wondered what he would do if *he* were in that situation. **Depersonalization** (a disturbance in the perception of oneself) is differentiated from **derealization,** which describes an alteration in the perception of the external environment. Both of these phenomena also occur in a variety of psychiatric illnesses, such as schizophrenia, depression, anxiety states, and neurocognitive disorders. As previously stated, the symptoms of depersonalization and derealization are very common. It is estimated that approximately half of all adults have experienced transient episodes of the symptoms. They are also identified as the third-most common reported psychiatric symptoms after depression and anxiety (Sadock et al., 2015). Diagnosis of the disorder is made only if the symptoms cause significant distress or impairment in functioning.

The *DSM-5* describes this disorder as the persistence or recurrence of episodes of depersonalization or derealization, or both (APA, 2013). There may be a mechanical or dreamlike feeling or a belief that the body's physical characteristics have changed. If derealization is present, objects in the environment are perceived as altered in size or shape. Other people in the environment may seem automated or mechanical.

These distorted perceptions are experienced as disturbing and often accompanied by anxiety, depression, fear of going insane, obsessive thoughts, somatic complaints, and an alteration in the subjective sense of time. The age of onset is typically late adolescence or early adulthood, and it is two to four times more common in women than in men (Sadock et al., 2015). The *DSM-5* diagnostic criteria for depersonalization-derealization disorder are presented in Box 20–6.

Predisposing Factors Associated With Dissociative Disorders

Genetics

The overwhelming majority of adults with DID (85 to 97 percent) have a history of physical and sexual abuse, and although genetic factors are being studied, preliminary research does not show evidence of a significant genetic contribution (Sadock et al., 2015).

Neurobiological

Some clinicians have suggested a possible correlation between neurological alterations and dissociative disorders. Although available information is inadequate, it is possible that dissociative amnesia may be related to neurophysiological dysfunction. Areas of the brain

---

BOX 20–6 Diagnostic Criteria for Depersonalization-Derealization Disorder

A. The presence of persistent or recurrent depersonalization, derealization, or both:
   1. **Depersonalization:** Experiences of unreality, detachment, or being an outside observer with respect to one's thoughts, feelings, sensations, body, or actions (e.g., perceptual alterations, distorted sense of time, unreal or absent self, emotional and/or physical numbing).
   2. **Derealization:** Experiences of unreality or detachment with respect to surroundings (e.g., individuals or objects are experienced as unreal, dreamlike, foggy, lifeless, or visually distorted).
B. During the depersonalization or derealization experiences, reality testing remains intact.
C. The symptoms cause clinically significant distress or impairment in social, occupational, or other important areas of functioning.
D. The disturbance is not attributable to the physiological effects of a substance (e.g., a drug of abuse, medication) or another medical condition (e.g., seizures).
E. The disturbance is not better explained by another mental disorder, such as schizophrenia, panic disorder, major depressive disorder, acute stress disorder, posttraumatic stress disorder, or another dissociative disorder.

Reprinted with permission from American Psychiatric Association. (2013). Diagnostic and statistical manual of mental disorders (5th ed.). Washington, DC: American Psychiatric Publishing.

---

that have been associated with memory include the hippocampus, amygdala, fornix, mammillary bodies, thalamus, and frontal cortex.

Depersonalization has been associated with migraines and with marijuana use; responds to selective serotonin reuptake inhibitors (SSRIs); and is seen in cases where L-tryptophan, a serotonin precursor, is depleted—these facts all suggest some level of serotonergic involvement in this dissociative symptom (Sadock et al., 2015). Some studies have suggested a possible link between DID and certain neurological conditions, such as temporal lobe epilepsy and severe migraine headaches. Electroencephalographic abnormalities have been observed in some clients with DID.

Psychodynamic Theory

Freud (1962) believed that dissociative behaviors occurred when individuals repressed distressing mental contents from conscious awareness. He believed that the unconscious was a dynamic entity in which repressed mental contents were stored and unavailable to conscious recall. Current psychodynamic explanations of dissociation are based on Freud's concepts. The repression of mental contents is believed to protect the client from extreme emotional pain triggered by either disturbing external circumstances or anxiety-provoking internal urges and feelings. In the case of depersonalization and derealization, the pain and anxiety are expressed as feelings of unreality or detachment from the environment of the painful situation.

Psychological Trauma

A growing body of evidence points to the etiology of dissociative disorders as a response to traumatic experiences that overwhelm the individual's capacity to cope by any means other than dissociation. In DID, these experiences are most often physical, sexual, or psychological abuse by a parent or significant other in the child's life. The most widely accepted explanation for DID is that it begins as a survival strategy that serves to help children cope with the horrifying sexual, physical, or psychological abuse and evolves into a fragmented identity as the victim struggles to meld conflicting aspects of personality into an integrated whole. Dissociative amnesia is frequently related to acute and extreme trauma but may also develop in the clinical presentation of DID. Dissociative amnesia is also often noted in response to combat trauma during wartimes.

Diagnosis and Outcome Identification

Nursing diagnoses are formulated from the data gathered during the assessment phase and with background knowledge regarding predisposing factors to the disorder. Table 20–1 presents a list of patient behaviors

TABLE 20–1	Assigning Nursing Diagnoses to Behaviors Commonly Associated With Somatic Symptom and Dissociative Disorders	
BEHAVIORS	**NURSING DIAGNOSES**
Verbalization of numerous physical complaints in the absence of any pathophysiological evidence; focus on the self and physical symptoms (somatic symptom disorder)	Ineffective coping; chronic pain
History of "doctor shopping" for evidence of organic pathology to substantiate physical symptoms; statements such as, "I don't know why the doctor put me on the psychiatric unit. I have a physical problem" (somatic symptom disorder)	Deficient knowledge (psychological causes for physical symptoms)
Preoccupation with and unrealistic interpretation of bodily signs and sensations (illness anxiety disorder)	Fear (of having a serious disease)
Loss or alteration in physical functioning without evidence of organic pathology (conversion disorder) Alteration in the perception or experience of the self or the environment (depersonalization-derealization disorder)	Disturbed sensory perception*
Need for assistance to carry out self-care activities such as eating, dressing, maintaining hygiene, and toileting due to alteration in physical functioning (conversion disorder)	Self-care deficit
History of numerous exacerbations of physical illness; inappropriate or exaggerated behaviors; denial of emotional problems (psychological factors affecting other medical conditions)	Deficient knowledge (psychological factors affecting medical condition); denial
Loss of memory (dissociative amnesia)	Impaired memory
Verbalizations of frustration over lack of control and dependence on others (dissociative amnesia)	Powerlessness
Unresolved grief; depression; self-blame associated with childhood abuse (DID)	Risk for suicide
Presence of more than one personality within the individual (DID)	Disturbed personality identity
Feigning of physical or psychological symptoms to gain attention (factitious disorder)	Ineffective coping

*This diagnosis has been resigned from the NANDA-I list of approved diagnoses. It is used in this instance because it is most compatible with the identified behaviors.

and the NANDA-I nursing diagnoses (Herdman & Kamitsuru, 2018) that correspond to those behaviors, which may be used in planning care for patients with somatic symptom and dissociative disorders.

Outcome Criteria

The following criteria may be used for measurement of outcomes in the care of the patient with somatic symptom and dissociative disorders.

The patient:

- Effectively uses adaptive coping strategies during stressful situations without resorting to physical symptoms (somatic symptom disorder).
- Interprets bodily sensations rationally, verbalizes understanding of the significance the irrational fear held for him or her, and has decreased the number and frequency of physical complaints (illness anxiety disorder and somatic symptom disorder).
- Is free of physical disability and verbalizes understanding of the possible correlation between the loss of or alteration in function and extreme emotional stress (conversion disorder).

- Recalls events associated with a traumatic or stressful situation (dissociative amnesia).
- Verbalizes the extreme anxiety that precipitated the dissociation (depersonalization- derealization disorder).
- Demonstrates more adaptive coping strategies to avert dissociative behaviors in the face of severe anxiety (depersonalization-derealization disorder).
- Verbalizes understanding of the existence of multiple personality states and the purposes they serve (dissociative identity disorder).
- Maintains a sense of reality during stressful situations (depersonalization-derealization disorder).

Planning and Implementation

Tables 20–2 and 20–3 provide plans of care for patients with somatic symptom disorders and dissociative disorders. Nursing diagnoses are presented along with outcome criteria, appropriate nursing interventions, and rationales for each.

Table 20–2 | CARE PLAN FOR THE PATIENT WITH A SOMATIC SYMPTOM DISORDER

NURSING DIAGNOSIS: INEFFECTIVE COPING/CHRONIC PAIN

RELATED TO: Repressed anxiety and unmet dependency needs

EVIDENCED BY: Verbalization of numerous physical complaints in the absence of any pathophysiological evidence; total focus on the self and physical symptoms

OUTCOME CRITERIA	NURSING INTERVENTIONS	RATIONALE
Short-Term Goal ■ Within (specified time), patient will verbalize understanding of correlation between physical symptoms and psychological problems. **Long-Term Goal** ■ By time of discharge from treatment, patient will demonstrate ability to cope with stress by means other than preoccupation with physical symptoms.	1. Monitor physician's ongoing assessments, laboratory reports, and other data to maintain assurance that possibility of organic pathology is clearly ruled out. Review findings with patient. 2. Recognize and accept that the physical complaint is real to the patient, even though no organic etiology can be identified. 3. Provide pain medication as prescribed by physician. 4. Identify gains that the physical symptoms are providing: increased dependency, attention, distraction from other problems. 5. Initially, fulfill the patient's most urgent dependency needs, but gradually withdraw attention to physical symptoms. Minimize time given in response to physical complaints.	1. Accurate medical assessment is vital for the provision of adequate and appropriate care. Honest explanation may help patient understand psychological implications. 2. Denial of the patient's feelings is nontherapeutic and interferes with establishment of a trusting relationship. 3. Patient comfort and safety are nursing priorities. 4. Identification of underlying motivation is important in assisting the patient with problem resolution. 5. Anxiety and maladaptive behaviors will increase if dependency needs are ignored initially. Gradual lack of positive reinforcement will discourage repetition of maladaptive behaviors.

Continued

Table 20–2 | CARE PLAN FOR THE PATIENT WITH A SOMATIC SYMPTOM DISORDER—cont'd

OUTCOME CRITERIA	NURSING INTERVENTIONS	RATIONALE
	6. Encourage patient to verbalize fears and anxieties. Explain that attention will be withdrawn if rumination about physical complaints begins. Follow through.	6. The possibility of organic pathology must always be considered. Failure to do so could jeopardize patient safety.
	7. Discuss possible alternative coping strategies patient may use in response to stress (e.g., relaxation exercises; physical activities; assertiveness skills). Give positive reinforcement for use of these alternatives.	7. Without consistency of limit setting, change will not occur.
	8. Help patient identify ways to achieve recognition from others without resorting to physical symptoms.	8. Patient may need help with problem-solving. Positive reinforcement encourages repetition.
		9. Positive recognition from others enhances self-esteem and minimizes the need for attention through maladaptive behaviors.

NURSING DIAGNOSIS: FEAR (OF HAVING A SERIOUS DISEASE)

RELATED TO: Past experience with life-threatening illness of self or significant others

EVIDENCED BY: Preoccupation with and unrealistic interpretation of bodily signs and sensations

OUTCOME CRITERIA	NURSING INTERVENTIONS	RATIONALE
Short-Term Goal ■ Patient will verbalize that fears associated with bodily sensations are irrational (within time limit deemed appropriate for specific individual). **Long-Term Goal** ■ Patient will interpret bodily sensations correctly.	1. Monitor physician's ongoing assessments and laboratory reports.	1. Organic pathology must be clearly ruled out.
	2. Refer all new physical complaints to physician.	2. To ignore all physical complaints could place patient's safety in jeopardy.
	3. Assess the function that patient's excessive concern is fulfilling for him or her (e.g., unfulfilled needs for dependency, nurturing, caring, attention, or control).	3. This information may provide insight into reasons for maladaptive behavior and provide direction for planning client care.
	4. Identify times during which preoccupation with physical symptoms is worse. Determine extent of correlation of physical complaints with times of increased anxiety.	4. Patient may be unaware of the psychosocial implications of the physical complaints. Knowledge of the relationship is the first step in the process for creating change.
	5. Convey empathy. Let patient know that you understand how a specific symptom may conjure up fears of previous life-threatening illness.	5. Unconditional acceptance and empathy promote a therapeutic nurse/client relationship.
	6. Initially provide patient a limited amount of time (e.g., 10 minutes each hour) to discuss physical concerns.	6. Because this has been his or her primary method of coping for so long, complete prohibition of this activity would likely raise patient's anxiety level significantly, further exacerbating the behavior.
	7. Help patient determine what techniques may be most useful for him or her to implement when fear and anxiety are exacerbated (e.g., relaxation techniques, mental imagery, thought-stopping techniques, physical exercise).	7. All of these techniques are effective to reduce anxiety and may assist patient in the transition from focusing on fear of physical illness to the discussion of honest feelings.

Table 20–2 | CARE PLAN FOR THE PATIENT WITH A SOMATIC SYMPTOM DISORDER–cont'd

OUTCOME CRITERIA	NURSING INTERVENTIONS	RATIONALE
	8. Gradually increase the limit on amount of time spent each hour in discussing physical concerns. If patient violates the limits, withdraw attention.	8. Lack of positive reinforcement may help to extinguish maladaptive behavior.
	9. Facilitate patient discussion of feelings associated with fear of serious illness.	9. Verbalization of feelings in a nonthreatening environment facilitates expression and resolution of disturbing emotional issues. When the patient can express feelings directly, there is less need to express them through physical symptoms.
	10. Role-play the patient's plan for dealing with the fear the next time it assumes control and before anxiety becomes disabling.	10. Anxiety and fears are minimized when patient has achieved a degree of comfort through practicing a plan for dealing with stressful situations in the future.

NURSING DIAGNOSIS: DISTURBED SENSORY PERCEPTION

RELATED TO: Repressed severe anxiety

EVIDENCED BY: Loss or alteration in physical functioning, without evidence of organic pathology

OUTCOME CRITERIA	NURSING INTERVENTIONS	RATIONALE
Short-Term Goal ■ Patient will verbalize understanding of emotional problems as a contributing factor to the alteration in physical functioning (within time limit appropriate for specific individual). **Long-Term Goal** ■ Patient will demonstrate recovery of lost or altered function.	1. Monitor physician's ongoing assessments, laboratory reports, and other data to ensure that possibility of organic pathology is clearly ruled out.	1. Failure to do so may jeopardize patient safety.
	2. Identify primary or secondary gains that the physical symptom may be providing (e.g., increased dependency, attention, protection from experiencing a stressful event).	2. Primary and secondary gains are often etiological factors and may be used to assist in problem resolution.
	3. Do not focus on the disability and encourage patient to be as independent as possible. Intervene only when patient requires assistance.	3. Positive reinforcement would encourage continual use of the maladaptive response for secondary gains, such as dependency.
	4. Maintain nonjudgmental attitude when providing assistance to the patient. The physical symptom is not within the patient's conscious control and is very real to him or her.	4. A judgmental attitude interferes with the nurse's ability to establish trust and provide therapeutic care for the patient.
	5. Identify the expectation and importance of patient attending therapeutic activities. Withdraw attention if patient continues to focus on physical limitations as a reason to avoid participation.	5. Somatization may be used to avoid addressing issues. Clarifying expectations facilitates follow-through. Lack of reinforcement may help to extinguish the maladaptive response.
	6. Encourage the patient to verbalize fears and anxieties. Help identify physical symptoms as a coping mechanism that is used in times of extreme stress.	6. Patients with conversion disorder are usually unaware of the psychological implications of their illness.

Continued

Table 20–2 | CARE PLAN FOR THE PATIENT WITH A SOMATIC SYMPTOM DISORDER–cont'd

OUTCOME CRITERIA	NURSING INTERVENTIONS	RATIONALE
	7. Help patient identify coping mechanisms that he or she could use when faced with stressful situations, rather than retreating from reality with a physical disability.	7. Educating and engaging the patient in identifying alternative coping strategies helps diminish the need for maladaptive responses.
	8. Give positive reinforcement for identification or demonstration of alternative, more adaptive coping strategies.	8. Positive reinforcement enhances self-esteem and encourages repetition of desirable behaviors.

NURSING DIAGNOSIS: DEFICIENT KNOWLEDGE

RELATED TO: Psychological factors affecting medical condition

EVIDENCED BY: Statements such as, "I don't know why the doctor thinks this could be psychological. I have a physical problem."

OUTCOME CRITERIA	NURSING INTERVENTIONS	RATIONALE
Short-Term Goal ■ Patient will cooperate with plan for teaching provided by primary nurse. **Long-Term Goal** ■ By time of discharge from treatment, patient will be able to verbalize psychological factors affecting his or her physical condition.	1. Assess level of knowledge regarding effects of psychological problems on the body. 2. Assess level of anxiety and readiness to learn. 3. Discuss physical examinations and laboratory tests that have been conducted. Explain purpose and results of each. 4. Explore feelings and fears. Go slowly. These feelings may have been suppressed or repressed for so long that their disclosure may be a very painful experience. Be supportive. 5. Have patient keep a diary of appearance, duration, and intensity of physical symptoms. A separate record of situations that the patient finds especially stressful should also be kept. 6. Help patient identify needs that are being met through the sick role. Together, formulate more adaptive means for fulfilling these needs. Practice by role-playing. 7. Provide instruction in assertiveness techniques, especially the ability to recognize the differences among passive, assertive, and aggressive behaviors and the importance of respecting the rights of others while protecting one's own basic rights. 8. Discuss adaptive methods of stress management, such as relaxation techniques, physical exercise, meditation, breathing exercises, and autogenics.	1. An adequate database is necessary for the development of an effective teaching plan. 2. Learning does not occur beyond the moderate level of anxiety. 3. Fear of the unknown may contribute to elevated level of anxiety. Patient has the right to know about and accept or refuse any medical treatment. 4. Expression of feelings in the presence of a trusted individual and in a nonthreatening environment may encourage the individual to confront unresolved issues. 5. Comparison of these records may provide objective data from which to observe the relationship between physical symptoms and stress. 6. Repetition through practice serves to reduce discomfort in the actual situation. 7. These skills will preserve patient's self-esteem while also improving his or her ability to form satisfactory interpersonal relationships. 8. Use of these adaptive techniques may decrease appearance of physical symptoms in response to stress.

Table 20–3 | CARE PLAN FOR THE PATIENT WITH A DISSOCIATIVE DISORDER

NURSING DIAGNOSIS: IMPAIRED MEMORY

RELATED TO: Severe psychological stress and repression of anxiety

EVIDENCED BY: Loss of memory

OUTCOME CRITERIA	NURSING INTERVENTIONS	RATIONALE
Short-Term Goal ■ Patient will verbalize understanding that loss of memory is related to a stressful situation and begin discussing the stressful situation with nurse or therapist. **Long-Term Goal** ■ Patient will recover deficits in memory and develop more adaptive coping mechanisms to deal with stressful situations.	1. Obtain as much information as possible about the patient from family and significant others if possible. Consider likes, dislikes, important people, activities, music, and pets. 2. Do not flood patient with data regarding his or her past life. 3. Instead, expose patient to stimuli that represent pleasant experiences from the past, such as smells associated with enjoyable activities, beloved pets, and music known to have been pleasurable to the patient. As memory begins to return, engage patient in activities that may provide additional stimulation. 4. Encourage patient to discuss situations that have been especially stressful and to explore the feelings associated with those times. 5. Identify specific conflicts that remain unresolved and assist patient to identify possible solutions. Provide instruction regarding more adaptive ways to respond to anxiety.	1. A comprehensive baseline assessment is important for the development of an effective plan of care. 2. Individuals who are exposed to painful information from which the amnesia is providing protection may decompensate even further into a psychotic state. 3. Recall may occur during activities that simulate life experiences. 4. Verbalization of feelings in a non-threatening environment may help patient come to terms with unresolved issues that may be contributing to the dissociative process. 5. Unless these underlying conflicts are resolved, any improvement in coping behaviors must be viewed as only temporary.

NURSING DIAGNOSIS: DISTURBED PERSONAL IDENTITY

RELATED TO: Childhood trauma/abuse

EVIDENCED BY: The presence of more than one personality within the individual

OUTCOME CRITERIA	NURSING INTERVENTIONS	RATIONALE
Short-Term Goals ■ Patient will verbalize understanding about the existence of multiple identities within the self. ■ Patient will be able to recognize stressful situations that precipitate transition from one identity to another.	1. The nurse must develop a trusting relationship with the patient regardless of which identities are being manifested. 2. Help patient understand the existence of the subpersonalities and the need each serves in the personal identity of the individual.	1. Trust is the basis of a therapeutic relationship. Each of the identities views itself as a separate entity and must initially be treated as such. 2. Patient may initially be unaware of the dissociative response. Knowledge of the needs each identity fulfills is the first step in the integration process.

Continued

Table 20–3 | CARE PLAN FOR THE PATIENT WITH A DISSOCIATIVE DISORDER—cont'd

OUTCOME CRITERIA	NURSING INTERVENTIONS	RATIONALE
Long-Term Goals ■ Patient will verbalize understanding of the reason for existence of each personality and the role each plays for the individual. ■ Patient will enter into and cooperate with long-term therapy, the ultimate goal being integration into one personality.	3. Help patient identify stressful situations that precipitate transition from one identity to another. Carefully observe and record these transitions. 4. Use nursing interventions necessary to deal with maladaptive behaviors associated with individual subpersonalities. For example, if one identity is suicidal, precautions must be taken to guard against patient's self-harm. If another identity has a tendency toward physical hostility, precautions must be taken to protect others. Note: It may be possible to seek assistance from one of the identities. For example, the patient's strong-willed identity may be able to help control the behaviors of a "suicidal" identity. 5. Help the patient recognize that intervention is intended to promote an integrated, unified identity within the individual. 6. Provide support during disclosure of painful experiences and reassurance when patient becomes discouraged with lengthy treatment.	3. Identification of stressors is required to assist patient in responding more adaptively and to eliminate the need for transition to other identities. 4. The safety of patient and others is a nursing priority. 5. Because subpersonalities function as separate entities, the idea of total elimination generates fear and defensiveness. 6. Positive reinforcement may encourage repetition of desirable behaviors.

NURSING DIAGNOSIS: DISTURBED SENSORY PERCEPTION (VISUAL/KINESTHETIC)

RELATED TO: Severe psychological stress and repression of anxiety

EVIDENCED BY: Alteration in the perception or experience of the self or the environment

OUTCOME CRITERIA	NURSING INTERVENTIONS	RATIONALE
Short-Term Goal ■ Patient will verbalize adaptive ways of coping with stress. **Long-Term Goal** ■ Patient will demonstrate the ability to perceive stimuli correctly and maintain a sense of reality during stressful situations.	1. Provide support and encouragement during times of depersonalization. 2. Explain the depersonalization behaviors and the purpose they usually serve for the patient. 3. Explain the relationship between severe anxiety and depersonalization behaviors. Help relate these behaviors to times of severe psychological stress that patient has experienced.	1. Patients manifesting these symptoms may express fear and anxiety at experiencing such behaviors. They do not understand the response and may express a fear of going insane. Support and encouragement from a trusted individual provide a feeling of security when fears and anxieties are manifested. 2. This knowledge may help to minimize fears and anxieties associated with their occurrence. 3. The patient may be unaware that the occurrence of depersonalization behaviors is related to severe anxiety. Knowledge of this relationship is the first step in the process of behavioral change.

Table 20–3 | CARE PLAN FOR THE PATIENT WITH A DISSOCIATIVE DISORDER–cont'd

OUTCOME CRITERIA	NURSING INTERVENTIONS	RATIONALE
	4. Explore past experiences and possibly repressed painful situations, such as trauma or abuse, as the patient demonstrates readiness.	4. Prompting patients to recall traumatic events and experiences before they are ready can be retraumatizing, and premature recounting of traumatic experiences may predispose individuals to dissociative disorders.
	5. Discuss these painful experiences with patient and encourage him or her to deal with the feelings associated with these situations. Work to resolve the conflicts these repressed feelings have nurtured.	5. Conflict resolution will serve to decrease the need for the dissociative response to anxiety.
	6. Discuss ways the patient may more adaptively respond to stress and use role-play to practice using these new methods.	6. Role-play helps to prepare the patient to face stressful situations by using these new behaviors when they occur in real life.

Concept Care Mapping

The concept map care plan is a diagrammatic teaching and learning strategy that allows visualization of interrelationships between medical diagnoses, nursing diagnoses, assessment data, and treatments. Examples of concept map care plans for patients with somatic symptom and dissociative disorders are presented in Figures 20–1 and 20–2.

Evaluation

Reassessment is conducted to determine if the nursing actions have been successful in achieving the objectives of care. Evaluation of the nursing actions for the patient with a somatic symptom disorder may be facilitated by gathering information using the following types of questions:

Does the patient:

■ Recognize signs and symptoms of escalating anxiety?
■ Intervene with adaptive coping strategies to interrupt the escalating anxiety before physical symptoms are exacerbated?
■ Verbalize an understanding of the correlation between physical symptoms and times of escalating anxiety?
■ Have a plan for dealing with increased stress to prevent exacerbation of physical symptoms?
■ Demonstrate a decrease in ruminations about physical symptoms?
■ Express that fears of serious illness have diminished?

■ Demonstrate full recovery from previous loss or alteration of physical functioning?

Evaluation of the nursing actions for the patient with a dissociative disorder may be facilitated by gathering information using the following types of questions:

Does the patient:

■ Recall memories accurately?
■ Connect occurrence of psychological stress to loss of memory?
■ Discuss fears and anxieties with members of the staff in an effort toward resolution?
■ Discuss the presence of various identities within the self?
■ Verbalize situations that precipitate transition from one identity to another?
■ Maintain a sense of reality during stressful situations?
■ Verbalize a correlation between stressful situations and the onset of depersonalization behaviors?
■ Demonstrate more adaptive coping strategies for dealing with stress without resorting to dissociation?

Treatment Modalities

Somatic Symptom Disorders

Individual Psychotherapy

The goal of psychotherapy is to help clients develop healthy and adaptive behaviors and to encourage them to move beyond their somatization and manage

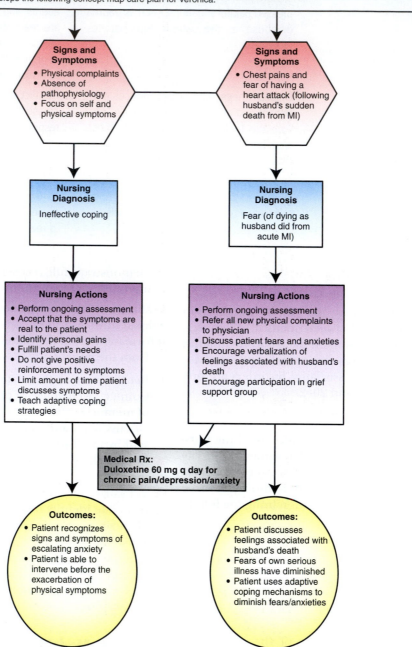

Clinical Vignette: Veronica, age 51, has a long history of "doctor shopping" for numerous complaints of gastrointestinal distress, daily headaches, and abdominal pain. She has undergone numerous tests that show no evidence of pathophysiology. Her husband of 25 years recently died of a myocardial infarction (MI). Yesterday, she began having chest pains and was certain she was having a heart attack. Her daughter called 911, and Veronica was transported to the emergency department. The staff performed diagnostic studies and laboratory tests, which were all negative for pathophysiology. She was referred for psychotherapeutic treatment with a diagnosis of Somatic Symptom Disorder. The nurse develops the following concept map care plan for Veronica.

Signs and Symptoms
- Physical complaints
- Absence of pathophysiology
- Focus on self and physical symptoms

Signs and Symptoms
- Chest pains and fear of having a heart attack (following husband's sudden death from MI)

Nursing Diagnosis

Ineffective coping

Nursing Diagnosis

Fear (of dying as husband did from acute MI)

Nursing Actions
- Perform ongoing assessment
- Accept that the symptoms are real to the patient
- Identify personal gains
- Fulfill patient's needs
- Do not give positive reinforcement to symptoms
- Limit amount of time patient discusses symptoms
- Teach adaptive coping strategies

Nursing Actions
- Perform ongoing assessment
- Refer all new physical complaints to physician
- Discuss patient fears and anxieties
- Encourage verbalization of feelings associated with husband's death
- Encourage participation in grief support group

Medical Rx:
Duloxetine 60 mg q day for chronic pain/depression/anxiety

Outcomes:
- Patient recognizes signs and symptoms of escalating anxiety
- Patient is able to intervene before the exacerbation of physical symptoms

Outcomes:
- Patient discusses feelings associated with husband's death
- Fears of own serious illness have diminished
- Patient uses adaptive coping mechanisms to diminish fears/anxieties

FIGURE 20–1 Concept map care plan for a patient with somatic symptom disorder.

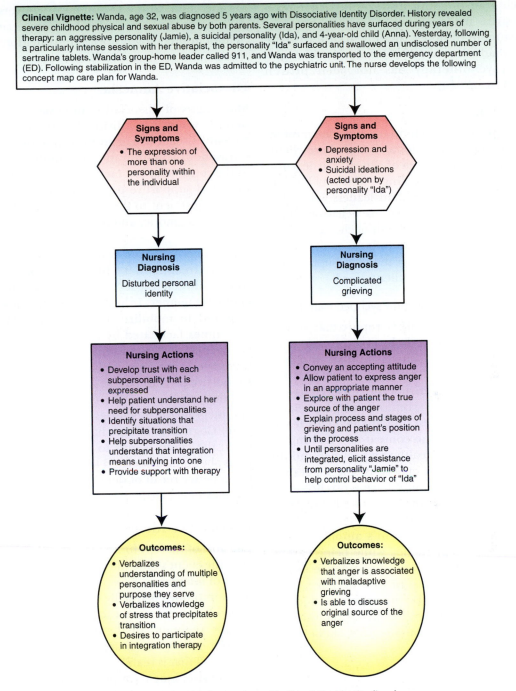

Clinical Vignette: Wanda, age 32, was diagnosed 5 years ago with Dissociative Identity Disorder. History revealed severe childhood physical and sexual abuse by both parents. Several personalities have surfaced during years of therapy: an aggressive personality (Jamie), a suicidal personality (Ida), and 4-year-old child (Anna). Yesterday, following a particularly intense session with her therapist, the personality "Ida" surfaced and swallowed an undisclosed number of sertraline tablets. Wanda's group-home leader called 911, and Wanda was transported to the emergency department (ED). Following stabilization in the ED, Wanda was admitted to the psychiatric unit. The nurse develops the following concept map care plan for Wanda.

Signs and Symptoms
- The expression of more than one personality within the individual

Signs and Symptoms
- Depression and anxiety
- Suicidal ideations (acted upon by personality "Ida")

Nursing Diagnosis

Disturbed personal identity

Nursing Diagnosis

Complicated grieving

Nursing Actions
- Develop trust with each subpersonality that is expressed
- Help patient understand her need for subpersonalities
- Identify situations that precipitate transition
- Help subpersonalities understand that integration means unifying into one
- Provide support with therapy

Nursing Actions
- Convey an accepting attitude
- Allow patient to express anger in an appropriate manner
- Explore with patient the true source of the anger
- Explain process and stages of grieving and patient's position in the process
- Until personalities are integrated, elicit assistance from personality "Jamie" to help control behavior of "Ida"

Outcomes:
- Verbalizes understanding of multiple personalities and purpose they serve
- Verbalizes knowledge of stress that precipitates transition
- Desires to participate in integration therapy

Outcomes:
- Verbalizes knowledge that anger is associated with maladaptive grieving
- Is able to discuss original source of the anger

FIGURE 20–2   Concept map care plan for a patient with dissociative identity disorder.

their lives more effectively. The focus is on personal and social difficulties that the client is experiencing in daily life as well as the achievement of practical solutions for these difficulties.

Treatment is initiated with a complete physical examination to rule out organic pathology. Clients

may be more amenable to psychotherapeutic treatment, particularly stress management, when it is conducted in a medical setting. Frequent, regular physical examinations are recommended to reassure clients that their concerns are being heard (Sadock et al., 2015; Yates, 2014) and may also provide an ongoing opportunity for education and stress management. Their use, however, in the treatment of illness anxiety disorder is controversial (Sadock et al., 2015). Individual insight-oriented psychotherapy has not been proven effective (Yates, 2014).

Group Psychotherapy

Group therapy may be helpful for somatic symptom disorders because it provides a setting where clients can share their experiences of illness, can learn to verbalize thoughts and feelings, and can be confronted by group members and leaders when they reject responsibility for maladaptive behaviors. It has been reported to be the treatment of choice for both somatic symptom disorder and illness anxiety disorder, in part because it provides the social support and anxiety reduction that these clients need.

Cognitive Behavior Therapy and Psychoeducation

Escobar and Dimsdale (2017) report that several studies support cognitive behavior therapy as an effective strategy for reducing symptoms in clients with somatic diseases. Psychoeducation has also been identified as beneficial and includes teaching the patient that the symptoms may be related to or exacerbated by stress and anxiety. This teaching should be done in the context of a trusting relationship between the healthcare provider and the client because the client may resist the suggestion that physical symptoms could have a psychological foundation. Psychoeducation for family members and other support systems focuses on teaching these individuals to reward the client's autonomy, self-sufficiency, and independence while being careful not to reinforce passivity and dependence associated with the sick role. This process becomes more difficult when the client is very regressed and the sick role is well established. In conversion disorder, symptoms usually abate spontaneously, but behavior therapy may be beneficial.

Psychopharmacology

In general, based on studies of somatization disorder, medication treatment is not effective unless it is being used to treat underlying depression or anxiety (Sadock et al., 2015; Yates, 2014). When antidepressant therapy is warranted, SSRIs are generally preferred. Anxiety may be treated in the short term with antianxiety agents such as benzodiazepines, but long-term use should be avoided because of the potential

for addiction. In the treatment of conversion disorders, parenteral amobarbital or lorazepam may be helpful in revealing historical information related to trauma.

Dissociative Amnesia

Many cases of dissociative amnesia resolve spontaneously when the individual is removed from the stressful situation. For more refractory conditions, intravenous administration of amobarbital is useful in the retrieval of lost memories. Most clinicians recommend supportive psychotherapy as well to reinforce adjustment to the psychological impact of the retrieved memories and the emotions associated with them.

In some instances, psychotherapy is used as the primary treatment. Techniques of persuasion and free or directed association are used to help the client remember. In other cases, hypnosis may be required to mobilize the memories. Hypnosis is sometimes facilitated by the use of pharmacological agents, such as sodium amobarbital. Once the memories have been obtained through hypnosis, supportive psychotherapy, group psychotherapy, and cognitive therapy may be employed to help the client integrate the memories into his or her conscious state. Cognitive therapy has an added benefit that when the client begins to correct cognitive distortions about the associated trauma, he or she may develop better recall of details about traumatic events (Sadock et al., 2015).

Dissociative Identity Disorder

The goal of therapy for the client with DID is to optimize the client's function and potential. The achievement of **integration** (a blending of all the personality states into one) is usually considered desirable, but some clients choose not to pursue this lengthy therapeutic regimen. In these cases, resolution, or a smooth collaboration among the subpersonalities, may be all that is realistic.

Intensive, long-term psychotherapy with the DID client is directed toward uncovering the underlying psychological conflicts, helping him or her gain insight into these conflicts, and striving to synthesize the various identities into one integrated personality. The therapist who engages in psychotherapy with this client must be skilled in various approaches, including insight-oriented psychotherapy, cognitive therapy, and especially trauma-informed and post-traumatic stress disorder (PTSD) treatment approaches. Clients are assisted to recall past traumas in detail. They must mentally reexperience the abuse that caused their illness. This process, called **abreaction,** or "remembering with feeling," is so painful that clients may actually cry, scream, and feel the pain that they felt at the time of the abuse.

During therapy, each personality state is actively explored and encouraged to become aware of the others across previously amnestic barriers. Traumatic memories associated with the different personality manifestations, especially those related to childhood abuse, are examined. The course of treatment is often difficult and anxiety provoking to client and therapist alike, especially when aggressive or suicidal personalities are in the dominant role. In these instances, brief periods of hospitalization may be necessary as an interim supportive measure. Escobar and Dimsdale (2017) identify that the standard of care for clients with DID (and dissociative amnesia) is a three-phase process, beginning first with stabilization in which the focus is on safety and symptom control; a second phase that involves an intensive focus on trauma issues; and a third phase that focuses on reintegration of the personality and a moving away from a framework of traumatization and victimization.

When integration is achieved, the individual is able to integrate all the feelings, experiences, memories, skills, and talents that were previously in the command of the various identities. He or she learns how to function effectively without the necessity for creating separate identities to cope with life. This is possible only after years of intense psychotherapy, and even then, recovery is often incomplete.

Depersonalization-Derealization Disorder

Information about the treatment of depersonalization-derealization disorder is sparse and inconclusive. Various psychiatric medications have been tried, both singly and in combination: antidepressants, mood stabilizers, anticonvulsants, and antipsychotics. Results have been sporadic at best. If other psychiatric disorders, such as schizophrenia, are evident, they too may be treated pharmacologically. For clients with evident intrapsychic conflict, analytically oriented insight psychotherapy may be useful. Some clients with depersonalization-derealization disorder have benefited from hypnotherapy or cognitive behavior therapy.

CASE STUDY AND SAMPLE CARE PLAN

NURSING HISTORY AND ASSESSMENT

Jake is a 54-year-old client of the psychiatric outpatient department of the VA Medical Center. At age 42, Jake was diagnosed with colon cancer and underwent a colon resection. Since that time, he has had regular follow-up examinations with no recurrence of the cancer and no residual effects. He did not require follow-up chemotherapy or radiation therapy. For 10 years, Jake has had yearly physical and laboratory examinations. He regularly complains to his family physician of mild abdominal pain, sensations of "fullness," "bowel rumblings," and what he calls a "firm mass," which he says he can sometimes feel in his lower left quadrant. The physician has performed x-rays of the entire gastrointestinal (GI) tract, an esophagoscopy, gastroscopy, and colonoscopy. All results were negative for organic pathology. Rather than being relieved, Jake appears to be resentful and disappointed that the physician has not been able to reveal a pathological problem. Jake's job is in jeopardy because of excessive use of sick leave. The family physician has referred Jake for psychiatric evaluation. Jake was admitted as an outpatient with the diagnosis of Illness Anxiety Disorder. He has been assigned to Lisa, a psychiatric nurse practitioner.

In her assessment, Lisa learns that Jake has lived most of his adult life in isolation. He was never close to his parents, who worked and seldom had time for Jake or his sister. Jake told Lisa, "My parents really didn't care about me. They were too busy taking care of the farm. Dad wanted me to take over the farm, but I was never interested. I liked working on cars and went to vocational school to learn how to be a mechanic. I thought they would be proud of me, but they never cared. I think they only had kids so they would have some help on the farm. When I left home, they really didn't care if they ever saw me again." He has never been married nor had a really serious relationship. "Women don't like me much. I spend most of my time alone. I guess I don't really like people, and they don't really like me."

Continued

CASE STUDY AND SAMPLE CARE PLAN—cont'd

NURSING DIAGNOSES AND OUTCOME IDENTIFICATION

From the assessment data, the nurse develops the following nursing diagnoses for Jake:

1. **Fear** (of cancer recurrence) related to history of colon cancer evidenced by numerous complaints of the GI tract and insistence that something is wrong despite objective tests that rule out pathophysiology
   a. **Short-Term Goal:** Jake will verbalize that fears associated with bodily sensations are irrational.
   b. **Long-Term Goal:** Jake interprets bodily sensations correctly.
2. **Chronic low self-esteem** related to unfulfilled childhood needs for nurturing and caring evidenced by transformation of internalized anger into physical complaints and hostility toward others
   a. **Short-Term Goal:** Within 2 weeks, Jake will verbalize aspects about self that he likes.
   b. **Long-Term Goal:** By discharge from treatment, Jake will demonstrate acceptance of self as a person of worth, as evidenced by setting realistic goals, limiting physical complaints and hostility toward others, and verbalizing positive prospects for the future.

PLANNING AND IMPLEMENTATION

FEAR (OF CANCER RECURRENCE)

The following nursing interventions have been identified for Jake.

1. Monitor the physician's ongoing assessments and laboratory reports to ensure that pathology is clearly ruled out.
2. Refer any new physical complaints to the physician.
3. Assess what function these physical complaints are fulfilling for Jake. Is it a way for him to get attention that he can't get in any other way?
4. Show empathy for Jake's feelings. Let him know that you understand how GI symptoms may bring about fears of the colon cancer recurring.
5. Encourage Jake to talk about his fears of cancer recurrence. What feelings did he have when it was first diagnosed? How did he deal with those feelings? What are his fears at this time?
6. Have Jake keep a diary of the appearance of the symptoms. In a separate diary, have Jake keep a record of situations that create stress for him. Compare these two records. Correlate whether symptoms appear at times of increased anxiety.
7. Help Jake determine what techniques may be useful for him to implement when fear and anxiety are exacerbated (e.g., relaxation techniques, mental imagery, thought-stopping techniques, physical exercise).

8. Offer positive feedback when Jake responds to stressful situations with coping strategies other than physical complaints.

CHRONIC LOW SELF-ESTEEM

The following nursing interventions have been identified for Jake.

1. Convey acceptance and unconditional positive regard and remain nonjudgmental at all times.
2. Encourage Jake to participate in decision making regarding his care as well as in life situations.
3. Help Jake to recognize and focus on strengths and accomplishments. Minimize attention given to past (real or perceived) failures.
4. Encourage Jake to talk about feelings related to his unsatisfactory relationship with his parents.
5. Discuss things in his life that Jake would like to change. Help him determine what *can* be changed and what changes are not realistic.
6. Encourage participation in group activities and in therapy groups that offer simple methods of achievement. Give recognition and positive feedback for actual accomplishments.
7. Teach assertiveness techniques and effective communication techniques.
8. Offer positive feedback for appropriate social interactions with others. Role-play with Jake situations that he finds particularly stressful. Help him to understand that ruminations about himself and his health may cause others to reject him socially.
9. Help Jake to set realistic goals for his future.

EVALUATION

Some of the outcome criteria for Jake have been met, and some are ongoing. He has come to realize that the fears about his "symptoms" are not rational. He understands that the physician has performed adequate diagnostic procedures to rule out illness. He still has fears of cancer occurrence and discusses these fears with the nurse practitioner on a weekly basis. He has kept his symptoms/stressful situations diary and has correlated the appearance of some of the symptoms to times of increased anxiety. Jake has started running and tries to use this exercise as a strategy to keep the anxiety from escalating out of proportion and bringing on new physical symptoms. He continues to discuss feelings associated with his childhood, and the nurse has helped him see that he has had numerous accomplishments in his life even though they were not recognized by his parents or others. He has joined a support group for depressed persons and states that he "has made a few friends." Jake has made a long-term goal of joining a church with the hope of meeting new people. He is missing fewer workdays because of illness, and his job is no longer in jeopardy.

Summary and Key Points

- Somatic symptom and related disorders and dissociative disorders are associated with anxiety that occurs at the severe level. The anxiety is repressed and manifested in the form of symptoms and behaviors associated with these disorders.

- Somatic symptom and related disorders affect about 4 to 8 percent (although statistics range from 0.1 percent to 11.6 percent) of the general population. Types of somatic disorders include somatic symptom disorder, illness anxiety disorder, conversion disorder, psychological factors affecting other medical conditions, factitious disorder, and other specified or unspecified somatic symptom and related disorders.

- Somatic symptom disorder is manifested by physical symptoms that may be vague, dramatized, or exaggerated in their presentation. No evidence of organic pathology can be identified.

- Illness anxiety disorder is an unrealistic preoccupation with fear of having a serious illness. This disorder may follow a personal experience or the experience of a close family member with serious or life-threatening illness.

- The individual with conversion disorder experiences a loss of or alteration in bodily functioning, unsubstantiated by medical or pathophysiological explanation. Psychological factors may be evident by the primary or secondary gains that the individual achieves from experiencing the physiological manifestation.

- With the diagnosis of psychological factors affecting medical condition, psychological or behavioral factors have been implicated in the development, exacerbation, or delayed recovery from a medical condition.

- In factitious disorder, the individual falsifies physical or psychological signs or symptoms or induces injury on the self or another person in order to receive attention from medical personnel.

- A dissociative response has been described as a defense mechanism to protect the ego in the face of overwhelming anxiety.

- Dissociative responses result in an alteration in the normally integrative functions of identity, memory, or consciousness.

- Classification of dissociative disorders includes dissociative amnesia, DID, depersonalization-derealization disorder, and other specified or unspecified dissociative disorders.

- The individual with dissociative amnesia is unable to recall important personal information that is too extensive to be explained by ordinary forgetfulness.

- The prominent feature of DID is the existence of two or more personality states within a single individual. An individual may have many personality states, each of which serves a purpose for that individual of enduring painful stimuli that the person's identity is too fragmented to integrate as one whole personality.

- Depersonalization-derealization disorder is characterized by an alteration in the perception of oneself and/or the environment. Depersonalization is described as a feeling of unreality or detachment from one's body. Derealization is an experience of unreality or detachment with respect to one's surroundings.

- Individuals with somatic symptom and dissociative disorders often receive healthcare initially in areas other than psychiatry.

- Nurses can assist patients with these disorders by helping them to understand the role of anxiety in symptom development and identify and establish new, more adaptive cognitive and behavior patterns.

- History of child abuse and other traumas is not uncommon in clients with these disorders. Nurses should provide trauma-informed care and be aware of resources for referral to specialists in trauma care and PTSD treatment.

Review Questions
Self-Examination/Learning Exercise

Select the answer that is most appropriate for each of the following questions:

1. Lorraine has been diagnosed with somatic symptom disorder. Which of the following symptom profiles would you expect when assessing Lorraine?
   a. Multiple somatic symptoms in several body systems
   b. Fear of having a serious disease
   c. Loss or alteration in sensorimotor functioning
   d. Belief that her body is deformed or defective in some way

Continued

Review Questions—cont'd
Self-Examination/Learning Exercise

2. Which of the following ego defense mechanisms describes the underlying psychodynamics of somatic symptom disorder?
   a. Denial of depression
   b. Repression of anxiety
   c. Suppression of grief
   d. Displacement of anger

3. Nursing care for Jenna, a patient with somatic symptom disorder, would focus on helping her to do which of the following?
   a. Eliminate the stress in her life.
   b. Discontinue her numerous physical complaints.
   c. Take her medication only as prescribed.
   d. Learn more adaptive coping strategies.

4. Lorraine, a client diagnosed with somatic symptom disorder, states, "My doctor thinks I should see a psychiatrist. I can't imagine why he would make such a suggestion." What is the most common basis for Lorraine's statement?
   a. She thinks her doctor wants to get rid of her as a client.
   b. She does not understand the correlation of symptoms and stress.
   c. She thinks psychiatrists are only for "crazy" people.
   d. She thinks her doctor has made an error in diagnosis.

5. Lorraine, a client diagnosed with somatic symptom disorder, tells the nurse about a pain in her side. She says she has not experienced it before. Which is the most appropriate response by the nurse?
   a. "I don't want to hear about another physical complaint. You know they are all in your head. It's time for group therapy now."
   b. "Let's sit down here together, and you can tell me about this new pain you are experiencing. You'll just have to miss group therapy today."
   c. "I will report this pain to your physician. In the meantime, group therapy starts in 5 minutes."
   d. "I will call your physician and see if he will order a new pain medication for your side. The one you have now doesn't seem to provide relief. Why don't you get some rest for now?"

6. Ellen has a history of childhood physical and sexual abuse. She was diagnosed with dissociative identity disorder (DID) 6 years ago. She has been admitted to the psychiatric unit following a suicide attempt. What is the primary nursing diagnosis for Ellen?
   a. Disturbed personal identity related to childhood abuse
   b. Disturbed sensory perception related to repressed anxiety
   c. Impaired memory related to disturbed thought processes
   d. Risk for suicide related to unresolved grief

7. In establishing trust with Ellen, a client with the diagnosis of DID, the nurse must do which of the following?
   a. Try to relate to Ellen as though she did not have multiple identities.
   b. Listen nonjudgmentally and respond empathically when Ellen transitions to different identity states.
   c. Ignore behaviors that Ellen attributes to other subpersonalities.
   d. Explain to Ellen that he or she will work with her only if she maintains the status of the primary identity.

Review Questions—cont'd
Self-Examination/Learning Exercise

8. What is the ultimate goal of therapy for a client with DID?
   a. Integration of the identities into one
   b. For the client to have the ability to switch from one identity to another voluntarily
   c. For the client to select which identity he or she wants to be the dominant self
   d. For the client to recognize that the various identities exist

9. The ultimate goal of therapy for a client with DID is most likely achieved through which of the following interventions?
   a. Crisis intervention and directed association
   b. Psychotherapy and hypnosis
   c. Psychoanalysis and free association
   d. Insight psychotherapy and dextroamphetamines

10. Lucille has a diagnosis of Illness Anxiety Disorder. Which of the following symptoms would be consistent with this diagnosis?
    a. Complains of a multitude of incapacitating physical symptoms
    b. Manifests with pseudoseizures or pseudocyesis
    c. Takes substances to induce vomiting in order to convince the nurse that she needs treatment
    d. Expresses persistent fears of having life-threatening disease
    e. All of the above

IMPLICATIONS OF RESEARCH FOR EVIDENCE-BASED PRACTICE

Stein, D. J., Koenen, K. C., Friedman, M. J., Hill, E., McLaughlin, K. A., Petukhova, M., . . . Kessler, R. C. (2013). Dissociation in posttraumatic stress disorder: Evidence from the world mental health surveys. *Biological Psychiatry, 73*(4), 302–312. doi:10.1016/j.biopsych.2012.08.022

DESCRIPTION OF THE STUDY: Interviews of 25,018 individuals from 16 countries were conducted in World Health Organization Mental Health Surveys to assess connections between PTSD and dissociative symptoms of depersonalization and derealization.

RESULTS OF THE STUDY: 14.4 percent of PTSD participants had dissociative symptoms, and these were associated with high counts of reexperiencing symptoms, childhood onset of post-traumatic stress disorder (PTSD),

high exposure to past traumatic events, childhood adversities, history of separation anxiety disorder and specific phobia, severe role impairment, and suicidality. The authors conclude that there should be a dissociative subtype for the diagnosis of PTSD to address these severe cases of PTSD.

IMPLICATIONS FOR NURSING PRACTICE: Being aware of evidence-based research is identified as an essential Quality and Safety in Education of Nurses competency. This study informs about linkages between various psychiatric illnesses and dissociative symptoms. Recognizing that reexperiencing of symptoms as well as other predisposing factors are associated with risk for dissociative symptoms underscores the importance of trauma-informed care as well.

TEST YOUR CRITICAL THINKING SKILLS

Tom was admitted to the psychiatric unit from the emergency department of a general hospital in the Midwest. The owner of a local bar called the police when Tom suddenly seemed to "lose control. He just went ballistic." The police reported that Tom did not know where he was or how he got there. He kept saying, "My name is John Brown, and I live in Philadelphia." When the police ran an identity check on Tom, they found that he was indeed John Brown from Philadelphia, and his wife had reported him missing a month ago. Mrs. Brown explained that about 12 months before his disappearance, her husband, who was a shop foreman at a large manufacturing plant, had been having considerable difficulty at work. He had been passed over for a promotion, and his supervisor had been very critical of his work. Several of his staff had left the company for other jobs, and without enough help, Tom had been unable to meet shop deadlines. Work stress made him very difficult to live with at home. Previously an easygoing, extroverted individual, he became withdrawn and extremely critical of his wife and children. Immediately preceding his disappearance, he had had a violent argument with his 18-year-old son, who called Tom a "loser." His son stormed out of the house to stay with some friends. It was the day after this argument that Tom disappeared. The psychiatrist assigns a diagnosis of Dissociative Amnesia, with dissociative fugue.

Answer the following questions related to Tom:

1. Describe the *priority* nursing intervention with Tom as he is admitted to the psychiatric unit.
2. What approach should be taken to help Tom with his problem?
3. What is the long-term goal of therapy for Tom?

🎦 MOVIE CONNECTIONS

Bandits (Illness anxiety disorder) • *Hanna and Her Sisters* (Illness anxiety disorder) • *Send Me No Flowers* (Illness anxiety disorder) • *Dead Again* (Amnesia) • *Mirage* (Amnesia) • *Suddenly Last Summer* (Amnesia) • *Sybil* (DID) • *The Three Faces of Eve* (DID) • *Identity* (DID)

References

American Psychiatric Association. (2013). *Diagnostic and statistical manual of mental disorders* (5th ed.). Washington, DC: Author.

Dimsdale, J. (2015). Illness anxiety disorder. *Merck manual: Professional version.* Retrieved from http://www.merckmanuals.com/professional/psychiatric-disorders/somatic-symptom-and-related-disorders/illness-anxiety-disorder

Escobar, J. I., & Dimsdale, J. E. (2017). Somatic symptom and related disorders. In B. J. Sadock, V. A. Sadock, & P. Ruiz (Eds.), *Comprehensive textbook of psychiatry* (10th ed., pp. 1827–1845). Philadelphia, PA: Wolters Kluwer.

Haberman, C. (2014). Debate persists over diagnosing mental disorders, long after "Sybil." *New York Times.* Retrieved from http://www.nytimes.com/2014/11/24/us/debate-persists-over-diagnosing-mental-health-disorders-long-after-sybil.html?_r=0

Herdman, T. H., & Kamitsuru, S. (Eds.). (2018). *NANDA-I nursing diagnoses: Definitions and classification, 2018–2020.* New York, NY: Thieme.

Lowenstein, R. J., Frewen, P., & Lewis-Fernandez, R. (2017). Dissociative disorders. In B. J. Sadock, V. A. Sadock, & P. Ruiz (Eds.), *Comprehensive textbook of psychiatry* (10th ed., pp. 1866–1952). Philadelphia, PA: Wolters Kluwer.

Sadock, B. J., Sadock, V. A., & Ruiz, P. (2015). *Synopsis of psychiatry: Behavioral sciences/clinical psychiatry* (11th ed.). Philadelphia, PA: Wolters Kluwer.

Soreff, S. (2018). *Fast five quiz: Are you prepared to treat patients with illness anxiety disorder?* Retrieved from https://reference.medscape.com/viewarticle/895692_2

Stein, D. J., Koenen, K. C., Friedman, M. J., Hill, E., McLaughlin, K. A., Petukhova, M., . . . Kessler, R. C. (2013). Dissociation in posttraumatic stress disorder: Evidence from the world mental health surveys. *Biological Psychiatry, 73*(4), 302–312. doi:10.1016/j.biopsych.2012.08.022

Venes, D. (2017). *Taber's medical dictionary* (23nd ed.). Philadelphia, PA: F.A. Davis.

Yates, W. (2014). Somatic symptom disorders. *Medscape.* Retrieved from http://emedicine.medscape.com/article/294908-overview

Classical References

Asher, R. (1951). Munchausen's syndrome. *Lancet, 257*(6650), 339–341.

Freud, S. (1962). The neuro-psychoses of defense. In J. Strachey (Ed.), *Standard edition of the complete psychological works of Sigmund Freud, Vol. 3 (1893–1899): Early psycho-analytic publications.* London, England: Hogarth Press.

Eating Disorders

21

CHAPTER OUTLINE

Objectives

Homework Assignment

Introduction

Epidemiological Factors

Application of the Nursing Process

Treatment Modalities

Summary and Key Points

Review Questions

Implications of Research for Evidence-Based Practice

Test Your Critical Thinking Skills

Communication Exercises

Movie Connections

CORE CONCEPTS

Anorexia

Body image

Bulimia

KEY TERMS

amenorrhea

anorexia nervosa

binging

binge eating disorder

bulimia nervosa

emaciated

lanugo

obesity

purging

OBJECTIVES
After reading this chapter, the student will be able to:

1. Identify and differentiate among several eating disorders.
2. Discuss epidemiological statistics related to eating disorders.
3. Describe symptomatology associated with anorexia nervosa, bulimia nervosa, and obesity, and use the information in patient assessment.
4. Identify predisposing factors in the development of eating disorders.
5. Formulate nursing diagnoses and outcomes of care for patients with eating disorders.
6. Describe appropriate interventions for behaviors associated with eating disorders.
7. Identify topics for patient and family teaching relevant to eating disorders.
8. Evaluate the nursing care of patients with eating disorders.
9. Discuss various modalities relevant to treatment of eating disorders.

HOMEWORK ASSIGNMENT
Please read the chapter and answer the following questions:

1. There is speculation that anorexia nervosa may be associated with a primary dysfunction of which brain structure?
2. What is the level of body mass index (BMI) that is associated with the definition of obesity?
3. Individuals with anorexia nervosa have a "distorted body image." What does this mean?
4. What physiological signs may be associated with the excessive vomiting of the purging syndrome?

Introduction

Nutrition is required to sustain life, and most individuals acquire nutrients from eating food; however, nutrition and life sustenance are not the only reasons most people eat food. In an affluent culture, life sustenance may not even be a consideration. It is sometimes difficult to remember that many people in this affluent American culture, as well as all over the world, are starving from lack of food.

The hypothalamus contains the appetite regulation center in the brain. This complex neural system regulates the body's ability to recognize when it is hungry and when it has been sated. Some studies have shown evidence of serotonin and norepinephrine dysfunction in individuals with eating disorders. These neurotransmitters both play a role in regulating eating behavior in the hypothalamus (Sadock, Sadock, & Ruiz, 2015).

Society and culture also have a great deal of influence on eating behaviors. Eating is a social activity; seldom does an event of any social significance occur without the presence of food. Yet, society and culture also influence how people (and in particular, women) must look. History reveals a regularity of fluctuation in what society has considered desirable in the human female body. Archives and historical paintings from the 16th and 17th centuries reveal that plump, full-figured women were considered fashionable and desirable. In the Victorian era, beauty was characterized by a slender, wan appearance that continued through the flapper era of the 1920s. During the Depression era and World War II, the full-bodied woman was again admired, only to be superseded in the late 1960s by the image of the super-thin model propagated by the media, which remains the ideal of today. As it has been said, "A woman can't be too rich or too thin." Eating disorders, as we know them, can refute this concept.

This chapter explores the disorders associated with undereating and overeating. Because psychological or behavioral factors play a potential role in the presentation of these disorders, they fall well within the realm of psychiatry and psychiatric nursing. Epidemiological statistics are presented along with factors that have been implicated in the etiology of anorexia nervosa, bulimia nervosa, and binge eating disorder. An explanation of the symptomatology is presented as background knowledge for assessing the patient with an eating disorder. Nursing care is described in the context of the nursing process. Various treatment modalities are explored.

Epidemiological Factors

The prevalence of **anorexia nervosa** has increased since the mid-20th century both in the United States and in Western Europe. Epidemiological studies have found that across all ages and genders, the lifetime prevalence for an episode of anorexia nervosa is 2.4 to 4.3 percent (Call, Attia, & Walsh, 2017). Once thought to be rare among males, more recent data (Woolridge & Lemberg, 2016) identify that men account for 25 percent of those with anorexia and bulimia and 36 percent of those with binge eating disorders. The authors also note that for the first time, the incidence in males may be increasing at a more rapid rate than in females. See "Real People, Real Stories" for more about Vic's experience with an eating disorder.

Social interests may also play a role in the prevalence of eating disorders. Among girls and women, ballet training carries a seven times greater risk of developing anorexia nervosa, and among boys and men, the evidence of eating disorders is more prevalent among those participating in wrestling sports; a minority continue to have symptoms beyond their involvement in the sport (Sadock et al., 2015). Anorexia nervosa was once believed to be more prevalent in the higher socioeconomic classes, but evidence is lacking to support this hypothesis.

Bulimia nervosa is decreasing in recent years with a lifetime prevalence of 2 percent among women (Call et al., 2017). Onset of bulimia nervosa occurs in late adolescence or early adulthood. Among college women, about 20 percent experience transient bulimic symptoms during their college years (Sadock et al., 2015). Cross-cultural research suggests that bulimia nervosa occurs primarily in societies that place emphasis on thinness as the model of attractiveness for women and where an abundance of food is available.

Binge eating disorder (BED) is defined in the *Diagnostic and Statistical Manual of Mental Disorders, Fifth Edition (DSM-5)* (American Psychiatric Association [APA], 2013) as recurrent episodes of eating significantly more than most people would eat in a similar period under similar circumstances, and these episodes occur at least once a week for 3 months. It is the most common eating disorder and affects women twice as often as men (Sadock et al., 2015). Its prevalence is estimated at 4 percent of the U.S. population (Balodis, Grilo, & Potenza, 2015). Weight gain and obesity are major health risks associated with this disorder. It is estimated that approximately 50 to 75 percent of people seeking medical attention for severe obesity have a BED (Sadock et al.,

Real People, Real Stories: Living With an Eating Disorder

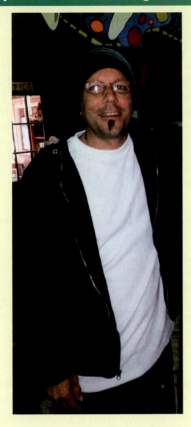

(Following is an excerpt of our conversation.)

Karyn: First of all, I appreciate your willingness to share your story.

Vic: I want to talk about this because there is such a stigma associated with being a guy and having an eating disorder. And it's hard for guys to find a support group of people who really "get it."

Karyn: What has your experience been with encountering stigma?

Vic: Well, my weight has sometimes been really high and sometimes very low. I fluctuate between anorexia and bulimia. So when my weight is really low, people have presumed I have AIDS. And in general, because eating disorders are presumed to be a female disorder, people have assumed I was gay. In high school, I was very heavy and the guys on the football team teased me a lot. I talked to my girlfriend at the time, and she suggested I try purging. I was using food and alcohol for comfort, but then I had to purge. I started working out a lot, and when I started getting compliments on my appearance, I began binging and purging every day and drinking alcohol. It was a stress relief for a while, but then it just wasn't working anymore and I still hated my appearance. To this day,

there's not one thing I like about my appearance even though my physician is happy with my current weight. I was hiding it from my family for some time: wearing baggy clothes and two sets of clothes so people wouldn't see my flaws. The behaviors are very isolating. When I tried to talk to my dad. he just told me to be a man . . . but there was a lot of physical and emotional abuse from him, so I didn't get support there.

Karyn: Where have you found support?

Vic: My mom and my fiancée are my biggest supports, but it's a struggle to find support with other guys who have eating disorders, and I feel like they would really understand. I tried to start a support group on Facebook, and no one responded. I have an individual counselor who knows a lot about eating disorders, and I have a family practice physician, and they are both helpful. It's just not the same as having the support of others who are having the same experiences that you are.

Karyn: Have you ever been engaged in group treatment specifically for eating disorders?

Vic: I tried, at one point, but most insurances don't cover eating disorder treatment, or the treatment program doesn't take insurance. I went into treatment in 2009 for alcohol rehabilitation, and they didn't address the eating disorder. In fact, they kind of force you to eat and tell you that you'll probably gain weight as you go through rehab, so the bulimia kicked in again for me because I didn't want to get fat like the other people in recovery. But I've been sober since 2009, and I take Vivitrol injections (to manage alcohol dependence) once a month; it blocks the pleasure centers.

Karyn: And has that been effective?

Vic: Oh yes, definitely. And my AA buddies are very supportive, but they don't see food as a similar issue to alcohol, so they don't really see a need to discuss that. Plus, you can't abstain from food like you can from alcohol. And society itself can be a trigger: television, all the messages that you need to be a certain way, picnics, going out to eat, grocery stores, talking about food, et cetera. And I think I have an element of "people pleasing" in my personality, so I'm always worried about what other people are thinking about me.

Karyn: It's not uncommon for people with eating disorders to also have depression and sometimes have suicide thoughts. Have you ever been in that place?

Vic: Yeah, once last year I took an overdose of pills with some alcohol, but I called some friends and they got me in to get help.

Karyn: Do you still have times when you have those thoughts?

Continued

Real People, Real Stories: Living With an Eating Disorder—cont'd

Vic: No. I'm doing really well right now. I still dabble from time to time with "the behavior" [Vic described this as his term for binging/purging or calorie restriction, stating that sometimes using the words can be a trigger for him], but not like before when I was taking up to 20 laxatives a day and my whole day was preoccupied with planning "the behaviors." I'm working in a setting that treats dual diagnosis clients, and I am hopeful that there may be opportunities to establish peer support groups for men with eating disorders, much like what exists in AA for alcohol recovery. As a guy, you just can't go to a group that is all women and talk about this stuff, especially what's going on with your body. And I don't want to be accused of "thirteen-steppin.'"

Karyn: "Thirteen steppin'"?

Vic: Yeah, that's the "thirteenth step" in the twelve-step program. It's the guys that go to AA meetings to pick up girls who are in recovery because they know they are more vulnerable when they're trying to stay sober. [Chuckles]

Karyn: [Chuckles] I didn't know that was a thing. But I understand what you're saying about the difficulty of finding support with other men who understand and are willing to acknowledge their eating disorder. I hope the peer support group works out, and in the meantime, I'm glad to hear that you are accessing resources to support your own health.

2015). **Obesity** has been defined as a body mass index (BMI) (weight/height^2) of 30 or greater. In the United States, statistics indicate that, among adults 20 years of age or older, the prevalence of obesity is 39.8 percent (Centers for Disease Control and Prevention [CDC], 2017). This percentage is higher among non-Hispanic black (46.8%) and Hispanic (47%) populations (CDC, 2017). The association between socioeconomics and obesity is complex, but one finding is a lower prevalence of obesity in both men and women from the highest income groups (CDC, 2017). Interestingly, the *DSM-5* does not include obesity as a mental health disorder with the rationale that "a range of genetic, physiological, behavioral, and environmental factors that vary across individuals contributes to the development of obesity; thus obesity is not considered a mental disorder" (APA, 2013, p. 329). The *DSM-5* also notes, however, that there are several mental disorders in which obesity is a significant problem (at least in part related to side effects of psychotropic medications) and that obesity may be a risk factor for the development of illnesses such as depression. BED, which *is* identified as a mental illness, carries a high risk for weight gain and obesity.

Application of the Nursing Process

Background Assessment Data: Anorexia Nervosa

CORE CONCEPT
Anorexia
Prolonged loss of appetite.

CORE CONCEPT
Body Image
A subjective concept of one's physical appearance based on the personal perceptions of self and the reactions of others.

Anorexia nervosa is characterized by a morbid fear of obesity. Symptoms include gross distortion of body image, preoccupation with food, and refusal to eat. The term *anorexia* is actually a misnomer. It was initially believed that individuals with anorexia nervosa did not experience sensations of hunger. However, research indicates that they do suffer from pangs of hunger, and it is only with food intake of less than 200 calories per day that hunger sensations actually cease.

The distortion in body image is manifested by the individual's perception of being "fat" when he or she is obviously underweight or even **emaciated** (excessively thin). Weight loss is usually accomplished by reduction in food intake and often extensive exercising. Self-induced vomiting and the abuse of laxatives or diuretics also may occur.

Weight loss is excessive. For example, the individual may present for healthcare services weighing less than 85 percent of expected weight. Other symptoms include hypothermia, bradycardia, hypotension with orthostatic changes, peripheral edema, **lanugo** (fine, neonatal-like hair growth), and a variety of metabolic changes. **Amenorrhea** (absence of menstruation) usually follows weight loss, but sometimes it happens early on in the disorder, even before severe weight loss has occurred.

Individuals with anorexia nervosa may be obsessed with food. For example, they may hoard or conceal food, talk about food and recipes at great length, or prepare elaborate meals for others, only to restrict themselves to a limited amount of low-calorie food intake. Compulsive behaviors, such as hand washing, may also be present.

Age at onset is usually early to late adolescence, and psychosexual development is often delayed. Feelings of depression and anxiety often accompany the disorder. Depression is strongly correlated with eating disorders, some of which may be secondary to malnutrition. However, even in those who have recovered from anorexia nervosa, there is a higher incidence of depression, anxiety, and obsessive thinking than in the general population (Uniacke & Broft, 2016). Box 21–1 outlines the *DSM-5* diagnostic criteria for anorexia nervosa.

Background Assessment Data: Bulimia Nervosa

CORE CONCEPT

Bulimia
Excessive, insatiable appetite.

Bulimia nervosa is an episodic, uncontrolled, compulsive, rapid ingestion of large quantities of food over a short period **(binging),** followed by inappropriate compensatory behaviors to rid the body of the excess calories. The food consumed during a binge often has a high caloric content, a sweet taste, and a soft or smooth texture that can be eaten rapidly, sometimes even without being chewed (Sadock et al., 2015). The binging episodes often occur in secret and are usually terminated by only abdominal discomfort, sleep, social interruption, or self-induced vomiting. Although the eating binges may bring pleasure while they are occurring, self-degradation and depressed mood commonly follow.

To rid the body of the excessive calories, the individual engages in **purging** behaviors (self-induced vomiting or the misuse of laxatives, diuretics, or enemas) or other inappropriate compensatory behaviors, such as fasting or excessive exercise. There is a persistent, excessive concern with personal appearance, particularly regarding how the individual believes others perceive them. Weight fluctuations are common because of the alternating binges and fasts. However, most individuals with bulimia are within a normal weight range—some slightly underweight, some slightly overweight.

BOX 21–1 Diagnostic Criteria for Anorexia Nervosa

A. Restriction of energy intake relative to requirements leading to a significantly low body weight in the context of age, sex, developmental trajectory, and physical health. Significantly low weight is defined as a weight that is less than minimally normal, or, for children and adolescents, less than that minimally expected.

B. Intense fear of gaining weight or becoming fat, or persistent behavior that interferes with weight gain, even though at a significantly low weight.

C. Disturbance in the way in which one's body weight or shape is experienced, undue influence of body weight or shape on self-evaluation, or persistent lack of recognition of the seriousness of the current low body weight.

Specify whether:

Restricting Type: During the last 3 months, the individual has not engaged in recurrent episodes of binge eating or purging behavior (i.e., self-induced vomiting or the misuse of laxatives, diuretics, or enemas). This subtype describes presentations in which weight loss is accomplished primarily through dieting, fasting, and/or excessive exercise.

Binge-Eating/Purging Type: During the last 3 months, the individual has engaged in recurrent episodes of binge eating or purging behavior (i.e., self-induced vomiting or the misuse of laxatives, diuretics, or enemas).

Specify if:

In partial remission
In full remission

Specify current severity:

Mild: BMI > 17 kg/m^2
Moderate: BMI 16–16.99 kg/m^2
Severe: BMI 15–15.99 kg/m^2
Extreme: BMI < 15 kg/m^2

Excessive vomiting and laxative or diuretic abuse may lead to problems with dehydration and electrolyte imbalance. Gastric acid in the vomitus also contributes to the erosion of tooth enamel. In rare instances, the individual may experience tears in the gastric or esophageal mucosa. Some individuals develop calluses on the dorsal surface of their hands, typically on knuckles, secondary to long-term, repeated self-induced vomiting. This feature is called *Russell's sign* after the British psychiatrist who first described it. It cannot be a reliable diagnostic symptom, however, because many individuals with purging behavior have developed skill in inducing vomiting without using their hands.

Common comorbidities include mood disorders, anxiety disorders, or substance abuse, most frequently involving central nervous system (CNS) stimulants or alcohol. About 50 percent of those with bulimia nervosa have had a history of anorexia nervosa (Sadock et al., 2015). The *DSM-5* diagnostic criteria for bulimia nervosa are presented in Box 21–2.

Background Assessment Data: Binge Eating Disorder

Individuals with BED have episodes of binge eating that may be similar to those with bulimia nervosa. However, one differential feature in BED is the absence of compensatory purging. As a result, this client is at risk for substantial weight gain. The episodes of eating are referred to as binges when they occur over a discrete period, usually defined as less than 2 hours (APA, 2013). Food consumption is rapid and often persists to the point that the individual feels uncomfortably full. Interpersonal stressors, low self-esteem, and boredom are identified as possible triggers. Typically, clients describe their eating as out of control (an important diagnostic clinical symptom) and, after an episode, report accompanying guilt and depression. As many as 50 percent of individuals with BED have a history of depression (WebMD, 2016). Another difference between bulimia nervosa and BED is that rates of improvement are consistently higher among individuals with BED than among those with bulimia nervosa (APA, 2013). The *DSM-5* diagnostic criteria for BED are presented in Box 21–3.

Predisposing Factors and Theories of Etiology Associated With Anorexia Nervosa, Bulimia Nervosa, and BED

Biological Influences

Genetics A hereditary predisposition to eating disorders has been hypothesized on the basis of family histories and an apparent association with other disorders for which the likelihood of genetic influences exists. Some studies identify higher concordance rates in monozygotic than in dizygotic twins (Sadock et al., 2015). Anorexia nervosa is more common

---

BOX 21–2 Diagnostic Criteria for Bulimia Nervosa

A. Recurrent episodes of binge eating. An episode of binge eating is characterized by both of the following:
1. Eating, in a discrete period of time (e.g., within any 2-hour period) an amount of food that is definitely larger than most individuals would eat during a similar period of time and under similar circumstances.
2. A sense of lack of control over eating during the episode (e.g., a feeling that one cannot stop eating or control what or how much one is eating).

B. Recurrent inappropriate compensatory behaviors in order to prevent weight gain, such as self-induced vomiting; misuse of laxatives, diuretics, or other medications; fasting; or excessive exercise.

C. The binge eating and inappropriate compensatory behaviors both occur, on average, at least once a week for 3 months.

D. Self-evaluation is unduly influenced by body shape and weight.

E. The disturbance does not occur exclusively during episodes of anorexia nervosa.

Specify if:

In partial remission
In full remission

Specify current severity:

Mild: An average of 1-3 episodes of inappropriate compensatory behaviors per week.

Moderate: An average of 4-7 episodes of inappropriate compensatory behaviors per week.

Severe: An average of 8-13 episodes of inappropriate compensatory behaviors per week.

Extreme: An average of 14 or more episodes of inappropriate compensatory behaviors per week.

Reprinted with permission from American Psychiatric Association (APA) (2013). Diagnostic and statistical manual of mental disorders, Fifth Edition (DSM-5). Washington, DC: American Psychiatric Publishing.

BOX 21–3 Diagnostic Criteria for Binge Eating Disorder

A. Recurrent episodes of binge eating. An episode of binge eating is characterized by both of the following:
 1. Eating, in a discrete period of time (e.g., within any 2-hour period), an amount of food that is definitely larger than what most people would eat in a similar period of time under similar circumstances
 2. A sense of lack of control over eating during the episode (e.g., a feeling that one cannot stop eating or control what or how much one is eating)
B. The binge-eating episodes are associated with 3 (or more) of the following:
 1. Eating much more rapidly than normal
 2. Eating until feeling uncomfortably full
 3. Eating large amounts of food when not feeling physically hungry
 4. Eating alone because of feeling embarrassed by how much one is eating
 5. Feeling disgusted with oneself, depressed, or very guilty after overeating

C. Marked distress regarding binge eating is present.
D. The binge eating occurs, on average, at least once a week for 3 months.
E. The binge eating is not associated with the recurrent use of inappropriate compensatory behavior as in bulimia nervosa and does not occur exclusively during the course of bulimia nervosa or anorexia nervosa.

Specify if:
In partial remission
In full remission

Specify current severity:
Mild: 1–3 binge-eating episodes per week
Moderate: 4–7 binge-eating episodes per week
Severe: 8–13 binge-eating episodes per week
Extreme: 14 or more binge-eating episodes per week

Reprinted with permission from American Psychiatric Association (APA) (2013). Diagnostic and statistical manual of mental disorders, Fifth Edition (DSM-5). Washington, DC: American Psychiatric Publishing.

among sisters and mothers of those with the disorder than among the general population, but social factors, such as modeling and mimicking, may influence these relationships. Family studies find that a history of anorexia nervosa confers up to 11 times the risk for family members (Call et al., 2017), and those with a family history of bulimia nervosa, mood disorders, substance use disorders, or obesity are at greater risk for developing bulimia.

Neurobiological Influences Neurochemical influences in bulimia and anorexia nervosa may be associated with the neurotransmitters serotonin and norepinephrine. Neurobiological changes that occur in starvation, including depression and obsessional thinking, may contribute to maintaining the illness (Call et al., 2017). This hypothesis has been supported by the positive response these individuals have shown to therapy with the selective serotonin reuptake inhibitors (SSRIs). Individuals with BED have manifested several neurobiological disturbances, including delayed gastric emptying, enlarged stomach capacity, and decreased secretion of cholecystokinin (CCK), which is a hormone responsible for signaling satiety (Call et al., 2017). Some studies have found high levels of endogenous opioids in the spinal fluid of clients with anorexia, which suggests that these chemicals may contribute to denial of hunger (Sadock et al., 2015). Some of these individuals have

been shown to gain weight when given naloxone, an opioid antagonist. Questions still remain as to whether neurochemical changes are causal or are an outcome of the body's reaction to changes in nutrition and mood.

The etiology of BED is unknown. Brain imaging studies of people with BED reveal increased activity in the orbitofrontal cortex, which is associated with reward and pleasure responses such as those seen in response to substances of abuse (Balodis et al., 2015). These studies support the hypothesis that BED may be an illness of addiction.

Psychodynamic Influences

Psychodynamic theories suggest that the development of an eating disorder is rooted in an unfulfilled sense of separation-individuation. When events occur that threaten the vulnerable ego, feelings of lack of control over one's body (self) emerge. Behaviors associated with food and eating serve to provide feelings of control over one's life.

Family Influences

Historically, parents of individuals with eating disorders have often been presumed to be overcontrolling and perfectionistic, which is then misconstrued as causing pathology in their children. This theory has been problematic, at least in part, because not all siblings in the same family develop eating disorders.

There is no sufficient evidence to support these claims, and, in fact, they may have contributed to a resistance to seeking healthcare based on parents' fear that they will be judged as "bad" or "the cause of the problem." The American Academy for Eating Disorders published a position statement (2009) that includes the following:

> The AED stands firmly against any model of eating disorders in which family influences are seen as the primary cause of eating disorders, condemns statements that blame families for their child's illness, and recommends that families be included in the treatment of younger patients, unless this is clearly ill-advised on clinical grounds.

Both perfectionistic and depressive tendencies do appear to be common in clients with anorexia nervosa, but Sadock and associates (2015) offer this explanation:

> Many anorexic patients feel that oral desires are greedy and unacceptable; therefore these desires are projectively disavowed . . . parents respond to the refusal to eat by becoming frantic about whether the patient is actually eating. The patient can then view the parents as the ones who have unacceptable desires and can projectively disavow them.

Certainly, conflicts arise in a family when a child is starving herself or himself, but it has become clear that family members need to be involved in treatment rather than shunned or blamed, and family-based approaches, such as the Maudsley approach, are supported by clinical evidence.

Background Assessment Data: Body Mass Index

Assessment for the presence of an eating disorder requires an understanding of the measurements for BMI. The following formula is used to determine an individual's BMI:

$$\text{Body mass index} = \frac{\text{Weight (kg)}}{\text{Height (m)}^2}$$

The BMI range for normal weight is 20 to 24.9. Studies by the National Center for Health Statistics indicate that *overweight* is defined as a BMI of 25 to 29.9 (based on U.S. Dietary Guidelines for Americans). Based on World Health Organization criteria, *obesity* is defined as a BMI of 30 or greater. These guidelines, which were released by the National Heart, Lung, and Blood Institute in July 1998, markedly increased the number of Americans considered to be overweight.

The average American woman has a BMI of 26, and fashion models typically have a BMI of 18. Anorexia nervosa is characterized by a BMI of 17 or lower. In extreme anorexia nervosa, the BMI may be less than 15. Table 21–1 presents an example of some BMIs based on weight (in pounds) and height (in inches).

Diagnosis and Outcome Identification

Nursing diagnoses are formulated from the data gathered during the assessment phase and with background knowledge regarding predisposing factors to the disorder. Table 21–2 presents a list of patient behaviors and the NANDA nursing diagnoses (Herdman & Kamitsuru, 2018) that correspond to those behaviors, which may be used in planning care for patients with eating disorders.

Outcome Criteria

The following criteria may be used for measurement of outcomes in the care of the patient with eating disorders:

The patient:

- Has achieved and maintained an expected BMI for age with consideration for body build, weight history, and any physiological disturbances (APA, 2013).
- Has vital signs, blood pressure, and laboratory serum studies within normal limits.
- Verbalizes importance of adequate nutrition.
- Verbalizes knowledge regarding consequences of fluid loss caused by self-induced vomiting (or laxative/diuretic abuse) and importance of adequate fluid intake (anorexia nervosa, bulimia nervosa).
- Verbalizes events that precipitate anxiety and demonstrates techniques for its reduction.
- Verbalizes ways in which he or she may gain more control of the environment and thereby reduce feelings of powerlessness.
- Expresses less preoccupation with own appearance (anorexia nervosa, bulimia nervosa).
- Demonstrates ability to take control of own life without resorting to maladaptive eating behaviors (anorexia nervosa, bulimia nervosa, BED).
- Establishes a healthy pattern of eating for weight control, and weight loss toward a desired goal is progressing (BED).
- Verbalizes plans for maintenance of weight control and relapse prevention (BED).

Planning and Implementation

In most instances, individuals with eating disorders are treated on an outpatient basis, but in some cases

TABLE 21–1 Body Mass Index (BMI) Chart

BMI HEIGHT (INCHES)	19	20	21	22	23	24	25	26	27	28	29	30	31	32	33	34	35	36	37	38	39	40
									BODY WEIGHT (POUNDS)													
58	91	96	100	105	110	115	119	124	129	134	138	143	148	153	158	162	167	172	177	181	186	191
59	94	99	104	109	114	119	124	128	133	138	143	148	153	158	163	168	173	178	183	188	193	198
60	97	102	107	112	118	123	128	133	138	143	148	153	158	163	168	174	179	184	189	194	199	204
61	100	106	111	116	122	127	132	137	143	148	153	158	164	169	174	180	185	190	195	201	206	211
62	104	109	115	120	126	131	136	142	147	153	158	164	169	175	180	186	191	196	202	207	213	218
63	107	113	118	124	130	135	141	146	152	158	163	169	175	180	186	191	197	203	208	214	220	225
64	110	116	122	128	134	140	145	151	157	163	169	174	180	186	192	197	204	209	215	221	227	232
65	114	120	126	132	138	144	150	156	162	168	174	180	186	192	198	204	210	216	222	228	234	240
66	118	124	130	136	142	148	155	161	167	173	179	186	192	198	204	210	216	223	229	235	241	247
67	121	127	134	140	146	153	159	166	172	178	185	191	198	204	211	217	223	230	236	242	249	255
68	125	131	138	144	151	158	164	171	177	184	190	197	203	210	216	223	230	236	243	249	256	262
69	128	135	142	149	155	162	169	176	182	189	196	203	209	216	223	230	236	243	250	257	263	270
70	132	139	146	153	160	167	174	181	188	195	202	209	216	222	229	236	243	250	257	264	271	278
71	136	143	150	157	165	172	179	186	193	200	208	215	222	229	236	243	250	257	265	272	279	286
72	140	147	154	162	169	177	184	191	199	206	213	221	228	235	242	250	258	265	272	279	287	294
73	144	151	159	166	174	182	189	197	204	212	219	227	235	242	250	257	265	272	280	288	295	302
74	148	155	163	171	179	186	194	202	210	218	225	233	241	249	256	264	272	280	287	295	303	311
75	152	160	168	176	184	192	200	208	216	224	232	240	248	256	264	272	279	287	295	303	311	319
76	156	164	172	180	189	197	205	213	221	230	238	246	254	263	271	279	287	295	304	312	320	328

Source: National Heart, Lung, and Blood Institute of the National Institutes of Health (n.d.). Clinical guidelines on the identification, evaluation, and treatment of overweight and obesity in adults: Body mass index tables. Retrieved from http://www.nhlbi.nih.gov/guidelines/obesity/bmi_tbl.htm

TABLE 21–2 Assigning Nursing Diagnoses to Behaviors Commonly Associated With Eating Disorders	
BEHAVIORS	**NURSING DIAGNOSES**
Refusal to eat; abuse of laxatives, diuretics, and/or diet pills; loss of 15 percent of expected body weight; pale conjunctiva and mucous membranes; poor muscle tone; amenorrhea; poor skin turgor; electrolyte imbalances; hypothermia; bradycardia; hypotension; cardiac irregularities; edema	**Imbalanced nutrition: Less than body requirements**
Decreased fluid intake; abnormal fluid loss caused by self-induced vomiting; excessive use of laxatives, enemas, or diuretics; electrolyte imbalance; decreased urine output; increased urine concentration; elevated hematocrit; decreased blood pressure; increased pulse rate; dry skin; decreased skin turgor; weakness	**Deficient fluid volume**
Minimizes symptoms; unable to admit impact of disease on life pattern; does not perceive personal relevance of symptoms; does not perceive personal relevance of danger	**Denial**
Compulsive eating; excessive intake in relation to metabolic needs; sedentary lifestyle; weight 20 percent over ideal for height and frame; BMI of 30 or more; reports the perception that eating is out of control	**Obesity**
Distorted body image; views self as fat, even in the presence of normal body weight or severe emaciation; denies that problem with low body weight exists; difficulty accepting positive reinforcement; self-destructive behavior (self-induced vomiting, abuse of laxatives or diuretics, refusal to eat); preoccupation with appearance and how others perceive it (anorexia nervosa, bulimia nervosa) Verbalization of negative feelings about the way he or she looks and the desire to lose weight (obesity) Lack of eye contact; depressed mood (all)	**Disturbed body image/Low self-esteem**
Increased tension; increased helplessness; overexcited; apprehensive; fearful; restlessness; poor eye contact; increased difficulty taking oral nourishment; inability to learn	**Anxiety (moderate to severe)**

hospitalization becomes necessary. Reasons for hospitalization include the following:

■ Malnutrition: Twenty percent below expected weight for height recommended for inpatient treatment; 30 percent below expected weight for height recommended for long-term intensive treatment (Sadock et al., 2015)

■ Dehydration: Assessment includes thirst, orthostatic hypotension, tachycardia, elevated sodium levels, and other symptoms

■ Severe electrolyte imbalance: Potassium levels below 3 mmol/L; phosphate levels below 3 mg/dL; magnesium levels below 1.4 mEq/L

■ Cardiac arrhythmias: ST segment and T wave changes usually related to electrolyte imbalances

■ Severe bradycardia: Below 50 beats per minute

■ Hypothermia: Body temperature below 96.8

■ Hypotension: A pattern of low blood pressure or orthostatic hypotension (20 mm Hg or greater drop in systolic blood pressure with positional changes and pulse rate increase by 20 or more beats per minute)

■ Suicidal ideation (see Chapter 11, Suicide Prevention, for an in-depth discussion of suicide risk assessment

In addition to the physical assessment parameters listed previously, when an eating disorder is suspected, a general assessment includes asking patients about their eating patterns and body image, their dieting patterns, whether or not they feel driven to be thin, exercise patterns, and any use of substances including diet pills, laxatives, or diuretics. Assess where the patient is getting information about weight loss, eating behaviors, and calorie restriction methods; several Web sites are established that teach others how to starve themselves and avoid detection. Although the individual may not be forthcoming with this information, asking the parents about their child's use of Internet resources may reveal the need for close monitoring and restrictions on Internet use. Evidence of calluses on the dorsum of the hands, parotid enlargement, mouth ulcers, dental caries, and edema may also be assessment findings in the patient with purging behaviors.

Tables 21–3 and 21–4 provide plans of care for patients with eating disorders. Nursing diagnoses are presented, along with outcome criteria, appropriate nursing interventions, and rationales.

Table 21–3 | CARE PLAN FOR PATIENT WITH EATING DISORDERS: ANOREXIA NERVOSA AND BULIMIA NERVOSA

NURSING DIAGNOSES: IMBALANCED NUTRITION: LESS THAN BODY REQUIREMENTS/DEFICIENT FLUID VOLUME (RISK FOR OR ACTUAL)

RELATED TO: Refusal to eat/drink; self-induced vomiting; abuse of laxatives/diuretics

EVIDENCED BY: Loss of weight; poor muscle tone and skin turgor; lanugo; bradycardia; hypotension; cardiac arrhythmias; pale, dry mucous membranes

OUTCOME CRITERIA	NURSING INTERVENTIONS	RATIONALE
Short-Term Goals ■ Patient will gain x pounds per week (amount to be established by the interdisciplinary team including the patient, nurse, and dietitian). ■ Patient will drink x mL of fluid each hour during waking hours. **Long-Term Goal** ■ By time of discharge from treatment, patient will exhibit no signs or symptoms of malnutrition or dehydration.	1. For the patient who is emaciated and is unable or unwilling to maintain an adequate oral intake, the physician may order a liquid diet to be administered via nasogastric tube. Nursing care of the individual receiving tube feedings should be administered according to established hospital protocol. 2. For the patient who is able and willing to consume an oral diet, collaborate with the dietitian to determine the appropriate amount of calories and fluids required to provide adequate nutrition and realistic weight gain. 3. Explain to the patient that privileges and restrictions will be based on compliance with treatment and direct weight gain. Minimize the focus on food and eating. 4. Weigh patient daily, immediately upon arising and following first voiding. Always use same scale, if possible. Keep strict record of intake and output. Assess skin turgor and integrity regularly. Assess moistness and color of oral mucous membranes. 5. Stay with patient during established time for meals (usually 30 min) and for at least 1 hour following meals. 6. If weight loss occurs, enforce restrictions. 7. Ensure that the patient and family understand that if nutritional status deteriorates, tube feedings will be initiated. This is implemented in a matter-of-fact, nonpunitive way. 8. Encourage the patient to explore and identify the true feelings and fears that contribute to maladaptive eating behaviors.	1. Without adequate nutrition, a life-threatening situation exists. 2. Adequate calories are required to allow a weight gain of 2–3 pounds per week. 3. The real issues have little to do with food or eating patterns. Focus on the control issues that have precipitated these behaviors. 4. These assessments are important measurements of nutritional status and provide guidelines for treatment. 5. Lengthy mealtimes put excessive focus on food and eating and provide patient with attention and reinforcement. The hour following meals may be used to discard food stashed from tray or to engage in self-induced vomiting. 6. Restrictions and limits must be established and carried out consistently to avoid power struggles, to encourage patient compliance with therapy, and to ensure patient safety. 7. This intervention is carried out for the patient's safety and protection from a life-threatening condition. 8. Emotional issues must be resolved if these maladaptive responses are to be eliminated.

Continued

Table 21–3 | CARE PLAN FOR PATIENT WITH EATING DISORDERS: ANOREXIA NERVOSA AND BULIMIA NERVOSA—cont'd

NURSING DIAGNOSIS: DENIAL

RELATED TO: Ineffective coping mechanisms, anxiety, fear of losing control

EVIDENCED BY: Inability to admit the impact of maladaptive eating behaviors on life pattern

OUTCOME CRITERIA	NURSING INTERVENTIONS	RATIONALE
Short-Term Goal ■ Patient will verbalize understanding of the correlation between emotional issues and maladaptive eating behaviors (within time deemed appropriate for individual patient). **Long-Term Goal** ■ By time of discharge from treatment, patient will demonstrate the ability to discontinue use of maladaptive eating behaviors and to cope with emotional issues in a more adaptive manner.	1. Establish a trusting relationship with the patient by being honest, accepting, and available, and by keeping all promises. Convey unconditional positive regard. 2. Acknowledge the patient's anger at feelings of loss of control brought about by the established eating regimen associated with the program of behavior modification. 3. Avoid arguing or bargaining with the patient who is resistant to treatment. State matter-of-factly which behaviors are unacceptable and how privileges will be restricted for noncompliance. 4. Encourage patient to verbalize feelings regarding role within the family and issues related to dependence/independence, the intense need for achievement, and sexuality. Help patient recognize how maladaptive eating behaviors may be related to these emotional issues. Discuss ways in which he or she can gain control over these problematic areas of life without resorting to maladaptive eating behaviors.	1. Trust and unconditional acceptance promote dignity and self-worth and provide a strong foundation for a therapeutic relationship. 2. Anger is a normal human response and should be expressed in an appropriate manner. Feelings that are not expressed remain unresolved and add an additional component to an already serious situation. 3. The person who is denying a problem and who also has a weak ego will use manipulation to achieve control. Consistency and firmness by staff will decrease use of these behaviors. 4. When patient feels control over major life issues, the need to gain control through maladaptive eating behaviors will diminish.

NURSING DIAGNOSIS: DISTURBED BODY IMAGE/LOW SELF-ESTEEM

RELATED TO: Ineffective coping, history of trauma, guilt or shame

EVIDENCED BY: Distorted body image, difficulty accepting positive reinforcement, depressed mood and self-deprecating thoughts

OUTCOME CRITERIA	NURSING INTERVENTIONS	RATIONALE
Short-Term Goal ■ Patient will verbally acknowledge misperception of body image as "fat" within specified time (depending on severity and chronicity of condition).	1. Help patient to develop a realistic perception of body image and relationship with food. Compare specific measurement of the patient's body with the patient's perceived calculations.	1. There may be a large discrepancy between the actual body size and the patient's perception of his or her body size.

Table 21–3 | CARE PLAN FOR PATIENT WITH EATING DISORDERS: ANOREXIA NERVOSA AND BULIMIA NERVOSA—cont'd

OUTCOME CRITERIA	NURSING INTERVENTIONS	RATIONALE
Long-Term Goal ■ By time of discharge from treatment, patient will demonstrate an increase in self-esteem as manifested by verbalizing positive aspects of self and exhibiting less preoccupation with own appearance as a more realistic body image is developed.		Patient needs to recognize that the misperception of body image is unhealthy and that maintaining control through maladaptive eating behaviors is dangerous—even life threatening.
	2. Promote feelings of control within the environment through participation and independent decision making. Through positive feedback, help patient learn to accept self as is, including weaknesses as well as strengths.	2. Patient must come to understand that he or she is a capable, autonomous individual who can perform outside the family unit and who is not expected to be perfect. Control of his or her life must be achieved in other ways besides dieting and weight loss.
	3. Help patient realize that perfection is unrealistic and explore this need with him or her.	3. As patient begins to feel better about self, identifies positive self-attributes, and develops the ability to accept certain personal inadequacies, the need for unrealistic achievement should diminish.
	4. Assess patient for history of trauma and other adverse childhood life events.	4. Assessing for trauma history is foundational to pursuing trauma-informed care.

Concept Care Mapping

The concept map care plan is a diagrammatic teaching and learning strategy that allows visualization of interrelationships between medical diagnoses, nursing diagnoses, assessment data, and treatments. Examples of concept map care plans for patients with eating disorders are presented in Figures 21–1 and 21–2.

Patient and Family Education

The role of patient teacher is important in the psychiatric area, as it is in all areas of nursing. It is essential to include the family in education and treatment unless there are overriding issues against it. A list of topics for patient and family education relevant to eating disorders is presented in Box 21–4.

Evaluation

Evaluation of the patient with an eating disorder requires a reassessment of the behaviors for which the patient sought treatment. Behavioral change will be required on the part of both the patient and family members. The following types of questions may provide assistance in gathering data required for evaluating whether the nursing interventions have been effective in achieving the goals of therapy.

For the Patient With Anorexia Nervosa or Bulimia Nervosa

Has the patient:

■ Steadily gained 2 to 3 pounds per week to at least 80 percent of expected body weight for age and size?
■ Demonstrated no signs or symptoms of malnutrition and dehydration?
■ Consistently consumed adequate calories as determined by the dietitian?
■ Attempted to stash food from the tray to discard later?
■ Attempted to self-induce vomiting?
■ Admitted that a problem exists and that eating behaviors are maladaptive?
■ Discontinued maladaptive behaviors to manipulate calorie restriction?
■ Discussed feelings related to family roles, sexuality, dependence/independence, and the need for achievement?
■ Verbalized understanding of how he or she has used maladaptive eating behaviors in an effort to achieve a feeling of some control over life events?
■ Acknowledged that perception of body image as "fat" is incorrect?

Table 21–4 | CARE PLAN FOR THE PATIENT WITH A BINGE EATING DISORDER: OBESITY

NURSING DIAGNOSIS: IMBALANCED NUTRITION: MORE THAN BODY REQUIREMENTS
RELATED TO: Compulsive overeating
EVIDENCED BY: Weight of more than 20 percent over expected body weight for age and height; BMI > 30

OUTCOME CRITERIA	NURSING INTERVENTIONS	RATIONALE
Short-Term Goal ■ Patient will identify desired weight loss plan. **Long-Term Goal** ■ Patient will demonstrate a change in eating patterns that results in the patient's desired weight loss.	1. Encourage the patient to keep a diary of food intake. 2. Discuss feelings and emotions associated with eating. 3. With input from the patient, formulate an eating plan that includes food from the required food groups with emphasis on low-fat intake. It is helpful to keep the plan as similar to patient's usual eating pattern as possible. 4. Identify realistic incremental goals for weekly weight loss. 5. Plan a progressive exercise program tailored to individual goals and choice. 6. Discuss the probability of reaching plateaus when weight remains stable for extended periods. 7. Provide instruction about medications to assist with weight loss if ordered by physician.	1. A food diary provides the opportunity for patient to gain a realistic picture of the amount of food ingested and provides a database on which to tailor the dietary program. 2. This helps to identify when patient is eating to satisfy an emotional need rather than a physiological one. 3. Diet must eliminate calories while maintaining adequate nutrition. Patient is more likely to stay on the eating plan if he or she is able to participate in its creation and it deviates as little as possible from usual types of foods. 4. Reasonable weight loss (1–2 pounds per week) results in more lasting effects. Excessive, rapid weight loss may result in fatigue and irritability and ultimately lead to failure in meeting goals for weight loss. Motivation is more easily sustained by meeting "stair-step" goals. 5. Exercise may enhance weight loss by burning calories and reducing appetite, increasing energy, toning muscles, and enhancing sense of well-being and accomplishment. Walking is an excellent choice for overweight individuals. 6. Patient should know that this is likely to happen as changes in metabolism occur. Plateaus cause frustration, and patient may need additional support during these times to remain on the weight loss program. 7. Appetite-suppressant drugs and others that have weight loss as a side effect may be helpful to someone who is severely overweight. They should be used for this purpose for only a short period while the individual attempts to adjust to the new pattern of eating.

Table 21–4 | CARE PLAN FOR THE PATIENT WITH A BINGE EATING DISORDER: OBESITY—cont'd

NURSING DIAGNOSIS: DISTURBED BODY IMAGE/LOW SELF-ESTEEM
RELATED TO: Dissatisfaction with appearance, trauma history
EVIDENCED BY: Verbalization of negative feelings about the way he or she looks and desire to lose weight

OUTCOME CRITERIA	NURSING INTERVENTIONS	RATIONALE
Short-Term Goal ■ Patient will begin to accept self, based on self-attributes rather than on appearance. **Long-Term Goal** ■ Patient will pursue loss of weight as desired.	1. Assess patient's feelings and attitudes about being obese. 2. Assess for history of trauma and adverse childhood life events. 3. Ensure that the patient has privacy during self-care activities. 4. Have patient recall coping patterns related to food in family of origin and explore how these may affect current situation. 5. Determine patient's motivation for weight loss and set goals. 6. Help patient identify positive self-attributes. Focus on strengths and past accomplishments unrelated to physical appearance. 7. Refer patient to support or therapy group.	1. Obesity and compulsive eating behaviors may have deep-rooted psychological implications, such as compensation for lack of love and nurturing or a defense against intimacy. 2. Assessing for trauma history is foundational to providing trauma-informed care. 3. The obese individual may be sensitive or self-conscious about his or her body. 4. Parents are role models for their children. Maladaptive eating behaviors may be learned within the family system and are supported through positive reinforcement. Food may be substituted by the parent for affection and love, and eating is associated with a feeling of satisfaction, becoming the primary defense. 5. The individual may harbor repressed feelings of hostility, which may be expressed inward on the self. Because of a poor self-concept, the person often has difficulty with relationships. When the motivation is to lose weight for someone else, successful weight loss is less likely to occur. 6. It is important that self-esteem not be tied solely to size of the body. Patient needs to recognize that obesity need not interfere with positive feelings regarding self-concept and self-worth. 7. Support groups can provide companionship, increase motivation, decrease loneliness and social ostracism, and give practical solutions to common problems. CBT has demonstrated effectiveness in treating eating disorders. Group therapy can be helpful in dealing with underlying psychological concerns.

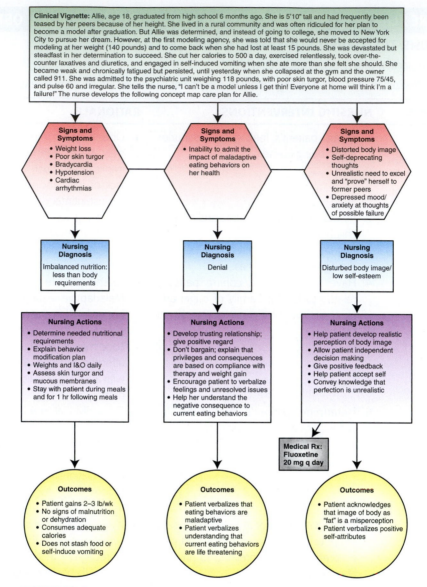

Clinical Vignette: Allie, age 18, graduated from high school 6 months ago. She is 5'10" tall and had frequently been teased by her peers because of her height. She lived in a rural community and was often ridiculed for her plan to become a model after graduation. But Allie was determined, and instead of going to college, she moved to New York City to pursue her dream. However, at the first modeling agency, she was told that she would never be accepted for modeling at her weight (140 pounds) and to come back when she had lost at least 15 pounds. She was devastated but steadfast in her determination to succeed. She cut her calories to 500 a day, exercised relentlessly, took over-the-counter laxatives and diuretics, and engaged in self-induced vomiting when she ate more than she felt she should. She became weak and chronically fatigued but persisted, until yesterday when she collapsed at the gym and the owner called 911. She was admitted to the psychiatric unit weighing 118 pounds, with poor skin turgor, blood pressure 75/45, and pulse 60 and irregular. She tells the nurse, "I can't be a model unless I get thin! Everyone at home will think I'm a failure!" The nurse develops the following concept map care plan for Allie.

Signs and Symptoms
- Weight loss
- Poor skin turgor
- Bradycardia
- Hypotension
- Cardiac arrhythmias

Signs and Symptoms
- Inability to admit the impact of maladaptive eating behaviors on her health

Signs and Symptoms
- Distorted body image
- Self-deprecating thoughts
- Unrealistic need to excel and "prove" herself to former peers
- Depressed mood/anxiety at thoughts of possible failure

Nursing Diagnosis
Imbalanced nutrition: less than body requirements

Nursing Diagnosis
Denial

Nursing Diagnosis
Disturbed body image/low self-esteem

Nursing Actions
- Determine needed nutritional requirements
- Explain behavior modification plan
- Weights and I&O daily
- Assess skin turgor and mucous membranes
- Stay with patient during meals and for 1 hr following meals

Nursing Actions
- Develop trusting relationship; give positive regard
- Don't bargain; explain that privileges and consequences are based on compliance with therapy and weight gain
- Encourage patient to verbalize feelings and unresolved issues
- Help her understand the negative consequence to current eating behaviors

Nursing Actions
- Help patient develop realistic perception of body image
- Allow patient independent decision making
- Give positive feedback
- Help patient accept self
- Convey knowledge that perfection is unrealistic

Medical Rx: Fluoxetine 20 mg q day

Outcomes
- Patient gains 2–3 lb/wk
- No signs of malnutrition or dehydration
- Consumes adequate calories
- Does not stash food or self-induce vomiting

Outcomes
- Patient verbalizes that eating behaviors are maladaptive
- Patient verbalizes understanding that current eating behaviors are life threatening

Outcomes
- Patient acknowledges that image of body as "fat" is a misperception
- Patient verbalizes positive self-attributes

FIGURE 21-1 Concept map care plan for a patient with anorexia nervosa.

For the Client With BED and Associated Obesity

Has the patient:

- Shown a steady weight loss since starting the new eating plan?
- Verbalized a relapse prevention plan to avoid triggers and abstain from binging?
- Verbalized positive self-attributes not associated with body size or appearance?

For the Client With Anorexia Nervosa, Bulimia Nervosa, or BED and Associated Obesity

Has the patient:

- Been able to develop a more realistic perception of body image?
- Acknowledged that past self-expectations may have been unrealistic?
- Verbalized improvement in self-acceptance?
- Developed adaptive coping strategies to deal with stress without resorting to maladaptive eating behaviors?

Quality and Safety Education for Nurses (QSEN)

The Institute of Medicine (IOM), in its 2003 report *Health Professions Education: A Bridge to Quality*, challenged faculties of medicine, nursing, and other health professions to ensure that their graduates have achieved a core set of competencies in order to

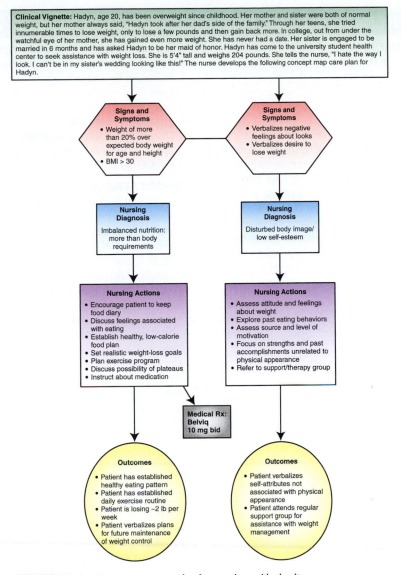

Clinical Vignette: Hadyn, age 20, has been overweight since childhood. Her mother and sister were both of normal weight, but her mother always said, "Hadyn took after her dad's side of the family." Through her teens, she tried innumerable times to lose weight, only to lose a few pounds and then gain back more. In college, out from under the watchful eye of her mother, she has gained even more weight. She has never had a date. Her sister is engaged to be married in 6 months and has asked Hadyn to be her maid of honor. Hadyn has come to the university student health center to seek assistance with weight loss. She is 5'4" tall and weighs 204 pounds. She tells the nurse, "I hate the way I look. I can't be in my sister's wedding looking like this!" The nurse develops the following concept map care plan for Hadyn.

Signs and Symptoms
• Weight of more than 20% over expected body weight for age and height
• BMI > 30

Signs and Symptoms
• Verbalizes negative feelings about looks
• Verbalizes desire to lose weight

Nursing Diagnosis
Imbalanced nutrition: more than body requirements

Nursing Diagnosis
Disturbed body image/low self-esteem

Nursing Actions
• Encourage patient to keep food diary
• Discuss feelings associated with eating
• Establish healthy, low-calorie food plan
• Set realistic weight-loss goals
• Plan exercise program
• Discuss possibility of plateaus
• Instruct about medication

Nursing Actions
• Assess attitude and feelings about weight
• Explore past eating behaviors
• Assess source and level of motivation
• Focus on strengths and past accomplishments unrelated to physical appearance
• Refer to support/therapy group

Medical Rx: Belviq 10 mg bid

Outcomes
• Patient has established healthy eating pattern
• Patient has established daily exercise routine
• Patient is losing ~2 lb per week
• Patient verbalizes plans for future maintenance of weight control

Outcomes
• Patient verbalizes self-attributes not associated with physical appearance
• Patient attends regular support group for assistance with weight management

FIGURE 21–2 Concept map care plan for a patient with obesity.

meet the needs of the 21st-century healthcare system. These competencies include *providing patient-centered care, maintaining safety, working in interdisciplinary teams, employing evidence-based practice, incorporating quality improvement,* and *utilizing informatics.* A QSEN teaching strategy is included in Box 21–5. The use of this type of activity is intended to arm the instructor and the student with guidelines for attaining the knowledge, skills, and attitudes necessary for achievement of quality and safety competencies in nursing.

Treatment Modalities

The immediate aim of treatment in eating disorders is to restore and stabilize the patient's nutritional status. Complications of emaciation, dehydration, and

electrolyte imbalance can lead to death. Once the physical condition is no longer life threatening, other treatment modalities may be initiated.

Behavior Modification

Efforts to change the maladaptive eating behaviors of clients with anorexia nervosa and bulimia nervosa have become the widely accepted treatment. The importance of instituting a behavior modification program with these clients is to ensure that the program does not "control" them. Issues of control are central in these disorders, and in order for the program to be successful, the client must perceive that he or she is in control of the treatment. The Maudsley approach, an evidence-based program for the treatment of adolescents with anorexia nervosa,

---

BOX 21–4 Topics for Patient and Family Education Related to Eating Disorders

NATURE OF THE ILLNESS
1. Symptoms of anorexia nervosa
2. Symptoms of bulimia nervosa
3. Symptoms of BED
4. What constitutes obesity
5. Causes of eating disorders
6. Effects of the illness or condition on the body
7. Behaviors that may reinforce unhealthy responses, such as television and social media, peer focus on clothing sizes, eating, and weight. Internet sources have become a means for sharing information among people with anorexia about how the individual can distract parents and healthcare providers from recognizing the extent of weight loss. Family members can learn more about some of these behaviors to look out for and may want to monitor their child's use of Internet and social media resources

MANAGEMENT OF THE ILLNESS
1. Principles of nutrition (foods for maintenance of wellness)
2. Ways patient may feel in control of life (aside from eating)
3. Importance of expressing fears and feelings, rather than holding them inside
4. Alternative coping strategies (to maladaptive eating behaviors)
5. For the obese patient:
    a. How to plan a reduced-calorie, nutritious diet
    b. How to read food content labels
    c. How to establish a realistic weight loss plan

d. How to establish a planned program of physical activity
6. Correct administration of prescribed medications
7. Indication for and side effects of prescribed medications
8. Relaxation techniques
9. Problem-solving skills
10. Discuss the Maudsley approach for treatment of anorexia nervosa as an evidence-based option for family involvement in the recovery program

SUPPORT SERVICES
1. Weight Watchers International
2. Overeaters Anonymous
3. National Association of Anorexia Nervosa and Associated Disorders (ANAD)
    220 N. Green St
    Chicago, IL 60607
    (630) 577-1330(helpline)
    www.anad.org
4. National Eating Disorders Association
    200 West 41th Street
    New York, NY 10036
    (212) 575-6200
    www.nationaleatingdisorders.org
5. National Association for Males with Eating Disorders
    2840 SW 3rd Ave.
    Miami, FL 33129
    Namedinc.org

---

modifies the traditional concept of the client being in control of their calorie intake: the first phase of treatment is designed to encourage *parental* control of eating, and control is returned to the adolescent after he or she demonstrates the readiness and ability to establish control in healthier ways.

Success has been observed when the client with anorexia nervosa is allowed to contract for privileges based on weight gain. The client has input into the care plan and can clearly see what the treatment choices are. The client has control over eating, over the amount of exercise pursued, and even over whether or not to induce vomiting. Goals of therapy, along with the responsibilities for achieving each goal, are agreed on by the client and staff.

Staff and the client also agree on a system of rewards and privileges that can be earned by the client, who is given ultimate control. He or she has a choice of whether or not to abide by the contract—a choice of whether or not to gain weight and whether or not to earn the desired privilege.

This method of treatment gives a great deal of autonomy to the client. It must be understood, however, that these behavior modification techniques are helpful for weight restoration only. Concomitant individual and/or family psychotherapy are required to prevent or reduce further morbidity. Cognitive behavior therapy (CBT) and dialectical behavior therapy (DBT) have demonstrated benefits in clients with anorexia nervosa, bulimia nervosa, and BED (Call et al., 2017; O'Melia, 2014).

By confronting irrational thinking patterns and associated feelings, CBT and DBT strive to eliminate the emotional components associated with unhealthy eating patterns.

Individual Therapy

Although individual psychotherapy is not the therapy of choice for eating disorders, it may be an adjunct to a comprehensive, multifaceted treatment approach when underlying comorbid psychological problems are contributing to the maladaptive behaviors. In

BOX 21–5 QSEN TEACHING STRATEGY

Assignment: Using Evidence to Address Clinical Problems
Intervention With a Patient Who Fears Gaining Weight (Anorexia Nervosa)

Competency Domain: Evidence-Based Practice

Learning Objectives: Student will:

- Differentiate clinical opinion from research and evidence summaries.
- Explain the role of evidence in determining the best clinical practice for intervening with clients who do not want to eat.
- Identify gaps between what is observed in the treatment setting to what has been identified as best practice.
- Discriminate between valid and invalid reasons for modifying evidence-based clinical practice based on clinical expertise or other reasons.
- Participate effectively in appropriate data collection and other research activities.
- Acknowledge own limitations in knowledge and clinical expertise before determining when to deviate from evidence-based best practices.

Strategy Overview

1. Investigate the research related to intervening with a patient who does not want to eat.
2. Identify best practices described in the literature. How were these best practices determined?
3. Compare and contrast staff intervention with best practices described in the literature.
4. Investigate staff perceptions related to intervening with a patient who is refusing to eat. How have they developed these perceptions?
5. Do staff members view any problems associated with their practice versus best practice described in the literature? If so, how would they like to see the problem addressed?
6. Describe ethical issues associated with intervening with a patient who does not want to eat.
7. What is your personal perception regarding the best evidence available to date related to intervening with a patient who has anorexia nervosa? Are there situations that you can think of when you might deviate from the best practice model?
8. What questions do you have about intervening with a patient who has anorexia nervosa that are not being addressed by current researchers?

Source: Adapted from teaching strategy submitted by Pamela M. Ironside, Associate Professor, Indiana University School of Nursing, Indianapolis, IN. © 2009 QSEN; http://qsen.org. With permission.

supportive psychotherapy, the therapist encourages the client to explore unresolved conflicts and to recognize the maladaptive eating behaviors as defense mechanisms used to ease the emotional pain. The goals are to resolve the personal issues and establish more adaptive coping strategies for dealing with stressful situations.

Family Treatment: The Maudsley Approach

The Maudsley approach is one of the few evidence-based treatment approaches for the treatment of teens with anorexia nervosa. This approach actively involves the family in each step of the process. In some of the first controlled studies of this method, 90 percent of the clients showed improvement compared to 36 percent of those in individual therapies (LeGrange, 2005). The treatment program is conducted in an intensive outpatient program, and it involves three phases of treatment. Phase I is focused on weight restoration, and in this phase, the parents are actively engaged in establishing the rules and guidelines around eating. Parents often need a lot of support during this phase because they typically encounter frequent power struggles with their child. When the patient accepts parental demands for increased food intake and demonstrates steady weight gain, and when there is a change in the mood of the family (i.e., relief at having taken charge of the eating disorder; both the adolescent and his or her parents identify reduced anxiety), phase II is ready to begin (LeGrange & Lock, n.d.). In this phase, control of maintaining weight gain is returned to the adolescent. Once he or she demonstrates the ability to maintain above 95 percent of ideal weight, the shift to phase III focuses on assisting the adolescent to develop a healthy self-identity. This phase includes incorporating CBT and DBT skills, which have also demonstrated effectiveness in treating this condition.

Psychopharmacology

Medication research has not yet identified a medication that results in definitive improvement of anorexia nervosa (Sadock et al., 2015). Trials of fluoxetine (Prozac) have shown some evidence of weight gain, and, in general, SSRIs may be beneficial in the treatment of comorbid depression, but they also carry a black-box warning about risk of increasing suicide ideation in adolescents. The anticholinergic side effects of tricyclic antidepressants, including orthostatic hypotension, may be problematic for patients who are already at risk for these symptoms. It is important to recognize that depression and other mood and cognitive symptoms can be a symptom of malnutrition and starvation. When nutrition is restored, those symptoms often improve.

Antidepressants, and particularly fluoxetine, have been found to be useful in the treatment of bulimia nervosa (Call et al., 2017) and appear to have benefits for patients with and without depressive symptoms. A dosage of 60 mg/day (triple the usual antidepressant dosage) was found to be most effective. It is possible that fluoxetine, an SSRI, may decrease the craving for carbohydrates, thereby decreasing the incidence of binge eating, which is often associated with consumption of large amounts of carbohydrates. Other antidepressants, such as imipramine (Tofranil), desipramine (Norpramin), amitriptyline (Elavil), nortriptyline (Aventyl), and phenelzine (Nardil), also have been shown to be effective in controlled treatment studies (Sadock et al., 2015).

High-dose SSRIs have demonstrated some effectiveness in promoting weight loss for those with BED, but the weight loss was temporary and weight *gain* typically occurred after the medication was discontinued (Sadock et al., 2015). Remember, too, that weight gain is a secondary symptom of BED. An effective medication needs to also manage the symptom of binging. Two medications, topiramate and lisdexamfetamine (a dopamine-norepinephrine reuptake inhibitor, originally used in the treatment of attention-deficit-hyperactivity/disorder) have demonstrated benefits in reducing both incidents of binge eating and weight gain (Balodis et al., 2015). Currently, lisdexamfetamine (Vyvanse) has been FDA approved specifically for short-term treatment of BED. Most studies reveal that medication in combination with CBT is more beneficial than medication alone (Sadock et al., 2015).

CASE STUDY AND SAMPLE CARE PLAN

NURSING HISTORY AND ASSESSMENT

When Katie fainted in history class, she was taken to the university health center by her roommate, Ashley. Ashley told the nurse that Katie had been taking a lot of over-the-counter laxatives and diuretics. She also said that Katie often self-induced vomiting when she felt that she had eaten too much. After an initial physical assessment, the nurse in the university health center referred Katie to the mental health clinic.

At the mental health clinic, Katie weighed 110 pounds and measured 5 feet 6 inches tall. She admitted to the psychiatric nurse that she tried to keep her weight down by dieting but sometimes she got so hungry that she would overeat, and then she felt the need to self-induce vomiting to get rid of the calories. "I really don't like doing it, but lots of the girls do. In fact, that is where I got the idea. I always thought I was too fat in high school, but the competition wasn't so great there. Here all the girls are so pretty . . . and so thin! It's the only way I can keep my weight down!"

Katie also admitted that she hoards food in her dorm room and that she eats when she is feeling particularly anxious and depressed (often during the night). She admitted to having eaten several bags of potato chips and whole packages of cookies in a single sitting. She sometimes drives to the local hamburger stand in the middle of the night, orders several hamburgers, fries, and milkshakes, and consumes them as she sits in her car alone. She stated that she feels so much better while she is eating these foods but then feels panicky after they have been consumed. That is when she self-induces vomiting. "Then I feel more depressed, and the only thing that helps is eating! I feel so out of control!"

NURSING DIAGNOSES AND OUTCOME IDENTIFICATION

From the assessment data, the nurse develops the following nursing diagnosis for Katie:

1. **Ineffective coping** related to feelings of helplessness, low self-esteem, and lack of control in life situation
   a. **Short-Term Goal:** Katie will identify and discuss fears and anxieties with the nurse.
   b. **Long-Term Goal:** Katie will identify adaptive coping strategies that can be realistically incorporated into her lifestyle, thereby eliminating binging and purging in response to anxiety.

CASE STUDY AND SAMPLE CARE PLAN—cont'd

PLANNING AND IMPLEMENTATION

INEFFECTIVE COPING

The following nursing interventions have been identified for Katie:

1. Establish a trusting relationship with Katie. Be honest and accepting. Show unconditional positive regard.
2. Help Katie identify the situations that produce anxiety and discuss how she coped with these situations before she began binging and purging.
3. Help Katie identify the emotions that precipitate binging (e.g., fear, boredom, anger, loneliness).
4. Once these high-risk situations have been identified, help her identify alternative behaviors, such as exercise, a hobby, or a warm bath.
5. Encourage Katie to express feelings that have been suppressed because they were considered unacceptable. Help her identify healthier ways to express those feelings.
6. Use role-play with Katie to deal with feelings and experiment with new behaviors.
7. Explore the dynamics of Katie's family. Intrafamilial conflicts may reinforce maladaptive eating behaviors.
8. Teach the concepts of good nutrition and the importance of healthy eating patterns in overall wellness.
9. Consult with the physician about a prescription for fluoxetine for Katie.
10. Help Katie find a support group for individuals with eating disorders. Encourage regular attendance in this group.

EVALUATION

The outcome criteria for Katie have been met. She discussed with the nurse the feelings that triggered binging episodes and the situations that precipitated those feelings. She has joined a support group of individuals with eating disorders and now has a "buddy" whom she may call (even in the middle of the night) when she is feeling like binging. She has started riding her bicycle regularly and goes to the fitness center when she is feeling especially anxious. Katie still sees the mental health nurse weekly and continues to discuss her fears and anxieties. The urges to binge at stressful times have not disappeared completely. However, they have decreased in frequency, and Katie is now able to choose more adaptive strategies for dealing with stress.

Summary and Key Points

- The incidence of eating disorders has continued to increase since the middle of the 20th century.
- Individuals with anorexia nervosa, a disorder that is characterized by a morbid fear of obesity and a gross distortion of body image, literally can starve themselves to death.
- The individual with anorexia nervosa believes he or she is fat even when emaciated. The disorder is commonly accompanied by depression and anxiety.
- Bulimia nervosa is an eating disorder characterized by the consumption of large amounts of food, usually in a short period and often in secret.
- With bulimia nervosa, tension is relieved and pleasure is felt during the time of the binge, but feelings of guilt and depression follow soon after the binge.
- Individuals with bulimia nervosa purge themselves of the excessive intake with self-induced vomiting or the misuse of laxatives, diuretics, or enemas. They also are subject to mood and anxiety disorders.
- BED is characterized by the consumption of huge amounts of food by an individual who feels a lack of control over the eating behavior. BED differs from bulimia nervosa in that the individual does not engage in behaviors to rid the body of the excess calories.
- Compulsive eating can result in obesity, which is defined by the National Institutes of Health as a BMI of 30 or more.
- Obesity predisposes the individual to many health concerns, and at the morbid level (a BMI of 40), weight alone can contribute to increases in morbidity and mortality.
- Predisposing factors to eating disorders include genetics, physiological factors, family dynamics, and environmental and lifestyle factors.
- Treatment modalities for eating disorders include behavior modification, individual psychotherapy, CBT, family treatment (such as the Maudsley approach), and psychopharmacology.

Review Questions
Self-Examination/Learning Exercise

Select the answer that is most appropriate for each of the following questions:

1. Some obese individuals take amphetamines to suppress appetite and help them lose weight. Which of the following is an adverse effect associated with use of amphetamines that makes this practice undesirable?
   a. Bradycardia
   b. Amenorrhea
   c. Tolerance
   d. Convulsions

2. The Maudsley approach to treatment of adolescents with anorexia nervosa advances which of the following fundamental concepts?
   a. Family should be actively involved in each phase of treatment.
   b. Parents should be prohibited from involvement in helping their child eat more because there are often control issues.
   c. Adolescents need to work on developing healthy self-identities before they can begin to gain weight.
   d. Individual psychotherapy is the most effective treatment for adolescents with anorexia nervosa.

3. John has sought help for his concern that he is binge eating, and he feels it has "gotten out of control." He asks the nurse what can be done to help him. Which of the following is the most accurate response?
   a. "There is nothing that can be done."
   b. "There are some medications and psychological treatments that have demonstrated effectiveness in reducing binge eating behaviors."
   c. "The primary problem is obesity. I can help you set up a calorie-restricted diet."
   d. "There are medications that can help with weight loss, but there are no medications effective for reducing binge eating."

4. Emma, age 14, has just been admitted to the psychiatric unit for anorexia nervosa. She is emaciated and refuses to eat. What is the primary nursing diagnosis for Emma?
   a. Complicated grieving
   b. Imbalanced nutrition: Less than body requirements
   c. Interrupted family processes
   d. Anxiety (severe)

5. Which of the following physical manifestations would you expect to assess in a patient suffering from anorexia nervosa?
   a. Tachycardia, hypertension, hyperthermia
   b. Bradycardia, hypertension, hyperthermia
   c. Bradycardia, hypotension, hypothermia
   d. Tachycardia, hypotension, hypothermia

6. The nurse is caring for a patient who has been hospitalized with anorexia nervosa and is severely malnourished. The patient continues to refuse to eat. What is the most appropriate response by the nurse?
   a. "You know that if you don't eat, you will die."
   b. "If you continue to refuse to take food orally, you will be fed through a nasogastric tube."
   c. "You might as well leave if you are not going to follow your therapy regimen."
   d. "You don't have to eat if you don't want to. It is your choice."

Review Questions—cont'd
Self-Examination/Learning Exercise

7. Which medication has been used with some success in clients with anorexia nervosa?
   a. Lorcaserin (Belviq)
   b. Diazepam (Valium)
   c. Fluoxetine (Prozac)
   d. Carbamazepine (Tegretol)

8. Marissa is hospitalized on the psychiatric unit. She has a history and current diagnosis of bulimia nervosa. Which of the following symptoms would be congruent with Marissa's diagnosis?
   a. Binging, purging, obesity, hyperkalemia
   b. Binging, purging, normal weight, hypokalemia
   c. Binging, laxative abuse, amenorrhea, severe weight loss
   d. Binging, purging, severe weight loss, hyperkalemia

9. A hospitalized patient with bulimia nervosa has stopped vomiting in the hospital and tells the nurse she is afraid she is going to gain weight. Which is the most appropriate response by the nurse?
   a. "Don't worry. The dietitian will ensure you don't get too many calories in your diet."
   b. "Don't worry about your weight. We are going to work on other problems while you are in the hospital."
   c. "I understand that you are concerned about your weight, and we will talk about the importance of good nutrition; but for now, I want you to tell me about your recent invitation to join the National Honor Society. That's quite an accomplishment."
   d. "You are not fat, and the staff will ensure that you do not gain weight while you are in the hospital, because we know that is important to you."

10. Mandy presents in the emergency department with complaints of suicidal ideation. The following data is collected by the nurse. Which of these assessment findings suggests that bulimia nervosa might be a health problem? (Select all that apply.)
    a. Mandy's parotid glands appear enlarged.
    b. Mandy's teeth have a "moth eaten" pattern of tooth decay.
    c. Mandy reports that she takes laxatives daily.
    d. Mandy's weight is within the expected range.

IMPLICATIONS OF RESEARCH FOR EVIDENCE-BASED PRACTICE

Bakalar, J. L., Barmine, M., Druskin, L., Olsen, C. H., Quinlan, J., Sbrocco, T., & Tanofsky-Kraff, M. (2018). Childhood adverse life events, disordered eating, and body mass index in US military service members. *International Journal of Eating Disorders, 51*(11). doi:10.1002/eat.22851

DESCRIPTION OF THE STUDY: The authors, noting a high prevalence of overweight and obesity and a high prevalence of childhood adverse life events among U.S. military personnel, conducted an online survey (N = 179) of active duty military personnel to explore the associations between these two phenomena.

RESULTS OF THE STUDY: Multiple indices of childhood adverse life events (both traumatic and subjective impact) were positively associated with a higher body mass index and were mediated by disordered eating.

IMPLICATIONS FOR NURSING PRACTICE: This study underscores the importance of trauma assessment and trauma-informed care for military personnel. Additionally, as the authors note, because there have been consistent links demonstrated between childhood adverse life events and eating disorders in the general population, assessment of trauma history should also be conducted for any client presenting with an eating disorder.

TEST YOUR CRITICAL THINKING SKILLS

Janice, a high school sophomore, wanted desperately to become a cheerleader. She practiced endlessly before tryouts, but she was not selected. A week later, her boyfriend, Roy, broke up with her to date another girl. Janice, who was 5 feet 3 inches tall and weighed 110 pounds, decided it was because she was too fat. She began to exercise at every possible moment. She skipped meals and tried to keep her daily consumption to no more than 300 calories. She lost a great deal of weight but became very weak. She felt cold all of the time and wore sweaters in the warm weather. Janice collapsed during her physical education class at school and was rushed to the emergency department. On admission, she weighed 90 pounds. She was emaciated and anemic. The physician admitted her with a diagnosis of Anorexia Nervosa.

Answer the following questions about Janice:

1. What will be the *primary* consideration in Janice's care?
2. How will treatment be directed toward helping her gain weight?
3. How will the nurse know if Janice is using self-induced vomiting to rid herself of food consumed at meals?

Communication Exercises

1. Helena was admitted to the psychiatric unit with a diagnosis of severe anorexia nervosa. After completing a meal, she asks the nurse to be excused so she can use the restroom.

   How would the nurse respond to Helena's request?

2. John has been seeking counseling for a binge eating disorder. When the nurse is weighing him, John states, "I hate myself. I should never have let myself get like this. I'm completely out of control."

   What would be the most empathic response by the nurse?

 MOVIE CONNECTIONS

The Best Little Girl in the World (Anorexia nervosa) • *Kate's Secret* (Bulimia nervosa) • *For the Love of Nancy* (Anorexia nervosa) • *Super Size Me* (Obesity). *To the Bone* (Anorexia nervosa)

References

American Academy for Eating Disorders. (2009). *Position statement: The role of the family in eating disorders.* Retrieved from https://www.aedweb.org/advocate/press-releases/role-of-the-family

American Psychiatric Association (APA). (2013). *Diagnostic and statistical manual of mental disorders, fifth edition (DSM-5).* Washington, DC: Author.

Bakalar, J. L., Barmine, M., Druskin, L., Olsen, C. H., Quinlan, J., Sbrocco, T., & Tanofsky-Kraff, M. (2018). Childhood adverse life events, disordered eating, and body mass index in US military service members. *International Journal of Eating Disorders, 51*(11). doi:10.1002/eat.22851

Balodis, I. M., Grilo, C. M., & Potenza, M. N. (2015). Neurobiological underpinnings of obesity and addiction: A focus on binge eating disorder and implications for treatment. *Psychiatric Times.* Retrieved from http://www.psychiatrictimes.com/cme/neurobiological-underpinnings-obesity-and-addiction-focus-binge-eating-disorder-and-implications/page/0/2#sthash.D9vZ5Ijs.dpuf

Call, C. C., Attia, E., & Walsh, B. T. (2017). Feeding and eating disorders. In B. J. Sadock, V. A. Sadock, & P. Ruiz (Eds.), *Comprehensive textbook of psychiatry* (10th ed., pp. 2065–2082). Philadelphia, PA: Wolters Kluwer.

Centers for Disease Control and Prevention (CDC). (2017). *Overweight and obesity.* Retrieved from http://www.cdc.gov/obesity/adult/index.html

Herdman, T. H., & Kamitsuru, S. (Eds.). (2018). *NANDA-I nursing diagnoses: Definitions and classification, 2018–2020.* New York, NY: Thieme.

Institute of Medicine (IOM). (2003). *Health professions education: A bridge to quality.* Washington, DC: National Academies Press.

LeGrange, D. (2005). The Maudsley family-based treatment for adolescent anorexia nervosa. *World Psychiatry, 4*(3), 142–146.

LeGrange, D., & Lock, J. (n.d.). *Family-based treatment of adolescent anorexia nervosa: The Maudsley approach.* Retrieved from http://www.maudsleyparents.org/whatismaudsley.html

National Heart, Lung, and Blood Institute. (n.d.). *Clinical guidelines on the identification, evaluation, and treatment of overweight and obesity in adults: Body mass index tables.* Retrieved from http://www.nhlbi.nih.gov/guidelines/obesity/bmi_tbl.htm

O'Melia, A. M. (2014). Binge eating disorder. *Current Psychiatry, 13*(4). Retrieved from http://www.currentpsychiatry.com/specialty-focus/eating-disorders/article/binge-eating-disorder/1e566fd65698cb7b06e0d2b355284392.html

Sadock, B. J., Sadock, V. A., & Ruiz, P. (2015). *Synopsis of psychiatry: Behavioral sciences/clinical psychiatry* (11th ed.). Philadelphia, PA: Wolters Kluwer.

Uniacke, B., & Broft, A. (2016). The interplay of mood disorders and eating disorders. *Psychiatric Times 33*(5). Retrieved from http://www.psychiatrictimes.com/special-reports/interplay-mood-disorders-and-eating-disorders

WebMD. (2016). *Symptoms of binge eating disorder.* Retrieved from https://www.webmd.com/mental-health/eating-disorders/binge-eating-disorder/binge-eating-symptoms#2

Woolridge, T., & Lemberg, R. (2016). Macho, bravado, and eating disorders in men: Special issues in diagnosis and treatment. *Psychiatric Times, 33*(5). Retrieved from http://www.psychiatrictimes.com/special-reports/macho-bravado-and-eating-disorders-men-special-issues-diagnosis-and-treatment

Personality Disorders

22

CORE CONCEPT

Personality

KEY TERMS

antisocial personality disorder

avoidant personality disorder

borderline personality disorder (BPD)

dependent personality disorder

histrionic personality disorder

narcissistic personality disorder

object constancy

obsessive-compulsive personality disorder

paranoid personality disorder

schizoid personality disorder

schizotypal personality disorder

splitting

OBJECTIVES
After reading this chapter, the student will be able to:

1. Define *personality*.
2. Compare stages of personality development according to Sullivan, Erikson, and Mahler.
3. Identify various types of personality disorders.
4. Discuss historical and epidemiological statistics related to various personality disorders.
5. Describe symptomatology associated with borderline personality disorder (BPD) and antisocial personality disorder and use these data in patient assessment.

6. Identify predisposing factors for BPD and antisocial personality disorder.
7. Formulate nursing diagnoses and goals of care for patients with BPD and antisocial personality disorder.
8. Describe appropriate nursing interventions for behaviors associated with BPD and antisocial personality disorder.
9. Evaluate nursing care of patients with BPD and antisocial personality disorder.
10. Discuss various modalities relevant to treatment of personality disorders.

561

Introduction

> **CORE CONCEPT**
>
> **Personality**
> The totality of emotional and behavioral characteristics that are particular to a specific person and that remain somewhat stable and predictable over time.

The word *personality* is derived from the Greek term *persona*. It was originally used to describe the theatrical mask worn by some dramatic actors at the time. Over the years, it lost its connotation of pretense and illusion and came to represent the person behind the mask—the "real" person.

Personality *traits* may be defined as characteristics with which an individual is born or develops early in life. They influence the way in which he or she perceives and relates to the environment and are quite stable over time. Personality *disorders* occur when these traits deviate markedly from the expectations of the individual's culture, become rigid and inflexible, contribute to maladaptive patterns of behavior or impairment in functioning, and lead to distress (American Psychiatric Association [APA], 2013). The most common symptoms occurring in personality disorders are impairment in interpersonal relationship functions (41 percent) and dysfunctions in cognition (30 percent), affect (18 percent), and impulse control (6 percent) (Bornstein et al., 2014). In specific types of personality disorders, such as paranoid and schizotypal personality disorders, cognitive symptoms may appear more prominently; and in other types, such as borderline personality and antisocial personality disorders, interpersonal dysfunctions may predominate (Bornstein et al., 2014). Virtually all individuals exhibit some behaviors associated with the various personality disorders from time to time. As previously stated, it is only when significant functional impairment occurs in response to these personality characteristics that the individual is thought to have a personality disorder.

Personality development occurs in response to a number of biological and psychological influences. These variables include (but are not limited to) heredity, temperament, experiential learning, and social interaction. Recent research on the psychobiology of human personality conducted through person-centered, functional brain imaging has broadened our understanding of healthy personality development and the factors that contribute to individual differences (Cloninger & Svrakic, 2017). For example, functional brain imaging and person-centered analysis has confirmed a model for human temperaments and character traits that is consistent among people from various cultures (Cloninger & Svrakic, 2017). These advances provide a firmer foundation for treatment of personality disorders based on a thorough assessment that includes laboratory findings, mental status, and clinical history.

A number of theorists have attempted to provide information about the psychological aspects of personality development. Most suggest that it occurs in an orderly, stepwise fashion. These stages overlap, however, as maturation occurs at different rates in different individuals. The theories of Sullivan (1953), Erikson (1963), and Mahler (Mahler, Pine, & Bergman, 1975) are presented at length in Chapter 29, Concepts of Personality Development, available online at Davis*Plus*. The stages of personality development according to these three theorists are compared in Table 22–1. The nurse should understand "normal" personality development before learning about what is considered maladaptive.

Individuals with personality disorders as their primary psychiatric diagnosis are not often treated in acute care settings. However, many clients with other psychiatric and medical diagnoses manifest symptoms of personality disorders. Nurses are likely to encounter clients with these personality characteristics in all healthcare settings.

TABLE 22–1 Comparison of Personality Development—Sullivan, Erikson, and Mahler

MAJOR DEVELOPMENTAL TASKS AND DESIGNATED AGES

SULLIVAN	ERIKSON	MAHLER
Birth to 18 months: Relief from anxiety through oral gratification of needs.	Birth to 18 months: To develop a basic trust in the mothering figure and be able to generalize it to others.	Birth to 1 month: Fulfillment of basic needs for survival and comfort
18 months to 6 years: Learning to experience a delay in personal gratification without undue anxiety.	18 months to 3 years: To gain some self-control and independence within the environment.	1 to 5 months: Developing awareness of external source of need fulfillment.
6 to 9 years: Learning to form satisfactory peer relationships.	3 to 6 years: To develop a sense of purpose and the ability to initiate and direct own activities.	5 to 10 months: Commencement of a primary recognition of separateness from the mothering figure.
9 to 12 years: Learning to form satisfactory relationships with persons of the same gender; the initiation of feelings of affection for another person.	6 to 12 years: To achieve a sense of self-confidence by learning, competing, performing successfully, and receiving recognition from significant others, peers, and acquaintances.	10 to 16 months: Increased independence through locomotor functioning; increased sense of separateness of self.
12 to 14 years: Learning to form satisfactory relationships with persons of the opposite gender; developing a sense of identity.	12 to 20 years: To integrate the tasks mastered in the previous stages into a secure sense of self.	16 to 24 months: Acute awareness of separateness of self; learning to seek "emotional refueling" from mothering figure to maintain feeling of security.
14 to 21 years: Establishing self-identity; experiences satisfying relationships; working to develop a lasting, intimate opposite-gender relationship.	20 to 30 years: To form an intense, lasting relationship or a commitment to another person, a cause, an institution, or a creative effort.	24 to 36 months: Sense of separateness established; on the way to object constancy: able to internalize a sustained image of loved object/person when it is out of sight; resolution of separation anxiety.
	30 to 65 years: To achieve the life goals established for oneself, while also considering the welfare of future generations.	
	65 years to death: To review one's life and derive meaning from both positive and negative events, while achieving a positive sense of self-worth. In late, older adulthood (80 years and beyond) an additional stage of development, *transcendence,* refers to a period in which one develops a broader sense of one's meaning and spirituality that transcends oneself.	

Nurses working in psychiatric settings are likely to encounter clients with borderline and antisocial personality characteristics. The behavior of clients with borderline personality disorder (BPD) is unstable, and hospitalization is often required as a result of attempts at self-injury, persistent suicide risk, substance abuse and dependence, or a combination of these behaviors. The client with antisocial personality disorder may enter psychiatric care as a result of judicially ordered evaluation. Psychiatric intervention may be an alternative to imprisonment for antisocial behavior if the intervention is deemed potentially helpful.

Historical and epidemiological aspects of personality disorders are discussed in this chapter.

Predisposing factors that have been implicated in the etiology of personality disorders are presented, and symptomatology is explained to provide background knowledge for assessing clients with personality disorders. Nursing care of patients with BPD or antisocial personality disorder is presented in the context of the nursing process. Various medical treatment modalities for personality disorders are also explored.

Historical Aspects

In the 4th century BC, Hippocrates concluded that all disease stemmed from an excess of or imbalance among four bodily humors: yellow bile, black bile, blood, and phlegm. Hippocrates identified four fundamental personality styles that he concluded stemmed from excesses in the four humors: the irritable and hostile choleric (yellow bile); the pessimistic melancholic (black bile); the overly optimistic and extraverted sanguine (blood); and the apathetic phlegmatic (phlegm).

The medical profession first acknowledged that personality disorders, apart from psychosis, were cause for their own special concern in 1801 with the recognition that an individual can behave irrationally even when the powers of intellect are intact. Nineteenth-century psychiatrists embraced the term *moral insanity,* the concept of which defines what we know today as personality disorders.

Historically, individuals with personality disorders have been labeled as "bad" or "immoral" and as deviants in the range of normal personality dimensions. The events and sequences that result in pathology of the personality are complicated and difficult to unravel. Continued study is needed to facilitate understanding of this complex behavioral phenomenon.

A major difficulty for psychiatrists has been the establishment of a classification of personality disorders. Ten specific types of personality disorders are identified in the *Diagnostic and Statistical Manual of Mental Disorders, Fifth Edition (DSM-5)* (APA, 2013). Looking toward the future, the APA has proposed a different and complex diagnostic system to identify impairments in personality functioning specifically related to the dimensions of *self* and *interpersonal relations* and to personality *trait domains and facets.* This diagnostic system is very specific and addresses symptoms that may differ not only among personality disorders but also among individuals with the same personality disorder. This trait-specific diagnostic methodology is described in the *DSM-5* as an alternative approach to diagnosis of personality disorder and is recommended for further study.

The current diagnostic system classifies the personality disorders into three clusters according to description of personality traits:

1. **Cluster A:** Behaviors described as odd or eccentric
   a. Paranoid personality disorder
   b. Schizoid personality disorder
   c. Schizotypal personality disorder
2. **Cluster B:** Behaviors described as dramatic, emotional, or erratic
   a. Antisocial personality disorder
   b. BPD
   c. Histrionic personality disorder
   d. Narcissistic personality disorder
3. **Cluster C:** Behaviors described as anxious or fearful
   a. Avoidant personality disorder
   b. Dependent personality disorder
   c. Obsessive-compulsive personality disorder

Types of Personality Disorders

Paranoid Personality Disorder

Definition and Epidemiological Statistics

Paranoid personality disorder is defined as a pattern of pervasive mistrust and suspicion of others and misinterpretation of others' motives as malevolent (APA, 2013). This pattern begins by early adulthood and remains present in a variety of contexts. Prevalence has been estimated at 1 to 4 percent of the general population. Symptoms are generally mild but interfere with occupational and social functioning (Cloninger & Svrakic, 2017). The disorder is more commonly diagnosed in men than in women.

Clinical Picture

Individuals with paranoid personality disorder are constantly on guard, hypervigilant, and ready for any real or imagined threat. They appear tense and irritable. They have developed a hard exterior and become insensitive to the feelings of others. They avoid interactions with other people lest they be forced to relinquish some of their own power. They always feel that others are there to take advantage of them.

They are overly sensitive and tend to misinterpret even minute cues within the environment, magnifying and distorting them into thoughts of trickery and deception. Because they trust no one, they are constantly "testing" the honesty of others. Their intimidating manner provokes exasperation and anger in almost everyone with whom they come in contact.

Individuals with paranoid personality disorder maintain their self-esteem by attributing their shortcomings to others. They do not accept responsibility for their own behaviors and feelings and project this responsibility onto others. They are envious and hostile toward others who are highly successful and believe that the only reason they are not as successful is because they have been treated unfairly. People who are paranoid are extremely vulnerable and constantly on the defensive. Any real or imagined threat can release hostility and anger that is fueled by animosities from the past. The desire for reprisal and vindication is so intense that a possible loss of control can result in aggression and violence. These outbursts are usually brief, and the paranoid person soon regains the external control, rationalizes the behavior, and reconstructs the defenses central to his or her personality pattern.

The *DSM-5* diagnostic criteria for paranoid personality disorder are presented in Box 22–1.

BOX 22–1 Diagnostic Criteria for Paranoid Personality Disorder

A. A pervasive distrust and suspiciousness of others such that their motives are interpreted as malevolent, beginning by early adulthood and present in a variety of contexts, as indicated by four (or more) of the following:

1. Suspects, without sufficient basis, that others are exploiting, harming, or deceiving him or her
2. Is preoccupied with unjustified doubts about the loyalty or trustworthiness of friends or associates
3. Is reluctant to confide in others because of unwarranted fear that the information will be used maliciously against him or her
4. Reads hidden demeaning or threatening meanings into benign remarks or events
5. Persistently bears grudges, (i.e., is unforgiving of insults, injuries, or slights)
6. Perceives attacks on his or her character or reputation that are not apparent to others and is quick to react angrily or to counterattack
7. Has recurrent suspicions, without justification, regarding fidelity of spouse or sexual partner

B. Does not occur exclusively during the course of schizophrenia, a bipolar disorder or depressive disorder with psychotic features, or another psychotic disorder and is not attributable to the physiological effects of another medical condition.

Reprinted with permission from American Psychiatric Association. (2013). Diagnostic and statistical manual of mental disorders (5th ed.). Washington, DC: American Psychiatric Publishing.

Predisposing Factors

Research has indicated a possible hereditary link in paranoid personality disorder. Studies have revealed a higher incidence of paranoid personality disorder among relatives of individuals with schizophrenia and delusional disorder, paranoid type (Sadock, Sadock, & Ruiz, 2015).

Psychological predisposing factors, as is the case with many personality disorders, include a history of childhood trauma, including neglect. People with paranoid personality disorder may have been subjected to parental antagonism and harassment. They learned to perceive the world as harsh and unkind, a place calling for protective vigilance and mistrust. They entered the world with a "chip-on-the-shoulder" attitude and were met with many rebuffs and rejections from others. Anticipating humiliation and betrayal by others, they learned to defend themselves by attacking first.

Schizoid Personality Disorder

Definition and Epidemiological Statistics

Schizoid personality disorder is characterized primarily by a profound defect in the ability to form personal relationships, and individuals with this disorder are often seen by others as eccentric, isolated, or lonely (Sadock et al., 2015). These individuals display a lifelong pattern of social withdrawal, and their discomfort with human interaction is apparent. The prevalence of schizoid personality disorder is difficult to determine because, as is the case with many other personality disorders, it may go undiagnosed unless it has been recognized when the individual seeks healthcare for other reasons. Estimates within the general population vary from 3 to 5 percent. Significant numbers of people with the disorder are never observed in a clinical setting. Gender ratio of the disorder is unknown, although it is diagnosed more frequently in men.

Clinical Picture

People with schizoid personality disorder appear cold, aloof, and indifferent to others. They typically have a long-standing history of engaging in primarily solitary activities or engaging more with animals than with people. They prefer to work in isolation and are unsociable with little need or desire for emotional ties. They are able to invest enormous affective energy in intellectual pursuits.

In the presence of others, they appear shy, anxious, or uneasy. They are inappropriately serious about everything and have difficulty acting in a light-hearted manner. Their behavior and conversation exhibit little or no spontaneity. Typically, they are unable to experience pleasure, and their affect is commonly bland and constricted.

The *DSM-5* diagnostic criteria for schizoid personality disorder are presented in Box 22–2.

Predisposing Factors

Although the role of heredity in the etiology of schizoid personality disorder is unclear, the feature of introversion appears to be a highly inheritable characteristic. Further studies are required before definitive statements can be made.

Psychosocially, the development of schizoid personality is probably influenced by early interactional patterns that the person found to be unsatisfying. The childhoods of these individuals have often been characterized as bleak, cold, and notably lacking empathy and nurturing. A child brought up with this type of parenting may develop schizoid personality traits if that child possesses a temperamental disposition that is shy, anxious, and introverted.

BOX 22–2 Diagnostic Criteria for Schizoid Personality Disorder

A. A pervasive pattern of detachment from social relationships and a restricted range of expression of emotions in interpersonal settings, beginning by early adulthood and present in a variety of contexts, as indicated by four (or more) of the following:

1. Neither desires nor enjoys close relationships, including being part of a family
2. Almost always chooses solitary activities
3. Has little, if any, interest in having sexual experiences with another person
4. Takes pleasure in few, if any, activities
5. Lacks close friends or confidants other than first-degree relatives
6. Appears indifferent to the praise or criticism of others
7. Shows emotional coldness, detachment, or flattened affectivity

B. Does not occur exclusively during the course of schizophrenia, a bipolar disorder or depressive disorder with psychotic features, another psychotic disorder, or autism spectrum disorder and is not attributable to the physiological effects of another medical condition.

Reprinted with permission from American Psychiatric Association. (2013). Diagnostic and statistical manual of mental disorders (5th ed.). Washington, DC: American Psychiatric Publishing.

Schizotypal Personality Disorder

Definition and Epidemiological Statistics

Individuals with **schizotypal personality disorder** were once described as "latent schizophrenics." Their behavior is odd and eccentric but does not decompensate to the level of schizophrenia. Schizotypal personality is marked by symptoms that look more like schizophrenia than do those in schizoid personality in that, in the former, individuals show significant peculiarities in thinking, behavior, and appearance. Studies indicate that schizotypal personality disorder has a prevalence of around 4 percent. More than one-half of these individuals have had at least one episode of comorbid major depressive disorder (Cloninger & Svrakic, 2017).

Clinical Picture

Individuals with schizotypal personality disorder are aloof and isolated and behave in a bland and apathetic manner. Magical thinking, ideas of reference, illusions, and depersonalization are part of their everyday world. Examples include superstitiousness; belief in clairvoyance, telepathy, or "sixth sense"; and beliefs that "others can feel my feelings."

The speech pattern is sometimes bizarre. People with this disorder often cannot orient their thoughts logically and become lost in personal irrelevancies and in tangential asides that seem vague, digressive, and not pertinent to the topic at hand. This feature of their personality only further alienates them from others.

Under stress, these individuals may decompensate and demonstrate psychotic symptoms, such as delusional thoughts, hallucinations, or bizarre behaviors, but they are usually of brief duration (Sadock et al., 2015). They often talk or gesture to themselves, as if "living in their own world." Their affect is bland or inappropriate, such as laughing at their own problems or at a situation that most people would consider sad.

The *DSM-5* diagnostic criteria for schizotypal personality disorder are presented in Box 22–3.

Predisposing Factors

Evidence suggests that schizotypal personality disorder is more common among the first-degree relatives of people with schizophrenia than among the general population. It is now considered as part of the genetic spectrum of schizophrenia (APA, 2013). Twin studies reveal a higher incidence in monozygotic twins than dizygotic twins (Sadock et al., 2015).

Psychological and environmental factors may also interact with genetic vulnerability in the development of schizotypal personality traits. For children with schizotypal personality disorder, their affective

BOX 22–3 Diagnostic Criteria for Schizotypal Personality Disorder

A. A pervasive pattern of social and interpersonal deficits marked by acute discomfort with, and reduced capacity for, close relationships as well as by cognitive or perceptual distortions and eccentricities of behavior, beginning by early adulthood and present in a variety of contexts, as indicated by five (or more) of the following:

1. Ideas of reference (excluding delusions of reference)
2. Odd beliefs or magical thinking that influences behavior and is inconsistent with subcultural norms (e.g., superstitiousness, belief in clairvoyance, telepathy, or "sixth sense"; in children and adolescents, bizarre fantasies or preoccupations)
3. Unusual perceptual experiences, including bodily illusions
4. Odd thinking and speech (e.g., vague, circumstantial, metaphorical, overelaborate, or stereotyped)
5. Suspiciousness or paranoid ideation
6. Inappropriate or constricted affect
7. Behavior or appearance that is odd, eccentric, or peculiar
8. Lack of close friends or confidants other than first-degree relatives
9. Excessive social anxiety that does not diminish with familiarity and tends to be associated with paranoid fears rather than negative judgments about self

B. Does not occur exclusively during the course of schizophrenia, a bipolar disorder or depressive disorder with psychotic features, another psychotic disorder, or autism spectrum disorder.

Reprinted with permission from American Psychiatric Association. (2013). Diagnostic and statistical manual of mental disorders (5th ed.). Washington, DC: American Psychiatric Publishing.

blandness, peculiar behaviors, and discomfort with interpersonal relationships may provoke other children to avoid relationships with them, or worse, to engage in bullying, which reinforces their withdrawal from others. Having failed repeatedly to cope with these adversities, they withdraw and reduce contact with individuals and situations that evoked sadness and humiliation. Their new inner world provides them with a more significant and potentially rewarding existence than the one experienced in reality.

Antisocial Personality Disorder

Definition and Epidemiological Statistics

Antisocial personality disorder is a pattern of socially irresponsible, exploitative, and guiltless behavior that reflects a general disregard for the rights of others. These individuals exploit and manipulate others for personal gain and are unconcerned with obeying the law. They have difficulty sustaining consistent employment and developing stable relationships. It is one of the oldest and best researched of the personality disorders and has been included in all editions of the *DSM*. In the United States, prevalence is estimated to be about 3 percent in the general population, but in prison populations, the prevalence is 50 percent or higher (Hatchett, 2015). It is more common in men than in women and in the lower socioeconomic classes, especially those highly mobile inhabitants of impoverished urban areas. The *DSM-5* currently identifies antisocial personality and psychopathy as synonymous terms, but recent research reveals that these are better understood as distinct disorders (Hatchett, 2015; Thompson, Ramos, & Willett, 2014). Substance use disorder is commonly identified as a comorbid disorder.

> **NOTE:** The clinical picture, predisposing factors, nursing diagnoses, and interventions for care of clients with antisocial personality disorder are presented later in this chapter.

Borderline Personality Disorder

Definition and Epidemiological Statistics

Borderline personality disorder (BPD) is characterized by a pattern of intense and chaotic relationships with affective instability and fluctuating attitudes toward other people. These individuals are impulsive, are directly and indirectly self-destructive, and lack a clear sense of identity. Prevalence of borderline personality is estimated at 1 to 2 percent of the population with impairment being frequent, severe, and influencing and characterized by job losses, education interruptions, and marriage breakups (Cloninger & Svrakic, 2017). It is generally estimated to be twice as common in women as in men (Sadock et al., 2015), and some researchers have estimated female-to-male ratios as high as 4 to 1 (Lubit, 2017).

> **NOTE:** The clinical picture, predisposing factors, nursing diagnoses, and interventions for care of clients with BPD are presented later in this chapter.

Histrionic Personality Disorder

Definition and Epidemiological Statistics

Histrionic personality disorder is characterized by colorful, dramatic, and extroverted behavior in excitable, emotional people. They have difficulty maintaining long-lasting relationships, although they require constant affirmation of approval and acceptance from others. This need often gives rise to seductive, flirtatious behavior in efforts to reassure themselves of their attractiveness and to gain approval. Prevalence of the disorder is thought to be about 2 to 3 percent, and it is more common in women than in men.

Clinical Picture

People with histrionic personality disorder tend to be self-dramatizing, attention seeking, overly gregarious, and seductive. They use manipulative and exhibitionistic behaviors in their demands to be the center of attention. People with histrionic personality disorder often demonstrate, to an extreme, what our society tends to foster and admire in its members: to be well liked, successful, popular, extroverted, attractive, and sociable. However, beneath these surface characteristics is a driven quality—an all-consuming need for approval and a desperate striving to be conspicuous and to evoke affection or attract attention at all costs. Failure to evoke the attention and approval they seek often results in feelings of dejection and anxiety.

Individuals with this disorder are highly distractible and flighty by nature. They have difficulty paying attention to detail. They can portray themselves as carefree and sophisticated on the one hand and as inhibited and naive on the other. They tend to be highly suggestible, impressionable, and easily influenced by others. They are strongly dependent.

Interpersonal relationships are fleeting and superficial. The person with histrionic personality disorder, having failed throughout life to develop the richness of inner feelings and lacking resources from which to draw, lacks the ability to provide another with genuinely sustained affection. Somatic complaints are not uncommon in these individuals, and fleeting episodes of psychosis may occur during periods of extreme stress.

The *DSM-5* diagnostic criteria for histrionic personality disorder are presented in Box 22–4.

Predisposing Factors

Heredity may be a factor in histrionic personality disorder because the disorder is apparently more common among first-degree biological relatives of people with the disorder than in the general population. Some traits may be inherited, whereas others are related to a combination of genetic predisposition and childhood experiences. At present, however, the exact cause is unknown.

BOX 22–4 Diagnostic Criteria for Histrionic Personality Disorder

A pervasive pattern of excessive emotionality and attention seeking, beginning by early adulthood and present in a variety of contexts, as indicated by five (or more) of the following:

1. Is uncomfortable in situations in which he or she is not the center of attention
2. Interaction with others is often characterized by inappropriate sexually seductive or provocative behavior
3. Displays rapidly shifting and shallow expression of emotions
4. Consistently uses physical appearance to draw attention to self
5. Has a style of speech that is excessively impressionistic and lacking in detail
6. Shows self-dramatization, theatricality, and exaggerated expression of emotion
7. Is suggestible (i.e., easily influenced by others or circumstances)
8. Considers relationships to be more intimate than they actually are

Reprinted with permission from American Psychiatric Association. (2013). Diagnostic and statistical manual of mental disorders (5th ed.). Washington, DC: American Psychiatric Publishing.

From a psychosocial perspective, learning experiences may contribute to the development of histrionic personality disorder. The child may have learned that positive reinforcement was contingent on the ability to perform parentally approved and admired behaviors. It is likely that the child rarely received either positive or negative feedback. Parental acceptance and approval came inconsistently and only when the behaviors met parental expectations.

Narcissistic Personality Disorder

Definition and Epidemiological Statistics

Persons with **narcissistic personality disorder** have an exaggerated sense of self-worth. They lack empathy and are hypersensitive to the evaluation of others. They believe that they have the inalienable right to receive special consideration and that their desire is sufficient justification for possessing whatever they seek.

This diagnosis appeared for the first time in the third edition of the *DSM*. However, the concept of narcissism has its roots in the 19th century. It was viewed by early psychoanalysts as a normal phase of psychosexual development. The prevalence of narcissistic personality disorder is estimated at 1 to 6 percent (Sadock et al., 2015). It is diagnosed more often in men than in women.

Clinical Picture

Individuals with narcissistic personality disorder appear to lack humility, being overly self-centered and exploiting others to fulfill their own desires. They often do not conceive of their behavior as being inappropriate or objectionable. Because they view themselves as "superior" beings, they believe they are entitled to special rights and privileges.

Although often grounded in grandiose distortions of reality, their mood is usually optimistic, relaxed, cheerful, and carefree. This mood can easily change, however, because of their fragile self-esteem. If they do not meet self-expectations, do not receive the positive feedback they expect from others, or draw criticism from others, they may respond with rage, shame, humiliation, or dejection. They may turn inward and fantasize rationalizations that convince them of their continued stature and perfection.

The exploitation of others for self-gratification results in impaired interpersonal relationships. In selecting a mate, narcissistic individuals frequently choose a person who will provide them with the praise and positive feedback that they require and who will not ask much from their partner in return.

The *DSM-5* diagnostic criteria for narcissistic personality disorder are presented in Box 22–5.

Predisposing Factors

Although the causes are unknown, psychodynamic theories have suggested that narcissistic personality disorder evolves from a parent-child dynamic of excessive pampering or excessive criticism (Mayo Clinic, 2017). Children may then grow to project an image of invulnerability and self-sufficiency that conceals their true sense of emptiness and contributes to their inability to feel deep emotion.

Sadock and associates (2015) identify the propensity for an increase in narcissistic personality disorders among children whose parents had the disorder. Children may evolve into adults with narcissistic personality disorder through role-modeling parent behavior, or as Sadock and associates suggest, these traits may be influenced by a narcissistic parent's imparting an unrealistic omnipotence, grandiosity, beauty, and talent to their children.

Narcissism may also develop from an environment in which parents attempt to live their lives vicariously through their child. They expect the child to achieve

BOX 22–5 Diagnostic Criteria for Narcissistic Personality Disorder

A pervasive pattern of grandiosity (in fantasy or behavior), need for admiration, and lack of empathy, beginning by early adulthood and present in a variety of contexts, as indicated by five (or more) of the following:

1. Has a grandiose sense of self-importance (e.g., exaggerates achievements and talents, expects to be recognized as superior without commensurate achievements)
2. Is preoccupied with fantasies of unlimited success, power, brilliance, beauty, or ideal love
3. Believes that he or she is "special" and unique and can only be understood by, or should associate with, other special or high-status people (or institutions)
4. Requires excessive admiration
5. Has a sense of entitlement (i.e., unreasonable expectations of especially favorable treatment or automatic compliance with his or her expectations)
6. Is interpersonally exploitative (i.e., takes advantage of others to achieve his or her own ends)
7. Lacks empathy: is unwilling to recognize or identify with the feelings and needs of others
8. Is often envious of others or believes that others are envious of him or her
9. Shows arrogant, haughty behaviors or attitudes

Reprinted with permission from American Psychiatric Association. (2013). Diagnostic and statistical manual of mental disorders (5th ed.). Washington, DC: American Psychiatric Publishing.

the things they did not achieve, possess that which they did not possess, and have a better and easier life than they had. The child is not subjected to the requirements and restrictions that may have dominated the parents' lives and thereby grows up believing that he or she is above that which is required for everyone else.

Genetics and environment may both have a role in the development of narcissistic personality disorder. Having an innately oversensitive temperament may be an associated factor. In addition, research has identified a decreased volume of gray matter in areas of the brain responsible for empathy, emotional regulation, compassion, and cognitive functions (Gregory, 2018).

Avoidant Personality Disorder

Definition and Epidemiological Statistics

The individual with **avoidant personality disorder** is extremely sensitive to rejection and consequently may lead a very socially withdrawn life. It is not that he or she is asocial; in fact, there may be a strong desire for companionship. The extreme shyness and fear of rejection, however, create needs for unusually strong assurances of unconditional acceptance. Prevalence of the disorder in the general population is about 2 to 3 percent, and it appears to be equally common in men and women.

Clinical Picture

Individuals with this disorder are awkward and uncomfortable in social situations. From a distance, others may perceive them as timid, withdrawn, or perhaps cold and strange. Those who have closer relationships with them, however, soon learn of their sensitivities, touchiness, evasiveness, and mistrustful qualities.

Their speech is usually slow and constrained with frequent hesitations, fragmentary thought sequences, and occasional confused and irrelevant digressions. They are often lonely and express feelings of being unwanted. They view others as critical, betraying, and humiliating. They desire to have close relationships but avoid them because of their fear of being rejected. Depression, anxiety, and anger at oneself for failing to develop social relations are commonly experienced.

The *DSM-5* diagnostic criteria for avoidant personality disorder are presented in Box 22–6.

Predisposing Factors

There is no clear cause of avoidant personality disorder. Contributing factors are most likely a combination of biological, genetic, and psychosocial influences. Some infants who exhibit hyperirritability, crankiness, tension, and withdrawal behaviors may possess a temperamental disposition toward an avoidant pattern.

Psychosocial influences may include childhood trauma or neglect leading to fears of abandonment or to viewing the world as a hostile and dangerous place.

Dependent Personality Disorder

Definition and Epidemiological Statistics

Dependent personality disorder is characterized by lack of self-confidence and extreme reliance on others to take responsibility for them, sometimes to the point of intense discomfort with being alone for even a brief period (Sadock et al., 2015). This mode of behavior is evident in the tendency to allow others to make decisions, to feel helpless when alone, to act submissively, to subordinate needs to others, to tolerate mistreatment by others, to demean oneself to gain acceptance, and to fail to function adequately in situations that require assertive or dominant behavior.

BOX 22–6 Diagnostic Criteria for Avoidant Personality Disorder

A pervasive pattern of social inhibition, feelings of inadequacy, and hypersensitivity to negative evaluation, beginning by early adulthood and present in a variety of contexts, as indicated by four (or more) of the following:

1. Avoids occupational activities that involve significant interpersonal contact, because of fears of criticism, disapproval, or rejection
2. Is unwilling to get involved with people unless certain of being liked
3. Shows restraint within intimate relationships because of the fear of being shamed or ridiculed
4. Is preoccupied with being criticized or rejected in social situations
5. Is inhibited in new interpersonal situations because of feelings of inadequacy
6. Views self as socially inept, personally unappealing, or inferior to others
7. Is unusually reluctant to take personal risks or to engage in any new activities because they may prove embarrassing

Reprinted with permission from American Psychiatric Association. (2013). Diagnostic and statistical manual of mental disorders (5th ed.). Washington, DC: American Psychiatric Publishing.

Clinical Picture

Individuals with dependent personality disorder have a notable lack of self-confidence that is often apparent in their posture, voice, and mannerisms. They are typically passive and acquiescent to the desires of others. They are overly generous and thoughtful and underplay their own attractiveness and achievements. They may appear to others to "see the world through rose-colored glasses," but when alone, they may feel pessimistic, discouraged, and dejected. Others are not made aware of these feelings; their "suffering" is done in silence.

Individuals with dependent personality disorder assume the passive and submissive role in relationships. They are willing to let others make their important decisions. Should the dependent relationship end, they feel fearful and vulnerable because they lack confidence in their ability to care for themselves. They may hastily and indiscriminately attempt to establish another relationship with someone they believe can provide them with the nurturance and guidance they need.

They avoid positions of responsibility and become anxious when forced into them. They have feelings of low self-worth and are easily hurt by criticism and disapproval. They will do almost anything, even if it is unpleasant or demeaning, to earn the acceptance of others.

The *DSM-5* diagnostic criteria for dependent personality disorder are presented in Box 22–7.

Predisposing Factors

An infant may be genetically predisposed to a dependent temperament. Twin studies measuring submissiveness have shown a higher correlation between identical twins than fraternal twins.

Psychosocially, dependency is fostered in infancy when stimulation and nurturance are experienced exclusively from one source. The infant becomes attached to one source to the exclusion of all others. If this exclusive attachment continues as the child grows, the dependency is nurtured. A problem may arise when parents become overprotective and discourage independent behaviors on the part of the child. Parents who make new experiences unnecessarily easy for the child and refuse to allow him or her to learn

---

BOX 22–7 Diagnostic Criteria for Dependent Personality Disorder

A pervasive and excessive need to be taken care of that leads to submissive and clinging behavior and fears of separation, beginning by early adulthood and present in a variety of contexts, as indicated by five (or more) of the following:

1. Has difficulty making everyday decisions without an excessive amount of advice and reassurance from others
2. Needs others to assume responsibility for most major areas of his or her life
3. Has difficulty expressing disagreement with others because of fear of loss of support or approval (**Note:** Do not include realistic fears of retribution.)
4. Has difficulty initiating projects or doing things on his or her own (because of a lack of self-confidence in judgment or abilities rather than a lack of motivation or energy)
5. Goes to excessive lengths to obtain nurturance and support from others, to the point of volunteering to do things that are unpleasant
6. Feels uncomfortable or helpless when alone because of exaggerated fears of being unable to care for himself or herself
7. Urgently seeks another relationship as a source of care and support when a close relationship ends
8. Is unrealistically preoccupied with fears of being left to take care of himself or herself

Reprinted with permission from American Psychiatric Association. (2013). Diagnostic and statistical manual of mental disorders (5th ed.). Washington, DC: American Psychiatric Publishing.

---

by experience encourage their child to give up efforts at achieving autonomy. Dependent behaviors may be subtly rewarded in this environment, and the child may come to fear a loss of love or attachment from the parental figure if independent behaviors are attempted.

Obsessive-Compulsive Personality Disorder

Definition and Epidemiological Statistics

Individuals with **obsessive-compulsive personality disorder** are very serious and formal and have difficulty expressing emotions. They are overly disciplined, perfectionistic, and preoccupied with rules. They are inflexible about the way in which things must be done and have a devotion to productivity to the exclusion of personal pleasure. An intense fear of making mistakes leads to difficulty with decision making. The disorder is relatively common and occurs more often in men than in women. Within the family constellation, it appears to be most common in oldest children. Recurrent obsessions and compulsions are absent in this personality disorder, and clients who present with such symptoms are diagnosed with obsessive-compulsive disorder rather than obsessive compulsive *personality* disorder (Sadock et al., 2015). Prevalence is estimated at anywhere from 2 to 8 percent.

Clinical Picture

Individuals with obsessive-compulsive personality disorder are inflexible and lack spontaneity. They are meticulous and work diligently and patiently at tasks that require accuracy and discipline. They are especially concerned with matters of organization and efficiency and tend to be rigid and unbending about rules and procedures.

Social behavior tends to be polite and formal. They are very "rank conscious," a characteristic that is reflected in their contrasting behaviors with "superiors" as opposed to "inferiors." They tend to be very solicitous to and ingratiating with authority figures. With subordinates, however, the compulsive person can become quite autocratic and condemnatory, often appearing pompous and self-righteous.

People with obsessive-compulsive personality disorder typify the "bureaucratic personality," the so-called company man. They see themselves as conscientious, loyal, dependable, and responsible and are contemptuous of people whose behavior they consider frivolous and impulsive. Emotional behavior is considered immature and irresponsible.

Although on the surface these individuals appear to be calm and controlled, underneath this exterior lies a great deal of ambivalence, conflict, and hostility. Individuals with this disorder commonly use the defense mechanism of reaction formation. Not daring to expose their true feelings of defiance and anger, they withhold these feelings so strongly that the opposite feelings come forth. The defenses of isolation, intellectualization, rationalization, and undoing are also commonly evident.

The *DSM-5* diagnostic criteria for obsessive-compulsive personality disorder are presented in Box 22–8.

Predisposing Factors

Genetic vulnerability may be a predisposing factor because it is noted to occur more frequently in first-degree biological relatives than in the general population (Sadock et al., 2015).

In the psychoanalytical view, the parenting style in which the individual with obsessive-compulsive personality disorder was reared is one of over-control.

BOX 22–8 Diagnostic Criteria for Obsessive-Compulsive Personality Disorder

A pervasive pattern of preoccupation with orderliness, perfectionism, and mental and interpersonal control, at the expense of flexibility, openness, and efficiency, beginning by early adulthood and present in a variety of contexts, as indicated by four (or more) of the following:

1. Is preoccupied with details, rules, lists, order, organization, or schedules to the extent that the major point of the activity is lost
2. Shows perfectionism that interferes with task completion (e.g., is unable to complete a project because his or her own overly strict standards are not met)
3. Is excessively devoted to work and productivity to the exclusion of leisure activities and friendships (not accounted for by obvious economic necessity)
4. Is overconscientious, scrupulous, and inflexible about matters of morality, ethics, or values (not accounted for by cultural or religious identification)
5. Is unable to discard worn-out or worthless objects even when they have no sentimental value
6. Is reluctant to delegate tasks or to work with others unless they submit to exactly his or her way of doing things
7. Adopts a miserly spending style toward both self and others; money is viewed as something to be hoarded for future catastrophes
8. Shows rigidity and stubbornness

Reprinted with permission from American Psychiatric Association. (2013). Diagnostic and statistical manual of mental disorders (5th ed.). Washington, DC: American Psychiatric Publishing.

These parents expect their children to live up to their imposed standards of conduct and condemn them if they do not. Praise for positive behaviors is bestowed on the child with much less frequency than punishment for undesirable behaviors. In this environment, individuals become experts in learning what they must *not* do to avoid punishment and condemnation rather than what they *can* do to achieve attention and praise. They learn to heed rigid restrictions and rules. Positive achievements are expected, taken for granted, and only occasionally acknowledged by their parents, whose comments and judgments are limited to pointing out transgressions and infractions of rules.

Application of the Nursing Process

Borderline Personality Disorder (Background Assessment Data)

Historically, there have been clients who did not classically conform to the standard categories of neuroses or psychoses. The designation "borderline" was introduced to identify clients who seemed to fall on the border between the two categories. Other terminology that has been used in an attempt to identify this disorder includes *ambulatory schizophrenia, pseudoneurotic schizophrenia,* and *emotionally unstable personality.* When the term *borderline* was first proposed for inclusion in the third edition of the *DSM,* some psychiatrists feared that it might be used as a "wastebasket" diagnosis for difficult-to-treat clients. However, a specific set of criteria, listed in Box 22–9, has been established for diagnosing what has been described as "a consistent and stable course of unstable behavior."

Clinical Picture

Individuals with borderline personality always seem to be in a state of crisis and have frequent mood swings (although there may also be comorbid bipolar disorder). Their affect is one of extreme intensity, and their behavior reflects frequent changeability. These changes can occur within days, hours, or even minutes. They are sometimes described as "thriving on chaos" because their behaviors frequently generate chaos, particularly in interpersonal relationships. Often, these individuals exhibit a single, dominant affective tone, such as depression, which may give way periodically to anxious agitation or inappropriate outbursts of anger.

Chronic Depression

Depression is so common in clients with this disorder that before the inclusion of BPD in the *DSM,* many of these clients were diagnosed with depressive

BOX 22–9 Diagnostic Criteria for Borderline Personality Disorder

A pervasive pattern of instability of interpersonal relationships, self-image, and affects, and marked impulsivity beginning by early adulthood and present in a variety of contexts, as indicated by five (or more) of the following:

1. Frantic efforts to avoid real or imagined abandonment (**Note:** Do not include suicidal or self-mutilating behavior covered in criterion 5.)
2. A pattern of unstable and intense interpersonal relationships characterized by alternating between extremes of idealization and devaluation
3. Identity disturbance: markedly and persistently unstable self-image or sense of self
4. Impulsivity in at least two areas that are potentially self-damaging (e.g., spending, sex, substance abuse, reckless driving, binge eating) (**Note:** Do not include suicidal or self-mutilating behavior covered in criterion 5.)
5. Recurrent suicidal behavior, gestures, or threats, or self-mutilating behavior
6. Affective instability due to marked reactivity of mood (e.g., intense episodic dysphoria, irritability, or anxiety, usually lasting a few hours and only rarely more than a few days)
7. Chronic feelings of emptiness
8. Inappropriate, intense anger or difficulty controlling anger (e.g., frequent displays of temper, constant anger, recurrent physical fights)
9. Transient, stress-related paranoid ideation or severe dissociative symptoms

Reprinted with permission from American Psychiatric Association. (2013). Diagnostic and statistical manual of mental disorders (5th ed.). Washington, DC: American Psychiatric Publishing.

disorder. Depression may be rooted in feelings of abandonment by the mother in early childhood (see "Predisposing Factors to Borderline Personality Disorder"). Underlying the depression is a sense of rage that is sporadically turned inward on the self and externally on the environment. Associated symptoms include uncontrolled anger and chronic feelings of emptiness. The individual is seldom aware of the true source of these feelings until well into long-term therapy.

Bipolar Disorder

Much has been written about the common comorbidity of BPD with bipolar disorder and the overlap of features. There are so many features in common that it has been suggested by some that BPD should be considered a disorder along a bipolar spectrum (Rodriguez, 2017). Supporting the concept that these two illnesses, although distinct, are very similar are the findings that both illnesses have a shared genetic variance, childhood parent loss, early trauma, and dysfunctional family environment as predisposing factors (Rodriguez, 2017). Affective instability, moods that shift from depression to irritability or anxiety, are so common (reported in over 90 percent of patients with BPD) that Zimmerman (2017) notes that if these symptoms are not present it is likely that BPD can be ruled out.

Inability to Be Alone

Because of this chronic fear of abandonment, clients with BPD have little tolerance for being alone. They prefer a frantic search for companionship, no matter how unsatisfactory, to sitting with feelings of loneliness, emptiness, and boredom (Sadock et al., 2015).

Patterns of Interaction

Clinging and Distancing

The client with BPD commonly exhibits a pattern of interaction with others that is characterized by clinging and distancing behaviors. When clients are clinging to another individual, they may exhibit helpless, dependent, or even childlike behaviors. They overidealize a single individual with whom they want to spend all their time, with whom they express a frequent need to talk, or from whom they seek constant reassurance. Impulsive behaviors, even self-mutilation, may result when they cannot be with this chosen individual. Distancing behaviors are characterized by hostility, anger, and devaluation of others, arising from a feeling of discomfort with closeness. Distancing behaviors also occur in response to separations, confrontations, or attempts to limit certain behaviors. Devaluation of others is manifested by discrediting or undermining their strengths and personal significance.

Splitting

Splitting is a primitive ego defense mechanism that is common in people with BPD. It arises from their lack of achievement of **object constancy** and is manifested by an inability to integrate and accept both positive and negative feelings. In their view, people—including themselves—and life situations are either all good or all bad. For example, a nurse-patient relationship may be perceived to be very intense and overvalued (e.g., "No one else in the world can help me the way you do") until the individual with BPD feels threatened in any way. The reason for feeling threatened could be as simple as a perception that the nurse looked at the individual with a different expression or that the nurse was not immediately available to spend time with him or her. Because this individual also struggles with emotional regulation, suddenly the nurse is devalued, valuing is shifted to another nurse, and the idealized image changes from beneficent caregiver to one of hateful and cruel persecutor. These shifting allegiances and valuing/devaluing responses can generate conflict, anger, and frustration in staff members (or in any interpersonal relationships) unless this dynamic is clearly understood and managed appropriately.

Manipulation

In their efforts to prevent the separation they so desperately fear, clients with this disorder become masters of manipulation. Virtually any behavior becomes an acceptable means of achieving the desired result: relief from separation anxiety. Playing one individual against another is a common ploy to allay these fears of abandonment.

Self-Destructive Behaviors

Repetitive, self-mutilative behaviors are classic manifestations of BPD. About 75 percent of individuals with BPD have a history of at least one deliberate act of self-harm, and about 1 in 10 die by suicide (Lubit, 2017). Although these acts can be fatal, most commonly they are manipulative gestures designed to elicit a rescue response from significant others. Suicide attempts are quite common and result from feelings of abandonment following separation from a significant other. The endeavor is often attempted, however, incorporating a measure of "safety" into the plan (e.g., swallowing pills in an area where the person will surely be discovered by others or swallowing pills and making a phone call to report the deed to someone).

Other types of destructive behaviors include cutting, scratching, and burning. Various theories abound regarding why these individuals are able to inflict pain on themselves. One hypothesis suggests that they may have higher levels of endorphins in their bodies than most people, thereby increasing their threshold for pain. Another theory relates to the individual's personal identity disturbance. It proposes that because many of the self-mutilating behaviors take place when the individual is in a state of depersonalization and derealization, he or she does not initially feel the pain. The mutilation continues until pain is felt in an attempt to counteract the feelings of unreality. Some clients with BPD have

reported that "to feel pain is better than to feel nothing." The pain validates their existence.

Impulsivity

Individuals with BPD have poor impulse control. Impulsive behaviors associated with BPD include substance abuse, gambling, promiscuity, reckless driving, and binging and purging. These behaviors often occur in response to real or perceived feelings of abandonment.

Predisposing Factors to Borderline Personality Disorder

Biological Influences

BPD, once thought to be an entirely psychodynamic illness, has been the focus of much current research revealing a wealth of information about the neurobiological underpinnings of this illness. Current research clearly shows that BPD evolves through a complex interplay of environmental factors, brain anatomy and function, genetics, and epigenetics (Pier et al., 2016).

Biochemical Clients with BPD have a high incidence of major depressive episodes, and antidepressants have demonstrated benefits in some cases (Sadock et al., 2015). This fact and supporting information from brain imaging studies have led to the hypothesis that serotonin and/or norepinephrine dysregulation may contribute to the development of BPD. As stated elsewhere, questions remain about whether these dysfunctions contribute to the development of such disorders or whether they are a neurochemical response to intense emotional states.

Genetic An increased prevalence of major depression and substance use disorders in first-degree relatives of individuals with borderline personality suggest that there are complex genetic vulnerabilities as well as environmental influences (Sadock et al., 2015). Clients with BPD are five times more likely than others to have a first-degree relative with BPD, and many studies have shown personality traits such as impulsivity, affect lability, and neuroticism to be heritable traits (MacIntosh, Godbout, & Dubash, 2015). In addition, BPD increases familial risk for antisocial personality disorder, substance abuse, and mood disorders (Cloninger & Svrakic, 2017). Epigenetic studies have identified changes to the oxytocin system (related to being a carrier of a specific allele) as associated with negative perceptions of others, increased stress markers, decreased empathy, confidence, and positivity (Pier et al., 2016). In this scenario, prosocial behaviors such as empathy, positivity, and confidence decrease. Treatment with oxytocin has demonstrated some benefits but requires more research.

Neurobiological Magnetic resonance imaging studies to assess anatomical and functional activities in the brain have identified several factors associated with BPD. The left amygdala, left hippocampus, and posterior cingulate cortex show heightened activation, and the prefrontal cortex shows decreased activation during the processing of negative emotions (Pier et al., 2016).

Psychosocial Influences

Childhood Trauma Research about specific types of trauma that predispose one to the development of BPD is inconsistent, but there is clear and strong evidence that they are linked (MacIntosh et al., 2015). One recent model describes BPD as influenced by a triad of factors that includes childhood trauma, a vulnerable temperament, and a series of triggering events (Cloninger & Svrakic, 2017). In some instances, this disorder has been likened to post-traumatic stress disorder (PTSD) in response to childhood trauma and abuse. In fact, BPD has been considered a controversial diagnosis because of the many apparent overlaps with PTSD (and bipolar disorder), but as MacIntosh and associates (2015) cite, other research (Hodges et al., 2013) demonstrates that the complexity of symptoms seen in BPD does not fit with general profiles of individuals with PTSD. Ford and Courtois (2014) cite several studies identifying a 30 to 40 percent comorbidity of PTSD and BPD and indicate that about 85 percent of those diagnosed with BPD were initially diagnosed with PTSD. In these cases, BPD symptoms persisted after remission of PTSD symptoms. Comorbid substance use disorders may also complicate the differentiation of symptoms and treatment needs. Thorough assessment to identify the multiple psychosocial influences in BPD is clearly essential.

Developmental Factors

Theory of Object Relations According to Mahler's theory of object relations (Mahler et al., 1975), infants pass through six phases from birth to 36 months, when a sense of separateness from the parenting figure is finally established. Between the ages of 16 and 24 months (phase 5, the rapprochement phase), children become acutely aware of their separateness, and because this is frightening, they look to the mother for "emotional refueling" and to maintain a sense of security while at the same time beginning to explore their separateness and independence. (See Table 22–1 for a more detailed outline of Mahler's theory.)

According to object relations theorists, the individual with BPD becomes fixed in the rapprochement phase of development. This occurs when the child shows increasing separation and autonomy. The mother, who feels secure in the relationship as long as the child is dependent, begins to feel threatened by the child's increasing independence. The mother may be experiencing her own fears of abandonment. In response to separation behaviors, the mother withdraws the emotional support or "refueling" that is so vitally needed during this phase for the child to feel secure. Instead, the mother rewards clinging, dependent behaviors and punishes (withholding emotional support) independent behaviors. With his or her sense of emotional survival at stake, the child learns to behave in a manner that satisfies the parental wishes. The child develops an internal conflict based on fear of abandonment. He or she wants to achieve independence common to this stage of development but fears that the mother will withdraw emotional support as a result. This unresolved fear of abandonment remains with the child into adulthood. Unresolved grief for the nurturing they failed to receive results in internalized rage that manifests itself in the depression so common in people with BPD.

Other research looking at attachment issues in childhood suggests that childhood maltreatment, particularly neglect, may be associated with reactive attachment disorder, which results in the development of neurocognitive deficits, particularly temporal limbic dysfunction; the symptoms of BPD with regard to unhealthy attachment in relationships may be related, at least in part, to these neurocognitive deficits rooted in childhood development disruptions (Mak & Lam, 2013; Pier et al., 2016).

Diagnosis and Outcome Identification

Nursing diagnoses are formulated from the data gathered during the assessment phase and with background knowledge regarding predisposing factors to the disorder. Table 22–2 presents a list of patient behaviors and the NANDA International nursing diagnoses that correspond to these behaviors, which may be used in planning care for patients with BPD.

Outcome Criteria

The following criteria may be used for measurement of outcomes in the care of patients with BPD.

TABLE 22–2 Assigning Nursing Diagnoses to Behaviors Commonly Associated With Borderline Personality Disorder

BEHAVIORS	NURSING DIAGNOSES
Risk factors: History of self-injurious behavior; history of inability to plan solutions; impulsivity; irresistible urge to damage self; feels threatened with loss of significant relationship	**Risk for self-mutilation**
Risk factors: History of suicide attempts; suicidal ideation; suicidal plan; impulsiveness; childhood abuse; fears of abandonment; internalized rage	**Risk for self-directed violence Risk for suicide**
Risk factors: Body language (e.g., rigid posture, clenching of fists and jaw, hyperactivity, pacing, breathlessness, threatening stances); history of childhood abuse; impulsivity; transient psychotic symptomatology	**Risk for other-directed violence**
Depression; persistent emotional distress; rumination; separation distress; traumatic distress; verbalizes feeling empty; inappropriate expression of anger	**Complicated grieving**
Alternating clinging and distancing behaviors; staff splitting; manipulation	**Impaired social interaction**
Feelings of depersonalization and derealization	**Disturbed personal identity**
Transient psychotic symptoms (disorganized thinking; misinterpretation of the environment); increased tension; decreased perceptual field	**Anxiety (severe to panic)**
Dependent on others; excessively seeks reassurance; manipulation of others; inability to tolerate being alone	**Chronic low self-esteem**

The patient:

■ Has not harmed self.
■ Seeks out staff when desire for self-mutilation is strong.
■ Is able to identify true source of anger.
■ Expresses anger appropriately.
■ Relates to more than one staff member.
■ Completes activities of daily living independently.
■ Does not manipulate one staff member against the other in order to fulfill own desires.

Planning and Implementation

In Table 22–3, selected nursing diagnoses common to the patient with borderline personality disorder are presented in a plan of care. Outcome criteria, along with appropriate nursing interventions and rationales, are included for each.

Concept Care Mapping

The concept map care plan is a diagrammatic teaching and learning strategy that allows visualization of interrelationships between medical diagnoses, nursing diagnoses, assessment data, and treatments. An example of a concept map care plan for a patient with BPD is presented in Figure 22–1.

Evaluation

Reassessment is conducted to determine if the nursing actions have been successful in achieving the objectives of care. Evaluation of the nursing actions for the patient with BPD may be facilitated by gathering information using the following types of questions:

Has the patient:

■ Been able to seek out staff when feeling the desire for self-harm?
■ Avoided self-harm?
■ Correlated times of desire for self-harm to times of elevation in level of anxiety?
■ Discussed feelings with staff (particularly feelings of depression and anger)?
■ Identified the true source toward which the anger is directed?
■ Verbalized understanding of the basis for his or her anger?
■ Expressed anger appropriately?
■ Demonstrated ability to function independently?
■ Related to more than one staff member?
■ Verbalized the knowledge that the staff members are not abandoning the patient when leaving for the day?
■ Separated from the staff in an appropriate manner?
■ Demonstrated ability to delay gratification and refrain from manipulating others in order to fulfill own desires?
■ Identified resources within the community from whom he or she may seek assistance in times of extreme stress?

Table 22–3 | CARE PLAN FOR THE PATIENT WITH BORDERLINE PERSONALITY DISORDER

NURSING DIAGNOSIS: RISK FOR SELF-INJURY/RISK FOR SELF-DIRECTED OR OTHER-DIRECTED VIOLENCE

RELATED TO: Parental emotional deprivation (unresolved fears of abandonment)

OUTCOME CRITERIA	NURSING INTERVENTIONS	RATIONALE
Short-Term Goals ■ Patient will seek out staff member if feelings of harming self or others emerge. ■ Patient will not harm self or others. **Long-Term Goal** ■ Patient will not harm self or others.	1. Observe patient's behavior frequently. Do this through routine activities and interactions; avoid appearing watchful and suspicious. 2. Encourage the patient to seek out a staff member when the urge for self-injury intensifies. 3. If self-mutilation occurs, care for patient's wounds in a matter-of-fact manner. Do not give positive reinforcement to this behavior by offering sympathy or additional attention. 4. Encourage patient to talk about feelings he or she was having just before this behavior occurred. 5. Act as a role model for appropriate expression of angry feelings and give positive reinforcement when attempts to conform are made. 6. Remove all dangerous objects from patient's environment. 7. Redirect violent behavior with physical outlets for the patient's anxiety (e.g., exercises, jogging). 8. Have sufficient staff available to indicate a show of strength to the patient if it becomes necessary. 9. Administer tranquilizing medications as ordered by the physician or obtain an order if necessary. Monitor the patient for effectiveness of the medication, for the appearance of adverse side effects, and to ensure that patient is not hoarding medication. 10. If patient is not calmed by "talking down" or by medication, use of mechanical restraints may be necessary.	1. Close observation is required so that intervention can occur if required to ensure patient's (and others') safety. 2. Discussing feelings of self-harm with a trusted individual may provide some relief to the patient. An attitude of acceptance of the patient as a worthwhile individual is conveyed. 3. Lack of attention to the maladaptive behavior may decrease repetition of its use. 4. To problem solve the situation with the patient, knowledge of the precipitating factors is important. 5. It is vital that the patient learns to express angry feelings in adaptive ways; suicide and other self-destructive behaviors are often viewed as a result of anger turned inward on the self. 6. Patient safety is a nursing priority. 7. Physical exercise is a safe and effective way of relieving pent-up tension. 8. This conveys to the patient evidence of control over the situation and provides some physical security for patient and staff. 9. Tranquilizing medications, such as anxiolytics or antipsychotics, may have a calming effect on the patient and may prevent aggressive behaviors. Close monitoring is important because impulsivity is a common symptom in BPD and may increase risk for an overdose attempt. 10. The avenue of the "least restrictive alternative" must be selected when planning interventions for a violent patient. Restraints should be used only as a last resort, after all other interventions have been unsuccessful, and the patient is clearly at risk of harm to self or others.

Continued

Table 22–3 | CARE PLAN FOR THE PATIENT WITH BORDERLINE PERSONALITY DISORDER–cont'd

OUTCOME CRITERIA	NURSING INTERVENTIONS	RATIONALE
	11. If restraint is deemed necessary, ensure that sufficient staff is available to assist. Follow protocol established by the institution. Provide care with consideration for patient's trauma history.	11. Restraints should be used only as a last resort, after all other interventions have been unsuccessful and the patient is clearly at imminent risk of harming self or others. The safety and protection of patient, staff, and other patients is a top priority. Trauma-informed care should always be the foundation for decisions about appropriateness of interventions.
	12. If warranted by high acuity of the situation, staff may need to be assigned on a one-to-one basis.	12. Because of their extreme fear of abandonment, patients with this disorder should not be left alone at a stressful time because it may cause an acute rise in anxiety and agitation levels.
	13. As agitation decreases, assess the patient's readiness for restraint removal or reduction. Remove one restraint at a time while assessing the patient's response.	13. This minimizes the risk of injury to patient and staff.

NURSING DIAGNOSIS: COMPLICATED GRIEVING

RELATED TO: Maternal deprivation during rapprochement phase of development (internalized as a loss, with fixation in anger stage of grieving process); possible childhood physical or sexual abuse

EVIDENCED BY: Depressed mood, maladaptive expressions of anger

OUTCOME CRITERIA	NURSING INTERVENTIONS	RATIONALE
Short-Term Goal ■ Within 5 days, the patient will discuss with nurse or therapist maladaptive patterns of expressing anger. **Long-Term Goal** ■ By time of discharge from treatment, the patient will be able to identify the true source of angry feelings, accept ownership of these feelings, and express them in a socially acceptable manner, in an effort to satisfactorily progress through the grieving process.	1. Convey an accepting attitude—one that creates a nonthreatening environment for the patient to express feelings. Be honest and keep all promises. 2. Identify the function that anger, frustration, and rage serve for the patient. Allow him or her to express these feelings within reason. 3. Encourage patient to discharge pent-up anger through participation in large motor activities (e.g., brisk walks, jogging, physical exercises, volleyball, exercise bike). 4. Explore with patient the true source of the anger. This is a painful therapy that often leads to regression as the patient deals with the feelings of early abandonment or issues of abuse. 5. Because anger may be displaced onto the nurse, caution must be taken to guard against the negative effects of countertransference.	1. An accepting attitude conveys to the patient that you believe he or she is a worthwhile person. Trust is enhanced. 2. Verbalization of feelings in a nonthreatening environment may help patient come to terms with unresolved issues. 3. Physical exercise provides a safe and effective method for discharging pent-up tension. 4. Reconciliation of the feelings associated with this stage is necessary before progression through the grieving process can continue. 5. Countertransference has the potential to generate an array of negative feelings from the nurse. The existence of negative feelings must be acknowledged, but they must not be allowed to interfere with the therapeutic process.

Table 22–3 | CARE PLAN FOR THE PATIENT WITH BORDERLINE PERSONALITY DISORDER—cont'd

OUTCOME CRITERIA	NURSING INTERVENTIONS	RATIONALE
	6. Explain the behaviors associated with the normal grieving process. Help the patient recognize his or her position in this process.	6. Knowledge of the acceptability of the feelings associated with normal grieving may help to relieve some of the guilt that these responses generate.
	7. Help the patient understand appropriate ways to express anger. Give positive reinforcement for behaviors used to express anger appropriately. Act as a role model. It is important to let the patient know when he or she has done something that has generated angry feelings in you.	7. Positive reinforcement enhances self-esteem and encourages repetition of desirable behaviors. Role-modeling ways to express anger in an appropriate manner is a powerful learning tool.
	8. Set limits on maladaptive behaviors and explain consequences of violation of those limits. Be supportive, yet consistent and firm in caring for this patient.	8. Patient lacks sufficient self-control to limit maladaptive behaviors, so assistance is required. Consistency on the part of all staff members working with this patient is essential for achieving positive outcomes.

NURSING DIAGNOSIS: IMPAIRED SOCIAL INTERACTION

RELATED TO: Extreme fears of abandonment and engulfment

EVIDENCED BY: Alternating clinging and distancing behaviors and staff splitting

OUTCOME CRITERIA	NURSING INTERVENTIONS	RATIONALE
Short-Term Goal ■ Within 5 days, patient will discuss with nurse or therapist behaviors that impede the development of satisfactory interpersonal relationships. **Long-Term Goal** ■ By time of discharge from treatment, patient will interact appropriately with others in the therapy setting in both social and therapeutic activities (evidencing a discontinuation of splitting and clinging and distancing behaviors).	1. Encourage patient to examine maladaptive behaviors (to recognize that they are occurring). 2. Reinforce that you will be available, without reinforcing dependent behaviors. 3. Rotate staff members who work with the patient in order to avoid patient's developing dependence on particular individuals. 4. Discuss with patient and other staff members when it is apparent that the patient is pitting one staff member against another. Do not listen as patient tries to degrade other staff members. Suggest instead that the patient discuss the problem directly with the staff person involved. 5. With the patient, explore feelings that relate to fears of abandonment and engulfment. Help him or her to understand that clinging and distancing behaviors are engendered by these fears.	1. Patient may be unaware of splitting or of clinging and distancing pattern of interaction with others. Recognition must occur before change can occur. 2. Knowledge of your availability may provide needed security for the patient. 3. Patient must learn to relate to more than one staff member in an effort to decrease use of splitting and to diminish fears of abandonment. 4. Splitting is the primary defense mechanism of patients with BPD, and the impressions they have of others as either "good" or "bad" are a manifestation of this defense. These interventions are intended to help the individual understand that staff splitting will not be tolerated, and to work toward diminishing clinging and distancing behaviors. 5. Exploration of feelings with a trusted individual may help patient come to terms with unresolved issues.

Continued

Table 22–3 | CARE PLAN FOR THE PATIENT WITH BORDERLINE PERSONALITY DISORDER—cont'd

OUTCOME CRITERIA	NURSING INTERVENTIONS	RATIONALE
	6. Help patient explore how these behaviors interfere with satisfactory relationships.	6. Patient may be unaware of how others perceive these behaviors and why they are not acceptable.
	7. Assist patient to work toward achievement of object constancy. Be available, without promoting dependency.	7. This may help patient resolve fears of abandonment in the process toward developing the ability to establish satisfactory intimate relationships.
	8. Provide education, support, and referral resources for family members and significant others who may also experience anger and frustration at failed attempts to navigate interpersonal relationships with this individual.	8. Research has found that family members often report feeling excluded and discriminated against by healthcare providers (Lawn, Diped, & McMahon, 2015).

NOTE: The patient with BPD has been identified as being at high risk for being stigmatized, even among healthcare professionals (Black, Pfhol, & Blum, 2011; McNee, Donogue, & Coppola, 2014; Weight & Kendal, 2013; Westwood & Baker, 2010).

Patient behaviors, such as manipulating, lying, and splitting, violate the nurse's sense of success in establishing a trusting relationship with this individual and may culminate in negative or distancing behaviors from the nurse. The following guidelines are helpful in decreasing negative attitudes and stigmatization of this client:

■ Understand the disorder and the impact of childhood trauma on the dynamics of the patient's behavior to develop an approach of compassion and convey hopefulness that this is a treatable rather than an untreatable condition.

■ Recognize that even brief encounters with a patient, during short hospital stays, provide an opportunity to convey connectedness and a sense that the patient is valued. This is particularly important because the patient with BPD is interpersonally hypersensitive, fears abandonment, and has had a history of instability in interpersonal relationships (Helleman et al., 2014).

■ Frequently reflect on your feelings in response to patient behavior. For example, self-harming behaviors by the patient frequently generate feelings of anger and frustration in nurses when the behavior seems to be manipulative rather than a sign of true

distress. These feelings may culminate in the nurse distancing himself or herself from the patient (Westwood & Baker, 2010). Indeed, self-harming behaviors may be used as a tool for manipulating others *and* they are a sign of true distress.

■ Develop a clear model of communication and intervention among team members for the hospitalized patient with BPD. Consistency in intervention helps to model healthy interpersonal skills for the patient and may minimize successful efforts at splitting staff members. In addition, when healthcare team members develop strong communication skills with each other, it provides a foundation for discussing and confronting negative attitudes toward the patient and promotes culture change. For example, McNee and associates (2014) developed a commitment among their team members that they would avoid using phrases such as "acting out" and "attention seeking" because these reinforced a culture of negativity toward the patient.

Antisocial Personality Disorder (Background Assessment Data)

In the *DSM-I*, antisocial behavior was categorized as a "sociopathic or psychopathic" reaction that was symptomatic of any of several underlying personality disorders. The *DSM-II* represented it as a separate personality type, a distinction that has been retained in subsequent editions. The *DSM-5* diagnostic criteria for antisocial personality disorder are presented in Box 22–10.

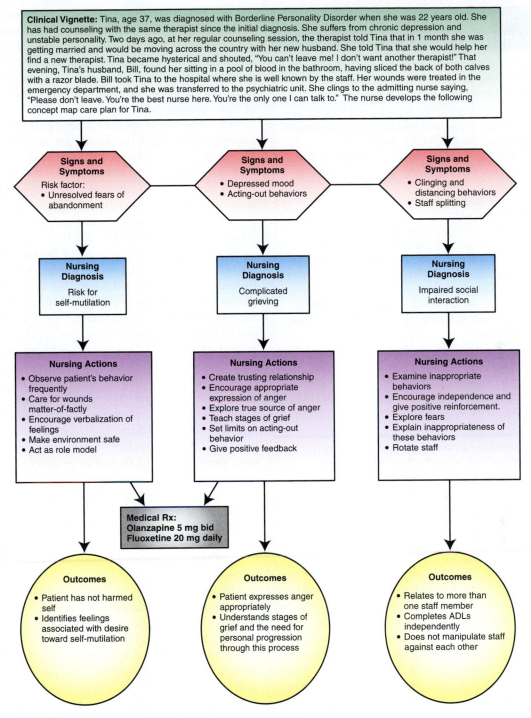

Clinical Vignette: Tina, age 37, was diagnosed with Borderline Personality Disorder when she was 22 years old. She has had counseling with the same therapist since the initial diagnosis. She suffers from chronic depression and unstable personality. Two days ago, at her regular counseling session, the therapist told Tina that in 1 month she was getting married and would be moving across the country with her new husband. She told Tina that she would help her find a new therapist. Tina became hysterical and shouted, "You can't leave me! I don't want another therapist!" That evening, Tina's husband, Bill, found her sitting in a pool of blood in the bathroom, having sliced the back of both calves with a razor blade. Bill took Tina to the hospital where she is well known by the staff. Her wounds were treated in the emergency department, and she was transferred to the psychiatric unit. She clings to the admitting nurse saying, "Please don't leave. You're the best nurse here. You're the only one I can talk to." The nurse develops the following concept map care plan for Tina.

Signs and Symptoms

Risk factor:
• Unresolved fears of abandonment

Signs and Symptoms
• Depressed mood
• Acting-out behaviors

Signs and Symptoms
• Clinging and distancing behaviors
• Staff splitting

Nursing Diagnosis

Risk for self-mutilation

Nursing Diagnosis

Complicated grieving

Nursing Diagnosis

Impaired social interaction

Nursing Actions
• Observe patient's behavior frequently
• Care for wounds matter-of-factly
• Encourage verbalization of feelings
• Make environment safe
• Act as role model

Nursing Actions
• Create trusting relationship
• Encourage appropriate expression of anger
• Explore true source of anger
• Teach stages of grief
• Set limits on acting-out behavior
• Give positive feedback

Nursing Actions
• Examine inappropriate behaviors
• Encourage independence and give positive reinforcement.
• Explore fears
• Explain inappropriateness of these behaviors
• Rotate staff

Medical Rx:
Olanzapine 5 mg bid
Fluoxetine 20 mg daily

Outcomes
• Patient has not harmed self
• Identifies feelings associated with desire toward self-mutilation

Outcomes
• Patient expresses anger appropriately
• Understands stages of grief and the need for personal progression through this process

Outcomes
• Relates to more than one staff member
• Completes ADLs independently
• Does not manipulate staff against each other

FIGURE 22–1   Concept map care plan for a patient with BPD.

Individuals with antisocial personality disorder are seldom seen in most clinical settings, and when they are, it is commonly a way to avoid legal consequences. Sometimes they are admitted to the healthcare system by court order for psychological evaluation. Most frequently, however, these individuals may be encountered in prisons, jails, and rehabilitation services.

Although the *DSM-5* continues to identify antisocial personality disorder as synonymous with psychopathy, recent evidence is beginning to distinguish these as separate entities (Anderson et al., 2014;

> **BOX 22–10 Diagnostic Criteria for Antisocial Personality Disorder**
>
> A. A pervasive pattern of disregard for and violation of the rights of others occurring since age 15 years, as indicated by three (or more) of the following:
>
>   1. Failure to conform to social norms with respect to lawful behaviors as indicated by repeatedly performing acts that are grounds for arrest
>   2. Deceitfulness, as indicated by repeated lying, use of aliases, or conning others for personal profit or pleasure
>   3. Impulsivity or failure to plan ahead
>   4. Irritability and aggressiveness, as indicated by repeated physical fights or assaults
>   5. Reckless disregard for safety of self or others
>   6. Consistent irresponsibility, as indicated by repeated failure to sustain consistent work behavior or honor financial obligations
>   7. Lack of remorse, as indicated by being indifferent to or rationalizing having hurt, mistreated, or stolen from another
>
> B. Individual is at least 18 years.
> C. There is evidence of conduct disorder with onset before age 15 years.
> D. The occurrence of antisocial behavior is not exclusively during the course of schizophrenia or bipolar disorder.
>
> *Reprinted with permission from American Psychiatric Association. (2013). Diagnostic and statistical manual of mental disorders (5th ed.). Washington, DC: American Psychiatric Publishing.*

APA, 2013; Thompson et al., 2014; Verona & Patrick, 2015). Antisocial personality disorder as a distinct entity is characterized by *behaviors* that are reactive to perceived threats, control, and a negative affect; psychopathy is described as *personality traits* that include low fear, low empathy, domination, callous cruelty, and emotional insensitivity (Thompson et al., 2015; Verona & Patrick, 2015). As separate entities, both may be considered prone to violence but with different etiologies and potentially different responses in treatment. For the purpose of discussion here, they are identified together as antisocial personality disorder.

Clinical Picture

Antisocial personality disorder is a pattern of socially irresponsible, exploitative, and guiltless behavior that reflects a general disregard for the rights of others. Individuals with this disorder exploit and manipulate others for personal gain and are unconcerned with obeying the law. They have difficulty sustaining consistent employment and in developing stable relationships. They appear cold and callous, often intimidating others with their brusque and belligerent manner. They tend to be argumentative and, at times, cruel and malicious. They lack warmth and compassion and are often suspicious of these qualities in others.

Individuals with antisocial personality have a very low tolerance for frustration, act impulsively, and are unable to delay gratification. They are restless and easily bored, often taking chances and seeking thrills, as if they were immune to danger. Their pattern of impulsivity may be manifested in failure to plan ahead, culminating in sudden job, residence, or relationship changes (APA, 2013).

When things go their way, individuals with this disorder act cheerful, even gracious and charming. Because of their low tolerance for frustration, this pleasant exterior can change very quickly. When what they desire at the moment is challenged, they are likely to become furious and vindictive. Easily provoked to attack, their first inclination is to demean and dominate. They believe that "good guys come in last," and they show contempt for the weak and underprivileged. They exploit others to fulfill their own desires, showing no trace of shame or guilt for their behavior. Individuals with antisocial personalities see themselves as victims, using projection, devaluing, and denial as primary ego defense mechanisms. They do not accept responsibility for the consequences of their behavior. In their own minds, the perception that they are being victimized by others justifies their malicious behavior, lest they be the recipient of unjust persecution and hostility from others. Physical attacks or other acts of aggression are not uncommon.

Satisfying interpersonal relationships are not possible because individuals with antisocial personalities have learned to place their trust only in themselves. They have a philosophy that "it's every man for himself" and that one should stop at nothing to avoid being manipulated by others. They may disregard the safety of themselves and others through reckless sexual activity, substance use, reckless driving, or child neglect (APA, 2013).

One of the most distinctive characteristics of individuals with antisocial personality disorder is their tendency to ignore conventional authority and rules. They act as though established social norms and guidelines for self-discipline and cooperative behavior do not apply to them. They are flagrant in their disrespect for the law and for the rights of others.

Predisposing Factors to Antisocial Personality Disorder

Biological Influences

Antisocial personality is more common among first-degree biological relatives of those with the disorder than among the general population. Twin and adoptive studies have implicated the role of genetics in antisocial personality disorder, especially for the personality traits of callousness and unemotional responses, which may be more definitive of psychopathy (Thompson et al., 2014). Interestingly, other antisocial behaviors among twins appear to be environmentally influenced and both biological and adoptive children of parents with antisocial personality disorder are at greater risk for this personality disorder (Cloninger & Svrakic, 2017), suggesting that this is a complex disorder with both genetic and environmental influences. Recent research has suggested that a particular gene, *MAOA*, may be moderated after exposure to violence such as child maltreatment, physical abuse, or sexual abuse (Ouellet-Morin et al., 2016). Mutations in this gene are believed to be associated with the eventual development of differential features of antisocial personality, although the authors note that more research is needed. Nonetheless, it adds support to the evidence that genetics and environment interact in the development of antisocial personality disorder and underscores the influence of childhood trauma.

Characteristics associated with temperament in the newborn may be significant in the predisposition to antisocial personality disorder. Parents who bring their children with behavior disorders to clinics often report that the child displayed temper tantrums from infancy and would become furious when awaiting a bottle or a diaper change. As these children mature, they commonly develop a bullying attitude toward other children. Parents report that they are undaunted by punishment and generally quite unmanageable.

The likelihood of developing antisocial personality disorder is increased if the individual had attention deficit-hyperactivity disorder and conduct disorder as a child that began under the age of 10 (APA, 2013). Brain imaging studies have identified deficits in prefrontal cortex gray matter, which regulates cognitive control and inhibition, and decreased activity in the amygdala, which is responsible for modulating fearful or threatening stimuli. Other studies have identified dysregulation of neurotransmitters (dopamine and serotonin), and endocrine abnormalities (testosterone and cortisol) as present in individuals with antisocial personality disorder, and these dysregulations may be related to the symptoms of impulsivity (Thompson et al., 2014). Neuropsychological studies have demonstrated an increased reactivity to environmental irritants and cues that may be triggers for disinhibition (Verona & Patrick, 2015).

Family Dynamics

Antisocial personality disorder frequently arises from a chaotic home environment. Parental deprivation during the first 5 years of life appears to be a critical predisposing factor in the development of antisocial personality disorder. Separation due to parental delinquency appears to be more highly correlated with the disorder than is parental loss from other causes.

Studies have shown that antisocial personality disorder in adulthood is highly associated with physical abuse and neglect, teasing, and lack of parental bonding in childhood (Cloninger & Svrikac, 2017; Kolla et al., 2013; Krastins et al., 2014). Severe physical abuse was found to be particularly correlated to violent offending, triggering the development of a pattern of reactive aggression that is persistent over one's lifetime (Kolla et al., 2013). The abuse also contributes to the development of antisocial behavior in that it provides a model for behavior, and it may result in injury to the child's central nervous system, thereby impairing the child's ability to function appropriately. Although a diagnosis of antisocial personality disorder is made only when the client is at least 18 years of age, these behavioral patterns are often seen earlier in childhood and adolescence. When they are identified in children and adolescents, the diagnosis is *conduct disorder,* and the common symptoms are bullying, fighting, physical cruelty to animals, destruction of property and theft, among others (APA, 2013). Whether better identification and early intervention might prevent more dangerous behavior in adulthood is yet to be determined through ongoing research.

Diagnosis and Outcome Identification

Nursing diagnoses are formulated from the data gathered during the assessment phase and with background knowledge regarding predisposing factors to the disorder. Table 22–4 presents a list of patient behaviors and the NANDA International nursing diagnoses that correspond to those behaviors, which may be used in planning care for patients with antisocial personality disorder.

TABLE 22–4	Assigning Nursing Diagnoses to Behaviors Commonly Associated With Antisocial Personality Disorder	
BEHAVIORS	**NURSING DIAGNOSES**	
Risk factors: Body language (e.g., rigid posture, clenching of fists and jaw, hyperactivity, pacing, breathlessness, threatening stances); cruelty to animals; rage reactions; history of childhood abuse; history of violence against others; impulsivity; substance abuse; negative role modeling; inability to tolerate frustration	**Risk for other-directed violence**	
Disregard for societal norms and laws; absence of guilty feelings; inability to delay gratification; denial of obvious problems; grandiosity; hostile laughter; projection of blame and responsibility; ridicule of others; superior attitude toward others	**Defensive coping**	
Manipulation of others to fulfill own desires; inability to form close, personal relationships; frequent lack of success in life events; passive-aggressiveness; overt aggressiveness (hiding feelings of low self-esteem)	**Chronic low-self esteem**	
Inability to form a satisfactory, enduring, intimate relationship with another; dysfunctional interaction with others; use of unsuccessful social interaction behaviors	**Impaired social interaction**	
Demonstration of inability to take responsibility for meeting basic health practices; history of lack of health-seeking behavior; demonstrated lack of knowledge regarding basic health practices; lack of expressed interest in improving health behaviors	**Ineffective health maintenance**	

Outcome Criteria

The following criteria may be used for measurement of outcomes in the care of the patient with antisocial personality disorder.

The patient:

- Discusses angry feelings with staff and in group sessions.
- Has not harmed self or others.
- Can rechannel hostility into socially acceptable behaviors.
- Follows rules and regulations of the therapy environment.
- Can verbalize which of his or her behaviors are not acceptable.
- Shows regard for the rights of others by delaying gratification of own desires when appropriate.
- Does not manipulate others in an attempt to increase feelings of self-worth.
- Verbalizes understanding of knowledge required to maintain basic health needs.

Planning and Implementation

The following section presents a group of selected nursing diagnoses common to patients with antisocial personality disorder with short- and long-term goals and nursing interventions for each.

Risk for Other-Directed Violence

An individual is defined as at *risk for other-directed violence* when he or she is "susceptible to behaviors in which an individual demonstrates that he or she can be physically, emotionally, and/or sexually harmful to others" (Herdman & Kamitsuru, 2018, p. 416).

Patient Goals

Outcome criteria include short- and long-term goals. Timelines are individually determined.

Short-Term Goals

- Within 3 days, patient will discuss angry feelings and situations that precipitate hostility.
- Patient will not harm others.

Long-Term Goal

- Patient will not harm others.

Interventions

- Convey an accepting attitude toward this patient. Feelings of rejection are undoubtedly familiar to him or her. Work on development of trust. Be honest, keep all promises, and convey the message to the patient that it is not *him* or *her* but the *behavior* that is unacceptable. An attitude of acceptance promotes feelings of self-worth. Trust is the basis of a therapeutic relationship. Be alert, however, to the tendency of this patient to manipulate others. Don't misconstrue charm or compliments as indicative of mutual trust. Maintaining clear, professional boundaries is essential.
- Maintain a low level of stimuli in the patient's environment (low lighting, few people, simple decor, low noise level). A stimulating environment may increase agitation and promote aggressive behavior.

- Observe the patient's behavior frequently. Do this through routine activities and interactions; avoid appearing watchful and suspicious. Close observation is required so that intervention can occur if needed to ensure the patient's (and others') safety.
- Remove all dangerous objects from the patient's environment so that he or she may not purposefully or inadvertently use them to inflict harm to self or others.
- Help the patient identify the true object of his or her hostility (e.g., "You seem to be upset with . . ."). Because of weak ego development, the patient may use the defense mechanism of displacement. Helping him or her recognize this in a nonthreatening manner may help reveal unresolved issues so that they may be confronted.
- Encourage the patient to gradually verbalize hostile feelings. Verbalization of feelings in a nonthreatening environment may help the patient come to terms with unresolved issues.
- Explore with the patient alternative ways of handling frustration (e.g., large motor skills that channel hostile energy into socially acceptable behavior). Physically demanding activities help to relieve pent-up tension.
- The staff should maintain and convey a calm attitude toward the patient. Anxiety is contagious and can be transferred from staff to patient. A calm attitude provides the patient with a feeling of safety and security.
- Have sufficient staff available to present a show of strength to the patient if necessary. This conveys to the patient evidence of control over the situation and provides some physical security for the staff.
- Administer tranquilizing medications as ordered by the physician or obtain an order if necessary. Monitor the patient for effectiveness of the medication as well as for appearance of adverse side effects. Antianxiety agents (e.g., lorazepam, chlordiazepoxide, oxazepam) produce a calming effect and may help to allay hostile behaviors.

(**NOTE:** Medications are not often prescribed for patients with antisocial personality disorder because of these individuals' strong susceptibility to addictions.)

- If the patient is not calmed by "talking down" or with medication and becomes an imminent threat to the safety of others, use of mechanical restraints may be necessary. The avenue of the "least restrictive alternative" must be selected when planning interventions for a violent patient. Restraints should be used only as a last resort,

after all other interventions have been unsuccessful, and the patient is clearly at risk of harm to self or others.
- If restraint is deemed necessary, ensure that sufficient staff is available to assist. Follow protocol established by the institution.
- As agitation decreases, assess the patient's readiness for restraint removal or reduction. Remove one restraint at a time while assessing the patient's response. This minimizes the risk of injury to patient and staff.

Defensive Coping

Defensive coping is defined as "repeated projection of falsely positive self-evaluation based on a self-protective pattern that defends against underlying perceived threats to positive self-regard" (Herdman & Kamitsuru, 2018, p. 326).

Patient Goals

Outcome criteria include short- and long-term goals. Timelines are individually determined.

Short-Term Goals

- Within 24 hours after admission, patient will verbalize understanding of treatment setting rules and regulations and the consequences for violation of them.
- Patient will verbalize personal responsibility for difficulties experienced in interpersonal relationships within (time period reasonable for patient).

Long-Term Goals

- By the time of discharge from treatment, patient will be able to cope more adaptively by delaying gratification of own desires and following rules and regulations of the treatment setting.
- By the time of discharge from treatment, patient will demonstrate ability to interact with others without becoming defensive, rationalizing behaviors, or expressing grandiose ideas.

Interventions

- From the onset, the patient should be made aware of which behaviors are acceptable and which are not. Explain consequences of violation of the limits. A consequence must involve something of value to the patient. All staff must be consistent in enforcing these limits. Consequences should be administered in a matter-of-fact manner immediately following the infraction. Because the patient cannot (or will not) impose own limits on maladaptive behaviors, these behaviors must be delineated and enforced by staff. Undesirable consequences may help to decrease repetition of these behaviors.

■ Explanations must be concise, concrete, and clear with little or no capacity for misinterpretation. The ideal goal would be for this patient to eventually internalize societal norms, beginning with a step-by-step, "either/or" approach on the unit (*either* you do [don't do] this, *or* this will occur).

> **CLINICAL PEARL** Do not attempt to coax or convince the patient to do the "right thing." Do not use the words "You should (or shouldn't) . . ."; instead, use the words "You will be expected to . . ."

■ Provide positive feedback or reward for acceptable behaviors. Positive reinforcement enhances self-esteem and encourages repetition of desirable behaviors.

■ In an attempt to assist the patient to delay gratification, begin to increase the length of time requirement for acceptable behavior in order to achieve the reward. For example, 2 hours of acceptable behavior may be exchanged for a phone call; 4 hours of acceptable behavior for 2 hours of television; 1 day of acceptable behavior for a recreational therapy bowling activity; 5 days of acceptable behavior for a weekend pass.

■ A milieu unit provides the appropriate environment for the patient with antisocial personality. The democratic approach with specific rules and regulations, community meetings, and group therapy sessions emulates the type of societal situation in which the patient must learn to live. Feedback from peers is often more effective than confrontation from an authority figure. The patient learns to follow the rules of the group as a positive step in the progression toward internalizing the rules of society.

■ Help the patient to gain insight into his or her own behavior. Often, these individuals rationalize to such an extent that they deny that their behavior is inappropriate. For example, thinking may be reflected in statements such as "The owner of this store has so much money, he'll never miss the little bit I take. He has everything, and I have nothing. It's not fair! I deserve to have some of what he has." The patient must come to understand that certain behaviors will not be tolerated within the society and that severe consequences will be imposed on those individuals who refuse to comply.

The patient must *want* to change behavior before he or she can be helped. One of the difficulties posed in interventions for personality disorders is that often the behaviors are ego-syntonic; in other words, the patient may not perceive these behaviors as requiring change.

■ Talk about past behaviors with the patient. Discuss which behaviors are acceptable by societal norms and which are not. Help the patient identify ways in which he or she has exploited others and the benefits versus consequences of previous behavior. Explore the patient's insight into feelings associated with his or her behavior. An attempt may be made to enlighten the patient to the sensitivity of others by promoting self-awareness in an effort to help the patient gain insight into his or her own behavior.

■ Throughout the relationship with the patient, maintain an attitude of "It is not *you* but *your behavior* that is unacceptable." An attitude of acceptance promotes feelings of dignity and self-worth.

Concept Care Mapping

The concept map care plan is a diagrammatic teaching and learning strategy that allows visualization of interrelationships between medical diagnoses, nursing diagnoses, assessment data, and treatments. An example of a concept map care plan for a patient with antisocial personality disorder is presented in Figure 22–2.

Evaluation

Reassessment is conducted to determine if the nursing actions have been successful in achieving the objectives of care. Evaluation of the nursing actions for the patient with antisocial personality disorder may be facilitated by gathering information using the following types of questions:

Has the patient:

■ Recognized when anger is getting out of control?
■ Sought out staff instead of expressing anger in an inappropriate manner?
■ Used other sources for rechanneling anger (e.g., physical activities)?
■ Expressed anger without physical aggression or harm to others?
■ Followed rules and regulations of the therapeutic milieu with little or no reminding?
■ Verbalized which behaviors are appropriate and which are not?
■ Expressed a desire to change?

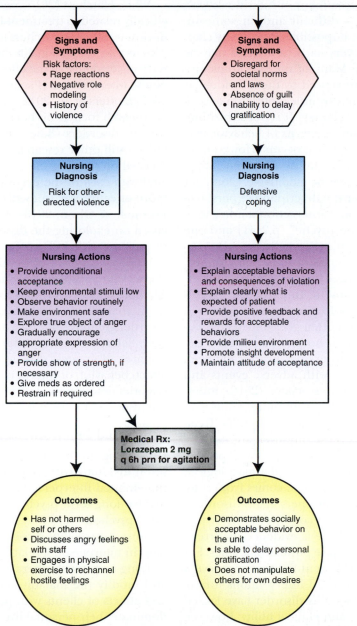

Clinical Vignette: Joey, age 32, is the oldest of five children of a single mother, each of whom had a different father. He was physically abused by his mother's boyfriends, did not attend school regularly, and eventually dropped out in 10th grade. He has a history of violence, always carries a weapon (gun or knife) on his person, and threatens to use it if he is challenged in his attempts to fulfill his own desires. He has had numerous skirmishes with the law: shoplifting, auto theft, possession and sale of heroin and cocaine, and, most recently, armed robbery of a liquor store. He was identified by his image on the store's surveillance camera. Because of his long history of criminal behavior, the judge has ordered that Joey undergo psychological testing before he is sentenced. On the psychiatric unit, he says to the nurse, "Why am I here? I'm not crazy! And I've never hurt anybody! I don't belong in this loony bin!" The nurse develops the following concept map care plan for Joey.

Signs and Symptoms

Risk factors:
• Rage reactions
• Negative role modeling
• History of violence

Signs and Symptoms

• Disregard for societal norms and laws
• Absence of guilt
• Inability to delay gratification

Nursing Diagnosis

Risk for other-directed violence

Nursing Diagnosis

Defensive coping

Nursing Actions

• Provide unconditional acceptance
• Keep environmental stimuli low
• Observe behavior routinely
• Make environment safe
• Explore true object of anger
• Gradually encourage appropriate expression of anger
• Provide show of strength, if necessary
• Give meds as ordered
• Restrain if required

Nursing Actions

• Explain acceptable behaviors and consequences of violation
• Explain clearly what is expected of patient
• Provide positive feedback and rewards for acceptable behaviors
• Provide milieu environment
• Promote insight development
• Maintain attitude of acceptance

Medical Rx:
Lorazepam 2 mg
q 6h prn for agitation

Outcomes

• Has not harmed self or others
• Discusses angry feelings with staff
• Engages in physical exercise to rechannel hostile feelings

Outcomes

• Demonstrates socially acceptable behavior on the unit
• Is able to delay personal gratification
• Does not manipulate others for own desires

FIGURE 22–2   Concept map care plan for a patient with antisocial personality disorder.

■ Demonstrated ability to delay gratifying own desires in deference to those of others when appropriate?

■ Refrained from manipulating others to fulfill own desires?

■ Fulfilled activities of daily living willingly and independently?

■ Verbalized methods of achieving and maintaining optimal wellness?

■ Identified community resources from which he or she can seek assistance with daily living and health-care needs when required?

Treatment Modalities

Few would argue that treatment of individuals with personality disorders is difficult and, in some instances, may even seem impossible. Personality characteristics are learned very early in life and may be genetically influenced. Many of the symptoms of a personality disorder are viewed by the individual as ego-syntonic, so there may be little motivation to seek treatment or to explore change. It is not surprising, then, that these enduring patterns of behavior may take years to change, if change occurs. However, we now understand the personality as a dynamic, adaptive system and, as such, may be modifiable. Cloninger and Svrakic (2017) offer the description of personality as a "multidimensional interaction among temperament, character, and psyche" (p.2141) and one that can undergo maturation through a complex process of developing awareness of those interactions. Zimmerman (2017) stresses that screening is imperative to appropriate treatment. In particular, BPD is a comorbid condition in 40 percent of hospitalized psychiatric patients, but it often goes undetected. Although extended inpatient hospitalization for treatment of personality disorders has historically been believed to be associated with adverse events and deterioration, Fowler and associates (2018) found that longer-term stays, of 40 days or more, resulted in significant improvement for patients with BPD. Treatment programs such as these, however, are in short supply. The main treatment modalities for all personality disorders are psychosocial and pharmacological, but most of the available evidence comes from studies of borderline and antisocial personality disorders.

Comorbid conditions are common in most personality disorders, and there is evidence that treating these conditions may have positive outcomes. For example, Hatchett (2015) identifies that, in a review of the literature, psychosocial interventions for clients with antisocial personality disorder have lacked both treatment efficacy and clinical utility; however, treatment of comorbid substance use disorder has demonstrated positive outcomes. Furthermore, when the individual with antisocial personality disorder has comorbid depression, he or she is more likely to persevere with treatment. This may be related to the fact that symptoms of depression are considered undesirable (not ego-syntonic) and therefore may promote interest in change or improvement. He notes that this review should not be interpreted as meaning that a client's personality disorder is untreatable. Instead, as Hatchett cites (Skeem et al., 2011), this client should be identified as "high risk" and requiring intensive treatment to maximize public safety.

While Hatchett (2015) reviewed the literature specifically related to treatment for antisocial personality disorders, other researchers identify in their literature reviews that, for personality disorders in general, there is strong evidence of the effectiveness of psychotherapeutic interventions (Papaioannou, Brazier, & Perry, 2013; Stoffers et al., 2012), although, again, the bulk of research focuses on borderline and antisocial personality disorders (Bateman, Gunderson, & Mulder, 2015). Still other researchers identify that treatment focused on tackling the defense mechanisms associated with each of the personality disorders may be a more effective way to mediate improvement (Perry, Presniak, & Olson, 2013). For example, therapy focused on exploring the dissociation that is common in patients with BPD or focusing on exploring the defense mechanism of devaluing others, as seen in clients with antisocial personality, may promote overall improvement in symptoms. There is general agreement that all treatment modalities for personality disorders require intensive and longer-term plans of care. Selection of intervention is generally based on the area of greatest dysfunction, such as cognition, affect, behavior, or interpersonal relations. Following is a brief description of various types of therapies and the disorders to which they are customarily suited.

Individual Psychotherapy

Depending on the therapeutic goals, psychotherapy for individuals with personality disorders may be time-limited interpersonal psychotherapy, or it may involve long-term psychoanalytic therapy. Interpersonal psychotherapy may be particularly appropriate because personality disorders largely reflect problems in interpersonal relationship skills.

Long-term psychotherapy attempts to understand and modify the maladjusted behaviors, cognition, and affects of clients with personality disorders that dominate their personal lives and relationships.

Milieu or Group Therapy

This treatment is especially appropriate for individuals with antisocial personality disorder who respond more adaptively to support and feedback from peers. In milieu or group therapy, feedback from peers is more effective than in one-to-one interaction with a therapist.

Group therapy—particularly homogenous supportive groups that emphasize the development of social skills—may be helpful in overcoming social anxiety and developing interpersonal trust and rapport in clients with avoidant personality disorder.

Cognitive Behavior Therapy

Behavioral strategies offer reinforcement for positive change. Social skills training and assertiveness training teach alternative ways to deal with frustration. Cognitive strategies help the client recognize and correct distorted and irrational thinking patterns. Davidson and colleagues (2009) found that the addition of cognitive behavior therapy to usual treatment for clients with antisocial personality disorders afforded a reduction in both verbal and physical aggression symptoms. There is also some limited evidence that cognitive therapy is beneficial for clients with schizotypal personality disorder (Bateman et al., 2015).

Dialectical Behavior Therapy

Dialectical behavior therapy (DBT) is a type of psychotherapy that was originally developed by Marsha Linehan, PhD, specifically as a treatment for the chronic self-injurious and parasuicidal behavior of clients with BPD (Sadock et al., 2015). It is rooted in a belief that the primary problem for this client is emotional dysregulation (a kind of emotional reactivity to perceived threats), and it has become a well-established treatment for clients with BPD. It is a complex, eclectic treatment that combines the concepts of cognitive, behavioral, and interpersonal therapies with Eastern mindfulness practices.

The four primary modes of treatment in DBT include the following:

1. **Group skills training:** These groups focus on teaching skills considered relevant to the particular problems experienced by people with BPD, such as core mindfulness skills, interpersonal effectiveness skills, emotion modulation skills, and distress tolerance skills.
2. **Individual psychotherapy:** Dysfunctional behavioral patterns, personal motivation, and skills strengthening are addressed in weekly sessions.
3. **Telephone contact:** The therapist is available to the client by telephone, usually on a 24-hour basis, but according to limits set by the therapist. Kiehn and Swales (2013) state, "Telephone contact is to give the patient help and support in applying the skills that she is learning to her real life situation between sessions and to help her find ways of avoiding self-injury."

4. **Therapist consultation and team meeting:** Therapists meet regularly to review their work with their clients. These meetings are focused specifically on providing support for each other, keeping the therapists motivated, and providing effective treatment to their clients. DBT has been well studied, and the evidence supports the benefits of this treatment for clients with BPD. O'Connell and Dowling (2014), citing a systematic review of seven studies (Binks et al., 2006), report that:

> Despite the difficulty in treating people with BPD, if the person with BPD is engaged in their treatment plan, there was a reduction in anxiety levels, depression, self-harm, hospital admission, and the use of prescribed medication. (p. 522)

This method of treatment is now being used with other disorders, including substance use disorders, eating disorders, schizophrenia, and PTSD (Sadock et al., 2015). Bateman and colleagues (2015) caution, however, that of the many interventions that have been specialized for the treatment of personality disorders, improvement is more often evidenced by symptom reduction; the interventions that have been specialized for the treatment of personality disorders have failed to produce significant improvements in social functioning.

Psychoanalytic Therapies

Two psychoanalytically oriented approaches that have demonstrated benefit in the treatment of BPD include mentalization therapy and transference therapy. Mentalization therapy focuses on assisting the client to improve their ability to reflect on and understand internal states (their own and others) and how those impact behavior so that the client can use mentalization when they are experiencing stressful situations and ultimately improve their ability to relate to others (Yasgur, 2017). Transference therapy seeks to use the transference that occurs in a client-therapist relationship to help the client improve self-perception and relationship skills.

Psychopharmacology

Psychopharmacology may be helpful in some instances. Although these medications have no effect in the direct treatment of the disorder itself, some symptomatic relief can be achieved. Among the cluster A disorders, there has been some limited evidence of the benefits of antipsychotic medication in the treatment of schizotypal personality disorder, but the risk-to-benefit ratio is unclear (Bateman et al., 2015).

For the treatment of BPD, symptom-targeted pharmacotherapy has been identified as an important adjunct. Antipsychotic medications show some benefits in treating cognitive-perceptual symptoms, selective serotonin reuptake inhibitors show some benefit in treating emotional dysregulation, and mood-stabilizing agents have shown some benefit in treating emotional dysregulation and impulsive aggressive symptoms (Bateman et al., 2015).

For antisocial personality disorder, pharmacotherapy is generally not recommended unless it is being used to treat a comorbid condition, and among the cluster C group of personality disorders, no randomized trials have been published that support pharmacological treatment for these disorders (Bateman et al., 2015).

Caution must be used when prescribing medications outside the structured setting because of the high risk for substance abuse in this population.

CASE STUDY AND SAMPLE CARE PLAN

NURSING HISTORY AND ASSESSMENT

Anthony, age 34, has been admitted to the psychiatric unit with a diagnosis of Antisocial Personality Disorder. He was recently arrested and convicted of armed robbery of a convenience store and attempted murder of the store clerk. Due to the actions of the store clerk, who quickly alerted police, and to the store surveillance camera, Anthony was identified and apprehended within hours of the crime. The judge has ordered physical, neurological, and psychiatric evaluations before sentencing Anthony.

Anthony was physically and psychologically abused as a child by his alcoholic father. He was suspended from high school because of failing grades and habitual truancy. He has a long history of arrests, beginning with shoplifting at age 7 and progressing in adolescence to burglary, auto theft, and sexual assault and finally to armed robbery and attempted murder. He was out on probation when he committed his latest crime.

On the psychiatric unit, Anthony is loud, belligerent, and uncooperative. When Carol, his admitting nurse, arrives to work the evening shift on Anthony's second hospital day, he says to her, "I'm so glad you are finally here. You are the best nurse on the unit. I can't talk to anyone but you. These people are nothing but a bunch of loonies around here . . . and that includes staff as well as patients! Maybe you and I could walk down to the coffee shop together later. Are you married? I'd sure like to get to know you better after I get out of this nut house!"

NURSING DIAGNOSES OUTCOME IDENTIFICATION

From the assessment data, the nurse develops the following nursing diagnoses for Anthony:

1. **Risk for other-directed violence** related to history of violence against others and history of childhood abuse
   a. **Short-Term Goals:**
      • Patient will discuss angry feelings and situations that precipitate hostility.
      • Patient will not harm others.
   b. **Long-Term Goal:** Patient will not harm others.

2. **Defensive coping** related to low self-esteem, dysfunctional nuclear family, underdeveloped ego and superego, evidenced by absence of guilt feelings, disregard for societal laws and norms, inability to delay gratification, superior attitude toward others, denial of problems, and projection of blame and responsibility
   a. **Short-Term Goal:** Patient will verbalize understanding of unit rules and regulations and consequences for violation of them.
   b. **Long-Term Goals:**
      • Patient will be able to delay gratification and follow rules and regulations of the unit.
      • Patient will verbalize personal responsibility for own actions and behaviors.

PLANNING AND IMPLEMENTATION

RISK FOR OTHER-DIRECTED VIOLENCE

The following nursing interventions have been identified for Anthony:

1. Develop a trusting relationship with Anthony by conveying an accepting attitude. Ensure that he understands it is not *him* but *his behavior* that is unacceptable.
2. Try to keep excess stimuli out of the environment. Speak to Anthony in a calm, quiet voice.
3. Observe Anthony's behavior regularly. Do so through routine activity so that he doesn't become suspicious and angry about being watched. This is important so that if hostile and aggressive behaviors are observed, intervention may prevent harm to Anthony, staff members, and/or other patients.
4. Sit with Anthony and encourage him to talk about his anger and hostile feelings. Help him understand where these feelings originate and who is the true target of the hostility.
5. Help him develop adaptive ways of dealing with frustration, such as exercise and other physical activities.
6. Administer tranquilizing medication, as ordered by the physician.
7. If Anthony should become out of control and mechanical restraints become necessary, ensure that sufficient staff is available to intervene. Do not use restraints as

CASE STUDY AND SAMPLE CARE PLAN—cont'd

a punishment but only as a protective measure for Anthony and the other patients.

DEFENSIVE COPING

The following nursing interventions have been identified for Anthony:

1. Explain to Anthony which of his behaviors are acceptable on the unit and which are not. Simply state that unacceptable behaviors will not be tolerated.
2. Determine appropriate consequences for violation of these limits (e.g., no TV or movies; no phone calls; time-out room). Ensure that all staff members follow through with these consequences.
3. Recognize that many of these patients use charm and compliments to manipulate others. Explain to Anthony that you will not accept these types of comments from him, and if they continue, impose consequences.
4. Encourage Anthony to talk about his past misdeeds. Try to help him understand how he would feel if someone treated him in the manner that he has treated others.

EVALUATION

The outcome criteria for Anthony have only partially been met. Personality characteristics such as those of Anthony's are deep-rooted and enduring. He is not likely to change. Unless testing reveals a serious medical problem, Anthony will no doubt go to prison for most of the rest of his life. During his time on the psychiatric unit, harm to self and others has been avoided. He has discussed his anger and hostile feelings with Carol and other staff members. He continues to become belligerent when told that he cannot smoke on the unit and must wait for someone to escort him to the smoking area. He yells at the other patients and calls them "nut cases." He refuses to take responsibility for his actions and blames negative behavioral outcomes on others. He has begun a regular exercise program in the fitness room and receives positive feedback from the staff for this attempt to integrate healthier coping strategies.

Summary and Key Points

■ Clients with personality disorders present with some of the most challenging symptoms that healthcare workers are likely to encounter.

■ Personality characteristics are formed very early in life and are difficult to change because they are complex in nature and the individual with personality disorder traits may not recognize the need to change. Some clinicians believe that the therapeutic approach is not to focus on changing the characteristics but rather to focus on decreasing the inflexibility of the maladaptive traits and reduce their interference with everyday functioning and meaningful relationships.

■ The concept of a personality disorder has been present throughout the history of medicine. Attempts to establish a classification system for these disorders have been problematic.

■ The *DSM-5* identifies 10 individual personality disorders: antisocial, avoidant, borderline, histrionic, dependent, narcissistic, obsessive-compulsive, paranoid, schizoid, and schizotypal.

■ Nursing care of the patient with a personality disorder is accomplished using the steps of the nursing process.

■ Other treatment modalities include interpersonal psychotherapy, psychoanalytical psychotherapy (including mentalization and transference therapy), milieu or group therapy, cognitive behavior therapy, DBT, and psychopharmacology.

■ Individuals with BPD may enter the healthcare system because of their instability and frequent attempts at self-destructive behavior.

■ The individual with antisocial personality disorder may become part of the healthcare system to avoid legal consequences or because of a court order for psychological evaluation.

■ Nurses who work in all types of clinical settings should be familiar with the characteristics associated with personality disorders.

■ Nurses working with patients who manifest symptoms of personality disorders, particularly BPD and antisocial personality disorder, must be skilled in clear and consistent communication, effective limit setting, and maintaining professional boundaries. Trauma-informed care is foundational in assessment and intervention.

Review Questions
Self-Examination/Learning Exercise

Select the answer that is most appropriate for each of the following questions:

1. Kim has a diagnosis of BPD. She often exhibits alternating clinging and distancing behaviors. Which of the following is the most appropriate nursing intervention with this type of behavior?
   a. Encourage Kim to establish trust in one staff person with whom all therapeutic interaction should take place.
   b. Secure a verbal contract from Kim that she will discontinue these behaviors.
   c. Withdraw attention if these behaviors continue.
   d. Rotate staff members who work with Kim so that she will learn to relate to more than one person.

2. Kim, a patient diagnosed with BPD, manipulates the staff in an effort to fulfill her own desires. All of the following may be examples of manipulative behaviors in the borderline client *except*:
   a. Refusal to stay in room alone, stating, "It's so lonely."
   b. Asking the nurse for cigarettes after 30 minutes, knowing that the assigned nurse has explained she must wait 1 hour.
   c. Stating to the nurse, "I really like having you for my nurse. You're the best one around here."
   d. Cutting arms with razor blade after discussing discharge plans with physician.

3. "Splitting" by the client with BPD denotes which of the following?
   a. Evidence of precocious development
   b. A primitive defense mechanism in which the client sees objects as all good or all bad
   c. A brief psychotic episode in which the client loses contact with reality
   d. Two distinct personalities within the borderline client

4. According to Margaret Mahler, predisposition to BPD occurs when developmental tasks go unfulfilled in which of the following phases?
   a. Autistic phase, during which the child's needs for security and comfort go unfulfilled
   b. Symbiotic phase, during which the child fails to bond with the mother
   c. Differentiation phase, during which the child fails to recognize a separateness between self and mother
   d. Rapprochement phase, during which the mother withdraws emotional support in response to the child's increasing independence

5. Jack is a new patient on the psychiatric unit with a diagnosis of antisocial personality disorder. Which of the following characteristics would you expect to assess in Jack?
   a. Lack of guilt for wrongdoing
   b. Insight into his own behavior
   c. Ability to learn from past experiences
   d. Compliance with authority

6. Milieu therapy is a good choice for patients with antisocial personality disorder because it:
   a. Provides a system of punishment and rewards for behavior modification.
   b. Emulates a social community in which the patient may learn to live harmoniously with others.
   c. Provides mostly one-to-one interaction between the patient and therapist.
   d. Provides a structured setting in which the patients have very little input into the planning of their care.

7. In evaluating the progress of Jack, a patient diagnosed with antisocial personality disorder, which of the following behaviors would be considered the most significant indication of positive change?
   a. Jack got angry only once in group this week.
   b. Jack tells the nurse how much he respects her work and that she has helped him immensely.
   c. On his own initiative, Jack sent a note of apology to a man he had injured in a recent fight.
   d. Jack stated that he would not start any more fights.

Review Questions—cont'd
Self-Examination/Learning Exercise

8. Which of the following behavioral patterns is characteristic of individuals with narcissistic personality disorder?
   a. Overly self-centered and exploitative of others
   b. Suspicious and mistrustful of others
   c. Rule conscious and disapproving of change
   d. Anxious and socially isolated

9. Jessica is a nurse who was floated to the psychiatric unit to cover for a staff nurse who called out sick. She encounters a patient who is diagnosed with BPD, and the patient states, "Thank goodness they sent you to the unit. No one else here has taken the time to listen to my concerns." This may be an example of which symptom common in BPD?
   a. Impulsivity
   b. Self-harming behaviors
   c. Dissociation
   d. Splitting

10. Which of the following behavioral patterns is characteristic of individuals with schizotypal personality disorder?
   a. Belittling themselves and their abilities
   b. A lifelong pattern of social withdrawal
   c. Suspiciousness and mistrust of others
   d. Overreacting inappropriately to minor stimuli

IMPLICATIONS OF RESEARCH FOR EVIDENCE-BASED PRACTICE

Brook, J., Lee. J. Y., Rubenstone, E., Brook, D., & Finch, S. (2014). Triple comorbid trajectories of tobacco, alcohol, and marijuana use as predictors of antisocial personality disorder and generalized anxiety disorder among urban adults. *American Journal of Public Health, 104*(8), 1413–1420.

DESCRIPTION OF THE STUDY: As part of the Harlem longitudinal development study, 816 urban youth of African American and Puerto Rican heritage were studied from the age of 19 until 32 years to evaluate the likelihood that those who were multi-substance users (alcohol, tobacco, and marijuana) were at greater risk for developing antisocial personality disorder (ASPD) and/or generalized anxiety disorder (GAD) in adulthood. The authors note that previous research has supported a relationship between multi-substance use and the development of ASPD. Evidence has also shown that psychosocial outcomes are worse when there is multi-substance abuse versus use of only one substance.

RESULTS OF THE STUDY: The concomitant use of tobacco, alcohol, and marijuana did significantly increase the likelihood of developing antisocial personality disorder in adulthood. A surprising finding was that, contrary to other research studies, this population did not show a decline in substance use after the mid-20s (as is typical of other populations), suggesting that these co-occurring problems may be more persistent for this population. The authors hypothesize that this may be related to less conventional ties (such as family or institutions) and more exposure to deviant peers, drug abusers, and antisocial behavior.

IMPLICATIONS FOR NURSING PRACTICE: Understanding the evidence base for treatment issues relevant to specific cultural and ethnic groups provides the nurse with a foundation for providing culturally sensitive and informed care. This study highlights risks for African American and Puerto Rican youth in urban settings, and the findings suggest that earlier intervention and treatment of comorbid substance use disorders may be effective in decreasing the likelihood of antisocial personality disorders in adulthood as well as decreasing their risk for longer-standing substance use disorders. Nursing assessment, particularly among adolescents, should include assessment for multi-substance use as well as assessment for evidence of conduct disorder behavior and treatment should focus on addressing all substances.

TEST YOUR CRITICAL THINKING SKILLS

Dana, age 32, was diagnosed with BPD when she was 26 years old. Her husband took her to the emergency department when he walked into the bathroom and found her cutting her legs with a razor blade. At that time, assessment revealed that Dana had a long history of self-mutilation, which she had carefully hidden from her husband and others. Dana began long-term psychoanalytical psychotherapy on an outpatient basis. Therapy revealed that Dana had been physically and sexually abused as a child by both her mother and her father, both now deceased. She admitted to having chronic depression and her husband related episodes of rage reactions. Dana has been hospitalized on the psychiatric unit for a week because of suicidal ideations. The psychiatrist has ordered that she is allowed to leave the unit on pass to keep a dental appointment that she made a number of weeks ago. She has just returned to the unit and says to her nurse, "I just took 20 Desyrel while I was sitting in my car in the parking lot."

Answer the following questions related to Dana:

1. The nurse is well acquainted with Dana and believes that her suicide attempt is a manipulative gesture. How should the nurse handle this situation?
2. What is the priority nursing diagnosis for Dana?
3. Dana likes to "split" the staff into "good guys" and "bad guys." What is the most important intervention for splitting by a person with BPD?

COMMUNICATION EXERCISES

1. Nathan, age 37, has been admitted to the hospital for a psychiatric evaluation after being arrested for armed robbery of a convenience store. He has a history of encounters with law enforcement since early adolescence. He has been diagnosed with Antisocial Personality Disorder. Nathan says to the nurse, "Hey pretty lady! Where have you been all my life?"

   How would the nurse respond appropriately to this statement by Nathan?

2. "I really got a bum rap! I had no intentions of hurting anyone. The gun only had one bullet in it! I just wanted to scare that clerk into giving me a few bucks! Just my bad luck an off-duty cop had to walk in about that time."

   How would the nurse respond appropriately to this statement by Nathan?

3. "You're really cute. Are you married? I'm pretty sure my lawyer can get me out of this rap, and I'll be a free man! Why don't you give me your phone number and I'll call you sometime. We could go out and have some fun!"

   How would the nurse respond appropriately to this statement by Nathan?

MOVIE CONNECTIONS

Taxi Driver (Schizoid personality) • *One Flew Over the Cuckoo's Nest* (Antisocial) • *The Boston Strangler* (Antisocial) • *Just Cause* (Antisocial) • *The Dream Team* (Antisocial) • *Goodfellas* (Antisocial) • *Fatal Attraction* (Borderline) • *Play Misty for Me* (Borderline) • *Girl, Interrupted* (Borderline) • *Gone With the Wind* (Histrionic) • *Wall Street* (Narcissistic) • *The Odd Couple* (Obsessive-compulsive)

References

American Psychiatric Association. (2013). *Diagnostic and statistical manual of mental disorders* (5th ed.). Washington, DC: Author.

Anderson, J. L., Sellbom, M., Wygant, D. B., Salekin, R. T., & Krueger, R. F. (2014). Examining the association between *DSM-5* section III antisocial personality traits and psychopathy in community and university samples. *Journal of Personality Disorders, 28*(5), 675–697.

Bateman, A. W., Gunderson, J., & Mulder, R. (2015). Treatment of personality disorder. *Lancet, 385,* 735–743.

Binks, C., Fenton, M., McCarthy, L., Lee, T., Adams, C., & Duggan, C. (2006). Psychological therapies for people with BPDs (review). *Cochrane Database of Systematic Reviews, 1.* doi:10.1002/14651858.CD005652

Black, D., Pfhol, B., & Blum, M. (2011). Attitudes towards BPD: A survey of 706 mental health clinicians. *CNS Spectrums, 16*(3), 67–74.

Bornstein, R. F., Bianucci, V., Fishman, D. P., & Biars, J. W. (2014). Toward a firmer foundation for *DSM-5.1*: Domains of impairment in *DSM IV/DSM-5* personality disorders. *Journal of Personality Disorders, 28*(2), 212–224.

Brook, J., Lee. J. Y., Rubenstone, E., Brook, D., & Finch, S. (2014). Triple comorbid trajectories of tobacco, alcohol, and marijuana use as predictors of antisocial personality disorder and generalized anxiety disorder among urban adults. *American Journal of Public Health, 104*(8), 1413–1420.

Cloninger, C. R., & Svrakic, D. M. (2017). Personality disorders. In B. J. Sadock, V. A. Sadock, & P. Ruiz (Eds.), *Comprehensive textbook of psychiatry* (10th ed., pp. 2126–2176). Philadelphia, PA: Wolters Kluwer.

Davidson, K. M., Tyrer, P., Tata, P., Cook, D., Gumely, A., Ford, I., . . . Crawford, M. J. (2009). Cognitive behaviour therapy for violent men with antisocial personality disorder in the community: An exploratory randomized controlled trial. *Psychological Medicine, 39*(4), 569–577. doi:10.1017/S00332910708004066

Ford, J. D., & Courtois, C. A. (2014). Complex PTSD, affect dysregulation, and borderline personality disorder. *Borderline Personality Disorder and Emotion Dysregulation, 1*(9), 1–7. doi:10.1186/2051-6673-1-9

Fowler, J. C., Clapp, J. D., Madan, A., Allen, J. G., Frueh, C., Fonagy, P., & Oldham, J. M. (2018). A naturalistic longitudinal study of extended inpatient treatment for adults with borderline personality disorder: An examination of treatment response, remission and deterioration. *Journal of Affective Disorders, 235,* 323–331. doi:https://doi.org/10.1016/j.jad.2017.12.054

Gregory, C. (2018). *Narcissistic personality disorder: A guide to signs, diagnosis, and treatment.* Retrieved from https://www.psycom.net/personality-disorders/narcissistic

Hatchett, G. (2015). Treatment guidelines for clients with antisocial personality disorder. *Journal of Mental Health Counseling, 37*(1), 15–27.

Helleman, M., Goossens, P. J., Kaasenbrood, A., & Van Achterberg, T. (2014). Experiences of patients with BPD with the brief admission intervention: A phenomenological study. *International Journal of Mental Health Nursing, 23,* 442–450.

Herdman, T. H., & Kamitsuru, S. (Eds.). (2018). *NANDA-I nursing diagnoses: Definitions and classification, 2018–2020.* New York, NY: Thieme.

Hodges, M., Godbout, N., Briere, J., Lanktree, C., Gilbert, A., & Kletzka, N. T. (2013). Cumulative trauma and symptom complexity in children: A path analysis. *Child Abuse and Neglect, 37,* 891–898.

Kiehn, B., & Swales, M. (2013). An overview of dialectical behaviour therapy in the treatment of BPD. *Psychiatry Online.* Retrieved from http://www.priory.com/dbt.htm

Kolla, N. J., Malcolm, C., Attard, S., Arenovich, T., Blackwood, N., & Hodgins, S. (2013). Childhood maltreatment and aggressive behavior in violent offenders with psychopathy. *Canadian Journal of Psychiatry, 58*(8), 487–494.

Krastins, A., Francis, A. J., Field, A. M., & Carr, S. N. (2014). Childhood predictors of adult antisocial personality disorder symptomatology. *Australian Psychologist, 49,* 142–150.

Lawn, S., Diped, B. A., & McMahon, J. (2015). Experience of family carers of people diagnosed with BPD. *Journal of Psychiatric and Mental Health Nursing, 22,* 234–243.

Lubit, R. H. (2017). BPD. *eMedicine Psychiatry.* Retrieved from http://emedicine.medscape.com/article/913575-overview

MacIntosh, H. B., Godbout, N., & Dubash, N. (2015). BPD: Disorder of trauma or personality, a review of the empirical literature. *Canadian Psychology, 56*(2), 227–241.

Mak, A. D., & Lam, L. C. (2013). Neurocognitive profiles of people with borderline personality disorder. *Current Opinion in Psychiatry, 26*(1), 90–96. doi:10.1097/YCO.0b013e32835b57a9

Mayo Clinic. (2017). *Narcissistic personality disorder.* Retrieved from https://www.mayoclinic.org/diseases-conditions/narcissistic-personality-disorder/symptoms-causes/syc-20366662

McNee, L., Donogue, C., & Coppola, A. M. (2014). A team approach to BPD. *Mental Health Practice, 17*(10), 33–35.

O'Connell, B., & Dowling, M. (2014). Dialectical behavior therapy (DBT) in the treatment of BPD. *Journal of Psychiatric and Mental Health Nursing, 21,* 518–525.

Ouellet-Morin, I., Côté, S. M., Vitaro, F., Hébert, M., Carbonneau, R., Lacourse, E., & Tremblay, R. E. (2016). Effects of the *MAOA* gene and levels of exposure to violence on antisocial outcomes. *British Journal of Psychiatry, 208*(1), 42–48. doi:10.1192/bjp.bp.114.162081

Papaioannou, D., Brazier, J., & Parry, G. (2013). How to measure quality of life for cost effectiveness analyses or personality disorders: A systematic review. *Journal of Personality Disorders, 27*(3), 383–401.

Perry, J. C., Presniak, M. D., & Olson, T. R. (2013). Defense mechanisms in schizotypal, borderline, antisocial, and narcissistic personality disorders. *Psychiatry, 76*(1), 32–52.

Pier, K., Marin, L. K., Wilsnack, J., & Goodman, M. (2016). The neurobiology of borderline personality disorder. *Psychiatric Times, 33*(3). Retrieved from http://www.psychiatrictimes.com/borderline-personality/neurobiology-borderline-personality-disorder/page/0/2

Rodriguez, T. (2017). *Bipolar disorder, borderline personality disorder may represent the same disorder.* Retrieved from http://www.psychiatryadvisor.com/bipolar-disorder/bipolar-disorder-same-as-borderline-personality-disorder/article/712397

Sadock, B. J., Sadock, V. A., & Ruiz, P. (2015). *Synopsis of psychiatry: Behavioral sciences/clinical psychiatry* (11th ed.). Philadelphia, PA: Wolters Kluwer.

Skeem, J. L., Polaschek, D. L., Patrick, C. J., & Lilienfeld, S. O. (2011). Psychopathic personality: Bridging the gap between scientific evidence and public policy. *Psychological Science in the Public Interest, 12,* 95–162. doi:10.1177/1529100611426707

Stoffers, J. M., Vollm, B., Rucker, G., Timmer, A., Huband, N., & Lieb, K. (2012). Psychological therapies for people with BPDs (review). *Cochrane Database of Systematic Reviews.* doi:10.1002/14651858.CD005652.pub2

Thompson, D. F., Ramos, C. L., & Willett, J. K. (2014). Psychopathy: Clinical features, developmental basis, and therapeutic challenges. *Journal of Clinical Pharmacology and Therapeutics, 39,* 485–495.

Verona, E., & Patrick, C. J. (2015). Psychobiological aspects of antisocial personality disorder, psychopathy, and violence. *Psychiatric Times,* 1–7. Retrieved from http://www.psychiatrictimes.com

Weight, J., & Kendal, S. (2013). Staff attitudes towards inpatients with BPD. *Mental Health Practice, 17*(3), 35–38.

Westwood, I., & Baker, J. (2010). Attitudes and perceptions of mental health nurses towards BPD clients in acute mental health settings: A review of the literature. *Journal of Psychiatric and Mental Health Nursing, 17*(7), 657–662.

Yasgur, B. S. (2017). Borderline personality disorder: Not just an adult condition. *Psychiatric Advisor.* Retrieved from http://www.psychiatryadvisor.com/childadolescent-psychiatry/borderline-personality-adult-adolescent/article/708450/2/

Zimmerman, M. (2017). Improving the recognition of borderline personality disorder. *Current Psychiatry, 16*(10), 13–19.

Classical References

Erikson, E. (1963). *Childhood and society* (2nd ed.). New York, NY: WW Norton.

Mahler, M., Pine, F., & Bergman, A. (1975). *The psychological birth of the human infant.* New York, NY: Basic Books.

Sullivan, H. S. (1953). *The interpersonal theory of psychiatry.* New York, NY: W W Norton.

Classical References

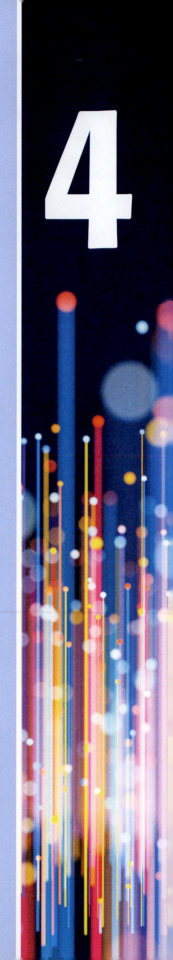

UNIT

4

Psychiatric Mental Health Nursing of Special Populations

23

Children and Adolescents

KEY TERMS

aggression
autism spectrum disorder
clinging
echolalia

impulsivity
negativism
palilalia

OBJECTIVES
After reading this chapter, the student will be able to:

1. Identify psychiatric disorders that most
   commonly have their onset in infancy,
   childhood, or adolescence.
2. Discuss predisposing factors implicated
   in the etiology of intellectual disability,
   autism spectrum disorder, attention-
   deficit/hyperactivity disorder, conduct
   disorder, oppositional defiant disorder,
   Tourette's disorder, and separation anxiety
   disorder.
3. Identify symptomatology and use
   the information in the assessment

   of clients with the aforementioned
   disorders.
4. Identify nursing diagnoses common to
   clients with these disorders and select
   appropriate nursing interventions for each.
5. Discuss relevant criteria for evaluating
   nursing care of clients with selected
   infant, childhood, and adolescent
   psychiatric disorders.
6. Describe treatment modalities relevant to
   selected disorders of infancy, childhood,
   and adolescence.

HOMEWORK ASSIGNMENT
Please read the chapter and answer the following questions:

1. What maternal prenatal activity has
   been associated with attention-deficit/
   hyperactivity disorder (ADHD) in children?
2. Which antidepressant medication has been
   used with some success in treating ADHD?
3. Neuroimaging brain studies in children
   with Tourette's disorder have been

   consistent in finding dysfunction in what
   area of the brain?
4. What are some family behaviors that
   have been implicated as influential in the
   development of separation anxiety disorder?

Introduction

This chapter examines various disorders in which the symptoms usually first become evident during infancy, childhood, or adolescence. It is important to note, however, that some of the disorders discussed in this chapter do appear later in life, and that symptoms associated with other disorders, such as major depressive disorder or bipolar disorder, also can appear in childhood or adolescence.

All nurses working with children or adolescents should be knowledgeable about "normal" stages of growth and development. Chapter 29, Concepts of Personality Development, available at DavisPlus, discusses this topic, and a summary of personality development theories appears in Chapter 22, Personality Disorders. The developmental process is one that is fraught with challenges. Behavioral responses are individual and idiosyncratic. They are, indeed, *human* responses.

Whether or not a child's behavior indicates emotional problems is often difficult to determine. Guidelines for making such a determination should consider appropriateness of the behavior regarding age and cultural norms and whether the behavior interferes with adaptive functioning. This chapter focuses on the nursing process in care of clients with intellectual disability, autism spectrum disorder (ASD), attention-deficit/hyperactivity disorder (ADHD), conduct disorder, oppositional defiant disorder (ODD), Tourette's disorder, and separation anxiety disorder. A discussion of treatment modalities is included.

Neurodevelopmental Disorders

Intellectual Disability (Intellectual Developmental Disorder)

The *Diagnostic and Statistical Manual of Mental Disorders, Fifth Edition (DSM-5)* (American Psychiatric Association [APA], 2013), defines *intellectual disability* as a "disorder with onset during the developmental period that includes both intellectual and adaptive functioning deficits in conceptual, social, and practical domains" (p. 33). The incidence rate in the general population is about 1 percent (APA, 2013). Onset of intellectual and adaptive deficits occurs during the developmental period. Level of impairment (mild, moderate, severe, or profound) is based on adaptive functioning within the three domains. General intellectual functioning is measured by both clinical assessment and an individual's performance on intelligence quotient (IQ) tests. Adaptive functioning refers to the person's ability to adapt to the requirements of daily living and the expectations of his or her age and cultural group. According to the *DSM-5* (APA, 2013), a diagnosis of intellectual disability requires the presence of deficits in intellectual (cognitive and learning functions) and adaptive (such as independent functioning, communication, and social) domains that began during the developmental period.

Predisposing Factors

The etiology of intellectual disability may be primarily biological or primarily psychosocial, or a combination of both, or in some instances, unknown. The common factors, regardless of etiology, are significant impairments in intellectual functions and social adaptation.

Genetic Factors

Genetic factors are implicated as the cause of intellectual disability in approximately 5 percent of the cases. These factors include inborn errors of metabolism, such as Tay-Sachs disease, phenylketonuria, and hyperglycinemia. Also included are chromosomal disorders such as Down syndrome and Klinefelter's syndrome and single-gene abnormalities such as fragile X syndrome, tuberous sclerosis, and neurofibromatosis.

Disruptions in Embryonic Development

Conditions affecting early (embryonic) development account for approximately 30 percent of intellectual disability cases. Damage may occur in response to toxicity associated with maternal ingestion of alcohol or other drugs. Fetal alcohol syndrome is an example, and this disorder has been identified as one of the leading preventable causes of intellectual disability. Maternal illnesses and infections during pregnancy (e.g., rubella, cytomegalovirus) and complications of pregnancy (e.g., pre-eclampsia, uncontrolled diabetes) may also play a role in causing congenital intellectual disability (Sadock, Sadock, & Ruiz, 2015).

Pregnancy and Perinatal Factors

Approximately 10 percent of cases of intellectual disability are the result of circumstances that occur during pregnancy (e.g., fetal malnutrition, viral and other infections, and prematurity) or during the birth process. Examples of the latter include trauma to the head incurred during the process of birth, placenta previa or premature separation of the placenta, and prolapse of the umbilical cord.

General Medical Conditions Acquired in Infancy or Childhood

General medical conditions acquired during infancy or childhood account for approximately 5 percent of cases of intellectual disability. They include infections, such as meningitis and encephalitis; poisonings, such as from insecticides, medications, and lead; and physical trauma, such as head injuries, asphyxiation, and hyperpyrexia (Sadock et al., 2015).

Sociocultural Factors and Other Mental Disorders

Between 15 and 20 percent of cases of intellectual disability may be attributed to deprivation of nurturance and social stimulation and to impoverished environments associated with poor prenatal and perinatal care and inadequate nutrition. Additionally, other mental disorders, such as ASD, can result in intellectual disability.

Recognition of the cause and period of inception provides information regarding what to expect in terms of behavior and potential. However, each child is different, and consideration must be given on an individual basis.

Application of the Nursing Process to Intellectual Disability

Background Assessment Data (Symptomatology)

The degree of severity of intellectual disability may be measured by the client's IQ level. Four levels have

been delineated: mild, moderate, severe, and profound. The various behavioral manifestations and abilities associated with each of these levels of severity are outlined in Table 23–1.

Nurses should assess and focus on each child's strengths and individual abilities. Knowledge regarding level of independence in the performance of self-care activities is essential to the development of an adequate plan for the provision of nursing care.

Nursing Diagnosis

Selection of appropriate nursing diagnoses for the patient with intellectual disability depends largely on the degree of severity of the condition and the patient's capabilities. Possible nursing diagnoses include the following:

■ Risk for injury related to altered physical mobility or aggressive behavior
■ Self-care deficit related to altered physical mobility or lack of maturity

TABLE 23–1	**Developmental Characteristics of Intellectual Developmental Disorder by Degree of Severity**			
LEVEL (IQ)	**ABILITY TO PERFORM SELF-CARE ACTIVITIES**	**COGNITIVE/EDUCATIONAL CAPABILITIES**	**SOCIAL/COMMUNICATION CAPABILITIES**	**PSYCHOMOTOR CAPABILITIES**
Mild (50–70)	Capable of independent living, with assistance during times of stress.	Capable of academic skills to sixth-grade level. As adult can achieve vocational skills for minimum self-support.	Capable of developing social skills. Functions well in a structured, sheltered setting.	Psychomotor skills usually not affected, although may have some slight problems with coordination.
Moderate (35–49)	Can perform some activities independently. Requires supervision.	Capable of academic skill to second-grade level. As adult may be able to contribute to own support in sheltered workshop.	May experience some limitation in speech communication. Difficulty adhering to social convention may interfere with peer relationships.	Motor development is fair. Vocational capabilities may be limited to unskilled gross motor activities.
Severe (20–34)	May be trained in elementary hygiene skills. Requires complete supervision.	Unable to benefit from academic or vocational training. Benefits from systematic habit training.	Minimal verbal skills. Wants and needs often communicated by acting-out behaviors.	Poor psychomotor development. Able to perform only simple tasks under close supervision.
Profound (below 20)	No capacity for independent functioning. Requires constant aid and supervision.	Unable to benefit from academic or vocational training. May respond to minimal training in self-help if presented in the close context of a one-to-one relationship.	Little, if any, speech development. No capacity for socialization skills.	Lack of ability for both fine and gross motor movements. Requires constant supervision and care. May be associated with other physical disorders.

Sources: Boat, T. F., & Wu, J. T. (2015). *Mental disorders and disabilities among low-income children.* Washington, DC: National Academies Press.; Sadock, B. J., Sadock, V. A., & Ruiz, P. (2015). *Synopsis of psychiatry: Behavioral sciences/clinical psychiatry* (11th ed.). Philadelphia, PA: Wolters Kluwer.

- Impaired verbal communication related to developmental alteration
- Impaired social interaction related to speech deficiencies or difficulty adhering to conventional social behavior
- Delayed growth and development related to isolation from significant others, inadequate environmental stimulation, genetic factors
- Anxiety (moderate to severe) related to hospitalization and absence of familiar surroundings
- Defensive coping related to feelings of powerlessness and threat to self-esteem
- Ineffective coping related to inadequate coping skills secondary to developmental delay

Outcome Identification

Outcome criteria include short- and long-term goals. Timelines are individually determined. The following criteria may be used for measurement of outcomes in the care of the patient with intellectual disability.

The patient:

- Has experienced no physical harm.
- Has self-care needs fulfilled.
- Interacts with others in a socially appropriate manner.
- Maintains anxiety at a manageable level.
- Is able to accept direction without becoming defensive.
- Demonstrates adaptive coping skills in response to stressful situations.

Planning and Implementation

Table 23–2 provides a plan of care for the child with intellectual disability using selected nursing diagnoses, outcome criteria, and appropriate nursing interventions and rationales.

Although this plan of care is directed toward the individual patient, it is essential that family members or primary caregivers participate in the ongoing care of the patient with intellectual disability. They need to receive information regarding the scope of the condition, realistic expectations and patient potentials, methods for modifying behavior as required, and community resources from which they may seek assistance and support.

Evaluation

Evaluation of care given to the patient with intellectual disability should reflect positive behavioral changes. Evaluation is accomplished by determining if the goals of care (previously identified) have been met through implementation of the nursing actions selected. The nurse reassesses the plan and makes changes as required. Reassessment data may include information gathered by asking the following questions:

Has the patient:

- Remained free from injury?
- Had self-care needs fulfilled? Been able to fulfill some of these needs independently?
- Been able to communicate needs and desires so that he or she can be understood?
- Learned to interact appropriately with others?
- Accepted constructive feedback and discontinued inappropriate behavior when regressive behavior surfaces?
- Maintained anxiety at a manageable level?
- Learned new coping skills through behavior modification?
- Demonstrated evidence of increased self-esteem because of the accomplishment of these new skills and adaptive behaviors?

Have primary caregivers:

- Demonstrated understanding of realistic expectations for patient's behavior and methods for attempting to modify unacceptable behaviors?
- Demonstrated awareness of various resources from which they can seek assistance and support within the community?

CORE CONCEPT

Autism spectrum disorder

A heterogenous group of neurodevelopmental syndromes characterized by a wide range of communication impairments and restricted, repetitive behaviors (Sadock et al., 2015).

Autism Spectrum Disorder

Clinical Findings

In the *Diagnostic and Statistical Manual of Mental Disorders, Fourth Edition, Text Revision (DSM-IV-TR)* (APA, 2000), the category of autism spectrum disorders encompassed a broad spectrum of diagnoses that included autistic disorder, Rett's disorder, childhood disintegrative disorder, pervasive developmental disorder not otherwise specified, and Asperger's disorder. The *DSM-5* groups these disorders into a single diagnostic category—**autism spectrum disorder** (ASD). The diagnosis is adapted to each individual by clinical specifiers (e.g., level of severity, verbal abilities) and associated features (e.g., known

Table 23–2 | CARE PLAN FOR THE CHILD WITH INTELLECTUAL DISABILITY

NURSING DIAGNOSIS: RISK FOR INJURY

RELATED TO: Altered physical mobility or aggressive behavior

OUTCOME CRITERIA	NURSING INTERVENTIONS	RATIONALE
Short- and Long-Term Goal ■ Patient will not experience injury.	1. Create a safe environment for the patient. 2. Ensure that small items are removed from area where patient will be ambulating and that sharp items are out of reach. 3. Store items that patient uses frequently within easy reach. 4. Pad side rails and headboard of patient with history of seizures. 5. Prevent physical aggression and acting-out behaviors by learning to recognize signs that patient is becoming agitated.	1–5. Patient safety is a nursing priority.

NURSING DIAGNOSIS: SELF-CARE DEFICIT

RELATED TO: Altered physical mobility or lack of maturity

OUTCOME CRITERIA	NURSING INTERVENTIONS	RATIONALE
Short-Term Goal ■ Patient will be able to participate in aspects of self-care. **Long-Term Goal** ■ Patient will have all self-care needs met.	1. Identify aspects of self-care that may be within patient's capabilities. Work on one aspect of self-care at a time. Provide simple, concrete explanations. Offer positive feedback for efforts. 2. When one aspect of self-care has been mastered to the best of patient's ability, move on to another. Encourage independence but intervene when patient is unable to perform.	1. Positive reinforcement enhances self-esteem and encourages repetition of desirable behaviors. 2. Patient comfort and safety are nursing priorities.

NURSING DIAGNOSIS: IMPAIRED VERBAL COMMUNICATION

RELATED TO: Developmental alteration

OUTCOME CRITERIA	NURSING INTERVENTIONS	RATIONALE
Short-Term Goal ■ Patient will establish trust with caregiver and a means of communication of needs. **Long-Term Goals** ■ Patient's needs are being met through established means of communication. ■ If patient cannot speak or communicate by other means, needs are met by caregiver's anticipation of patient's needs.	1. Maintain consistency of staff assignment over time. 2. Anticipate and fulfill patient's needs until satisfactory communication patterns are established. Learn (from family, if possible) special words client uses that are different from the norm. Identify nonverbal gestures or signals that patient may use to convey needs if verbal communication is absent. Practice these communications skills repeatedly.	1. Consistency of staff assignments facilitates trust and the ability to understand patient's actions and communications. 2. Some children with intellectual disability, particularly at the severe level, can learn only by systematic habit training.

Table 23–2 | CARE PLAN FOR THE CHILD WITH INTELLECTUAL DISABILITY—cont'd		
NURSING DIAGNOSIS: IMPAIRED SOCIAL INTERACTION		
RELATED TO: Speech deficiencies or difficulty adhering to conventional social behavior		
OUTCOME CRITERIA	**NURSING INTERVENTIONS**	**RATIONALE**
Short-Term Goal ■ Patient will attempt to interact with others in the presence of trusted caregiver. **Long-Term Goal** ■ Patient will be able to interact with others using behaviors that are socially acceptable and appropriate to developmental level.	1. Remain with patient during initial interactions with others on the unit. 2. Explain to other patients the meaning behind some of client's nonverbal gestures and signals. Use simple language to explain to patient which behaviors are acceptable and which are not. Establish a procedure for behavior modification with rewards for appropriate behaviors and aversive reinforcement for inappropriate behaviors.	1. Presence of a trusted individual provides a feeling of security. 2. Positive, negative, and aversive reinforcements can contribute to desired changes in behavior. These privileges and penalties are individually determined as staff learns the likes and dislikes of the patient.

genetic disorders, epilepsy, intellectual disability) (APA, 2013). ASD is characterized by a withdrawal of the child into the self and into a fantasy world of his or her own creation. The child has abnormal or impaired development in social interaction and communication and a restricted repertoire of activity and interests, some of which may be considered somewhat bizarre.

Epidemiology and Course

The Centers for Disease Control and Prevention (CDC) Autism and Developmental Disabilities Monitoring (ADDM) Network estimates that 1 in 59 children in the United States is identified with ASD and more than doubling since 2000 (CDC, 2018a). It occurs about four times more often in boys than in girls. Almost half (44 percent) of individuals with ASD have an average or above average IQ. Onset of the disorder occurs in early childhood, and in most cases it runs a chronic course with symptoms persisting into adulthood.

Predisposing Factors

Neurological Implications

Imaging studies have revealed a number of alterations in major brain structures of individuals with ASD. Total brain volume, the size of the amygdala, and the size of the striatum have all been identified as enlarged in very young children (under 4 years of age), and there is evidence of a decrease in size over time (Hazlett et al., 2011; Kranjac, 2016: Sadock et al., 2015). Sadock and associates identify that this dynamic pattern of change in total brain volume over time lends support for the hypothesis that there are critical periods in the brain's plasticity that, when disrupted, may contribute to the development of ASD. These findings related to brain plasticity also support that early recognition and intervention can be meaningful in improving functional abilities over time. Volkmar and associates (2017) report that The Infant Brain Imaging Study, a national study of developmental changes in at-risk infants has repeatedly demonstrated abnormal organizational properties in white matter within the first year of life that accentuate over time. Recent in vitro stem cell reprogramming research is beginning to identify the cellular mechanisms responsible for early brain overgrowth and the subsequent disruptions in neural connectivity that may yield valuable information about causes and treatment options (Marchetto et al., 2016).

Genetics

Research has revealed strong evidence that genetic factors play a significant role in the etiology of ASD. About 15 percent of ASD cases are related to a known genetic mutation; in most cases, its expression is related to multiple genes (Sadock et al., 2015). Genetic studies have identified genes that confer risk for autism and schizophrenia, suggesting that these conditions are related (Gilman et al., 2012), but the same genetic variations also appear to confer risk for some other neurodevelopmental disorders as well (Volkmar et al., 2017). Kranjac (2016) reports that rare genetic variants such as copy number variations increase the risk for autism by 20 to 60 percent. Familial and twin studies have also supported genetic influences. DNA studies have implicated areas on several chromosomes that contain genes that may contribute to the development of ASD. Genetic studies have also identified disruptions in serotonin (5-HT), and because 5-HT is important in brain development, it is postulated that changes in 5-HT may be associated with enlargement in the brain (Sadock et al., 2015).

Prenatal and Perinatal Influences

Some of the prenatal risk factors that have been associated with development of ASD include advanced parental age, fetal exposure to valproate, gestational diabetes, and gestational bleeding (APA, 2013; Sadock et al., 2015). Perinatal influences include low birth weight, obstetrical complications (particularly those associated with neonatal hypoxia), hyperbilirubinemia, congenital malformation, and ABO or Rh factor incompatibilities (Sadock et al., 2015). Exposure to environmental toxins, including air pollution and pesticides, showed the strongest links to ASD when it occurred during preconception, gestational, and early childhood stages (Rossignol & Frye, 2016). Volkmar and associates (2017) note that "despite multiple focused investigations, there is no evidence that vaccinations play a role in the environmental liability for ASD" (p. 3576).

Application of the Nursing Process to Autism Spectrum Disorder

Background Assessment Data (Symptomatology)

The symptomatology presented here is common among children with ASD, but it is important to understand these disorders along a spectrum and with varying levels of functionality. Some individuals who meet criteria for ASD may be highly functional and highly intelligent in spite of communication impairments and repetitive or restrictive behaviors. The dramatic increase in prevalence of ASD has led to research focused on differential and common features along the continuum as well as etiological factors. This information is important in creating an accurate plan of care for the patient. Because ASD is a *spectrum* disorder, the symptomatology described here should be understood on a continuum ranging from milder to more severe.

Impairment in Social Interaction Children with ASD have difficulty forming interpersonal relationships with others. They show little interest in people and often do not respond to others' attempts at interaction. As infants, they may have an aversion to affection and physical contact. As toddlers, the attachment to a significant adult may be either absent or manifested as exaggerated adherence behaviors. In childhood, there is a lack of spontaneity manifested in less cooperative play, less imaginative play, and fewer friendships. Those children with minimal handicaps may progress to the point of recognizing other children

as part of their environment but struggle nonetheless in interpersonal relationships. Social interaction is further impaired by deficits in ability to accurately process others' feelings or affect. Higher functioning children may recognize their difficulty with social skills even though they may desire friendship. In one study (Strunz et al., 2015), the researchers noted that as these relational struggles unfold into adulthood, it is difficult at times to distinguish ASD from personality disorders because there are disruptions in interpersonal relationships within both groups. They found that the differential features in ASD were less extroversion, less openness to experience, increased inhibition, and increased compulsivity than among those with personality disorders.

Impairment in Communication and Imaginative Activity Both verbal and nonverbal skills are affected. In more severe levels of ASD, language may be totally absent or characterized by immature structure or idiosyncratic utterances whose meaning is clear only to those who are familiar with the child's past experiences. Nonverbal communication, such as facial expression or gestures, may be absent or socially inappropriate. Some children with autism spectrum disorder are misinterpreted as being deaf as a result of their lack of response to sounds, whereas other children may overreact to sound or other stimuli. In some cases, children with ASD demonstrate special abilities, such as fluent reading skills while still in preschool (Sadock et al., 2015). The pattern of play is often restricted and repetitive.

Restricted Activities and Interests Even minor changes in the environment are often met with resistance or sometimes with agitated irritability. Attachment to, or extreme fascination with, objects that move or spin (e.g., fans) is common. Stereotyped body movements (hand-clapping, rocking, whole-body swaying) and verbalizations (repetition of words or phrases) are typical. Diet abnormalities may include eating only a few specific foods or consuming an excessive amount of fluids. Behaviors that are self-injurious, such as head banging or biting the hands or arms, may be evident. Harrop and associates (2014) studied children with ASD compared to children without this disorder and found that all children demonstrated some repetitive behaviors as part of their development of skill mastery, but children with ASD displayed a wider range of repetitive behaviors in many different circumstances.

The *DSM-5* (APA, 2013) diagnostic criteria for ASD are presented in Box 23–1. The criteria specify a range of behaviors, thus addressing the spectrum of symptomatology associated with this diagnosis.

BOX 23–1 Diagnostic Criteria for Autism Spectrum Disorder

A. Persistent deficits in social communication and social interaction across multiple contexts, as manifested by the following, currently or by history (examples are illustrative, not exhaustive):

1. Deficits in social-emotional reciprocity, ranging, for example, from abnormal social approach and failure of normal back-and-forth conversation; to reduced sharing of interests, emotions, or affect; to failure to initiate or respond to social interactions.
2. Deficits in nonverbal communicative behaviors used for social interaction, ranging, for example, from poorly integrated verbal and nonverbal communication; to abnormalities in eye contact and body language or deficits in understanding and use of gestures; to a total lack of facial expressions and nonverbal communication.
3. Deficits in developing, maintaining, and understanding relationships, ranging, for example, from difficulties adjusting behavior to suit various social contexts; to difficulties in sharing imaginative play or in making friends; to absence of interest in peers.

Specify current severity:

Severity is based on social communication impairments and restricted, repetitive patterns of behavior.

A. Restricted, repetitive patterns of behavior, interests, or activities, as manifested by at least two of the following, currently or by history (examples are illustrative, not exhaustive):

1. Stereotyped or repetitive motor movements, use of objects, or speech (e.g., simple motor stereotypes lining up toys or flipping objects, echolalia, idiosyncratic phrases).
2. Insistence on sameness, inflexible adherence to routines, or ritualized patterns of verbal or nonverbal behavior (e.g., extreme distress at small changes, difficulties with transitions, rigid thinking patterns, greeting rituals, need to take same route or eat same food every day).
3. Highly restricted, fixated interests that are abnormal in intensity or focus (e.g., strong attachment to or preoccupation with unusual objects, excessively circumscribed or perseverative interests).
4. Hyper- or hypo-reactivity to sensory input or unusual interest in sensory aspects of environment (e.g., apparent indifference to pain/temperature, adverse response to specific sounds or textures, excessive smelling or touching of objects, visual fascination with lights or movement).

Specify current severity:

Severity is based on social communication impairments and restricted, repetitive patterns of behavior.

A. Symptoms must be present in the early developmental period (but may not become fully manifest until social demands exceed limited capacities, or may be masked by learned strategies in later life).
B. Symptoms cause clinically significant impairment in social, occupational, or other important areas of current functioning.
C. These disturbances are not better explained by intellectual disability (intellectual developmental disorder) or global developmental delay. Intellectual disability and autism spectrum disorder frequently co-occur; to make comorbid diagnoses of autism spectrum disorder and intellectual disability, social communication should be below that expected for general developmental level.

Specify if:

With or without accompanying intellectual impairment

With or without accompanying language impairment

Associated with a known medical or genetic condition or environmental factor

Associated with another neurodevelopmental, mental, or behavioral disorder

With catatonia

Reprinted with permission from American Psychiatric Association. (2013). Diagnostic and statistical manual of mental disorders (5th ed.). Washington, DC: American Psychiatric Publishing.

Nursing Diagnosis

Based on data collected during the nursing assessment, possible nursing diagnoses for the patient with ASD include the following:

■ Risk for self-mutilation or self-injury related to neurological, cognitive, or social deficits.

■ Impaired social interaction related to inability to trust; neurological alterations, evidenced by lack of responsiveness to or interest in people

■ Impaired verbal communication related to withdrawal into the self; neurological alterations, evidenced by inability or unwillingness to speak; lack of nonverbal expression

■ Disturbed personal identity related to neurological alterations; delayed developmental stage, evidenced by difficulty separating own physiological and emotional needs and personal boundaries from those of others

Outcome Identification

Outcome criteria include short- and long-term goals. Timelines are individually determined. The following criteria may be used for measurement of outcomes in the care of the patient with ASD.

The patient:

■ Exhibits no evidence of self-harm.
■ Interacts appropriately with at least one staff member.
■ Demonstrates trust in at least one staff member.
■ Is able to communicate so that he or she can be understood by at least one staff member.
■ Demonstrates behaviors that indicate he or she has begun the separation/individuation process.

Planning and Implementation

Table 23–3 provides a plan of care for the child with ASD, including selected nursing diagnoses, outcome criteria, and appropriate nursing interventions and rationales.

Table 23–3 | CARE PLAN FOR THE CHILD WITH AUTISM SPECTRUM DISORDER

NURSING DIAGNOSIS: RISK FOR SELF-MUTILATION

RELATED TO: Neurological alterations; history of self-mutilative behaviors; hysterical reactions to changes in the environment

OUTCOME CRITERIA	NURSING INTERVENTIONS	RATIONALE
Short-Term Goal ■ Patient will demonstrate alternative behavior (e.g., initiating interaction between self and nurse) in response to anxiety within specified time. (Length of time required for this objective will depend on severity and chronicity of the disorder.) **Long-Term Goal** ■ Patient will not harm self.	1. Work with the child on a one-to-one basis. 2. Try to determine if the self-mutilative behavior occurs in response to increasing anxiety, and if so, to what the anxiety may be attributed. 3. Try to intervene with diversion or replacement activities and offer self to the child as anxiety level starts to rise. 4. Protect the child when self-mutilative behaviors occur. Devices such as a helmet, padded hand mitts, or arm covers may provide protection when the risk for self-harm exists.	1. One-to-one interaction facilitates trust. 2. Self-mutilation behaviors may be averted if the cause can be determined and alleviated. 3. Diversion and replacement activities may provide needed feelings of security and substitute for self-mutilative behaviors. 4. Patient safety is a priority nursing intervention.

NURSING DIAGNOSIS: IMPAIRED SOCIAL INTERACTION

RELATED TO: Inability to trust; neurological alterations

EVIDENCED BY: Lack of responsiveness to, or interest in, people

OUTCOME CRITERIA	NURSING INTERVENTIONS	RATIONALE
Short-Term Goal ■ Patient will demonstrate trust in one caregiver (as evidenced by facial responsiveness and eye contact) within specified time (depending on severity and chronicity of disorder). **Long-Term Goal** ■ Patient will initiate social interactions (physical, verbal, nonverbal) with caregiver by time of discharge from treatment.	1. Assign a limited number of caregivers to the child. Ensure that warmth, acceptance, and availability are conveyed. 2. Provide child with familiar objects, such as familiar toys or a blanket. Support child's attempts to interact with others. 3. Give positive reinforcement for eye contact with something acceptable to the child (e.g., food, familiar object). Gradually replace with social reinforcement (e.g., touch, smiling, hugging).	1. Warmth, acceptance, and availability, along with consistency of assignment, enhance the establishment and maintenance of a trusting relationship. 2. Familiar objects and presence of a trusted individual provide security during times of distress. 3. Being able to establish eye contact is essential to the child's ability to form satisfactory interpersonal relationships.

Table 23–3 | CARE PLAN FOR THE CHILD WITH AUTISM SPECTRUM DISORDER–cont'd

NURSING DIAGNOSIS: IMPAIRED VERBAL COMMUNICATION

RELATED TO: Withdrawal into the self; neurological alterations

EVIDENCED BY: Inability or unwillingness to speak; lack of nonverbal expression

OUTCOME CRITERIA	NURSING INTERVENTIONS	RATIONALE
Short-Term Goal ■ Patient will establish trust with one caregiver (as evidenced by facial responsiveness and eye contact) by specified time (depending on severity and chronicity of disorder). **Long-Term Goal** ■ Patient will establish a means of communicating needs and desires to others.	1. Maintain consistency in assignment of caregivers. 2. Anticipate and fulfill the child's needs until communication can be established. 3. Seek clarification and validation. 4. Give positive reinforcement when eye contact is used to convey nonverbal expressions.	1. Consistency facilitates trust and enhances the caregiver's ability to understand the child's attempts to communicate. 2. Anticipating needs helps to minimize frustration while the child is learning communication skills. 3. Validation ensures that the intended message has been conveyed. 4. Positive reinforcement increases self-esteem and encourages repetition.

NURSING DIAGNOSIS: DISTURBED PERSONAL IDENTITY

RELATED TO: Neurological alterations; delayed developmental stage

EVIDENCED BY: Difficulty separating own physiological and emotional needs and personal boundaries from those of others

OUTCOME CRITERIA	NURSING INTERVENTIONS	RATIONALE
Short-Term Goal ■ Patient will name own body parts as separate and individual from those of others. **Long-Term Goal** ■ Patient will develop ego identity (evidenced by ability to recognize physical and emotional self as separate from others) by time of discharge from treatment.	1. Assist child to recognize separateness during self-care activities, such as dressing and feeding. 2. Assist the child in learning to name own body parts. This can be facilitated by the use of mirrors, drawings, and pictures of the child. Encourage appropriate touching of, and being touched by, others.	1. Recognition of body parts during dressing and feeding increases the child's awareness of self as separate from others. 2. All of these activities may help increase the child's awareness of self as separate from others.

Evaluation

Evaluation of care for the child with ASD reflects whether the nursing actions have been effective in achieving the established goals. The nursing process calls for reassessment of the plan. Questions for gathering reassessment data may include the following:

Has the child:

■ Been able to establish trust with at least *one* caregiver?
■ Remained free from mutilative behaviors or other self-harm?
■ Attempted to interact with others?

■ Improved in his or her ability to maintain eye contact?
■ Established a means of communicating his or her needs and desires to others? Have all self-care needs been met?
■ Demonstrated an awareness of self as separate from others?
■ Accepted touch from others and been appropriate in touching others?

Psychopharmacological Intervention for ASD

Pharmacological interventions are directed toward relief of targeted irritability symptoms, such as

aggression, hyperactivity, self-harm, impulsivity, and temper tantrums. There are no medications that treat the core symptoms of ASD. The U.S. Food and Drug Administration (FDA) has approved two medications for the treatment of irritability associated with ASD: risperidone (Risperdal; in children and adolescents 5 to 16 years) and aripiprazole (Abilify; in children and adolescents 6 to 17 years). When administering risperidone, caution must be maintained concerning less common but more serious side effects, including neuroleptic malignant syndrome, tardive dyskinesia, hyperglycemia, and diabetes.

In clinical studies with aripiprazole, the most frequently reported adverse events included sedation, fatigue, weight gain, vomiting, somnolence, and tremor. The most common reasons for discontinuation of aripiprazole were sedation, drooling, tremor, vomiting, and extrapyramidal disorder.

CORE CONCEPT

Hyperactivity

Excessive psychomotor activity that may be purposeful or aimless, accompanied by physical movements and verbal utterances that are usually more rapid than normal. Inattention and distractibility are common with hyperactive behavior.

Attention-Deficit/Hyperactivity Disorder

Clinical Findings, Epidemiology, and Course

The essential behavior pattern of a child with attention-deficit/hyperactivity disorder (ADHD) is one of inattention and/or hyperactivity and **impulsivity.** These children are highly distractible and unable to contain stimuli. Motor activity is excessive, and movements are random and impulsive. Onset of the disorder is difficult to diagnose in children younger than age 4 years because their characteristic behavior is much more variable than that of older children. Frequently, the disorder is not recognized until the child enters school. It is more common in boys (14.2 percent) than girls (6.4 percent), and the overall prevalence among school-age children is 10.4 percent (CDC, 2017). It is estimated that in 50 to 70 percent of the cases, ADHD persists into young adulthood and beyond, and unlike other psychiatric disorders that are typically episodic, the adult with

ADHD has symptoms that are chronic and unrelenting (McGough, 2017). Without prompt diagnosis and treatment the child with ADHD is at higher risk for substance abuse and negative consequences associated with risky behavior; the adult, with restlessness and functional impairment, occupation difficulties, and disorganization (Mathews-Wilson & Daitch, 2016). See "Real People, Real Stories" to learn more about Myrle's experience as an adult living with ADHD.

In making the diagnosis of ADHD, the *DSM-5* criteria are further specified according to current clinical presentation. These subtypes include a combined presentation (meeting the criteria for both inattention and hyperactivity/impulsivity), a predominantly inattentive presentation, and a predominantly hyperactive/impulsive presentation.

CORE CONCEPT

Impulsiveness

The trait of acting without reflection and without thought to the consequences of the behavior. An abrupt inclination to act (and the inability to resist acting) on certain behavioral urges.

Predisposing Factors

Biological Influences

Genetics A number of studies have revealed supportive evidence of genetic influences in the etiology of ADHD. Twin and family studies showed that the heritability for ADHD exceeds 75 percent (McGough, 2017). Adoption studies reveal that biological parents of children with ADHD have more psychopathology than the adoptive parents.

Studies of genetic evidence for ADHD found copy number variants on a specific region of chromosome 16 (Acosta et al., 2016; Williams et al., 2010). Researchers have also found that these copy number variants overlap with chromosomal regions previously linked to ASD and schizophrenia.

Biochemical Theory Hypotheses about the impact of neurotransmitters have been based on benefits associated with taking stimulant medications, which are known to affect dopamine and norepinephrine levels. But several studies, using single photon emission computed tomography (SPECT), have now demonstrated

Real People, Real Stories: Attention-Deficit/Hyperactivity Disorder

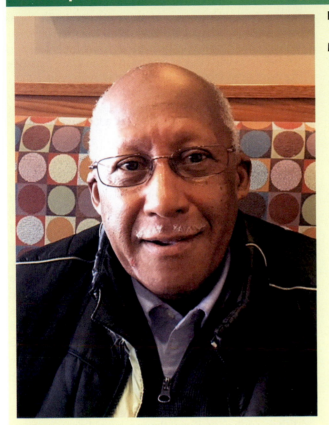

Karyn: When did you first become aware that you had ADHD?

Myrle: I had symptoms as a child but I didn't get diagnosed or treated until I was 50 years old. They put me on Ritalin first and then on Ritalin-XR. When I first started to take it I got very high and very talkative, then after a little while I could focus better and then it wears off.

Karyn: What symptoms do you remember having as a child?

Myrle: I guess I thought of myself as selfish; I was easily distracted, I couldn't handle noise; like the noise at a basketball game was unmanageable and agitating. I was the youngest child but even so, I wanted my way right now. No one else had anything important to say. Later I realized it wasn't that I was so smart but that everyone else seemed to go too slow.

Karyn: How did you get along in school?

Myrle: I didn't have any trouble. I went to school in the country and the classrooms were very small and very quiet so that helped me. When I graduated from high school I went into the military and that was when I really realized I had a problem. I got into fights a lot because the noise and the talking and all the activity really agitated me.

Karyn: Impulsivity is a common symptom in ADHD. Did you experience that?

Myrle: I don't think so. I was pretty forward, outgoing, and I liked to take the lead but I had trouble paying attention. I did become hypersexual as I got older and as an adult, I started smoking pot because it improved my sexual performance and I started drinking alcohol because it helped me sleep. Then those became problems, too. I always wanted to be a lawyer so I went to law school after I got out of the military but I was on probation because I got involved in too many things and couldn't focus on my studies. I eventually did graduate with a PhD but then I took the bar exam four times and couldn't pass it; sometimes I would get sick and couldn't study; even after I got accommodations when I had less noise and twice the time, I would second guess myself and change my answers. I had a lot of anxiety. Then I got fired from a job I had at the sewer department and since I had admitted to lying, I was unable to take the bar exam for another five years. I never was able to pass.

I got a job at the Department of Education as a disabilities investigator and I was good at handling these cases. I had cases of people with attention-deficit disorders that were being discriminated against. I was very detailed but it took me a lot longer to get things done. I collected a lot of information but I was unable to shorten the process compared to my coworkers. It was there that I had the epiphany that I had a lot of the same symptoms that my clients were describing. In general, I've always had a lot of trouble separating myself from the noise and other distractions.

Karyn: How would you describe your ability to function now that you are being treated with medication?

Myrle: Well, just like I'm doing now, I can go on and on talking about nothing.

(There were several subject changes and refocusings; at times Myrle had difficulty refocusing, stating that he just had to finish one more point.)

Myrle: I'm still very disorganized and sometimes have trouble with attention. The meds help somewhat but I still can't stop talking. My current medical record says I also have OCD, hoarding disorder, and depression. I see a psychiatrist for medications but I still have symptoms. I never feel very confident and I can't seem to get all my ducks in a row. The medication helps me not get quite so agitated as I used to. So I am able to conduct my current role as a minister and I am better able to listen.

Karyn: Yes, I heard you preach a sermon and it sounded like a very focused message.

Myrle: Well, I do better with structured time limits and I let the Spirit take over when I preach. I know this is what I was called to do and I serve a congregation that has a lot of disabilities so I understand their needs because of my own experiences.

Continued

increased dopamine transporter-binding densities in the striatal regions (McGough, 2017) (Fig. 23–1).

Anatomical Changes Brain imaging studies show decreased volume and activity in the prefrontal cortex, anterior cingulated, globus pallidus, caudate, thalamus, and cerebellum (Sadock et al., 2015). Several alterations occur in neural connectivity with evidence of decreased activation in frontoparietal areas and overactivation in visual, dorsal attention, and default networks (McGough, 2017). A recent study by Humphreys and associates (2018) found a correlation between brain volume changes, elevated ADHD symptoms, and the number of childhood stressors. This finding underscores the interaction between genetics and environmental influences and reinforces the need for trauma-informed care.

Prenatal, Perinatal, and Postnatal Factors Maternal smoking during pregnancy has been linked to hyperkinetic-impulsive behavior in offspring (ADHD Institute, 2016; Froehlich et al., 2009). Intrauterine exposure to toxic substances, including alcohol, can produce effects on behavior. Fetal alcohol syndrome includes hyperactivity, impulsivity, and inattention as well as physical anomalies. Maternal infections during pregnancy have also been associated with higher risks for ADHD.

Perinatal and postnatal influences that may contribute to ADHD are low birth weight, trauma, early infancy infections, or other insults to the brain during this period (Sadock et al., 2015). Maternal hypertension has also been implicated as a risk factor for both ADHD and ASD (Maher et al., 2018). Prematurity has, in the past, been identified as posing an increased risk for ADHD, but in a large research study (Heinonen et al., 2010) cited by the ADHD Institute (2016), this was not found to be the case.

Environmental Influences

Environmental Lead Studies continue to provide evidence of the adverse effects of elevated serum levels of lead on cognitive and behavioral development in children (Froehlich et al., 2009; Nigg et al., 2010; Rossignol & Frye, 2016). Research by Froehlich and associates showed a direct link to ADHD. The government has placed tighter restrictions on the substance in recent years, making exposure to toxic levels less prevalent than it once was. However, reports indicate that at least 4 million households in the United States include children who are being exposed to lead and that approximately 500,000 U.S. children ages 1 to 5 have blood lead levels above 5 micrograms per deciliter, the reference level at which the initiation of public health actions are recommended (CDC, 2018b).

Diet Factors The possible link between food dyes and additives, such as artificial flavorings and preservatives, and sugar was introduced in the mid-1970s. Studies on these possibilities have failed to confirm a clear link.

Psychosocial Influences

Disorganized or chaotic environments or a disruption in family equilibrium may contribute to ADHD in some individuals. Galéra and colleagues (2011) identified several psychosocial influences associated with the development of ADHD, including nonintact family, young maternal age at birth of the target child, paternal history of antisocial behavior, and maternal depression.

Application of the Nursing Process to ADHD

Background Assessment Data (Symptomatology)

A major portion of the hyperactive child's problems relate to difficulties in performing age-appropriate tasks. Hyperactive children are highly distractible and have extremely limited attention spans. They often shift from one uncompleted activity to another. Impulsivity, or deficit in inhibitory control, is also common.

Hyperactive children have difficulty forming satisfactory interpersonal relationships. They demonstrate behaviors that inhibit acceptable social

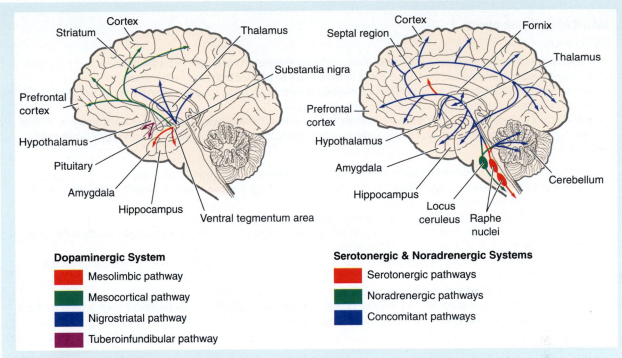

Dopaminergic System
- Mesolimbic pathway
- Mesocortical pathway
- Nigrostriatal pathway
- Tuberoinfundibular pathway

Serotonergic & Noradrenergic Systems
- Serotonergic pathways
- Noradrenergic pathways
- Concomitant pathways

FIGURE 23–1   Neurobiology of attention-deficit/hyperactivity disorder.

NEUROTRANSMITTERS

The major neurotransmitters implicated in the pathophysiology of ADHD are dopamine, norepinephrine, and possibly serotonin. Dopamine and norepinephrine appear to be depleted in ADHD. Serotonin in ADHD has been studied less extensively, but recent evidence suggests that it also is reduced in children with ADHD.

NEUROTRANSMITTER FUNCTIONS

- Norepinephrine is thought to play a role in the ability to perform executive functions, such as analysis and reasoning, and in the cognitive alertness essential for processing stimuli and sustaining attention and thought.
- Dopamine is thought to play a role in sensory filtering, memory, concentration, controlling emotions, locomotor activity, and reasoning.
- Deficits in norepinephrine and dopamine have both been implicated in the inattention, impulsiveness, and hyperactivity associated with ADHD.
- Serotonin appears to play a role in ADHD, although possibly less significant than norepinephrine and dopamine. It has been suggested that alterations in serotonin may be related to the disinhibition and impulsivity observed in children with ADHD. It may play a role in mood disorders, particularly depression, which is a common comorbid disorder associated with ADHD.

FUNCTIONAL AREAS OF THE BRAIN AFFECTED

- **Prefrontal cortex:** Associated with maintaining attention, organization, and executive function. Also serves to modulate behavior inhibition with serotonin as the predominant central inhibiting neurotransmitter for this function.
- **Basal ganglia** (particularly the caudate nucleus and globus pallidus): Involved in the regulation of high-level movements. In association with its connecting circuits to the prefrontal cortex, may also be important in cognition. Interruptions in these circuits may result in inattention or impulsivity.
- **Hippocampus:** Plays an important role in learning and memory.
- **Limbic System** (composed of the amygdala, hippocampus, mammillary body, hypothalamus, thalamus, fornix, cingulate gyrus, and septum pellucidum): Regulation of emotions. A neurotransmitter deficiency in this area may result in restlessness, inattention, or emotional volatility.
- **Reticular activating system** (composed of the reticular formation [located in the brain stem] and its connections): It is the major relay system among the many pathways that enter and leave the brain. It is thought to be the center of arousal and motivation and is crucial for maintaining a state of consciousness.

Continued

MEDICATIONS FOR ADHD

CNS Stimulants

- Amphetamines (dextroamphetamine, lisdexamfetamine, methamphetamine, and mixtures): Cause the release of norepinephrine from central noradrenergic neurons. At higher doses, dopamine may be released in the mesolimbic system.
- Methylphenidate and dexmethylphenidate: Block the reuptake of norepinephrine and dopamine into the presynaptic neuron and increase the release of these monoamines into the extraneuronal space.
- Side effects of CNS stimulants include restlessness, insomnia, headache, palpitations, weight loss, suppression of growth in children (with long-term use), increased blood pressure, abdominal pain, anxiety, tolerance, and physical and psychological dependence.

Others

- Atomoxetine: Selectively inhibits the reuptake of norepinephrine by blocking the presynaptic transporter.
  - Side effects include headache, upper abdominal pain, nausea and vomiting, anorexia, cough, dry mouth, constipation, increase in heart rate and blood pressure, and fatigue.
- Bupropion: Inhibits the reuptake of norepinephrine and dopamine into presynaptic neurons.
  - Side effects include headache, dizziness, insomnia or sedation, tachycardia, increased blood pressure, dry mouth, nausea and vomiting, weight gain or loss, seizures (dose dependent).
- Alpha agonists (clonidine, guanfacine): Stimulate central alpha-adrenoreceptors in the brain, resulting in reduced sympathetic outflow from the CNS.
  - Side effects include palpitations, bradycardia, constipation, dry mouth, and sedation.
- Tricyclic antidepressants, escitalopram, and sertraline (SSRIs), and venlafaxine (SSNRI) have demonstrated some benefits for those not responding to stimulants and for those with comorbid depression.

interaction. They are disruptive and intrusive in group endeavors. They have difficulty complying with social norms. Some children with ADHD are very aggressive or oppositional, whereas others exhibit more regressive and immature behaviors. Low frustration tolerance and outbursts of temper are common.

Children with ADHD have boundless energy, exhibiting excessive levels of activity, restlessness, and fidgeting. They have been described as "perpetual motion machines," continuously running, jumping, wiggling, or squirming. They experience a greater than average number of accidents, from minor mishaps to more serious incidents that may lead to physical injury or the destruction of property. The *DSM-5* diagnostic criteria for ADHD are presented in Box 23–2.

Comorbidity The prevalence of comorbid psychiatric disorders with ADHD is common, with up to 30 percent experiencing comorbid depression and 20 percent experiencing a comorbid anxiety disorder (Sherman & Tarnow, 2013). The APA (2013) reports that in children with ADHD who have symptoms of both inattention and hyperactivity/impulsivity, oppositional defiant disorder co-occurs about 50 percent of the time. They further identify that most children and adolescents with disruptive mood dysregulation disorder also meet criteria for ADHD. Other comorbidities include conduct disorder, specific learning disorder, anxiety, depression, and intermittent explosive disorder. Sadock

and associates (2015) identify that although bipolar mania and ADHD share many core features, such as distractibility, excessive talking, and hyperactivity, children with bipolar I disorder exhibit symptoms that wax and wane; children with ADHD have more persistent continuous symptoms. They note that bipolar disorder and ADHD can coexist and that when certain features of ADHD occur, they do appear to predict future mania. Sherman and Tarnow (2013) estimate the prevalence of comorbid bipolar disorder and ADHD at around 20 percent. These authors also note that because ADHD is associated with frontal lobe abnormalities, it is not surprising that 89.4 percent of children with frontal lobe epilepsy also have comorbid ADHD.

Nursing Diagnosis

Based on the data collected during the nursing assessment, possible nursing diagnoses for the child with ADHD include the following:

- Risk for injury related to impulsive and accident-prone behavior and the inability to perceive self-harm
- Impaired social interaction related to intrusive and immature behavior
- Low self-esteem related to dysfunctional family system and negative feedback
- Noncompliance with task expectations related to low frustration tolerance and short attention span

BOX 23–2 Diagnostic Criteria for Attention-Deficit/Hyperactivity Disorder

A. A persistent pattern of inattention and/or hyperactivity-impulsivity that interferes with functioning or development, as characterized by (1) and/or (2):

1. **Inattention:** Six (or more) of the following symptoms have persisted for at least 6 months to a degree that is inconsistent with developmental level and that negatively impacts directly on social and academic/occupational activities. **Note:** The symptoms are not solely a manifestation of oppositional behavior, defiance, hostility, or failure to understand tasks or instructions. For older adolescents and adults (age 17 and older), at least five symptoms are required.

   a. Often fails to give close attention to details or makes careless mistakes in schoolwork, at work, or during other activities (e.g., overlooks or misses details, work is inaccurate).

   b. Often has difficulty sustaining attention in tasks or play activities (e.g., has difficulty remaining focused during lectures, conversations, or lengthy reading).

   c. Often does not seem to listen when spoken to directly (e.g., mind seems elsewhere, even in the absence of any obvious distraction).

   d. Often does not follow through on instructions and fails to finish schoolwork, chores, or duties in the workplace (e.g., starts tasks but quickly loses focus and is easily sidetracked).

   e. Often has difficulty organizing tasks and activities (e.g., difficulty managing sequential tasks; difficulty keeping materials and belongings in order; messy, disorganized, work; has poor time management; fails to meet deadlines).

   f. Often avoids, dislikes, or is reluctant to engage in tasks that require sustained mental effort (e.g., schoolwork or homework; for older adolescents and adults, preparing reports, completing forms, reviewing lengthy papers).

   g. Often loses things necessary for tasks or activities (e.g., school materials, pencils, books, tools, wallets, keys, paperwork, eyeglasses, or mobile telephones).

   h. Is often easily distracted by extraneous stimuli (for older adolescents and adults, may include unrelated thoughts).

   i. Is often forgetful in daily activities (e.g., chores, running errands; for older adolescents and adults, returning calls, paying bills, keeping appointments).

2. *Hyperactivity and Impulsivity:* Six (or more) of the following symptoms have persisted for at least 6 months to a degree that is inconsistent with developmental level and that negatively impacts directly on social and academic/occupational activities.

   NOTE: The symptoms are not solely a manifestation of oppositional behavior, defiance, hostility, or a failure to understand tasks or instructions. For older adolescents and adults (age 17 and older), at least five symptoms are required.

   a. Often fidgets with or taps hands or feet or squirms in seat.

   b. Often leaves seat in situations when remaining seated is expected (e.g., leaves his or her place in the classroom, in the office or other workplace, or in other situations that require remaining in place).

   c. Often runs about or climbs in situations where it is inappropriate. (**Note:** In adolescents or adults, may be limited to feeling restless.)

   d. Often unable to play or engage in leisure activities quietly.

   e. Is often "on the go," acting as if "driven by a motor" (e.g., is unable to be or uncomfortable being still for extended time, as in restaurants, meetings; may be experienced by others as being restless and difficult to keep up with).

   f. Often talks excessively.

   g. Often blurts out an answer before a question has been completed (e.g., completes people's sentences; cannot wait for turn in conversation).

   h. Often has difficulty waiting his or her turn (e.g., while waiting in line).

   i. Often interrupts or intrudes on others (e.g., butts into conversations, games, or activities; may start using other people's things without asking or receiving permission; for adolescents or adults, may intrude into or take over what others are doing).

B. Several inattentive or hyperactive-impulsive symptoms were present prior to age 12 years.

C. Several inattentive or hyperactive-impulsive symptoms are present in two or more settings (e.g., at home, school or work; with friends or relatives; in other activities).

D. There is clear evidence that the symptoms interfere with or reduce the quality of social, academic, or occupational functioning.

E. The symptoms do not occur exclusively during the course of schizophrenia or another psychotic disorder and are not better explained by another mental disorder (e.g., mood disorder, anxiety disorder, dissociative disorder, personality disorder, substance intoxication or withdrawal).

Continued

BOX 23–2 Diagnostic Criteria for Attention-Deficit/Hyperactivity Disorder—cont'd

Specify whether:

Combined presentation: If both Criterion A1 (inattention) and Criterion A2 (hyperactivity-impulsivity) are met for the past 6 months.

Predominantly inattentive presentation: If Criterion A1 (inattention) is met but Criterion A2 (hyperactivity-impulsivity) is not met for the past 6 months.

Predominantly hyperactive/impulsive presentation: If Criterion A2 (hyperactivity-impulsivity) is met and Criterion A1 (inattention) is not met for the past 6 months.

Specify if:

In partial remission

Specify current severity:

Mild

Moderate

Severe

Reprinted with permission from American Psychiatric Association. (2013). Diagnostic and statistical manual of mental disorders (5th ed.). Washington, DC: American Psychiatric Publishing.

Outcome Identification

Outcome criteria include short- and long-term goals. Timelines are individually determined. The following criteria may be used for measurement of outcomes in the care of the child with ADHD.

The patient:

■ Experiences no physical harm.
■ Interacts with others appropriately.
■ Verbalizes positive aspects about self.
■ Demonstrates fewer demanding behaviors.
■ Cooperates with staff in an effort to complete assigned tasks.

Planning and Implementation

Table 23–4 provides a plan of care for the child with ADHD using nursing diagnoses common to the disorder, outcome criteria, and appropriate nursing interventions and rationales.

Concept Care Mapping

The concept map care plan is a diagrammatic teaching and learning strategy that allows visualization of interrelationships between medical diagnoses, nursing diagnoses, assessment data, and treatments. An example of a concept map care plan for a client with ADHD is presented in Figure 23–2.

Evaluation

Evaluation of the care of a patient with ADHD involves examining client behaviors following implementation of the nursing actions to determine if the goals of therapy have been achieved. Collecting data by using the following types of questions may provide appropriate information for evaluation.

Has the child:

■ Remained free from injury?
■ Been able to establish a trusting relationship with the primary caregiver?
■ Responded to limits set on unacceptable behaviors?
■ Been able to interact appropriately with others?
■ Been able to verbalize positive statements about self?
■ Been able to complete tasks independently or with a minimum of assistance? Can he or she follow through after listening to simple instructions?
■ Been able to apply self-control to decrease motor activity?

Psychopharmacological Intervention for ADHD

Indications

Pharmacological intervention, and particularly stimulants, are considered first-line treatment for ADHD (Sadock et al., 2015). For a list of agents to treat ADHD, see Table 23–5. The mechanism of action is unclear, but because these drugs are known to elevate dopamine and norepinephrine levels, it has been hypothesized that their effectiveness is in response to neurotransmitter dysregulation. They have generally mild side effects, but they are contraindicated in anyone with cardiac problems or risks for cardiac problems. There is a high potential for abuse, tolerance, and dependence.

One study (Van den Ban et al., 2014) explored whether use of stimulants had an impact on reducing injuries and hospital admissions for children with ADHD. This study is relevant because these children have a high incidence of injury and hospital admissions related to hyperactivity and

Table 23–4 | CARE PLAN FOR THE CHILD WITH ATTENTION-DEFICIT/HYPERACTIVITY DISORDER

NURSING DIAGNOSIS: RISK FOR INJURY

RELATED TO: Impulsive and accident-prone behavior and the inability to perceive self-harm

OUTCOME CRITERIA	NURSING INTERVENTIONS	RATIONALE
Short- and Long-Term Goal ■ Patient will be free of injury.	1. Ensure that patient has a safe environment. Remove from immediate area objects on which patient could injure self as a result of random, hyperactive movements. 2. Identify deliberate behaviors that put the child at risk for injury. Institute consequences for repetition of this behavior. 3. If there is risk of injury associated with specific therapeutic activities, provide adequate supervision and assistance, or limit patient's participation if adequate supervision is not possible.	1. Objects that are appropriate to the normal living situation can be hazardous to the child whose motor activities are out of control. 2. Behavior can be modified with aversive reinforcement. 3. Patient safety is a nursing priority.

NURSING DIAGNOSIS: IMPAIRED SOCIAL INTERACTION

RELATED TO: Intrusive and immature behavior

OUTCOME CRITERIA	NURSING INTERVENTIONS	RATIONALE
Short-Term Goal ■ Patient will interact in age-appropriate manner with nurse in one-to-one relationship within 1 week. **Long-Term Goal** ■ Patient will observe limits set on intrusive behavior and will demonstrate ability to interact appropriately with others.	1. Develop a trusting relationship with the child. Convey acceptance of the child separate from the unacceptable behavior. 2. Discuss with patient those behaviors that are and are not acceptable. Describe in a matter-of-fact manner the consequences of unacceptable behavior. Follow through. 3. Provide group situations for patient.	1. Unconditional acceptance increases feelings of self-worth. 2. Aversive reinforcement can alter undesirable behaviors. 3. Appropriate social behavior is often learned from the positive and negative feedback of peers.

NURSING DIAGNOSIS: LOW SELF-ESTEEM

RELATED TO: Dysfunctional family system and negative feedback

OUTCOME CRITERIA	NURSING INTERVENTIONS	RATIONALE
Short-Term Goal ■ Patient will independently direct own care and activities of daily living within 1 week.	1. Ensure that goals are realistic. 2. Plan activities that provide opportunities for success. 3. Convey unconditional acceptance and positive regard.	1. Unrealistic goals set patient up for failure, which diminishes self-esteem. 2. Success enhances self-esteem. 3. Affirmation of patient as worthwhile human being may increase self-esteem.

Continued

Table 23–4 | CARE PLAN FOR THE CHILD WITH ATTENTION-DEFICIT/HYPERACTIVITY DISORDER–cont'd

OUTCOME CRITERIA	NURSING INTERVENTIONS	RATIONALE
Long-Term Goal ■ Patient will demonstrate increased feelings of self-worth by verbalizing positive statements about self and exhibiting fewer demanding behaviors.	4. Offer recognition of successful endeavors and positive reinforcement for attempts made. Give immediate positive feedback for acceptable behavior.	4. Positive reinforcement enhances self-esteem and may increase the desired behaviors.

NURSING DIAGNOSIS: NONCOMPLIANCE (WITH TASK EXPECTATIONS)

RELATED TO: Low frustration tolerance and short attention span

OUTCOME CRITERIA	NURSING INTERVENTIONS	RATIONALE
Short-Term Goal ■ Patient will participate in and cooperate during therapeutic activities. **Long-Term Goal** ■ Patient will be able to complete assigned tasks independently or with a minimum of assistance.	1. Provide an environment for task efforts that is as free as possible of distractions. 2. Provide assistance on a one-to-one basis, beginning with simple, concrete instructions. 3. Ask patient to repeat instructions to you. 4. Establish goals that allow patient to complete a part of the task, rewarding completion of each step with a break for physical activity. 5. Gradually decrease the amount of assistance given, while assuring patient that assistance is still available if deemed necessary.	1. Patient is highly distractible and is unable to perform in the presence of even minimal stimulation. 2. Patient lacks the ability to assimilate information that is complicated or has abstract meaning. 3. Repetition of the instructions helps to determine client's level of comprehension. 4. Short-term goals are not so overwhelming to one with such a short attention span. The positive reinforcement (physical activity) increases self-esteem and provides incentive for patient to pursue the task to completion. 5. This intervention encourages patient to perform independently while providing a feeling of security with the presence of a trusted individual.

impulsivity, and about 60 percent show suboptimal motor performance, which may also increase their risks for injury. The researchers found that children treated with ADHD drugs (mostly stimulants) had a twofold higher risk of injury-related hospital admissions than those not treated with ADHD drugs. They also found that children taking ADHD drugs and psychotropic drugs such as antipsychotics and benzodiazepines had five times increased risk for injuries and hospital admissions than those who were on ADHD medication alone. Some of these findings may reflect the severity of ADHD in children on medication, but it is significant that these

medications, while mediating other core symptoms of ADHD, may not reduce risks for injury. Amphetamines are a common substance of abuse and demonstrate high risk for dependence, and similar concerns have been identified for clients with ADHD. The recent FDA approval of Adzenys XR-ODT, a flavored chewable amphetamine mixture tablet, has raised concerns that it may increase use or abuse in children and become a gateway drug (Grohol, 2016). See Chapter 4, Psychopharmacology, for a complete discussion of the medications used in the treatment of ADHD, including safety and education issues.

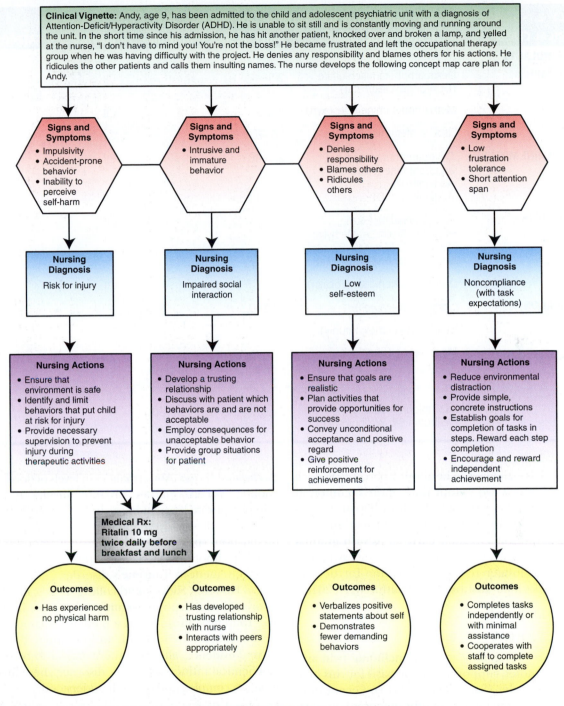

FIGURE 23–2   Concept map care plan for a patient with attention-deficit/hyperactivity disorder.

Tourette's Disorder

Clinical Findings, Epidemiology, and Course

Tourette's disorder is characterized by the presence of multiple motor tics and one or more vocal tics, which may appear simultaneously or at different periods during the illness (APA, 2013). The disturbance may cause distress or interfere with social, occupational, or other important areas of functioning. The age at onset of Tourette's disorder can be as early as 2 years, but the disorder occurs most commonly during childhood (around age 6 to 7 years). Prevalence of the disorder is estimated at 3 to 8 per 1,000 in school-age children (APA, 2013). The lifetime

TABLE 23–5	**Agents for Attention-Deficit/Hyperactivity Disorder**		
CHEMICAL CLASS	**GENERIC (TRADE) NAME**	**DAILY DOSAGE RANGE (MG)**	**CONTROLLED CATEGORIES**
CNS STIMULANTS			
AMPHETAMINES	Dextroamphetamine sulfate (Dexedrine; Dextrostat)	2.5–40	CII
	Methamphetamine (Desoxyn)	5–25	CII
	Lisdexamfetamine (Vyvanse)	20–70	CII
AMPHETAMINE MIXTURES	Dextroamphetamine/ amphetamine (Adderall; Adderall XR)	2.5–40	CII
	Adderall XR-ODT	6.3–18.8	CII
MISCELLANEOUS	Methylphenidate (Ritalin; Ritalin-SR; Ritalin LA; Methylin; Methylin ER; Metadate ER; Metadate CD; Concerta; Daytrana)	10–60	CII
	Dexmethylphenidate (Focalin)	5–20	CII
ALPHA AGONISTS	Clonidine (Catapres)	0.05–0.3	—
	Guanfacine (Tenex; Intuniv)	1–4	—
MISCELLANEOUS	Atomoxetine (Strattera)	>70 kg: 40–100; <70 kg: 0.5–1.4 mg/kg (or 100 mg–whichever is less)	—
	Bupropion (Wellbutrin; Wellbutrin SR; Wellbutrin XL)	3 mg/kg (ADHD); 100–300 (depression)	—

prevalence is estimated to be about 1 percent (Sadock et al., 2015). It is two to four times more common in boys than in girls. Although the disorder can be lifelong, most people with this condition experience the worst tic symptoms in their early teens with gradual improvement thereafter; some may become symptom free and no longer require medication for tic suppression (National Institutes of Health [NIH], 2018).

Predisposing Factors

Biological Factors

Genetics Various genetic studies, including twin and adoption studies, support a genetic basis for this neurological disorder (Sadock et al., 2015). Recent studies suggest that the pattern of inheritance is complex, probably involving several genes influenced by environmental factors (NIH, 2018). In addition, genetic studies suggest that ADHD and obsessive-compulsive disorder are genetically related to Tourette's disorder; as many as 50 percent of patients with Tourette's disorder also have ADHD, and up to 40 percent have obsessive-compulsive disorder (NIH, 2018; Sadock et al., 2015).

Biochemical Factors Abnormalities in levels of dopamine, choline, *N*-acetylaspartate, creatine, myoinositol, and norepinephrine have all been demonstrated in neuroimaging studies, and the effectiveness of antipsychotic medication (particularly haloperidol and fluphenazine) in suppressing tics, also support neurotransmitter involvement in Tourette's disorder (Sadock et al., 2015). However, Sadock and colleagues add that there is variability in response to antipsychotic medications, and Tourette's disorder has sometimes emerged while a client is being treated with antipsychotics. Based on current evidence, although there appear to be several biochemical influences in this disorder, these interactions are complex and not well understood.

Structural Factors Neuroimaging brain studies have been consistent in finding dysfunction in the area of the basal ganglia. Abnormalities in the frontal lobes, cortex, and circuits that connect these regions have also been implicated in the pathology of this disorder (NIH, 2018). Although many influences have been identified, the direct cause is not yet known. It is probably a complex interaction of genetics, biochemistry, and environmental influences.

Environmental Factors

Some studies have shown that environmental influences, such as maternal alcohol use during pregnancy, low birth weight, complications during childbirth, and infection may be associated with the development of Tourette's disorder (CDC, 2018c). Further research is needed to confirm these influences. Sadock and colleagues (2015) report that studies inferring beta-hemolytic streptococcal infections as a mechanism in Tourette's disorder have been "conflicting and controversial, and this mechanism appears to be unlikely as an etiology of Tourette's disorder in most cases" (p. 1198).

Application of the Nursing Process to Tourette's Disorder

Background Assessment Data (Symptomatology)

The motor tics of Tourette's disorder may involve the head, torso, and upper and lower limbs. Initial symptoms may begin with a single motor tic, most commonly eye blinking, or with multiple symptoms. Initially, tics tend to occur in the face and neck and progress downward to the torso and lower limbs over time (Sadock et al., 2015). Simple motor tics include movements such as eye blinking, neck jerking, shoulder shrugging, and facial grimacing. The more complex motor tics include squatting, hopping, skipping, tapping, and retracing steps.

Vocal tics include various words or sounds such as squeaks, grunts, barks, sniffs, snorts, coughs and, in rare instances, a complex vocal tic involving the uttering of obscenities. Vocal tics may include repeating certain words or phrases out of context, repeating one's own sounds or words **(palilalia),** or repeating what others say **(echolalia).**

The movements and vocalizations are experienced as compulsive and irresistible, but they can be suppressed for varying lengths of time. Many report a buildup of tension as they attempt to suppress tics to the point where they feel the tic must be expressed against their will. Tics are often worse during periods of stress or excitement and better during periods of calm, focused activity (NIH, 2018). In most cases, tics are diminished during sleep. Neurobehavioral disorders that are common in conjunction with Tourette's disorder (and may be more troublesome than the tics themselves) are inattention, hyperactivity, and impulsivity as are seen in ADHD; and obsessive-compulsive disorder, depression, and anxiety. Many children with Tourette's disorder also manifest difficulty with reading, writing, and arithmetic (NIH, 2018). The *DSM-5* diagnostic criteria for Tourette's disorder require that both motor and vocal tics have been present at some time during the illness and are persistent for more than one year.

Nursing Diagnosis

Based on data collected during the nursing assessment, possible nursing diagnoses for the patient with Tourette's disorder include the following:

■ Risk for self-directed or other-directed violence related to low tolerance for frustration
■ Impaired social interaction related to impulsiveness, oppositional and aggressive behavior
■ Low self-esteem related to embarrassment associated with tic behaviors

Outcome Identification

Outcome criteria include short- and long-term goals. Timelines are individually determined. The following criteria may be used for measurement of outcomes in the care of the patient with Tourette's disorder.

The patient:

■ Has not harmed self or others.
■ Interacts with staff and peers in an appropriate manner.
■ Demonstrates self-control by managing tic behavior.
■ Follows rules without becoming defensive.
■ Verbalizes positive aspects about self.

Planning and Implementation

Table 23–6 provides a plan of care for the child or adolescent with Tourette's disorder using selected nursing diagnoses, outcome criteria, and appropriate nursing interventions and rationales.

Evaluation

Evaluation of care for the child with Tourette's disorder reflects whether or not the nursing actions have been effective in achieving the established goals. The nursing process calls for reassessment of the plan. Questions for gathering reassessment data may include the following:

Has the patient:

■ Refrained from causing harm to self or others during times of increased tension?
■ Developed adaptive coping strategies for dealing with frustration to prevent resorting to self-destruction or aggression to others?
■ Been able to interact appropriately with staff and peers?
■ Been able to suppress tic behaviors when he or she chooses to do so?

Table 23–6 | CARE PLAN FOR THE CHILD OR ADOLESCENT WITH TOURETTE'S DISORDER

NURSING DIAGNOSIS: RISK FOR SELF-DIRECTED OR OTHER-DIRECTED VIOLENCE

RELATED TO: Low tolerance for frustration

OUTCOME CRITERIA	NURSING INTERVENTIONS	RATIONALE
Short-Term Goal ■ Patient will seek out staff or support person at any time if thoughts of harming self or others should occur. **Long-Term Goal** ■ Patient will not harm self or others.	1. Observe patient's behavior frequently through routine activities and interactions. Become aware of behaviors that indicate a rise in agitation. 2. Monitor for self-destructive behavior and impulses. A staff member may need to stay with patient to prevent self-mutilation. 3. Provide hand coverings and other restraints that prevent patient from self-mutilative behaviors. 4. Redirect violent behavior with physical outlets for frustration.	1. Stress commonly increases tic behaviors. Recognition of behaviors that precede the onset of aggression may provide the opportunity to intervene before violence occurs. 2. Patient safety is a nursing priority. 3. For patient's protection, provide immediate external controls against self-aggressive behaviors. 4. Excess energy is released through physical activities and a feeling of relaxation is induced.

NURSING DIAGNOSIS: IMPAIRED SOCIAL INTERACTION

RELATED TO: Impulsiveness; oppositional and aggressive behavior

OUTCOME CRITERIA	NURSING INTERVENTIONS	RATIONALE
Short-Term Goal ■ Patient will develop a one-to-one relationship with a nurse or support person within 1 week. **Long-Term Goal** ■ Patient will be able to interact with staff and peers using age-appropriate, acceptable behaviors.	1. Develop a trusting relationship with patient. Convey acceptance of the person separate from the unacceptable behavior. 2. Discuss with patient which behaviors are and are not acceptable. Describe in matter-of-fact manner the consequences of unacceptable behavior. Follow through. 3. Provide group situations for patient.	1. Unconditional acceptance increases feelings of self-worth. 2. Aversive reinforcement can alter undesirable behaviors. 3. Appropriate social behavior is often learned from the positive and negative feedback of peers.

NURSING DIAGNOSIS: LOW SELF-ESTEEM

RELATED TO: Embarrassment associated with tic behaviors

OUTCOME CRITERIA	NURSING INTERVENTIONS	RATIONALE
Short-Term Goal ■ Patient will verbalize positive aspects about self not associated with tic behaviors.	1. Convey unconditional acceptance and positive regard. 2. Set limits on manipulative behavior. Take caution not to reinforce manipulative behaviors by providing desired attention. Identify the consequences of manipulation. Administer consequences in a matter-of-fact manner when manipulation occurs.	1. Communicating a perception of patient as a worthwhile human being may increase self-esteem. 2. Aversive consequences may work to decrease unacceptable behaviors.

Table 23–6 | CARE PLAN FOR THE CHILD OR ADOLESCENT WITH TOURETTE'S DISORDER—cont'd

OUTCOME CRITERIA	NURSING INTERVENTIONS	RATIONALE
Long-Term Goal ■ Patient will exhibit increased feeling of self-worth as evidenced by verbal expression of positive aspects about self, past accomplishments, and future prospects.	3. Help patient understand that he or she uses manipulation to try to increase own self-esteem. Interventions should reflect other actions to accomplish this goal. 4. If patient chooses to suppress tics in the presence of others, provide a specified "tic time" during which he or she "vents" tics, feelings, and behaviors (alone or with staff). 5. Ensure that patient has regular one-to-one time with nursing staff.	3. When patient feels better about self, the need to manipulate others will diminish. 4. Allows for release of tics and assists in sense of control and management of symptoms. 5. One-to-one time gives the nurse the opportunity to provide patient with information about the illness and healthy ways to manage it. Exploring feelings about the illness helps patient incorporate the illness into a healthy sense of self.

■ Set a time for "release" of the suppressed tic behaviors?

■ Verbalized positive aspects about self, particularly as they relate to his or her ability to manage the illness?

■ Complied with treatment in a nondefensive manner?

Psychopharmacological Intervention for Tourette's Disorder

Systematic review of current evidence supports the efficacy of antipsychotic agents, both typical and atypical agents, and the use of alpha$_2$-adrenergic agonist agents (such as clonidine) in treating tics (Weisman et al., 2013). However, nonpharmacological treatments have demonstrated the same effectiveness as psychopharmacological agents and cognitive behavior therapy is now first-line treatment for mild to moderate tics (Jummani & Coffey, 2017). Medications are reserved for those with significant impairment and unresponsive to psychological therapies. The researchers note that alpha$_2$ agonists are more efficacious in treating tics among patients with ADHD. Pharmacotherapy is most effective when it is combined with psychosocial therapy, such as behavioral therapy, individual counseling or psychotherapy, and/or family therapy. Medications that are used in the treatment of Tourette's disorder include antipsychotics and alpha agonists.

Antipsychotics

The conventional antipsychotics, haloperidol (Haldol) and pimozide (Orap), have been approved by the FDA for control of tics and vocal utterances associated with Tourette's disorder. These drugs have been widely investigated and have proved to be highly effective in alleviating these symptoms. They are often not the first-line choice of therapy, however, because of their propensity for severe adverse effects, such as extrapyramidal symptoms, neuroleptic malignant syndrome, tardive dyskinesia, and electrocardiographic changes. Haloperidol is not recommended for children younger than 3 years of age, and pimozide should not be administered to children younger than 12 years.

Although not presently approved by the FDA for use in Tourette's disorder, some clinicians prefer to prescribe atypical antipsychotics, such as risperidone (Risperdal), olanzapine (Zyprexa), or ziprasidone (Geodon), because of their more favorable side-effect profiles. Sadock and associates (2015) identify risperidone as the most well-studied atypical antipsychotic for the treatment of tics and report that there is considerable evidence for its efficacy. These medications have a lower incidence of neurological side effects than the typical antipsychotics, although extrapyramidal symptoms have been observed with risperidone. Common side effects include weight gain, metabolic side effects, and hyperprolactinemia (Sadock et al., 2015). Ziprasidone has been associated with increased risk of QTc interval prolongation. Hyperglycemia has also been reported in some patients taking atypical antipsychotics.

Alpha Agonists

Clonidine (Catapres) and guanfacine (Tenex; Intuniv) are alpha-adrenergic agonists that are approved for use as antihypertensive agents. The extended-release forms have been approved by the FDA for the treatment of ADHD. These medications may be used for treatment of Tourette's disorder because of their favorable side-effect profile and because they are often effective for comorbid symptoms of ADHD, anxiety, and insomnia. Common side effects include dry mouth, sedation, headaches, fatigue, and dizziness or postural hypotension. Guanfacine is longer lasting and less sedating than clonidine; however, its efficacy in reducing tics is controversial (Sadock et al., 2015). Alpha agonists should not be prescribed for children and adolescents with pre-existing cardiac or vascular disease. They should not be discontinued abruptly; to do so could result in symptoms of nervousness, agitation, tremor, and a rapid rise in blood pressure.

Disruptive Behavior Disorders

Oppositional Defiant Disorder

Clinical Findings, Epidemiology, and Course

Oppositional defiant disorder (ODD) is characterized by a persistent pattern of angry mood and defiant behavior that occurs more frequently than is usually observed in individuals of comparable age and developmental level and interferes with social, educational, occupational, or other important areas of functioning (APA, 2013). It must be understood as distinct, pervasive, and more disruptive than the sometimes negativistic and oppositional behavior that is typical in childhood and adolescence. The disorder typically begins by 8 years of age and usually not later than early adolescence. Prevalence estimates range from 2 to 16 percent, and common comorbid disorders include ADHD, anxiety, major depressive disorder, conduct disorder, and substance use disorders (APA, 2013). It is more prevalent in boys than in girls before puberty, but the rates are more closely equal after puberty. The *DSM-5* identifies that ODD often precedes conduct disorder, especially in children with onset of conduct disorder prior to 10 years of age (APA, 2013).

Predisposing Factors

Biological Influences

What role, if any, genetics, temperament, or biochemical alterations play in the etiology of ODD is still unclear. Some studies have identified genetic influences in the establishment of a child's temperament, but there is no clear evidence of this connection in ODD. However, having a temperament in which the child has difficulty regulating emotions and has low frustration tolerance is an identified risk factor for ODD (Mayo Clinic, 2018).

Family Influences

Opposition during various developmental stages is both normal and healthy. Children first exhibit oppositional behaviors at around 10 or 11 months of age, again as toddlers between 18 and 36 months of age, and finally during adolescence. Pathology is considered only when the developmental phase is prolonged or when there is overreaction in the child's environment to his or her behavior.

Some children exhibit these behaviors in a more intense form than others. Sadock and colleagues (2015) report, "Epidemiological studies of negativistic traits in nonclinical populations found such behavior in 16 to 22 percent of school-age children" (p. 1245).

Some parents interpret average or increased level of developmental oppositional behavior as hostility and a deliberate effort on the part of the child to be in control. If power and control are issues for parents, or if they exercise authority for their own needs, a power struggle can be established between the parents and the child that sets the stage for the development of ODD. Lubit (2015) suggested the following pattern of family dynamics:

■ There is the combination of a strong-willed child with a reactive and high-energy temperament and parents who are authoritarian rather than authoritative.
■ The parents become frustrated with the strong-willed child who does not obey and increase their attempts to enforce authority.
■ The child reacts to the excessive parental control with anger and increased self-assertion.

Lubit (2015) stated:

These patterns develop when parents inadvertently reinforce disruptive and deviant behaviors in a child by giving those behaviors a significant amount of negative attention. At the same time, the parents, who are often exhausted by the struggle to obtain compliance with simple requests, usually fail to provide positive attention; often, the parents have infrequent positive interactions with their children. The pattern of negative interactions evolves quickly as the result of repeated, ineffective, emotionally expressed commands and comments; ineffective harsh punishments; and insufficient attention and modeling of appropriate behaviors.

A childhood history of trauma can be influential in the appearance of oppositional defiant behaviors so it is essential to assess the child for history of abuse, neglect, or other traumas.

BOX 23–3 Diagnostic Criteria for Oppositional Defiant Disorder

A. A pattern of angry/irritable mood, argumentative/defiant behavior, or vindictiveness lasting at least 6 months as evidenced by at least four symptoms from any of the following categories and exhibited during interaction with at least one individual that is not a sibling.

ANGRY/IRRITABLE MOOD

1. Often loses temper.
2. Is often touchy or easily annoyed.
3. Is often angry and resentful.

ARGUMENTATIVE/DEFIANT BEHAVIOR

1. Often argues with authority figures or, for children and adolescents, with adults.
2. Often actively defies or refuses to comply with requests from authority figures or with rules.
3. Often deliberately annoys others.
4. Often blames others for his or her mistakes or misbehavior.

VINDICTIVENESS

1. Has been spiteful or vindictive at least twice within the past 6 months.

   Note: The persistence and frequency of these behaviors should be used to distinguish a behavior that is within normal limits from a behavior that is symptomatic. For children younger than 5 years, the behavior should occur on most days for a period of at least 6 months unless otherwise noted (Criterion A8). For individuals 5 years or older, the behavior should occur at least once per week for at least 6 months, unless otherwise noted (Criterion A8). While these frequency criteria provide guidance on a minimal level of frequency to define symptoms, other factors should also be considered, such as whether the frequency and intensity of the behaviors are outside a range that is normative for the individual's developmental level, gender, and culture.

B. The disturbance in behavior is associated with distress in the individual or others in his or her immediate social context (e.g., family, peer group, work colleagues), or it impacts negatively on social, educational, occupational, or other important areas of functioning.
C. The behaviors do not occur exclusively during the course of a psychotic, substance use, depressive, or bipolar disorder. Also, the criteria are not met for disruptive mood dysregulation disorder.

Specify current severity:

Mild: Symptoms are confined to only one setting (e.g., at home, at school, at work, with peers).

Moderate: Some symptoms are present in at least two settings.

Severe: Some symptoms are present in three or more settings.

Reprinted with permission from American Psychiatric Association. (2013). Diagnostic and statistical manual of mental disorders (5th ed.). Washington, DC: American Psychiatric Publishing.

Application of the Nursing Process to ODD

Background Assessment Data (Symptomatology)

ODD is characterized by passive-aggressive behaviors such as stubbornness, procrastination, disobedience, carelessness, **negativism,** testing of limits, resistance to directions, deliberately ignoring the communication of others, and unwillingness to compromise. Other symptoms that may be evident are running away, school avoidance, school underachievement, temper tantrums, fighting, and argumentativeness.

Initially, the oppositional attitude is directed toward the parents, but in time, relationships with peers and teachers become affected. These impairments in social interaction often lead to depression, anxiety, and additional problematic behavior (Lubit, 2015).

Usually, these children do not see themselves as being oppositional but view the problem as arising from others whom they believe are making unreasonable demands on them. These children are often friendless, perceiving human relationships as negative and unsatisfactory. School performance is usually poor because of their refusal to participate and their resistance to external demands.

The *DSM-5* (APA, 2013) diagnostic criteria for ODD are presented in Box 23–3.

Nursing Diagnosis

Based on the data collected during the nursing assessment, possible nursing diagnoses for the patient with ODD include the following:

■ Noncompliance with therapy related to negative temperament, denial of problems, underlying hostility
■ Defensive coping related to retarded ego development, low self-esteem, unsatisfactory parent-child relationship
■ Low self-esteem related to lack of positive feedback, retarded ego development
■ Impaired social interaction related to negative temperament, underlying hostility, manipulation of others

Outcome Identification

Outcome criteria include short- and long-term goals. Timelines are individually determined. The following criteria may be used for measurement of outcomes in the care of the patient with ODD.

The patient:

- Complies with treatment by participating in therapies without negativism.
- Accepts responsibility for his or her part in the problem.

- Takes direction from staff without becoming defensive.
- Does not manipulate other people.
- Verbalizes positive aspects about self.
- Interacts with others in an appropriate manner.

Planning and Implementation

Table 23–7 provides a plan of care for the child with ODD using nursing diagnoses common to the disorder, outcome criteria, and appropriate nursing interventions and rationales.

Table 23–7 | CARE PLAN FOR THE CHILD/ADOLESCENT WITH OPPOSITIONAL DEFIANT DISORDER

NURSING DIAGNOSIS: NONCOMPLIANCE WITH THERAPY

RELATED TO: Negative temperament; denial of problems; underlying hostility

OUTCOME CRITERIA	NURSING INTERVENTIONS	RATIONALE
Short-Term Goal ■ Patient will participate in and cooperate during therapeutic activities. **Long-Term Goal** ■ Patient will complete assigned tasks willingly and independently or with a minimum of assistance.	1. Set forth a structured plan of therapeutic activities. Start with minimum expectations and increase as patient begins to manifest evidence of compliance. 2. Establish a system of rewards for compliance with therapy and consequences for noncompliance. Ensure that the rewards and consequences are concepts of value to patient. 3. Convey acceptance of patient separate from the undesirable behaviors being exhibited ("It is not *you* but your *behavior* that is unacceptable").	1. Structure provides security and one or two activities may not seem as overwhelming as the whole schedule of activities presented at one time. 2. Positive, negative, and aversive reinforcements can contribute to desired changes in behavior. 3. Unconditional acceptance enhances self-worth and may contribute to a decrease in the need for passive-aggression toward others.

NURSING DIAGNOSIS: DEFENSIVE COPING

RELATED TO: Retarded ego development; low self-esteem; unsatisfactory parent-child relationship

OUTCOME CRITERIA	NURSING INTERVENTIONS	RATIONALE
Short-Term Goal ■ Patient will verbalize personal responsibility for difficulties experienced in interpersonal relationships within (time period reasonable for patient). **Long-Term Goal** ■ Patient will accept responsibility for own behaviors and interact with others without becoming defensive.	1. Teach patient that feelings of inadequacy provoke may defensive behaviors, such as blaming others for problems and the need to "get even." 2. Provide immediate, nonthreatening feedback for passive-aggressive behavior. 3. Help identify situations that provoke defensiveness, and practice through role-play more appropriate responses. 4. Provide immediate positive feedback for acceptable behaviors.	1. Recognition of the problem is the first step toward initiating change. 2. When the patient denies responsibility for problems, he or she is denying the inappropriateness of behavior. 3. Role-playing provides confidence to deal with difficult situations when they actually occur. 4. Positive feedback encourages repetition, and immediacy is significant for these children who respond to immediate gratification.

Table 23–7 | CARE PLAN FOR THE CHILD/ADOLESCENT WITH OPPOSITIONAL DEFIANT DISORDER–cont'd

NURSING DIAGNOSIS: LOW SELF-ESTEEM

RELATED TO: Lack of positive feedback; retarded ego development

OUTCOME CRITERIA	NURSING INTERVENTIONS	RATIONALE
Short-Term Goal ■ Patient will participate in own self-care and discuss with nurse aspects of self about which he or she feels good. **Long-Term Goal** ■ Patient will demonstrate increased feelings of self-worth by verbalizing positive statements about self and exhibiting fewer manipulative behaviors.	1. Ensure that goals are realistic. 2. Plan activities that provide opportunities for success. 3. Convey unconditional acceptance and positive regard. 4. Set limits on manipulative behavior. Take caution not to reinforce manipulative behaviors by providing desired attention. Identify the consequences of manipulation. Administer consequences matter-of-factly when manipulation occurs. 5. Help patient understand that he or she uses this behavior to try to increase own self-esteem. Interventions should reflect other actions to accomplish this goal.	1. Unrealistic goals set patient up for failure, which diminishes self-esteem. 2. Success enhances self-esteem. 3. Affirmation of patient as a worthwhile human being promotes positive self-esteem. 4. Aversive reinforcement may work to decrease unacceptable behaviors. 5. When patient feels better about self, the need to manipulate others will diminish.

NURSING DIAGNOSIS: IMPAIRED SOCIAL INTERACTION

RELATED TO: Negative temperament; underlying hostility; manipulation of others

OUTCOME CRITERIA	NURSING INTERVENTIONS	RATIONALE
Short-Term Goal ■ Patient will interact in age-appropriate manner with nurse in one-to-one relationship within 1 week. **Long-Term Goal** ■ Patient will be able to interact with staff and peers using age-appropriate, acceptable behaviors.	1. Develop a trusting relationship. Convey acceptance of the person separate from the unacceptable behavior and listen to the patient's perceptions about relationships and behaviors. 2. Explain to patient about passive-aggressive behavior. Explain how these behaviors are perceived by others. Describe which behaviors are not acceptable, and role-play more adaptive responses. Give positive feedback for acceptable behaviors. 3. Provide peer group situations for patient.	1. Unconditional acceptance increases feelings of self-worth and may serve to diminish feelings of rejection that have accumulated over a long period. 2. Role-playing is a way to practice behaviors that do not come readily to patient, making it easier when the situation actually occurs. Positive feedback enhances repetition of desirable behaviors. 3. Appropriate social behavior is often learned from the positive and negative feedback of peers. Groups also provide an atmosphere for using the behaviors rehearsed in role-play.

Evaluation

The evaluation step of the nursing process calls for reassessment of the plan of care to determine if the nursing actions have been effective in achieving the goals of therapy. The following questions can be used with the child or adolescent with ODD to gather information for the evaluation.

Is the patient:

- Cooperating with schedule of therapeutic activities? Is level of participation adequate?
- Manifesting a less negative attitude toward therapy?
- Accepting responsibility for problem behavior?
- Verbalizing the unacceptability of his or her passive-aggressive behavior?
- Able to identify which behaviors are unacceptable and substitute more adaptive behaviors?
- Able to interact with staff and peers without defending behavior in an angry manner?
- Able to verbalize positive statements about self?
- Manifesting fewer manipulative behaviors?
- Able to make compromises with others when issues of control emerge?
- Expressing anger and hostility appropriately and verbalizing ways of releasing anger adaptively?
- Able to verbalize true feelings instead of allowing them to emerge through use of passive-aggressive behaviors?

Conduct Disorder

Clinical Findings, Epidemiology, and Course

With conduct disorder (CD), there is a repetitive and persistent pattern of behavior in which the basic rights of others or major age-appropriate societal norms or rules are violated (APA, 2013). This feature distinguishes it from ODD. Physical aggression is common, and peer relationships are disturbed. This is one of the most frequent reasons that children and adolescents are referred for psychiatric intervention (Sadock et al., 2015). Prevalence estimates range from 2 percent to more than 10 percent, the prevalence rises from childhood to adolescence, and it is more common in males than females (APA, 2013). There is a higher male predominance among those with the childhood-onset subtype. A number of comorbidities are common with CD, including ADHD, mood disorders, learning disorders, and substance use disorders. The symptoms of ODD are generally considered less severe than those of CD but ODD

may progress to CD and both ODD and CD confer greater risk for antisocial personality disorder in adulthood (Connor, 2017). When the disorder begins in childhood, there is more likely to be a history of ODD and a greater likelihood of antisocial personality disorder in adulthood than if the disorder is diagnosed in adolescence.

> **CORE CONCEPT**
> **Temperament**
> Personality characteristics that define an individual's mood and behavioral tendencies. The sum of physical, emotional, and intellectual components that affect or determine a person's actions and reactions.

Predisposing Factors
Biological Influences

Genetics Family, twin, and adoptive studies have revealed a significantly higher number of individuals with CD among those who have family members with the disorder. Although genetic factors appear to be involved in the etiology of CD, little is yet known about the actual mechanisms involved in genetic transmission. There is some evidence though, of the distinction between behaviors that appear to be genetic versus environmental risk factors. In a large study of male twins (N = 2,769), researchers attempted to determine the structure of genetic and environmental influences in CD and found that the familial risk to CD is composed of two discrete dimensions of genetic risk: rule breaking (such as truancy) and overt aggression (harming other people) and one dimension of shared environmental risk, reflecting covert delinquency (such as stealing and hurting animals) (Kendler, Aggen, & Patrick, 2013). Studies such as these support a complex dynamic of both genetic and environmental factors in the development of conduct disorder.

Temperament The term *temperament* refers to personality traits that become evident very early in life and may be present at birth. As early as 2 years of age, children who show signs of an irritable temperament, poor compliance, inattentiveness, and impulsivity can begin to show signs of CD at later ages (Bernstein, 2016).

Bernstein adds that children with severe temperamental disturbances, including poor attachment, may develop ODD and CD despite good parental intervention, but it is more common that these children come from unstable families with frequent changes in residence and economic stress. Evidence suggests a genetic influence in temperament and an association between temperament and behavioral problems later in life.

Neurobiological Factors Sadock and associates (2015) identify three neurobiological findings relevant to CDs. First, neuroimaging studies identify decreased gray matter in limbic structures, bilateral insula (an area of the cortex that plays a role connecting emotional responses to pain), and the left amygdala. Second, studies have found high plasma concentration of serotonin and low levels in cerebrospinal fluid, both of which are correlated with aggression and violence. The third finding is that aggressive children had "significantly greater relative right frontal brain activity at rest than healthy controls" (p. 1250).

Psychosocial Influences

Peer Relationships Poor academic performance and social maladaptation often lead to affiliations with a deviant peer group. "Considerable research indicates that the deviant peer group provides training in criminal and delinquent behavior including substance abuse" (Bernstein, 2016). In addition, there is some evidence that engaging in risk-taking behaviors can yield reinforcement on a social level (acceptance within a peer group), and as Bernstein cites, "Studies of neural processing show that risk-taking may be associated with reward-related brain activation."

Family Influences

The following factors related to family dynamics have been implicated as contributors in the predisposition to CD and are typically in combination with one another to create a pattern of chaotic disruption in family life (Bernstein, 2016; Mayo Clinic, 2018; Sadock et al., 2015):

■ Parental rejection, neglect, or severe physical and verbal aggression
■ Inconsistent or harsh punitive discipline
■ Parental sociopathy
■ Lack of parental supervision
■ Frequent changes in residence
■ Economic stressors
■ Parents with antisocial personality disorder, severe psychopathology, and/or alcohol or other substance dependence

■ Marital conflict and divorce (particularly where there is persistence of hostility)

Application of the Nursing Process to Conduct Disorder

Background Assessment Data (Symptomatology)

The classic characteristic of CD is the use of physical aggression in the violation of the rights of others. The behavior pattern manifests itself in virtually all areas of the child's life (home, school, with peers, and in the community). Stealing, lying, and truancy are common problems. The child lacks feelings of guilt or remorse.

The use of tobacco, liquor, or nonprescribed drugs, as well as the participation in sexual activities, occurs earlier than at the expected age for the peer group. Projection is a common defense mechanism.

Low self-esteem is manifested by a "tough guy" image. Characteristics include poor frustration tolerance, irritability, and frequent temper outbursts. Symptoms of anxiety and depression are not uncommon.

Level of academic achievement may be low in relation to age and IQ. Manifestations associated with ADHD (e.g., attention difficulties, impulsiveness, and hyperactivity) are common in children with CD.

The *DSM-5* diagnostic criteria for CD are presented in Box 23–4.

Nursing Diagnosis

Based on the data collected during the nursing assessment, possible nursing diagnoses for the patient with CD include the following:

■ Risk for other-directed violence related to characteristics of temperament, peer rejection, negative parental role models, dysfunctional family dynamics
■ Impaired social interaction related to negative parental role models, impaired peer relations leading to inappropriate social behaviors
■ Defensive coping related to low self-esteem and dysfunctional family system
■ Low self-esteem related to lack of positive feedback and unsatisfactory parent-child relationship.

Outcome Identification

Outcome criteria include short- and long-term goals. Timelines are individually determined. The following

BOX 23–4 Diagnostic Criteria for Conduct Disorder

A. A repetitive and persistent pattern of behavior in which the basic rights of others or major age-appropriate societal norms or rules are violated, as manifested by the presence of at least three of the following 15 criteria in the past 12 months from any of the categories below, with at least one criterion present in the past 6 months:

AGGRESSION TO PEOPLE AND ANIMALS
1. Often bullies, threatens, or intimidates others.
2. Often initiates physical fights.
3. Has used a weapon that can cause serious physical harm to others (e.g., a bat, brick, broken bottle, knife, gun).
4. Has been physically cruel to people.
5. Has been physically cruel to animals.
6. Has stolen while confronting a victim (e.g., mugging, purse snatching, extortion, armed robbery).
7. Has forced someone into sexual activity.

DESTRUCTION OF PROPERTY
8. Has deliberately engaged in fire setting with the intention of causing serious damage.
9. Has deliberately destroyed others' property (other than by fire setting).

DECEITFULNESS OR THEFT
10. Has broken into someone else's house, building, or car.
11. Often lies to obtain goods or favors or to avoid obligations (i.e., "cons" others).
12. Has stolen items of nontrivial value without confronting a victim (e.g., shoplifting, but without breaking and entering; forgery).

SERIOUS VIOLATIONS OF RULES
13. Often stays out at night despite parental prohibitions, beginning before age 13 years.
14. Has run away from home overnight at least twice while living in parental or parental surrogate home, or once without returning for a lengthy period.
15. Is often truant from school, beginning before age 13 years.

B. The disturbance in behavior causes clinically significant impairment in social, academic, or occupational functioning.
C. If the individual is age 18 years or older, criteria are not met for antisocial personality disorder.

Specify whether:

Childhood-Onset Type: Individuals show at least one symptom characteristic of conduct disorder prior to age 10 years.

Adolescent-Onset Type: Individuals show no symptom characteristic of conduct disorder prior to age 10 years.

Unspecified Onset: Criteria for a diagnosis of conduct disorder are met, but there is not enough information available to determine whether the onset of the first symptom was before or after age 10 years.

Specify if:

With limited prosocial emotions

Specify current severity:

Mild

Moderate

Severe

Reprinted with permission from American Psychiatric Association. (2013). Diagnostic and statistical manual of mental disorders (5th ed.). Washington, DC: American Psychiatric Publishing.

criteria may be used for measurement of outcomes in the care of the patient with CD.

The patient:

■ Has not harmed self or others.
■ Interacts with others in a socially appropriate manner.
■ Accepts direction without becoming defensive.
■ Demonstrates evidence of increased self-esteem by discontinuing exploitative and demanding behaviors toward others.

Planning and Implementation

Table 23–8 provides a plan of care for the child with CD using nursing diagnoses common to the disorder,

outcome criteria, and appropriate nursing interventions and rationales.

Evaluation

Following the planning and implementation of care, evaluation is made of the behavioral changes in the child with CD. This is accomplished by determining if the goals of therapy have been achieved. Reassessment, the next step in the nursing process, may be initiated by gathering information using the following questions.

Has the patient:

■ Been able to manage aggressive impulses?
■ Been able to prevent harm to others or others' property?

Table 23–8 | CARE PLAN FOR CHILD/ADOLESCENT WITH CONDUCT DISORDER

NURSING DIAGNOSIS: RISK FOR OTHER-DIRECTED VIOLENCE

RELATED TO: Characteristics of temperament, peer rejection, negative parental role models, dysfunctional family dynamics

OUTCOME CRITERIA	NURSING INTERVENTIONS	RATIONALE
Short-Term Goal ■ Patient will discuss feelings of anger with nurse or therapist. **Long-Term Goal** ■ Patient will not harm others or others' property.	1. Observe patient's behavior frequently through routine activities and interactions. Become aware of behaviors that indicate a rise in agitation. 2. Redirect violent behavior with physical outlets for suppressed anger and frustration. 3. Encourage patient to express anger, and act as a role model for appropriate expression of anger. 4. Ensure that a sufficient number of staff is available to indicate a show of strength if necessary. 5. Administer tranquilizing medication, if ordered, or use mechanical restraints or isolation room only if situation cannot be controlled with less restrictive means.	1. Recognition of behaviors that precede the onset of aggression may provide the opportunity to intervene before violence occurs. 2. Excess energy is released through physical activities, inducing a feeling of relaxation. 3. Discussion of situations that create anger may lead to more effective ways of dealing with them. 4. This conveys evidence of control over the situation and provides physical security for staff and others. 5. Medications, mechanical restraint, and seclusion are only used if less restrictive measures have been unsuccessful and the patient is an imminent danger to the safety of self or others.

NURSING DIAGNOSIS: IMPAIRED SOCIAL INTERACTION

RELATED TO: Negative parental role models; impaired peer relations leading to inappropriate social behavior

OUTCOME CRITERIA	NURSING INTERVENTIONS	RATIONALE
Short-Term Goal ■ Patient will interact in age-appropriate manner with nurse in one-to-one relationship within 1 week. **Long-Term Goal** ■ Patient will be able to interact with staff and peers using age-appropriate, acceptable behaviors.	1. Develop a trusting relationship. Convey acceptance of the person separate from the unacceptable behavior. 2. Discuss which behaviors are and are not acceptable. Describe in matter-of-fact manner the consequence of unacceptable behavior. Follow through. 3. Provide group situations for patient.	1. Unconditional acceptance increases feeling of self-worth. 2. Aversive reinforcement can alter or extinguish undesirable behaviors. 3. Appropriate social behavior is often learned from the positive and negative feedback of peers.

NURSING DIAGNOSIS: DEFENSIVE COPING

RELATED TO: Low self-esteem and dysfunctional family system

OUTCOME CRITERIA	NURSING INTERVENTIONS	RATIONALE
Short-Term Goal ■ Patient will verbalize personal responsibility for difficulties experienced in interpersonal relationships within a time period reasonable for patient.	1. Explain to patient the correlation between feelings of inadequacy and the need for acceptance from others and how these feelings provoke defensive behaviors, such as blaming others for own behaviors.	1. Recognition of the problem is the first step in the change process toward resolution.

Continued

Table 23–8 | CARE PLAN FOR CHILD/ADOLESCENT WITH CONDUCT DISORDER—cont'd

OUTCOME CRITERIA	NURSING INTERVENTIONS	RATIONALE
Long-Term Goal ■ Patient will accept responsibility for own behaviors and interact with others without becoming defensive.	2. Provide immediate, matter-of-fact, nonthreatening feedback for unacceptable behaviors. 3. Help identify situations that provoke defensiveness, and practice through role-play more appropriate responses. 4. Provide immediate positive feedback for acceptable behaviors.	2. Patient may not realize how these behaviors are being perceived by others. 3. Role-playing provides confidence to deal with difficult situations when they actually occur. 4. Positive feedback encourages repetition, and immediacy is significant for these children, who respond to immediate gratification.

NURSING DIAGNOSIS: LOW SELF-ESTEEM

RELATED TO: Lack of positive feedback and unsatisfactory parent/child relationship

OUTCOME CRITERIA	NURSING INTERVENTIONS	RATIONALE
Short-Term Goal ■ Patient will participate in own self-care and discuss with nurse aspects of self about which he or she feels good. **Long-Term Goal** ■ Patient will demonstrate increased feelings of self-worth by verbalizing positive statements about self and exhibiting fewer manipulative behaviors.	1. Ensure that goals are realistic. 2. Plan activities that provide opportunities for success. 3. Convey unconditional acceptance and positive regard. 4. Set limits on manipulative behavior. Take caution not to reinforce manipulative behaviors by providing desired attention. Identify the consequences of manipulation. Administer consequences matter-of-factly when manipulation occurs. 5. Help patient understand that he or she uses this behavior in order to try to increase own self-esteem. Interventions should reflect other actions to accomplish this goal.	1. Setting goals that the patient can realistically accomplish, promotes self-esteem. 2. Success promotes self-esteem. 3. Communicating that patient is a worthwhile human being promotes positive self-esteem. 4. Aversive consequences may work to decrease unacceptable behaviors. 5. When patient feels better about self, the need to manipulate others will diminish.

- Been able to express anger in an appropriate manner?
- Developed more adaptive coping strategies to deal with anger and feelings of aggression?
- Demonstrated the ability to trust others and interact with staff and peers in an appropriate manner?
- Been able to accept responsibility for his or her own behavior? Is there less blaming of others?
- Been able to accept feedback from others without becoming defensive?
- Been able to verbalize positive statements about self?
- Been able to interact with others without engaging in manipulation?

Anxiety Disorders

Separation Anxiety Disorder

Clinical Findings, Epidemiology, and Course

Separation anxiety disorder is characterized by excessive fear or anxiety concerning separation from those to whom the individual is attached (APA, 2013). The anxiety is beyond that which would be expected for the individual's developmental level and interferes with social, academic, occupational, or other areas of functioning. In children, onset may occur any time before age 18 years, but the disorder is most commonly diagnosed around age 5 or 6, when the child goes to school. Diagnosis at this time may be related to the surfacing of symptoms when the child faces new stressors. Typically schoolteachers and counselors are the first to recognize anxiety and associated behavioral disturbances. Because there is also a high prevalence of separation anxiety disorders (43 percent) with onset after the age of 18, the *DSM-5* removed the diagnostic criteria that specified this disorder as one that occurs only in children and adolescents. Prevalence estimates for the disorder average about 4 percent, and it is more common in girls than in boys. Over 50 percent experience remission of symptoms within 10 years of onset, but there are several common comorbidities, including panic disorder, social anxiety disorders, specific phobias, depression, and bipolar disorders (Kimmel & Roy-Byrne, 2017).

Predisposing Factors

Biological Influences

Genetics A greater number of children with relatives who manifest anxiety problems develop anxiety disorders themselves than do children with no such family patterns. The results are significant enough to speculate that there is a hereditary influence in the development of separation anxiety disorder, but the mode of genetic transmission has not been determined. Sadock and associates (2015) state:

> Current consensus on the genetics of anxiety disorders suggests that what is inherited is a general predisposition toward anxiety, with resulting heightened levels of arousability, emotional reactivity, and increased negative affect, all of which increase the risk for the development of separation anxiety disorder [and other anxiety disorders]. (p. 1255)

Temperament It is well established that children differ from birth, or shortly thereafter, on a number of temperamental characteristics. "The temperamental traits of shyness and withdrawal in unfamiliar situations have been shown to be associated with a higher risk of developing separation anxiety disorder [as well as other anxiety disorders]" (Sadock et al. 2015, p. 1255).

Environmental Influences

Stressful Life Events Studies have shown a relationship between life events and the development of anxiety disorders. Significant changes or losses often coincide with the development of the disorder (Sadock et al., 2015). Children of mothers who were stressed during pregnancy also appear to be at greater risk for developing separation anxiety disorder (Dryden-Edwards, 2016).

Family Influences

Various theories expound on the idea that anxiety disorders in children are related to attachment issues with the mother. Three family influences that have demonstrated an increased risk for anxiety disorders in children include parental overprotection, insecure parent-child attachment, and maternal depression (Sadock et al., 2015).

Some parents may also transfer their fears and anxieties to their children through role modeling. For example, a parent who becomes significantly fearful and apprehensive when confronted with unfamiliar circumstances, such as a job or residence change, teaches the child that this is an appropriate response.

Application of the Nursing Process to Separation Anxiety Disorder

Background Assessment Data (Symptomatology)

Onset of this disorder may occur as early as preschool age; it rarely begins as late as adolescence. In most cases, the child has difficulty separating from the mother. Occasionally, the separation reluctance is directed toward the father, siblings, or other significant individual to whom the child is attached. Anticipation of separation may result in tantrums, crying, screaming, complaints of physical problems, and **clinging** behaviors.

Reluctance or refusal to attend school occurs in the majority of these children. Up to 80 percent of children with school refusal meet criteria for separation anxiety disorder (Dryden-Edwards, 2016). Younger children may "shadow," or follow around the person from whom they are afraid to be separated. During middle childhood or adolescence, they may refuse to sleep away from home (e.g., at a friend's house or at camp). Interpersonal peer relationships are usually not a problem with these children. They are generally well liked by their peers and are reasonably socially skilled.

Worrying is common and relates to the possibility of harm coming to self or to the attachment figure. Younger children may even have nightmares to this effect.

Specific phobias are not uncommon (e.g., fear of the dark, ghosts, animals). Depressed mood is frequently present and often precedes the onset of the anxiety symptoms, which commonly occur following a major stressor. The *DSM-5* diagnostic criteria for separation anxiety disorder are presented in Box 23–5.

BOX 23–5 Diagnostic Criteria for Separation Anxiety Disorder

A. Developmentally inappropriate and excessive fear or anxiety concerning separation from those to whom the individual is attached, as evidenced by at least three of the following:
   1. Recurrent excessive distress when anticipating or experiencing separation from home or major attachment figures.
   2. Persistent and excessive worry about losing major attachment figures or about possible harm to them, such as illness, injury, disasters, or death.
   3. Persistent and excessive worry about experiencing an untoward event (e.g., getting lost, being kidnapped, having an accident, becoming ill) that causes separation from a major attachment figure.
   4. Persistent reluctance or refusal to go out, away from home, to school, to work, or elsewhere because of fear of separation.
   5. Persistent and excessive fear of or reluctance about being alone or without major attachment figures at home or in other settings.
   6. Persistent reluctance or refusal to sleep away from home or to go to sleep without being near a major attachment figure.

   7. Repeated nightmares involving the theme of separation.
   8. Repeated complaints of physical symptoms (e.g., headaches, stomachaches, nausea, vomiting) when separation from major attachment figures occurs or is anticipated.

B. The fear, anxiety, or avoidance is persistent, lasting at least 4 weeks in children and adolescents and typically 6 months or more in adults.

C. The disturbance causes clinically significant distress or impairment in social, academic, occupational, or other important areas of functioning.

D. The disturbance is not better accounted for by another mental disorder, such as refusing to leave home because of excessive resistance to change in autism spectrum disorder; delusions or hallucinations concerning separation in psychotic disorders; refusal to go outside without a trusted companion in agoraphobia; worries about ill health or other harm befalling significant others in generalized anxiety disorder; or concerns about having an illness in illness anxiety disorder.

Reprinted with permission from American Psychiatric Association. (2013). Diagnostic and statistical manual of mental disorders (5th ed.). Washington, DC: American Psychiatric Publishing.

Nursing Diagnosis

Based on the data collected during the nursing assessment, possible nursing diagnoses for the patient with separation anxiety disorder include the following:

- Anxiety (severe) related to family history, temperament, overattachment to parent, negative role modeling
- Ineffective coping related to unresolved separation conflicts and inadequate coping skills evidenced by numerous somatic complaints
- Impaired social interaction related to reluctance to be away from attachment figure

Outcome Identification

Outcome criteria include short- and long-term goals. Timelines are individually determined. The following criteria may be used for measurement of outcomes in the care of the patient with separation anxiety disorder.

The patient:

- Is able to maintain anxiety at manageable level.
- Demonstrates adaptive coping strategies for dealing with anxiety when separation from attachment figure is anticipated.

- Interacts appropriately with others and spends time away from attachment figure to do so.

Planning and Implementation

Table 23–9 provides a plan of care for the child or adolescent with separation anxiety, using nursing diagnoses common to this disorder, outcome criteria, and appropriate nursing interventions and rationales.

Evaluation

Evaluation of the child or adolescent with separation anxiety disorder requires reassessment of the behaviors for which the family sought treatment. Both the patient and the family members may need to change their behavior. The following types of questions may provide assistance in gathering data required for evaluating whether the nursing interventions have been effective in achieving the goals of therapy.

Has the patient:

- Been able to maintain anxiety at a manageable level (i.e., without temper tantrums, screaming, or clinging)?
- Had fewer complaints of physical symptoms?
- Demonstrated the ability to cope in more adaptive ways in the face of escalating anxiety?

Table 23–9 | CARE PLAN FOR THE CHILD WITH SEPARATION ANXIETY DISORDER

NURSING DIAGNOSIS: ANXIETY (SEVERE)

RELATED TO: Family history; temperament; overattachment to parent; negative role modeling

OUTCOME CRITERIA	NURSING INTERVENTIONS	RATIONALE
Short-Term Goal ■ Patient will discuss fears of separation with trusted individual. **Long-Term Goal** ■ Patient will maintain anxiety at no higher than moderate level in the face of events that formerly have precipitated panic.	1. Establish an atmosphere of calmness, trust, and genuine positive regard. 2. Assure patient of his or her safety and security. 3. Explore the child's or adolescent's fears of separating from the parents. Explore with the parents possible fears they may have of separation from the child. 4. Help parents and child initiate realistic goals (e.g., child to stay with sitter for 2 hours with minimal anxiety; or child to stay at friend's house without parents until 9 p.m. without experiencing panic or anxiety). 5. Give, and encourage parents to give, positive reinforcement for desired behaviors.	1. Trust and unconditional acceptance are necessary for satisfactory nurse–patient relationship. Calmness is important because anxiety is easily transmitted from one person to another. 2. Symptoms of panic and anxiety are very frightening. 3. Some parents may have an underlying fear of separation from the child of which they are unaware and which they are unconsciously transferring to the child. 4. Parents may be so frustrated with child's clinging and demanding behaviors that assistance with problem-solving may be required. 5. Positive reinforcement encourages repetition of desirable behaviors.

NURSING DIAGNOSIS: INEFFECTIVE COPING

RELATED TO: Unresolved separation conflicts and inadequate coping skills

EVIDENCED BY: Numerous somatic complaints

OUTCOME CRITERIA	NURSING INTERVENTIONS	RATIONALE
Short-Term Goal ■ Patient will verbalize relationship of somatic symptoms to fear of separation. **Long-Term Goal** ■ Patient will demonstrate use of more adaptive coping strategies (than physical symptoms) in response to stressful situations.	1. Encourage child or adolescent to discuss specific situations in life that produce the most distress and to describe his or her response to these situations. Include parents in the discussion. 2. Help the child or adolescent who is perfectionistic to recognize that self-expectations may be unrealistic. Connect times of unmet self-expectations to the exacerbation of physical symptoms. 3. Encourage parents and child to identify more adaptive coping strategies that the child could use in the face of anxiety that feels overwhelming. Practice through role-play.	1. Patient and family may be unaware of the correlation between stressful situations and the exacerbation of physical symptoms. 2. Recognition of maladaptive patterns is the first step in the change process. 3. Practice facilitates the use of the desired behavior when the individual is actually faced with the stressful situation.

Continued

Table 23–9 | CARE PLAN FOR THE CHILD WITH SEPARATION ANXIETY DISORDER–cont'd

NURSING DIAGNOSIS: IMPAIRED SOCIAL INTERACTION

RELATED TO: Reluctance to be away from attachment figure

OUTCOME CRITERIA	NURSING INTERVENTIONS	RATIONALE
Short-Term Goal ■ Patient will spend time with staff or other support person, without presence of attachment figure, without excessive anxiety. **Long-Term Goal** ■ Patient will be able to spend time with others (without presence of attachment figure) without excessive anxiety.	1. Develop a trusting relationship. 2. Attend groups with the child, and support efforts to interact with others. Give positive feedback. 3. Convey to the child the acceptability of his or her not participating in group in the beginning. Gradually encourage small contributions until patient is able to participate more fully. 4. Help patient set small personal goals (e.g., "Today I will speak to one person I don't know").	1. This is the first step in helping the child learn to interact with others. 2. Presence of a trusted individual provides security during times of distress. Positive feedback encourages repetition. 3. Small successes will gradually increase self-confidence and decrease self-consciousness so that client will feel less anxious in the group situation. 4. Simple, realistic goals provide opportunities for success that increase self-confidence and may encourage the patient to attempt more difficult objectives in the future.

■ (Parents) Identified more adaptive coping strategies?
■ Verbalized an intention to return to school?
■ Been able to sleep without nightmares?
■ Been able to interact with others away from the attachment figure?

Quality and Safety Education for Nurses (QSEN)

The Institute of Medicine, in its 2003 report *Health Professions Education: A Bridge to Quality,* challenged faculties of medicine, nursing, and other health professions to ensure that their graduates have achieved a core set of competencies in order to meet the needs of the 21st-century healthcare system. These competencies include *providing patient-centered care, working in interdisciplinary teams, employing evidence-based practice, applying quality improvement,* and *utilizing informatics.* A QSEN teaching strategy is presented in Box 23–6. The use of this type of activity is intended to arm the instructor and the student with guidelines for attaining the knowledge, skills, and attitudes necessary for achievement of quality and safety competencies in nursing.

General Therapeutic Approaches

Treatment for neurodevelopmental disorders, disruptive behavior disorders, and anxiety disorders poses many challenges and requires a comprehensive treatment plan that may include individual, group, and family therapies; family education; pharmacotherapy; and psychotherapeutic interventions specifically designed for the unique clinical issues presented in each disorder. The following general therapeutic approaches are described.

Behavior Therapy

Behavior therapy is based on the concepts of classical conditioning and operant conditioning. Behavior therapy is a common and effective treatment with disruptive behavior disorders such as ADHD, ODD, and CD. With this approach, rewards are given for appropriate behaviors and withheld when behaviors are disruptive or otherwise inappropriate. The principle behind behavior therapy is that positive reinforcements encourage repetition of desirable behaviors, and aversive reinforcements (punishments) discourage repetition of undesirable behaviors. Behavior modification techniques—the system of rewards and

BOX 23–6 QSEN TEACHING STRATEGY

Assignment: Patient-Centered Care: Kleinman's Mini-Ethnography
Interviewing Families of Children With Psychiatric Disorders

Competency Domain: Patient-Centered Care

Learning Objectives: Student will:
• Demonstrate skills in hearing patients' and family members' stories of living with the disorder.
• Identify their own explanatory models of the disorder.
• Demonstrate attitudes that reflect a desire to cultivate cultural humility and cultural competence in nursing practice.

Strategy Overview

1. Read the article *Anthropology in the Clinic: The Problem of Cultural Competency and How to Fix it* by A. Kleinman and P. Benson. The article is available online at www.plosmedicine.org/article/info:doi/10.1371/ journal.pmed.0030294

2. Based on the "mini ethnography" described by Kleinman and Benson, interview a family member of a child with a psychiatric disorder and elicit a narrative of his or her experience in living with the disorder.

3. Drawing on notes from the interview, write one paper that is the narrative of the illness from the perspective of the interviewee and another paper that describes the student's own explanatory model.

Source: Adapted from Day, L., & Smith, E. L. (2007). Integrating quality and safety content into clinical teaching in the acute care setting. Nursing Outlook, 55(3), 138–143. With permission.

consequences—can be taught to parents to be used in the home environment. Consistency is an essential component. In the treatment setting, individualized behavior modification programs are designed for each client.

Family Therapy

Therapy for children and adolescents must involve the entire family if problems are to be resolved. Parents should be involved in designing and implementing the treatment plan for the child and should be involved in all aspects of the treatment process.

The genogram can be used to identify problem areas between family members. It provides an overall picture of the life of the family over several generations, including roles that various family members play and emotional distance between specific individuals. Areas for change can be easily identified.

The impact of family dynamics on disruptive behavior disorders has been identified. The impact of disruptive behavior on family dynamics cannot be ignored. Family coping can become severely compromised by the chronic stress of dealing with a child with a behavior disorder. It is therefore imperative that the treatment plan for the identified patient be instituted within the context of family-centered care.

Group Therapy

Group therapy provides children and adolescents with the opportunity to interact within an association of their peers. This interaction can be both gratifying and overwhelming, depending on the child.

Group therapy provides a number of benefits. Appropriate social behavior often is learned from the positive and negative feedback of peers. Opportunity is provided to learn to tolerate and accept differences in others, to learn that it is acceptable to disagree, to learn to offer and receive support from others, and to practice these new skills in a safe environment. It provides a way to learn from the experiences of others.

Group therapy with children and adolescents can take several forms. Music therapy groups provides the opportunity to express feelings through; some children may be unable to express themselves in any other way. Art and activity/craft therapy groups allow individual expression through artistic means.

Group play therapy is the treatment of choice for many children between the ages of 3 and 9 years. The Association for Play Therapy (2016) states:

Play therapy builds on the natural way that children learn about themselves and their relationships in the world around them. Through play therapy, children learn to communicate with others, express feelings, modify behavior, develop problem-solving skills, and learn a variety of ways of relating to others. Play provides a safe psychological distance from their problems and allows expression of thoughts and feelings appropriate to their development.

Psychoeducational groups are very beneficial for adolescents. The only drawback to this type of group is that it works best when the group is closed-ended; that is, once the group has been formed, no one is allowed to join until the group has reached its pre-established closure. Members are allowed to propose topics for discussion. The leader serves as teacher much of the time and facilitates discussion of the proposed topic. Members may from time to time be presenters and serve as discussion leaders. Sometimes, psychoeducation groups evolve into traditional therapy discussion groups.

Cognitive behavior therapy (CBT) has demonstrated benefit in the treatment of tic disorders (Tourette's); separation anxiety disorder; and the disruptive behavior disorders including ADHD, ODD, and CD. It has also been identified as beneficial for clients with ASD to treat secondary issues such as depression, anger, anxiety, and social skills deficits (Creed, 2015). Creed notes that because people on the autism spectrum are typically concrete thinkers CBT may be adapted to meet their individual needs and level of functioning.

Psychopharmacology

Several of the disorders presented in this chapter are treated with medications. The appropriate pharmacology is presented following the section in which the disorder is discussed. Medication should never be the sole method of treatment. It is undeniable that medication can and does improve quality of life for families of children and adolescents with these disorders. However, research has indicated that medication alone is not as effective as a combination of medication and psychosocial therapy. It is important for families to understand that there is no way to "give him a pill and make him well." The importance of the psychosocial therapies cannot be overstressed. Some clinicians will not prescribe medications for a patient unless he or she also participates in concomitant psychotherapy sessions. The beneficial effects of the medications promote improved coping ability, which in turn enhances the intent of the psychosocial therapy.

Summary and Key Points

- Intellectual disability is defined by deficits in general intellectual functioning and adaptive functioning.

- Four levels of intellectual disability—mild, moderate, severe, and profound—are associated with various behavioral manifestations and abilities.

- ASD is characterized by a withdrawal of the child into the self and into a fantasy world of his or her own creation.

- It is generally accepted that ASD is caused by abnormalities in brain structures or functions. Genetic factors are also thought to play a significant role in ASD.

- Children with ADHD may exhibit symptoms of inattention or hyperactivity and impulsiveness or a combination of the two.

- Genetics plays a role in the etiology of ADHD. Neurotransmitters that have been implicated include dopamine, norepinephrine, and serotonin. Maternal smoking and alcohol use during pregnancy has been linked to hyperactive behavior in offspring.

- CNS stimulants, alpha agonists, atomoxetine, and bupropion are commonly used to treat ADHD.

- The essential feature of Tourette's disorder is the presence of multiple motor tics and one or more vocal tics.

- Common medications used with Tourette's disorder include haloperidol; pimozide; clonidine; guanfacine; and atypical antipsychotics such as risperidone, olanzapine, and ziprasidone. CBT, however, is considered the first-line treatment for mild to moderate tics.

- ODD is characterized by a pattern of negativistic, defiant, disobedient, and hostile behavior toward authority figures that occurs more frequently than is usually observed in individuals of comparable age and developmental level.

- Conduct disorder is distinguished by a repetitive and persistent pattern of behavior in which the basic rights of others or major age-appropriate societal norms or rules are violated.

- The essential feature of separation anxiety disorder is excessive anxiety concerning separation from the home or from those to whom the person is attached.

- Children with separation anxiety disorder may have temperamental characteristics present at birth that predispose them to the disorder.

- General therapeutic approaches for child and adolescent psychiatric disorders include behavior therapy, family therapy, group therapies (including music, art, crafts, play, and psychoeducation), cognitive behavior therapy, and psychopharmacology.

Review Questions
Self-Examination/Learning Exercise

Select the answer that is most appropriate for each of the following questions:

1. In an effort to help the child with mild to moderate intellectual developmental disorder develop satisfying relationships with others, which of the following nursing interventions is most appropriate?
   a. Interpret the child's behavior for others.
   b. Set limits on behavior that is socially inappropriate.
   c. Allow the child to behave spontaneously, for he or she has no concept of right or wrong.
   d. This child is not capable of forming social relationships.

2. The child with autism spectrum disorder (ASD) has difficulty with trust. With this in mind, which of the following nursing actions would be most appropriate?
   a. Encourage all staff to hold the child as often as possible, conveying trust through touch.
   b. Assign a different staff member each day so child will learn that everyone can be trusted.
   c. Assign same staff person as often as possible to promote feelings of security and trust.
   d. Avoid eye contact, because this is extremely uncomfortable for the child, and may even discourage trust.

3. Which of the following nursing diagnoses would be considered the *priority* in planning care for the child with a severe ASD?
   a. Risk for self-mutilation evidenced by banging head against wall
   b. Impaired social interaction evidenced by unresponsiveness to people
   c. Impaired verbal communication evidenced by absence of verbal expression
   d. Disturbed personal identity evidenced by inability to differentiate self from others

4. Which of the following activities would be most appropriate for the child with attention-deficit/hyperactivity disorder (ADHD)?
   a. Monopoly
   b. Volleyball
   c. Pool
   d. Checkers

5. Which of the following drug classes is most commonly used for management of the child with ADHD?
   a. CNS depressants (e.g., diazepam [Valium])
   b. CNS stimulants (e.g., methylphenidate [Ritalin])
   c. Anticonvulsants (e.g., phenytoin [Dilantin])
   d. Major tranquilizers (e.g., haloperidol [Haldol])

6. The child with ADHD has a nursing diagnosis of impaired social interaction. Which of the following nursing interventions are appropriate for this child? (Select all that apply.)
   a. Socially isolate the child when interactions with others are inappropriate.
   b. Set limits with consequences on inappropriate behaviors.
   c. Provide rewards for appropriate behaviors.
   d. Provide group situations for the child.

7. The nursing history and assessment of an adolescent with a conduct disorder might reveal all of the following behaviors *except:*
   a. Manipulation of others for fulfillment of own desires.
   b. Chronic violation of rules.
   c. Feelings of guilt associated with the exploitation of others.
   d. Inability to form close peer relationships.

Continued

Review Questions—cont'd
Self-Examination/Learning Exercise

8. Certain family dynamics often predispose adolescents to the development of conduct disorder. Which of the following patterns is thought to be a contributing factor?
   a. Parents who are overprotective
   b. Parents who have high expectations for their children
   c. Parents who consistently set limits on their children's behavior
   d. Parents who are alcohol dependent

9. Which of the following is *least* likely to predispose a child to Tourette's disorder?
   a. Absence of parental bonding
   b. Family history of the disorder
   c. Abnormalities of brain neurotransmitters
   d. Structural abnormalities of the brain

10. Which of the following medications is used to treat Tourette's disorder?
    a. Methylphenidate (Ritalin)
    b. Haloperidol (Haldol)
    c. Imipramine (Tofranil)
    d. Phenytoin (Dilantin)

IMPLICATIONS OF RESEARCH FOR EVIDENCE-BASED PRACTICE

Melagari, M. G., Nanni, V., Lucidi, F., Russo, P., Donfrancesco, R., & Cloninger, C. R. (2015). Temperamental and character profiles of preschool children with ODD, ADHD, & anxiety disorders. *Comprehensive Psychiatry, 58,* 94–101.

DESCRIPTION OF THE STUDY: This study evaluated the reports of 120 parents of preschool children with AHDH, ODD, or anxiety disorders to identify whether their reports of child temperament and character accurately predicted their child's diagnostic picture using a specific assessment inventory (the Preschool Temperament and Character Inventory).

RESULTS OF THE STUDY: The researchers found that three dimensions of temperament (harm avoidance, novelty seeking, and persistence) enabled correct identification of ADHD, ODD, or anxiety disorders 75 percent of the time.

Specifically, children with ADHD showed high scores on novelty seeking and low scores on reward dependence and persistence, children with anxiety disorders showed high scores on harm avoidance, and children with ODD had higher scores on novelty seeking, persistence, and harm avoidance.

IMPLICATIONS FOR NURSING PRACTICE: This study has implications for nurses who work with children and particularly those who work in schools. Early identification of these childhood disorders enables intensive and comprehensive intervention to be initiated at the earliest signs of a developing disorder. If temperament profiles can accurately differentiate among these disorders, then screening as early as preschool is justified and may help to mediate longer-term consequences of these disorders by enabling targeted intervention.

Jimmy, age 9, has been admitted to the child psychiatric unit with a diagnosis of attention-deficit/hyperactivity disorder. He has been unmanageable at school and at home and has had several suspensions from school for continuous disruption of his class. He refuses to sit in his chair or do his work. He yells out in class, interrupts the teacher and the other students, and lately has become physically aggressive when he cannot have his way. Most recently, he was suspended after hitting his teacher when she asked him to return to his seat.

Jimmy's mother describes him as a restless and demanding baby who grew into a restless and demanding toddler. He has never gotten along well with his peers. Even as a small child, he would take his friends' toys away from them or bite them if they tried to hold their own with him. His 5-year-old sister is afraid of him and refuses to be alone with him.

During the nurse's intake assessment, Jimmy paced the room or rocked in his chair. He talked incessantly on a superficial level and jumped from topic to topic. He told the nurse that he did not know why he was there. He acknowledged that he had some problems at school but said that was only because the other kids picked on him and the teacher did not like him. He said he got into trouble at home sometimes but that was because his parents liked his little sister better than they liked him.

The physician has ordered methylphenidate 5 mg twice a day for Jimmy. His response to this order is, "I'm not going to take medicine. I'm not sick!"

Answer the following questions related to Jimmy:

1. What are the pertinent assessment data to be noted by the nurse?
2. What is the primary nursing diagnosis for Jimmy?
3. Aside from patient safety, to what problems would the nurse want to direct intervention with Jimmy?

 MOVIE CONNECTIONS

Bill (Intellectual disability) • *Bill, On His Own* (Intellectual disability) • *Sling Blade* (Intellectual disability) • *Forrest Gump* (Intellectual disability) • *Rain Man* (Autism spectrum disorder [ASD]) • *Mercury Rising* (ASD) • *Niagara, Niagara* (Tourette's disorder) • *Toughlove* (Conduct disorder)

References

Acosta, M. T., Swanson, J., Stehli, A., Molina, B., Martinez, A. F., Arcos-Burgos, . . . MTA Team. (2016). ADGRL3 (LPHN3) variants are associated with a refined phenotype of ADHD in the MTA study. *Molecular Genetics and Genomic Medicine, 4*(5), 540–547. doi:10.1002/mgg3.230

ADHD Institute. (2016). *Environmental risk factors.* Retrieved from http://www.adhd-institute.com/burden-of-adhd/aetiology/environmental-risk-factors

American Psychiatric Association (APA). (2000). *Diagnostic and statistical manual of mental disorders* (4th ed., text rev.). Washington, DC: Author.

American Psychiatric Association (APA). (2013). *Diagnostic and statistical manual of mental disorders* (5th ed.). Washington, DC: Author.

Association for Play Therapy. (2016). *Play therapy makes a difference.* Retrieved from http://www.a4pt.org/?page=PTMakesADifference

Bernstein, B. E. (2016). *Conduct disorder.* Retrieved from http://emedicine.medscape.com/article/918213-over view#a3

Boat, T. F., & Wu, J. T. (Eds.). (2015). *Mental disorders and disabilities among low-income children.* Washington, DC: National Academies Press.

Centers for Disease Control and Prevention (CDC). (2017). *FastStats: Attention deficit hyperactivity disorder.* Retrieved from http://www.cdc.gov/nchs/fastats/adhd.htm

Centers for Disease Control and Prevention (CDC). (2018a). *Autism spectrum disorders. Autism and Developmental Disabilities Monitoring Network.* Retrieved from http://www.cdc.gov/ncbddd/autism/addm.html

Centers for Disease Control and Prevention (CDC). (2018b). *Lead.* Retrieved from http://www.cdc.gov/nceh/lead

Centers for Disease Control and Prevention (CDC). (2018c). *Tourette syndrome: Risk factors and causes.* Retrieved from http://www.cdc.gov/ncbddd/tourette/riskfactors.html

Connor, D. (2017). Disruptive behavior disorders in children and adolescents. In B. J. Sadock, V. A. Sadock, & P. Ruiz (Eds.), *Comprehensive textbook of psychiatry* (10th ed., pp. 3605–3621). Philadelphia, PA: Wolters Kluwer.

Creed, T. (2015). *An introduction to CBT for people with autism spectrum disorder.* Retrieved from https://beckinstitute.org/an-introduction-to-cbt-for-people-with-an-autism-spectrum-disorder/

Day, L., & Smith, E. L. (2007). Integrating quality and safety content into clinical teaching in the acute care setting. *Nursing Outlook, 55*(3), 138–143.

Dryden-Edwards, R. (2016). *Separation anxiety.* Retrieved from http://www.medicinenet.com/separation_anxiety/page4.htm

Froehlich, T. E., Lanphear, B. P., Auinger, P., Hornung, R., Epstein, J. N., Braun, J., & Kahn, R. S. (2009). Association of tobacco and lead exposures with attention-deficit/hyperactivity disorder. *Pediatrics, 124,* 1054–1063. Retrieved from http://www.ncbi.nlm.nih.gov/pmc/articles/PMC2853804/

Galéra, C., Côté, S. M., Bouvard, M. P., Pingault, J. B., Melchior, M., Michel, G., . . . Tremblay R. E. (2011). Early risk factors for hyperactivity-impulsivity and inattention trajectories from age 17 months to 8 years. *Archives of General Psychiatry, 68*(12), 1267–1275. doi:10.1001/archgenpsychiatry.2011.138

Gilman, S.R., Chang, J., Xu, B., Bawa, T.S., Gogos, J.A., Karayiorgou, M., & Vitkup, D. (2012). Diverse types of genetic variation converge on functional gene networks involved in schizophrenia. *Nature Neuroscience, 15*(12), 1723–1728. doi:10.1038/nn.3261

Grohol, J. (2016). New chewable ADHD medication, Adzenys, has some worried. *Psych Central.* Retrieved from http://psychcentral.com/news/2016/05/31/new-chewableadhd-medication-adzenys-has-some-worried/104077.html

Harrop, C., McConachie, H., Emsly, R., Leadbitter, K., Green, J., & PACT Consortium. (2014). Restricted and repetitive behaviors in autism spectrum disorders and typical development: Cross sectional and longitudinal comparisons. *Journal of Autism and Developmental Disorders, 44,* 1207–1219. doi:10.1007/s10803-13-1986-5

Hazlett, H. C., Poe, M. D., Gerig, G., Styner, M., Chappell, C., Smith, R. G., . . . Piven, J. (2011). Early brain overgrowth in autism associated with an increase in cortical surface area before age 2 years. *Archives of General Psychiatry, 68*(5), 467–476.

Heinonen, K., Räikkönen, K., Pesonen, A. K., Andersson, S., Kajantie, E., Eriksson, J. G., . . . Lano. (2010). Behavioural symptoms of attention deficit/hyperactivity disorder in preterm and term children born small and appropriate for gestational age: A longitudinal study. *BMC Pediatrics, 10*, 91. doi: 10.1186/1471-2431-10-91

Humphreys, K. L., Watts, E. L., Dennis, E. L., King, L. S., Thompson, P. M., Gotlib, I. H. (2018). Stressful life events, ADHD symptoms, and brain structure in early adolescence. *Journal of Abnormal Child Psychology.* doi:10.1007/s10802-018-0443-5

Institute of Medicine. (2003). *Health professions education: A bridge to quality.* Washington, DC: Author.

Jummani, R., & Coffey, B. J. (2017). Tic disorders. In B. J. Sadock, V. A. Sadock, & P. Ruiz (Eds.), *Comprehensive textbook of psychiatry* (10th ed., pp. 3635–3649). Philadelphia, PA: Wolters Kluwer.

Kendler, K. S., Aggen, S. H., & Patrick, C. J. (2013). Familial influences on conduct disorder reflect 2 genetic factors and 1 shared environmental factor. *JAMA Psychiatry, 70*(1), 78–86. doi: 10.1001/jamapsychiatry.2013.267

Kimmel, R. J., & Roy-Byrne, P. (2017). Clinical features of anxiety disorders. In B. J. Sadock, V. A. Sadock, & P. Ruiz (Eds.), *Comprehensive textbook of psychiatry* (10th ed., pp. 1723–1730). Philadelphia, PA: Wolters Kluwer.

Kranjac, D. (2016). *In vitro modeling of early brain overgrowth in autism.* Retrieved from http://www.psychiatryadvisor.com/neurodevelopmental-disorder/modeling-early-brainovergrowth-in-autism/article/508852/

Lubit, R. H. (2015). *Oppositional defiant disorder.* Retrieved from http://emedicine.medscape.com/article/918095-overview

Maher, G. M., O'Keeffe, G. W., Kearney, P. M., Kenny, L. C., Dinan, T. G., Mattsson, M., & Khashan, A. S. (2018). Association of hypertensive disorders of pregnancy with risk of neurodevelopmental disorders in offspring: A systematic review and meta-analysis. *JAMA Psychiatry.* doi: 10.1001/jamapsychiatry.2018.0854

Marchetto, M. C., Belinson, H., Tian, Y., Freitas, B. C., Fu, C., Vadodaria, K. C., . . . Muotri, A. R. (2016). Altered proliferation and networks in neural cells derived from idiopathic autistic individuals. *Molecular Psychiatry.* doi:10.1038/mp.2016.95

Mathews-Wilson, L., & Daitch, L. (2016). *The psychosocial implications of ADHD in adults.* Retrieved from http://nursing.advanceweb.com/the-psychosocial-implications-of-adhd-in-adults/

Mayo Clinic. (2018). *Oppositional defiant disorder.* Retrieved from http://www.mayoclinic.org/diseases-conditions/oppositional-defiant-disorder/basics/risk-factors/con-20024559

McGough, J. J. (2017). Adult manifestations of attention-deficit/hyperactivity disorder. In B. J. Sadock, V. A. Sadock, & P. Ruiz (Eds.), *Comprehensive textbook of psychiatry* (10th ed., pp. 3598–3604). Philadelphia, PA: Wolters Kluwer.

Melagari, M. G., Nanni, V., Lucidi, F., Russo, P., Donfrancesco, R., & Cloninger, C. R. (2015). Temperamental and character profiles of preschool children with ODD, ADHD, & anxiety disorders. *Comprehensive Psychiatry, 58,* 94–101.

National Institutes of Health (NIH). (2018). *Tourette's syndrome information page.* Retrieved from https://www.ninds.nih.gov/Disorders/All-Disorders/Tourette-Syndrome-Information-Page

Nigg, J. T., Nikolas, M., Mark Knottnerus, G., Cavanagh, K., & Friderici, K. (2010). Confirmation and extension of association of blood lead with attention-deficit/hyperactivity disorder (ADHD) and ADHD symptom domains at population-typical exposure levels. *Journal of Child Psychology and Psychiatry, 51*(1), 58–65.

Rossignol, D. A., & Frye, R. E. (2016). Environmental toxicants and autism spectrum disorder. Retrieved from http://www.psychiatrictimes.com/special-reports/environmentaltoxicants-and-autism-spectrum-disorder

Sadock, B. J., Sadock, V. A., & Ruiz, P. (2015). *Synopsis of psychiatry: Behavioral sciences/clinical psychiatry* (11th ed.). Philadelphia, PA: Wolters Kluwer.

Sherman, J., & Tarnow, J. (2013). What are common comorbidities in ADHD? *Psychiatric Times.* Retrieved from http://www.psychiatrictimes.com/adhd/what-are-common-comorbidities-in-adhd

Strunz, S., Westphal, L., Ritter, K., Heuser, I., Dziobek, I., & Roepke, S. (2015). Personality pathology of adults with autism spectrum disorder without accompanying intellectual impairment in comparison to adults with personality disorders. *Journal of Autism and Developmental Disorders, 45,* 4026–4038. doi: 10.1007/s10803-14-2183-x

Van den Ban, E., Souverein, P., Meijer, W., van Engeland, H., Swaab, H., Egber, T., & Heerdinle, E. (2014). Association between ADHD drug use and injuries among children and adolescents. *European Child and Adolescent Psychiatry, 23,* 95–102. doi:10.1007/s00787-013-0432-8

Volkmar, F. R., Klin, A., Schultz, R. T., & State, M. W. (2017). Autism spectrum and social communication disorder. In B. J. Sadock, V. A. Sadock, & P. Ruiz (Eds.), *Comprehensive textbook of psychiatry* (10th ed., pp. 3571–3586). Philadelphia, PA: Wolters Kluwer.

Weisman, H., Qureshi, I. A., Leckman, J. F., Scahill, L., & Bloch M. H. (2013). Systematic review: Pharmacological treatment of tic disorders—Efficacy of antipsychotic and alpha-2 adrenergic agonist agents. *Neuroscience and Biobehavioral Reviews, 37*(6), 1162–1171. doi: 10.1016/j.neubiorev.2012.09.008

Williams, N. M., Zaharieva, I., Martin, A., Langley, K., Mantripragada, K., Fossdal, R., . . . Thapar, A. (2010). Rare chromosomal deletions and duplications in attention-deficit hyperactivity disorder: A genome-wide analysis. *Lancet, 376*(9750), 1401–1408.

CHAPTER OUTLINE

KEY TERMS

attachment

bereavement overload

disengagement theory

geriatrics

gerontology

geropsychiatry

"granny-dumping"

long-term memory

Medicaid

Medicare

menopause

osteoporosis

reminiscence therapy

short-term memory

transcendence

OBJECTIVES
After reading this chapter, the student will be able to:

1. Discuss societal perspectives on aging.
2. Describe an epidemiological profile of aging in the United States.
3. Discuss various theories of aging.
4. Describe biological, psychological, sociocultural, and sexual aspects of the normal aging process.
5. Discuss retirement as a special concern to the aging individual.
6. Explain personal and sociological perspectives of long-term care of the aging individual.
7. Describe the problem of elder abuse as it exists in today's society.
8. Discuss the implications of the increasing number of suicides among the elderly population.
9. Apply the steps of the nursing process to the care of aging individuals.

HOMEWORK ASSIGNMENT
Please read the chapter and answer the following questions:

1. Which theory of aging postulates that life span and longevity changes are predetermined?
2. How is the ability to learn affected by aging?
3. What are the most common causes of psychopathology in the elderly?
4. What are some factors that are thought to contribute to elder abuse?

Introduction

What is it like to grow old? It is not likely that many people in the American culture would state that it is something they want to do. Most would agree, however, that it is "better than the alternative."

Roberts (1991) tells the following often-told tale of Supreme Court Justice Oliver Wendell Holmes, Jr. In the year before he retired at the age of 91 as the oldest justice ever to sit on the Supreme Court of the United States, Holmes and his close friend Justice Louis Brandeis, then a mere 74 years old, were out for one of their frequent walks on Washington's Capitol Hill. On this particular day, the justices spotted a very attractive young woman approaching them. As she passed, Holmes paused, sighed, and said to Brandeis, "Oh, to be 70 again!" Obviously, being old is relative to the individual experiencing it.

Growing old has not been popular among the youth-oriented American culture. However, with 66 million adults reaching their 65th birthdays by the year 2030, greater emphasis is being placed on the needs of an aging population. The disciplines of **gerontology** (the study of the aging process), **geriatrics** (the branch of clinical medicine specializing in problems of the elderly), and **geropsychiatry** (the branch of clinical medicine specializing in psychopathology of the elderly population) are expanding rapidly in response to this predictable demand.

Growing old in a society that has been obsessed with youth may have a critical impact on the mental health of many people. This situation has serious implications for psychiatric nursing.

What is it like to grow old? Increasing numbers of people will be able to answer this question as the 21st century progresses. Perhaps they will also be asking the question that Roberts (1991) asks: "How did I get here so fast?"

This chapter focuses on physical and psychological changes associated with the aging process as well as on special concerns of the elderly population, such as retirement, long-term care, elder abuse, and high suicide rates. The nursing process is presented as the vehicle for delivery of nursing care to elderly individuals.

How Old Is *Old*?

The concept of "old" has changed drastically over the years. Our prehistoric ancestors probably had a life span of 40 years with the average individual living around 18 years. As civilization developed, mortality rates remained high as a result of periodic famine and frequent malnutrition. Improvement in the standard of living was not truly evident until about the middle of the 17th century. Since that time, ensured food supply, changes in food production, better housing conditions, and more progressive medical and sanitation facilities have contributed to population growth, declining mortality rates, and substantial increases in longevity.

In 1900, the average life expectancy in the United States was 47 years, and only 4 percent of the population was aged 65 or over. In 2016, the average life expectancy at birth was 78.8 years (76.3 years for men and 81.2 years for women) (National Center for Health Statistics [NCHS], 2017).

The U.S. Census Bureau has created a system for classification of older Americans:

- Older: 55 through 64 years
- Elderly: 65 through 74 years
- Aged: 75 through 84 years
- Very old: 85 years and older

Some gerontologists use a simpler classification system:

- Young old: 60 through 74 years
- Middle old: 75 through 84 years
- Old old: 85 years and older

So how old is *old*? Obviously, the term cannot be defined by a number. Myths and stereotypes of aging have long obscured our understanding of the aged and the process of aging. Ideas that all elderly individuals are sick, depressed, obsessed with death, senile, and incapable of change affect the way elderly people are treated. They even shape the pattern of aging of the people who believe them. They can become self-fulfilling prophecies—people start to believe they should behave in certain ways and therefore act according to those beliefs. Generalized assumptions can be demeaning and interfere with the quality of life for older individuals.

Just as there are many differences in individual adaptation at earlier stages of development, so it is in the elderly population. Erikson (1963) suggested that the mentally healthy older person possesses a sense of ego integrity and self-acceptance that will help in adapting to the ambiguities of the future with a sense of security and optimism.

Murray, Zentner, and Yakimo (2009) describe the mentally healthy older adult as such:

> [Having accomplished the earlier developmental tasks], the person accepts life as his or her own and as the only life for the self. He or she would wish for none other and would defend the meaning and the dignity of the lifestyle. The person has further refined the characteristics of maturity described for the middle-aged adult, achieving both wisdom and an enriched perspective about life and people. (p. 662)

Everyone, particularly healthcare workers, should see aging people as individuals, each with specific needs and abilities, rather than as a stereotypical group. Some individuals may seem old at 40, whereas others may not seem old at 70. Variables such as attitude, mental health, physical health, and degree of independence strongly influence how an individual perceives himself or herself. Surely, in the final analysis, whether one is considered old must be self-determined.

Epidemiological Statistics

The Population

In 1980, Americans 65 years of age or older numbered 25.5 million. By 2016, these numbers had increased to 49.2 million, and this number is expected to double by 2060 to 98 million (Administration on Aging [AoA], 2018). In 2015, that number represented 15.2 percent of the population, and it is projected that by 2040, the number of Americans over 65 will reach 21.7 percent of the population.

Marital Status

In 2016, of individuals aged 65 and older, 70 percent of men and 46 percent of women were married (AoA, 2018). Thirty-three percent of all women in this age group were widowed. There were more than three times as many widows as widowers, which is consistent with the longer life expectancy for women.

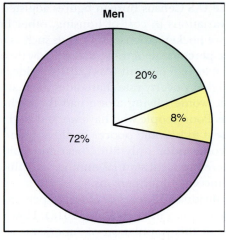

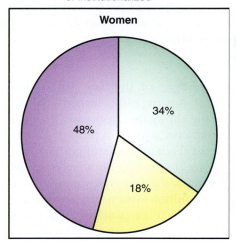

FIGURE 24–1 Living arrangements of noninstutionalized persons age 65 and older (AoA 2018).

Living Arrangements

The majority of individuals aged 65 or older live alone, with a spouse, or with relatives (AoA, 2018). In 2016, 1 million adults over 60 were caregivers to one or more grandchildren living with them. A small percentage, 3.1 percent of people over the age of 65, live in institutions. This percentage increases dramatically with age, ranging from 1 percent for persons 65 to 74 years to 3 percent for persons 75 to 84 years, and 9 percent for persons 85 and older. See Figure 24–1 for a distribution of living arrangements for persons aged 65 and older.

Economic Status

More than 4.6 million (9.5 percent) persons aged 65 or older were below the poverty level in 2016, and when the U.S Census Bureau figures adjusted for regional variations in cost of housing, other benefits, and out-of-pocket expenses for needs such as medical care, the percentage of those living below the poverty level rose to 14.5 percent (AoA, 2018). Older women had a higher poverty rate than older men, and older Hispanic women living alone had the highest poverty rate. Poor people who have worked all their lives can expect to become poorer in old age, and others will become poor only after becoming old. However, there are a substantial number of affluent and middle-income older persons.

Of individuals 75 years or older, 76 percent owned their own homes in 2016 (AoA, 2018). However, the housing of this population of Americans is usually older and less adequate than that of the younger population; therefore, a higher percentage of income must be spent on maintenance and repairs. The AoA reports that in 2016, 44 percent of older adults living in houses spent more than 33 percent of their income on housing costs.

Employment

With the passage of the Age Discrimination in Employment Act in 1967, forced retirement has been virtually eliminated in the workplace. It is well accepted that involvement in purposeful activity is vital to successful adaptation and perhaps even to survival at any age. Increasing numbers of adults over 65 are remaining active in employment environments. In 2016, 9.6 million Americans aged 65 and older were in the labor force (working or actively seeking work), and that number represents a steady increase for both men and women since around the year 2000; the number of older women in particular has increased from 9.7percent in 2000 to 15.7 percent in 2017 (AoA, 2018). The data do not clarify whether this tendency to remain in the workforce during older adulthood is related to the desire to remain active and productive through the labor force or whether it is based in necessity for income.

Health Status

The number of days in which usual activities are restricted because of illness or injury increases with age. The Centers for Disease Control and Prevention (CDC) (2018) reports that approximately 80 percent of older adults have at least one chronic condition, and 50 percent have two or more. The most commonly occurring conditions among the elderly population are hypertension (58 percent), hyperlipidemia (48 percent), arthritis (31 percent),

ischemic heart disease (29 percent), and diabetes (27 percent) (AoA, 2018).

Emotional and mental illnesses increase over the life cycle. Depression is particularly prevalent, and suicide is a serious problem among elderly Americans. Prevalence of major depression is estimated at between 1 and 5 percent for the general population of older adults but that may rise to as high as 13.5 percent for older adults requiring hospitalization or home health care (CDC, 2018). The CDC adds that depression in this age group is particularly underdiagnosed and undertreated by both healthcare providers and older adults themselves, perhaps related to a misperception that this is a normal part of aging or a natural reaction to illnesses. Neurocognitive disorders increase dramatically in old age.

Theories of Aging

A number of theories related to the aging process have been described. These theories are grouped into two broad categories: biological and psychosocial.

Biological Theories

Biological theories attempt to explain the physical process of aging, including molecular and cellular changes in the major organ systems and the body's ability to function adequately and resist disease. They also attempt to explain why people age differently and what factors affect longevity and the body's ability to resist disease.

Genetic Theory

According to one genetic theory, aging is an involuntarily inherited process that operates over time to alter cellular or tissue structures. This theory suggests that life span and longevity changes are predetermined. The theory is supported by the finding that there are similar life spans among identical twins and children of parents with a long life span (Rogers, Guarente, & Simic, 2018).

A second genetic theory identifies aging as a process of genetic mutations that essentially create "errors" in transmission of information, resulting in malfunction of specific proteins. Epigenetics, which involves the study of changes in the way genes are expressed in the absence of changes in the sequence of nucleic acids (Venes, 2017), has confirmed some fascinating findings that have implications for aging and illness. First, it was discovered that DNA methylation (the addition of a methyl group to a DNA base) is a mechanism responsible for gene regulation.

Genome studies of aging cells and tissues have shown that a variable "DNA methylation drift" creates changes in aging stem cells culminating in reduced stem cell plasticity, stem cell exhaustion, and focal defects that can lead to illnesses such as cancer (Issa, 2014). Issa describes that "aging pathologies in turn accelerate methylation drift by promoting chronic inflammation and uncontrolled proliferation which creates a vicious cycle that may explain why some illnesses increase . . . exponentially . . . with age" (p. 28). It is possible, with ongoing research, that we may discover what aging will look like for an individual and what his or her disease risks are. If epigenetic drift can be prevented, it may be possible to prevent diseases associated with aging.

Wear-and-Tear Theory

Proponents of this theory believe that the body wears out on a scheduled basis. Because animals have some ability to repair themselves, it would seem that this theory does not fit what we know about biological systems (Rogers et al., 2018). A related theory suggests that free radicals, which are the waste products of metabolism, accumulate and cause damage to important biological structures. Free radicals are molecules with unpaired electrons that exist normally in the body; they also are produced by ionizing radiation, ozone, and chemical toxins. According to this theory, these free radicals cause DNA damage, cross-linkage of collagen, and the accumulation of age pigments.

Environmental Theory

According to this theory, factors in the environment (e.g., industrial carcinogens, sunlight, trauma, and infection) bring about changes in the aging process. Although these factors are known to accelerate aging, the impact of the environment is a secondary rather than a primary factor in aging. Science is only beginning to uncover the many environmental factors that affect aging.

Autoimmune Theory

The autoimmune theory describes an age-related decline in the immune system. As people age, their ability to defend against foreign organisms decreases, resulting in susceptibility to diseases such as cancer and infection. Aging immune cells become unable to distinguish between "self" proteins and foreign proteins and begin to attack the body's own cells. A rise in the body's autoimmune response occurs, leading to the development of autoimmune diseases such as rheumatoid arthritis and allergies to food and environmental agents. This theory, however, is based on clinical rather than experimental evidence (Rogers et al., 2018).

Neuroendocrine Theory

The neuroendocrine theory was first developed in 1954 by Vladimir Dilman, MD. Dilman subsequently worked with another physician, Ward Dean, to update this theory in the early 1990s. The theory suggests that as humans age, the hypothalamus declines in its ability to regulate hormones and becomes less sensitive to them. Consequently, hormone secretion and hormone effectiveness decline. Dilman identified several hypotheses to explain why the hypothalamus becomes less sensitive, including reduced neurotransmitter levels (serotonin in particular), decline in the secretion of pineal gland hormones, reduced glucose utilization and fat accumulation, neuronal lesions caused by chronically elevated cortisol levels secondary to stress, and accumulation of cholesterol in plasma membranes of neurons (Dean, 2018). Some believe that hormone replacements impacted by the hypothalamus may be a future treatment to counter the effects of aging, but more research is needed.

Psychosocial Theories

Psychosocial theories focus on social and psychological changes that accompany advancing age rather than on the biological implications of anatomic deterioration. Several theories have attempted to describe how attitudes and behavior in the early phases of life affect people's reactions during the late phase. This work is called the process of "successful aging."

Personality Theory

Personality theories address aspects of psychological growth without delineating specific tasks or expectations of older adults. Some evidence suggests that personality characteristics in old age are highly correlated with early life characteristics. Murray and associates (2009) state:

> No specific personality changes occur as a result of aging. The older person becomes more of what he or she was. The older person continues to develop emotionally and in personality and adds on characteristics instead of making drastic changes. (p. 663)

In extreme old age, however, people show greater similarity in certain characteristics, probably because of similar declines in biological functioning and societal opportunities.

In one study of personality traits, Srivastava, John, Gosling, and Potter (2003) examined the big five personality traits (conscientiousness, agreeableness, neuroticism, openness, and extraversion) in a large sample to determine how personality changes over the life span. Age range of the participants was 21 to 60 years. The researchers found that conscientiousness (being organized and disciplined) increased throughout the age range studied with the biggest increases during the 20s. Agreeableness (being warm, generous, and helpful) increased most during a person's 30s. Neuroticism (being anxious and emotionally labile) declined with age for women but did not decline for men. Openness (being acceptable to new experiences) showed small declines with age for both men and women. Extroversion (being outwardly expressive and interested in the environment) declined for women but did not show changes in men. This study contradicts the view that personality traits tend to stop changing in early adulthood. These researchers suggest that personality traits change gradually but systematically throughout the life span. Their research has been foundational in understanding the adult population, although the elderly were not evaluated in that study.

In a review of research on personality and aging that studied people between 60 and 80 years of age, Srivastava and Das (2013) identify support for the premise that personality traits are relatively stable but do change somewhat over the long term related to aging and possibly in response to intervention. The personality trait of conscientiousness, for example, when viewed over the course of a lifetime, was found to be relatively stable.

As the population of older adults continues to grow, research has focused not only on what constitutes aging but more specifically on what constitutes successful aging. Srivastava and Das stress that personality is undeniably influential in successful aging (they note that the term *successful aging* is often used but is controversial to some). Rowe and Kahn (1997) provide the classic paradigm for successful aging, identifying three criteria that must be met: (1) absence of disease, disability, and risk factors; (2) maintaining physical and mental functioning; and (3) active engagement in life.

What role do personality factors play in these aspects of successful aging? The research of Kern and Friedman (2008) identified the personality trait of conscientiousness as most linked to health-promoting behaviors. More recent research (Terracciano et al., 2010) studied the genetic underpinnings of each of the big five personality traits and, among other findings, identified a gene associated with the trait of conscientiousness. They found that this personality trait gene was associated with the same gene that has been linked to some neurodegenerative diseases, including Alzheimer's disease. Several studies have found that the personality trait of conscientiousness is protective against dementia and the facets of conscientiousness most protective against cognitive impairment are one's sense of personal responsibility, one's belief in one's ability to control his or her behavior, and one's sense of himself or herself as hard working (Sutin, Stephan, & Terracciano, 2018). This research suggests that personality may indeed play a significant role in aging and age-related illness. What all of this means for intervention in and possible improvement of the aging process is still unknown. Future research may begin to reveal the intricate interaction between genetic and environmental influences such that personality traits might become alterable to promote healthier, more successful aging.

Developmental Task Theory

In contrast to the personality trait theories of aging, which discuss a largely stable process that continues into old age, developmental task theory holds that there are activities and challenges that one must accomplish at predictable, changing stages in life to achieve successful aging. Erikson (1963) described the primary task of old age as being able to see one's life as having been lived with integrity. In the absence of achieving that sense of having lived well, the older adult is at risk for becoming preoccupied with feelings of regret or despair. As noted previously, the life span was significantly different when Erikson's developmental tasks and stages were first identified, and in the late 1990s, Erikson expanded the concept of **transcendence** as an additional stage that occurs after the stage of integrity versus despair (Erikson & Erikson, 1997). McCarthy, Ling, and Carini (2013) identify transcendence as a concept within the spiritual domain, and they cite McCarthy and Bockweg's (2012) definition:

> Transcendence [is] an inherent developmental process, resulting in a shift from a rational, materialistic view to a wider world view characterized by broadened personal boundaries, within interpersonal, intrapersonal, transpersonal, and temporal dimensions resulting in an increased sense of meaning in life, well-being, and life satisfaction. (p. 180)

McCarthy and associates' research on transcendence supports that transcendence is a significant contributor to successful aging. McCarthy adds that even in the face of chronic illness and functional limitations, individuals can age successfully depending on their ability to cope and adapt while maintaining a sense of connectedness and meaning in life (News Medical, 2014).

Disengagement Theory

Disengagement theory describes the process of withdrawal by older adults from societal roles and responsibilities. According to this theory, this withdrawal process is predictable, systematic, inevitable, and necessary for the proper functioning of a growing society. Older adults were said to be happy when social contacts diminished and responsibilities were assumed by a younger generation. The benefit to the older adult is thought to be in providing time for reflecting on life's accomplishments and for coming to terms with unfulfilled expectations. The benefit to society is thought to be an orderly transfer of power from old to young.

There have been many critics of this theory, and the postulates have been challenged. For many healthy and productive older individuals, the prospect of a slower pace and fewer responsibilities is undesirable.

Activity Theory

In direct opposition to the disengagement theory is the activity theory of aging, which holds that the way to age successfully is to stay active.

Sadock, Sadock, and Ruiz (2015) report that growing evidence supports the importance of remaining socially active for both physical and emotional well-being. Cultural expectations are influential, and as more older Americans are identified as reaping the benefits of physical and social activity, cultural expectations begin to shift. Many fitness classes, for example, are now finding a membership of people in their 80s and beyond.

Continuity Theory

This theory, also known as the developmental theory, is a follow-up to the disengagement and activity theories. It emphasizes the individual's previously established coping abilities and personal character traits as a basis for predicting how the person will adjust to the changes of aging. Basic lifestyle characteristics are likely to remain stable in old age, barring physical or other types of complications that necessitate change. A person who has enjoyed the company of others and an active social life will continue to enjoy this lifestyle into old age. One who has preferred solitude and a limited number of activities will probably find satisfaction in a continuation of this lifestyle.

Maintenance of internal continuity is motivated by the need for preservation of self-esteem, ego integrity, cognitive function, and social support. As they age, individuals maintain their self-concept by reinterpreting their current experiences so that old values can take on new meanings in keeping with present circumstances. Internal self-concepts and beliefs are not readily vulnerable to environmental change, and external continuity in skills, activities, roles, and relationship styles can remain remarkably stable into the 70s and beyond.

The Normal Aging Process

Biological Aspects of Aging

Individuals are unique in their physical and psychological aging processes, as influenced by their predisposition or resistance to illness; the effects of their external environment and behaviors; their exposure to trauma, infections, and past diseases; and the health and illness practices they have adopted during their life span. As the individual ages, there is a quantitative loss of cells and changes in many of the enzymatic activities within cells, resulting in a diminished responsiveness to biological demands made on the body. Age-related changes occur at different rates for different individuals, although in actuality, when growth stops, aging begins. This section presents a brief overview of the normal biological changes that occur with the aging process.

Skin

One of the most dramatic changes that occurs in aging is the loss of elastin in the skin. This effect, as well as changes in collagen, causes aged skin to wrinkle and sag. Excessive exposure to sunlight compounds these changes and increases the risk of developing skin cancer.

Fat redistribution results in a loss of the subcutaneous cushion of adipose tissue. Thus, older people lose "insulation," their skin appears thinner, and they are more sensitive to extremes of ambient temperature than are younger people. A diminished supply of blood vessels to the skin results in a slower rate of healing.

Cardiovascular System

The age-related decline in the cardiovascular system is thought to be the major determinant of decreased tolerance for exercise and loss of conditioning and the overall decline in energy reserve. The aging heart is characterized by modest hypertrophy and loss of pacemaker cells, resulting in a decrease in maximal heart rate and diminished cardiac output. This results in a decrease in response to work demands and some diminishment of blood flow to the brain, kidneys, liver, and muscles. Heart rate also slows with time. If arteriosclerosis is present, cardiac function is further compromised.

Respiratory System

Thoracic expansion is diminished by an increase in fibrous tissue and loss of elastin. Pulmonary vital capacity decreases, and the amount of residual air increases. Scattered areas of fibrosis in the alveolar septa interfere with exchange of oxygen and carbon dioxide. These changes are accelerated by the use of cigarettes or other inhaled substances. Cough and laryngeal reflexes are reduced, causing decreased ability to defend the airway. Decreased pulmonary blood flow and diffusion ability result in reduced efficiency in responding to sudden respiratory demands.

Musculoskeletal System

Skeletal aging involving the bones, muscles, ligaments, and tendons probably generates the most frequent limitations on activities of daily living experienced by aging individuals. Loss of muscle mass is significant, although this occurs more slowly in men than in women. Demineralization of the bones occurs at a rate of about 1 percent per year throughout the life span in both men and women. However, this increases to approximately 10 percent in women around **menopause,** making them particularly vulnerable to **osteoporosis.**

Individual muscle fibers become thinner and less elastic with age. Muscles become less flexible following disuse. There is diminished storage of muscle glycogen, resulting in loss of energy reserve for increased activity. These changes are accelerated by nutritional deficiencies and inactivity.

Gastrointestinal System

In the oral cavity, the teeth show a reduction in dentine production, shrinkage and fibrosis of root pulp, gingival retraction, and loss of bone density in the alveolar ridges. There is some loss of peristalsis in the stomach and intestines, and gastric acid production decreases. Levels of intrinsic factor may also decrease, resulting in vitamin B_{12} malabsorption in some aging individuals. A significant decrease in absorptive surface area of the small intestine may be associated with some decline in nutrient absorption. Motility slowdown of the large intestine, combined with poor dietary habits, dehydration, lack of exercise, and some medications, may give rise to problems with constipation.

A modest decrease in size and weight of the liver results in losses in enzyme activity required to deactivate certain medications by the liver. These age-related changes can influence the metabolism and excretion of these medications. These changes, along with the

pharmacokinetics of the drug, must be considered when giving medications to aging individuals.

Endocrine System

A decreased level of thyroid hormones causes a lowered basal metabolic rate. Decreased amounts of adrenocorticotropic hormone may result in less efficient stress response.

Impairments in glucose tolerance are evident in aging individuals. Glucose challenge studies show that insulin levels are equivalent to or slightly higher than those in younger individuals, although peripheral insulin resistance appears to play a significant role in carbohydrate intolerance. The observed glucose clearance abnormalities and insulin resistance in older people may be related to many factors other than biological aging (e.g., obesity, family history of diabetes) and may be influenced substantially by diet or exercise.

Genitourinary System

Age-related declines in renal function occur because of a steady attrition of nephrons and sclerosis within the glomeruli over time. Vascular changes affect blood flow to the kidneys, which results in reduced glomerular filtration and tubular function. Elderly people have an increased risk of developing the syndrome of inappropriate antidiuretic hormone secretion, and levels of blood urea nitrogen and creatinine may be elevated slightly. The overall decline in renal functioning has serious implications for physicians who prescribe medications for elderly individuals.

In men, enlargement of the prostate gland is common as aging occurs. Prostatic hypertrophy is associated with an increased risk for urinary retention and may also be a cause of urinary incontinence (Johnston, Harper, & Landefeld, 2013). Loss of muscle and sphincter control, as well as the use of some medications, may cause urinary incontinence in women. Not only is this problem a cause of social stigma, but also, if left untreated, it increases the risk of urinary tract infection and local skin irritation. Normal changes in the genitalia are discussed in the section "Sexual Aspects of Aging."

Immune System

Aging results in changes in both cell-mediated and antibody-mediated immune responses. The size of the thymus gland declines continuously from just beyond puberty to about 15 percent of its original size by age 50. The consequences of these changes include a greater susceptibility to infections and a diminished inflammatory response that results in delayed healing. There is also evidence of an increase in various autoantibodies as a person ages, increasing the risk of autoimmune disorders, such as rheumatoid arthritis (National Institutes of Health [NIH], 2018).

Because of the overall decrease in efficiency of the immune system, the proliferation of abnormal cells is facilitated in the elderly individual. Cancer is the best example of aberrant cells allowed to proliferate due to the ineffectiveness of the immune system.

Nervous System

With aging, there is an absolute loss of neurons, which correlates with decreases in brain weight of about 10 percent by age 90 (Murray et al., 2009). Gross morphological examination reveals gyral atrophy in the frontal, temporal, and parietal lobes; widening of the sulci; and ventricular enlargement. However, it must be remembered that these changes have been identified in careful study of adults with normal intellectual function.

The brain has enormous reserve and little cerebral function is lost over time, although greater functional decline is noted in the periphery. There appears to be a disproportionately greater loss of cells in the cerebellum, the locus ceruleus, the substantia nigra, and olfactory bulbs, accounting for some of the more characteristic aging behaviors such as mild gait disturbances, sleep disruptions, and decreased smell and taste perception.

Some of the age-related changes within the nervous system may be due to alterations in neurotransmitter release, uptake, turnover, catabolism, or receptor functions (Galasko, 2017). Decreases in dopamine and acetylcholine are of particular interest because of their significance in cognition and mood. These biochemical changes may be responsible for the altered responses of many older persons to stressful events and some biological treatments.

Sensory Systems

Vision

Visual acuity begins to decrease in midlife. Presbyopia (blurred near vision) is the standard marker of aging of the eye. It is caused by a loss of elasticity of the crystalline lens and results in compromised accommodation.

Cataract development is inevitable if the individual lives long enough for the changes to occur. Cataracts occur when the lens of the eye becomes less resilient (due to compression of fibers) and increasingly opaque (as proteins lump together), ultimately resulting in a loss of visual acuity.

The color in the iris may fade, and the pupil may become irregular in shape. A decrease in production of secretions by the lacrimal glands may cause dryness and result in increased irritation and infection. The pupil may become constricted, requiring an increase in the amount of light needed for reading.

Hearing

Hearing changes significantly with the aging process. Gradually over time, the ear loses its sensitivity to discriminate sounds because of damage to the hair cells of the cochlea. The most dramatic decline appears to be in perception of high-frequency sounds.

Age-related hearing loss, called *presbycusis,* is common and affects more than one-half of all adults by age 75 years and most adults over the age of 80 (Blevins, 2018). It is more common in men than it is in women, a fact that may be related to differences in levels of lifetime noise exposure.

Taste and Smell

Beyond 70 years of age, taste sensitivity begins to decline related to atrophy and loss of taste buds (Shock, 2018). Taste discrimination decreases, and bitter taste sensations predominate. Sensitivity to sweet and salty tastes is diminished.

The deterioration of the olfactory bulbs is accompanied by loss of smell acuity. The effect of aging on the sense of smell has not been precisely identified, though, and is difficult to evaluate because so many environmental factors influence sensitivity to smell (Shock, 2018). However, some decreased sensitivity may be related to loss of nerve endings in the nose and less mucus production (MedlinePlus, 2018).

Touch and Pain

Although the primary sensory changes that occur specifically related to aging are in hearing and vision, sensitivity to touch and pain may also decline or change with age related to less blood flow to nerve endings, in the spinal cord, or to the brain (MedlinePlus, 2018). These changes have critical implications for the elderly in their potential inability to use sensory warnings to escape serious injury.

Psychological Aspects of Aging

Memory Functioning

Age-related memory deficiencies and slower response times have been extensively reported in the literature. Although **short-term memory** seems to deteriorate with age, perhaps because of poorer sorting strategies, **long-term memory** does not show similar changes. However, in nearly every instance, well-educated, mentally active people do not exhibit the same decline in memory functioning as their age peers who lack similar opportunities to flex their minds. Nevertheless, with few exceptions, the time required for memory scanning is longer for both recent and remote recall among older people. This can sometimes be attributed to social or health factors (e.g., stress, fatigue, illness), but it can also occur because of certain normal physical changes associated with aging (e.g., decreased blood flow to the brain).

Intellectual Functioning

There appears to be a high degree of regularity in intellectual functioning across the adult age span. Crystallized abilities, or knowledge acquired in the course of the socialization process, tend to remain stable over the adult life span. Fluid abilities, or abilities involved in solving novel problems, tend to decline gradually from young to old adulthood. In other words, intellectual abilities of older people do not decline but do become obsolete. The age of their formal educational experiences is reflected in their intelligence scoring.

Learning Ability

The ability to learn is not diminished by age. Studies, however, have shown that some aspects of learning do change with age. The ordinary slowing of reaction time with age for nearly all tasks or the overarousal of the central nervous system may account for lower performance levels on tests requiring rapid responses. Under conditions that allow for self-pacing by the participant, differences in accuracy of performance diminish. Ability to learn continues throughout life, although it is strongly influenced by interests, activity, motivation, health, and experience. Adjustments need to be made in teaching methodology and time allowed for learning.

Adaptation to the Tasks of Aging

Loss and Grief

Individuals experience losses from the very beginning of life. By the time individuals reach their 60s and 70s, they have experienced numerous losses, and mourning has become a lifelong process. Unfortunately, with the aging process comes a convergence of losses, the timing of which makes it impossible for the aging individual to complete the grief process in response to one loss before another occurs. Because grief is cumulative, this can result in **bereavement overload,** which has been implicated in the predisposition to depression in the elderly.

Attachment to Others

Many studies have confirmed the importance of interpersonal relationships at all stages in the life cycle. Murray and associates (2009) state:

> [Social networks] contribute to well-being of the elder by (a) promoting socialization and companionship, (b) elevating morale and life satisfaction, (c) buffering the effects of stressful events, (d) providing a confidant, and (e) facilitating coping skills and mastery. (p. 620)

This need for **attachment** is consistent with the activity theory of aging that correlates the importance of social integration with successful adaptation in later life. Evidence supports that in addition to psychosocial benefits, social engagement is also correlated with physical and cognitive health in older adulthood (Thomas, 2011).

Maintenance of Self-Identity

Maintaining a positive self-concept and identity is important in successful aging. Individuals who tend toward a rigid self-identity and a negative self-concept will no doubt struggle with any changes and adaptations faced in the process of aging. For example, individuals whose identity centers entirely around their job may struggle more with their identity in retirement than those whose identity includes job, family, travel, and so on. Researchers in one study found that maintaining a youthful age identity and positive perceptions and experiences related to aging had a self-enhancing function for self-esteem and identity (Westerhof, Whitbourne, & Freeman, 2012). The authors compared citizens in the United States with citizens in the Netherlands and found that this self-enhancing function was stronger for Americans than for Netherlanders. Their conclusion was that factors influencing self-identity and self-concept in older age need to be considered within the cultural context.

Dealing With Death

Death anxiety is a universal phenomenon, and attitudes about death are a result of cumulative life experiences (Lehto & Stein, 2009). As more people are living longer there has been a resurgence of interest in research about death anxiety. Lehto and Stein conducted an extensive review of the research to lay a foundation for an emerging understanding of this concept. Kübler-Ross's (1969) pioneering research on attitudes about death and the experience of dying paved the way for discussions of this issue, but as Lehto and Stein (2009) identify in their review of literature, death anxiety is largely denied or repressed. They cited several studies confirming that religious beliefs reduced death anxiety and suggest that these were beneficial because they provide a context for meaning about life and death. Positive self-esteem mediates death anxiety or at least "assists in preventing overt manifestations of death anxiety" (p. 27). Other researchers found similarly that fear of the dying process among elderly individuals in care institutions was correlated with low self-esteem, purposelessness, and poor mental health (Missler et al., 2012). These authors also found that, in their sample, death anxiety was more correlated with fears for significant others than fear of the unknown.

Interestingly, death anxiety seems to be the highest during middle age and, by later adulthood, stabilizes. But as Lehto and Stein (2009) identified, maladaptive consequences of death anxiety include mental illnesses such as depression and anxiety disorders, so assessing and intervening with regard to death anxiety may be beneficial in preventing longer-term consequences. Self-esteem interventions, for example, may be beneficial in preventing older adult depression secondary to death anxiety. Some research has shown that death education is beneficial in reducing anxiety associated with fear of death (McClatchey & King, 2015). Addressing these issues with middle-aged clients may be in the interest of primary or secondary prevention in the aging process.

Psychiatric Disorders in Later Life

Cognitive disorders, depressive disorders, phobias, and alcohol use disorders are among the most common psychiatric illnesses in later life (Sadock et al., 2015). Many factors, including medical conditions and medications, may influence symptomatology. One should never assume that psychiatric symptoms are a usual part of aging. For example, as Sadock and colleagues, identify, "Age itself is not a risk factor for depression, but being widowed and having a chronic medical illness are associated with vulnerability to depressive disorders" (p. 1346). A thorough assessment is essential to distinguish the multiple factors that may concurrently influence symptomatology.

Neurocognitive Disorder

Neurocognitive disorders (NCDs) are common causes of psychopathology in the elderly and expected to increase over the next few decades as the population of older adults increases and research on early identification of NCDs improves (Jeste, 2017). About one-half of these disorders are of the Alzheimer's type, which is characterized by an insidious onset and a gradually progressive course of cognitive impairment. No curative treatment is currently available. Symptomatic treatments, including pharmacological interventions, attention to the environment, and family support, can help to maximize the client's level of functioning.

Delirium

Delirium is one of the most common and critical forms of psychopathology in later life. A number of factors have been identified that predispose elderly people to delirium, including structural brain disease, reduced capacity for homeostatic regulation, impaired vision and hearing, a high prevalence of chronic disease, reduced resistance to acute stress, and age-related changes in the pharmacokinetic and pharmacodynamics of drugs. Delirium needs to be recognized and the underlying condition treated as soon as possible. A high mortality rate is associated with this condition.

Depression

Depressive disorders are the most common affective illnesses occurring after the middle years. The incidence of increased depression among elderly people is influenced by many variables, particularly physical illness and losses. Somatic symptoms such as changes in appetite and complaints of pain are common in the depressed elderly but should always be assessed to rule out other illnesses. Symptomatology often mimics that of NCD, a condition that is referred to as *pseudodementia*. (See Table 13–1 for a comparison of the symptoms of NCD and pseudodementia.) Suicide is prevalent in the elderly, with declining health and decreased economic status being considered important influencing factors. Studies have noted that depression, depression-related suicide, and substance abuse are higher in the baby boomer generation than those prior to World War II (Jeste, 2017) although the reasons are unclear. Treatment of depression in the elderly individual may include psychotropic medications or electroconvulsive therapy. Tricyclic antidepressants pose a risk for orthostatic hypotension and other anticholinergic effects, and selective serotonin reuptake inhibitors (SSRIs) pose a higher risk for hyponatremia in the elderly, so risks and benefits of medication use should be carefully reviewed.

Schizophrenia

Schizophrenia is an illness that typically begins in young adulthood. In most instances, individuals who manifest psychotic disorders early in life show a decline in psychopathology as they age. Late-onset schizophrenia (after age 60) is rare, and when it does occur, it is more common in women and is often characterized by paranoid delusions or hallucinations. Antipsychotic agents may be beneficial for the older adult with schizophrenia but should be used judiciously and at lower than usual doses (Sadock et al., 2015).

Anxiety Disorders

Anxiety disorders are the second most common mental disorders in older adults (Jeste, 2017). Most anxiety disorders begin in early to middle adulthood, but some appear for the first time after age 60. Because the autonomic nervous system is more fragile in older persons, the response to a major stressor is often quite intense. The presence of physical disability frequently compounds the situation, resulting in a more severe post-traumatic stress response than is commonly observed in younger persons. In older adults, symptoms of anxiety and depression often accompany each other, making it difficult to determine which disorder is dominant.

Substance Use Disorders

It is believed that the incidence of substance abuse and addiction in older adults may have been underdiagnosed, but nationwide attention to the epidemic use and abuse of opioid pain medication has shed light on this problem in the elderly population. Older adults use prescription and over-the-counter (OTC) medications at least three times as frequently as the general population (Jeste, 2017) and may have more difficulty tolerating some drugs, particularly some long-acting drugs, sedative hypnotics, and benzodiazepines. For these reasons (and others), older adults are an at-risk population for substance use disorders and should be screened for prescription, OTC, and other substance use to identify an emerging problem.

Sleep Disorders

Sleep disorders are very common in the aging individual. Roughly 50 percent of older adults report difficulty initiating or maintaining sleep (Crowley, 2011), and these disorders may contribute to cognitive changes. Contributing factors include medical conditions, medications, age-related changes in circadian rhythms, sleep disordered breathing, and restless leg syndrome. Sedative-hypnotics, along with nonpharmacological approaches, are often used as sleep aids with the elderly. Changes in aging associated with metabolism and elimination must be considered when maintenance medications are administered for chronic insomnia in the aging client.

Sociocultural Aspects of Aging

Old age brings many important socially induced changes, some of which have the potential for negative effect on both the physical and mental well-being of older persons. In American society, *old age* is defined arbitrarily as being 65 years or older because that is the age when most people have been able to retire with full Social Security and other pension benefits. Recent legislation has increased the age beyond 65 years for full Social Security benefits. Currently, the age increases yearly (based on year of birth) until 2027, when the age for full benefits will be 67 years for all individuals.

Elderly people in virtually all cultures share some basic needs and interests. There is little doubt that most individuals choose to live the most satisfying life possible for as long as possible. They want protection from hazards and release from the weariness of everyday tasks. They want to be treated with the respect and dignity they deserve as individuals who have reached this pinnacle in life; and they want to die with the same respect and dignity.

Historically, the aged have had a special status in society. Even today, in some cultures, the aged are the most powerful, the most engaged, and the most respected members of society. This has not been the case in the modern industrial societies, although trends in the status of the aged differ widely among industrialized countries. For example, the status and integration of the aged in Japan have remained relatively high when compared with other industrialized nations, such as the United States.

Many negative stereotypes influence the perspective on aging in the United States. Ideas that elderly individuals are always tired or sick, slow and forgetful, isolated and lonely, unproductive, and angry determine the way younger individuals relate to the elderly in this society. Increasing disregard for the elderly has resulted in a type of segregation, as aging individuals voluntarily seek out or are involuntarily placed in special residences for the aged.

Assisted living centers, retirement apartment complexes, and even entire retirement communities intended solely for individuals over age 50 are becoming increasingly common. Geographic distribution of the elder populations is clustered in certain areas of the country; in 2016, more than half (54 percent) of persons aged 65 and older lived in 10 states with the largest numbers in California, Florida, Texas, New York, and Pennsylvania (AoA, 2018). Older adults may be migrating to these areas in an effort to achieve integration with others in their age group. This phenomenon provides additional corroboration for the activity theory of aging and the importance of attachment to others.

Employment is another area in which the elderly have experienced discrimination. Although compulsory retirement has been virtually eliminated, discrimination still exists in hiring and promotion practices. Many employers are not eager to retain or hire older workers. It is difficult to determine how much of the failure to hire and promote results from discrimination based on age alone and how much of it is related to a realistic and fair appraisal of the aged employee's ability and efficiency. It is true that some elderly individuals are no longer capable of doing as good a job as a younger worker; however, there are many who likely can do a *better* job than their younger counterparts if given the opportunity. Nevertheless, surveys have shown that some employers accept the negative stereotypes about elderly individuals and believe that older workers are hard to please, set in their ways, less productive, frequently absent, and involved in more accidents.

The status of the elderly may improve with time and as their numbers increase with the aging of the baby boomers. As older individuals gain political power and increase in number, the benefits and privileges designed for the elderly will increase.

Sexual Aspects of Aging

Sexuality and the sexual needs of elderly people are frequently misunderstood, condemned, stereotyped, ridiculed, repressed, and ignored. Americans have grown up in a society that has liberated sexual expression for all other age groups but still maintains old-fashioned standards for sexual expression by the elderly. Negative stereotyped notions concerning sexual interest and activity of the elderly are common. Some of these include ideas that older people have no sexual interests or desires, that they are sexually undesirable, or that they are too fragile or too ill to engage in sexual activity. Some people even believe that it is disgusting or comical to consider elderly individuals as sexual beings.

These cultural stereotypes undoubtedly play a large part in the misperception that many people

hold regarding sexuality of the aged, and they may be reinforced by the common tendency of the young to deny the inevitability of aging. With reasonably good health and an interesting and interested partner, there is no inherent reason that individuals should not enjoy an active sexual life well into late adulthood.

Physical Changes Associated With Sexuality

Many of the changes in sexuality that occur in later years are related to the physical changes that are taking place at that time of life.

Changes in Women

Menopause may begin anytime during the 40s or early 50s. During this time, there is a gradual decline in the functioning of the ovaries and the subsequent production of estrogen, which results in a number of changes. The walls of the vagina become thin and inelastic, the vagina itself shrinks in both width and length, and the amount of vaginal lubrication decreases noticeably. Orgastic uterine contractions may become spastic. All of these changes can result in painful penetration, vaginal burning, pelvic aching, or irritation on urination. In some women, the discomfort may be severe enough to result in an avoidance of intercourse. Paradoxically, these symptoms are more likely to occur with infrequent intercourse of only one time a month or less. Regular and more frequent sexual activity results in a greater capacity for sexual performance (King & Regan, 2013). Other symptoms that are associated with menopause in some women include hot flashes, night sweats, sleeplessness, irritability, mood swings, migraine headaches, urinary incontinence, and weight gain.

Some menopausal women elect to take hormone therapy (HT) for relief of these changes and symptoms. With estrogen therapy, the symptoms of menopause are minimized or do not occur at all. Women who have a uterus must take a second hormone, progesterone, to decrease the risk of endometrial cancer that is associated with estrogen use. Progesterone may be prescribed cyclically (7 to 10 days during the month) or continuously throughout the entire month. A combination pill, taken in this manner, is also available.

Results of the Women's Health Initiative (WHI), as reported in the *Journal of the American Medical Association,* indicated that the combination pill is associated with an increased risk of cardiovascular disease and breast cancer. Benefits related to colon cancer and osteoporosis were reported; however, investigators stopped this arm of the study and suggested discontinuation of this type of therapy. In a 3-year follow-up study of the participants, the results showed that the increased risk for cardiovascular disease dissipated with discontinuation of the hormone therapy (Heiss et al., 2008). Yang and Reckelhoff's (2011) review of the literature cites studies that suggest that the cardiovascular risks versus benefits may be associated with the age at which HT is initiated, and that HT may be cardioprotective when it is started earlier in menopause. A more recent WHI study reported that their findings do not support use of HT for chronic disease prevention but that it may be beneficial in management of certain menopause symptoms (Manson et al., 2013). As the Mayo Clinic (2018) summarizes, the decision to use HT should be individualized and be based on a careful assessment of the risks and benefits.

Changes in Men

Testosterone production declines gradually over the years, beginning between ages 40 and 60. A major change resulting from this hormone reduction is that erections occur more slowly and require more direct genital stimulation to achieve. There may also be a modest decrease in the firmness of the erection in men older than age 60. The refractory period lengthens with age, increasing the amount of time following orgasm before the man may achieve another erection. The volume of ejaculate gradually decreases, and the force of ejaculation lessens. The testes become somewhat smaller, but most men continue to produce viable sperm well into old age. Prolonged control over ejaculation in middle-aged and elderly men may bring increased sexual satisfaction for both partners. Adverse effects of some medications and circulatory problems may increase risks for erectile dysfunction in older adult men. Vasodilator medications such as sildenafil (Viagra) and tadalafil (Cialis) are treatment options.

Sexual Behavior in the Elderly

Coital frequency in early marriage and the overall quantity of sexual activity between ages 20 and 40 correlate significantly with frequency patterns of sexual activity during aging (Masters, Johnson, & Kolodny, 1995). Although sexual interest and behavior do appear to decline somewhat with age, studies show that significant numbers of elderly men and women have active and satisfying sex lives well into their 80s. A survey commissioned by the American Association of Retired Persons (AARP) provided some revealing information regarding the sexual attitudes and behavior of senior citizens. Some statistics from the survey are summarized in Table 24–1. The information from this survey clearly indicates that sexual activity can and does continue well past the 70s for healthy, active individuals who have regular opportunities for sexual expression. King and Regan (2013) identify that if an individual has healthy attitudes about sexuality and healthy sexual relationships in younger adulthood, those will probably continue into older adulthood.

Special Concerns of the Elderly Population

Retirement

Statistics reflect that a larger percentage of Americans are living longer and that many of them are retiring earlier. Reasons often given for the increasing pattern of early retirement include health problems, Social Security and other pension benefits, attractive "early out" packages offered by companies, and long-held plans (e.g., turning a hobby into a money-making situation). Although many Americans are retiring earlier, the Bureau of Labor Statistics notes that the growth rates of older adults continuing to work into their 70s, 80s, and beyond are increasing rapidly. They estimate that in the decade from 2014 to 2024, the growth rate will increase 55 percent for those 65 to 75 years old and 86 percent for those 75 and older (Toossi and Torpey, 2017).

Studies have shown that about 10 to 20 percent of individuals reenter the workforce following retirement (Cahill, Giandrea, & Quinn, 2011). Reentry is more common among men than women and among those individuals who are at a younger age and in good health at the time of their retirement. Some reasons people give for returning to work following retirement include negative reactions to being retired, feelings of being unproductive, economic hardship, and loneliness.

Retirement has both social and economic implications for elderly individuals. The role is fraught with a great deal of ambiguity and is one that requires many adaptations on the part of those involved.

Social Implications

Retirement is often anticipated as an achievement in principle but met with a great deal of ambiguity when it actually occurs. Our society places a great deal of importance on productivity, making as much money as possible, and doing it at as young an age

TABLE 24–1 **Sexuality at Midlife and Beyond**			
	AGES	**MEN (%)**	**WOMEN (%)**
Have sex at least once a week	45–49 50–59 60–69 70+	50 41 24 15	26 32 24 5
Report very satisfied with physical relationship	45–49 50–59 60–69 70+	60 50 52 26	48 40 41 27
Report very satisfied with emotional relationship	45–49 50–59 60–69 70+	26 32 28 20	37 23 29 24
Report sexual activity is important to their overall quality of life	45–49 50–59 60–69 70+	69 65 55 46	33 28 33 12
Believe non-marital sex is okay	45–49 50–59 60–69 70+	88 91 80 68	86 75 71 61
Describe their partners as physically attractive	45–49 50–59 60–69 70+	50 53 58 51	60 48 58 48
Report always or usually having an orgasm with sexual intercourse	45–49 50–59 60–69 70+	95 88 91 82	70 64 59 61
Report being impotent	45–49 50–59 60–69 70+	6 16 29 48	— — — —
Report having used medicine, hormones, or other treatments to improve sexual functioning	45–49 50–59 60–69 70+	7 12 14 13	9 16 14 13
What would most improve your sex life?	All	Better health for self; partner initiates sex more often; less stress	Less stress; better health for self and partner; finding a partner

Source: Adapted from American Association of Retired Persons (AARP). (2010). *Sex, romance, and relationships: AARP survey of midlife and older adults.* Washington, DC: AARP.

as possible. These types of values contribute to the ambiguity associated with retirement. Although leisure has been acknowledged as a legitimate reward for workers, leisure during retirement historically has lacked the same social value. Adjustment to this life-cycle event becomes more difficult in the face of societal values that are in direct conflict with the new lifestyle.

Historically, many women have derived a good deal of their self-esteem from their children—giving birth to them, rearing them, and being a "good mother." Likewise, many men have achieved self-esteem through work-related activities—creativity, productivity, and earning money. With the termination of these activities may come a loss of self-worth, resulting in depression in some individuals who are unable to adapt satisfactorily. Well-being in retirement is linked to factors such as stable health status and access to healthcare services, adequate income, the ability to pursue new goals or activities, extended social network of family and friends, and satisfaction with current living arrangements (Murray et al., 2009).

American society often identifies an individual by his or her occupation. This is reflected in the conversation of people who are meeting each other for the first time. Undoubtedly, most people have either asked or been asked at some point in time, "What do you do?" or "Where do you work?" Occupation determines status, and retirement represents a significant change in status. The basic ambiguity of retirement occurs in an individual's or society's definition of this change. Is it undertaken voluntarily or involuntarily? Is it desirable or undesirable? Is one's status made better or worse by the change? It is a major life event that requires planning and realistic expectations of life changes.

Economic Implications

Because retirement is generally associated with 20 to 40 percent reduction in personal income, the standard of living after retirement may be adversely affected. Most older adults derive post-retirement income from a combination of Social Security benefits, public and private pensions, and income from savings or investments.

The Social Security Act of 1935 promised assistance with financial security for the elderly. Since then, the original legislation has been modified, yet the basic philosophy remains intact. Its effectiveness, however, is now being questioned. Faced with deficits, the program is forced to pay benefits to those currently retired from both the reserve funds and monies being collected at present. There is genuine concern about paying Social Security benefits to future generations, when there may be no reserve funds from which to draw. Because many of the programs that benefit older adults depend on contributions from the younger population, the growing ratio of older Americans to younger people may affect society's ability to supply the goods and services necessary to meet this expanding demand.

Medicare and **Medicaid** were established by the government to provide medical care benefits for elderly and indigent Americans. The Medicaid program is jointly funded by state and federal governments, and coverage varies significantly from state to state. Medicare covers only a percentage of healthcare costs; therefore, to reduce risk related to out-of-pocket expenditures, many older adults purchase private "Medigap" policies designed to cover charges in excess of those approved by Medicare.

The magnitude of retirement earnings depends almost entirely on preretirement income. The poor will remain poor and the wealthy are unlikely to lower their status during retirement; however, for many in the middle classes, the relatively fixed income sources may be inadequate, possibly forcing them to face financial hardship for the first time in their lives.

Long-Term Care

Long-term care facilities are defined by the level of care they provide. They may be skilled nursing facilities or intermediate care facilities, or a combination of the two. Some institutions provide convalescent care for individuals recovering from acute illness or injury, some provide long-term care for individuals with chronic illness or disabilities, and still others provide both types of assistance.

Most elderly individuals prefer to remain in their own homes or in the homes of family members for as long as this arrangement can meet their needs without deterioration of family or social patterns. Many elderly individuals are placed in institutions as a last resort only after heroic efforts have been made to keep them in their own or a relative's home. The increasing emphasis on home healthcare has extended the period of independence for aging individuals.

Fewer than 4 percent of the population aged 65 and older live in nursing homes. The percentage increases dramatically with age, ranging from 1 percent for persons aged 65 to 74, 3 percent for persons aged 75 to 84, to 9 percent for persons aged 85 and older (AoA, 2018). A profile of the "typical" elderly nursing home resident is about 80 years of age, white, female, widowed with multiple chronic health conditions.

Risk Factors for Institutionalization

In determining who in our society will need long-term care, several factors have been identified that appear to place people at risk. The following risk factors are taken into consideration to predict potential need for services and to estimate future costs.

Age

Because people grow older in different ways, and the range of differences becomes greater with the passage of time, age is becoming a less relevant characteristic than it was historically. However, because of the high prevalence of chronic health conditions and disabilities, as well as the greater chance of diminishing social supports associated with advancing age, the 65-and-older population is often viewed as an important long-term care target group.

Health

Level of functioning, as determined by ability to perform various behaviors or activities—such as bathing, eating, mobility, meal preparation, handling finances, judgment, and memory—is a measurable risk factor. The need for ongoing assistance from another person is critical in determining the need for long-term care.

Mental Health Status

Mental health problems are risk factors in assessing need for long-term care. Many of the symptoms associated with certain mental disorders (especially NCDs) such as memory loss, impaired judgment, impaired intellect, and disorientation would render the individual incapable of meeting the demands of daily living independently.

Socioeconomic and Demographic Factors

Low income generally is associated with greater physical and mental health problems among the elderly. Because many elderly individuals have limited finances, they are less able to purchase care resources available outside of institutions (e.g., home healthcare), although Medicare and Medicaid now contribute a limited amount to this type of noninstitutionalized care.

Women are at greater risk of being institutionalized than men, not because they are less healthy but because they tend to live longer and thus reach the age at which more functional and cognitive impairments occur. They are also more likely to be widowed. Whites have a higher rate of institutionalization than nonwhites, which may be related to cultural and financial influences.

Marital Status, Living Arrangement, and the Informal Support Network

Individuals who are married and live with a spouse are the least likely of all disabled people to be institutionalized. Those who live alone without resources for home care and with few or no relatives living nearby to provide informal care are at higher risk for institutionalization.

Attitudinal Factors

Many people dread the thought of even visiting a nursing home, let alone moving to one or placing a relative in one. Negative perceptions exist of nursing homes as "places to go to die." The media picture and subsequent reputation of nursing homes has not been positive. Stories of substandard care and patient abuse have scarred the industry, making it difficult for those facilities that are clean and well-managed and that provide innovative, quality care to their residents to rise above the stigma.

State and national licensing boards perform periodic inspections to ensure that standards set forth by the federal government are being met. These standards address quality of patient care as well as adequacy of the nursing home facility. Yet, many elderly individuals and their families perceive nursing homes as a place to go to die, and the fact that many of these institutions are poorly equipped, understaffed, and disorganized keeps this societal perception alive. There are, however, many excellent nursing homes that strive to go beyond the minimum federal regulations for Medicaid and Medicare reimbursement. In addition to medical, nursing, rehabilitation, and dental services, social and recreational services are provided to increase the quality of life for elderly people living in nursing homes. These activities include playing cards, bingo, and other games; parties; church activities; books; television; movies; and arts, crafts, and other classes. Some nursing homes provide occupational and professional counseling. These facilities strive to enhance opportunities for improving quality of life and for becoming places to *live* rather than to die.

Elder Abuse

Abuse of elderly individuals is a serious form of family violence. Statistics regarding the prevalence of elder abuse are difficult to determine. It is estimated that 1 in 10 older adults in the United States is a victim of abuse (National Council on Aging, 2018). However, a study in 2015 found that only 45 percent of older adult (over 65) victims of violence reported those crimes to the police (National Crime Justice Reference Center, 2017). The abuser is often a relative who lives with the elderly person and may be the assigned caregiver. Typical caregivers who are likely to be abusers of the elderly were described by Murray and associates (2009) as being under economic stress, substance abusers, themselves the victims of previous family violence, and exhausted and frustrated by the caregiver role. Identified risk factors for victims of abuse included being a white female age 70 or older, being mentally or physically impaired, being unable to meet daily self-care needs, and having care needs that exceeded the caretaker's ability.

Abuse of elderly individuals may be psychological, physical, or financial. Neglect may be intentional or unintentional. Psychological abuse includes yelling, insulting, harsh commands, threats, silence, and social isolation. Physical abuse is described as striking, shoving, beating, or restraint. Financial abuse refers to misuse or theft of finances, property, or material possessions. Neglect implies failure to fulfill the physical needs of an individual who cannot do so independently. Unintentional neglect is inadvertent, whereas intentional neglect is deliberate. In addition, elderly individuals may be the victims of sexual abuse, which is sexual intimacy between two persons that occurs without the consent of one of the persons involved. Another type of abuse, dubbed **"granny-dumping"** by the media, involves abandoning elderly individuals at emergency departments, nursing homes, or other facilities—literally leaving them in the hands of others when the strain of caregiving becomes intolerable. Types of elder abuse are summarized in Box 24–1.

Elder victims often minimize the abuse or deny that it has occurred. The elderly person may be unwilling to disclose information because of fear of retaliation, embarrassment about the existence of abuse in the family, protectiveness toward a family member, or unwillingness to institute legal action. Adding to this unwillingness to report is the fact that infirm elders are often isolated, so their mistreatment is less likely to be noticed by those who might be alert to symptoms of abuse. For these reasons, detection of abuse in the elderly is difficult at best.

Factors That Contribute to Abuse

A number of contributing factors have been implicated in the abuse of elderly individuals.

Longer Life

The 65-and-older age group has become the fastest-growing segment of the population. Within this segment, the number of elderly persons older than age 75 has increased most rapidly. This trend is expected to continue well into the 21st century. The 75-and-older age group is the one most likely to be physically or mentally impaired, requiring assistance and care from family members. This group also is the most vulnerable to abuse from caregivers.

Dependency

Dependency appears to be the most common precondition in domestic abuse. Changes associated with normal aging or induced by chronic illness

---

BOX 24–1 Examples of Elder Abuse

PHYSICAL ABUSE
Striking, hitting, beating
Shoving
Bruising
Cutting
Restraining

PSYCHOLOGICAL ABUSE
Yelling
Insulting, name-calling
Harsh commands
Threats
Ignoring, silence, social isolation
Withholding of affection

NEGLECT (INTENTIONAL OR UNINTENTIONAL)
Withholding food and water
Inadequate heating

Unclean clothes and bedding
Lack of needed medication
Lack of eyeglasses, hearing aids, false teeth

FINANCIAL ABUSE OR EXPLOITATION
Misuse of the elderly person's income by the caregiver
Forcing the elderly person to sign over financial affairs to another person against his or her will or without sufficient knowledge about the transaction

SEXUAL ABUSE
Sexual molestation; rape
Any type of sexual contact against the elderly person's will

often result in loss of self-sufficiency in the elderly person, requiring that he or she become dependent on another for assistance with daily functioning. Long life may also consume finances to the point that the elderly individual becomes financially dependent on another as well. This type of dependency also increases the elderly person's vulnerability to abuse.

Stress

The stress inherent in the caregiver role is a factor in most abuse cases. Some clinicians believe that elder abuse results from individual or family psychopathology. Others suggest that even psychologically healthy family members can become abusive as the result of the exhaustion and acute stress caused by overwhelming caregiving responsibilities. This is compounded in an age group that has been dubbed the "sandwich generation"—those individuals who elected to delay childbearing so that they are now at a point in their lives when they are "sandwiched" between providing care for their children and providing care for their aging parents.

Learned Violence

Children who have been abused or have witnessed abusive and violent parents are more likely to evolve into abusive adults. In some families, abusive behavior is the normal response to tension or conflict, and this type of behavior can be transmitted from one generation to another. There may be some unresolved family conflicts or retaliation for previous maltreatment that foster and promote abuse of the elderly person.

Identifying Elder Abuse

Because so many elderly individuals are reluctant to report personal abuse, healthcare workers need to be able to detect signs of mistreatment when they are in a position to do so. Box 24–1 lists a number of *types* of elder abuse. The following *manifestations* of the various categories of abuse have been identified (Koop, 2012; Murray et al., 2009):

- Indicators of psychological abuse include a broad range of behaviors such as the symptoms associated with depression, withdrawal, anxiety, sleep disorders, and increased confusion or agitation.
- Indicators of physical abuse may include bruises, welts, lacerations, burns, punctures, evidence of hair pulling, and skeletal dislocations and fractures.

- Neglect may be manifested as consistent hunger, poor hygiene, inappropriate dress, consistent lack of supervision, consistent fatigue or listlessness, unattended physical problems or medical needs, or abandonment.
- Sexual abuse may be suspected when the elderly person is presented with pain or itching in the genital area; bruising or bleeding in external genitalia, vaginal, or anal areas; or unexplained sexually transmitted disease.
- Financial abuse may be occurring when there is an obvious disparity between assets and satisfactory living conditions or when the elderly person complains of a sudden lack of sufficient funds for daily living expenses.

Healthcare workers often feel intimidated when confronted with cases of elder abuse. In these instances, referral to an individual experienced in management of victims of such abuse may be the most effective approach to evaluation and intervention. Healthcare workers are responsible for reporting any suspicions of elder abuse. An investigation is then conducted by regulatory agencies, whose job it is to determine if the suspicions are corroborated. Every effort must be made to ensure the client's safety, but it is important to remember that a competent elderly person has the right to choose his or her healthcare options. As inappropriate as it may seem, some elderly individuals choose to return to the abusive situation. In this instance, he or she should be provided with names and phone numbers to call for assistance if needed. A follow-up visit by an adult protective services representative should be conducted.

Increased efforts need to be made to ensure that healthcare providers have comprehensive training in the detection of and intervention in elder abuse. More research is needed to increase knowledge and understanding of the phenomenon of elder abuse and ultimately to effect more sophisticated strategies for prevention, intervention, and treatment.

Suicide

In 2016, the highest rates of suicide occurred in those aged 45 to 54, but the second highest rates were among those aged 85 and older (American Foundation for Suicide Prevention [AFSP], 2018). The AFSP also reports that men, and particularly white men (in all age groups), die by suicide more often than do women. Predisposing factors include loneliness, financial problems, physical illness, loss, and depression.

It has been suggested that increased social isolation may be a contributing factor to suicide among the elderly. The number of elderly individuals who are divorced, widowed, or otherwise living alone has increased, and being a widow is associated with higher risk for depression and suicide (Sadock et al., 2015).

Many elderly individuals express symptoms associated with depression that are never recognized as such, particularly somatic symptoms. Any sign of helplessness or hopelessness should prompt an assessment for suicide risk using clear and, often, closed-ended questions to elicit a specific response, such as the following:

■ Have you thought of hurting yourself or taking your own life?
■ Do you have a plan for hurting yourself?
■ Have you ever acted on that plan?
■ Have you ever attempted suicide?

Components of intervention with a suicidal elderly person should include demonstrations of genuine concern, interest, and caring; indications of empathy for their fears and concerns; and help in identifying, clarifying, and formulating a plan of action to deal with the unresolved issue. If the elderly person's behavior seems particularly lethal, additional family or staff coverage and contact should be arranged to prevent isolation.

Application of the Nursing Process

Assessment

Assessment of the elderly individual may follow the same framework used for all adults but with consideration of the possible biological, psychological, sociocultural, and sexual changes that occur in the normal aging process described previously in this chapter. In no other area of nursing is it more important for nurses to practice holistic nursing than with the elderly. Older adults are likely to have multiple physical problems that contribute to problems in other areas of their lives. Obviously, these components cannot be addressed as separate entities. Nursing the elderly is a multifaceted, challenging process because of the multiple changes occurring at this time in the life cycle and the way in which each change affects every aspect of the individual.

Several considerations are unique to assessment of the elderly. Assessment of the older person's thought processes is a primary responsibility. Knowledge about the presence and extent of disorientation or confusion will influence the way in which the nurse approaches elder care.

Information about sensory capabilities is also extremely important. Because hearing loss is common, the nurse should lower the pitch and loudness of his or her voice when addressing the older person. Looking directly into the face of the older person when talking facilitates communication. Questions that require a declarative sentence in response should be asked; in this way, the nurse is able to assess the client's ability to use words correctly. Visual acuity can be determined by assessing adaptation to the dark, color matching, and the perception of color contrast. Knowledge about these aspects of sensory functioning is essential in the development of an effective care plan.

The nurse should be familiar with the normal physical changes associated with the aging process. Examples of some of these changes include the following:

■ Less effective response to changes in environmental temperature, resulting in hypothermia
■ Decreases in oxygen use and the amount of blood pumped by the heart, resulting in cerebral anoxia or hypoxia
■ Skeletal muscle wasting and weakness, resulting in difficulty in physical mobility
■ Limited cough and laryngeal reflexes, resulting in risk of aspiration
■ Demineralization of bones, resulting in spontaneous fracturing
■ Decrease in gastrointestinal motility, resulting in constipation
■ Decrease in the ability to interpret painful stimuli, resulting in risk of injury

Common psychosocial changes associated with aging include the following:

■ Prolonged and exaggerated grief, resulting in depression
■ Physical changes, resulting in disturbed body image
■ Changes in status, resulting in loss of self-worth

This list is by no means exhaustive. The nurse should consider many other alterations in his or her assessment of the patient. Knowledge of the patient's functional capabilities is essential for determining the physiological, psychological, and sociological needs of the elderly individual. Age alone does not preclude the occurrence of all these changes. The aging process progresses at a wide range of variance, and each client must be assessed as a unique individual.

Diagnosis and Outcome Identification

Virtually any nursing diagnosis may be applicable to the aging patient, depending on individual needs for assistance. Based on normal changes that occur in the elderly, the following nursing diagnoses may be considered.

Physiologically related diagnoses:

- Risk for trauma related to confusion, disorientation, muscular weakness, spontaneous fractures, falls
- Hypothermia related to loss of adipose tissue under the skin, evidenced by increased sensitivity to cold and body temperature below 98.6°F
- Decreased cardiac output related to decreased myocardial efficiency secondary to age-related changes, evidenced by decreased tolerance for activity and decline in energy reserve
- Ineffective breathing pattern related to increase in fibrous tissue and loss of elasticity in lung tissue, evidenced by dyspnea and activity intolerance
- Risk for aspiration related to diminished cough and laryngeal reflexes
- Impaired physical mobility related to muscular wasting and weakness, evidenced by need for assistance in ambulation
- Imbalanced nutrition, less than body requirements, related to inefficient absorption from gastrointestinal tract, difficulty chewing and swallowing, anorexia, difficulty in feeding self, evidenced by wasting syndrome, anemia, weight loss
- Constipation related to decreased motility; inadequate diet; insufficient activity or exercise, evidenced by decreased bowel sounds; hard, formed stools; or straining at stool
- Stress urinary incontinence related to degenerative changes in pelvic muscles and structural supports associated with increased age, evidenced by reported or observed dribbling with increased abdominal pressure or urinary frequency
- Urinary retention related to prostatic enlargement, evidenced by bladder distention, frequent voiding of small amounts, dribbling, or overflow incontinence

- Disturbed sensory perception related to age-related alterations in sensory transmission, evidenced by decreased visual acuity, hearing loss, diminished sensitivity to taste and smell, or increased touch threshold. (This diagnosis has been retired by NANDA-I but retained in this text because of its appropriateness to the specific behaviors described.)
- Insomnia related to age-related cognitive decline, decrease in ability to sleep ("sleep decay"), or medications, evidenced by interrupted sleep, early awakening, or falling asleep during the day
- Chronic pain related to degenerative changes in joints, evidenced by verbalization of pain or hesitation to use weight-bearing joints
- Self-care deficit (specify) related to weakness, confusion, or disorientation, evidenced by inability to feed self, maintain hygiene, dress/groom self, or toilet self without assistance
- Risk for impaired skin integrity related to alterations in nutritional state, circulation, sensation, or mobility

Psychosocially related diagnoses:

- Disturbed thought processes related to age-related changes that result in cerebral anoxia, evidenced by short-term memory loss, confusion, or disorientation. (This diagnosis has been retired by NANDA-I but retained in this text because of its appropriateness to the specific behaviors described.)
- Complicated grieving related to bereavement overload, evidenced by symptoms of depression
- Risk for suicide related to depressed mood and feelings of low self-worth
- Powerlessness related to lifestyle of helplessness and dependency on others, evidenced by depressed mood, apathy, or verbal expressions of having no control or influence over life situation
- Low self-esteem related to loss of preretirement status, evidenced by verbalization of negative feelings about self and life
- Fear related to nursing home placement, evidenced by symptoms of severe anxiety and statements such as "Nursing homes are places to go to die"
- Disturbed body image related to age-related changes in skin, hair, and fat distribution, evidenced by verbalization of negative feelings about body

- Ineffective sexuality pattern related to pain associated with vaginal dryness, evidenced by reported dissatisfaction with decrease in frequency of sexual intercourse
- Sexual dysfunction related to medications (e.g., antihypertensives) evidenced by inability to achieve an erection
- Social isolation related to total dependence on others, evidenced by expression of inadequacy in or absence of significant purpose in life
- Risk for trauma (elder abuse) related to caregiver role strain
- Caregiver role strain related to severity and duration of the care receiver's illness; lack of respite and recreation for the caregiver, evidenced by feelings of stress in relationship with care receiver; feelings of depression and anger; or family conflict around issues of providing care

Outcome Criteria

The following criteria may be used for measurement of outcomes in the care of the elderly patient.

The patient:

- Has not experienced injury.
- Maintains reality orientation consistent with cognitive level of functioning.
- Manages self-care with assistance.
- Expresses positive feelings about self, past accomplishments, and hope for the future.
- Compensates adaptively for diminished sensory perception.

Caregivers:

- Can problem solve effectively regarding care of the elderly patient.
- Demonstrate adaptive coping strategies for dealing with stress of caregiver role.
- Openly express feelings.
- Express desire to join a support group of other caregivers.

Planning and Implementation

In Table 24–2, selected nursing diagnoses are presented for the elderly patient. Outcome criteria are included along with appropriate nursing interventions and rationale for each.

Reminiscence therapy is especially helpful with elderly patients. This therapeutic intervention is highlighted in Box 24–2.

Evaluation

Reassessment is conducted to determine if the nursing actions have been successful in achieving the objectives of care. Evaluation of the nursing actions for the elderly patient may be facilitated by gathering information using the following types of questions.

Has the patient:

- Remained free from injury from falls, burns, or other means to which he or she is vulnerable because of age?
- Maintained reality orientation at an optimum for his or her cognitive functioning?
- Distinguished between reality-based and non-reality-based thinking?
- Accomplished self-care activities independently to his or her optimum level of functioning?
- Sought assistance for aspects of self-care that he or she is unable to perform independently?
- Expressed positive feelings about himself or herself?
- Reminisced about accomplishments that have occurred in his or her life?
- Expressed some hope for the future?
- Used eyeglasses or a hearing aid, if needed, to compensate for sensory deficits?
- Consistently looked others in the face to facilitate hearing when they are talking to him or her?
- Used helpful aids, such as signs identifying various rooms, to help maintain orientation?

Have the caregivers:

- Verbalized the means to provide a safe environment for the patient?
- Verbalized strategies for reality orientation, if needed?
- Worked through problems and made decisions regarding care of the elderly patient?
- Included the elderly family member in the decision-making process, if appropriate?
- Demonstrated adaptive coping strategies for dealing with the strain of long-term caregiving?
- Been open and honest in expression of feelings?
- Verbalized community resources to which they can go for assistance with their caregiving responsibilities?
- Joined a support group?

Table 24–2 | CARE PLAN FOR THE ELDERLY PATIENT

NURSING DIAGNOSIS: RISK FOR TRAUMA

RELATED TO: Confusion, disorientation, muscular weakness, spontaneous fractures, falls

OUTCOME CRITERIA	NURSING INTERVENTIONS	RATIONALE
Short-Term Goals ■ Patient will call for assistance when ambulating or carrying out other activities. ■ Patient will not experience injury. **Long-Term Goal** ■ Patient will not experience injury.	1. The following measures may be instituted: a. Arrange furniture and other items in the room to accommodate patient's disabilities. b. Store frequently used items within easy access. c. Keep bed in unelevated position. Pad side rails and headboard if patient has history of seizures. Keep bed rails up when patient is in bed (if permitted by institutional policy). d. Assign room near nurses' station; observe frequently. e. Assist patient with ambulation. f. Keep a dim light on at night. g. Frequently orient patient to place, time, and situation.	1. Patient safety is a priority.

NURSING DIAGNOSIS: DISTURBED THOUGHT PROCESSES

RELATED TO: Age-related changes that result in cerebral anoxia

EVIDENCED BY: Short-term memory loss, confusion, or disorientation

OUTCOME CRITERIA	NURSING INTERVENTIONS	RATIONALE
Short-Term Goal ■ Patient will accept explanations of inaccurate interpretations of the environment within (time to be determined based on patient condition). **Long-Term Goal** ■ Patient will interpret the environment accurately and maintain reality orientation to the best of his or her cognitive ability.	1. Frequently orient patient to reality. Use clocks and calendars with large numbers that are easy to read. Notes and large, bold signs may be useful as reminders. Allow patient to have personal belongings. 2. Keep explanations simple. Use face-to-face interaction. Speak slowly, and do not shout. 3. Discourage rumination of delusional thinking. Talk about real events and real people. 4. Monitor for medication side effects.	1. To help maintain orientation and aid in memory and recognition. 2. To facilitate comprehension. Shouting may create discomfort and, in some instances, provoke anger. 3. Rumination promotes disorientation. Reality orientation increases sense of self-worth and personal dignity. 4. Physiological changes in the elderly can alter the body's response to certain medications. Toxic effects may intensify altered thought processes.

Continued

Table 24–2 | CARE PLAN FOR THE ELDERLY PATIENT–cont'd

NURSING DIAGNOSIS: SELF-CARE DEFICIT (SPECIFY)

RELATED TO: Weakness, disorientation, confusion, or memory deficits

EVIDENCED BY: Inability to fulfill activities of daily living (ADLs)

OUTCOME CRITERIA	NURSING INTERVENTIONS	RATIONALE

Short-Term Goal
■ Patient will participate in ADLs with assistance from caregiver.
 	
Long-Term Goals
■ Patient will accomplish ADLs to the best of his or her ability.
■ Unfulfilled needs will be met by caregivers.
	1. Provide a simple, structured environment:
	  a. Identify self-care deficits and provide assistance as required. Promote independent actions as able.
	  b. Allow plenty of time for patient to perform tasks.
	  c. Provide guidance and support for independent actions by talking patient through the task one step at a time.
	  d. Provide a structured schedule of activities that do not change from day to day.
	  e. ADLs should follow home routine as closely as possible.
	  f. Allow consistency in assignment of daily caregivers.
		1. To minimize confusion.

NURSING DIAGNOSIS: CAREGIVER ROLE STRAIN

RELATED TO: Severity and duration of the care receiver's illness; lack of respite and recreation for the caregiver

EVIDENCED BY: Feelings of stress in relationship with care receiver; feelings of depression and anger; family conflict around issues of providing care

OUTCOME CRITERIA	NURSING INTERVENTIONS	RATIONALE
Short-Term Goal ■ Caregivers will verbalize understanding of ways to facilitate the caregiver role. **Long-Term Goal** ■ Caregivers will achieve effective problem-solving skills and develop adaptive coping mechanisms to regain equilibrium.	1. Assess prospective caregivers' ability to anticipate and fulfill client's unmet needs. Provide information to assist caregivers with this responsibility. Ensure that caregivers are aware of available community support systems from which they can seek assistance when required. Examples include adult day-care centers, housekeeping and homemaker services, respite care services, or a local chapter of the Alzheimer's Association. This organization sponsors a nationwide 24-hour hot line to provide information and link families who need assistance with nearby chapters and affiliates. The hot-line number is 800-272-3900.	1. Caregivers require relief from the pressures and strain of providing 24-hour care for their loved one. Studies have shown that elder abuse arises out of caregiving situations that place overwhelming stress on the caregivers.

Table 24–2 | CARE PLAN FOR THE ELDERLY PATIENT–cont'd

OUTCOME CRITERIA	NURSING INTERVENTIONS	RATIONALE
	2. Encourage caregivers to express feelings, particularly anger.	2. Release of these emotions can serve to prevent psychopathology, such as depression or psychophysiological disorders, from occurring.
	3. Encourage participation in support groups composed of members with similar life situations.	3. Hearing others who are experiencing the same problems discuss ways in which they have coped may help caregiver adopt more adaptive strategies. Individuals with similar life experiences provide empathy and support for each other.

NURSING DIAGNOSIS: LOW SELF-ESTEEM

RELATED TO: Loss of preretirement status; early stages of cognitive decline

EVIDENCED BY: Verbalization of negative feelings about self and life

OUTCOME CRITERIA	NURSING INTERVENTIONS	RATIONALE
Short-Term Goal ■ Patient will verbalize positive aspects of self and past accomplishments. **Long-Term Goal** ■ Patient will participate in group activities in which he or she can experience a feeling of enjoyment and accomplishment (to the best of his or her ability).	1. Encourage patient to express honest feelings in relation to loss of prior status. Acknowledge pain of loss. Support patient through process of grieving. 2. If lapses in memory are occurring, devise methods for assisting patient with memory deficit. Examples: a. Name sign on door identifying client's room. b. Identifying sign on outside of dining room door. c. Identifying sign on outside of restroom door. d. Large clock, with oversized numbers and hands, appropriately placed. e. Large calendar, indicating one day at a time, with month, day, and year in bold print. f. Printed, structured daily schedule, with one copy for client and one posted on unit wall. g. "News board" on unit wall where current news of national and local interest may be posted.	1. Patient may be fixed in anger stage of grieving process, which is turned inward on the self, resulting in diminished self-esteem. 2. These aids may assist patient to function more independently, thereby increasing self-esteem.

Continued

Table 24–2 | CARE PLAN FOR THE ELDERLY PATIENT—cont'd

OUTCOME CRITERIA	NURSING INTERVENTIONS	RATIONALE
	3. Encourage patient's attempts to communicate. If verbalizations are not understandable, express to client what you think he or she intended to say. It may be necessary to reorient patient frequently.	3. The ability to communicate effectively with others may enhance self-esteem.
	4. Encourage reminiscence and discussion of life review (see Box 24–2). Sharing picture albums, if possible, is especially good. Also discuss present-day events.	4. Reminiscence and life review help patient resume progression through the grief process associated with disappointing life events and increase self-esteem as successes are reviewed.
	5. Encourage participation in group activities. May need to accompany patient at first until he or she feels secure that the group members will be accepting, regardless of limitations in verbal communication.	5. Positive feedback from group members will increase self-esteem.
	6. Encourage patient to be as independent as possible in self-care activities. Provide written schedule of tasks to be performed. Provide assistance in areas where patient is unable to perform tasks independently.	6. The ability to perform independently preserves self-esteem.

NURSING DIAGNOSIS: DISTURBED SENSORY PERCEPTION

RELATED TO: Age-related alterations in sensory transmission

EVIDENCED BY: Decreased visual acuity, hearing loss, diminished sensitivity to taste and smell, and increased touch threshold

OUTCOME CRITERIA	NURSING INTERVENTIONS*	RATIONALE
Short-Term Goal ■ Patient will not experience injury due to diminished sensory perception. **Long-Term Goals** ■ Patient will attain optimal level of sensory stimulation. ■ Patient will not experience injury due to diminished sensory perception.	1. The following nursing strategies are indicated: a. Provide meaningful sensory stimulation to all special senses through conversation, touch, music, or pleasant smells. b. Encourage wearing of glasses, hearing aids, prostheses, and other adaptive devices. c. Use bright, contrasting colors in the environment. d. Provide large-print reading materials, such as books, clocks, calendars, and educational materials. e. Maintain room lighting that distinguishes day from night and that is free of shadows and glare.	1. Patient safety is a priority.

Table 24–2 | CARE PLAN FOR THE ELDERLY PATIENT–cont'd

OUTCOME CRITERIA	NURSING INTERVENTIONS*	RATIONALE
	f. Teach patient to scan the environment to locate objects. g. Help patient to locate food on plate using "clock" system, and describe food if patient is unable to visualize; assist with feeding as needed. h. Arrange physical environment to maximize functional vision. i. Place personal items and call light within patient's field of vision. j. Teach patient to watch the person who is speaking. k. Reinforce wearing of hearing aid; if patient does not have an aid, may consider a communication device (e.g., amplifier). l. Communicate clearly, distinctly, and slowly, using a low-pitched voice and facing patient; avoid overarticulation. m. Remove as much unnecessary background noise as possible. n. Do not use slang or extraneous words. o. As speaker, position self at eye level and no farther than 6 feet away. p. Get the patient's attention before speaking. q. Avoid speaking directly into the patient's ear. If the patient does not understand what is being said, rephrase the statement rather than simply repeating it. r. Help patient select foods from the menu that will ensure discrimination between various tastes and smells. s. Ensure that food has been properly cooled so that patient with diminished pain threshold is not burned. t. Ensure that bath or shower water is appropriate temperature. u. Use backrubs and massage as therapeutic touch to stimulate sensory receptors.	

*The interventions for this nursing diagnosis were adapted from Rogers-Seidl, F. F. (1997). *Geriatric nursing care plans* (2nd ed). St. Louis: Mosby Year Book.

BOX 24–2 Reminiscence Therapy and Life Review With the Elderly

Studies have indicated that *reminiscence*, or thinking about the past and reflecting on it, may promote better mental health in old age. *Life review* is related to reminiscence but differs from it in that it is a more guided or directed cognitive process that constructs a history or story in an autobiographical way (Murray et al., 2009).

Elderly individuals who spend time thinking about the past experience an increase in self-esteem and are less likely to suffer depression. Some psychologists believe that life review may help some people adjust to memories of an unhappy past. Others view reminiscence and life review as ways to bolster feelings of well-being, particularly in older people who can no longer remain active.

Reminiscence therapy can take place on a one-to-one basis or in a group setting. In reminiscence groups, elderly individuals share significant past events with peers. The nurse leader facilitates the discussion of topics that deal with specific life transitions, such as childhood, adolescence, marriage, childbearing, grandparenthood, and retirement. Members share both positive and negative aspects, including personal feelings, about these life-cycle events.

Reminiscence on a one-to-one basis can provide a way for elderly individuals to work through unresolved issues from the past. Painful issues may be too difficult to discuss in the group setting. As the individual reviews his or her life process, the nurse can validate feelings and help the elderly patient come to terms with painful issues that may have been long suppressed. This process is necessary if the elderly individual is to maintain (or attain) a sense of positive identity and self-esteem and ultimately achieve the goal of ego integrity, as described by Erikson (1963).

A number of creative measures can be used to facilitate life review with the elderly individual. Having the patient keep a journal for sharing may be a way to stimulate discussion (as well as provide a permanent record of past events for significant others). Pets, music, and special foods have a way of provoking memories from the patient's past. Photographs of family members and past significant events are an excellent way of guiding the elderly patient through his or her autobiographical review.

Care must be taken in the life review to assist clients to work through unresolved issues. Anxiety, guilt, depression, and despair may result if the individual is unable to work through the problems and accept them. Life review can work in a negative way if the individual comes to believe that his or her life was meaningless. However, it can be a very positive experience for the person who can take pride in past accomplishments and feel satisfied with his or her life, resulting in a sense of serenity and inner peace in the older adult.

Summary and Key Points

- Care of the aging individual presents one of the greatest challenges for nursing.
- The growing population of individuals aged 65 and older suggests that the trend will progress well into the 21st century.
- America is a youth-oriented society. It is not desirable to be old in mainstream American culture.
- In some cultures, the elderly are revered and hold a special place of honor within the society, but in highly industrialized countries such as the United States, status declines with the decrease in productivity and participation in the mainstream of society.
- Individuals experience many changes as they age. Physical changes occur in virtually every body system.
- Psychologically, there may be age-related memory deficiencies, particularly for recent events.
- Intellectual functioning does not decline with age, but length of time required for learning increases.
- Aging individuals experience many losses, potentially leading to bereavement overload. They are vulnerable to depression and to feelings of low self-worth.
- The elderly population, especially those older than age 85, represents a disproportionately high percentage of individuals who die by suicide.
- Neurocognitive disorders are the most frequent causes of psychopathology in the elderly. Anxiety disorders are the second most common. Sleep disorders, depression, and substance use disorders are also common.
- The need for sexual expression by the elderly is often misunderstood within our society. Although many physical changes occur at this time of life that alter an individual's sexuality, if he or she has reasonably good health and a willing partner, sexual activity can continue well past the 70s for most people.
- Retirement has both social and economic implications for elderly individuals. Society often equates an individual's status with occupation, and loss of employment may result in the need for adjustment in the standard of living because retirement

income may be reduced by 20 to 40 percent of preretirement earnings.

■ Less than 4 percent of the population aged 65 and older live in nursing homes. A profile of the typical elderly nursing home resident is a white woman about 80 years old, widowed, with multiple chronic health conditions. Much stigma is attached to what some still call "rest homes" or "old age homes," and many elderly people still equate them with a place to go to die.

■ The strain of the caregiver role has become a major dilemma in our society. Elder abuse is sometimes inflicted by caregivers for whom the role has become overwhelming and intolerable. There is an intense need to find assistance for family caregivers, who must provide care for their loved ones on a 24-hour basis. Home healthcare, respite care, support groups, and financial assistance are needed to ease the burden of this role strain.

■ Caring for elderly individuals requires a special kind of inner strength and compassion. The poem on page 670 conveys a vital message for nurses.

What Do You See, Nurse?

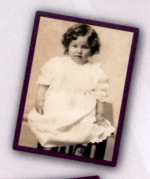

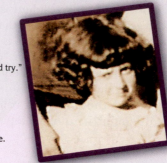

What do you see, nurse, what do you see?
　　What are you thinking when you look at me?
A crabbed old woman, not very wise.
　　Uncertain of habit, with faraway eyes.
Who dribbles her food and makes no reply
　　When you say in a loud voice, "I do wish you'd try."
Who seems not to notice the things that you do
　　And forever is losing a stocking or shoe.
Who unresisting or not, lets you do as you will
　　With bathing and feeding, the long day to fill.
Is that what you're thinking, is that what you see?
　　Then open your eyes, you're not looking at me.
I'll tell you who I am as I sit there so still.
　　As I move at your bidding, as I eat at your will.
I'm a small child of ten with a father and a mother,
　　Brothers and sisters who love one another.

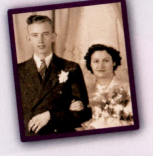

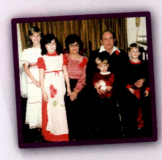

A young girl at sixteen with wings on her feet
　　Dreaming that soon now a lover she'll meet.
A bride soon at twenty—my heart gives a leap
　　Remembering the vows that I promised to keep.
At twenty-five, now, I have young of my own
　　Who need me to build a secure happy home.
A woman of thirty, my young now grow fast
　　Bound to each other with ties that should last.

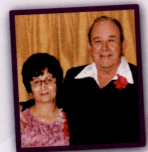

At forty my young will now soon be gone,
　　But my man stays beside me to see I don't mourn.
At fifty once more babies play round my knee.
　　Again we know children, my loved one and me.

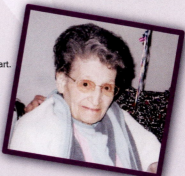

Dark days are upon me, my husband is dead.
　　I look at the future, I shudder with dread.
For my young are all busy rearing young of their own.
　　And I think of the years and the love I have known.

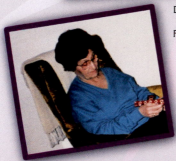

I'm an old woman now and nature is cruel.
　　Tis her jest to make old age look like a fool.
The body it crumbles, grace and vigor depart.
　　There is now just a stone where I once had a heart.
But inside this old carcass a young girl still dwells.
　　And now and again my battered heart swells.

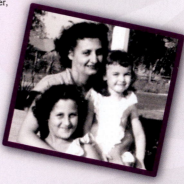

I remember the joys, I remember the pain.
　　And I'm loving and living life all over again.
I think of the years all too few—gone so fast.
　　And accept the stark fact that nothing can last.
So open your eyes, nurse, open and see.
　　Not a crabbed old woman—look closer—SEE ME.

Author Unknown

Review Questions
Self-Examination/Learning Exercise

Select the answer that is most appropriate for each of the following questions:

1. Stanley, age 72, is admitted to the hospital for depression. His son reports that he has periods of confusion and forgetfulness. In her admission assessment, the nurse notices an open sore on Stanley's arm. When she questions him about it he says, "I scraped it on the fence two weeks ago. It's smaller than it was." How might the nurse analyze these data?
   a. Consider that Stanley may have been attempting self-harm.
   b. The delay in healing may indicate that Stanley has developed skin cancer.
   c. A diminished inflammatory response in the elderly increases healing time.
   d. Age-related skin changes and distribution of adipose tissue delay healing in the elderly.

2. What is the most appropriate way to communicate with an elderly person who is deaf in his right ear?
   a. Speak loudly into his left ear.
   b. Speak to him from a position on his left side.
   c. Speak face-to-face in a high-pitched voice.
   d. Speak face-to-face in a low-pitched voice.

3. Why is it important for the nurse to check the temperature of the water before an elderly individual gets into the shower?
   a. The client may catch cold if the water temperature is too low.
   b. The client may burn himself because of a higher pain threshold.
   c. Elderly clients have difficulty discriminating between hot and cold.
   d. The water must be exactly 98.6°F.

4. Mr. B, age 79, is admitted to the psychiatric unit for depression. He has lost weight and has become socially isolated. His wife died 5 years ago, and his son tells the nurse, "He did very well when Mom died. He didn't even cry." Which would be the priority nursing diagnosis for Mr. B?
   a. Complicated grieving
   b. Imbalanced nutrition: Less than body requirements
   c. Social isolation
   d. Risk for injury

5. Mr. B, age 79, is admitted to the psychiatric unit for depression. He has lost weight and has become socially isolated. His wife died 5 years ago, and he lives alone. A suicide assessment is conducted. Why is Mr. B at high risk for suicide?
   a. All depressed people are at high risk for suicide.
   b. Mr. B is in the age group in which the highest percentage of suicides occur.
   c. Mr. B is a white man, recently bereaved, living alone.
   d. His son reports that Mr. B owns a gun.

6. Mr. B, age 79, is admitted to the psychiatric unit for depression. He has lost weight and has become socially isolated. His wife died 5 years ago, and his son tells the nurse, "He did very well when Mom died. He didn't even cry." Which would be the priority nursing intervention for Mr. B?
   a. Take blood pressure once each shift.
   b. Ensure that Mr. B attends group activities.
   c. Encourage Mr. B to eat all of the food on his food tray.
   d. Encourage Mr. B to talk about his wife's death.

7. In group exercise, Mr. B, a 79-year-old man with major depression, reports feeling tired and states "Nothing is going to help." Which nursing action should take priority?
   a. Assess Mr. B. for suicide risk.
   b. Encourage Mr. B. to get more sleep.
   c. Give Mr. B. prn antianxiety medication.
   d. Instruct Mr. B. that if he doesn't participate in the activity he will have to leave the group.

Continued

Review Questions—cont'd
Self-Examination/Learning Exercise

8. Clara, an 80-year-old woman, says to the nurse, "I'm all alone now. My husband is gone. My best friend is gone. My daughter is busy with her work and family. I might as well just go, too." Which is the best response by the nurse?
   a. "Are you thinking that you want to die, Clara?"
   b. "You have lots to live for, Clara."
   c. "Cheer up, Clara. You have so much to be thankful for."
   d. "Tell me about your family, Clara."

9. An elderly patient says to the nurse, "I don't want to go to that crafts class. I'm too old to learn anything." Based on knowledge of the aging process, which of the following is a true statement?
   a. Memory functioning in the elderly most likely reflects loss of long-term memories of remote events.
   b. Intellectual functioning declines with advancing age.
   c. Learning ability remains intact, but time required for learning increases with age.
   d. Cognitive functioning is rarely affected in aging individuals.

10. According to the literature, which of the following is most important for individuals to maintain a healthy, adaptive old age?
    a. To remain socially interactive
    b. To disengage slowly in preparation of the last stage of life
    c. To move in with family
    d. To maintain total independence and accept no help from anyone

IMPLICATIONS OF RESEARCH FOR EVIDENCE-BASED PRACTICE

Jeste, D. V., Savla, G. N., Thompson, W. K., Vahia, I. V., Glorioso, D. K., Martin, A. S., . . . Depp, C. (2013). Association between older age and successful aging: Critical role of resilience and depression. *American Journal of Psychiatry, 170*, 188–196.

DESCRIPTION OF THE STUDY: This study was a Successful Aging Evaluation (SAGE) study of 1,006 community-dwelling adults between 55 and 99 years of age. The mean age of respondents was 77.3 years. Telephone interviews were conducted for 25 minutes followed by a comprehensive mail-in survey in which physical, cognitive, and psychological domains were assessed. In addition, participants completed a self-reported rating of successful aging.

RESULTS OF THE STUDY: Contrary to the researchers' hypothesis, older age was associated with higher reported ratings of successful aging in spite of worsening physical and cognitive functions. The two factors contributing most to successful aging were higher scores on resilience and lower scores on depression. These were similar in strength to physical disability as an influential factor in successful aging. The authors

identify, therefore, that interventions focused on increasing resilience and decreasing depression might be factors as strong as decreasing physical disability in contributing to successful aging. They add that the study highlighted the benefits of self-measurement tools. This is supported by the fact that when people were asked about their own perceptions, information was revealed that was contrary to what was expected.

IMPLICATIONS FOR NURSING PRACTICE: First, this study underscores the importance of thorough assessment to rule out depression in the elderly and to initiate intervention as soon as possible when it is identified. Historically, depression has been underrecognized and undertreated in this population, and we are learning that reducing depression may have a significant impact on successful aging. Second, nurses can play an active role in assessing, educating, and initiating other interventions to promote resilience in the elderly. Finally, as the authors suggest, using self-reporting measures provides a valuable tool for identifying the abilities and needs of this population. Stated more simply, when healthcare providers listen to what the patient has to say, there is much to be learned, and it lays the foundation for patient-centered care.

TEST YOUR CRITICAL THINKING SKILLS

Mrs. M, age 76, is seeing her primary physician for her regular 6-month physical examination. Mrs. M's husband died 2 years ago, at which time she sold her home in Kansas and came to live in California with her only child, a daughter. The daughter is married and has three children (one in college and two teenagers at home). The daughter reports that her mother is becoming increasingly withdrawn, stays in her room, and eats very little. She has lost 13 pounds since her last 6-month visit. The primary physician refers Mrs. M to a psychiatrist, who hospitalizes her for evaluation. He diagnoses Mrs. M with Major Depressive Disorder.

Mrs. M tells the nurse, "I didn't want to leave my home, but my daughter insisted. I would have been all right. I miss my friends and my church. Back home I drove my car everywhere. But there's too much traffic out here. They sold my car, and I have to depend on my daughter or grandkids to take me places. I hate being so dependent! I miss my husband so much. I just sit and think about him and our past life all the time. I don't have any interest in meeting new people. I want to go home!"

Mrs. M admits to having some thoughts of dying, although she denies feeling suicidal. She denies having a plan or means for taking her life. "I really don't want to die, but I just can't see much reason for living. My daughter and her family are so busy with their own lives. They don't need me—or even have time for me!"

Answer the following questions about Mrs. M:

1. What would be the *primary* nursing diagnosis for Mrs. M?
2. Formulate a short-term goal for Mrs. M.
3. From the assessment data, identify the major problem that may be a long-term focus of care for Mrs. M.

 MOVIE CONNECTIONS

The Hiding Place • On Golden Pond • To Dance With the White Dog • 5 Flights Up • Still Alice • The Second Best Exotic Marigold Hotel

References

Administration on Aging (AoA). (2018). *2017 Profile of older Americans.* Retrieved from https://www.acl.gov/sites/default/files/Aging%20and%20Disability%20in%20America/2017OlderAmericansProfile.pdf

American Association of Retired Persons (AARP). (2010). *Sex, romance, and relationships: AARP survey of midlife and older adults.* Washington, DC: Author.

American Foundation for Suicide Prevention (AFSP). (2018). *Suicide statistics.* Retrieved from https://afsp.org/about-suicide/suicide-statistics/

Blevins, N. H. (2018). *Presbycusis.* Waltham, MA: UpToDate Inc. Retrieved from http://www.uptodate.com/contents/presbycusis

Cahill, K. E., Giandrea, M. D., & Quinn, J. F. (2011). Reentering the labor force after retirement. Bureau of Labor Statistics. *Monthly Labor Review, 134*(6), 34–42.

Centers for Disease Control and Prevention (CDC). (2018). *Depression is not a normal part of growing older.* Retrieved from http://www.cdc.gov/aging/mentalhealth/depression.htm

Crowley, K. (2011). Sleep and sleep disorders in older adults. *Neuropsychology Review, 21*(1), 41–53. doi:10.1007/s11065-010-9154-6

Dean, W. (2018). *Neuroendocrine theory of aging: Chapter 1.* Retrieved from http://warddeanmd.com/articles/neuroendocrine-theory-of-aging-chapter-1

Dilman, V. (1954). *Data regarding the origin of climacteric and the role of age-associated "perestroika" in the elevation of blood pressure, blood cholesterol levels, and body weight* (Master's thesis, Leningrad).

Galasko, D. R. (2017). The aging brain. In B. J. Sadock, V. A. Sadock, & P. Ruiz (Eds.), *Comprehensive textbook of psychiatry* (10th ed., pp. 3986–3995). Philadelphia, PA: Wolters Kluwer.

Heiss, G., Wallace, R., Anderson, G. L., Aragak, A., Beresford, S. A. A., Brzyski, R., . . . Stefanick, M. L. (2008). Health risks and benefits three years after stopping randomized treatment with estrogen and progestin. *Journal of the American Medical Association, 299*(9), 1036–1045.

Issa, J. P. (2014). Aging and epigenetic drift: A vicious cycle. *Journal of Clinical Investigation, 124*(1), 24–29.

Jeste, D. V. (2017). Introduction to geriatric psychiatry. In B. J. Sadock, V. A. Sadock, & P. Ruiz (Eds.), *Comprehensive textbook of psychiatry* (10th ed., pp. 3947–3955). Philadelphia, PA: Wolters Kluwer.

Jeste, D. V., Savla, G. N., Thompson, W. K., Vahia, I. V., Glorioso, D. K., Martin, A. S., . . . Depp, C. (2013). Association between older age and successful aging: Critical role of resilience and depression. *American Journal of Psychiatry, 170*, 188–196.

Johnston, C. B., Harper, G. M., & Landefeld, C. S. (2013). Geriatric disorders. In S. J. McPhee & M. A. Papadakis (Eds.), *Current medical diagnosis and treatment* (pp. 57–73). New York, NY: McGraw Hill Medical.

Kern, M. L., & Friedman, H. S. (2008). Do conscientious individuals live longer? A quantitative review. *Health Psychology, 27*(5), 505–512. doi:10.1037/0278-6133.27.5.505

King, B. M., & Regan, P. (2013). *Human sexuality today* (8th ed.). Upper Saddle River, NJ: Pearson Prentice Hall.

Koop, P. M. (2012). Older adults as caregivers and care recipients. In J. W. Lange (Ed.), *The nurse's role in promoting optimal health of older adults* (pp. 295–305). Philadelphia, PA: F. A. Davis.

Lehto, R. H., & Stein, K. I. (2009). Death anxiety: An analysis of an evolving concept. *Research and Theory for Nursing Practice, 23*(1), 23–41.

Manson, A. E., Chlebowski, R. T., Stefanick, M. L., Aragaki, A. K., Rossouw, J. E., Prentice, R. L., & Wallace, R. B. (2013). Menopausal hormone therapy and health outcomes during the intervention and extended poststopping phases of the Women's Health Initiative randomized trials. *Journal of the American Medical Association, 310*(13), 1353–1368. doi:10.1001/jama.2013.278040

Mayo Clinic. (2018). *Hormone therapy: Is it right for you?* Retrieved from https://www.mayoclinic.org/diseases-conditions/menopause/in-depth/hormone-therapy/art-20046372

McCarthy, V. L., & Bockweg, M. (2012). The role of transcendence in a holistic view of successful aging: A concept analysis and model of transcendence in maturation and aging. *Journal of Holistic Nursing, 31*(2), 84–92. doi:10.1177/0898010112463492

McCarthy, V. L., Ling, J., & Carini, R. M. (2013). The role of self-transcendence: A missing variable in the pursuit of successful aging? *Research in Gerontological Nursing, 6*(3), 178–186.

McClatchey, I. S., & King, S. (2015). The impact of death education on fear of death and death anxiety among human services students. *Omega (Westport), 71*(4), 343–361.

MedlinePlus. (2018). *Aging changes in the senses.* Retrieved from https://medlineplus.gov/ency/article/004013.htm

Missler, M., Stroebe, M., Geurtsen, L., Mastenbroek, M., Chmoun, S., & van der Houwen, K. (2012). Exploring death anxiety among elderly people: A literature review and empirical investigation. *Omega (Westport), 64*(4), 357–379.

Murray, R. B., Zentner, J. P., & Yakimo, R. (2009). *Health promotion strategies through the life span* (8th ed.). Upper Saddle River, NJ: Prentice Hall.

National Center for Health Statistics (NCHS). (2017). *Health, United States, 2016: With chartbook on long-term trends in Health.* Hyattsville, MD. Retrieved from https://www.cdc.gov/nchs/data/hus/hus16.pdf#015

National Crime Justice Reference Center. (2017). *Elder victimization fact sheet.* Retrieved from https://ovc.ncjrs.gov/ncvrw2017/images/en_artwork/Fact_Sheets/2017NCVRW_ElderVictimization_508.pdf

National Council on Aging. (2018). *Elder abuse facts.* Retrieved from https://www.ncoa.org/public-policy-action/elder-justice/elder-abuse-facts/

National Institutes of Health (NIH). (2018). *Aging changes in immunity.* Retrieved from https://www.nlm.nih.gov/ medlineplus/ency/article/004008.htm

News Medical. (2014). *Transcendence is the best predictor of positive aging, study show.* Retrieved from https://www.news-medical.net/news/20140521/Transcendence-is-the-best-predictor-of-positive-aging-shows-study.aspx

Rogers, K., Guarente, L. P., & Simic, P. (2018). *Aging: Life process.* Retrieved from http://www.britannica.com/science/aging-life-process

Sadock, B. J., Sadock, V. A., & Ruiz, P. (2015). *Synopsis of psychiatry: Behavioral sciences/clinical psychiatry* (11th ed.). Philadelphia, PA: Wolters Kluwer.

Shock, N. W. (2018). *Human aging: Physiology and sociology.* Retrieved from http://www.britannica.com/science/human-aging

Srivastava, S., & Das, R. C. (2013). Personality pathways of successful ageing. *Industrial Psychiatry Journal, 22*(1), 1–3. doi:10.4103/0972-6748.123584

Srivastava, S., John, O. P., Gosling, S. D., & Potter, J. (2003). Development of personality in early and middle adulthood: Set like plaster or persistent change? *Journal of Personality and Social Psychology, 84*(5), 1041–1053.

Sutin, A. R., Stephan, Y., & Terracciano, A. (2018). Facets of conscientiousness and risk of dementia. *Psychological Medicine, 48,* 974–982. https://doi.org/10.1017/S0033291717002306

Terracciano, A., Sanna, S., Uda, M., Deiana, B., Usala, G., Busonero, F., . . . Costa, P. T. (2010). Genome-wide association scan for five major dimensions of personality. *Molecular Psychiatry, 15*(6), 647–656. doi:10.1038/mp.2008.113

Thomas, P. A. (2011). Trajectories of social engagement and limitations in late life. *Journal of Health and Social Behavior, 52*(4), 430–443. doi:10.1177/0022146511411922

Toossi, M., & Torpey, E. (2017). *Older workers: Labor force trends and career options.* Retrieved from https://www.bls.gov/careeroutlook/2017/article/older-workers.htm

Westerhof, G. J., Whitbourne, S. K., & Freeman, J. P. (2012). The aging self in a cultural context: The relation of conceptions of aging to identity processes and self-esteem in the United States and the Netherlands. *Journals of Gerontology. Series B, Psychological Sciences and Social Sciences. 67*(1), 52–60. doi:10.1093/geronb/gbr075

Venes, D. (Ed.). (2017). *Taber's cyclopedic medical dictionary* (23rd ed.). Philadelphia. PA: F. A. Davis.

Yang, X., & Reckelhoff, J. F. (2011). Estrogen, hormonal replacement therapy and cardiovascular disease. *Current Opinion in Nephrology and Hypertension, 20*(2), 133–138. doi:10.1097/MNH.0b013e3283431921

Classical References

Erikson, E. H. (1963). *Childhood and society* (2nd ed.). New York, NY: WW Norton.

Erikson, E. H., & Erikson, J. M. (1997). *The life cycle completed: Extended version with new chapters on the ninth stage of development.* New York, NY: Norton.

Kübler-Ross, E. (1969). *On death and dying.* New York, NY: Macmillan.

Masters, W. H., Johnson, V. E., & Kolodny, R. C. (1995). *Human sexuality* (5th ed.). New York, NY: Addison-Wesley Longman.

Roberts, C. M. (1991). *How did I get here so fast?* New York, NY: Warner Books.

Rogers-Seidl, F. F. (1997). *Geriatric nursing care plans* (2nd ed.). St. Louis, MO: Mosby Year Book.

Rowe, J. W., & Kahn, R. L. (1997). Successful aging. *Gerontology, 37*(4), 433–440.

Survivors of Abuse or Neglect

25

CORE CONCEPTS

Abuse

Battering

Incest

Neglect

Rape

KEY TERMS

acquaintance rape

child sexual abuse

compounded rape reaction

controlled response pattern

cycle of battering

date rape

emotional abuse

emotional neglect

expressed response pattern

intimate partner violence

marital rape

physical neglect

rape trauma syndrome

safe houses or shelters

sexual exploitation of a child

silent rape reaction

statutory rape

OBJECTIVES
After reading this chapter, the student will be able to:

1. Describe epidemiological statistics associated with intimate partner violence, child abuse, and sexual assault.
2. Discuss characteristics of victims and victimizers.
3. Identify predisposing factors to abusive behaviors.
4. Describe physical and psychological effects on the survivors of intimate partner violence, child abuse, and sexual assault.
5. Identify nursing diagnoses, goals of care, and appropriate nursing interventions for care of survivors of intimate partner violence, child abuse, and sexual assault.
6. Evaluate nursing care of survivors of intimate partner violence, child abuse, and sexual assault.
7. Discuss various modalities relevant to treatment of survivors of abuse.

Introduction

> **CORE CONCEPT**
> **Abuse**
> The maltreatment of one person by another.

Abuse is a significant and frightening public health problem. Books, newspapers, movies, and television inundate their readers and viewers with stories of "man's inhumanity to man" (no gender bias intended).

The most recent Centers for Disease Control and Prevention (CDC, 2018) report on intimate partner and sexual violence identified that

> during their lifetime, 1 in 5 women experienced completed or attempted rape; 1 in 6 women were stalked; and 1 in 4 experienced contact sexual violence, physical violence, and/or stalking by an intimate partner and reported some form of intimate partner violence-related impact. Results indicate that many males are also experiencing these forms of violence. For example, during their lifetime, 1 in 14 men were made to sexually penetrate someone else; 1 in 17 men were stalked; and 1 in 10 experienced contact sexual violence, physical violence, and/or stalking by an intimate partner and reported some form of intimate partner violence-related impact.

The evidence also supports that these forms of violence most often occur before the age of 25 for both men and women. Child abuse and related fatalities continue to be a significant health concern. It is well documented that adverse childhood experiences (ACEs) such as abuse and neglect can have a major impact on health and well-being throughout one's life. ACE studies have found that as the number of ACE events increases, so do risks for myocardial infarction, asthma, diabetes, coronary heart disease, depression, disability, unemployment, mental distress, and other health problems (CDC, 2016). Child abuse includes physical or sexual abuse, psychological maltreatment, and neglect. Data from the U.S.

Department of Health and Human Services (2018) identifies that the majority of abused children (74.8 percent) are neglected, whereas a smaller percentage are physically or sexually abused. Nationally, in 2016, an estimated 1,750 children died of abuse or neglect. Human trafficking, which includes sex trafficking is another form of child abuse that is a significant public health concern. Federal law defines human trafficking as:

> a commercial sex act [that] is induced by force, fraud, or coercion, or in which the person induced to perform such act has not attained 18 years of age or, the recruitment, harboring, transportation, provision, or obtaining of a person for labor or services, through the use of force, fraud, or coercion for the purpose of subjection to involuntary servitude, peonage, debt bondage, or slavery. (U.S. Department of Education, 2013)

Prevalence statistics are difficult to compile, but sex trafficking of children has been reported in all 50 U.S. states, and traffickers have been known to prey on children as young as 9 years of age.

Elder abuse and neglect are also a significant problem. The CDC (2017a) estimates that 1 in 10 people over the age of 60 and living at home is a victim of physical or sexual abuse, neglect (the most common form of elder abuse), abandonment, and/or financial exploitation. *Institutional abuse* refers to elder adults who live in residential facilities and are victimized by any of the above-mentioned forms of abuse. There is general agreement that statistics underestimate the scope of the problem. Despite mandatory reporting laws in most states and the recent trend toward more reporting of abuse, adult protective services vary markedly from state to state. One study found that for every 1 case that came to the attention of these agencies, 24 had not been reported (National Center on Elder Abuse [NCEA], n.d.).

Abuse affects all populations equally. It occurs among all races, religions, economic classes, ages, and educational backgrounds. Many abusers were themselves victims of abuse as children.

Family violence is not a new problem; in fact, it is probably as old as humankind and has been documented as far back as Biblical times. Child abuse became a mandatory reportable occurrence in the United States in 1968. Responsibility for the protection of elders from abuse rests primarily with the states. In 1987, Congress passed amendments to the Older Americans Act of 1965 that provide for state Area Agencies on Aging to assess the need for elder abuse prevention services. These events have made it possible for individuals who once felt powerless to stop the abuse against them to come forward and seek advice, support, and protection.

This chapter discusses intimate partner violence, child abuse (including neglect), and sexual assault. Elder abuse is discussed in Chapter 24, The Aging Individual. Factors that predispose individuals to commit acts of abuse against others, as well as the physical and psychological effects on the survivors, are examined.

Nursing of individuals who have experienced abusive behavior from others is presented within the context of the nursing process. Various treatment modalities are described.

Predisposing Factors

What predisposes individuals to be abusive? Although no one really knows for sure, several theories have been espoused. As researchers have sought to better understand aggression and violence, two distinct forms of aggression have been identified: *reactive* aggression, which is associated with impulsivity and is more common among people who have a history of being abused, and *proactive* aggression, which is initiated rather than provoked and is more common in psychopathy (Rosell & Siever, 2015). Most research is associated with reactive aggression, and the following is a brief discussion of current evidence associated with biological, psychological, and sociocultural influences.

Biological Theories

Neurophysiological Influences

Research demonstrates consistently that lower volume of the amygdala plays a role in aggression (Rosell & Siever, 2015). The amygdala, which is responsible for impulse control and affective processing, appears to be less well modulated in people with aggression, and responses to fear are reduced. The limbic prefrontal cortex also has a primary role in aggression; smaller volumes of left-sided gray matter and greater right-sided volume have been noted in people with aggressive traits. Evidence has also demonstrated lowered

connectivity between the amygdala and the prefrontal cortex as associated with increased aggression. The striatum, an area of the brain that plays a critical role in selection and inhibition of affective, cognitive, and motor responses, has been identified as dysfunctional in aggression (Rosell & Siever, 2015).

Biochemical Influences

Studies have associated increased dopamine release with aggression, and low levels of striatal serotonin have been associated with increases in impulsivity and aggression (Rosell & Siever, 2015). Evidence supports that high plasma (and low cerebrospinal fluid) concentrations of 5-hydroxyindoleacetic acid (5-HIAA) serotonin are associated with aggression (Sadock, Sadock, & Ruiz, 2015). Finally, research is showing that a complex interaction between testosterone and cortisol levels is associated with aggression. Research is ongoing to explore these mechanisms, their interactions in the brain, and the influence of environmental factors. An explanation of these biochemical influences on violent behavior is presented in Figure 25–1.

Genetic Influences

Various genetic components related to aggressive behavior have been investigated. Studies have found a potential role for the X-linked monoamine oxidase A gene in the etiology of antisocial behaviors (Sadock et al., 2015). Mutations in this gene may have implications for impulsivity and aggression, but further research is needed. Human and animal genetics studies show a strong role for 5-HT transporter genes in aggression. It has also been demonstrated that stressful life events can influence some gene variants in the development of aggressive tendencies.

Disorders of the Brain

Organic brain syndromes associated with various cerebral disorders have been implicated in the predisposition to aggressive and violent behavior (Sadock et al., 2015). Brain tumors, particularly in the areas of the limbic system and the temporal lobes; trauma to the brain, resulting in cerebral changes; and diseases, such as encephalitis (or medications that may effect this syndrome) and epilepsy, particularly temporal lobe epilepsy, have all been implicated.

Psychological Theories

Psychodynamic Theory

Psychodynamic theorists suggest that unmet needs for satisfaction and security result in an underdeveloped ego and a weak superego. It is thought that

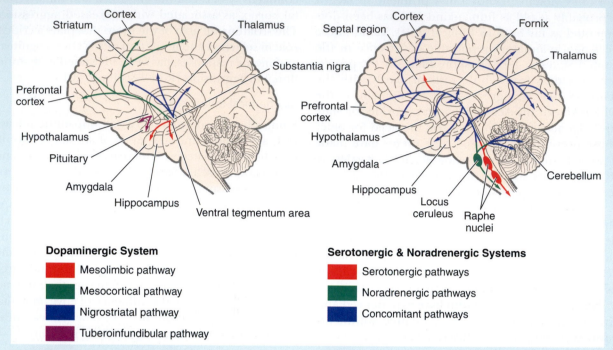

FIGURE 25-1 Neurobiology of violence.

NEUROTRANSMITTERS

Neurotransmitters that have been implicated in the etiology of aggression and violence include decreases in serotonin and increases in norepinephrine and dopamine.

ASSOCIATED AREAS OF THE BRAIN

- Limbic structures: Emotional alterations
- Prefrontal and frontal cortices: Modulation of social judgment
- Amygdala: Anxiety, rage, fear
- Hypothalamus: Stimulates sympathetic nervous system in "fight-or-flight" response
- Hippocampus: Learning and memory

MEDICATIONS USED TO MODULATE AGGRESSION

1. Studies have suggested that selective serotonin reuptake inhibitors (SSRIs) may reduce irritability and aggression consistent with the hypothesis of reduced serotonergic activity in aggression.
2. Mood stabilizers that dampen limbic irritability may be important in reducing the susceptibility to react to provocation or threatening stimuli by overactivation of limbic system structures such as the amygdala (Rosell & Siever, 2015). Carbamazepine (Tegretol), phenytoin (Dilantin), and divalproex sodium (Depakote) have yielded positive results. Lithium has also been used effectively in violent individuals (Schatzberg, Cole, & DeBattista, 2010).
3. Antiadrenergic agents such as beta blockers (e.g., propranolol) have been shown to reduce aggression in some individuals, presumably by dampening excessive noradrenergic activity (Schatzberg et al., 2015).

In their ability to modulate excessive dopaminergic activity, antipsychotics—both typical and atypical—have been helpful in the control of aggression and violence, particularly in individuals with comorbid psychosis.

when frustration occurs, aggression and violence supply this individual with a dose of power and prestige that boosts the self-image and validates a significance to his or her life that is lacking. The immature ego cannot prevent dominant id behaviors from occurring, and the weak superego is unable to produce feelings of guilt.

Learning Theory

Children learn to behave by imitating their role models, which are usually their parents. Models are more likely to be imitated when they are perceived as prestigious or influential or when the behavior is followed by positive reinforcement. Children may have an idealistic perception of their parents during the very early developmental stages but as they mature may begin to imitate the behavior patterns of their teachers, friends, and others. Individuals who were abused as children or who witnessed domestic violence as children are more likely to manifest reactive aggression as adults (Rosell & Siever, 2015).

Adults and children alike model many of their behaviors after individuals they observe on television and in movies. Unfortunately, modeling can result in maladaptive as well as adaptive behavior, particularly when children view heroes triumphing over villains by using violence. It is also possible that individuals who have a biological predisposition toward aggressive behavior may be more susceptible to negative role modeling.

Sociocultural Theories

Societal Influences

Although they agree that some biological and psychological aspects are influential, social scientists believe that aggressive behavior is primarily a product of one's culture and social structure.

Historically, American society has accepted some forms of aggression and violence as the means to solve problems (e.g., engaging in war, physical disciplining of children). However, there is widespread general acceptance that aggression or violence in certain situations is wrong (e.g., child abuse). The concept of relative deprivation has been shown to have a profound effect on collective violence within a society. Poverty, prolonged unemployment, family breakdown, emotional distress, lack of access to resources, and exposure to violence in the community and in the family have all been linked to increases in aggression (American Psychological Association, 2018; Espolage et al., 2013).

Application of the Nursing Process

Background Assessment Data

Data related to **intimate partner violence,** child abuse and neglect, and sexual assault are presented in this section. Characteristics of both victim and abuser are addressed. This information may be used as background knowledge in designing plans of care for these clients.

Intimate Partner Violence

> ### CORE CONCEPT
> **Battering**
> A pattern of coercive control founded on and supported by physical and/or sexual violence or threat of violence of an intimate partner.

Various terms are used to describe the pattern of violence between intimate partners, including intimate partner violence (IPV), domestic violence, and battering.

Tracy (2016) adds to the definition of battering as follows:

> Battering is also known by the term "domestic violence" and refers to acts of violence between two parties in an intimate relationship. Battering happens in heterosexual and homosexual relationships and either a male or a female can be the batterer or victim. Battering may occur in a marriage or in any other form of relationship.

The CDC (2017b) defines intimate partner violence as follows:

> Intimate partner violence includes physical violence, sexual violence, stalking and psychological aggression (including coercive tactics) by a current or former intimate partner (i.e., spouse, boyfriend/girlfriend, dating partner, or ongoing sexual partner). An intimate partner is a person with whom one has a close personal relationship that may be characterized by the partners' emotional connectedness, regular contact, ongoing physical contact and sexual behavior, identity as a couple, and familiarity and knowledge about each other's lives. The relationship need not involve all of these dimensions.

The U.S. Department of Justice (2011) defines *intimate partner violence* as:

> A pattern of abusive behavior that is used by an intimate partner to gain or maintain power and control over the other intimate partner. [Intimate partner] violence can be physical, sexual, emotional, economic, or psychological actions or threats of actions that influence another person. This includes any behaviors that intimidate, manipulate, humiliate, isolate, frighten, terrorize, coerce, threaten, blame, hurt, injure, or wound someone.

Physical abuse between domestic partners may be known as spouse abuse, domestic or family violence, wife or husband battering, or intimate partner violence (IPV). Data from the U.S. Bureau of Justice Statistics (2014a) reflect that over the period from 2003 to 2012: (1) 76 percent of victims of intimate violence were women and 24 percent were men; (2) women ages 18 to 24 years experienced the highest per capita rates of intimate violence; and (3) most of the perpetrators were current or former boyfriends or girlfriends. During the same period, 35.5 percent of domestic violence incidents were identified as "serious violent crime" that included rape or sexual assault, robbery, and/or aggravated assault, and around 9 percent involved serious injuries. Many of the victimizations are not reported to the police, and the main reason given for not reporting is that it was "considered a personal matter."

Profile of the Victim

For the purposes of this chapter, women are identified as the victim (and men as the victimizer) because the largest percentage of victims are women and most of the available data speak specifically about female victims. It should be noted that men may also be victims and victimized in similar ways. Likewise, female perpetrators of IPV may share many of the characteristics that are commonly identified as the profile of male victimizers.

Battered women represent all age, racial, religious, cultural, educational, and socioeconomic groups. They may be married or single, housewives or business executives. Many women who are battered have low self-esteem, commonly adhere to feminine sex-role stereotypes, and often accept the blame for the batterer's actions. Feelings of guilt, anger, fear, and shame are common. They may be isolated from family and support systems.

Some women who are in violent relationships grew up in abusive homes and may have left those homes and have even gotten married at a very young age in order to escape the abuse. The battered woman views her relationship as male dominant, and as the battering continues, her ability to see the options available to her and to make decisions concerning her life (and possibly those of her children) decreases. The phenomenon of *learned helplessness* may be applied to the woman's progressing inability to act on her own behalf. Learned helplessness occurs when an individual comes to understand that regardless of his or her behavior, the outcome is unpredictable and usually undesirable.

Profile of the Victimizer

Men who batter usually are characterized as persons with low self-esteem. Pathologically jealous, they present a "dual personality," one to the partner and one to the rest of the world (Meskill & Conner, 2013). They are often under a great deal of stress but have limited ability to cope with the stress. The typical abuser is very possessive and perceives his spouse as a possession. He becomes threatened when she shows any sign of independence or attempts to share herself and her time with others. Small children are often ignored by the abuser; however, they may also become the targets of abuse as they grow older, particularly if they attempt to protect their mother from abuse. The abuser also may use threats of taking the children away as a tactic of emotional abuse.

The abusive man typically wages a continuous campaign of degradation against his female partner. He insults and humiliates her and everything she does at every opportunity. He strives to keep her isolated from others and totally dependent on him. He demands to know where she is at every moment, and when she tells him, he challenges her honesty. He achieves power and control through intimidation.

The Cycle of Battering

In her classic studies of battered women and their relationships, Walker (1979) identified a cycle of predictable behaviors that are repeated over time. The behaviors can be divided into three distinct phases that vary in time and intensity both within the same relationship and among different couples. Figure 25–2 depicts a graphic representation of the **cycle of battering.**

Phase I. The Tension-Building Phase During this phase, the woman senses that the man's tolerance for frustration is declining. He becomes angry with little provocation but, after lashing out at her, may be quick to apologize. The woman may become very nurturing and compliant, anticipating his every whim in an effort to prevent his anger from escalating. She may just try to stay out of his way.

Minor battering incidents may occur during this phase, and in a desperate effort to avoid more serious confrontations, the woman accepts the abuse as legitimately directed toward her. She denies her anger and rationalizes his behavior (e.g., "I need to do better," "He's under so much stress at work," "It's the alcohol—if only he didn't drink"). She assumes the guilt for the abuse, even reasoning that perhaps she *did* deserve the abuse, just as her aggressor suggests.

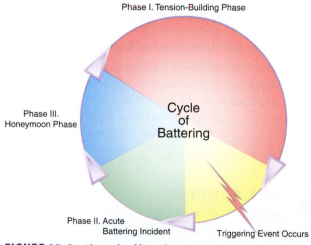

FIGURE 25–2 The cycle of battering.

The minor battering incidents continue, and the tension mounts as the woman waits for the impending explosion. The abuser begins to fear that his partner will leave him. His jealousy and possessiveness increase, and he uses threats and brutality to keep her in his captivity. Battering incidents become more intense, after which the woman becomes less and less psychologically capable of restoring equilibrium. She withdraws from him, which he misinterprets as rejection, further escalating his anger toward her. Phase I may last from a few weeks to many months or even years.

Phase II. The Acute Battering Incident This phase is the most violent and the shortest, usually lasting up to 24 hours. It most often begins with the batterer justifying his behavior to himself. By the end of the incident, however, he cannot understand what has happened, only that in his rage he has lost control over his behavior.

This incident may begin with the batterer wanting to "just teach her a lesson." In some instances, the woman may intentionally provoke the behavior. Having come to a point in phase I in which the tension is unbearable, long-term battered women know that once the acute phase is behind them, things will be better.

During phase II, women feel their only option is to find a safe place to hide from the batterer. The beating is severe, and many women can describe the violence in great detail, almost as if dissociation from their bodies had occurred. The batterer generally minimizes the severity of the abuse. Help is usually sought only in the event of severe injury or if the woman fears for her life or the lives of her children.

Phase III. Calm, Loving, Respite ("Honeymoon") Phase In this phase, the batterer becomes extremely loving, kind, and contrite. He promises that the abuse will never recur and begs her forgiveness. He is afraid she will leave him and uses every bit of charm he can muster to ensure this does not happen. He believes he now can control his behavior, and because now that he has "taught her a lesson," he believes she will not "act up" again.

He plays on her feelings of guilt, and she desperately wants to believe him. She wants to believe that he *can* change, and that she will no longer have to suffer abuse. During this phase, the woman relives her original dream of ideal love and chooses to believe that *this* is what her partner is *really* like.

This loving phase becomes the focus of the woman's perception of the relationship. She bases her reason for remaining in the relationship on this "magical" ideal phase and hopes against hope that the previous phases will not be repeated. This hope is evident even in those women who have lived through a number of horrendous cycles.

Although phase III usually lasts somewhere between the lengths of time associated with phases I and II, it can be so short as to almost pass undetected. In most instances, the cycle soon begins again with renewed tensions and minor battering incidents. In an effort to "steal" a few precious moments of the phase III kind of loving, the battered woman becomes a collaborator in her own abusive lifestyle. Victim and batterer become locked together in an intense, symbiotic relationship.

Why Do They Stay?

Probably the most common response that battered women give for staying is that they fear for their life and/or the lives of their children. As the battering progresses, the man gains power and control through intimidation and instilling fear with threats such as, "I'll kill you and the kids if you try to leave." Challenged by these threats and dealing with her low self-esteem and sense of powerlessness, the woman sees no way out. In fact, she may try to leave only to return when confronted by her partner and the psychological power he holds over her.

Women have been known to stay in an abusive relationship for many reasons, some of which include the following (Dockterman, 2014; Malkin, 2013; Meskill & Conner, 2013):

- **Fear of retaliation:** A woman may have been threatened with murder of herself and her children. Other acts that Dockterman (2014) describes as psychological terrorism are sleep deprivation, blackmail, and murdering pets. Each act may be used to increase fear of retaliation. In the lesbian, gay, bisexual, and transgender community, fear of being outed is sometimes used to manipulate the victim.
- **Fear of losing custody of the children:** Women are sometimes threatened by the spouse that he or she will take away the children. There may have been attempts to convince the woman that she is an unfit mother.
- **Physical or financial dependence:** Victims may fear that they are unable to care for themselves without the victimizer. Victims with disabilities may also be physically dependent on the victimizer for caregiving and financial support.

■ **Lack of a support network:** The victim may be under pressure from family members to stay in the marriage and try to work things out. In addition, the victimizer may have isolated the victim from family and friends.

■ **Cultural/Religious reasons:** Cultural or religious convictions against divorce may dictate trying to save the marriage at all costs.

■ **Hopefulness:** The victim remembers good times and love in the relationship and has hope that her partner will change his behavior and they can have good times again.

■ **Lack of attention to the danger:** Malkin (2013) describes the dissociation that accompanies post-traumatic stress disorder (PTSD), which may contribute to the victim's numbness or lack of awareness of the reality of the situation. Or, as Leslie Morgan Steiner poignantly states in a TED Talk (cited by Dockterman, 2014):

> Why did I stay? I didn't know he was abusing me. Even though he held those loaded guns to my head, pushed me down stairs, threatened to kill our dog, pulled the key out of the car ignition as I drove down the highway, poured coffee grinds on my head as I dressed for a job interview, I never once thought of myself as a battered wife. Instead I was a very strong woman in love with a deeply troubled man, and I was the only person on earth who could help [him] face his demons.

It is important to recognize that when a victim leaves an abusive relationship, the victim is at a 75 percent greater risk of being killed by the partner, and the abuse often does not stop once she has left (Center for Relationship Abuse Awareness, 2018). Clients should be empowered to make that decision and provided with resources and referrals to maximize their safety if they choose to leave, but nonetheless, the decision must be theirs to make.

Child Abuse

Erik Erikson (1963) stated, "The worst sin is the mutilation of a child's spirit." Children are vulnerable and relatively powerless, and the effects of maltreatment are deep and long lasting. Child maltreatment typically includes physical or emotional injury, physical or emotional neglect, or sexual acts inflicted upon a child by a caregiver. The Child Abuse Prevention and Treatment Act (CAPTA), as amended and reauthorized in 2010, identifies a minimum set of acts or behaviors that characterize maltreatment (Child Welfare Information Gateway [CWIG], 2013). States may use these definitions as foundations on which to establish state legislation.

Physical Abuse

Physical abuse of a child includes "any nonaccidental physical injury (ranging from minor bruises to severe fractures or death) as a result of punching, beating, kicking, biting, shaking, throwing, stabbing, choking, hitting (with a hand, stick, strap, or other object), burning, or otherwise harming a child, that is inflicted by a parent, caregiver, or other person who has responsibility for the child" (CWIG, 2013). Maltreatment is considered whether or not the caretaker intended to cause harm or even if the injury resulted from discipline or physical punishment. The most obvious way to detect it is by outward physical signs. However, behavioral indicators also may be evident.

Signs of Physical Abuse Physical abuse may include any of the following (CWIG, 2013). The child:

■ Has unexplained burns, bites, bruises, broken bones, or black eyes.

■ Has fading bruises or other marks noticeable after an absence from school.

■ Seems frightened of the parents and protests or cries when it is time to go home.

■ Shrinks at the approach of adults.

■ Reports injury by a parent or another adult caregiver.

■ Abuses animals or pets.

Physical abuse may be suspected when the parent or other adult caregiver (CWIG, 2013):

■ Offers conflicting, unconvincing, or no explanation for the child's injury.

■ Describes the child as "evil" or in some other very negative way.

■ Uses harsh, physical discipline with the child.

■ Has a history of abuse as a child.

■ Has a history of abusing animals or pets.

Emotional Abuse

Emotional abuse involves a pattern of behavior on the part of the parent or caretaker that results in serious impairment of the child's social, emotional, or intellectual functioning. Examples of emotional injury include belittling or rejecting the child, ignoring the child, blaming the child for things over which he or she has no control, isolating the child from normal social experiences, and using harsh and inconsistent discipline. Emotional maltreatment may be indicated if the child (CWIG, 2013):

■ Shows extremes in behavior, such as overly compliant or demanding behavior, extreme passivity, or aggression.

- Is either inappropriately adult (e.g., parenting other children) or inappropriately infantile (e.g., frequently rocking or head-banging).
- Is delayed in physical or emotional development.
- Has attempted suicide.
- Reports a lack of attachment to the parent.

Emotional abuse may be suspected when the parent or other adult caregiver (CWIG, 2013):

- Constantly blames, belittles, or berates the child.
- Is unconcerned about the child and refuses to consider offers of help for the child's problems.
- Overtly rejects the child.

Physical and Emotional Neglect

> ## CORE CONCEPT
>
> **Neglect**
> **Physical neglect** of a child includes refusal of or delay in seeking healthcare, abandonment, expulsion from the home or refusal to allow a runaway to return home, and inadequate supervision.
>   **Emotional neglect** refers to a chronic failure by the parent or caretaker to provide the child with the hope, love, and support necessary for the development of a sound, healthy personality.

Indicators of Neglect The possibility of neglect may be considered when the child (CWIG, 2013):

- Is frequently absent from school.
- Begs or steals food or money.
- Lacks needed medical or dental care, immunizations, or glasses.
- Is consistently dirty and has severe body odor.
- Lacks sufficient clothing for the weather.
- Abuses alcohol or other drugs.
- States that there is no one at home to provide care.

The possibility of neglect may be considered when the parent or other adult caregiver (CWIG, 2013):

- Appears to be indifferent to the child.
- Seems apathetic or depressed.
- Behaves irrationally or in a bizarre manner.
- Is abusing alcohol or other drugs.

Sexual Abuse of a Child

Various definitions of **child sexual abuse** are available in the literature. CAPTA defines *sexual abuse* as

> Employment, use, persuasion, inducement, enticement, or coercion of any child to engage in, or assist any other person to engage in, any sexually explicit conduct or simulation of such conduct for the purpose

of producing any visual depiction of such conduct; or the rape, and in cases of caretaker or inter-familial relationships, statutory rape, molestation, prostitution, or other form of sexual exploitation of children, or incest with children. (CWIG, 2013)

Included in the definition is **sexual exploitation of a child,** in which a child is induced or coerced into engaging in sexually explicit conduct for the purpose of promoting any performance, and child sexual abuse, in which a child is being used for the sexual pleasure of an adult (parent or caretaker) or any other person.

> ## CORE CONCEPT
>
> **Incest**
> The occurrence of sexual contacts or interaction between, or sexual exploitation of, close relatives or between participants who are related to each other by a kinship bond that is regarded as a prohibition to sexual relations (e.g., caretakers, stepparents, stepsiblings) (Sadock et al., 2015).

Indicators of Sexual Abuse Child sexual abuse may be considered a possibility when the child (CWIG, 2013):

- Has difficulty walking or sitting.
- Suddenly refuses to change for gym or to participate in physical activities.
- Reports nightmares or bedwetting.
- Experiences a sudden change in appetite.
- Demonstrates bizarre, sophisticated, or unusual sexual knowledge or behavior.
- Becomes pregnant or contracts a venereal disease, particularly if under age 14.
- Runs away.
- Reports sexual abuse by a parent or another adult caregiver.
- Attaches very quickly to strangers or new adults in their environment.

Sexual abuse may be considered a possibility when the parent or other adult caregiver (CWIG, 2013):

- Is unduly protective of the child or severely limits the child's contact with other children, especially of the opposite sex.
- Is secretive and isolated.
- Is jealous or controlling with family members.

Characteristics of the Abuser

A number of factors have been associated with adults who abuse or neglect their children. Sadock and associates (2015) report that parents who abuse their children were often victims of abuse in their own early lives and have impaired attachment with their child. Substance use disorders also increase the risk for child abuse and neglect. Hosier (2015) identifies additional characteristics that may be associated with abusive parents:

- Experiencing a stressful life situation (e.g., unemployment, poverty)
- Having few, if any, support systems; commonly isolated from others
- Lacking understanding of child development or care needs
- Lacking adaptive coping strategies; angers easily; has difficulty trusting others
- Expecting the child to be perfect; may exaggerate any mild difference the child manifests from the "usual"

Flaherty and Stirling (2010) identify a number of characteristics of children, their parents, and the environment that increase a child's risk for maltreatment. For example, when a child has a chronic illness, disabilities, or behavioral problems and when parents are ill-equipped to parent, related to their own emotional, behavioral, or substance-use issues, children may become the victim of abuse or neglect. Environmental factors including social isolation, poverty, IPV, and a nonbiologically related male living in the household have also been linked to increased risk. Although individual risk factors don't necessarily predict that a child is in danger, when multiple factors coexist, the risk of child abuse increases.

The Incestuous Relationship

A great deal of attention has been given to the study of father-daughter incest. In these cases, there is usually an impaired sexual relationship between the parents. Communication between the parents is ineffective, which prevents them from correcting their problems. Typically, the father is domineering, impulsive, and physically abusing, whereas the mother is passive and submissive and denigrates her role as wife and mother. She is often aware of, or at least strongly suspects, the incestuous behavior between the father and daughter but may believe in or fear her husband's absolute authority over the family. She may deny that her daughter is being harmed and may actually be grateful that her husband's sexual demands are being met by someone other than herself.

Onset of the incestuous relationship typically occurs when the daughter is 8 to 10 years of age and commonly begins with genital touching and fondling. In the beginning, the child may accept the sexual advances from her father as signs of affection. As the incestuous behavior continues and progresses, the daughter usually becomes more bewildered, confused, and frightened, never knowing whether her father will be paternal or sexual in his interactions with her.

The relationship may become a love-hate situation on the part of the daughter. She continues to strive for the ideal father-daughter relationship but is fearful and hateful of the sexual demands he places on her. The mother may be alternately caring and competitive as she witnesses her husband's possessiveness and affections directed toward her daughter. Out of fear that his daughter may expose their relationship, the father may attempt to interfere with her normal peer relationships (Sadock et al., 2015).

Although the oldest daughter in a family is most vulnerable to becoming a participant in father-daughter incest, some fathers form sequential relationships with several daughters. If incest has been reported with one daughter, it should be suspected with all of the other daughters.

The Adult Survivor of Incest

Several common characteristics have been identified in adults who have experienced incest as children. Basic to these characteristics is a fundamental lack of trust resulting from an unsatisfactory parent-child relationship, which contributes to low self-esteem and a poor sense of identity. Children of incest often feel trapped, for they have been admonished not to talk about the experience and may be afraid, or even fear for their lives, if they are exposed. If they do muster the courage to report the incest, particularly to the mother, they sometimes are not believed. This is confusing to the child, who is then left with a sense of self-doubt, inability to trust his or her own feelings, and inability to trust either parent for protection. The child develops feelings of guilt with the realization over the years that the parents are using him or her in an attempt to solve their own problems.

Childhood sexual abuse commonly disrupts the development of a normal association of pleasure with sexual activity. Peer relationships are often delayed, altered, inhibited, or perverted. In some instances, individuals who were sexually abused as children completely retreat from sexual activity and avoid all close interpersonal relationships throughout life, whereas others may engage in high-risk and frequent sexual activity. Other adult manifestations of childhood sexual abuse in women include diminished libido, pain/penetration disorder, hypersexuality, and promiscuity. In male survivors of childhood sexual abuse, erectile disorder, premature ejaculation, exhibitionistic disorder, and compulsive sexual conquests may occur. Sadock and associates (2015) report that child maltreatment, including repeated sexual abuse, causes changes in a child's brain that are evident on magnetic resonance imaging (MRI) in adult survivors. They add that a robust finding from 20 studies indicates that childhood maltreatment culminates in future increased levels of C-reactive protein, fibrinogen, and pro-inflammatory cytokines. These inflammatory markers increase the adult survivor's risk for multiple physical illnesses. Depression, anxiety, substance use, eating disorders, suicidal behaviors, and a pattern of unstable relationships are also identified as risks that are increased by a history of child maltreatment (Sadock et al., 2015). ACE studies have been instrumental in linking these adverse childhood experiences to future mental, psychosocial, and physical illness.

The conflicts associated with pain (either physical or emotional) and sexual pleasure experienced by children who are sexually abused are often repeated in adult relationships. Betrayal of trust and violations of personal boundaries in childhood contribute to trust issues and interpersonal difficulties in adulthood that increase risk for re-victimization (Cashmore & Shackel, 2013). Women who were abused as children often enter into relationships with men who abuse them physically, sexually, or emotionally. In addition, studies have shown that childhood sexual abuse victims are at greater risk for instability in adult relationships, more sexual partners and sexual problems, and greater negativity toward partners (Cashmore & Shackel, 2013). The researchers add that, although most childhood abuse victims do not become sex offenders in adulthood, of those who are known to be offenders, as many as 75 percent report childhood sexual victimization.

Adult survivors of incest who decide to come forward with their stories usually are estranged from nuclear family members. They may be blamed by family members for disclosing the "family secret" and often are accused of overreacting to the incest. Frequently, the estrangement becomes permanent when family members continue to deny the behavior and the individual is accused of lying. In recent years, a number of celebrities have come forward with stories of their childhood sexual abuse. Some have chosen to make the disclosure only after the death of their parents. Revelation of these past activities can be one way of

contributing to the healing process for which incest survivors so desperately strive.

Sexual Violence

Sexual violence is often equated with rape, but that is only one type of sexual assault. It is important for nurses and other healthcare providers to be aware that sexual violence includes any act of sexual coercion, including penetration, unwanted sexual contact, and noncontact unwanted sexual experiences (CDC, 2018). All of these experiences can result in trauma, and assessment for history of these events is foundational to providing trauma-informed care. Read about Diana's experiences in this chapter's "Real People, Real Stories" feature.

Sexual assault is any type of sexual act in which an individual is threatened or coerced to submit against his or her will. Rape, a type of sexual assault, occurs over a broad spectrum of experiences ranging from the surprise attack by a stranger to insistence on sexual intercourse by an acquaintance or spouse. Regardless of the defining source, one common theme always emerges: rape is an act of aggression, not one of passion.

CORE CONCEPT

Rape

The expression of power and dominance by means of sexual violence, most commonly by men over women, although men may also be rape victims.

Acquaintance rape (called **date rape** if the encounter is a social engagement agreed to by the victim) is a term applied to situations in which the rapist is acquainted with the victim. They may be out on a first date, may have been dating for a number of months, or merely may be acquaintances or schoolmates. College campuses are the location for a staggering number of these types of rapes, a great many of which go unreported. An increasing number of colleges and universities are establishing programs for rape prevention and counseling for survivors of rape.

Marital rape, which has been recognized only in recent years as a legal category, is the case in which a spouse may be held liable for sexual abuse directed at a marital partner against that person's will. Historically, with societal acceptance of the concept of women as marital property, the legal definition of rape held an exemption within the marriage relationship. In 1993, marital rape became a crime in all 50 states, under at least one section of the sexual offenses code. In 17 states and the District of Columbia,

Real People, Real Stories: Diana's Journey

This individual wished to remain anonymous. Diana is not her real name. Her story is a poignant lesson in the various ways that one can be victimized, the long-term impact of such experiences on one's sense of self-esteem and personal safety, and the importance of nurses' understanding of trauma-informed care.

Karyn: I appreciate your willingness to talk about your experiences. If at any time you become uncomfortable discussing these events we don't need to continue. All right?

Diana: I've had a lot of therapy, and I feel like it's important to tell and keep on telling so that, hopefully, something good will come out of it. When I was 6 years old, I had a crush on my best friend's brother. He was 12 years old, and when he started giving me attention, I thought he liked me; until he took me into a room, took my clothes off, and was touching me. He wanted me to take his clothes off, and I said no. I told my mom, and she intervened with his parents, but when a second incident occurred, my mother stopped me from going to my friend's house. I felt a lot of shame and embarrassment, but I never really talked about my feelings. For a long time, I carried around the belief that it was somehow my fault because I had a crush on him. I found out later that there were several other children who he molested and that his mom had implied they were "making it up."

When I was around 8 years old, I was in a toy store and a man came up from behind me and rubbed my rear end under my dress. I ran to get my father, but the perpetrator ran out of the store, and my parents decided not to call the police. They felt like I'd been scared enough. As an adult, I can understand that. But as a child, I felt like someone did a bad thing to me, and I wished that someone had defended me. As a middle schooler, one of the neighborhood girls wanted to play Truth or Dare. I think she did this with a lot of girls. The dare was to take off my clothes after which she put her hands on me. I said no but felt paralyzed with fear when she touched me anyway. She was a year older, and again, I remember feeling powerless and thinking I didn't know what to do.

In another incident in middle school, one of the boys jumped out in front of me in the school hallway and grabbed my breasts. A teacher saw him do it and was going to send him to the principal's office, but the boy looked scared and I somehow thought it must be my job to protect him . . . or maybe I was trying to act like it was no big deal, so I told the teacher to just let him go. I didn't want to get the boy in trouble, and I was so embarrassed and humiliated, I just wanted it to go away. Part of me wishes the teacher hadn't listened to me, though. I don't think that boy had any idea how much he hurt me and how awful it was.

Karyn: I think that may be a common reaction by girls or women; even though someone has offended against us, we don't want to hurt them in return. And it minimizes the fact that we have been hurt.

Diana: Yes, and my parents were knee deep in the Catholic training that if someone hurts you, you should just walk away or turn the other cheek. That influenced my own thinking, that you don't defend yourself—you should just walk away and avoid conflict. But that's a misunderstanding of the "turn the other cheek" teaching, which is really about showing forgiveness when people demonstrate remorse. It doesn't mean letting people hurt you without consequences. Around this time, I started putting on a lot of weight. I've always felt it was, in part, a reaction meant to keep people at a distance, so they couldn't hurt me.

Karyn: I've heard other people share a similar coping or defense mechanism; doing something simply to keep people away. Was that effective?

Diana: It only added to my self-esteem issues. I struggled with the question of why these things were happening to me. I felt like I must be doing something wrong. As a teenager, I struggled with anxiety and depression, and I was sent to a psychiatrist, but it wasn't helpful. Then when I moved to New York City for college, there were a couple of incidents on the subway. One was a frail-looking elderly man who stuck his hand between my legs, and when I turned around to confront him, he was laughing at me. I felt very powerless. I thought about kicking him, but, again, I didn't want to injure this shriveled-up old man, and I also didn't know if he had a knife, a gun. . . . So there's the fear, the powerlessness, and the anger that someone was touching me and laughing at me, and I could do nothing. I wondered if I was sending out some vibe—i.e., it must be my fault. My friend told me I needed to learn how to put on an angry face and carry an umbrella to better defend myself. I knew I had anxiety and self-esteem issues, and that's when I decided I needed therapy.

Karyn: That took a lot of courage to identify what you needed to do to take some control back. What has been most helpful about that process?

Diana: I explored the underpinnings of my self-esteem issues and identified coping skills, but nonetheless, as an adult many things can trigger the feelings of vulnerability, anxiety, and low self-esteem: news stories about rape or abuse, or times when women or children are demeaned in the media, especially from people manipulating their power or authority. That brings up a lot of "stuff" for me. When my counselor challenged me to identify what was in the way of being able to set all this stuff aside—that's when I had the insight that I just wanted to know something good could come out of all this pain.

Karyn: One of the things you've told me is that you've been able to teach your daughters how to respond in such situations.

Diana: Yes, that was important and felt like a victory. I'm better able to identify potentially harmful situations. I've taught them to listen to that inner voice, where you get

Real People, Real Stories: Diana's Journey—cont'd

that "bad feeling" you can get that warns you when you're in a situation that may require defending or protecting yourself, and I taught my daughters how to be prepared. I've told them that if someone tries to touch them, it's okay to fight back. It's okay to tell me, school officials, tell anyone, and to keep telling until someone believes them and responds. I want them to know that it's safe to talk to me about their feelings and that they are not powerless.

Karyn: I think that's an important message for healthcare professionals as well: to listen, to not brush off someone's experiences but rather to explore the events, thoughts, and feelings and identify coping strategies.

Diana: Yes, I think sometimes adults who thought it was less traumatizing for me to walk away or try to forget about it thought they were helping, but that's not the answer. Even now, after all these years, I wasn't sure if you would think my story was important enough to tell, I mean, to some people, it might not seem so bad. I wasn't raped, it wasn't a family member—but it still left me feeling awful.

Karyn: I think your story is very important to tell. You are taking the opportunity to teach others that victimization can occur in a variety of ways, that it can have long-term effects on self-esteem, and that it is important to find ways to regain a sense of control and self-worth. I really appreciate your sharing this. What do you think are the most important things that nurses need to know about your and others' experience with victimization and trauma?

Diana: First of all, that 40 years later, those incidents still affect me. I saw a picture of the boy who molested me

on a friend's Facebook page, and I felt sick and afraid all over again. And I beat myself up for still letting it get to me. Nurses need to know that even events that happened years ago can influence one's emotional responses in the present.

Second, the idea of "getting closure," even so many years later, is a misnomer. Certain things can trigger those memories and anxieties, and when they come back, all you can do is drag them out and talk about them again and again and again. It's another version of "you tell and you tell and you don't stop telling" until you remember that you survived it, that it wasn't your fault, and that you don't need to feel ashamed or embarrassed or humiliated (even if part of you still does).

Third, I want nurses to know that they are the front lines, and no matter what clinical area they practice in, a history of sexual trauma or abuse can affect how their patients experience and receive healthcare. I had a lot of trouble as an adult fertility patient, having to dress and undress so many times and deal with so many invasive procedures. It was important to tell my healthcare providers why my heart was pounding, why I seemed so nervous, why I hated mammographies and regular GYN exams a little bit more than the average woman. . . . That, as always, a nurse's ability to care and offer compassion can make the biggest difference, and it all begins with trust and helping your patient to "tell." And I wanted to say thank you for the times those nurses held my hand, and squeezed tight, and told me that I would be okay.

---

there are no exemptions from rape prosecution granted to husbands. However, in 33 states, there are still some exemptions given to husbands from rape prosecution, and in all states where husbands can be prosecuted, the criteria for proving marital rape are very stringent.

Statutory rape is defined as unlawful intercourse between a person who is over the age of consent with a person who is under the age of consent. In the United States, legal age of consent varies from state to state, ranging from age 16 to 18 (Barnett, 2016). An adult who has intercourse with a person who is under the age of consent can be arrested for statutory rape, even if the interaction occurred between consenting individuals.

Profile of the Victimizer

It is difficult to profile a rapist because rapists comprise a heterogenous group and are not distinguished by looks or intelligence. Sadock and associates (2015)

identify that the underlying motives of rape perpetrators can be classified into four groups: sexual sadists who are aroused by inflicting pain, exploitative predators who are using the victim to gratify needs such as dominance and power, inadequate men who are obsessed with fantasies of sex that they believe cannot be achieved without force, and those who are displacing anger and rage. They add that victims of childhood abuse show increased likelihood of perpetrating violence of all kinds in adulthood.

The majority of rapes are premeditated, and some behavioral characteristics that have been identified as associated with premeditation include the perpetrator seeking out a victim who appears to be vulnerable (capable of being overpowered or in an opportunistic position such as being alone or isolated from others); alcohol and drugs such as Rohypnol (flunitrazepam) may serve the purpose of increasing victim vulnerability. The perpetrator may also violate or ignore others' rights in a way that gives them information about whether a potential victim is passive or tolerant of those behaviors. But again, although these behaviors might be observed more commonly, they do not clearly define the complete profile of these perpetrators. Feminist theories suggest that rape is most common in societies that encourage aggressiveness in males, that have distinct gender roles, and in which men regard women's roles as inferior. Male aggressiveness as a cultural norm, however, does not explain why some men become perpetrators of criminal aggression and violence whereas others do not.

In 80 percent of the cases of rape and sexual assault among college-aged females, the offender was known to the victim, and 1 in 10 rapes involved the use of a weapon (U.S. Bureau of Justice Statistics, 2014b). Although statistics such as these help to describe aspects of the problem, understanding the essence of what defines the perpetrator of aggression and violence is the subject of ongoing research.

The Victim

Rape can occur at any age; however, the most recent statistics suggest that the highest-risk age group is females younger than age 34 and that most victims tend to have lower incomes and have never married (U.S. Bureau of Justice Statistics, 2017). Rapes are less likely to be reported than other violent crimes; only 23 percent of rapes or sexual assaults are reported to the police (U.S. Bureau of Justice Statistics, 2017). Most sexual assault victims are single women, and the attack frequently occurs in or close to the victim's own neighborhood.

Although women are at highest risk for being victims of rape perpetrated by males, males may also be victimized by women or other men. Sadock and associates (2015) describe the dynamics as identical and state that in all cases,

> the crime enables the rapist to discharge aggression and aggrandize himself [or herself]. The victim is usually smaller than the rapist, perceived as passive . . . and is used as an object. (p. 826)

Rape survivors who present themselves for care shortly after the crime has occurred likely may be experiencing an overwhelming sense of violation and helplessness that began with the powerlessness and intimidation experienced during the rape. Burgess and Holmström (1974), who developed the classical definition of what has been described as **rape trauma syndrome,** identified two emotional patterns of response that may occur within hours after a rape and with which healthcare workers may be confronted

in the emergency department or rape crisis center. In the **expressed response pattern,** the survivor expresses feelings of fear, anger, and anxiety through such behaviors as crying, sobbing, restlessness, and tension. In the **controlled response pattern,** the feelings are masked or hidden, and a calm, composed, or subdued affect is seen.

The following manifestations may be evident in the days and weeks after the attack (Burgess, 2010):

■ Contusions and abrasions on various parts of the body
■ Headaches, fatigue, sleep pattern disturbances
■ Stomach pains, nausea, and vomiting
■ Vaginal discharge and itching, burning upon urination, rectal bleeding and pain
■ Rage, humiliation, embarrassment, desire for revenge, and self-blame
■ Fear of physical violence and death

The long-term effects of sexual assault depend largely on the individual's ego strength, social support system, and the way he or she was treated as a victim (Burgess, 2010). Various long-term effects include increased restlessness, dreams and nightmares, and phobias (particularly those having to do with sexual interaction). Some women report that it takes years to get over the experience; they describe a sense of vulnerability and a loss of control over their own lives during this period. They feel defiled and unable to wash themselves clean, and some women are unable to remain living alone in their home or apartment.

Some survivors develop a **compounded rape reaction** in which additional symptoms such as depression and suicide, substance abuse, and even psychotic behaviors may be noted (Burgess, 2010). Another variation has been called the **silent rape reaction** in which the survivor tells no one about the assault. Anxiety is suppressed and the emotional burden may become overwhelming. The unresolved sexual trauma may not be revealed until the woman is forced to face another sexual crisis in her life that reactivates the previously unresolved feelings.

Diagnosis and Outcome Identification

Nursing diagnoses are formulated from the data gathered during the assessment phase and with background knowledge regarding predisposing factors to the situation. Some common nursing diagnoses for survivors of abuse include the following:

■ Rape trauma syndrome related to sexual assault evidenced by verbalizations of the attack; bruises and lacerations over areas of body; severe anxiety

- Powerlessness related to cycle of battering evidenced by verbalizations of abuse; bruises and lacerations over areas of body; fear for her safety and that of her children; verbalizations of no way to get out of the relationship
- Risk for delayed development related to abusive family situation

Outcome Criteria

The following criteria may be used to measure outcomes in the care of abuse survivors:

The patient who has been sexually assaulted:

- Is no longer experiencing panic anxiety.
- Demonstrates a degree of trust in the primary nurse.
- Has received immediate attention to physical injuries.
- Has initiated behaviors consistent with the grief response.

The patient who has been physically battered:

- Has received immediate attention to physical injuries.
- Verbalizes assurance of his or her immediate safety.
- Discusses life situation with primary nurse.
- Can verbalize choices from which he or she may receive assistance.

The child who has been abused:

- Has received immediate attention to physical injuries.
- Demonstrates trust in primary nurse by discussing abuse through the use of play therapy.
- Is demonstrating a decrease in regressive behaviors.

Planning and Implementation

Table 25–1 provides a plan of care for the patient who is a survivor of abuse. Nursing diagnoses are presented, along with outcome criteria, appropriate nursing interventions, and rationales for each.

Concept Care Mapping

The concept map care plan (see Chapter 6, The Nursing Process in Psychiatric Mental Health Nursing) is a diagrammatic teaching and learning strategy that allows visualization of interrelationships between medical diagnoses, nursing diagnoses, assessment data, and treatments. An example of a concept map care plan for a patient who is a survivor of abuse is presented in Figure 25–3.

Evaluation

Evaluation of nursing actions to assist survivors of abuse must be considered on both a short- and a long-term basis.

Short-term evaluation may be facilitated by gathering information using the following types of questions:

- Has the individual been reassured of his or her safety?
- Is this evidenced by a decrease in panic anxiety?
- Have wounds been properly cared for and provision made for follow-up care?
- Have emotional needs been attended to?
- Has trust been established with at least one person to whom the patient feels comfortable relating the abusive incident?
- Have available support systems been identified and notified?
- Have options for immediate circumstances been presented?

Long-term evaluation may be conducted by healthcare workers who have an ongoing professional relationship with the individual long after the immediate crisis has passed.

- Is the individual able to conduct activities of daily living satisfactorily?
- Have physical wounds healed properly?
- Is the patient appropriately progressing through the behaviors of grieving?
- Is the patient free of sleep disturbances (nightmares, insomnia); psychosomatic symptoms (headaches, stomach pains, nausea/vomiting); regressive behaviors (enuresis, thumb sucking, phobias); and psychosexual disturbances?
- Is the individual free from problems with interpersonal relationships?
- Has the individual considered the alternatives for change in his or her personal life?
- Has a decision been made relative to the choices available?
- Is he or she satisfied with the decision that has been made?

Treatment Modalities

Crisis Intervention

The focus of the initial interview and follow-up with the patient who has been sexually assaulted is on the rape incident alone. Problems not associated with the rape are not dealt with at this time. The goal of crisis

Table 25–1 | CARE PLAN FOR SURVIVORS OF ABUSE

NURSING DIAGNOSIS: RAPE-TRAUMA SYNDROME
RELATED TO: Sexual assault
EVIDENCED BY: Verbalizations of the attack; bruises and lacerations over areas of body; severe anxiety

OUTCOME CRITERIA	NURSING INTERVENTIONS	RATIONALE
Short-Term Goal ▪ Patient's physical wounds will heal without complication. **Long-Term Goal** ▪ Patient will begin a healthy grief resolution, initiating the process of physical and psychological healing (time to be individually determined).	1. It is important to communicate the following to the individual who has been sexually assaulted: • You are safe here. • I'm sorry that it happened. • I'm glad you survived. • It's not your fault. No one deserves to be treated this way. • You did the best that you could. 2. Explain every assessment procedure that will be conducted and why it is being conducted. Ensure that data collection is conducted in a caring, nonjudgmental manner. 3. Ensure that patient has adequate privacy for all immediate postcrisis interventions. Try to have as few people as possible providing the immediate care or collecting immediate evidence. 4. Encourage patient to give an account of the assault. Listen, but do not probe. 5. Discuss with patient whom to call for support or assistance. Provide information about referrals for aftercare.	1. The victim of rape or sexual assault is often frightened and must be reassured of his or her safety. He or she may also be overwhelmed with self-doubt and self-blame, and these statements instill trust and validate self-worth. 2. This may serve to decrease fear/anxiety and increase trust. 3. The post-trauma patient typically feels extremely vulnerable. Additional people in the environment increase this feeling of vulnerability and serve to escalate anxiety. 4. Nonjudgmental listening provides an avenue for catharsis to begin healing. A detailed account may be required for legal follow-up, and a caring nurse, as patient advocate, may help to lessen the trauma of evidence collection. 5. Because of severe anxiety and fear, patient may need assistance from others during this immediate postcrisis period. Provide referral information in writing for later reference (e.g., psychotherapist, mental health clinic, community advocacy group).

Table 25–1 │ CARE PLAN FOR SURVIVORS OF ABUSE–cont'd

NURSING DIAGNOSIS: POWERLESSNESS

RELATED TO: Cycle of battering

EVIDENCED BY: Verbalizations of abuse; bruises and lacerations over areas of body; fear for own safety and that of children; verbalizations of no way to get out of the relationship

OUTCOME CRITERIA	NURSING INTERVENTIONS	RATIONALE
Short-Term Goal ■ Patient will recognize and verbalize choices available, thereby perceiving some control over life situation. **Long-Term Goal** ■ Patient will exhibit control over life situation by making decision about how to maintain personal safety.	1. In collaboration with physician, ensure that all physical wounds, fractures, and burns receive immediate attention. Take photographs if the individual will permit. 2. Take patient to a private area to do the interview. 3. If patient has come alone or with children, reassure them of their safety. Encourage to discuss the battering incident. Ask questions about whether this has happened before, whether the abuser takes drugs, whether the victim has a safe place to go, and whether he or she is interested in pressing charges. 4. Ensure that "rescue" efforts are not attempted by the nurse. Offer support but remember that the final decision must be made by patient. 5. Stress to patient the importance of safety. Provide information about available resources. These may include crisis hot lines, community groups for victims of abuse, shelters, counseling services, and information regarding the victim's rights in the civil and criminal justice system. Respect the patient's decision about whether to stay or leave the home or marriage.	1. Patient safety is a nursing priority. Photographs may be called in as evidence if charges are filed. 2. If patient is accompanied by the person who did the battering, he or she is not likely to be truthful about the injuries. 3. Some victims attempt to keep secret how their injuries occurred in an effort to protect the partner or because they are fearful that the partner will kill them if they tell. 4. Making one's own decision promotes the patient's sense of control over his or her life situation. Imposing judgments and giving advice are nontherapeutic. 5. Knowledge of available choices decreases the individual's sense of powerlessness. Respecting the patient's decision empowers critical thinking and decision making.

Continued

Table 25–1 | CARE PLAN FOR SURVIVORS OF ABUSE–cont'd

NURSING DIAGNOSIS: RISK FOR DELAYED DEVELOPMENT
RELATED TO: Child abuse

OUTCOME CRITERIA	NURSING INTERVENTIONS	RATIONALE
Short-Term Goal ■ Patient will develop trusting relationship with nurse and report how evident injuries were sustained. **Long-Term Goal** ■ Patient will demonstrate behaviors consistent with age-appropriate growth and development.	1. Perform complete physical assessment of the child. Take particular note of bruises (in various stages of healing), lacerations, and client complaints of pain in specific areas. Do not overlook or discount the possibility of sexual abuse. Assess for nonverbal signs of abuse: aggressive conduct, excessive fears, extreme hyperactivity, apathy, withdrawal, age-inappropriate behaviors. 2. Conduct an in-depth interview with the parent or adult who accompanies the child. Consider: If the injury is being reported as an accident, is the explanation reasonable? Is the injury consistent with the explanation? Is the injury consistent with the child's developmental capabilities? 3. Use games or play therapy to gain child's trust. Use these techniques to assist in describing his or her side of the story.	1. An accurate and thorough physical assessment is required to provide appropriate care for client. 2. Fear of imprisonment or loss of child custody may place the abusive parent on the defensive. Discrepancies may be evident in the description of the incident and lying to cover up involvement is a common defense that may be detectable in an in-depth interview. 3. Establishing a trusting relationship with an abused child is extremely difficult. He or she may not even want to be touched. These types of play activities can provide a nonthreatening environment that may enhance the child's attempt to discuss these painful issues.

intervention is to help survivors return to their previous lifestyle as quickly as possible.

The patient should be involved in the intervention and decision making from the beginning. This involvement promotes a sense of competency, control, and empowerment in decision making. It is the essence of patient-centered care. Because an overwhelming sense of powerlessness accompanies the rape experience, active involvement by the survivor is both a validation of personal worth and the beginning of the recovery process. Crisis intervention is time limited—usually 6 to 8 weeks. If problems resurface beyond this time, the individual is referred for assistance from other agencies (e.g., long-term psychotherapy from a psychiatrist or mental health clinic).

During the crisis period, attention is given to coping strategies for dealing with the symptoms common to the post-trauma client. Initially, the individual undergoes a period of disorganization during which there is difficulty making decisions, extreme or irrational fears, and general mistrust. Observable manifestations may range from stark hysteria to expression of anger and rage to silence and withdrawal. Guilt and feelings of responsibility for the rape, as well as numerous physical manifestations, are common. The crisis counselor will attempt to help the individual draw upon previous successful coping strategies to regain control over his or her life.

If the patient is a victim of domestic violence, the counselor ensures that various resources and options

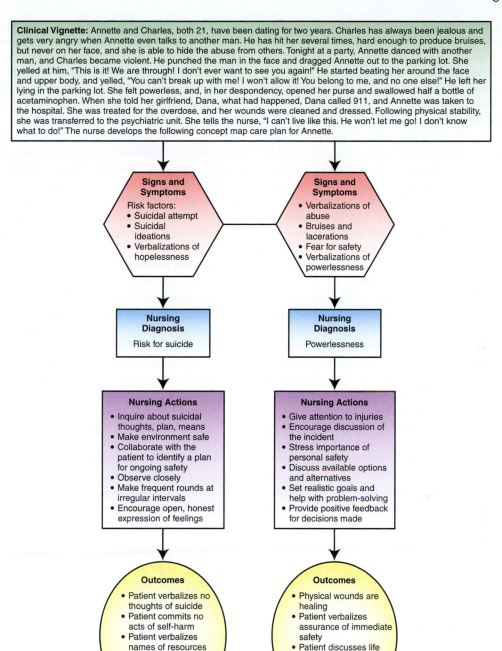

Clinical Vignette: Annette and Charles, both 21, have been dating for two years. Charles has always been jealous and gets very angry when Annette even talks to another man. He has hit her several times, hard enough to produce bruises, but never on her face, and she is able to hide the abuse from others. Tonight at a party, Annette danced with another man, and Charles became violent. He punched the man in the face and dragged Annette out to the parking lot. She yelled at him, "This is it! We are through! I don't ever want to see you again!" He started beating her around the face and upper body, and yelled, "You can't break up with me! I won't allow it! You belong to me, and no one else!" He left her lying in the parking lot. She felt powerless, and, in her despondency, opened her purse and swallowed half a bottle of acetaminophen. When she told her girlfriend, Dana, what had happened, Dana called 911, and Annette was taken to the hospital. She was treated for the overdose, and her wounds were cleaned and dressed. Following physical stability, she was transferred to the psychiatric unit. She tells the nurse, "I can't live like this. He won't let me go! I don't know what to do!" The nurse develops the following concept map care plan for Annette.

Signs and Symptoms

Risk factors:
• Suicidal attempt
• Suicidal ideations
• Verbalizations of hopelessness

Signs and Symptoms

• Verbalizations of abuse
• Bruises and lacerations
• Fear for safety
• Verbalizations of powerlessness

Nursing Diagnosis

Risk for suicide

Nursing Diagnosis

Powerlessness

Nursing Actions

• Inquire about suicidal thoughts, plan, means
• Make environment safe
• Collaborate with the patient to identify a plan for ongoing safety
• Observe closely
• Make frequent rounds at irregular intervals
• Encourage open, honest expression of feelings

Nursing Actions

• Give attention to injuries
• Encourage discussion of the incident
• Stress importance of personal safety
• Discuss available options and alternatives
• Set realistic goals and help with problem-solving
• Provide positive feedback for decisions made

Outcomes

• Patient verbalizes no thoughts of suicide
• Patient commits no acts of self-harm
• Patient verbalizes names of resources outside the hospital that may provide help

Outcomes

• Physical wounds are healing
• Patient verbalizes assurance of immediate safety
• Patient discusses life situation with nurse
• Patient verbalizes available choices and plan of action

FIGURE 25–3   Concept map care plan for a patient with physical abuse.

are made known to the individual so that she or he may make a personal decision regarding next steps. Support groups provide a valuable forum for reducing isolation and learning new strategies for coping with the aftermath of physical or sexual abuse. Particularly for the survivor of rape, the peer support group provides a therapeutic forum for reducing the sense of isolation she may feel in the aftermath of predictable social and interpersonal responses to her experience.

The Safe House or Shelter

Most major cities in the United States now have **safe houses or shelters** where women can go to be assured of protection for them and their children. These shelters provide a variety of services, and the women receive emotional support from staff and each other. Most shelters provide individual and group counseling; help with bureaucratic institutions such as the police, legal representation, and social services; child care and children's programming; and aid for the woman in making future plans, such as employment counseling and linkages with housing authorities. Safe houses have historically catered exclusively to the needs of female victims but recently more safe houses for male victims of domestic violence are surfacing in the United States (Silverman, 2017) and in other countries.

Shelters are usually run by a combination of professional and volunteer staff, including nurses, psychologists, lawyers, and others. Individuals who themselves have been previously abused are often among the volunteer staff members.

Group work is an important part of the service of shelters. Victims in residence range from those in the immediate crisis phase to those who have progressed through a variety of phases of the grief process. Newer members can learn a great deal from those who have successfully resolved similar problems. Length of stay varies and depends on a number of factors, such as outside support network, financial situation, and personal resources.

The shelter provides a haven of physical safety for the victim and promotes expression of the intense emotions he or she may be experiencing. Emotions may include depression, extreme fear, or even violent expressions of anger and rage. In the shelter, one learns that these feelings are normal and that others have also experienced these same emotions in similar situations. The victim is allowed to grieve for what has been lost and for what was expected but not achieved. Help is provided in overcoming the tremendous guilt associated with self-blame. This is a difficult step for someone who has accepted responsibility for another's behavior over a long period.

New arrivals at the shelter are given time to experience the relief from the safety and security provided. Making decisions is discouraged during the period of immediate crisis and disorganization. Once the victim's emotions have become more stable, planning for the future begins. Through information from staff and peers, he or she learns what resources are available within the community. Feedback is provided, but the individual makes his or her own decision about "where to go from here." An individual's decision is accepted and respected.

Family Therapy

The focus of therapy with families who experience violence is to help them develop democratic (respectful,

interactive) ways of solving problems. Studies show that the more a family uses the democratic means of conflict resolution, the less likely they are to engage in physical violence. Families need to learn to deal with problems in ways that can produce mutual benefits for all concerned rather than engaging in power struggles among family members.

Parents also need to learn effective methods of disciplining children that do not include physical punishment. Time-out techniques and methods that emphasize the importance of positive reinforcement for acceptable behavior can be very effective. Family members must be committed to consistent use of this behavior modification technique for it to be successful.

Teaching parents about expectations for various developmental levels may alleviate some of the stress that accompanies these changes. Knowing what to expect from individuals at various stages of development may provide needed anticipatory guidance to deal with the crises commonly associated with these stages.

Therapy sessions with all family members together may focus on problems with family communication. Members are encouraged to express honest feelings in a manner that is nonthreatening to other family members. Active listening, assertiveness techniques, and respecting the rights of others are taught and encouraged. Barriers to effective communication are identified and resolved.

Referrals to agencies that promote effective parenting skills (e.g., parent effectiveness training) may be made. Alternative agencies that may relieve the stress of parenting (e.g., "Mom's Day Out" programs, sitter-sharing organizations, and day-care institutions) also may be considered. Support groups for abusive parents may also be helpful, and assistance in locating or initiating such a group may be provided.

Summary and Key Points

- Abuse is the maltreatment of one person by another.
- Intimate partner violence, child abuse, and sexual assault are widespread.
- Various factors have been theorized as influential in the predisposition to violent behavior. Physiological and biochemical influences within the brain have been suggested, as has the possibility of a direct genetic link.
- Organic brain syndromes associated with various cerebral disorders and traumatic brain injury have been implicated in the predisposition to aggressive and violent behavior.

- Psychoanalytical theorists relate the predisposition to violent behavior to underdeveloped ego and a poor self-concept.
- Learning theorists suggest that children imitate the abusive behavior of their parents. This theory has been substantiated by studies that show that individuals who were abused as children or whose parents disciplined them with physical punishment are more likely to be abusive as adults.
- Societal influences, such as general acceptance of violence as a means of solving problems, also have been implicated.
- Although domestic violence is more frequently perpetrated by men against women, about 24 percent of victims are men.
- Victims who are battered often blame themselves for their situation. They may have been reared in abusive families and have come to expect this type of behavior.
- Battered women commonly see no way out of their present situation and may be encouraged by their social support network to remain in the abusive relationship.
- Child abuse includes physical and emotional abuse, physical and emotional neglect, and sexual abuse.

- A child may experience many years of abuse without reporting it because of fear of retaliation by the abuser.
- Some children report incest experiences to their mothers only to be rebuffed and told to remain secretive about the abuse.
- Research has identified a strong link between adverse childhood experiences (ACEs) (including abuse and neglect) and physical, psychosocial, and mental illness in adulthood.
- Sexual assault is identified as an act of aggression, not passion.
- A history of abuse and neglect in childhood increases one's risk of perpetrating abuse and neglect upon others in adulthood.
- Rape is a traumatic experience, and many victims experience flashbacks, nightmares, rage, physical symptoms, depression, and thoughts of suicide for many years after the occurrence.
- Treatment modalities for survivors of abuse include crisis intervention with the sexual assault victim, safe shelters for battered women (and limited numbers available for men), and therapy for families who use violence.

Review Questions
Self-Examination/Learning Exercise

Select the answer that is most appropriate for each of the following questions:

1. Sharon, a woman with multiple cuts and abrasions, arrives at the emergency department with her three small children. She tells the nurse that her husband inflicted these wounds on her. She says, "I didn't want to come. I'm really okay. He only does this when he has too much to drink. I just shouldn't have yelled at him." Which of the following is the best response by the nurse?
   a. "How often does he drink too much?"
   b. "It is not your fault. You did the right thing by coming here."
   c. "How many times has he done this to you?"
   d. "He is not a good husband. You have to leave him before he kills you."

2. Sharon, a woman with multiple cuts and abrasions, arrives at the emergency department with her three small children. She tells the nurse that her husband inflicted these wounds on her. In the interview, Sharon tells the nurse, "He's been getting more and more violent lately. He's been under a lot of stress at work the last few weeks, so he drinks a lot when he gets home. He always gets mean when he drinks. I was getting scared. So I just finally told him I was going to take the kids and leave. He got furious when I said that and began beating me with his fists." With knowledge about the cycle of battering, what does this situation represent?
   a. Phase I. Sharon was desperately trying to stay out of his way and keep everything calm.
   b. Phase I. A minor battering incident for which Sharon assumes all the blame.
   c. Phase II. The acute battering incident that was provoked by her threat to leave.
   d. Phase III. The honeymoon phase when the husband believes that he has "taught her a lesson and she won't act up again."

Continued

3. A battered woman presents to the emergency department with multiple cuts and abrasions. Her right eye is swollen shut. She says that her husband did this to her. Which of the following is the *priority* nursing intervention?
   a. Tending to the immediate care of her wounds
   b. Providing her with information about a safe place to stay
   c. Administering the prn tranquilizer ordered by the physician
   d. Explaining how she may go about bringing charges against her husband

4. A woman who has a long history of being battered by her husband is staying at the woman's shelter. She has received emotional support from staff and peers and has been made aware of the alternatives open to her. Nevertheless, she decides to return to her home and marriage. Which of the following is the best response by the nurse to the woman's decision?
   a. "I just can't believe you have decided to go back to that horrible man."
   b. "I'm just afraid he will kill you or the children when you go back."
   c. "What makes you think things have changed with him?"
   d. "I hope you have made the right decision. Call this number if you need help."

5. Jana, age 5, is sent to the school nurse's office with an upset stomach. She has vomited and soiled her blouse. When the nurse removes her blouse, she notices that Jana has numerous bruises on her arms and torso in various stages of healing. She also notices some small scars. Jana's abdomen protrudes on her small, thin frame. From the objective physical assessment, the nurse suspects that:
   a. Jana is experiencing physical and sexual abuse.
   b. Jana is experiencing physical abuse and neglect.
   c. Jana is experiencing emotional neglect.
   d. Jana is experiencing sexual and emotional abuse.

6. A school nurse notices bruises and scars on a child's body, but the child refuses to say how she received them. What is another way in which the nurse can get information from the child?
   a. Have her evaluated by the school psychologist.
   b. Tell her she may select a "treat" from the treat box (e.g., sucker, balloon, junk jewelry) if she answers the nurse's questions.
   c. Explain to her that if she answers the questions, she may stay in the nurse's office and not have to go back to class.
   d. Use a "family" of dolls to role-play the child's family with her.

7. A school nurse notices bruises and scars on Jana's body. The nurse suspects that the child is being physically abused. How should the nurse proceed with this information?
   a. As a healthcare worker, report the suspicion to child protective services.
   b. Check Jana again in a week and see if there are any new bruises.
   c. Meet with Jana's parents and ask them how Jana got the bruises.
   d. Initiate paperwork to have Jana placed in foster care.

Review Questions—cont'd
Self-Examination/Learning Exercise

8. Kate is an 18-year-old freshman at the state university. She was extremely flattered when Don, a senior star football player, invited her to a party. On the way home, he parked the car in a secluded area by the lake. He became angry when she refused his sexual advances. He began to beat her and finally raped her. She tried to fight him, but his physical strength overpowered her. He dumped her in the dorm parking lot and left. The dorm supervisor rushed Kate to the emergency department. Kate says to the nurse, "It's all my fault. I shouldn't have allowed him to stop at the lake." Which of the following is the nurse's best response?
   a. "Yes, you're right. You put yourself in a very vulnerable position when you allowed him to stop at the lake."
   b. "You are not to blame for his behavior. You obviously made some right decisions, because you survived the attack."
   c. "There's no sense looking back now. Just look forward, and make sure you don't put yourself in the same situation again."
   d. "You'll just have to see that he is arrested so he won't do this to anyone else."

9. A young woman who was a recent victim of a sexual assault is brought into the emergency department by a friend. Which of the following is the *priority* nursing intervention?
   a. Help her to bathe and clean herself up.
   b. Provide physical and emotional support during evidence collection.
   c. Provide her with a written list of community resources for survivors of rape.
   d. Discuss the importance of a follow-up visit to evaluate for sexually transmitted diseases.

10. A woman who was sexually assaulted 6 months ago by a man with whom she was acquainted has since been attending a support group for survivors of rape. From this group, she has learned that the most likely reason the man raped her was:
    a. Because he had been drinking, he was not in control of his actions.
    b. He had not had sexual relations with a girl in many months.
    c. He was predisposed to become a rapist by virtue of the poverty conditions under which he was reared.
    d. He was expressing power and dominance by means of sexual aggression and violence.

IMPLICATIONS OF RESEARCH FOR EVIDENCE-BASED PRACTICE

Bowland, S., Edmond, T., & Fallot, R. D. (2012). Evaluation of a spiritually focused intervention with older trauma survivors. *Social Work, 57*(1), 73–82.

DESCRIPTION OF THE STUDY: The purpose of this study was to evaluate a spiritually focused group intervention for a sample of women trauma survivors over 55 years of age (*n* = 21, control group *n* = 22). The authors cite research supporting that older women value spirituality more than men or younger adults, and more often this was correlated to personal growth, well-being, and involvement in creative activities. They also cited research linking personal violation (trauma) to spiritual crisis. Inclusion criteria sought a homogenous group of participants who all had a background in Christian tradition. They randomly assigned participants into treatment and control groups, and they chose a treatment intervention that was a "manualized, psychoeducational, cognitive restructuring and skill building approach to addressing spiritual struggles in recovery." They evaluated for changes in symptoms of depression, anxiety, post-traumatic stress disorder (PTSD), and physical symptoms.

RESULTS OF THE STUDY: The treatment group in this study was found to have fewer symptoms of depression, anxiety, and PTSD and fewer physical symptoms than the control group at the completion of the intervention, and these gains were still evident at 3-month follow-up.

IMPLICATIONS OF RESEARCH FOR EVIDENCE-BASED PRACTICE—cont'd

IMPLICATIONS FOR NURSING PRACTICE: Holistic nursing practice includes addressing the spiritual needs of clients in recovery, particularly because spiritual crisis has been identified as a risk for trauma survivors. This study supported that interventions focused on spiritual needs can have an impact on symptom reduction for several disorders common to this population. Use of structured interventions, consideration for homogeneity of belief traditions, and individual assessment of the client's interest in such interventions are important variables to consider.

IMPLICATIONS OF RESEARCH FOR EVIDENCE-BASED PRACTICE

McClean, C. P., Morris, S. H., Conklin, P., Jayawickreme, N., & Foa, E. B. (2014). Trauma characteristics and post-traumatic stress disorder among adolescent survivors of childhood sexual abuse. *Journal of Family Violence, 29,* 559–566.

DESCRIPTION OF THE STUDY: This study examined the relationship between specific characteristics of childhood sexual abuse and the severity of consequent post-traumatic stress disorder (PTSD), depression, suicide ideation, and substance use symptoms. The risk for illness subsequent to trauma is well documented in the literature, but these researchers wanted to know if specific characteristics, such as the relationship of the perpetrator to the victim, the duration or frequency of abuse, and the type of abuse, could predict the severity of the future PTSD or other symptoms. The participants ($N = 83$) were a culturally diverse sample of female adolescents who were already seeking treatment. The researchers note that there have been conflicting findings in existing research about these relationships in previous studies of adolescents.

RESULTS OF THE STUDY: One significant finding in this study was that the frequency of sexual abuse victimization was correlated with an increase in suicide ideation. Contrary to what the researchers expected to find, the type of trauma, the relationship of the perpetrator, and the duration of victimization did not predict severity of other future illness symptoms, including depression, PTSD, and substance use. They acknowledge that two influential variables include that, in their sample, all participants had already identified themselves as having moderate to high PTSD. The researchers also note that the severity of symptoms may be more distinctive in adulthood, so the relationships that are not clear in a study of adolescents may become clearer as the adolescent moves through adulthood.

IMPLICATIONS FOR NURSING PRACTICE: The finding that frequency of victimization was linked to increased suicide ideation suggests that nurses who conduct victim assessment should assess for suicide ideation and evaluate risks for suicide attempts, especially in adolescents who have experienced sustained, frequent sexual abuse.

The other findings of this research (including their review of studies with conflicting results) highlight that it is important for nurses to explore available research on any issue to increase confidence in their clinical judgments.

TEST YOUR CRITICAL THINKING SKILLS

Sandy is a psychiatric registered nurse who works at a safe house for battered women. Lisa has just been admitted with her two small children after she was treated in the emergency department. She had been beaten severely by her husband while he was intoxicated last night. She escaped with her children after he passed out in their bedroom.

In her initial assessment, Sandy learns from Lisa that she has been battered by her husband for 5 years, beginning shortly after their marriage. She explained that she "knew he drank quite a lot before we were married but thought he would stop after we had kids." Instead, the drinking has increased. Sometimes, he does not even get home from work until 11 o'clock or midnight after stopping to drink at the bar with his buddies.

Lately, he has begun to express jealousy and a lack of trust in Lisa, accusing her of numerous infidelities and indiscretions, none of which are true. Lisa says, "If only he wasn't under so much stress on his job, then maybe he wouldn't drink so much. Maybe if I tried harder to make everything perfect for him at home—I don't know. What do you think I should do to keep him from acting this way?"

Answer the following questions related to Lisa:

1. What is an appropriate response to Lisa's question?
2. Identify the priority psychosocial nursing diagnosis for Lisa.
3. What must the nurse ensure that Lisa learns from this experience?

Communication Exercises

1. Sarah is being treated in the emergency department for wounds inflicted by her husband. Sarah says to the nurse, "He's really not a bad person. He's just under so much stress right now. His company is laying people off, and he thinks he will be next. He drinks a lot when he comes home from work. I just need to make things easier for him at home. I shouldn't have asked him to mow the lawn."

    How would the nurse respond appropriately to this statement by Sarah?

2. Sarah tells the nurse, "I don't know what to do. I'm afraid he will hurt the kids."

    How would the nurse respond appropriately to this statement by Sarah?

3. Sarah also states, "I don't want to press charges. I just want to go home!"

    How would the nurse respond appropriately to this statement by Sarah?

👤 MOVIE CONNECTIONS

The Burning Bed (Domestic violence) • *Life With Billy* (Domestic violence) • *Two Story House* (Child abuse) • *The Prince of Tides* (Domestic violence) • *Radio Flyer* (Child abuse) • *Flowers in the Attic* (Child abuse) • *A Case of Rape* (Sexual assault) • *The Accused* (Sexual assault) • *Spotlight* (Child molestation)

References

American Psychological Association. (2018). *Violence and socioeconomic status.* Retrieved from http://www.apa.org/pi/ses/resources/publications/violence.aspx

Barnett, B. (2016). *What is the age of consent in the United States?* Retrieved from https://www.bhwlawfirm.com/legal-age-consent-united-states-map/

Bowland, S., Edmond, T., & Fallot, R. D. (2012). Evaluation of a spiritually focused intervention with older trauma survivors. *Social Work, 57*(1), 73–82.

Burgess, A. (2010). Rape violence. *Gannett Education Course #60025.* Retrieved from http://ce.nurse.com/60025/Rape-Violence

Cashmore, J., & Shackel, R. (2013). *The long-term effects of child sexual abuse.* Retrieved from https://aifs.gov.au/cfca/publications/long-term-effects-of-child-sexual-abuse/introduction

Center for Relationship Abuse Awareness. (2018). *Barriers to leaving an abusive relationship.* Retrieved from http://stoprelationshipabuse.org/educated/barriers-to-leaving-an-abusive-relationship/

Centers for Disease Control and Prevention (CDC). (2016). *Violence prevention: About behavioral risk factor surveillance system ACE data.* Retrieved from https://www.cdc.gov/violenceprevention/acestudy/ace_brfss.html

Centers for Disease Control and Prevention (CDC). (2017a). *Elder abuse prevention.* Retrieved from http://www.cdc.gov/features/elderabuse

Centers for Disease Control and Prevention (CDC). (2017b). *Intimate partner violence: Definitions.* Retrieved from https://www.cdc.gov/violenceprevention/intimatepartnerviolence/definitions.html

Centers for Disease Control and Prevention (CDC). (2018). *Violence prevention: National Intimate Partner and Sexual Violence Survey: 2015 Data Brief.* Retrieved from https://www.cdc.gov/violenceprevention/nisvs/2015NISVSdatabrief.html

Child Welfare Information Gateway (CWIG). (2013). *What is child abuse and neglect? Recognizing the signs and symptoms.* Retrieved from https://www.childwelfare.gov/pubs/factsheets/whatiscan

Dockterman, E. (2014). *Why women stay: The paradox of abusive relationships.* Retrieved from http://time.com/3309687/why-women-stay-in-abusive-relationships

Espolage, D. L., Low, S., Mrinalini, A. R., Hong, J. S., & Little, T. D. (2013). Family violence, bullying, fighting, and substance use among adolescents: A longitudinal mediational model. *Journal of Research on Adolescence.* doi.org/10.1111/jora.12060

Flaherty, E. G., Stirling, J., & American Academy of Pediatrics, Committee on Child Abuse and Neglect. (2010). Clinical report—The pediatrician's role in child maltreatment prevention. *Pediatrics, 126*(4), 833–841.

Hosier, D. (2015). *Characteristics of abusive mothers.* Retrieved from http://childhoodtraumarecovery.com/2015/10/21/characteristics-of-abusive-mothers

Malkin, C. (2013). *Why do people stay in abusive relationships?* Retrieved from https://www.psychologytoday.com/blog/romance-redux/201303/why-do-people-stay-in-abusiverelationships

McClean, C. P., Morris, S. H., Conklin, P., Jayawickreme, N., & Foa, E. B. (2014). Trauma characteristics and posttraumatic stress disorder among adolescent survivors of childhood sexual abuse. *Journal of Family Violence, 29,* 559–566. doi:10.1007/s10896-014-9613-6

Meskill, J., & Conner, M. (2013). *Understanding and dealing with domestic violence against women.* Retrieved from http://www.oregoncounseling.org/Handouts/DomesticViolenceWomen.htm

National Center on Elder Abuse (NCEA). (n.d.). *Elder abuse: Frequently asked questions.* U.S. Administration on Aging. Retrieved from https://ncea.acl.gov/faq/index.html#faq5

Rosell, D. R., & Siever, L. J. (2015). The neurobiology of aggression and violence. *CNS Spectrum, 20*(3), 254–279. doi:10.1017/S109285291500019X

Sadock, B. J., Sadock, V. A., & Ruiz, P. (2015). *Synopsis of psychiatry: Behavioral sciences/clinical psychiatry* (11th ed.). Philadelphia, PA: Wolters Kluwer.

Schatzberg, A. F., Cole, J. O., & DeBattista, C. (2015). *Manual of clinical psychopharmacology* (8th ed.). Arlington, VA: American Psychiatric.

Silverman, L. (2017). *More domestic violence shelters for men opening.* [Transcript]. Retrieved from https://www.npr.org/2017/07/15/537381161/more-domestic-violence-shelters-for-men-opening

Tracy, N. (2016). *What is battering?* Retrieved from http://www.healthyplace.com/abuse/domestic-violence/what-is-battering

U.S. Bureau of Justice Statistics (2014a). *Nonfatal domestic violence, 2003–2012.* Retrieved from https://www.bjs.gov/content/pub/ndv0312.pdf

U.S. Bureau of Justice Statistics. (2014b). *Rape and sexual assault among college-age females, 1995–2013.* Retrieved from http://www.bjs.gov/index.cfm?ty=pbdetail&iid=5176

U.S. Bureau of Justice Statistics. (2017). *Criminal victimization, 2016.* Retrieved from https://www.bjs.gov/content/pub/pdf/cv16.pdf

U.S. Department of Education. (2013). *Human trafficking of children in the United States.* Retrieved from http://www2.ed.gov/about/offices/list/oese/oshs/factsheet.html

U.S. Department of Health & Human Services, Administration for Children and Families, Administration on Children, Youth and Families, Children's Bureau. (2018). *Child maltreatment 2016.* Retrieved from https://www.acf.hhs.gov/cb/research-data -technology/statistics-research/child-maltreatment

U.S. Department of Justice. (2011). *OJP fact sheet: Domestic violence.* Retrieved from https://ojp.gov/newsroom/factsheets/ojpfs_ domesticviolence.html

Classical References

Burgess, A. W., & Holmström, L. L. (1974). Rape trauma syndrome. *American Journal of Psychiatry, 131*(9), 981–986. doi:10.1176/ appi.ajp.131.9.981. PMID 4415470

Erikson, E. H. (1963). *Childhood and society* (2nd ed.). New York, NY: WW Norton.

Walker, L. E. (1979). *The battered woman.* New York, NY: Harper & Row.

Community Mental Health Nursing

CORE CONCEPTS

Community
Primary prevention
Secondary prevention
Tertiary prevention

KEY TERMS

case management
case manager
deinstitutionalization
diagnosis-related groups (DRGs)

mobile outreach units
prospective payment
shelters
storefront clinics

OBJECTIVES
After reading this chapter, the student will be able to:

1. Discuss the changing focus of care in the field of mental health.
2. Define the concepts of care associated with the public health model.
3. Discuss primary prevention of mental illness within the community.
4. Identify populations at risk for mental illness within the community.
5. Discuss nursing intervention in primary prevention of mental illness within the community.
6. Discuss secondary prevention of mental illness within the community.
7. Describe treatment alternatives related to secondary prevention within the community.

8. Discuss tertiary prevention of mental illness within the community as it relates to the seriously mentally ill and homeless mentally ill.
9. Relate historical and epidemiological factors associated with caring for the seriously mentally ill and homeless mentally ill within the community.
10. Identify treatment alternatives for care of the seriously mentally ill and homeless mentally ill within the community.
11. Apply steps of the nursing process to care of the seriously mentally ill and homeless mentally ill within the community.

HOMEWORK ASSIGNMENT
Please read the chapter and answer the following questions:

1. What are *diagnosis-related groups* (DRGs)?
2. Describe and differentiate how interventions at the primary, secondary, and tertiary prevention levels are implemented.
3. Name three common client populations that benefit from psychiatric home health nursing.
4. What is the most common psychiatric diagnosis among homeless people with mental illness?

Introduction

This chapter explores the concepts of primary and secondary prevention of mental illness within communities. Additional focus is placed on tertiary prevention of mental illness: use of community resources to treat individuals with severe and persistent mental illness and homeless persons with mental illness. Emphasis is given to the role of the psychiatric nurse in the various treatment alternatives in the community setting.

The Changing Focus of Care

Before 1840, there was no known treatment for individuals with mental illness. Because mental illness was perceived as incurable, the only "reasonable" intervention was thought to be removing these individuals from the community to a place where they would do no harm to themselves or others.

In 1841, Dorothea Dix, a former schoolteacher, began a personal crusade across the land on behalf of institutionalized individuals with mental illness. Her efforts resulted in more humane treatment of these clients and the establishment of a number of psychiatric hospitals.

Following the movement initiated by Dix, the number of hospitals for persons with mental illness increased, although unfortunately not as rapidly as did the population with mental illness. The demand soon outgrew the supply, and hospitals became overcrowded and understaffed with conditions that would have sorely distressed Dorothea Dix.

The community mental health movement had its impetus in the 1940s. With establishment of the National Mental Health Act of 1946, the U.S. government awarded grants to the states to develop mental health programs outside of state hospitals. Outpatient clinics and psychiatric units in general hospitals were inaugurated. Then, in 1949, as an outgrowth of the National Mental Health Act, the National Institute of Mental Health (NIMH) was established. The U.S. government has charged this agency with the responsibility for mental health in the United States.

In 1955, the Joint Commission on Mental Health and Illness was established by Congress to identify the nation's mental health needs and to make recommendations for improvement in psychiatric care. In 1961, the Joint Commission published the report *Action for Mental Health* in which recommendations were made for treatment of clients with mental illness, training for caregivers, and improvements in

education and research on mental illness. With consideration given to these recommendations, Congress passed the Mental Retardation Facilities and Community Mental Health Centers Construction Act (often called the Community Mental Health Centers Act) of 1963. This act called for the construction of comprehensive community mental health centers, the cost of which would be shared by federal and state governments. The **deinstitutionalization** movement (the closing of state mental hospitals and discharging of individuals with mental illness) had begun.

Unfortunately, many state governments did not have the capability to match the federal funds required for the establishment of these mental health centers. Some communities found it difficult to follow the rigid requirements for services required by the legislation that provided the grant.

In 1980, the Community Mental Health Systems Act, which was to have played a major role in renovation of mental healthcare, was established. Funding was authorized for community mental health centers, for services to high-risk populations, and for rape research and services. Approval was also granted for the appointment of an associate director for minority concerns at NIMH. However, before this plan could be enacted, the newly inaugurated administration set forth its intention to diminish federal involvement. Budget cuts reduced the number of mandated services, and federal funding for community mental health centers was terminated in 1984.

Meanwhile, costs of care for hospitalized psychiatric clients continued to rise. The problem of the "revolving door" began to intensify. Individuals with severe and persistent mental illness had no place to go when their symptoms exacerbated, except back to the hospital. Individuals without support systems remained in the hospital for extended periods because of lack of appropriate community services. Hospital services were paid for by cost-based, retrospective reimbursement: Medicaid, Medicare, and private health insurance. Retrospective reimbursement encouraged hospital expenditure; the more services provided, the more payment received.

This system of healthcare delivery was interrupted in 1983 with the advent of **prospective payment—** the Reagan administration's proposal of cost containment. It was directed at control of Medicare costs by setting forth pre-established amounts that would be reimbursed for specific diagnoses, or **diagnosis-related groups (DRGs).** Since that time, prospective payment has also been integrated by the states (Medicaid) and by some private insurance companies, drastically affecting the amount of reimbursement for healthcare services.

Mental health services have been influenced by prospective payment. General hospital services to psychiatric clients have been severely restricted. Clients who present with acute symptoms, such as acute psychosis, suicidal ideations or attempts, or manic exacerbations, constitute the largest segment of the psychiatric hospital census. Clients with less serious illnesses (e.g., moderate depression or adjustment disorders) may be hospitalized, but length of stay has been shortened considerably by the reimbursement guidelines. Clients are being discharged from the hospital with a greater need for aftercare than in the past, when hospital stays were longer.

A positive outgrowth of efforts to reduce costly hospital stays and implement restricted reimbursement has been the development of a broader continuum of outpatient treatment options than what has been available historically. In the past, people who needed psychiatric treatment saw an outpatient therapist or were hospitalized, but today there are partial hospitalization programs, intensive outpatient programs, aftercare programs, and a host of other community-based services available to clients with mental health disorders. For those with health insurance, inroads have been made to eliminate discrimination against those with mental illness and substance use disorders; The Paul Wellstone and Pete Domenici Mental Health Parity and Addictions Equity Act (2008) required that, for health insurance plans that provide mental health and substance use disorder benefits, the plan cannot provide less favorable benefits than those provided for medical/surgical issues. The Affordable Care Act also required some insurance plans to include mental health and substance use disorder benefits. In reality, however, many people with chronic mental illnesses are uninsured, undertreated, and homeless.

Deinstitutionalization continues to be the changing focus of mental healthcare in the United States. Care for the client in the hospital has become cost-prohibitive, whereas care for the client in the community is considered cost-effective. However, as experience with the community mental health movement lengthens, it has also been criticized for being a continuation of an "overly narrow biomedical model" (Vanderplasschen et al., 2013). Ironically, the prison populations of homeless persons and those with mental illnesses have risen dramatically during this same time period—one of the problems that Dorothea Dix fought so adamantly against in the first place. The

reality of the provision of healthcare services today is often more of a political and funding issue than providers would care to admit. Decisions about how to treat are rarely made without consideration of cost and method of payment.

The recovery model (see Chapter 10, The Recovery Model) promises the hope of integrating the support of community mental health services, peer support, and client empowerment to improve interventions and outcomes as we look to the future. We must serve the consumer by working collaboratively to provide the essential services for health promotion, for early intervention, and to promote improvement in quality of life for this population.

The Public Health Model

The premise of the model of public health is based largely on the concepts set forth by Gerald Caplan (1964) during the initial community mental health movement. They include primary prevention, secondary prevention, and tertiary prevention. These concepts have expanded beyond mental health treatment and are now widely accepted as guiding principles in clinical and community settings over a wide range of medical and nursing specialties.

CORE CONCEPT
Primary prevention
Services aimed at reducing the incidence of mental disorders within the population.

Primary prevention targets both individuals and the environment. Emphasis is twofold:

1. Assisting individuals to increase their ability to cope effectively with stress
2. Targeting and diminishing harmful forces (stressors) within the environment

Nursing in primary prevention is focused on the targeting of groups at risk and the provision of educational programs. Examples include the following:

- Teaching parenting skills and child development to prospective new parents
- Teaching physical and psychosocial effects of alcohol/drugs to elementary school students
- Teaching techniques of stress management to virtually anyone who desires to learn
- Teaching groups of individuals ways to cope with the changes associated with various maturational stages

■ Teaching concepts of mental health to various groups within the community

■ Providing education and support to unemployed or homeless individuals

■ Providing education and support to other individuals in various transitional periods (e.g., widows and widowers, new retirees, and women entering the workforce in middle life)

These are only a few examples of the types of services that nurses provide in primary prevention. Such services can be offered in a variety of settings that are convenient for the public (e.g., churches, schools, colleges, community centers, YMCAs and YWCAs, workplaces of employee organizations, meetings of women's groups, or civic or social organizations such as parent-teacher associations, health fairs, and community shelters).

CORE CONCEPT

Secondary prevention

Interventions aimed at minimizing early symptoms of psychiatric illness and directed toward reducing the prevalence and duration of the illness.

Secondary prevention is accomplished through early identification of problems and prompt initiation of effective treatment. Nursing in secondary prevention focuses on recognition of symptoms and provision of, or referral for, treatment. Examples include:

■ Ongoing assessment of individuals at high risk for illness exacerbation (e.g., during home visits, day care, community health centers, or in any setting where screening of high-risk individuals might occur).

■ Provision of care for individuals in whom illness symptoms have been assessed (e.g., individual or group counseling, medication administration, education and support during periods of increased stress [crisis intervention], staffing rape crisis centers, suicide hotlines, homeless shelters, shelters for abused persons, or mobile mental health units).

■ Referral for treatment of individuals in whom illness symptoms have been assessed. Referrals may come from support groups, community mental health centers, emergency services, psychiatrists or psychologists, and day or partial hospitalization. Inpatient therapy on a psychiatric unit of a general hospital or in a private psychiatric hospital may be necessary. Psychopharmacology and various adjunct therapies may be initiated as part of the treatment.

Secondary prevention is addressed extensively in Unit 3, Care of Patients With Psychiatric Disorders. Nursing assessment, diagnosis and outcome identification, planning and implementation, and evaluation are discussed for many of the mental illnesses identified in the *Diagnostic and Statistical Manual of Mental Disorders, Fifth Edition (DSM-5)* (American Psychiatric Association [APA], 2013). These concepts may be applied in any setting where nursing is practiced.

CORE CONCEPT

Tertiary prevention

Services aimed at reducing the residual challenges that are associated with severe and persistent mental illness.

Tertiary prevention is accomplished in two ways:

1. Preventing complications of the illness
2. Promoting rehabilitation that is directed toward achievement of each individual's maximum level of functioning

Historically, individuals with severe and persistent mental illness often experienced long hospitalizations that resulted in loss of social skills and increased dependency. With deinstitutionalization, many of these individuals may never have experienced hospitalization, but they still do not possess adequate skills to live productive lives within the community.

Nursing in tertiary prevention focuses on helping clients learn or relearn socially appropriate behaviors so that they may achieve a satisfying role in the community. Examples include:

■ Consideration of the rehabilitation process at the time of initial diagnosis and treatment planning.

■ Teaching the client daily living skills and encouraging independence to his or her maximum ability.

■ Referring clients for various aftercare services (e.g., support groups, day treatment programs, partial hospitalization programs, psychosocial rehabilitation programs, group home or other transitional housing).

■ Monitoring effectiveness of aftercare services (e.g., through home health visits or follow-up appointments in community mental health centers).

■ Making referrals for support services when required (e.g., some communities have programs linking individuals with serious mental disorders to volunteers who serve to develop friendships with the individuals and who may assist with household chores, shopping, and other activities of daily living with which the individual is having difficulty, in addition to participating in social activities with the individual).

Nursing care at the tertiary level of prevention can be administered on an individual or a group basis and in a variety of settings, such as inpatient hospitalization, day or partial hospitalization, group home or halfway house, shelters, home healthcare, nursing homes, and community mental health centers.

The Community as Client

Primary Prevention

> ### CORE CONCEPT
> **Community**
> A group, population, or cluster of people with at least one common characteristic, such as geographic location, occupation, ethnicity, or health concern.

Primary prevention within communities encompasses the twofold emphasis defined earlier in this chapter:

1. Identifying stressful life events that precipitate crises and targeting the relevant populations at high risk
2. Intervening with these high-risk populations to prevent or minimize harmful consequences

Populations at Risk

One way to view populations at risk is to focus on types of crises that individuals experience in their lives. Two broad categories are maturational crises and situational crises.

Maturational Crises

Maturational crises are crucial experiences that are associated with various stages of growth and development. Erikson (1963) described eight stages of the life cycle during which individuals struggle with developmental "tasks." Crises can occur during any of these stages, although several developmental periods and life-cycle events have been recognized as having increased crisis potential: adolescence, marriage, parenthood, midlife, and retirement.

Adolescence The task for adolescence, according to Erikson (1963), is *identity versus role confusion*. This is the time in life when individuals ask questions such as "Who am I?" "Where am I going?" and "What is life all about?"

Adolescence is a transition into young adulthood. It is a very volatile time in most families. Commonly, there is conflict over issues of control. Parents sometimes have difficulty relinquishing even a minimal amount of the control they have had throughout their child's infancy, toddler, and school-age years at this time when the adolescent is seeking increased independence. It may seem that the adolescent is 25 years old one day and 5 years old the next. An often-quoted definition of an adolescent, by an anonymous author, is "a toddler with hormones and wheels."

At this time, adolescents are "trying out their wings," although they possess an essential need to know that the parents (or surrogate parents) are available if support is required. In fact, it is believed that the most frequent immediate precipitant to adolescent suicide is loss, or threat of loss, or abandonment by parents or closest peer relationship.

Adolescents have many issues to deal with and many choices to make. Some of these include issues that relate to self-esteem and body image (in a body that is undergoing rapid changes), peer relationships (with both genders), education and career selection, establishing a set of values and ideals, sexuality and sexual experimentation (including issues of birth control and prevention of sexually transmitted diseases), drug and alcohol use, and physical appearance.

Nursing interventions with adolescents at the primary level of prevention focus on providing support and accurate information to ease the difficult transition they are undergoing. Educational offerings can be presented in schools, churches, youth centers, or any location in which groups of teenagers gather. Types of programs may include (but are not limited to) the following:

■ Alateen groups for adolescents with alcoholic parent(s)
■ Other support groups for teenagers who are in need of assistance to cope with stressful situations (e.g., children dealing with divorce of their parents, pregnant teenagers, teenagers coping with abortion, adolescents coping with the death of a parent)
■ Educational programs that inform about and validate body changes and the emotions that may accompany these changes
■ Educational programs that inform about positive self-esteem and resilience

- Educational programs that inform about sexuality, pregnancy, contraception, and sexually transmitted diseases
- Educational programs that inform about the use of alcohol and other drugs

Marriage The "American dream" of the 1950s— especially that of the American woman—was to marry, have two or three children, buy a house in the suburbs, and drive a station wagon. To not be at least betrothed by their mid-20s caused many women to fear becoming an "old maid." Living together without the benefit of marriage was an unacceptable and rarely considered option.

Times have changed considerably since the middle of the 20th century. Today's young women are choosing to pursue careers before marriage, to continue their careers after marriage, or to not marry at all. Many couples are deciding to live together without being married, and, as with most trends, the practice now receives more widespread societal acceptance than it once did. Although there are far more culturally accepted choices about the nature of relationships and living arrangements in today's society, crises may develop related to conflicting values between generations within a family and related to the many factors influencing those choices, including economic concerns. Ideological changes that stress personal freedom, self-fulfillment, and individual choice have contributed to an increase in people delaying marriage to fulfill career aspirations or leaving marriages that don't fulfill their expectations (Casper & Coritz, 2018).

When young adults do decide to enter into marriage, crisis may develop associated with unrealistic or uninformed expectations about this institution. It is well understood, too, that children raised in abusive, dysfunctional families are at higher risk for subconsciously choosing partners who perpetuate the experiences they were accustomed to while they were growing up. Both of these circumstances can increase the risk for crisis in a marriage. Nursing interventions at the primary level of prevention with individuals in this stage of development involve education regarding what to expect at various stages of marriage. Many high schools offer courses in marriage and family living in which students role-play through anticipatory marriage and family situations. Nurses could offer these kinds of classes within the community to individuals considering marriage. Educating young adults about factors to consider when choosing a spouse and, particularly, the risks associated with

choosing a partner that perpetuates a cycle of violence is a form of primary prevention at the level of basic survival. Many people enter marriage with the idea that their soon-to-be husband or wife will discontinue his or her "undesirable" traits and change into the perceived ideal spouse. Primary prevention with these individuals involves:

- Encouraging honest communication
- Determining what each person expects from the relationship
- Discerning whether or not each individual can accept compromise

This type of intervention can be effective in individual or couple's therapy and in support or educational groups of couples experiencing similar circumstances.

Parenthood There is perhaps no developmental stage that creates an upheaval equal to that of the arrival of a child. Even when the child is desperately wanted and pleasurably anticipated, his or her arrival usually results in some degree of chaos within the family.

Because the family operates as a system, the addition of a new member influences all parts of the system as a whole. If it is a first child, the relationship between the spouses is likely to be affected by the demands of caring for the infant on a 24-hour basis. If there are older children, they may resent the attention showered on the new arrival and show their resentment in a variety of creative ways.

The concept of having a child (particularly the first one) is often romanticized with little or no consideration given to the realities and responsibilities that accompany this "bundle of joy." Many parents are shocked to realize that such a tiny human can create so many changes in so many lives. It is unfortunate that although parenting is one of the most important positions an individual will hold in life, it is one for which he or she is often least prepared.

Nursing intervention at the primary level of prevention with those in the developmental stage of parenthood must begin long before the child is born. How do we prepare individuals for parenthood? *Anticipatory guidance* is a term used to describe the interventions used to help new parents know what they might expect. Volumes have been written on the subject, but it is also important for expectant parents to have a support person or network with whom they can talk and express feelings, excitement, and fears. Nurses can provide the following type of information to help ease the transition into parenthood (Spock & Needlman, 2018; Veltri, Wilson-Mitchell, & O'Mahony, 2018).

■ **Prepared childbirth classes:** These classes present what most likely will happen along with information about possible variations from that which is expected.

■ **What to expect after the baby arrives**:

■ *Parent-infant bonding.* Expectant parents should know that it is common for parent-infant bonding not to occur immediately. The strong attachment will occur as parent and infant get to know each other.

■ *Changing communication patterns and relationship styles.* The couple should be encouraged to engage in open, honest communication with each other. Education should be offered about expected changes in communication patterns and the challenges of establishing communication with an infant as well as resources for referral if communication patterns are creating significant role strain. Frustrated attempts to adapt to these challenges can have consequences for the infant as well. In some cases, an infant's need may be neglected if the parents lack skills or resources to navigate communication challenges. "Abusive head trauma, which includes shaken baby syndrome, is an extreme example of an inability to adapt to changed communication patterns with an infant" (Veltri et al., p. 367). Discuss strategies that family members may consider using to maintain motivation and morale as well as provide for comfort, rest, and self-care for each member.

■ *Clothing and equipment.* Expectant parents need to know what is required to care for a newborn child. Financing childbearing and child rearing, arranging space for a child, and lifestyle should be considered.

■ *Feeding.* Advantages and disadvantages of breastfeeding and formula feeding should be presented. The couple should be supported in whatever method is chosen. Anticipatory guidance related to technique should be provided for one or both methods, as the expectant parents request.

■ *Other expectations.* It is important for expectant parents to receive anticipatory guidance about the infant's sleeping and crying patterns, bathing the infant, care of the circumcision and cord, toys that provide stimulation of the newborn's senses, aspects of providing a safe environment, and when to call the physician.

■ **Stages of growth and development:** It is very important for parents to understand what behaviors should be expected at what stage of development.

It is also important to know that their child may not necessarily follow the age guidelines associated with these stages. However, a substantial deviation from these guidelines should be reported to their physician.

Midlife What is middle age? A colleague once remarked that upon turning 50 years of age, she stated, "'Now I can say I am officially middle aged' . . . until I began thinking about how few individuals I really knew who were 100!"

Midlife crises are not defined by a specific number. Various sources in the literature identify these conflicts as occurring anytime between ages 35 and 65 years.

What is a midlife crisis? This, too, is very individual, but a number of patterns have been identified within three broad categories:

1. **An alteration in perception of the self.** One's perception of self may occur slowly. One may suddenly become aware of being "old" or "middle aged." Other biological changes that occur naturally with the aging process may also affect the crises that occur at this time. In women, a gradual decrease in the production of estrogen initiates the menopause, which results in a variety of physical and emotional symptoms. Some physical symptoms include hot flashes, vaginal dryness, cessation of menstruation, loss of reproductive ability, night sweats, insomnia, headaches, and minor memory disturbances. Emotional symptoms include anxiety, depression, crying for no reason, and temper outbursts.

   Some men experience hot flashes, sweating, chills, dizziness, and heart palpitations, whereas others may experience severe depression and an overall decline in physical vigor (Sadock, Sadock, & Ruiz, 2015). An alteration in sexual functioning is not uncommon.

2. **An alteration in perception of others.** A change in relationship with adult children requires a sensitive shift in caring. Wright and Leahey (2013) state:

   > The family of origin must relinquish the primary roles of parent and child. They must adapt to the new roles of parent and adult child. This involves renegotiation of emotional and financial commitments. The key emotional process during this stage is for family members to deal with a multitude of exits from and entries into the family system. (p. 107)

These experiences are particularly difficult when parents' values conflict with the relationships and types of lifestyles their children choose. An alteration in perception of one's parents also begins to occur during this time. Having always looked to parents for support and comfort, the middle-aged individual may suddenly find that the roles are beginning to reverse. Aging parents may look to their children for assistance with making decisions regarding their everyday lives and for assistance with chores that they have previously accomplished independently. When parents die, middle-aged individuals must come to terms with their own mortality. The process of recognition and resolution of one's own finitude begins in earnest at this time.

3. **An alteration in perception of time.** *Middle age* has been defined as the end of youth and the beginning of old age. Individuals often experience a sense that time is running out: "I haven't done all I want to do or accomplished all I intended to accomplish!" Depression and a sense of loss may occur as individuals realize that some of the goals established in their youth may go unmet.

The term *empty nest syndrome* has been used to describe the adjustment period parents experience when the last child leaves home to establish an independent residence. The crisis is often more profound for the mother who has devoted her life to nurturing her family. As the last child leaves, she may perceive her future as uncertain and meaningless.

Some women who have devoted their lives to rearing their children decide to develop personal interests and pursue personal goals once the children are grown. This occurs at a time when many husbands have begun to decrease what may have been a compulsive drive for occupational security during the earlier years of their lives. This disparity in common goals may create conflict between husband and wife. At a time when she is experiencing more value in herself and her own life, he may begin to feel less valued. This may also relate to a decrease in the amount of time and support from the wife to which the husband has become accustomed. This type of role change will require numerous adaptations on the part of both spouses.

Finally, an alteration in one's perception of time may be related to the societal striving for eternal youth. The individual may try to delay the external changes that come with aging by the use of cosmetics, hormone creams, or even surgery. This yearning for youth may take the form of sexual promiscuity or extramarital affairs with much younger individuals in an effort to prove that one "still has what it takes." Some individuals reach for the trappings of youth with regressive-type behaviors, such as the middle-aged man who buys a motorcycle and joins a motorcycle club or the 50-year-old woman who wears miniskirts and flirts with her daughter's boyfriends. These individuals may be denying their own past and experience. With a negative view of self, they strongly desire to relive their youth.

Nursing intervention at the primary level of prevention with those in the developmental stage of midlife involves providing accurate information regarding changes that occur during this time of life and support for adapting to these changes effectively. These interventions might include the following:

■ Nutrition classes to inform individuals in this age group about the essentials of diet and exercise and the importance of good nutrition. Educational materials on how to avoid obesity or reduce weight can be included.

■ Assistance with ways to improve health (e.g., quit smoking, cease or reduce alcohol consumption, reduce fat intake).

■ Discussions of the importance of having regular physical examinations, including Pap and breast examinations for women and prostate examinations for men. Monthly breast self-examinations should be taught and yearly mammograms encouraged.

■ Classes on menopause should be given. Provide information about what to expect. Myths that abound regarding this topic should be expelled. Support groups for women (and men) undergoing the menopausal experience could be formed.

■ Support and information related to physical changes occurring in the body during this time of life. Assist with the grief response that some individuals will experience in relation to loss of youth, "empty nest," and sense of identity.

■ Support and information related to care of aging parents should be given. Individuals should be referred to community resources for respite and assistance before strain of the caregiver role threatens to disrupt the family system.

Retirement Retirement, which is often anticipated as an achievement in principle, may be met with a great deal of ambivalence when it actually occurs. Our society places a great deal of importance on productivity and on earning as much money as possible at as young an age as possible. These types of values contribute to the ambivalence associated with retirement. Although leisure has been acknowledged as a legitimate reward for workers, leisure during retirement has never been accorded the same social value. Adjustment to this life-cycle event becomes more difficult in the face of societal values that are in direct conflict with the new lifestyle.

Historically, many women have derived much of their self-esteem from having children, rearing children, and being a "good mother." Likewise, many men have achieved self-esteem through work-related activities—creativity, productivity, and earning money. Termination of these activities can result in a loss of self-worth, and individuals who are unable to adapt satisfactorily may become depressed.

It would appear that retirement is becoming, and will continue to become, more accepted by societal standards. With increasing numbers of individuals retiring earlier and living longer, the growing number of aging persons will spend a significantly longer time in retirement. At present, retirement has become more of an institutionalized expectation, and there appears to be increasing acceptance of it as a marker of social status. At the same time, an emerging trend is growth in the rate of older adults remaining in the workforce or returning post-retirement.

Nursing intervention at the primary level of prevention with the developmental task of retirement involves providing information and support to individuals who have retired or are considering retirement and assessing individual needs with regard to continuing employment in older adulthood. Support can be on a one-to-one basis to assist these individuals to sort out their feelings regarding retirement. Well-being in retirement is linked to factors such as stable health status, adequate income, the ability to pursue new goals or activities, extended social network of family and friends, and satisfaction with current living arrangements.

One trend that has been a hallmark of change for many older adults is the increasing numbers of grandparents who are caring for grandchildren and, in many cases, assuming primary responsibility for their care (Casper & Coritz, 2018). Nurses can promote primary prevention of crisis through education about resources for caregiving assistance and sharing what the evidence is teaching us about this new role. In fact, evidence shows that in spite of grief and burdens associated with caregiving, many grandparents identify that this role revealed their inner strength and gave them a sense of accomplishment (White & Cartwright, 2018).

Support can also be provided in a group environment. Support groups of individuals undergoing the same types of experiences can be extremely helpful. Nurses can form and lead these types of groups to assist retiring individuals through this critical period. These groups can also serve to provide information about available resources that offer assistance to individuals in or nearing retirement, such as information concerning Medicare, Social Security, and Medicaid; information related to organizations that specialize in hiring retirees; and information regarding ways to use newly acquired free time constructively.

Situational Crises

Situational crises are acute responses that occur as a result of an external circumstantial stressor. The number and types of situational stressors are limitless and may be real or exist only in the perception of the individual. Some types of situational crises that put individuals at risk for mental illness include the following:

■ Poverty: A number of studies have identified poverty as a direct correlation to emotional illness. This may have to do with the direct consequences of poverty, such as inadequate and crowded living conditions, nutritional deficiencies, medical neglect, unemployment, or being homeless.

■ High rate of life change events: Many studies have found that changes in life patterns due to a large number of significant events occurring in close proximity tend to decrease a person's ability to deal with stress, and physical or emotional illness may be the result (McLeod, 2010). These include life change events such as death of a loved one, divorce, being fired from a job, a change in living conditions, a change in place of employment or residence, physical illness, or a change in body image caused by the loss of a body part or function.

■ Environmental conditions: Environmental conditions can create situational crises. Tornados, floods, hurricanes, and earthquakes have wreaked devastation on thousands of individuals and families in recent years.

■ Trauma: Individuals who have encountered traumatic experiences must be considered at risk for emotional illness. These include traumatic experiences usually considered outside the range of usual human experience, such as rape, war, physical attack, torture, or natural or manmade disaster.

Nursing intervention at the primary level of prevention with individuals experiencing situational crises is aimed at maintaining the highest possible level of functioning while offering support and assistance with problem-solving during the crisis period. Interventions for nursing of patients in crisis include the following:

■ Use a reality-oriented approach. The focus of the problem is on the here and now.

■ Remain with the individual who is experiencing panic anxiety.

■ Establish a rapid working relationship by showing unconditional acceptance, by active listening, and by attending to immediate needs.

■ Discourage lengthy explanations or rationalizations of the situation; promote an atmosphere for verbalization of true feelings.

■ Set firm limits on aggressive, destructive behaviors. At high levels of anxiety, behavior is likely to be impulsive and regressive. Establish at the outset what is acceptable and what is not and maintain consistency.

■ Clarify the problem that the individual is facing. The nurse does this by describing his or her perception of the problem and comparing it with the individual's perception of the problem.

■ Help the individual determine what he or she believes precipitated the crisis.

■ Acknowledge feelings of anger, guilt, helplessness, and powerlessness while taking care not to provide positive feedback for these feelings.

■ Guide the individual through a problem-solving process by which he or she may move in the direction of positive life change:

▪ Help the individual confront the source of the problem that is creating the crisis response.

▪ Encourage the individual to discuss changes that he or she would like to make. Jointly determine whether desired changes are realistic.

▪ Encourage exploration of feelings about aspects that cannot be changed and explore alternative ways of coping more adaptively in these situations.

▪ Discuss alternative strategies for creating change in situations that can realistically be changed.

▪ Weigh benefits and consequences of each alternative.

▪ Assist the individual to select alternative coping strategies that will help alleviate future crises.

■ Identify external support systems and new social networks from which the individual may seek assistance in times of stress.

Nursing at the level of primary prevention focuses largely on education of the consumer to prevent initiation or exacerbation of mental illness. An example of one type of teaching tool for use in primary prevention is presented in Table 26–1. This particular tool provides organized information that may be used to educate adolescents and parents about the effects of commonly abused substances.

Secondary Prevention
Populations at Risk

Secondary prevention within communities relates to using early detection and prompt intervention with individuals experiencing mental illness symptoms. The same maturational and situational crises that are presented in the previous section on primary prevention are used to discuss intervention at the secondary level of prevention.

Maturational Crises

Adolescence The need for intervention at the secondary level of prevention in adolescence occurs when disruptive and age-inappropriate behaviors become the norm, and the family can no longer cope adaptively with the situation. All levels of dysfunction are considered—from dysfunctional family coping to the need for hospitalization of the adolescent.

Nursing intervention with the adolescent at the secondary level of prevention may occur in the community setting at community mental health centers, physician's offices, schools, public health departments, and crisis intervention centers. Nurses may work with families to problem solve and improve coping and communication skills, or they may work on a one-to-one basis with the adolescent in an attempt to modify behavior patterns.

Adolescents may be hospitalized for a variety of problems, including (but not limited to) conduct disorders, adjustment disorders, eating disorders, substance-related disorders, depression, and anxiety disorders. Inpatient care is determined by severity of symptomatology. Nursing care of adolescents in the hospital setting focuses on problem identification and stabilizing a crisis situation. Once stability has been achieved, patients are commonly discharged to outpatient care. If an adolescent's home situation has been deemed unsatisfactory, the state may take custody, and the child is then discharged to a group or foster home.

Marriage Problems that are not uncommon to the disruption of a marriage relationship include substance abuse on the part of one or both partners and

TABLE 26–1 Patient Education for Primary Prevention: Drugs of Abuse

CLASS OF DRUGS	EFFECTS	SYMPTOMS OF OVERDOSE	TRADE NAMES	COMMON NAMES	EFFECTS OF THE BODY (CHRONIC OR HIGH-DOSE USE)
CNS DEPRESSANTS					
Alcohol	Relaxation, loss of inhibitions, lack of concentration, drowsiness, slurred speech, sleep	Nausea, vomiting; shallow respirations; cold, clammy skin; weak, rapid pulse; coma; possible death	Ethyl alcohol, beer, gin, rum, vodka, bourbon, whiskey, liqueurs, wine, brandy, sherry, champagne	Booze, alcohol, liquor, drinks, cocktails, high-balls, nightcaps, moonshine, white lightning, firewater	Peripheral nerve damage, skeletal muscle wasting, encephalopathy, psychosis, cardiomyopathy, gastritis, esophagitis, pancreatitis, hepatitis, cirrhosis of the liver, leukopenia, thrombocytopenia, sexual dysfunction
Other (barbiturates and nonbarbiturates)	Same as alcohol	Anxiety, fever, agitation, hallucinations, disorientation, tremors, delirium, convulsions, possible death	Seconal Nembutal Amytal Valium Librium Chloral hydrate Miltown Rohypnol GHB (gamma-hydroxybutyric acid)	Red birds Yellow birds Blue birds Blues/yellows Green & whites Mickies Downers Circles, Forget Pill, Forget-Me-Pill, La Rocha, Lunch Money Drug, Roofies Easy Lay, G, Georgia Home Boy, GHB, Goop, Grievous Bodily Harm, Liquid Ecstasy, Liquid X, and Scoop	Decreased REM sleep, respiratory depression, hypotension, possible kidney or liver damage, sexual dysfunction Slurred speech, loss of motor coordination, weakness, headache, and respiratory depression Unconsciousness, seizures, slowed heart rate, greatly slowed breathing, lower body temperature, vomiting, nausea, coma, and death
CNS STIMULANTS					
Amphetamines and related drugs	Hyperactivity, agitation, euphoria, insomnia, loss of appetite	Cardiac arrhythmias, headache, convulsions, hypertension, rapid heart rate, coma, possible death	Dexedrine, Didrex, Tenuate, Bontril, Ritalin, Focalin, Provigil Khat (amphetamine-like plant)	Uppers, pep pills, wakeups, bennies, eye-openers, speed, black beauties, sweet A's, Abyssinian tea, arabian tea, chaat, gat, kat	Aggressive, compulsive behavior; paranoia; hallucinations; hypertension
Cocaine	Euphoria, hyperactivity, restlessness, talkativeness, increased pulse, dilated pupils	Hallucinations, convulsions, pulmonary edema, respiratory failure, coma, cardiac arrest, possible death	Cocaine hydrochloride	Coke, flake, snow, dust, happy dust, gold dust, girl, Cecil, C, toot, blow, crack	Pulmonary hemorrhage, myocardial infarction, ventricular fibrillation

Continued

TABLE 26–1 Patient Education for Primary Prevention: Drugs of Abuse—cont'd

CLASS OF DRUGS	EFFECTS	SYMPTOMS OF OVERDOSE	TRADE NAMES	COMMON NAMES	EFFECTS OF THE BODY (CHRONIC OR HIGH-DOSE USE)
Synthetic stimulants	Agitation, insomnia, irritability, dizziness, decreased ability to think clearly, increased heart rate, chest pains	Depression, paranoia, delusions, suicidal thoughts, seizures, panic attacks, nausea, vomiting, heart attack, stroke	Mephedrone, MDPV (3–4 methylene-dioxy-pyrovalerone) Flakka	Bath salts, bliss, vanilla sky, ivory wave, purple wave Gravel, the zombie drug	Increased heart rate, increased blood pressure, nosebleeds, hallucinations, aggressive behavior
Opioids	Euphoria, lethargy, drowsiness, lack of motivation, constricted pupils	Shallow breathing, slowed pulse, clammy skin, pulmonary edema, respiratory arrest, convulsions, coma, possible death	Heroin Morphine Codeine Dilaudid Demerol Dolophine Percodan Talwin Opium Fentanyl (synthetic) Carfentanyl (synthetic) U47700 (synthetic) Kratom (plant with opioid and stimulant effects)	Snow, stuff, H, Harry, horse M, morph, Miss Emma Schoolboy Lords Doctors Dollies Perkies T's Big O, black stuff Apache, China Girl, China White, Dance Fever, Friend, Goodfella, Jackpot, Murder 8, TNT, and Tango and Cash Gray death Pinky, Pink Blak, Ketum, Ithang, Kakuam, Thom	Respiratory depression, constipation, fecal impaction, hypotension, decreased libido, retarded ejaculation, impotence, orgasm failure
Hallucinogens	Visual hallucinations, disorientation, confusion, paranoid delusions, euphoria, anxiety, panic, increased pulse	Agitation, extreme hyperactivity, violence, hallucinations, psychosis, convulsions, possible death	LSD PCP Mescaline DMT STP, DOM MDMA Ketamine	Acid, cube, big D Angel dust, hog, peace pill Mesc Businessman's trip Serenity and peace Ecstasy, XTC Special K, Vitamin K, Kit Kat	Panic reaction, acute psychosis, flashbacks
Cannabinols	Relaxation, talkativeness, lowered inhibitions, euphoria, mood swings	Fatigue, paranoia, delusions, hallucinations, possible psychosis	Cannabis Hashish	Marijuana, pot, grass, joint, Mary Jane, MJ Hash, rope, Sweet Lucy	Tachycardia, orthostatic hypotension, chronic bronchitis, problems with infertility, amotivational syndrome

disagreements on issues of sex, money, children, gender roles, and infidelity, among others.

Nursing intervention at the secondary level of prevention with individuals encountering marriage problems may include one or more of the following:

- Counseling with the couple or with one of the spouses on a one-to-one basis
- Referral to a couples' support group
- Identification of the problem and possible solutions; support and guidance as changes are undertaken
- Referral to a sex therapist
- Referral to a financial advisor
- Referral to parent effectiveness training

When a marriage fails, individuals often experience a spectrum of troubling emotions including anger, mistrust, depression, and grief (even among individuals who initiate divorce). In community health settings, nurses can lead support groups for newly divorced individuals. They can also provide one-to-one counseling for individuals experiencing the emotional chaos engendered by the dissolution of a marriage relationship.

Divorce also has an impact on the children involved. Nurses can intervene with the children of divorce in an effort to prevent dysfunctional behaviors associated with the break-up of a marriage.

Parenthood Intervention at the secondary level of prevention with parents can be required for a number of reasons, such as:

- Physical, emotional, or sexual abuse of a child
- Physical or emotional neglect of a child
- Birth of a child with special needs
- Diagnosis of a terminal illness in a child
- Death of a child

Nursing intervention at the secondary level of prevention includes being able to recognize the physical and behavioral signs that indicate possible abuse of a child. The child may be cared for in the emergency department or as an inpatient on the pediatric unit or child psychiatric unit of a general hospital.

Nursing intervention with parents may include teaching effective methods of disciplining children, aside from physical punishment. Methods that emphasize the importance of positive reinforcement for acceptable behavior can be very effective. Family members must be committed to consistent use of this behavior modification technique for it to be successful.

Parents should also be informed about behavioral expectations at the various levels of development.

Knowledge of what to expect from children at these various stages may provide needed anticipatory guidance to deal with the crises commonly associated with each stage.

Therapy sessions with all family members together may focus on problems with family communications. Members are encouraged to express honest feelings in a manner that is nonthreatening to other family members. Active listening, assertiveness techniques, and respect for the rights of others are taught and encouraged. Barriers to effective communication are identified and resolved.

Referrals to agencies that promote effective parenting skills may be made (e.g., parent effectiveness training). Alternative agencies that may provide relief from the stress of parenting may also be considered (e.g., "Mom's Day Out" programs, sitter-sharing organizations, and day-care institutions). Support groups for abusive parents may also be helpful, and assistance in locating or initiating such a group may be provided.

The nurse can assist parents who are grieving the loss of a child or the birth of a child with special needs by helping them to express their feelings associated with the loss. Feelings such as shock, denial, anger, guilt, powerlessness, and hopelessness need to be expressed in order for the parents to progress through the grief response.

Home healthcare assistance can be provided for the family of a child with special needs. This can be done by making referrals to other professionals, such as speech, physical, and occupational therapists; medical social workers; psychologists; and nutritionists. If the child with special needs is hospitalized, the home health nurse can provide specific information to hospital staff that may be helpful in providing continuity of care for the client and help in the transition for the family.

Nursing intervention also includes providing assistance in the location of and referral to support groups that deal with loss of a child or birth of a child with special needs. Some nurses may serve as leaders of these types of groups in the community.

Midlife Nursing care at the secondary level of prevention during midlife becomes necessary when the individual is unable to integrate all of the changes that are occurring during this period. An inability to accept the physical and biological changes, the changes in relationships between themselves and their adult children and aging parents, and the loss of the perception of youth may result in depression for which the individual may require help to resolve.

Retirement Retirement can also result in depression for individuals who are unable to satisfactorily grieve for the loss of this aspect of their lives. Depression is more likely to occur when individuals have not planned for retirement or when they have derived most of their self-esteem from their employment.

Nursing intervention at the secondary level of prevention with depressed individuals takes place in both inpatient and outpatient settings. Severely depressed patients with suicidal ideations will need close observation in the hospital setting, whereas those with mild to moderate depression may be treated in the community. A plan of care for the patient with depression is found in Chapter 16, Depressive Disorders. These concepts apply to the secondary level of prevention and may be used in all nursing care settings.

The physician may elect to use pharmacotherapy with antidepressants. Nurses may intervene by providing information to the patient about what to expect from the medication, possible side effects, adverse effects, and how to self-administer the medication.

Situational Crises

Nursing care at the secondary level of prevention with patients undergoing situational crises occurs only if crisis intervention at the primary level failed and the individual is unable to function socially or occupationally. Exacerbation of mental illness symptoms requires intervention at the secondary level of prevention. These disorders are addressed in pertinent chapters throughout Unit 3, Care of Patients With Psychiatric Disorders. Nursing assessment, diagnosis and outcome identification, planning and implementation, and evaluation are discussed for many of the mental illnesses identified in the *DSM-5* (APA, 2013). These skills may be applied in any setting where nursing is practiced.

A case study situation of nursing care at the secondary level of prevention in a community setting is presented in Box 26–1.

Tertiary Prevention

Individuals With Severe and Persistent Mental Illness

Various terms such as *chronic mental illness, severe and persistent mental illness,* or *serious mental illness*" have been used to describe disorders that contribute to significant functional impairment. The term *chronic* has been replaced by the latter two descriptors because "chronic" may have a negative connotation suggesting recovery is not possible (Substance Abuse and Mental Health Services Administration [SAMHSA], 2016). In fact, those with serious mental illness can respond to treatment, services, and recovery-oriented support (SAMHSA, 2016). Furthermore, not all serious mental illnesses are severe *and* persistent.

The NIMH (2017) defines *serious mental illness* as "a mental, behavioral, or emotional disorder resulting in serious functional impairment, which substantially interferes with or limits one or more major life activities." Those that are identified as "severe and persistent" are characterized by significant, ongoing, functional impairment, and major disability. These disorders are identified by criteria listed in the *DSM-5.* Diagnoses may include schizophrenia and related disorders, bipolar disorder, autism spectrum disorders, major depressive disorder, panic disorder, obsessive-compulsive disorder, post-traumatic stress disorder, borderline personality disorder, and attention deficit-hyperactivity disorder. Based on 2016 statistics, serious mental illness affects about 4.2 percent of the population residing in the United States (NIMH, 2017). The actual number may be significantly higher because this research did not attempt to include the homeless or those who were in correctional facilities for the entire year.

Historical and Epidemiological Aspects

In 1955, more than one-half million individuals resided in public mental hospitals. Estimates suggest that this number is fewer than 100,000 today.

Deinstitutionalization of persons with serious mental illness began in the 1960s as national policy change and with a strong belief in the individual's right to freedom. Other considerations included the deplorable conditions of some of the state hospitals, the introduction of psychotropic medications, and the cost-effectiveness of caring for these individuals in the community setting.

Deinstitutionalization began to occur rapidly and without sufficient planning for the needs of these individuals as they reentered the community. Individuals with support systems that could provide assistance with living arrangements and sheltered employment experiences most often received the outpatient treatment they required. Those without adequate support, however, either managed to survive at a subsistence level or were forced to join the ranks of the homeless. Some ended up in nursing homes meant to provide care for individuals with physical disabilities.

Among certain segments of our population—the elderly, the working poor, the homeless, and individuals previously covered by funds that have been cut by various social reforms, including persons with severe and persistent mental illness—have been left

BOX 26–1 Secondary Prevention Case Study: Parenthood

The identified patient was a petite, doll-like 4-year-old girl named Tanya. She was the older of two children in a Latino American family. The other child was a boy named Joseph, aged 2. The mother was 5 months pregnant with their third child. The family had been referred to the nurse after Tanya was placed in foster care following a report to child protective services by her nursery school teacher that the child had marks on her body suspicious of child abuse.

The parents, Paulo and Annette, were in their mid-20s. Paulo had lost his job at an aircraft plant 3 months ago and had been unable to find work since. Annette brought in a few dollars from cleaning houses for other people, but the family was struggling to survive.

Paulo and Annette were angry at having to see the nurse. After all, "Parents have the right to discipline their children." The nurse did not focus on the *intent* of the behavior but instead looked at factors in the family's life that could be viewed as stressors. This family had multiple stressors: poverty, the father's unemployment, the age and spacing of the children, the mother's chronic fatigue from work at home and in other people's homes, and finally, having a child removed from the home against the parents' wishes.

During therapy with this family, the nurse discussed the behaviors associated with various developmental levels. She also discussed possible deviations from these norms and when they should be reported to the physician. The nurse and the family discussed Tanya's behavior and how it compared with the norms.

The parents also discussed their own childhoods. They were able to relate some of the same types of behaviors that they observed in Tanya. But they both admitted that they came from families whose main method of discipline was physical punishment. Annette had been the oldest child in her large family and had been expected to "keep the younger ones in line." When she had not done so, she was punished with her father's belt. She expressed anger toward her father, although she had never been allowed to express it at the time.

Paulo's father had died when he was a small boy, and Paulo had been expected to be the "man of the family." From the time he was very young, he worked at odd jobs to bring money into the home. Because of this, he had little time for the usual activities of childhood and adolescence. He held much resentment toward the young men who "had everything and never had to work for it."

Paulo and Annette had high expectations for Tanya. In effect, they expected her to behave in a manner well beyond her developmental level. These expectations were based on the reflections of their own childhoods. They were uncomfortable with the spontaneity and playfulness of childhood because they had had little personal experience with these behaviors. When Tanya balked and expressed the verbal assertions common to early childhood, Paulo and Annette interpreted these behaviors as defiance toward them and retaliated with anger in the manner in which they had been parented.

With the parents, the nurse explored feelings and behaviors from their past so that they were able to understand the correlation to their current behaviors. They learned to negotiate ways to deal with Tanya's age-appropriate behaviors. In combined therapy with Tanya, they learned how to relate to her childishness and even how to enjoy playing with both of their children.

The parents ceased blaming each other for the family's problems. Annette had spent a good deal of her time deprecating Paulo for his lack of support of his family, and Paulo blamed Annette for being "unable to control her daughter." Communication patterns were clarified, and life in the family became more peaceful.

Without a need to "prove himself" to his wife, Paulo's efforts to find employment met with success because he no longer felt the need to turn down jobs that he believed his wife would perceive to be beneath his capabilities. Annette no longer works outside the home, and both she and Paulo participate in the parenting chores. Tanya and her siblings continue to demonstrate age-appropriate developmental progression.

---

untreated. In individuals with severe and persistent mental illness, these circumstances have promoted a greater number of crisis-oriented emergency department visits and hospital admissions and repeated confrontations with law enforcement officials.

In 2002, President George W. Bush established the New Freedom Commission on Mental Health. This commission was charged with the task of conducting a comprehensive study of the United States mental health service delivery system. Members were to identify unmet needs and barriers to services and recommend steps for improvement in services and support

for individuals with serious mental illness. In July 2003, the commission presented its final report (President's New Freedom Commission on Mental Health, 2003). The commission identified the following five barriers:

1. **Fragmentation and gaps in care for children.** About 7 to 9 percent of all children (ages 9 to 17) have a serious emotional disturbance (SED). The commission found that services for children are even more fragmented than those for adults with more uncoordinated funding and differing eligibility requirements. Only a fraction of children with SED appear to have access to school-based

or school-linked mental health services. Children with SED who are identified for special education services have higher levels of absenteeism, higher drop-out rates, and lower levels of academic achievement than students with other disabilities.

2. **Fragmentation and gaps in care for adults with serious mental illness.** The commission expressed concern that so many adults with serious mental illness are homeless, dependent on alcohol or drugs, unemployed, and go without treatment. The commission identified public attitudes and the stigma associated with mental illness as major barriers to treatment. Stigma is often internalized by individuals with mental illness, leading to hopelessness, lower self-esteem, and isolation. Stigma deprives these individuals of the support they need to recover.

3. **High unemployment and disability for people with serious mental illness.** Undetected, untreated, and poorly treated mental disorders interrupt careers, leading many individuals into lives of disability, poverty, and long-term dependence. The commission found a 90 percent unemployment rate among adults with serious mental illness—the worst level of employment of any group of people with disabilities. Some surveys have shown that many individuals with serious mental illness *want* to work—and could with modest assistance. However, the largest "program" of assistance the United States offers for people with mental illness is disability payments. Sadly, societal stigma is also reflected in employment discrimination against people with mental illness.

4. **Older adults with mental illnesses are not receiving care.** The commission reported that about 5 to 10 percent of older adults have major depression, yet most are not properly recognized and treated. The report stated:

> Older people are reluctant to get care from specialists. They feel more comfortable going to their primary care physician. Still, they are often more sensitive to the stigma of mental illness, and do not readily bring up their sadness and despair. If they acknowledge problems, they are more likely than young people to describe physical symptoms. Primary care doctors may see their suffering as "natural" aging or treat their reported physical distress instead of the underlying mental disorder. What is often missed is the deep impact of depression on older people's capacity to function in ways that are seemingly effortless for others.

5. **Mental health and suicide prevention are not yet national priorities.** The United States' failure to prioritize mental health puts many lives at stake. Families struggle to maintain equilibrium while communities try (and often fail) to provide needed assistance for adults and children with mental illness. The report noted that over 30,000 lives are lost annually to suicide. About 90 percent of those who take their own lives have a mental disorder. Many individuals who die by suicide have not had the care in the months before their death that would have helped them. Both the APA and the National Mental Health Association called on the U.S. Congress to pass parity legislation.

In 2008, a federal law known as the Paul Wellstone and Pete Domenici Mental Health Parity and Addiction Equity Act was enacted that generally prevents group health plans and health insurance issuers that provide mental health or substance use disorder benefits from imposing less favorable limitations on those benefits than on medical/surgical benefits. In 2010, the Affordable Care Act amended this provision to include individual insurance plans, and in 2014, a final regulation clarified and expanded the parity law (Centers for Medicare & Medicaid Services [CMS], n.d.). Many recent national initiatives since the commission's report have attempted to bridge the gaps, particularly with efforts to address the still climbing national suicide rates and the opiate overdose epidemic. In 2014, the National Alliance on Mental Illness reported that unemployment rates among the seriously mentally ill were approximately 80 percent. Clearly, there is still much work to be done.

The commission outlined the following goals and recommendations for mental health reform:

Goal 1. Americans will understand that mental health is essential to overall health.
Advance and implement a national campaign to reduce the stigma of seeking care and a national strategy for suicide prevention.
- Address mental health with the same urgency as physical health.

Goal 2. Mental healthcare will be consumer and family driven.
- Develop an individualized plan of care for every adult with a serious mental illness and child with a serious emotional disturbance.
- Involve consumers and families fully in orienting the mental health system toward recovery.

- Align relevant federal programs to improve access and accountability for mental health services.
- Create a comprehensive state mental health plan.
- Protect and enhance the rights of people with mental illness.

Goal 3. Disparities in mental health services will be eliminated.

- Improve access to quality care that is culturally competent.
- Improve access to quality care in rural and geographically remote areas.

Goal 4. Early mental health screening, assessment, and referral to services will be common practice.

- Promote the mental health of young children.
- Improve and expand school mental health programs.
- Screen for co-occurring mental and substance use disorders and link with integrated treatment strategies.
- Screen for mental disorders in primary healthcare, across the life span, and connect to treatment and supports.

Goal 5. Excellent mental healthcare will be delivered and research will be accelerated.

- Accelerate research to promote recovery and resilience and ultimately to cure and prevent mental illnesses.
- Advance evidence-based practices using dissemination and demonstration projects and create a public-private partnership to guide their implementation.
- Improve and expand the workforce providing evidence-based mental health services and supports.
- Develop the knowledge base in four understudied areas: mental health disparities, long-term effects of medications, trauma, and acute care.

Goal 6. Technology will be used to access mental healthcare and information.

- Use health technology and telehealth to improve access and coordination of mental healthcare, especially for Americans in remote areas or in underserved populations.
- Develop and implement integrated electronic health record and personal health information systems.

SAMHSA, in collaboration with a number of other federal agencies, currently identifies about 311 federal action agenda initiatives to address mental health issues for specific, underserved populations, for suicide prevention, and a host of other community and public health concerns (SAMHSA, 2018). In 2016, the surgeon general released a landmark report identifying substance abuse as a national health priority in response to the rising death toll from opiate overdoses. In 2018, the National Institutes of Health launched the HEAL (Helping End Addictions Long-term) effort that includes 15 initiatives geared toward better treatment of opiate addiction and pain management. There is no doubt much current national attention to mental health and addiction concerns particularly related to epidemic levels of suicide and opiate-related deaths. The solutions to the multitude of serious mental illness and substance use-related issues that affect individuals and communities are complex and will require ongoing individual, local, and nationwide efforts.

Many nurse leaders see this period of healthcare reform as an opportunity for nurses to expand their roles and assume key positions in education, prevention, assessment, and referral. Nurses are, and will continue to be, in key positions to assist individuals with severe and persistent mental illness to remain as independent as possible, to manage their illness within the community setting, and to strive to minimize the number of hospitalizations required.

Treatment Alternatives

In the current *Scope and Standards of Practice: Psychiatric Mental Health Nursing* (American Nurses Association, American Psychiatric Nurses Association, & International Society of Psychiatric-Mental Health Nurses, 2014) community-based care is identified as within the scope of practice for psychiatric mental health registered nurses. They define *community-based care* as potentially including "care delivered in partnership with health care consumers in their homes, worksites, mental health clinics and programs, health maintenance organizations, shelters and clinics for the homeless, crisis centers, senior centers, group homes, and other community settings" (p. 24). It is clear that psychiatric nurses can and should play an active role in mental healthcare in the community.

Community Mental Health Centers The goal of community mental health centers in caring for individuals with severe and persistent mental illness is to improve coping ability and prevent exacerbation of acute symptoms. A major obstacle in meeting this goal has been the lack of advocacy or sponsorship for clients who require services from a variety of sources. This has placed responsibility for healthcare on an individual with mental illness who is often barely able to cope with everyday life. **Case management** (which is discussed in Chapter 6, The Nursing Process in Psychiatric Mental Health Nursing) has become a recommended method of treatment for individuals with severe and persistent mental illness. Ling and Ruscin (2013) state:

> Nurses may be uniquely qualified to be case managers because of their holistic and broad-based background, understanding of health care, and role in patient education and referrals. Case management is an area of practice that offers nurses an opportunity to build on their clinical knowledge, communication, and nursing process skills to function in an expanded patient care role.

In its standards of practice, the Case Management Society of America (2016) defines case management as "a collaborative process of assessment, planning, facilitation, care coordination, evaluation and advocacy for options and services to meet an individual's and family's comprehensive health needs through communication and available resources to promote patient safety, quality of care, and cost effective outcomes"(p. 11).

Ling and Ruscin (2013) identify six essential activities and nursing role functions that blend with the steps of the nursing process to form a framework for nursing case management:

1. **Assessment.** During the assessment process, the nurse gathers pertinent information about a client's situation and ability to function. Information may be obtained through physical examination, client interview, medical records, and reports from significant others. Ling and Ruscin state, "The case manager's goal is to obtain accurate information about the patient's status and identify factors that may significantly affect the patient's recovery and care."

2. **Planning.** A service care plan is devised with client participation. The plan should include mutually agreed-on goals, specific actions directed toward goal achievement, and selection of essential resources and services through collaboration among healthcare professionals, the client, and the family or significant others.

3. **Implementation.** In this phase, the client receives the needed services from the appropriate providers. In some instances, the nursing **case manager** is also a provider of care, whereas in others, he or she is only the coordinator of care.

4. **Coordination.** The case manager deliberately organizes care between two or more participants,

including the patient, to facilitate delivery of healthcare services and to ensure that patient care needs and preferences and appropriate sharing of information among resources occurs over time (Case Management Society of America [CMSA], 2016). This coordination effort involves the client, the physician, any other pertinent healthcare providers, and family members or significant others concerned with the client's care. The case manager ensures that all tests and treatments are conducted according to schedule and maintains close communication with all healthcare providers to ensure that client care is proceeding according to the plan.

5. **Monitoring.** The case manager monitors the effectiveness of the care plan by gathering pertinent information from various sources at regular intervals to determine the client's response and progress (CMSA, 2016). If problems are identified, immediate adjustments are made.

6. **Evaluation.** The case manager evaluates the client's responses to interventions and progress toward pre-established goals. Regular contact is maintained with client, family or significant others, and direct service providers. Ongoing coordination of care continues until outcomes have been achieved. If the expected outcomes are not achieved, the case manager reevaluates the plan to determine the reason and takes steps to intervene and modify the existing plan.

A case study of nursing case management within a community mental health center is presented in Box 26–2.

Assertive Community Treatment (ACT) The National Alliance on Mental Illness (NAMI, 2018) defines *ACT* as:

> a team-based treatment model that provides multidisciplinary, flexible treatment and support to people with mental illness 24/7. ACT is based around the idea that people receive better care when their mental health care providers work together. ACT team members help the person address every aspect of their life, whether it be medication, therapy, social support, employment or housing.

This approach includes members from psychiatry, social work, nursing, and substance abuse and vocational rehabilitation. The ACT team provides these services 24 hours a day, 7 days a week, 365 days a year.

The ACT team provides treatment, rehabilitation, and support services to individuals with severe and persistent mental illness who are unable on their own to receive treatment from a traditional model of case

BOX 26–2 Nursing Case Management in the Community Mental Health Center: A Case Study

William is a 63-year-old man with chronic schizophrenia who came into the community mental health center upon the recommendation of a local church where he sometimes attends their meal program. The nurse begins a comprehensive assessment and assures William that she wants to collaborate with him to identify how to best meet his needs. She assesses his basic physical health, management of daily living, family involvement, work history, involvement with any other social agencies, finances, medications, and other concerns identified by William. She determines that William has not been taking antipsychotic medication for at least 3 months. Prior to that, he had been living in a house with several other individuals, most of whom were abusing substances. They were helping him access medications from a community medication program but were often taking or reselling most of his prescription.

When the house was raided by police, William became homeless. He is currently disorganized in his thinking and actively hallucinating. He expresses desire to take medication but feels that finding a place to live is his most important priority. There is no family involvement, and William is unable to identify any support systems.

The nurse contacts the social worker for assistance with housing options and social resources such as food stamps and contacts the physician to schedule an appointment for medication evaluation. The nurse recommends that William attend the partial hospitalization program offered at the community mental health center, and he agrees but says he does not have transportation. The local church has offered to help William in any way they can, so the nurse contacts them and asks about their availability to provide transportation. The church informs her that they can provide transportation on Tuesdays and Thursdays.

During the assessment, William identified that sometimes the "people start fighting" in his mind and when he starts to scream back someone nearby always calls the police because they "don't get that I'm just trying to defend myself." The nurse then engages a peer support specialist who introduces William to Alfonzo, a 65-year-old man with chronic schizophrenia who is willing to provide support to William regarding symptom management. Alfonzo is also willing to provide transportation to the partial hospitalization program on the days when the church resources are not available. The nurse notices that William has some open sores on his feet. She cleans and bandages his feet, orders bloodwork to assess for infection, and accesses socks and footwear from the clothes bank offered through the Salvation Army. She continues to meet regularly with William once a month on a day that he attends PHP and administers the injectable antipsychotic medication (fluphenazine [Prolixin]) ordered by the physician. During her reassessment, William identifies that he has been "hanging out" with Alfonzo and states "he really understands me." He expresses that he still hears people fight sometimes in his head but is not as bothered by them. The social worker has facilitated group home placement, which is not available for another 3 months, but in the meantime the local homeless shelter has arranged for William to stay there. The local church has offered William a small stipend to help with stuffing envelopes, and when the nurse asks him how that job is going, William says, "They are nice people at the church, and they say I really help them, too."

---

management. The team is usually able to provide most services with minimal referrals to other mental health programs or providers. Services are provided within community settings, such as a person's home, local restaurants, parks, nearby stores, and any other place that the individual requires assistance with living skills. NAMI (2018) reports, "Studies have shown that ACT is more effective than traditional treatment for people experiencing mental illnesses such as schizophrenia and schizoaffective disorder and can reduce hospitalizations by 20%."

Partial Hospitalization Programs Partial hospitalization programs (also called day or evening treatment programs) are designed to prevent institutionalization or to ease the transition from inpatient hospitalization to community living. Various types of treatment are offered. Many include therapeutic community (milieu) activities; individual, group, and family therapies; psychoeducation; alcohol and drug education; crisis intervention; therapeutic recreational activities; and occupational therapy. Many programs offer medication administration and monitoring as part of their care. Some programs have established medication clinics for individuals on long-term psychopharmacological therapy. These clinics may include educational classes and support groups for individuals with similar conditions and treatments.

Partial hospitalization programs generally offer a comprehensive treatment plan formulated by an interdisciplinary team of psychiatrists, psychologists, nurses, occupational and recreational therapists, and social workers. Nurses take a leading role in the administration of partial hospitalization programs. They lead groups, provide crisis intervention, conduct individual counseling, act as role models, and make necessary referrals for specialized treatment. Use of the nursing process provides continual evaluation of the program, and modifications can be made as necessary.

Partial hospitalization programs are an effective method of preventing hospitalization for many individuals with severe and persistent mental illness. They are a way of transitioning individuals from the acute care setting back into the mainstream of the community. For some individuals who have been deinstitutionalized, they provide structure, support, opportunities for socialization, and an improvement in their overall quality of life.

Community Residential Facilities Community residential facilities for persons with severe and persistent mental illness are known by many names: group homes, halfway houses, foster homes, boarding homes, sheltered care facilities, transitional housing, independent living programs, social rehabilitation residences, and others. These facilities differ by the purpose for which they exist and the activities that they offer.

Some of these facilities provide food, shelter, housekeeping, and minimal supervision and assistance with activities of daily living. Others may also include a variety of therapies and serve as a transition between hospital and independent living. In addition to the basics, services might include individual and group counseling, medical care, job training or employment assistance, and leisure-time activities.

A wide variety of personnel staff these facilities. Some facilities have live-in professionals who are available at all times; some have professional staff who are on call for intervention during crisis situations; and some are staffed by volunteers and individuals with little knowledge or background for understanding and treating persons with severe and persistent mental illness.

The concept of transitional housing for individuals with serious mental illness is sound and has often been a successful means of therapeutic support and intervention to facilitate residence within the community. However, without guidance and planning, transition to the community may not be successful. Individuals may be ridiculed and rejected by the community. They may be targets of unscrupulous individuals who take advantage of their inability to care for themselves satisfactorily. These behaviors may increase maladaptive responses to the demands of community living and exacerbate the mental illness. A period of structured reorientation to the community in a living situation that is supervised and monitored by professionals is more likely to result in a successful transition for the individual with severe and persistent mental illness. Since 2013, transitional housing beds have declined in favor of rapid

rehousing and permanent supportive housing; rapid rehousing capacity more than tripled between 2013 and 2016 (U.S. Conference of Mayors [USCM], 2016). Yet, the USCM (2016) reports that even if every emergency shelter and transitional housing bed were filled, there would still be 34,000 people without shelter on a given night. Clearly, affordable and supportive housing continue to be significant needs in the struggle to end homelessness.

Psychiatric Home Healthcare For the individual with serious mental illness who no longer lives in a structured, supervised setting, home healthcare may be the element that helps to keep him or her living independently. To receive home healthcare, individuals must validate their homebound status for the prospective payer (Medicare, Medicaid, most insurance companies, and Department of Veterans Affairs [VA] benefits). An acute psychiatric diagnosis is not enough to qualify for the service. The client must show that he or she is unable to leave the home without considerable difficulty or the assistance of another person. The plan of treatment and subsequent charting must explain why the client's psychiatric disorder keeps him or her at home and justify the need for home services.

Homebound clients most often have a diagnosis of depressive disorder, neurocognitive disorder, anxiety disorder, bipolar disorder, or schizophrenia. Many elderly clients are homebound because of medical conditions that impair mobility and necessitate home care.

Nurses who provide psychiatric home care must have an in-depth knowledge of psychopathology, psychopharmacology, and how medical and physical problems can be influenced by psychiatric impairments. These nurses must be highly adept at performing biopsychosocial assessments. They must be sensitive to changes in behavior that signal that the client is decompensating psychiatrically or medically so that early intervention may be implemented.

Another important job of the psychiatric home health nurse is monitoring the patient's adherence to the regimen of psychotropic medications. Some patients who are receiving injectable medications remain on home healthcare only until they can be placed on oral medications. Those receiving oral medications require close monitoring for adherence and assistance with the uncomfortable side effects of some of these drugs. Lack of adherence to the medication regimen is responsible for approximately two-thirds of psychiatric hospital readmissions. Home health nurses can assist patients with this problem by helping them to see the relationship between control of their psychiatric symptoms and adherence to their medication regimen.

Patient populations that benefit from psychiatric home health nursing include:

- **Elderly:** These individuals may not have a psychiatric diagnosis, but they may be experiencing emotional difficulties that have arisen from medical, sociocultural, or developmental factors. Depressed mood and social isolation are common.
- **Persons with severe and persistent mental illness:** These individuals have a history of psychiatric illness and hospitalization. They require long-term medications and continual supportive care. Common diagnoses include recurrent major depressive disorder, schizophrenia, and bipolar disorder.
- **Individuals in acute crisis situations:** These individuals are in need of crisis intervention and/or short-term psychotherapy.

Medicare requires that psychiatric home nursing care be provided by "psychiatrically trained nurses," which the CMS defines as "nurses who have special training and/or experience beyond the standard curriculum required for a registered nurse" (CMS, 2017).

The guidelines that cover psychiatric nursing services are not well defined by the CMS. This has presented some reimbursement problems for psychiatric nurses in the past. The CMS statement regarding psychiatric nursing services is presented in Box 26–3.

Preparation for psychiatric home health nursing, in addition to the registered nurse licensure, should include several years of psychiatric inpatient treatment experience. It is also recommended that the nurse have medical-surgical nursing experience

---

BOX 26–3 CMS Guidelines for Psychiatric Home Nursing Care

PSYCHIATRIC EVALUATION, THERAPY, AND TEACHING

The evaluation, psychotherapy, and teaching needed by a patient suffering from a diagnosed psychiatric disorder that requires active treatment by a psychiatrically trained nurse and the costs of the psychiatric nurse's services may be covered as a skilled nursing service. Psychiatrically trained nurses are nurses who have special training and/or experience beyond the standard curriculum required for a registered nurse. The services of the psychiatric nurse are to be provided under a plan of care established and reviewed by a physician.

Source: Centers for Medicare & Medicaid Services. (2017). Medicare Benefit Policy Manual. *Baltimore, MD.*

---

because of common comorbidities and to provide holistic nursing care. Additional training and experience in psychotherapy is viewed as an asset. However, psychotherapy is not the primary focus of psychiatric home nursing care. In fact, most reimbursement sources do not pay for exclusively insight-oriented therapy. Crisis intervention, patient education, and hands-on care are common interventions in psychiatric home nursing care.

The psychiatric home health nurse provides comprehensive nursing care, incorporating interventions for physical and psychosocial problems into the treatment plan. The interventions are based on the patient's mental and physical health status, cultural influences, and available resources. The nurse is accountable to the patient at all times during the therapeutic relationship. Nursing interventions are carried out with appropriate knowledge and skill, and referrals are made when the need is outside the scope of nursing practice. Continued collaboration with other members of the healthcare team (e.g., psychiatrist, social worker, psychologist, occupational therapist, and/or physical therapist) is essential for maintaining continuity of care.

See the following case study on psychiatric home healthcare and the nursing process. A plan of care for Mrs. C (the client in the case study) is presented in Table 26–2. Nursing diagnoses are presented, along with outcome criteria, appropriate nursing interventions, and rationale for each.

Care for the Caregivers Another aspect of psychiatric home healthcare is to provide support and assistance to primary caregivers. When family is the provider of care on a 7-day-a-week, 24-hour-a-day schedule for a loved one with a severe and persistent mental disorder, it can be very exhausting and very frustrating. A care plan for primary caregivers is presented in Table 26–3.

The Homeless Population

Historical and Epidemiological Aspects

In 1993, Dr. Richard Lamb, a recognized expert in the field of severe and persistent mental illness, wrote:

> Alec Guinness, in his memorable role as a British Army colonel in *Bridge on the River Kwai*, exclaims at the end of the film when he finally realizes he has been working to help the enemy, "What have I done?" As a vocal advocate and spokesman for deinstitutionalization and community treatment of severely mentally ill patients for well over two decades, I often find myself asking that same question. (p. 1209)

PSYCHIATRIC HOME HEALTHCARE AND THE NURSING PROCESS: A CASE STUDY

ASSESSMENT

Mrs. C, aged 76, has been living alone in her small apartment for 6 months since the death of her husband to whom she had been married for 51 years. Mrs. C had been an elementary school teacher for 40 years, retiring at age 65 with an adequate pension. She and her husband had no children. A niece looks in on Mrs. C regularly. It was she who contacted Mrs. C's physician when she observed that Mrs. C was not eating properly, was losing weight, and seemed to be isolating herself more and more. She had not left her apartment in weeks. Her physician referred her to psychiatric home healthcare.

On her initial visit, Renee, the psychiatric home health nurse, conducted a preliminary assessment, revealing the following information about Mrs. C:

1. Blood pressure 90/60 mm Hg
2. Height 5 ft 5 in.; weight 102 lb
3. Poor skin turgor; dehydration
4. Subjective report of occasional dizziness
5. Subjective report of loss of 20 pounds since the death of her husband
6. Oriented to time, place, person, and situation
7. Memory (remote and recent) intact
8. Flat affect
9. Mood is dysphoric and tearful at times, but client is cooperative
10. Denies thoughts to harm self but states, "I feel so alone; so useless."
11. Subjective report of difficulty sleeping
12. Subjective report of constipation

DIAGNOSIS AND OUTCOME IDENTIFICATION

The following nursing diagnoses were formulated for Mrs. C:
1. Complicated grieving related to death of husband evidenced by symptoms of depression such as withdrawal, anorexia, weight loss, difficulty sleeping, dysphoric/tearful mood
2. Risk for injury related to dizziness and weakness from lack of activity, low blood pressure, and poor nutritional status
3. Social isolation related to depressed mood and feelings of worthlessness, evidenced by staying home alone, refusing to leave her apartment

Outcome Criteria
The following criteria were selected as measurement of outcomes in the care of Mrs. C:

■ Experiences no physical harm/injury
■ Is able to discuss feelings about husband's death with nurse

■ Sets realistic goals for self
■ Is able to participate in problem-solving regarding her future
■ Eats a well-balanced diet with snacks to restore nutritional status and gain weight
■ Drinks adequate fluids daily
■ Sleeps at least 6 hours per night and verbalizes feeling well rested
■ Shows interest in personal appearance and hygiene and is able to accomplish self-care independently
■ Seeks to renew contact with previous friends and acquaintances
■ Verbalizes interest in participating in social activities

PLAN AND IMPLEMENTATION

A plan of care for Mrs. C is presented in Table 26–2.

EVALUATION

Mrs. C started the second week taking trazodone (Desyrel) 150 mg at bedtime. Her sleep was enhanced, and within 2 weeks she showed a noticeable improvement in mood. She began to discuss how angry she felt about being all alone in the world. She admitted that she had felt anger toward her husband but experienced guilt and tried to suppress that anger. As she was assured that these feelings were normal, they became easier for her to express.

The nurse arranged for a local teenager to do some weekly grocery shopping for Mrs. C and contacted the local Meals on Wheels program, which delivered her noon meal to her every day. Mrs. C began to eat more and slowly to gain a few pounds. She still has an occasional problem with constipation but verbalizes improvement with the addition of vegetables, fruit, and a daily stool softener prescribed by her physician.

Mrs. C used her walker until she felt she was able to ambulate without assistance. She reports that she no longer experiences dizziness, and her blood pressure has stabilized at around 100/70 mm Hg.

Mrs. C has joined a senior citizens group and attends activities weekly. She has renewed previous friendships and formed new acquaintances. She sees her physician monthly for medication management and visits a local adult day health center for regular blood pressure and weight checks. Her niece still visits regularly, but her favorite relationship is the one she has formed with her constant canine companion, Molly, whom Mrs. C rescued from the local animal shelter and who continually demonstrates her unconditional love and gratitude.

Table 26–2 | CARE PLAN FOR PSYCHIATRIC HOME HEALTHCARE OF DEPRESSED ELDERLY (MRS. C)

NURSING DIAGNOSIS: COMPLICATED GRIEVING

RELATED TO: Death of husband

EVIDENCED BY: Symptoms of depression such as withdrawal, anorexia, weight loss, difficulty sleeping, and dysphoric/tearful mood

OUTCOME CRITERIA	NURSING INTERVENTIONS	RATIONALE
Short-Term Goal ■ Mrs. C will discuss any angry feelings she has about the loss of her husband. **Long-Term Goal** ■ Mrs. C will demonstrate adaptive grieving behaviors and evidence of progression toward resolution.	1. Assess Mrs. C's position in the grief process. 2. Develop a trusting relationship by showing empathy and caring. Be honest and keep all promises. Show genuine positive regard. 3. Explore feelings of anger and help Mrs. C direct them toward the source. Help her understand it is appropriate and acceptable to have feelings of anger and guilt about her husband's death. 4. Encourage Mrs. C to review honestly the relationship she had with her husband. With support and sensitivity, point out reality of the situation in areas where misrepresentations may be expressed. 5. Determine if Mrs. C has spiritual needs that are going unfulfilled. If so, contact spiritual leader for intervention with Mrs. C. 6. Refer Mrs. C to physician for medication evaluation.	1. Accurate baseline data are required to plan accurate care for Mrs. C. 2. These interventions provide the basis for a therapeutic relationship. 3. Knowledge of acceptability of the feelings associated with normal grieving may help to relieve some of the guilt that these responses generate. 4. Mrs. C must give up an idealized perception of her husband. Only when she is able to see both positive and negative aspects about the relationship will the grieving process be complete. 5. Recovery may be blocked if spiritual distress is present and care is not provided. 6. Antidepressant therapy may help Mrs. C to function while confronting the dynamics of her depression.

NURSING DIAGNOSIS: RISK FOR INJURY

RELATED TO: Dizziness and weakness from lack of activity, low blood pressure, and poor nutritional status

OUTCOME CRITERIA	NURSING INTERVENTIONS	RATIONALE
Short-Term Goals ■ Mrs. C will use walker when ambulating. ■ Mrs. C will not experience physical harm or injury. **Long-Term Goal** ■ Mrs. C will not experience physical harm or injury.	1. Assess vital signs at every visit. Report to physician should they fall below baseline. 2. Encourage Mrs. C to use walker until strength has returned. 3. Visit Mrs. C during mealtimes and sit with her while she eats. Encourage her niece to do the same. Ensure that easy-to-prepare, nutritious foods for meals and snacks are available in the house and that they are items that Mrs. C likes.	1. Client safety is a nursing priority. 2. The walker will help prevent Mrs. C from falling. 3. She is more likely to eat what is convenient and what she enjoys.

Continued

Table 26–2 | CARE PLAN FOR PSYCHIATRIC HOME HEALTHCARE OF DEPRESSED ELDERLY (MRS. C)—cont'd

OUTCOME CRITERIA	NURSING INTERVENTIONS	RATIONALE
	4. Contact local meal delivery service (e.g., Meals on Wheels) to deliver some of Mrs. C's meals.	4. This would ensure that she receives at least one complete and nutritious meal each day.
	5. Weigh Mrs. C each week.	5. Weight gain is a measurable, objective means of assessing whether Mrs. C is eating.
	6. Ensure that diet contains sufficient fluid and fiber.	6. Adequate dietary fluid and fiber will help to alleviate constipation. She may also benefit from a daily stool softener.

NURSING DIAGNOSIS: SOCIAL ISOLATION

RELATED TO: Depressed mood and feelings of worthlessness

EVIDENCED BY: Staying home alone, refusing to leave apartment

OUTCOME CRITERIA	NURSING INTERVENTIONS	RATIONALE
Short-Term Goal ■ Mrs. C will discuss with nurse feelings about past social relationships and those she may like to renew. **Long-Term Goal** ■ Mrs. C will renew contact with friends and participate in social activities.	1. As nutritional status improves and strength is gained, encourage Mrs. C to become more active. Take walks with her; help her perform simple tasks around her house. 2. Assess lifelong patterns of relationships. 3. Help her identify present relationships that are satisfying and activities that she considers interesting. 4. Assess mental status for mood changes and risk for suicide. 5. Consider the feasibility of a pet. 6. Suggest possible alternatives that Mrs. C may consider as she seeks to participate in social activities. These may include foster grandparent programs, senior citizens centers, church activities, craft groups, and volunteer activities. Help her to locate individuals with whom she may attend some of these activities.	1. Increased activity enhances both physical and mental status. 2. Basic personality characteristics will not change. Mrs. C will very likely keep the same style of relationship development that she had in the past. 3. She is the person who truly knows what she likes, and these personal preferences will facilitate success in reversing social isolation. 4. Mrs. C has expressed feelings of depression and worthlessness so her mental status should be assessed regularly to identify any worsening of symptoms and risk for suicide. 5. There are many documented studies of the benefits to elderly individuals of companion pets. 6. She is more likely to attend and participate if she does not have to do so alone.

Table 26–3 | CARE PLAN FOR PRIMARY CAREGIVER OF INDIVIDUAL WITH SEVERE AND PERSISTENT MENTAL ILLNESS

NURSING DIAGNOSIS: CAREGIVER ROLE STRAIN

RELATED TO: Severity and duration of the care receiver's illness and lack of respite and recreation for the caregiver

EVIDENCED BY: Feelings of stress in relationship with care receiver, feelings of depression and anger, family conflict around issues of providing care

OUTCOME CRITERIA	NURSING INTERVENTIONS	RATIONALE

Short-Term Goal
■ Caregivers will verbalize understanding of ways to facilitate the caregiver role.
 	
Long-Term Goal
■ Caregivers will demonstrate effective problem-solving skills and develop adaptive coping mechanisms to regain equilibrium.
	1. Assess caregivers' abilities to anticipate and fulfill the individual's unmet needs. Provide information to assist caregivers with this responsibility. Ensure that caregivers encourage individual to be as independent as possible.
	2. Ensure that caregivers are aware of available community support systems from which they may seek assistance when required. Examples include respite care services, day treatment centers, and adult day-care centers.
	3. Encourage caregivers to express feelings, particularly anger.
	
	4. Encourage participation in support groups comprised of members with similar life situations. Provide information about support groups that may be helpful:
	    a. National Alliance on Mental Illness (NAMI) (800) 950-NAMI
	    b. American Association on Intellectual and Developmental Disabilities (AAIDD) (202) 387-1968
	    c. Alzheimer's Association (800) 272-3900
		1. Caregivers may be unaware of what their loved one can realistically accomplish. They may be unaware of the nature of the illness.
		
		2. Caregivers require relief from the pressures and strain of providing 24-hour care for their loved one. Studies have shown that abuse arises out of caregiving situations that place overwhelming stress on the caregivers.
		3. Release of these emotions can serve to prevent psychopathology, such as depression or psychophysiological disorders, from occurring.
		4. Hearing others who are experiencing the same problems discuss ways in which they have coped may help caregiver adopt more adaptive strategies. Individuals who are experiencing similar life situations provide empathy and support for each other.

Mental illness is the third largest reason for homelessness and substance use disorders are a common comorbidity (National Coalition for the Homeless [NCH], 2017). It is difficult to determine the true scope of the problem because even the statisticians who collect the data have difficulty defining *homeless persons*. They have sometimes been identified as "those people who sleep in shelters or public spaces."

This approach results in underestimates because available shelter services are insufficient to meet the numbers of homeless people (USCM, 2016).

According to the Stewart B. McKinney Homeless Assistance Act (govtrack, 1987), a person is considered homeless when he or she

lacks a fixed, regular, and adequate night-time residence; and . . . has a primary night-time residency that is: (A) a supervised publicly or privately operated shelter designed to provide temporary living accommodations, (B) an institution that provides a temporary residence for individuals intended to be institutionalized, or (C) a public or private place not designed for, or ordinarily used as, a regular sleeping accommodation for human beings.

The National Alliance to End Homelessness (2018) reports that from 2007 to 2017, homelessness overall declined by 14.4 percent with the most dramatic decreases among veterans. However, about 33 percent of the current homeless population have some form of severe mental illness (NCH, 2017) and one of the cited contributing factors is limited access to inpatient psychiatric treatment. Homelessness among the mentally ill continues to be a significant concern for this vulnerable population.

Many homeless individuals are children and young adults. Some are homeless because of their dependence on a parent who is homeless, but many are trauma victims who have left their homes to avoid physical or sexual abuse and neglect. Some are LGBTQ (lesbian, gay, bisexual, transgender, or questioning) youth who have become homeless secondary to family intolerance about their sexual orientation and identity (Safe Horizon, 2018). In 2017, there were approximately 40,799 unaccompanied homeless youth, representing just over 7 percent of the total homeless population, and 55 percent of those youth were unsheltered (U.S. Department of Housing and Urban Development [HUD], 2017). Many initiatives have sought to reduce these numbers and to provide resources to minimize disruptions posed by homelessness. In October 2016, amendments to the McKinney-Vento Act went into effect that include provisions for homeless children and young adults to receive adequate and accessible education. However, these provisions do not address the child who is "on the run." These children remain a high-risk, vulnerable population who often have a history of trauma as well as additional trauma posed by homelessness and sex trafficking.

Mental Illness and Homelessness

Demographics The prevalence of severe mental illness among the homeless population is difficult to clarify. SAMHSA (2016) provides the following demographics through statistics gathered from Projects for Assistance in Transition from Homelessness (PATH), which was specifically established for funding services to people with severe mental illness. Thus, these statistics are based on the makeup of PATH clients:

■ Age: Thirty-nine percent of clients with severe mental illness are younger than age 30; individuals between the ages of 31 and 61 make up the bulk of this population at 70 percent; about 5 percent are older than age 61.

■ Gender: Fifty-nine percent of homeless individuals are male, and 41 percent are female.

■ Ethnicity: The homeless severe mental illness population is estimated to be 57 percent Caucasian, 34 percent African American, 13 percent Hispanic, 3 percent of other single races/ethnic groups, and 5 percent of multiple races (SAMHSA, 2016). The ethnic makeup of homeless populations varies according to geographic location.

The USCM (2016) survey revealed that approximately 33 percent of the homeless population suffers from some form of mental illness. Who are these individuals, and why are they homeless? Some blame the deinstitutionalization movement. Persons with mental illness who were released from state and county mental hospitals and who did not have families with whom they could reside sought residence in board and care homes of varying quality. Halfway houses and supportive group living arrangements were helpful but scarce. Many of those with families returned to their homes, but because families received little, if any, instruction or support, the consequences of their mentally ill loved one returning to live at home were often turbulent, resulting in the individual frequently leaving home.

Types of Mental Illness Among the Homeless A number of studies have been conducted, primarily in large, urban areas that have addressed the most common types of mental illness identified among homeless individuals. Schizophrenia is frequently described as the most common diagnosis. Other prevalent disorders include bipolar disorder, substance addiction, depression, personality disorders, and neurocognitive disorders. Many who exhibit psychotic symptoms are former residents of long-term care institutions for the mentally ill and have such a strong desire for independence that they isolate themselves in an effort to avoid being identified as a part of the mental health system. Many are clearly a danger to themselves or others, yet they often do not even see themselves as ill. SAMHSA (2016) identifies that in 2015, 53 percent of clients receiving PATH services had a co-occurring substance use disorder.

Contributing Factors to Homelessness Among Individuals With Mental Illness

Deinstitutionalization As previously stated, deinstitutionalization is frequently implicated as a contributing factor to homelessness among individuals with mental illness. Deinstitutionalization began out of expressed concern by mental health professionals and others who described the "deplorable conditions" under which mentally ill individuals were housed.

The advent of psychotropic medications and the community mental health movement began a growing philosophical view that individuals with mental illness receive better and more humanitarian treatment in the community than in state hospitals far removed from their homes. It was believed that commitment and institutionalization in many ways deprived these individuals of their civil rights. Not the least of the motivating factors for deinstitutionalization was the financial burden these clients placed on state governments.

Although the deinstitutionalization movement has prompted an expansion of community mental health resources, the number of people with mental illness being incarcerated in correctional facilities has skyrocketed and is now estimated to be two to four times that of the general population (National Institute of Corrections, n.d.). Supporters of the community mental health movement have argued that ongoing problems for those with severe mental illness are related to lack of compliance with medications, but critics have argued that the community mental health model has been too narrowly focused on a biomedical approach and must revise and expand its model of services to meet the complex needs of this population going forward.

Deinstitutionalization has been criticized for contributing to both homelessness rates and criminalization of people with mental illnesses, but several other factors have been implicated as well.

Poverty Cuts in various government entitlement programs have depleted the allotments available for individuals with severe and persistent mental illness living in the community. The job market is prohibitive for individuals whose behavior is incomprehensible or even frightening to many. The stigma and discrimination associated with mental illness may be diminishing slowly, but it is highly visible to those who suffer from its effects.

Scarcity of Affordable Housing Not only is there a scarcity of affordable housing, but the number of single-room-occupancy (SRO) hotels has diminished drastically. These SRO hotels provided a means of relatively inexpensive housing, and although some people believe that these facilities nurtured isolation, they provided adequate shelter from the elements for their occupants. Because so many mentally ill individuals rely on homeless shelters, there is concern that shelters are becoming mini-institutions for individuals with serious mental illness.

Other Factors Several other factors that may contribute to homelessness have been identified:

- **Lack of affordable healthcare:** For families barely able to pay for their day-to-day living expenses, a catastrophic illness can start the downward spiral to homelessness.
- **Domestic violence:** According to a Family and Youth Services Report (2016) up to 57 percent of homeless women identify domestic violence as the primary reason for homelessness. Other research has found that 93 percent of homeless mothers had a history of trauma, 79 percent experienced trauma as children, and 81 percent experienced multiple traumatic events (NCH, 2015). The need for trauma-informed care in this population cannot be overstated.
- **Addiction disorders:** For individuals with alcohol or drug addictions, in the absence of appropriate treatment, the chances increase for being forced into life on the street. The following have been cited as obstacles to addiction treatment for homeless persons: lack of health insurance, lack of documentation, waiting lists, scheduling difficulties, daily contact requirements, lack of transportation, ineffective treatment methods, lack of supportive services, and cultural insensitivity.

Community Resources for the Homeless

Interfering Factors Among the many issues that complicate service planning for homeless individuals with mental illness is this population's penchant for mobility. Frequent relocation confounds service delivery and interferes with providers' efforts to ensure appropriate care. Some individuals with serious mental illness may be affected by homelessness only temporarily or intermittently. These individuals are sometimes called the "episodically homeless."

Others move around within neighborhoods or cities as needs change and based on whether or not they can obtain needed services. A large number of the homeless mentally ill population exhibits continuous unbounded movement over wide geographical areas.

Not all homeless individuals with mental illness are mobile. Some studies have indicated that a large percentage remain in the same location over a number of years. Healthcare workers must identify movement patterns of homeless people in their area to at least try to bring the best care possible to this unique population. This effort may mean delivering services to those individuals who do not seek out services on their own.

Health Issues Life as a homeless person can have severe consequences in terms of health. Exposure to the elements, poor diet, sleep deprivation, risk of violence, injuries, and little or no healthcare lead to a precarious state of health and exacerbate any pre-existing illnesses. One of the major problems is alcoholism. It has been estimated that about 40 percent of homeless individuals abuse alcohol. Compared with other homeless individuals, those who abuse alcohol are at greater risk for neurological impairment, heart disease and hypertension, chronic lung disease, gastrointestinal disorders, hepatic dysfunction, and trauma.

Thermoregulation is a health problem for all homeless individuals because of their exposure to all kinds of weather. It is a compounded problem for the homeless alcoholic who spends much time in an altered level of consciousness.

It is difficult to determine whether mental illness is a cause or an effect of homelessness. Some behaviors that may seem deviant may be adaptations to life on the street. It has been suggested that some homeless individuals may even seek hospitalization in psychiatric institutions in an attempt to get off the streets for a short time.

Whereas tuberculosis (TB) rates in the United States have been on the decline for several years, the homeless remain an at-risk population; 5 percent of those with TB reported homelessness within the prior year (Centers for Disease Control and Prevention, 2018). Crowded **shelters** provide ideal conditions for spread of respiratory infections among their inhabitants. The risk of acquiring TB is also increased by the prevalence of alcoholism, drug addiction, HIV infection, poor nutrition, and lack of access to medical care among homeless individuals.

Dietary deficiencies are a continuing problem for homeless individuals. Not only is the homeless person commonly in a poor nutritional state, but also the condition itself exacerbates a number of other health problems. Homeless people have higher mortality rates and a greater number of serious disorders than their counterparts in the general population.

Sexually transmitted infections (STIs), such as gonorrhea and syphilis, are a serious problem for the homeless. One of the most serious STIs prevalent among homeless individuals is HIV infection. Street life is precarious for individuals who are immunosuppressed by HIV. Rummaged food scraps are often spoiled, and exposure to the elements is a continuous threat. Individuals with HIV disease who stay in shelters often are exposed to the infectious diseases of others, which can be life threatening in their vulnerable condition.

Homeless children have special health needs. Children without a home are more vulnerable to asthma, ear infections, stomach problems, and speech problems than their counterparts who are not homeless. They also experience more mental health problems, such as anxiety, depression, and withdrawal. They are twice as likely to experience hunger and four times as likely to have delayed development.

A growing problem, which has captured national attention, is the increasing number of hate crimes perpetrated against the homeless. These attacks do not appear to be specifically directed toward the mentally ill but rather reflect a primary bias against homeless people. Based on the most recent report by NCH (2016), most of the victims (77 percent) are male, 57 percent are 40 years of age or older, 35 percent of the attacks are fatal, and 73 percent of the perpetrators were younger than age 30. The NCH adds that there is a documented correlation between criminalization laws and increases in attacks on the homeless, possibly because it sends a message to the public that "'Homeless people do not matter and are not worthy of living in our city.' This message is blatant in the attitudes many cities have toward homeless people" (2016, p. 68). Community mental health nurses have an opportunity and a responsibility to assess and intervene for homeless people, who are a vulnerable population on so many levels.

Types of Resources Available

Homeless Shelters The system of shelters for the homeless in the United States varies widely from converted warehouses that provide cots or floor space on which to sleep overnight to significant operations that provide a multitude of social and healthcare services. They are run by volunteers and paid professionals and are sponsored by churches, community governments, and a variety of social agencies.

It is impossible, then, to describe a "typical" shelter. One profile may be described as the provision of lodging, food, and clothing to individuals who are in need of these services. Some shelters also provide medical and psychiatric evaluations, first aid and other healthcare services, and referral for case management services by nurses or social workers.

Individuals who seek services from the shelter are generally assigned a bed or cot, issued a set of clean linen, provided a place to shower, given access to laundry facilities, and offered a meal in the shelter kitchen or dining hall. Most shelters attempt to separate dormitory areas for men and women with various consequences for those who violate the rules.

Shelters cover expenses through private and corporate donations, church sponsorships, and government grants. From the outset, shelters were conceptualized as "temporary" accommodations for individuals who needed a place to spend the night. Realistically, they have become permanent lodging for homeless individuals with little hope for improving their situation. Some individuals use shelters for their mailing address.

Shelters provide a safe and supportive environment for homeless individuals who have no other place to go. Some homeless people who inhabit shelters use the resources offered to improve their lot in life, whereas others become hopelessly dependent on the shelter's provisions. To a few, the availability of a shelter may even mean the difference between life and death.

Healthcare Centers and Storefront Clinics Some communities have established "street clinics" to serve the homeless population. Many of these clinics are operated by nurse practitioners who work in consultation with physicians in the area. In recent years, some of these clinics have provided clinical sites for nursing students in their community health rotation. Some have been staffed by faculties of nursing schools that have established group practices in the community setting.

A wide variety of services are offered at these clinics, including administering medications, assessing vital signs, screening for tuberculosis and other communicable diseases, giving immunizations and flu shots, changing dressings, and administering first aid. Physical and psychosocial assessments, health education, and supportive counseling are also frequent interventions.

Nursing in **storefront clinics** for the homeless provides many special challenges, not the least of which is poor working conditions. These clinics often operate under severe budgetary constraints with inadequate staffing, supplies, and equipment in rundown facilities located in high-crime neighborhoods. Frustration is often high among nurses who work in these clinics because they are seldom able to see measurable progress in their homeless patients. Maintenance of health management is virtually impossible for many individuals who have no resources outside the healthcare setting. When return appointments for preventive care are made, the lack of follow-through is high.

Mobile Outreach Units Outreach programs literally reach out to the homeless in their own environment in an effort to provide healthcare. Volunteers and paid professionals form teams to drive or walk around and seek out homeless individuals who are in need of assistance. They offer coffee, sandwiches, and blankets in an effort to show concern and establish trust. If assistance can be provided at the site, it is done so. If not, every effort is made to ensure that the individual is linked with a source that can provide the necessary services.

Mobile outreach units provide assistance to homeless individuals who are in need of physical or psychological care. The emphasis of outreach programs is to accommodate the homeless who refuse to seek treatment elsewhere. Most target the mentally ill segment of the population. When trust has been established and the individual agrees to come to the team's office, medical and psychiatric treatment is initiated. Involuntary hospitalization is initiated when an individual is deemed harmful to self or others or otherwise meets the criteria for being considered "gravely disabled."

The Homeless Client and the Nursing Process

Following is a case study demonstrating nursing process with a homeless client.

CASE STUDY: NURSING PROCESS WITH A HOMELESS CLIENT

ASSESSMENT

Joe, age 68, is brought to the community health clinic by two of his peers, who report: "He just had a fit. He needs a drink bad!" Joe is dirty and unkempt, has visible tremors of the upper extremities, and is weak enough to require assistance when ambulating. He is cooperative as the nurse completes the intake assessment. He is coherent, although thought processes are slow. He is disoriented to time and place. He appears somewhat frightened as he scans the unfamiliar surroundings. He is unable to tell the nurse when he had his last drink. He reports no physical injury, and none is observable.

Joe carries a small bag with a few personal items inside, including a Department of Veterans Affairs (VA) benefit card, identifying him as a veteran of the Vietnam War. The nurse finds a cot for Joe to lie down, ensures that his vital signs are stable, and telephones the number on the VA card. The clinic nurse discovers that Joe is well known to the admissions personnel at the VA. He has a 35-year history of schizophrenia with numerous hospitalizations. At the time of his last discharge, he was taking fluphenazine (Prolixin) 10 mg twice a day. He told the clinic nurse that he took the medication for a few months after he got out of the hospital but then did not have the prescription refilled. He could not remember when he had last taken fluphenazine.

Joe also has a long history of alcohol-related disorders and has participated in the VA substance rehabilitation program three times. He has no home address and receives his VA disability benefit checks at a shelter address. He reports that he has no family. The nurse makes arrangements for VA personnel to drive Joe from the clinic to the VA hospital, where he is admitted for detoxification. She sets up a case management file for Joe and arranges with the hospital to have Joe return to the clinic after discharge.

DIAGNOSIS AND OUTCOME IDENTIFICATION

The following nursing diagnosis was formulated for Joe:

Ineffective health maintenance related to ineffective coping skills evidenced by abuse of alcohol, lack of follow-through with antipsychotic medication, and lack of personal hygiene Ongoing criteria were selected as outcomes for Joe:

■ Follows the rules of the group home and maintains his residency status
■ Attends weekly sessions of group therapy at the VA day treatment program
■ Attends weekly sessions of Alcoholics Anonymous and maintains sobriety
■ Reports regularly to the health clinic for injections of fluphenazine
■ Volunteers at the VA hospital 3 days a week
■ Secures and retains permanent employment

PLAN AND IMPLEMENTATION

During Joe's hospitalization, the clinic nurse remained in contact with his case. Joe received complete physical and dental examinations and treatment during his hospital stay. The clinic nurse attended the treatment team meeting for Joe as his outpatient case manager. It was decided at the meeting to try giving Joe injections of fluphenazine decanoate because of his history of lack of adherence to his daily oral medication regimen. The clinic nurse would administer the injection every 4 weeks.

At Joe's follow-up clinic visit, the nurse explains to Joe that she has found a group home where he may live with others who have personal circumstances similar to his. At the group home, meals will be provided and the group home manager will ensure that Joe's basic needs are fulfilled. A criterion for remaining at the residence is for Joe to remain alcohol free. Joe is agreeable to these living arrangements.

With Joe's concurrence, the clinic nurse also performs the following interventions:

■ Goes shopping with Joe to purchase some new clothing, allowing Joe to make decisions as independently as possible
■ Helps Joe move into the group home and introduces him to the manager and residents
■ Helps Joe change his address from the shelter to the group home so that he may continue to receive his VA benefits
■ Enrolls Joe in the weekly group therapy sessions of the day treatment facility connected with the VA hospital
■ Helps Joe locate the nearest Alcoholics Anonymous group and identifies a sponsor who will ensure that Joe gets to the meetings
■ Sets up a clinic appointment for Joe to return in 4 weeks for his fluphenazine injection; telephones Joe 1 day in advance to remind him of his appointment
■ Instructs Joe to return to or call the clinic if any of the following symptoms occur: sore throat, fever, nausea and vomiting, severe headache, difficulty urinating, tremors, skin rash, or yellow skin or eyes
■ Assists Joe in securing transportation to and from appointments
■ Encourages Joe to set realistic goals for his life and offers recognition for follow-through
■ When Joe is ready, discusses employment alternatives with him; suggests the possibility of starting with a volunteer job (perhaps as a VA hospital volunteer)

EVALUATION

Evaluation of the nursing process with homeless individuals who have mental illness must be highly individualized. Statistics show that chances for relapse with this population are high. Therefore, it is extremely important that outcome criteria be realistic so as not to set the client up for failure.

Summary and Key Points

■ The trend in psychiatric care is shifting from that of inpatient hospitalization to a focus on outpatient care within the community. This trend is largely due to the need for greater cost-effectiveness in the provision of medical care to the masses.

■ The community mental health movement began in the 1960s with the closing of state hospitals and the deinstitutionalization of many individuals with severe and persistent mental illness.

■ Mental healthcare within the community targets primary prevention (reducing the incidence of mental disorders within the population), secondary prevention (reducing the prevalence of psychiatric illness by shortening the course of the illness), and tertiary prevention (reducing the residual defects that are associated with severe and persistent mental illness).

■ Primary prevention focuses on identification of populations at risk for mental illness, increasing their ability to cope with stress, and targeting and diminishing harmful forces within the environment.

■ Secondary prevention is accomplished through early identification of problems and prompt initiation of effective treatment.

■ Tertiary prevention focuses on preventing complications of the illness and promoting rehabilitation that is directed toward achievement of the individual's maximum level of functioning.

■ Registered nurses serve as providers of psychiatric mental healthcare in the community setting.

■ Nurses provide outpatient care for individuals with severe and persistent mental illness in community mental health centers, partial hospitalization programs, community residential facilities, and through psychiatric home healthcare.

■ Homeless persons with mental illness provide a special challenge for the community mental health nurse. Care is provided within homeless shelters, at healthcare centers or storefront clinics, and through mobile outreach programs.

Review Questions
Self-Examination/Learning Exercise

Select the answer that is most appropriate for each of the following questions:

1. Which of the following represents a nursing intervention at the primary level of prevention?
   a. Teaching a class in parental effectiveness training
   b. Leading a group of adolescents in drug rehabilitation
   c. Referring a married couple for sex therapy
   d. Leading a support group for battered women

2. Which of the following represents a nursing intervention at the secondary level of prevention?
   a. Teaching a class about menopause to middle-aged women
   b. Providing support in the emergency department to a rape victim
   c. Leading a support group for women in transition
   d. Making monthly visits to the home of a client with schizophrenia to ensure medication compliance

3. Which of the following represents a nursing intervention at the tertiary level of prevention?
   a. Serving as case manager for a mentally ill homeless client
   b. Leading a support group for newly retired men
   c. Teaching prepared childbirth classes
   d. Caring for a depressed widow in the hospital

4. John, a homeless person, has just come to live in the shelter. The shelter nurse is assigned to his care. Which of the following is a *priority* intervention on the part of the nurse?
   a. Referring John to a social worker
   b. Developing a plan of care for John
   c. Conducting a behavioral and needs assessment on John
   d. Helping John apply for Social Security benefits

Continued

Review Questions—cont'd
Self-Examination/Learning Exercise

5. John, a homeless person, has a history of schizophrenia and nonadherence to his medication regimen. Which of the following medications might be the best choice for John?
   a. Haldol
   b. Navane
   c. Lithium carbonate
   d. Prolixin decanoate

6. Ann is a psychiatric home health nurse. She has just received an order to begin regular visits to Mrs. W, a 78-year-old widow who lives alone. Mrs. W's primary care physician has diagnosed her as depressed. Which of the following criteria would qualify Mrs. W for home health visits?
   a. Mrs. W never learned to drive and has to depend on others for her transportation.
   b. Mrs. W is physically too weak to travel without risk of injury.
   c. Mrs. W refuses to seek assistance as suggested by her physician because "I don't have a psychiatric problem."
   d. Mrs. W says she would prefer to have home visits than go to the physician's office.

7. Ann is a psychiatric home health nurse. She has just received an order to begin regular visits to Mrs. W, a 78-year-old widow who lives alone. Mrs. W's primary care physician has diagnosed her as depressed. Which of these potential problems is a priority to evaluate during the first home visit?
   a. Complicated grieving
   b. Social isolation
   c. Risk for injury
   d. Sleep pattern disturbance

8. Mrs. W, a 78-year-old depressed widow, says to her home health nurse, "What's the use? I don't have anything to live for anymore." Which is the best response on the part of the nurse?
   a. "Of course you do, Mrs. W. Why would you say such a thing?"
   b. "You seem so sad. I'm going to do my best to cheer you up."
   c. "Let's talk about why you are feeling this way."
   d. "Have you been thinking about harming yourself in any way?"

9. The physician orders trazadone (Desyrel) for Mrs. W, a 78-year-old widow with depression, 150 mg to take at bedtime. Which of the following statements about this medication would be appropriate for the home health nurse to make in teaching Mrs. W about trazadone?
   a. "You may feel dizzy when you stand up, so go slowly when you get up from sitting or lying down."
   b. "You must be sure and not eat any chocolate while you are taking this medicine."
   c. "We will need to draw a sample of blood to send to the lab every month while you are on this medication."
   d. "If you don't feel better right away with this medicine, the doctor can order a different kind for you."

10. Which of the following issues have been identified as contributing to the rise in the population of those who are homeless? (Select all that apply.)
   a. Poverty
   b. Lack of affordable healthcare
   c. Substance abuse
   d. Severe and persistent mental illness
   e. Growth in the number of family members living together

IMPLICATIONS OF RESEARCH FOR EVIDENCE-BASED PRACTICE

Raymond, K. Y., Willis, D. G., & Sullivan-Bolyai, S. (2017). Parents caring for adult children with serious mental illness. *Journal of the American Psychiatric Nurses Association* 23(2), 119–132. https://doi.org/10.1177/1078390316685404

DESCRIPTION OF THE STUDY: Noting that parents are often engaged in caregiving for adult children with serious mental illness, this qualitative study sought to identify current coping strategies among parent caregivers and to identify their perspectives on the most supportive community-based mental health interventions. Semistructured interviews were conducted with 30 parent caregivers. The majority of the participants were female, Caucasian, married, college-educated, and with a mean age of 63 years. The most common diagnosis of the adult child was schizoaffective disorder.

RESULTS OF THE STUDY: Four themes emerged with regard to coping issues faced by parents of a child with severe mental illness:

1. Recognition of a serious problem requiring a decision to act
2. Scrambling for a diagnosis to understand what illness their child has
3. Learning to maneuver family life and access to mental health systems
4. Enduring the illness, including fears for the future and implications for family life

IMPLICATIONS FOR NURSING PRACTICE: The authors cite studies supporting the importance of the parent role in care and recovery of adult children with serious mental illness. Consistent with theme #1, parents identified a need for more information; even though there was an abundance of information on the Internet they needed to know where to go next. The authors note that "Mental health resources need to be connected to primary care providers, elementary and secondary school systems, college mental health services, community mental health services, mental health hospitals, legal advocacy groups, police departments, and social service organizations. This is a vital intervention to increase public awareness of available services, reduce fragmentation of services in the community, and minimize the number of people falling through the holes within the mental health system." Community mental health nurses can play a significant role in disseminating intervention to these community agencies. A second identified need was difficulty accessing psychiatric evaluation and the authors note that this may have important implications for advanced practice nurses who can provide a significant bridge in quicker access to services. A third identified need and one that community mental health nurses could address is to include parents in each aspect of intervention so they become more knowledgeable about available resources, better equipped to provide ongoing care, and how to prevent or manage violence risks. A study such as this informs community mental health nurses about the needs of the family directly from the source and enables nurses to structure services to meet those identified needs.

References

American Nurses Association, American Psychiatric Nurses Association, & International Society of Psychiatric-Mental Health Nurses. (2014). *Scope and standards of practice: Psychiatric-mental health nursing* (2nd ed.). Silver Spring, MD: American Nurses Association.

American Psychiatric Association. (2013). *Diagnostic and statistical manual of mental disorders* (5th ed.). Washington, DC: Author.

Case Management Society of America (CMSA). (2016). *Standards of practice for case management*. Little Rock, AR: Author.

Casper, L. M., & Coritz, A. (2018). Family demography: Continuity and change in north American families. In J. R. Kaakinen, D. P. Coehlo, R. Steele, & M. Robinson (Eds.), *Family health care nursing* (6th ed., pp. 53–81). Philadelphia, PA: F.A. Davis.

Centers for Disease Control and Prevention (CDC). (2018). *TB in the homeless population*. Retrieved from https://www.cdc.gov/tb/topic/populations/Homelessness/default.htm

Centers for Medicare & Medicaid Services (CMS). (n.d.). *The mental health parity and addiction equity act*. Retrieved from https://www.cms.gov/CCIIO/Programs-and-Initiatives/Other-Insurance-Protections/mhpaea_factsheet.html

Centers for Medicare & Medicaid Services (CMS). (2017). *Medicare benefit policy manual*. Baltimore, MD: Author.

Family and Youth Services Bureau. (2016). *Domestic violence and homelessness: Statistics (2016)*. Retrieved from https://www.acf.hhs.gov/fysb/resource/dv-homelessness-stats-2016

Ling, C., & Ruscin, C. (2013). *Case management basics*. Gannett Education Course #60102. Retrieved from http://ce.nurse.com/60102/Case-Management-Basics

McLeod, S. A. (2010). *SRRS—Stress of life events*. Retrieved from http://www.simplypsychology.org/SRRS.html

National Alliance on Mental Illness (NAMI). (2014). *Mental illness: NAMI report deplores 80 percent unemployment rate; state rates and ranks listed—model legislation proposed*. Retrieved from https://www.nami.org/Press-Media/Press-Releases/2014/Mental-Illness-NAMI-Report-Deplores-80-Percent-Un

National Alliance on Mental Illness (NAMI). (2018). *Psychosocial treatments: Assertive community treatment*. Retrieved from https://www.nami.org/Learn-More/Treatment/Psychosocial-Treatments

National Alliance to End Homelessness. (2018). *The state of homelessness in America*. Retrieved from https://endhomelessness.org/homelessness-in-america/homelessness-statistics/state-of-homelessness-report/

National Coalition for the Homeless (NCH). (2015). *How trauma-informed care is helping homeless families*. Retrieved from http://nationalhomeless.org/category/domestic-violence/

National Coalition for the Homeless (NCH). (2016). *No safe street: A survey of hate crimes and violence committed against homeless people in 2014 & 2015*. Retrieved from http://nationalhomeless.org/wp-content/uploads/2016/07/HCR-2014-151.pdf

National Coalition for the Homeless (NCH). (2017). *Mental illness and homelessness*. Retrieved from http://nationalhomeless.org/wp-content/uploads/2017/06/Mental-Illness-and-Homelessness.pdf

National Institute of Corrections. (n.d.). *Mentally ill persons in corrections*. Retrieved from http://nicic.gov/mentalillness

National Institute of Mental Health (NIMH). (2017). *Serious mental illness (SMI) among U.S. adults*. Retrieved from http://www.nimh.nih.gov/health/statistics/prevalence/serious-mental-illness-smi-among-us-adults.shtml

President's New Freedom Commission on Mental Health. (2003). *Achieving the promise: Transforming mental health care in America*. Retrieved from http://govinfo.library.unt.edu/mentalhealthcommission/reports/reports.htm

Raymond, K. Y., Willis, D. G., & Sullivan-Bolyai, S. (2017). Parents caring for adult children with serious mental illness. *Journal of the American Psychiatric Nurses Association, 23*(2), 119–132. https://doi.org/10.1177/1078390316685404

Sadock, B. J., Sadock, V. A., & Ruiz, P. (2015). *Synopsis of psychiatry: Behavioral sciences/clinical psychiatry* (11th ed.). Philadelphia, PA: Wolters Kluwer.

Safe Horizon. (2018). *Youth homelessness statistics and facts*. Retrieved from https://www.safehorizon.org/get-informed/homeless-youth-statistics-facts/#definition/

Spock, B., & Needlman, R. (2018). *Dr. Spock's baby and child care* (10th ed.). New York, NY: Gallery Books.

Substance Abuse and Mental Health Services Administration (SAMHSA). (2016). *Behind the term serious mental illness*. Retrieved from https://nrepp.samhsa.gov/Docs/Literatures/Behind_the_Term_Serious%20%20Mental%20Illness.pdf

Substance Abuse and Mental Health Services Administration (SAMHSA). (2018). *Federal action agenda (search)*. Retrieved from https://search.samhsa.gov/search?q=federal+action+agenda+initiatives&sort=date%3AD%3AL%3Ad1&output=xml_no_dtd&ie=UTF-8&oe=UTF-8&client=beta_frontend_drupal&proxystylesheet=beta_frontend_drupal&filter=1&site=data%7CSAMHSA_Beta_Drupal%7Cdefault_collection%7CNewsletter&collectionator=data%7CSAMHSA_Beta_Drupal%7Cdefault_collection%7CNewsletter

U.S. Conference of Mayors (USCM). (2016). *A status report on hunger and homelessness in America's cities: 2016*. Washington, DC: Author.

U.S. Department of Housing and Urban Development (HUD). (2017). *The 2017 Annual Homeless Assessment Report (AHAR) to Congress*. Retrieved from https://www.hudexchange.info/resources/documents/2017-AHAR-The 2017 Annual Homeless Assessment Report (AHAR) to CongressPart-1.pdf

Vanderplasschen, W., Rapp, R. C., Pearce, S., Vandevelde, S., & Broekaert, E. (2013). Mental health, recovery, and the community. *Scientific World Journal, 2013*(4), 1–3. doi:10.1155/2013/926174

Veltri, L., Wilson-Mitchell, K., & O'Mahony, J. M. (2018). Family nursing with childbearing families. In J. R. Kaakinen, D. P. Coehlo, R. Steele, & M. Robinson (Eds.), *Family health care nursing* (6th ed., pp. 357–387). Philadelphia, PA: F.A. Davis.

White, D. L., & Cartwright, J. C. (2018). Family health in mid- and later life. In J. R. Kaakinen, D. P. Coehlo, R. Steele, & M. Robinson (Eds.), *Family health care nursing* (6th ed., pp. 457–496). Philadelphia, PA: F.A. Davis.

Wright, L. M., & Leahey, M. (2013). *Nurses and families: A guide to family assessment and intervention* (6th ed.). Philadelphia, PA: F.A. Davis.

Classical References

Caplan, G. (1964). *Principles of preventive psychiatry*. New York, NY: Basic Books.

Erikson, E. (1963). *Childhood and society* (2nd ed.). New York, NY: WW Norton.

Govtrack. (1987). *H.R. 558 (100th): Stewart B. McKinney Homeless Assistance Act*. Retrieved from https://www.govtrack.us/congress/bills/100/hr558/text

Lamb, H. R. (1993). Perspectives on effective advocacy for homeless mentally ill persons. *Hospital and Community Psychiatry, 43*(12), 1209–1212.

The Bereaved Individual

27

CORE CONCEPTS

Grief

Loss

KEY TERMS

advance directive

anticipatory grieving

bereavement

bereavement overload

delayed grief

hospice

mourning

OBJECTIVES

After reading this chapter, the student will be able to:

1. Describe various types of loss that trigger the grief response in individuals.
2. Discuss theoretical perspectives of grieving as proposed by Elisabeth Kübler-Ross, John Bowlby, George Engel, and J. William Worden.
3. Differentiate between normal and maladaptive responses to loss.
4. Discuss grieving behaviors common to individuals at various stages across the life span.
5. Formulate nursing diagnoses and goals of care for individuals experiencing the grief response.
6. Describe appropriate nursing interventions for individuals experiencing the grief response.
7. Identify relevant criteria for evaluating nursing care of individuals experiencing the grief response.
8. Describe the concept of hospice care for people who are dying and their families.
9. Discuss the use of advance directives for individuals to provide directions about their future medical care.

Introduction

> ### CORE CONCEPT
> **Loss**
> The experience of separation from something of personal importance.

Loss is anything that is perceived as such by the individual. The separation from loved ones or the giving up of treasured possessions for whatever reason; the experience of failure, either real or perceived; or life events that create change in a familiar pattern of existence—all can be experienced as loss, and all can trigger behaviors associated with the grieving process. Loss and bereavement are universal events encountered by all beings that experience emotions. Following are examples of some notable forms of loss:

■ A significant other (person or pet), through death, divorce, or separation for any reason.
■ Illness or debilitating conditions. Examples include (but are not limited to) diabetes, stroke, cancer, rheumatoid arthritis, multiple sclerosis, Alzheimer's disease, hearing or vision loss, and spinal cord or head injuries. Some of these conditions not only incur a loss of physical and/or emotional wellness but may also result in the loss of personal independence.
■ Developmental/maturational changes or situations, such as menopause, andropause, infertility, "empty nest," aging, impotence, or hysterectomy.
■ A decrease in self-esteem due to inability to meet self-expectations or the expectations of others (even if these expectations are only perceived by the individual as unfulfilled). This includes a loss of potential hopes and dreams.
■ Personal possessions that symbolize familiarity and security in a person's life. Separation from these familiar and personally valued external objects represents a loss of material extensions of the self.

> ### CORE CONCEPT
> **Grief**
> Deep mental and emotional anguish that is a response to the subjective experience of loss of something significant.

Some texts differentiate the terms **mourning** and *grief* by describing mourning as the psychological process (or stages) through which the individual passes on the way to successful adaptation to the loss of a valued object. Grief may be viewed as the subjective states that accompany mourning or the emotional work involved in the mourning process. Similarly, **bereavement** is described as the period of grief and sadness that is the normal process of reacting to a loss and may include mental, physical, social, and emotional reactions (MedlinePlus, 2018). For purposes of this text, grief work, bereavement, and the process of mourning are collectively referred to as the *grief response*.

This chapter examines human responses to the experience of loss. Care of bereaved individuals is presented in the context of the nursing process.

Theoretical Perspectives on Loss and Bereavement

Stages of Grief

Behavior patterns associated with the grief response include many individual variations. However, sufficient similarities have been observed to warrant characterization of the grief response as a syndrome that has a predictable course with an expected resolution. Early theorists, including Kübler-Ross (1969), Bowlby (1961), and Engel (1964), described behavioral stages through which individuals advance in their progression toward resolution. A number of variables influence one's progression through the grief process, and it should not be understood as a linear process. Some individuals may reach acceptance only to revert back to an earlier stage, some may never complete the sequence, and some may never progress beyond the initial stage.

A more contemporary grief specialist, J. William Worden (2009), offers a set of tasks that must be processed in order to complete the grief response. He suggests that it is possible for a person to accomplish some of these tasks and not others, resulting in an incomplete bereavement and thus impairing further growth and development. A comparison of the similarities among these four models is presented in Table 27–1.

Elisabeth Kübler-Ross

These well-known stages of the grief process were identified by Kübler-Ross in her extensive work with dying patients. Behaviors associated with each of these stages can be observed in individuals experiencing the loss of any concept of personal value.

Stage I: Denial. In this stage, the individual has difficulty believing that the loss has occurred. He or she may say, "No, it can't be true!" or "It's just not possible." This stage may protect the individual against the psychological pain of reality.

Stage II: Anger. This is the stage when reality sets in. Feelings associated with this stage include sadness, guilt, shame, helplessness, and hopelessness. Self-blame or blaming of others may lead to feelings of anger toward the self and others. The anxiety level may be elevated, and the individual may experience confusion and a decreased ability to function independently. He or she may be preoccupied with an idealized image of what has been lost. Numerous somatic complaints are common.

Stage III: Bargaining. At this stage in the grief response, the individual attempts to strike a bargain with God for a second chance or for more time. The person acknowledges the loss, or impending loss, but holds out hope for additional alternatives, as evidenced by statements such as, "If only I could. . ." or "If only I had. . . ."

Stage IV: Depression. In this stage, the individual mourns for that which has been or will be lost. This is a very painful stage during which the individual must confront feelings associated with having lost someone or something of value (called *reactive* depression). An example might be the individual who is mourning a change in body image. Feelings associated with an impending loss (called *preparatory* depression) are also confronted. Examples include permanent lifestyle changes related to the altered body image or even an impending loss of life itself. Regression, withdrawal, and social isolation may be observed behaviors with this stage. Therapeutic intervention should be available, but not imposed, and with guidelines for implementation based on client readiness.

Stage V: Acceptance. At this time, the individual has worked through the behaviors associated with the other stages and accepts or is resigned to the loss. Anxiety decreases, and methods for coping with the loss have been established. The client is less preoccupied with what has been lost and increasingly interested in other aspects of the environment. If this is an impending death of self, the individual is ready to die. The person may become very quiet and withdrawn, seemingly devoid of feelings. These behaviors are an attempt to facilitate the passage by slowly disengaging from the environment.

John Bowlby

John Bowlby hypothesized four stages in the grief process. He implies that these behaviors can be observed in all individuals who have experienced the loss of something or someone of value, even in babies as young as 6 months of age.

Stage I: Numbness or protest. This stage is characterized by a feeling of shock and disbelief that the loss has occurred. Reality of the loss is not acknowledged.

Stage II: Disequilibrium. During this stage, the individual has a profound urge to recover what has been lost. Behaviors associated with this stage include a preoccupation with the loss, intense weeping and expressions of anger toward the self and others, and feelings of ambivalence and guilt associated with the loss.

Stage III: Disorganization and despair. Feelings of despair occur in response to realization that the loss has occurred. Activities of daily living become increasingly disorganized, and behavior is characterized by restlessness and aimlessness. Efforts to regain productive patterns of behavior are ineffective, and the individual experiences fear, helplessness, and hopelessness. Somatic complaints are common. Perceptions of visualizing or being in the presence of that which has been lost may occur. Social isolation is common, and the individual may feel a great deal of loneliness.

TABLE 27–1 Stages and Tasks of the Normal Grief Response

A COMPARISON OF MODELS BY ELISABETH KÜBLER-ROSS, JOHN BOWLBY, GEORGE ENGEL, AND WILLIAM WORDEN

STAGES/TASKS KÜBLER-ROSS	BOWLBY	ENGEL	WORDEN	POSSIBLE TIME DIMENSION	BEHAVIORS
I. Denial	I. Numbness/ protest	I. Shock/ disbelief	I. Accepting the reality of the loss	Occurs immediately on experiencing the loss. Usually lasts no more than a few weeks.	Individual has difficulty believing that the loss has occurred.
II. Anger	II. Disequilibrium	II. Developing awareness		In most cases begins within hours of the loss. Peaks within a few weeks.	Anger is directed toward self or others. Ambivalence and guilt may be felt toward the lost entity.
III. Bargaining					The individual fervently seeks alternatives to improve current situation.
		III. Restitution			Attends to various rituals associated with the culture in which the loss has occurred.
IV. Depression	III. Disorganization and despair	IV. Resolution of the loss	II. Processing the pain of grief	Very individual. Commonly 6 to 12 months. Longer for some.	The actual work of grieving. Preoccupation with the lost entity. Feelings of helplessness and loneliness occur in response to realization of the loss. Feelings associated with the loss are confronted.
			III. Adjusting to a world without the lost entity	Ongoing.	How the environment changes depends on the roles the lost entity played in the life of the bereaved person. Adaptations will have to be made as the changes are presented in daily life. New coping skills will have to be developed.
IV. Acceptance	IV. Reorganization	V. Recovery	IV. Finding an enduring connection with the lost entity in the midst of embarking on a new life		Resolution is complete. The bereaved person experiences a reinvestment in new relationships and new goals. The lost entity is not purged or replaced but relocated in the life of the bereaved. At this stage, terminally ill persons express a readiness to die.

Stage IV: Reorganization. The individual accepts or becomes resigned to the loss. New goals and patterns of organization are established. The individual begins a reinvestment in new relationships and indicates a readiness to move forward within the environment. Grief subsides and recedes into valued remembrances.

George Engel

Stage I: Shock and Disbelief. The initial reaction to a loss is a stunned, numb feeling and refusal by the individual to acknowledge the reality of the loss. Engel states that this stage is an attempt by the individual to protect the self "against the effects of the overwhelming stress by raising the threshold against its recognition or against the painful feelings evoked thereby."

Stage II: Developing Awareness. This stage begins within minutes to hours of the loss. Behaviors associated with this stage include excessive crying and regression to a state of helplessness and a childlike manner. Awareness of the loss creates feelings of emptiness, frustration, anguish, and despair. Anger may be directed toward the self or toward others in the environment who are held accountable for the loss.

Stage III: Restitution. In this stage, the various rituals associated with loss within a culture are performed. Examples include funerals, wakes, special attire, a gathering of friends and family, and religious practices customary to the spiritual beliefs of the bereaved. Participation in these rituals is thought to assist the individual to accept the reality of the loss and to facilitate the recovery process.

Stage IV: Resolution of the loss. This stage is characterized by a preoccupation with the loss. The concept of the loss is idealized, and the individual may even imitate admired qualities of the lost entity. Preoccupation with the loss gradually decreases over a year or more, and the individual eventually begins to reinvest feelings in others.

Stage V: Recovery. Obsession with the loss has ended, and the individual is able to go on with his or her life.

J. William Worden

Worden views the bereaved person as active and self-determining rather than a passive participant in the grief process. He proposes that bereavement includes a set of tasks that must be reconciled in order to complete the grief process. Worden's four tasks of mourning include the following:

Task I. Accepting the reality of the loss. When something of value is lost, it is common for individuals to refuse to believe that the loss has occurred. Behaviors include misidentifying individuals in the environment as their lost loved one, retaining possessions of the lost loved one as though he or she has not died, and removing all reminders of the lost loved one so as not to have to face the reality of the loss. Worden (2009) stated:

> Coming to an acceptance of the reality of the loss takes time since it involves not only an intellectual acceptance but also an emotional one. The bereaved person may be intellectually aware of the finality of the loss long before the emotions allow full acceptance of the information as true. (p. 42)

Belief and denial are intermittent while grappling with this task. It is thought that traditional rituals such as the funeral help some individuals move toward acceptance of the loss.

Task II. Processing the pain of grief. Pain associated with a loss includes both physical and emotional pain. This pain must be acknowledged and worked through. To avoid or suppress it serves only to delay or prolong the grieving process. People do this by refusing to allow themselves to think painful thoughts, by idealizing or avoiding reminders of the lost entity, and by using alcohol or drugs. The intensity of the pain and the manner in which it is experienced are different for all individuals. However, the commonality is that it *must* be experienced. Failure to do so generally results in some form of depression that commonly requires therapy, which then focuses on working through the pain of grief that the individual failed to work through at the time of the loss. In this very difficult task II, individuals must "allow themselves to process the pain—to feel it and to know that one day it will pass" (Worden, 2009, p. 45).

Task III. Adjusting to a world without the lost entity. It usually takes a number of months for a bereaved person to realize what his or her world will be like without the lost entity. In the case of a lost loved one, how the environment changes will depend on the types of roles that person fulfilled in life. In the case of a changed lifestyle, the individual will be required to make adaptations to his or her environment in terms of the changes as they are presented in daily life. In addition, those individuals who had defined their identity through the lost entity will require an adjustment to their own sense of self. Worden identifies that successful completion of task III entails redefining the loss in a way that is beneficial to the survivor.

If the bereaved person experiences failures in his or her attempt to adjust in an environment without the lost entity, feelings of low self-esteem may result. Regressed behaviors and feelings of helplessness and inadequacy are not uncommon. Worden states:

> [Another] area of adjustment is to one's sense of the world. Loss through death can challenge one's fundamental life values and philosophical beliefs—beliefs that are influenced by our families, peers, education, and religion as well as life experiences. The bereaved person searches for meaning in the loss and its attendant life changes in order to make sense of it and to regain some control of his or her life. (pp. 48–49)

To be successful in task III, bereaved individuals must develop new skills to cope and adapt to their new environment without the lost entity. Successful achievement of this task determines the outcome of the mourning process—that of continued growth or a state of arrested development.

Task IV. Finding an enduring connection with the lost entity in the midst of embarking on a new life. This task allows the bereaved person to identify a special place for the lost entity. Individuals need not purge from their history or find a replacement for that which has been lost. Instead, there is a kind of continued presence of the lost entity that only becomes *relocated* in the life of the bereaved. Successful completion of task IV involves letting go of past attachments and forming new ones. However, there is also the recognition that although the relationship between the bereaved and what has been lost is changed, it is nonetheless still a relationship. Worden suggested that one never loses memories of a significant relationship. He states:

> For many people, Task IV is the most difficult one to accomplish. They get stuck at this point in their grieving and later realize that their life in some way stopped at the point the loss occurred. (p. 52)

Worden related the story of a teenaged girl who had a difficult time adjusting to the death of her father. After 2 years, when she began to finally fulfill some of the tasks associated with successful grieving, she wrote these words that express rather clearly what bereaved people in task IV are struggling with: "There are other people to be loved, and it doesn't mean that I love Dad any less" (p. 52).

Length of the Grief Process

Stages of grief allow bereaved persons an orderly approach to the resolution of mourning. Each stage presents tasks that must be overcome through a painful experiential process. Engel (1964) stated that successful resolution of the grief response is thought to have occurred when a bereaved individual is able "to remember comfortably and realistically both the pleasures and disappointments of [that which is lost]." The length of the grief process depends on the individual and can last for a number of years without being maladaptive. The acute phase of normal grieving usually lasts about 6 to 8 weeks—longer in older adults—but complete resolution of the grief response may take much longer. Sadock, Sadock, and Ruiz (2015) stated:

> Ample evidence suggests that the bereavement process does not end within a prescribed interval; certain aspects persist indefinitely for many otherwise high-functioning, normal individuals. Common manifestations of protracted grief occur intermittently . . . most grief does not fully resolve or permanently disappear; rather grief becomes circumscribed and submerged only to reemerge in response to certain triggers. (p. 1355)

A number of factors influence the eventual outcome of the grief response. The grief response can be more difficult if:

- The bereaved person was strongly dependent on or perceived the lost entity as an important means of physical and/or emotional support.
- The relationship with the lost entity was highly ambivalent. A love-hate relationship may instill feelings of guilt that can interfere with the grief work.
- The individual has experienced a number of recent losses. Grief tends to be cumulative, and if previous losses have not been resolved, each succeeding grief response becomes more difficult.
- The loss is that of a young person. Grief over loss of a child is often more intense than it is over the loss of an elderly person. Traumatic death, in general, increases the likelihood of abnormal grief, but when a child dies a violent death, studies have found an increased incidence of post-traumatic stress disorder (PTSD) in parents (Kearns, 2014). One study found PTSD symptoms in over 25 percent of the mothers up to 5 years after the death (Parris, 2011).

- The state of the person's physical or psychological health is unstable at the time of the loss.
- The bereaved person perceives (whether real or imagined) some responsibility for the loss.
- The loss is secondary to suicide.
- The loss is a traumatic death such as murder.

The grief response may be facilitated if:

- The individual has the support of significant others to assist him or her through the mourning process.
- The individual has the opportunity to prepare for the loss. Grief work is more intense when the loss is sudden and unexpected. The experience of *anticipatory grieving* is thought to facilitate the grief response that occurs at the time of the actual loss.

Worden (2009) states:

> There is a sense in which mourning can be finished, when people regain an interest in life, feel more hopeful, experience gratification again, and adapt to new roles. There is also a sense in which mourning is never finished. [People must understand] that mourning is a long-term process and that the culmination will not be a pre-grief state. (p. 77)

Anticipatory Grief

Anticipatory grieving is the experiencing of the feelings and emotions associated with the normal grief response before the loss actually occurs. One dissimilar aspect relates to the fact that conventional grief tends to diminish in intensity with the passage of time. Anticipatory grief can become more intense as the expected loss becomes imminent.

Although anticipatory grief is thought to facilitate the actual mourning process following the loss, problems may occur. In the case of a dying person, difficulties can arise when the family members complete the process of anticipatory grief, and detachment from the dying person occurs prematurely. The person who is dying experiences feelings of loneliness and isolation as the psychological pain of imminent death is faced without family support. Another example of difficulty associated with premature completion of the grief response is one that can occur on the return of persons long absent and presumed dead (e.g., soldiers missing in action or prisoners of war). In this instance, resumption of the previous relationship may be difficult for the bereaved person.

Anticipatory grieving may serve as a defense for some individuals to ease the burden of loss when it actually occurs. It may prove to be less functional for others who, because of interpersonal, psychological, or sociocultural variables, are unable in advance of the actual loss to express the intense feelings that accompany the grief response.

One qualitative study examined the unique process of grief for family caregivers of a relative who has dementia. One common theme was that in addition to anticipatory grief related to the final loss, these family members were, at the same time, grieving actual losses throughout the journey of their family member's illness (Peacock, Hammond-Collins, & Ford, 2014). These included grieving the loss of the ill person's personality, companionship, social self, and cognition as the disease progressed. The grief reactions of these active caregivers were similar to those of bereaved caregivers, although their family member was still alive. This study highlights the multiplicity of factors that can influence the grieving process.

Maladaptive Responses to Loss

When, then, is the grieving response considered to be maladaptive? Three types of pathological grief reactions have been described. These include delayed or inhibited grief, an exaggerated or distorted grief response, and chronic or prolonged grief.

Delayed or Inhibited Grief

Delayed or inhibited grief refers to the absence of evidence of grief when it ordinarily would be expected. Many times, cultural influences, such as the expectation to keep a "stiff upper lip," contribute to the delayed response.

Delayed or inhibited grief is potentially pathological because the person is simply not dealing with the reality of the loss. He or she remains fixed in the denial stage of the grief process, sometimes for many years. When this occurs, the grief response may be triggered, sometimes many years later, when the individual experiences a subsequent loss. Sometimes the grief process is triggered spontaneously or in response to a seemingly insignificant event. Overreaction to another person's loss may be one manifestation of **delayed grief.**

The recognition of delayed grief is critical because, depending on the profundity of the loss, the lack of mourning may prevent assimilation of the loss and thereby delay a return to satisfying living. Without the understanding and assimilation that the grief process can provide, subsequent losses may be compounded by previously unresolved grief work. Delayed grieving most commonly occurs because of ambivalent feelings toward the lost entity, outside pressure to resume normal function, or perceived lack of internal and external resources to cope with a profound loss.

Distorted (Exaggerated) Grief Response

In the distorted grief reaction, all of the symptoms associated with normal grieving are exaggerated. Feelings of sadness, helplessness, hopelessness, powerlessness, anger, and guilt, as well as numerous somatic complaints, render the individual dysfunctional in terms of management of daily living. Morrow (2016) describes this as a state of feeling "trapped" in one's grief during which the grief response either stays the same or intensifies over a prolonged period.

When the exaggerated grief reaction occurs, the individual remains fixed in the anger stage of the grief response. This anger may be directed toward others in the environment to whom the individual may be attributing the loss. However, many times the anger is turned inward on the self. When this occurs, depression is the result. Depressive mood disorder is a type of exaggerated grief reaction. This should be distinguished, though, from the depression that is considered part of the normal grieving process (see Table 27–2).

Chronic or Prolonged Grieving

Some authors have discussed a chronic or prolonged grief response as a type of maladaptive grief response. Care must be taken in making this determination

because, as was stated previously, length of the grief response depends on the individual. An adaptive response may take years for some people. A prolonged process may be considered maladaptive when certain behaviors are exhibited. Prolonged grief may be a problem when behaviors such as those that prevent the bereaved from adaptively performing activities of daily living are in evidence. An example is of a widow who refused to participate in family gatherings following the death of her husband. For many years until her own death, she took a sandwich to the cemetery on holidays, sat on the tombstone, and ate her "holiday meal" with her husband. Whether one's behaviors constitute prolonged or chronic grieving must be considered in a cultural context. In some cultures, establishing a memorial ritual to the deceased is the norm, whereas in other cultures, it might be perceived as prolonged grieving.

Normal Versus Maladaptive Grieving

Several authors have identified one crucial difference between normal and maladaptive grieving: the loss of self-esteem. Marked feelings of worthlessness are indicative of depression rather than uncomplicated bereavement. Corr and Corr (2013) state, "Normal grief reactions do not include the loss of self-esteem commonly found in most clinical depression" (p. 241).

Pies (2013) affirmed,

Unlike the person with [major depressive disorder] MDD, most recently bereaved individuals are usually not preoccupied with feelings of worthlessness,

TABLE 27–2 **Normal Grief Reactions Versus Symptoms of Clinical Depression**	
NORMAL GRIEF	**CLINICAL DEPRESSION**
Self-esteem intact	Self-esteem is disturbed
May openly express anger	Usually does not directly express anger
Experiences a mixture of "good and bad days"	Persistent state of dysphoria
Able to experience moments of pleasure	Anhedonia is prevalent
Accepts comfort and support from others	Does not respond to social interaction and support from others
Maintains feeling of hope	Feelings of hopelessness prevail
May express guilt feelings over some aspect of the loss	Has generalized feelings of guilt
Relates feelings of depression to specific loss experienced	Does not relate feelings to a particular experience
May experience transient physical symptoms	Expresses chronic physical complaints

Sources: Corr, C. A., & Corr, D. M. (2013). *Death and dying: Life & living* (7th ed.). Belmont, CA: Wadsworth; Pies, R. W. (2013). Grief and depression: The sages knew the difference. *Psychiatric Times, 30*(6); Sadock, B. J., Sadock, V. A., & Ruiz, P. (2015). *Synopsis of psychiatry: Behavioral sciences/clinical psychiatry* (11th ed.). Philadelphia, PA: Wolters Kluwer.

hopelessness, or unremitting gloom; rather, self-esteem is usually preserved; the bereaved person can envision a "better day;" and positive thoughts and feelings are often interspersed with negative ones.

Hensley and Clayton (2013) add that when depressed inpatients were compared with individuals who were experiencing depression associated with bereavement, four symptoms were absent in the bereavement population: suicide thoughts, feeling they were a burden to others, feeling they would rather be dead, and psychomotor retardation. These may be considered associated symptoms of low self-esteem and feelings of worthlessness.

It is thought that this major difference between normal grieving and a maladaptive grieving response (the feeling of worthlessness or low self-esteem) ultimately precipitates depression, which can be a progressive situation for some individuals. Studies have identified the incidence of major depressive disorder among the bereaved to be at around 35 percent at 1 month following a loss, and although the incidence tends to decrease over time, 8 to 11 percent develop chronic depression (Hensley & Clayton, 2013). The authors add that factors such as poor physical health, poor mental health, and substance use disorders prior to a loss increase the risk for chronic depression following loss. A summary of differences between normal grieving and clinical depression is presented in Table 27–2.

Application of the Nursing Process

Background Assessment Data: Concepts of Death—Developmental Issues

All individuals have their own unique concept of death, which is influenced by past experiences with death as well as age and level of emotional development. This section addresses the various perceptions of death according to developmental age.

Children

Birth to Age 2

Infants are unable to recognize and understand death, but they can experience the feelings of loss and separation. Infants who are separated from their mother may become quiet, lose weight, and sleep less. Children at this age will likely sense changes in the atmosphere of the home where a death has occurred. They often react to the emotions of adults by becoming irritable and crying more than usual.

Ages 3 to 5

Preschoolers and kindergartners have some understanding about death but often have difficulty distinguishing between fantasy and reality. They believe death is reversible, and their thoughts about death may include magical thinking. For example, they may believe that their thoughts or behaviors caused a person to become sick or to die.

Children of this age are capable of understanding at least some of what they see and hear from adult conversations or media reports. They become frightened if they feel a threat to themselves or their loved ones. They are concerned with safety issues and require a great deal of personal reassurance that they will be protected. Regressive behaviors, such as loss of bladder or bowel control, thumb sucking, and temper tantrums are common. Changes in eating and sleeping patterns may also occur.

Ages 6 to 9

Children at this age are beginning to understand the finality of death. They are able to understand a more detailed explanation of why or how a person died, although the concept of death is often associated with old age or with accidents. They may believe that death is contagious and avoid association with individuals who have experienced a loss by death. Death is often personified in the form of a "bogey man" or a monster—someone who takes people away or someone whom they can avoid if they try hard enough. It is difficult for them to perceive their own death. Normal grief reactions at this age include regressive and aggressive behaviors, withdrawal, school phobias, somatic symptoms, and clinging behaviors.

Ages 10 to 12

Preadolescent children are able to understand that death is final and eventually affects everyone, including themselves. They are interested in the physical aspects of dying and the final disposition of the body. They may ask questions about how the death will affect them personally. Feelings of anger, guilt, and depression are common. Peer relationships and school performance may be disrupted. There may be a preoccupation with the loss and a withdrawal into the self. Adams (2014) states that evidence supports that young people who are bereaved are more likely to be poor school attenders, change schools, and be excluded and are less likely to be involved in activities both in and out of school, which puts them at higher risk for underperformance, health problems, and feelings of hopelessness. They will require support, flexibility in management of anger responses, and reassurance of their own safety and self-worth.

Adolescents

Adolescents are usually able to view death on an adult level. They understand death to be universal and inevitable; however, they have difficulty tolerating the intense feelings associated with the death of a loved one. They may or may not cry. They may withdraw into themselves or attempt to go about usual activities in an effort to avoid dealing with the pain of the loss. Some teens exhibit acting-out behaviors, such as aggression and defiance. It is often easier for adolescents to discuss their feelings with peers than with their parents or other adults. Some adolescents may show regressive behaviors, whereas others react by trying to take care of their loved ones who are also grieving. In general, individuals of this age group have an attitude of immortality. Although they understand that their own death is inevitable, the concept is so far-reaching as to be imperceptible.

Adults

The adult's concept of death is influenced by experiential, cultural, and religious backgrounds. Behaviors associated with grieving in the adult are discussed in the section "Theoretical Perspectives on Loss and Bereavement."

Older Adults

Philosophers and poets have described late adulthood as the "season of loss." By the time individuals reach their 60s and 70s, they have experienced numerous losses, and mourning has become a life-long process. Those who are most successful at adapting earlier in life will similarly cope better with the losses and grief inherent in aging. Unfortunately, with the aging process comes a convergence of losses, the timing of which makes it impossible for the aging individual to complete the grief process in response to one loss before another occurs. Because grief is cumulative, multiple losses can result in **bereavement overload.** The person is less able to adapt and reintegrate, complicated grief responses ensue, and mental and physical health may be jeopardized (Tousley, 2013). Bereavement overload has been implicated as a predisposing factor in the development of depressive disorder in older adults.

Some believe that bereavement among elderly couples is also associated with increased risk for mortality. Although many variables influence mortality in this population, evidence suggests that, in cases where the loss is anticipated, there is not an increased risk for mortality; conversely, when the loss is unexpected, there is an increased risk (King et al., 2013; Shah et al., 2013). This research highlights the need for additional assessment and support during the bereavement period when loss, particularly of a spouse, is unexpected.

Background Assessment Data: Bereavement Risk Assessment

Several tools have been developed to assess the risk for maladaptive grief responses. They incorporate many of the issues previously discussed and are framed to identify multiple risk factors commonly associated with complicated grief reactions that may require additional resources and intervention. Some potential indicators of increased risk for maladaptive grief follow:

- Additional financial problems posed by the loss
- Lack of coping skills or lack of experience in responding to loss
- Emotional or physical dependence on the lost person or item
- History of mental illness or substance abuse
- History of trauma, including abuse
- Multiple losses within a short time frame

Although formalized tools are more often used in palliative care settings, they constitute an important aspect of assessment for all nurses responding to the needs of the bereaved client.

Background Assessment Data: Concepts of Death—Cultural Issues

As previously stated, bereavement practices are greatly influenced by cultural and religious backgrounds. It is important for healthcare professionals to have an understanding of these individual differences in order to provide culturally sensitive care to their clients. Clinicians must be able to identify and appreciate what is culturally expected or required, because failure to carry out expected rituals may hinder the grief process and result in unresolved grief for some bereaved individuals. Box 27–1 provides a set of guidelines for assessing individual preferences and practices with regard to death rituals.

Nursing Diagnosis and Outcome Identification

From analysis of the assessment data, appropriate nursing diagnoses are formulated for the patient and family experiencing grief and loss. From these identified diagnoses, accurate planning of nursing care is executed. Possible nursing diagnoses for grieving persons include the following:

■ Risk for complicated grieving related to loss of a valued entity/concept; loss of a loved one
■ Risk for spiritual distress related to complicated grief process

The following criteria may be used for measurement of outcomes in the care of the grieving patient:

The patient

■ Acknowledges awareness of the loss.
■ Is able to express feelings about the loss.
■ Verbalizes stages of the grief process and behaviors associated with each.
■ Expresses personal satisfaction and support from spiritual practices.

Planning and Implementation

Table 27–3 provides a plan of care for the grieving person. Selected nursing diagnoses are presented, along with outcome criteria, appropriate nursing interventions, and rationales for each.

Evaluation

In the final step of the nursing process, a reassessment is conducted to determine if the nursing actions have been successful in achieving the objectives of care. Evaluation of the nursing actions for the grieving patient may be facilitated by gathering information using the following types of questions:

■ Has the patient discussed the recent loss with staff and family members?
■ Is the patient able to verbalize feelings and behaviors associated with each stage of the grieving

process and recognize his or her own position in the process?
■ Has obsession with and idealization of the lost entity subsided?
■ Is anger toward the loss expressed appropriately?
■ Is the patient able to participate in usual religious practices and feel satisfaction and support from them?
■ Is the patient seeking out interaction with others in an appropriate manner?
■ Is the patient able to verbalize positive aspects about his or her life, past relationships, and prospects for the future?

Additional Assistance

Hospice

Hospice is a program that provides palliative and supportive care to meet the special needs of people who are dying and their families. Hospice care provides physical, psychological, spiritual, and social care for the person for whom aggressive treatment is no longer appropriate. Various models of hospice exist, including freestanding institutions that provide both inpatient and home care, those affiliated with hospitals and nursing homes in which hospice services are provided in the institutional setting, and hospice organizations that provide home care only. Historically, the hospice movement in the United States has evolved mainly as a system of home-based care.

Hospice helps patients achieve physical and emotional comfort so that they can concentrate on living life as fully as possible. Patients are urged to stay active for as long as they are able—to take part in activities they enjoy and to focus on the quality of life.

Hospice follows an interdisciplinary team approach to provide care for the terminally ill individual in the familiar surroundings of the home environment. The interdisciplinary team consists of nurses, attendants (homemakers, home health aides), physicians, social workers, volunteers, and other healthcare workers from other disciplines as required for individual patients.

The hospice approach is based on seven components:

1. The interdisciplinary team
2. Pain and symptom management
3. Emotional support to patient and family
4. Pastoral and spiritual care
5. Bereavement counseling
6. 24-hour on-call nurse/counselor
7. Staff support

Table 27–3 | CARE PLAN FOR THE GRIEVING PERSON

NURSING DIAGNOSIS: RISK FOR COMPLICATED GRIEVING

RELATED TO: Loss of a valued entity/concept; loss of a loved one

OUTCOME CRITERIA	NURSING INTERVENTIONS	RATIONALE

Short-Term Goals
■ Patient will acknowledge awareness of the loss.
■ Patient will express feelings about the loss.
■ Patient will verbalize own position in the grief process.
 	
Long-Term Goal
■ Patient will progress through the grief process in a healthful manner toward resolution.
	1. Assess the patient's stage in the grief process.
	2. Develop trust. Show empathy, concern, and unconditional positive regard.
	3. 💬 Help patient actualize the loss by talking about it. "When did it happen?" "How did it happen?" and so forth.
	4. Help the patient identify and express feelings. Some of the more problematic feelings include:
	  a. Anger. The anger may be directed at the deceased, at God, displaced onto others, or retroflected inward on the self. Encourage client to examine this anger and validate the appropriateness of this feeling.
	  b. Guilt. The patient may feel that he or she did not do enough to prevent the loss. Help patient by reviewing the circumstances of the loss and the reality that it could not be prevented.
	  c. Anxiety and helplessness. Help patient to recognize the way that life was managed before the loss. Help the patient to put the feelings of helplessness into perspective by pointing out ways that he or she managed situations effectively without help from others. Role-play life events and assist with decision-making situations.
	5. Interpret normal behaviors associated with grieving and provide patient with adequate time to grieve.
		1. Accurate baseline data are required to provide appropriate assistance.
		2. Developing trust provides the basis for a therapeutic relationship.
		3. Reviewing the events of the loss can help the patient come to full awareness of the loss.
		
		4. Until the patient can recognize and accept personal feelings regarding the loss, grief work cannot progress.
		  a. Many people will not admit to angry feelings, believing it is inappropriate and unjustified. Expression of this emotion is necessary to prevent fixation in this stage of grief.
		
		  b. Feelings of guilt prolong resolution of the grief process.
		
		  c. The patient may have fears that he or she may not be able to carry on alone.
		
		5. Understanding of the grief process will help prevent feelings of guilt generated by these responses. Individuals need adequate time to adjust to the loss and all its ramifications. This involves getting past birthdays and anniversaries of which the deceased was a part.

Table 27–3 | CARE PLAN FOR THE GRIEVING PERSON–cont'd

OUTCOME CRITERIA	NURSING INTERVENTIONS	RATIONALE
	6. Provide continuing support. If this is not possible by the nurse, then offer referrals to support groups. Support groups of individuals going through the same experiences can be very helpful for the grieving individual.	6. The availability of emotional support systems facilitates the grief process.
	7. Identify pathological defenses that patient may be using (e.g., drug/alcohol use, somatic complaints, social isolation). Educate the patient as to how these unhealthy defense mechanisms delay the process of grieving.	7. The bereavement process is impaired by behaviors that mask the pain of the loss.
	8. Encourage the patient to make an honest review of the relationship with the lost entity. Journal keeping is a facilitative tool with this intervention.	8. Only when the patient is able to see both positive and negative aspects related to the loss will the grieving process be complete.

NURSING DIAGNOSIS: RISK FOR SPIRITUAL DISTRESS

RELATED TO: Complicated grief process

OUTCOME CRITERIA	NURSING INTERVENTIONS	RATIONALE
Short-Term Goal ■ Patient will identify meaning and purpose in life, moving forward with hope for the future. **Long-Term Goal** ■ Patient will express achievement of support and personal satisfaction from spiritual practices.	1. Be accepting and nonjudgmental when patient expresses anger and bitterness toward God. Stay with the patient. 2. Encourage patient to ventilate feelings related to meaning of own existence in the face of current loss. 3. Encourage the patient as part of grief work to reach out to previously used religious practices for support. Encourage the patient to discuss these practices and how they provided support in the past. 4. Assure patient that he or she is not alone when feeling inadequate in the search for life's answers. 5. Contact spiritual leader of patient's choice if he or she requests.	1. The nurse's presence and nonjudgmental attitude increase patient's feelings of self-worth and promote trust in the relationship. 2. The patient may believe he or she cannot go on living without lost object. Catharsis can provide relief and put life back into realistic perspective. 3. The patient may find comfort in religious rituals with which he or she is familiar. 4. Validation of the patient's feelings and assurance that they are shared by others offer encouragement and an affirmation of acceptability. 5. These individuals serve to provide relief from spiritual distress and often can do so when other support persons cannot.

These are the ideal, and some hospice programs may not include all of these services. The National Hospice and Palliative Care Organization (NHPCO) is an organization that publishes standards of care based on principles that are directed at the hospice program concept.

Interdisciplinary Team

Nurses

A registered nurse usually acts as case manager for care of hospice patients. The nurse assesses the patient's and family's needs, establishes the goals of care, supervises and assists caregivers, evaluates care, serves as patient advocate, and provides educational information as needed to patient, family, and caregivers. He or she also provides physical care when needed, including IV therapy.

Attendants

These individuals are usually the members of the team who spend the most time with the client. They assist with personal care and all activities of daily living. Without these daily attendants, many individuals would be unable to spend their remaining days in their home. Attendants may be noncertified and provide basic housekeeping services; they may be certified nursing assistants who assist with personal care; or they may be licensed vocational or practical nurses who provide more specialized care, such as dressing changes or tube feedings.

Physicians

The patient's primary physician and the hospice medical consultant have input into the care of the hospice patient. Orders may continue to come from the primary physician, whereas pain and symptom management may come from the hospice consultant. Ideally, these physicians attend weekly patient care conferences and provide in-service education for hospice staff as well as others in the medical community.

Social Workers

The social worker assists the patient and family members with psychosocial issues, including those associated with the patient's condition, financial issues, legal needs, and bereavement concerns. The social worker provides information on community resources from which patient and family may receive support and assistance. Some of the functions of the nurse and social worker may overlap at times.

Trained Volunteers

Volunteers are vital to the hospice concept. They provide services that may otherwise be financially impossible. They are specially selected and extensively trained, and they provide services such as transportation, companionship, respite care, recreational activities, and light housekeeping, and in general, they are sensitive to the needs of families in stressful situations.

Rehabilitation Therapists

Physical therapists may assist hospice patients in an effort to minimize physical disability. They may assist with strengthening exercises and provide assistance with special equipment needs. Occupational therapists may help the debilitated patient learn to accomplish activities of daily living as independently as possible. Other consultants, such as speech therapists, may be called upon for the patient with special needs.

Dietitian

A nutritional consultant may be helpful to the hospice patient who is experiencing nausea and vomiting, diarrhea, anorexia, and weight loss. A nutritionist can ensure that the patient is receiving the proper balance of calories and nutrients.

Counseling Services

The hospice patient may require the services of a psychiatrist or psychologist if there is a history of mental illness or if neurocognitive disorder or depression has become a problem. Other types of counseling services are available to provide assistance in dealing with the special needs of each patient.

Pain and Symptom Management

Improved quality of life at all times is a primary goal of hospice care. Thus, a major intervention for all caregivers is to ensure that the patient is as comfortable as possible, whether experiencing pain or other types of symptoms common in the terminal stages of an illness.

Emotional Support

Members of the hospice team encourage patients and families to discuss the eventual outcome of the disease process. Some individuals find discussing issues associated with death and dying uncomfortable, and if so, their decision is respected. However, honest discussion of these issues provides a sense of relief for some people, and they are more realistically prepared for the future. It may even draw some families closer together during this stressful time.

Pastoral and Spiritual Care

Hospice philosophy supports the individual's right to seek guidance or comfort in the spiritual practices most suited to that person. The hospice team members help the patient obtain the spiritual support and guidance for which he or she expresses a preference.

Bereavement Counseling

Hospice provides a service to surviving family members or significant others after the death of their loved one. This service is usually provided by a bereavement counselor, but when one is not available, volunteers with special training in bereavement care may be of service. A grief support group may be helpful for the bereaved and provide a safe place for them to discuss their own fears and concerns about the death of a loved one.

Twenty-Four-Hour On-Call

The standards of care set forth by NHPCO state that care shall be available 24 hours a day, 7 days a week. A nurse or counselor is usually available by phone or for home visits around the clock. The knowledge that emotional or physical support is available at any time, should it be required, provides considerable support and comfort to significant others or family caregivers.

Staff Support

Team members (all of those who work closely and frequently with the patient) often experience emotions similar to those of the patient or their family and/or significant others. They may experience anger, frustration, or fears of death and dying—all of which must be addressed through staff support groups, team conferences, time off, and adequate and effective supervision. Burnout is a common concern among hospice staff. Stress can be reduced, trust enhanced, and team functioning made more effective if lines of communication are kept open among all members (medical director through volunteer), if information is readily accessible through staff conferences and in-service education, and if staff know they are appreciated and feel good about what they are doing.

Advance Directives

The term **advance directive** refers to either a living will or a durable power of attorney for healthcare (also called a *healthcare proxy*). Either document allows an individual to provide directions about his or her future medical care.

A living will is a written document made by a competent individual that provides instructions that should be used when that individual is no longer able to express his or her wishes for healthcare treatment. The durable power of attorney for healthcare is a written form that gives another person legal power to make decisions regarding healthcare when an individual is no longer capable of making such decisions. Some states have adopted forms that combine the intent of the durable power of attorney for healthcare (i.e., to have a proxy) and the intent of the living will (i.e., to state choices for end-of-life medical treatment).

Doctors usually follow clearly stated directives. It is important that the physician be informed that an advance directive exists and what the specific wishes of the patient are. Advance directives are legally binding in all 50 states in the United States (Sadock et al., 2015). In 1991, the U.S. Congress passed the *Patient Self-Determination Act*. This legislation mandates that all healthcare facilities must advise patients of their rights to refuse treatment, must make advance directives available to patients on admission, and must keep records of whether a patient has an advance directive or a designated healthcare proxy (Sadock et al., 2015). State laws also define how and under what circumstances individuals can refuse life-sustaining medical interventions. These are generally referred to as *natural death acts*. Nurses need to be aware of both federal law and the applicable state laws in the state where they practice nursing.

Despite the existence of laws allowing for an advance directive document, many people have not established this document for themselves, and even when advance directives exist they may not be honored when the circumstances are confusing or unclear. Catalano and Catalano (2015) identify additional reasons why advance directives are sometimes not honored:

- Advance directives that were formulated long before their implementation may call into question whether the client understood the ramifications of his or her decisions for future medical problems and interventions at that time.
- In general, the language used in standard living will documents is not specific enough to cover all healthcare circumstances. Consequently, healthcare providers may lack clarity about how to proceed because the advance directive lacks clarity.
- Because state laws vary, when a patient is in a state other than the one where the advance directive was established, it may raise questions about the document's legality.

Advance directives are designed to allow the patient to be in control of decisions about his or her right to live or die. It is also a way to spare family and loved ones the burden of making choices without knowing the wishes of the person who is dying. Nurses can play an active role in discussing advance directives within a culturally sensitive framework and encouraging patients who have advance directives to review and update them periodically to ensure that their wishes remain clear.

Summary and Key Points

■ Loss is the experience of separation from something of personal importance.

■ Loss is anything that is perceived as such by the individual.

■ Loss of any concept of value to an individual can trigger the grief response.

■ Elisabeth Kübler-Ross identified five stages that individuals pass through on their way to resolution of a loss: denial, anger, bargaining, depression, and acceptance.

■ John Bowlby described similar stages that he identified in the following manner: stage I, numbness or protest; stage II, disequilibrium; stage III, disorganization and despair; and stage IV, reorganization.

■ George Engel's stages include shock and disbelief, developing awareness, restitution, resolution of the loss, and recovery.

■ J. William Worden, a more contemporary clinician, has proposed that bereaved individuals must accomplish a set of tasks in order to complete the grief process. These four tasks include accepting the reality of the loss, processing the pain of grief, adjusting to a world without the lost entity, and finding an enduring connection with the lost entity in the midst of embarking on a new life.

■ The length of the grief process is highly individual, and it can last for a number of years without being maladaptive.

■ The acute stage of the grief process typically lasts a couple of months, but resolution usually takes much longer.

■ Anticipatory grieving is the experiencing of the feelings and emotions associated with the normal grief process in response to anticipation of the loss.

■ Anticipatory grieving is thought to facilitate the grief process when the actual loss occurs.

■ Three types of pathological grief reactions have been described:

1. Delayed or inhibited grief in which there is absence of evidence of grief when it ordinarily would be expected

2. Distorted or exaggerated grief response in which the individual remains fixed in the anger stage of the grief process and all of the symptoms associated with normal grieving are exaggerated

3. Chronic or prolonged grieving in which the individual is unable to let go of grieving behaviors after an extended period and in which behaviors are evident that indicate the bereaved individual is not accepting that the loss has occurred

■ Several authors have identified one crucial difference between normal and maladaptive grieving: the loss of self-esteem.

■ Feelings of worthlessness, feeling that one is a burden to others, suicide ideas, and psychomotor retardation are indicative of clinical depression rather than uncomplicated bereavement.

■ Very young children do not understand death but often react to the emotions of adults by becoming irritable and crying more than usual. They often believe death is reversible.

■ School-age children understand the finality of death. Grief behaviors may reflect regression or aggression, school phobias, or sometimes a withdrawal into the self.

■ Adolescents are usually able to view death on an adult level. Grieving behaviors may include withdrawal or acting out. Although they understand that their own death is inevitable, the concept is so far-reaching as to be imperceptible.

■ By the time a person reaches the 60s or 70s, he or she has experienced numerous losses. Because grief is cumulative, multiple losses can result in bereavement overload. Depression is a common response.

■ Nurses should assess a patient's bereavement needs within a culturally sensitive context.

■ Hospice is a program that provides palliative and supportive care to meet the special needs of people who are dying and their families.

■ The term *advance directive* refers to either a living will or a durable power of attorney for healthcare. Advance directives allow patients to be in control of decisions at the end of life and spare family and loved ones the burden of making choices without knowing what is most important to the person who is dying.

Review Questions
Self-Examination/Learning Exercise

Select the answer that is most appropriate for each of the following questions:

1. Which of the following is most likely to initiate a grief response in an individual? (Select all that apply.)
   a. Death of a pet dog
   b. Being told by her doctor that she has begun menopause
   c. Failing an examination
   d. Losing a spouse through divorce

2. Nancy, who is dying of cancer, says to the nurse, "I just want to see my new grandbaby. If only God will let me live until she is born. Then I'll be ready to go." This is an example of which of Kübler-Ross's stages of grief?
   a. Denial
   b. Anger
   c. Bargaining
   d. Acceptance

3. Gloria, a recent widow, states, "I'm going to have to learn to pay all the bills. Hank always did that. I don't know if I can handle all of that." This is an example of which of the tasks described by Worden?
   a. Task I. Accepting the reality of the loss
   b. Task II. Processing the pain of grief
   c. Task III. Adjusting to a world without the lost entity
   d. Task IV. Finding an enduring connection with the lost entity in the midst of embarking on a new life

4. Engel identifies which of the following as successful resolution of the grief process?
   a. When the bereaved person can talk about the loss without crying
   b. When the bereaved person no longer talks about the lost entity
   c. When the bereaved person puts all remembrances of the loss out of sight
   d. When the bereaved person can discuss both positive and negative aspects about the lost entity

5. Which of the following is thought to facilitate the grief process?
   a. The ability to grieve in anticipation of the loss
   b. The ability to grieve alone without interference from others
   c. Having recently grieved for another loss
   d. Taking personal responsibility for the loss

6. When Frank's wife of 34 years dies, he is very stoic, handles all the funeral arrangements, doesn't cry or appear sad, and comforts all of the other family members in their grief. Two years later, when Frank's best friend dies, Frank has sleep disturbances, difficulty concentrating, loss of weight, and difficulty performing on his job. This is an example of which of the following maladaptive responses to loss?
   a. Delayed grieving
   b. Distorted grieving
   c. Prolonged grieving
   d. Exaggerated grieving

7. A major difference between normal and maladaptive grieving has been identified by which of the following?
   a. There are no feelings of depression in normal grieving.
   b. There is no loss of self-esteem in normal grieving.
   c. Normal grieving lasts no longer than 1 year.
   d. In normal grief, the person does not show anger toward the loss.

Continued

Review Questions—cont'd
Self-Examination/Learning Exercise

8. Which grief reaction can the nurse anticipate in a 10-year-old child?
   a. Statements that the deceased person will soon return
   b. Regressive behaviors, such as loss of bladder control
   c. A preoccupation with the loss
   d. Thinking that he or she may have done something to cause the death

9. Which of the following is a correct statement when attempting to distinguish normal grief from clinical depression?
   a. In clinical depression, anhedonia is prevalent.
   b. In normal grieving, the person has generalized feelings of guilt.
   c. The person who is clinically depressed relates feelings of depression to a specific loss.
   d. In normal grieving, there is a persistent state of dysphoria.

10. Which of the following is *not* true regarding grieving by an adolescent?
    a. Adolescents may not show their true feelings about the death.
    b. Adolescents tend to have an immortal attitude.
    c. Adolescents do not perceive death as inevitable.
    d. Adolescents may exhibit acting-out behaviors as part of their grief.

IMPLICATIONS OF RESEARCH FOR EVIDENCE-BASED PRACTICE

Moriarty, J., Maguire, A., O'Reilly, D., & McCann, M. (2015). Bereavement after informal caregiving: Assessing mental health burden using linked population data. *American Journal of Public Health, 105*(8), 1630–1637.

DESCRIPTION OF THE STUDY: The researchers linked prescription records for antidepressant and antianxiety medications to characteristics and life-event data for members of a longitudinal study in Northern Ireland to assess comparative mental health burdens for nonprofessional (family/household) bereaved caregivers, bereaved noncaregivers, and nonbereaved caregivers ($N = 317,264$). Their expressed intent was to identify who suffers most after the death of someone close to them so that resources for intervention can be targeted appropriately.

RESULTS OF THE STUDY: The first significant finding was that both caregivers and bereaved individuals were at 20 to 50 times greater risk for mental health problems than noncaregivers in similar circumstances. Another significant finding was that among working-age people who were bereaved caregivers, mental health issues were greater than those of other caregivers, and the greater the hours of caregiving, the greater were their risks for sustained mental health issues in bereavement. The researchers identify that this finding was contrary to other studies, which have found increased resilience among bereaved caregivers. This resilience has been thought to be, among other things, a positive outcome of anticipatory grief. The idea that bereavement might provide a relief, of sorts, from the caregiving burden, was also found to be not true for working-age adults. Older adult bereaved caregivers, on the other hand, seemed to recover more quickly from caregiver bereavement.

IMPLICATIONS FOR NURSING PRACTICE: The bereavement process for caregivers of a family member who was ill may carry some additional risk for mental health problems in the bereavement process, but this study highlights the particular burden of working-age caregivers and the potential impact on bereavement and their mental health. The researchers suggest that this prolonged risk may be related to disrupted work schedules, employability, and disrupted social networks. For nurses working with bereaved caregivers, these findings suggest the importance of assessing for mental health issues during bereavement and particularly for working-age adults. Education and provision of resources for ongoing support may be beneficial in reducing long-term, sustained mental health problems for this subgroup.

Communication Exercises

1. Jane's husband has been hospitalized for several days in end-stage congestive heart failure and she has just been told that her husband has died. She begins sobbing and screams at the nurse "You killed my husband! I should have never brought him to the hospital!"
What would be an appropriate, empathic response by the nurse?

2. The doctor has shared test results with John revealing that his terminal cancer is not responding to treatment. John looks to the nurse and asks, "Am I dying?"
What would be an appropriate response by the nurse?

3. Nancy has been told that she has a terminal illness. She says to the nurse, "Why would God do this to me?" What response by the nurse would demonstrate sensitivity to Nancy's spiritual distress?

References

Adams, J. (2014). Death and bereavement: A whole-school approach. *Community Practitioner, 87*(8), 35–36.

Catalano, J. T., & Catalano, S. (2015). Bioethical issues. In J. T. Catalano, *Nursing now! Today's issues, tomorrow's trends.* Philadelphia, PA: F.A. Davis.

Corr, C. A., & Corr, D. M. (2013). *Death and dying: Life & living* (7th ed.). Belmont, CA: Wadsworth.

Hensley, P. L., & Clayton, P. J. (2013). Why the bereavement exclusion was introduced in DSM-III. *Psychiatric Annals, 43*(6), 256–260.

Kearns, C. (2014). *PTSD and the bereaved parent.* Retrieved from http://carolkearns.com/columns/col_ptsd-bereaved.html

King, M., Vasanthan, M., Petersen, I., Jones, L., Marston, L., & Nazareth, I. (2013). Mortality and medical care after bereavement: A practical cohort study. *PloS ONE, 8*(1), 1–7. doi:10.1371/journal.pone.0052561

MedlinePlus. (2018). *Bereavement.* Retrieved from https://medlineplus.gov/bereavement.html

Moriarty, J., Maguire, A., O'Reilly, D., & McCann, M. (2015). Bereavement after informal caregiving: Assessing mental health burden using linked population data. *American Journal of Public Health, 105*(8), 1630–1637.

Morrow, A. (2016). *Grief and mourning: What's normal and what's not?* Retrieved from https://www.verywell.com/grief-and-mourning-process-1132545

Parris, R. J. (2011). Initial management of bereaved relatives following trauma. *Trauma, 14*(2), 139–155.

Peacock, S. C., Hammond-Collins, K., & Ford, D. A. (2014). The journey with dementia from the perspective of bereaved caregivers: A qualitative descriptive study. *BioMed Central Nursing, 13*(42), 1–10.

Pies, R. W. (2013). Grief and depression: The sages knew the difference. *Psychiatric Times, 30*(6). Retrieved from http://www.psychiatrictimes.com/display/article/10168/2140230

Sadock, B. J., Sadock, V. A., & Ruiz, P. (2015). *Synopsis of psychiatry: Behavioral sciences/clinical psychiatry* (11th ed.). Philadelphia, PA: Wolters Kluwer.

Shah, S. M., Carey, I. M., Harris, T., DeWilde, S., Victor, C. R., & Cook, D. G. (2013). The effect of unexpected bereavement on mortality in older couples. *American Journal of Public Health, 103*(6), 1140–1145.

Tousley, M. (2013). Coping with cumulative losses. *Grief Healing.* Retrieved from http://www.griefhealingblog.com/2013/02/coping-with-cumulative-losses.html

Worden, J. W. (2009). *Grief counseling and grief therapy: A handbook for the mental health practitioner* (4th ed.). New York, NY: Springer.

Classical References

Bowlby, J. (1961). Processes of mourning. *International Journal of Psychoanalysis, 42*, 22.

Engel, G. (1964). Grief and grieving. *American Journal of Nursing, 64*, 93.

Kübler-Ross, E. (1969). *On death and dying.* New York, NY: Macmillan.

28

Military Families

KEY TERMS

deployment
post-traumatic stress disorder

traumatic brain injury
veterans

OBJECTIVES

After reading this chapter, the student will be able to:

1. Discuss historical aspects and epidemiological statistics related to members and veterans of the U.S. military.
2. Describe the lifestyle of career military families.
3. Discuss the impact of deployment on families of service members.
4. Discuss concerns of women in the military.
5. Describe combat-related illnesses common in members and veterans of the U.S. military.
6. Apply steps of the nursing process in care of veterans with traumatic brain injury and post-traumatic stress disorder.
7. Discuss various modalities relevant to treatment of traumatic brain injury and post-traumatic stress disorder.

HOMEWORK ASSIGNMENT

Please read the chapter and answer the following questions:

1. Name some positive and negative aspects associated with the military lifestyle.
2. Describe some behaviors exhibited by school-age children in response to the deployment of a parent.
3. How do the feelings about leaving their children during a deployment differ between men and women service members?
4. Name some symptoms of post-traumatic stress disorder.

Introduction

Because of U.S. involvement in Iraq and Afghanistan, perhaps at no time in modern history has so much attention been given to what individuals and families experience as a result of their lives in the military.

There is an ongoing effort by organizations that provide services for active-duty military personnel and **veterans** of military combat to keep up with the growing demand, and resources for these services will be required for many years to come. The need for mental healthcare practitioners will rise as the increasing

754

number of veterans and their family members struggle to cope with their combat-related experiences.

This chapter addresses issues associated with the lives of military families and veterans of military combat. A discussion of nursing care for these individuals is presented and selected medical treatment modalities are described.

Historical Aspects

> *To care for him who shall have borne the battle and for his widow and his orphan.*
> —Abraham Lincoln, 1865

There is little doubt that individuals who survive military combat return from battle with scars—physical or psychological, or both. Reports of war-related psychological symptoms have existed in writing throughout the centuries and have been identified by terms such as *shell shock* and *battle fatigue*. Many veterans of World War I and World War II were expected to be stoic, to lock up their feelings, and to never speak of the scenes of carnage and combat that they witnessed. Abusing alcohol became a common way to deal with the uncomfortable emotions and experiences. **Post-traumatic stress disorder** (PTSD) has been associated with high rates of alcoholism among veterans, particularly those who have experienced active-duty combat. Only in recent history have the invisible wounds of combat veterans received the attention they desperately require.

Very little was written about PTSD during the years between 1950 and 1970. This absence was followed in the 1970s and 1980s with an explosion in the amount of research and writing on the subject. Many of the papers written during this time were about Vietnam veterans. Clearly, the renewed interest in PTSD was linked to the psychological casualties of the Vietnam War. The diagnostic category of PTSD did not appear until the third edition of the *Diagnostic and Statistical Manual of Mental Disorders* (*DSM-III*) in 1980, after a need was indicated by increasing numbers of problems experienced by Vietnam veterans and victims of multiple disasters.

Epidemiological Statistics

Currently, the military comprises more than 1.3 million individuals on active duty in the U.S. armed forces in more than 150 countries around the world, 742,000 civilian personnel, another 826,000 serving in the National Guard and Reserve forces, and over 2 million military retirees (Department of Defense [DoD], 2017a). Approximately 16.1 percent of those in active duty are women. Veterans currently number more than 20 million, about 9 percent of whom are women (U.S. Census Bureau, 2016). Since the beginning of the wars in Afghanistan and Iraq in 2001, more than 2.2 million U.S. military personnel have been deployed in 3 million tours of duty lasting more than 30 days as part of Operation Enduring Freedom (OEF) and Operation Iraqi Freedom (OIF) (Institute of Medicine [IOM], 2013). According to the IOM report *Returning Home from Iraq and Afghanistan*, 44 percent of these military personnel identify difficulty readjusting to daily living upon return from deployment, and 30 percent report unemployment, which is twice the percentage of their nonveteran counterparts. The cost in deaths and physical and psychological injuries cannot be measured.

Application of the Nursing Process

Assessment

The Military Family

The military lifestyle offers both positive and negative aspects to those who choose this way of life. Hall (2011) summarizes several pros and cons about what has come to be known as the Warrior Society. Some advantages include the following:

- Early retirement compared to civilian counterparts
- The security of a vast system to meet family needs
- Job security with a guaranteed paycheck
- Healthcare benefits
- Opportunities to see different areas of the world
- Educational opportunities

Some disadvantages include the following:

- Frequent separations and reunions
- Regular household relocations
- Living life under the maxim of "the mission must always come first"
- A pattern of rigidity, regimentation, and conformity in family life
- Feelings of detachment from nonmilitary community
- The social effects of "rank"
- The lack of control over pay, promotion, and other benefits

Mary Wertsch (1996), who conducted a vast amount of research on the culture of the military family, stated, "The great paradox of the military is that its members, the self-appointed front-line guardians of our cherished American democratic values, do not live in democracy themselves" (p. 15). The military is maintained by a rigid authoritarian structure, and these characteristics often extend into the structure of the home.

A class system is strikingly evident in the military with two distinct subcultures: that of the officer and that of the enlisted ranks. Hall (2011) states:

> The United States has made great strides in the past five decades to affirm and equalize the differences in society, but the assumption of all military systems in the world is that it is essential for the functioning of the organization to maintain a rigid hierarchical system based on dominance and subordination. (p. 38)

Isolation and alienation are common facets of military life. To compensate for the extreme mobility, the focus of this lifestyle turns inward to the military world rather than outward to the local community. Children of military families almost always report that no matter what school they attend, they feel "different" from the other students (Wertsch, 1996).

These descriptions apply principally to "career" military families. Another type of military family, those in the all-volunteer military, have become a familiar part of the American culture in recent years. The military campaigns of OEF and OIF together make up the longest sustained U.S. military operation since the Vietnam War, and they are the first extended conflicts to depend on an all-volunteer military (IOM, 2013). There has been heavy dependence on the National Guard and Reserves and an escalation in the pace, duration, and number of deployments and redeployments experienced by these individuals. Many had joined the National Guard or Reserves as a second job for financial reasons or for the educational opportunities available to them. Little thought had been given to the possibility of actually fighting in a war. As one anonymous reservist posted on his blog,

> The active forces have the harder role. They're required to be fully ready 24/7/365, and to deploy and fight on much shorter notice than the Reserve [forces] . . . it's their livelihood and (for many) their career. They're serving full-time; reservists aren't. But is that really quite true anymore? . . . Many reservists have already served multiple years on active duty since 9/11, away from home/job/family. And this situation doesn't look to change anytime soon.(Kelly Temps in Uniform, 2012)

In recent years, enlistees in the National Guard and Reserves are being told that they should expect to serve an interval of active duty. The Iraq and Afghanistan conflicts have engaged more National Guard and Reserve forces members than previous conflicts, and perhaps associated with this is the finding that more women and parents of young children are being deployed as well (IOM, 2013). Most individuals in the National Guard and Reserves are willing to serve when and where they are needed. However, they consider themselves "part-timers." The extended campaigns of OEF and OIF have changed this part-time concept for many who have served multiple tours of duty, creating a hardship on their families and their civilian careers. The IOM reports that recent military tours of duty, in general, are marked by longer deployments and shorter intervals at home. Many of these "temporary citizen soldiers," as well as their full-time military counterparts, now carry the physical and psychological scars of battle.

Military Spouses and Children

A military spouse inherently knows and lives with the concept of "mission first." Devries and colleagues (2012) state, "While the military works hard to value the family lives of service members and their welfare, the nature of the job is that the mission trumps all other concerns" (p. 11). However, times have changed from the days when life in the military was viewed as a two-person career, in which a woman was expected to "create the right family setting so that her husband's work reflected his life at home, by staying positive, being interested in his duty, and being flexible and adaptable" (Hall, 2012, p. 148). Many of today's military spouses have their own careers or are pursuing higher levels of education. They do not view the military as a joint career with their service member spouse.

The lives of military spouses and children are clearly affected when the service member's active-duty assignments require frequent family moves. Wakefield (2007) stated, "The many short-term relationships, complications of spousal employment, university transfer issues, escalated misbehavior of the children, day care arrangements, spousal loneliness, and increased financial obligations are just some of the issues military personnel face that can lead to frustration." In most instances, when the service member receives orders for a new geographical assignment, the spouse's education or career, or both, is put on hold and the entire family is relocated. Other occasions may arise when the family is unable to immediately follow the service member to the new location. In certain instances, such as when a student may be about to complete a semester or is about to graduate, the service member may proceed to the new assignment without the family. This is difficult for the military spouse who is left alone to care for the children as well as to deal with all aspects of the move. Among active-duty members, 59 percent have children (DoD, 2017b).

Military children face unique challenges. There are over 1.7 million children and youth in military families, and almost one-half of the children of active-duty members (48.8 percent) are 6 years of age or younger (DoD, 2017b). They primarily attend civilian public schools where they form a unique subculture among staff and peers who often do not understand their life experiences. Children who grow up in a career military family learn to adapt to changing situations very quickly and to hide a certain level of fear associated with the nomadic lifestyle. Hall (2008) states:

> It is not just a fear of what might happen to their family or their military parents but a fear of the unknown, of not being accepted, of being behind, of not finding friends, or of not being cool. One of the most common concerns expressed by students when they arrive in a new school is who they will eat lunch with. Another reality for student athletes is that a student could be the star of the basketball team in one school and be sitting on the bench at the next. (p. 103)

The Impact of Deployment

Not since the Vietnam War have so many U.S. military families been affected by deployment-related family separation, combat injury, and death. Many service members have been deployed multiple times. Those who are deployed most frequently describe their greatest fear as that of having to leave their spouse and children. Lengthy separations pose many challenges to all members of the family. Spouses undertake all the challenges of managing the household in addition to assuming the role of the singular parent. The pressure and stress are intense as the spouse attempts to maintain an atmosphere of strength for the children while experiencing the fears and anxiety associated with the life-threatening conditions facing his or her service member partner.

Approximately 2 million American children have experienced the **deployment** of a parent to Iraq or Afghanistan. More than 48,000 children have either lost a parent or have a parent who was wounded in these conflicts. Smith (2012) states:

> The stress that comes when a family member is deployed is significant, and that stress is multiplied when a loved one is wounded or killed. When parents return from deployment, they are not always the same as they were before. Major injuries, such as loss

of a limb, traumatic brain injury, or posttraumatic stress disorder are life-altering, and children often have a hard time understanding the reason for a significant change in the appearance, personality, or behavior of a parent.

The following behaviors have been reported in children in response to the deployment of a parent (American Academy of Child & Adolescent Psychiatry, 2017):

- Infants (birth to 12 months) may respond to disruptions in their schedule with decreased appetite, weight loss, irritability, and/or apathy.
- Toddlers (1 to 3 years) may become sullen, tearful, throw temper tantrums, or develop sleep problems.
- Preschoolers (3 to 6 years) may regress in areas such as toilet training, sleep, separation fears, physical complaints, or thumb sucking. They may assume blame for parent's departure.
- School-age children (6 to 12 years) are more aware of potential dangers to parent. They may exhibit irritable behavior, aggression, or whininess and may become more regressed and fearful about parent's safety.
- Adolescents (13 to 18 years) may be rebellious, irritable, or more challenging of authority. Parents need to be alert to high-risk behaviors, such as problems with the law, sexual acting out, and drug or alcohol abuse.

Pincus and associates (2013) describe the cycle of deployment in five distinct stages: predeployment, deployment, sustainment, redeployment, and postdeployment.

Predeployment The time frame for this stage is variable, beginning with the receipt of the orders and ending when the service member departs. Family members alternate with feelings of denial and anticipation of loss. The soldier and family get their affairs in order, extended training periods result in long hours apart, and the anxiety of the anticipated departure promotes stress and irritability among family members.

Deployment This stage includes the time from actual deployment through the first month of separation. Military spouses report feeling disoriented and overwhelmed, and they experience a range of emotions, including numbness, sadness, loneliness, and abandonment. It is a time of disorganization as the spouse struggles to take charge of the details of living without his or her partner.

Sustainment Sustainment begins about 1 month into the deployment until about a month before the service member's expected return. During this stage, the spouse and children establish new support systems and institute new family routines. Technology makes it possible for the family and service member to keep in touch with each other by phone, video, and e-mail. Despite the difficulties and obstacles encountered, most military families successfully negotiate this stage and anxiously anticipate their loved one's return.

Redeployment This stage is defined as the month before the service member is scheduled to return home. There is excitement and apprehension associated with the homecoming. Pincus and associates (2013) identify concerns such as, "Will he (she) agree with the changes I have made?" "Will I have to give up my independence?" "Will we get along?"

Postdeployment This stage typically lasts 3 to 6 months and begins with the return of the service member to the home station. There is a period of adjustment beginning with the "honeymoon" period when the spouses reconnect physically but not necessarily emotionally. The returning service member may desire to "pick up where he or she left off," only to encounter resistance from the spouse, who expresses a reluctance to relinquish the degree of independence and autonomy to which he or she has become accustomed during the separation. Pincus and associates (2013) state:

> Postdeployment is probably the most important stage for both soldier and spouse. Patient communication, going slow, lowering expectations, and taking time to get to know each other again is critical to the task of successful reintegration of the soldier back into the family.

Counseling may be required if the service member has been injured or experiences a traumatic stress reaction.

Women in the Military

Women make up approximately 16 percent of the U.S. military and 19 percent of National Guard and Reserve members (DoD, 2017b). Women have been serving in the military since the time of the Civil War, mostly in the roles of nurses, spies, and support persons. More recently the Pentagon relaxed its ban on women serving in combat roles, and "women began to fly combat aircraft, staff missile placements, drive convoys in the desert, and participate in other roles that involved potential combat exposure" (Mathewson, 2011, p. 217). Early in 2013, the Secretary of Defense lifted the ban on combat jobs to women, gradually opening direct combat units to female troops. At the present time, certain specialty positions continue to remain off limits, although the plan is to integrate women into these positions. Flexibility in the new law exists for exemptions to occur if further assessment reveals that some jobs are inappropriate for women.

Special Concerns of Women in the Military

There are several issues of special concern to women in the military, including sexual harassment, sexual assault, differential treatment and conditions, and being a parent.

Sexual Harassment Sexual harassment includes "unwelcome sexual advances, requests for sexual favors, and other verbal or physical harassment of a sexual nature (U.S. Equal Employment Opportunity Commission [EEOC], n.d.). In addition to overt sexual behavior, sexual harassment includes making offensive comments about a person's sex/gender. From statements such as "You look nice this morning" or "Hey, you smell good" to blatant suggestions or requests for sexual interactions, Wolfe and associates (1998), in a study of women on active duty during the Persian Gulf War, found that rates of both physical and sexual harassment were higher than are typically found in peacetime military samples. Reports by military therapists conveyed that women who were sexually harassed while in the military suffer high rates of a range of problems following discharge, including poor self-image, relationship problems, drug use, depression, and PTSD.

Sexual Assault The DoD (2017c) reported 14,900 cases of sexual assault in 2016 (down from 20,200 in 2015), which represents 4.3 percent incidence of assault against women and 0.6 percent against men. The DoD defines *sexual assault* as "unwanted sexual contact," and they are now tracking reports annually. In each subsequent year for the past several reporting periods, there has been an increase in reporting. Despite more incidents being reported, 62 percent of those reporting an incident believed that there would be professional or social retaliation as a result of reporting an incident. Reasons for not reporting include being afraid of causing trouble in their unit, fear that their commanders and fellow soldiers would turn against them, fear that they would be passed over for well-deserved promotions, and fear that they would be transferred and removed from duty altogether (Vlahos, 2012). Some women who have reported an incident to their commanding officers have been told to "forget about it," "buckle up," or "pretend it didn't happen," and they are made to feel as though they are the perpetrator instead of the victim. Wolf (2018) describes the military's way of dealing with rape as "a culture of cover-up."

In 2000, following incidents of military sexual assault that were made public, the Veterans Health Administration mandated universal health screening for sexual trauma among military personnel. But despite the efforts within the DoD to identify and correct this problem, incidents continue, suggesting that sexual assault remains a part of military culture (Burgess, Slattery, & Herlihy, 2013).

Some women who report their sexual assaults are discharged from the service with psychiatric diagnoses of personality disorder or adjustment disorder. Vlahos (2012) reports:

> For the veteran, getting a personality disorder or adjustment disorder discharge can be catastrophic. Not only does it carry a stigma for future employers, it cuts the veteran off from a series of benefits, including health care and service-related disability compensation.

Although they comprise only 16 percent of military personnel, women constitute almost one-fourth of all personality disorder discharges. Survivors of sexual assault in the military report long-lasting effects, including PTSD, depression, suicidal ideation and attempts, eating disorders, anxiety disorders, relationship difficulties, and substance abuse. Wolf (2012) notes that, among military veterans, the leading cause of PTSD for men is combat trauma, whereas for women it is sexual trauma. She states, "Our women veterans are more likely to be traumatized by a sexual assault by a fellow soldier, or a commander, than by their own battlefield or war experiences."

Differential Treatment and Conditions Although their numbers have increased, women still constitute a minority in the military. One female officer stated that because of the small number of women in any given unit, officers and enlisted personnel are often housed together. She indicated that she missed being with other officers to discuss work and being able to spend time with her peers. She also reported that the enlisted women were uncomfortable with an officer in their presence. Burgess and colleagues (2013) add that when sexual trauma occurs among military personnel, it is occurring in the workplace and, consequently, the victim is often in a position of having ongoing contact with the perpetrator and may also be in a dependent position if the perpetrator is in a supervisory role.

Women's military careers are often limited by their exclusions from occupational specialties. These sanctions often preclude female officers and enlisted personnel from the most prestigious units and occupations in the military, their participation in which is essential to ascending in the ranks should they choose to make the military a career. Fears of additional occupational discrimination may prevent women from reporting incidents of sexual harassment and assault. Many bans have been lifted, and occupations that historically have been off limits are now open to women. However, the manner in which the culture within the military responds to those changes remains to be seen.

Parenting Issues Women's feelings associated with leaving their children often differ from those of men. Women seem to struggle more with guilt feelings for "abandoning" their children, whereas men have stronger emotions tied to a sense of doing their duty. Although men also experience regret at leaving their children, they often rely on the assurance that the children have their mothers to care for them.

Veterans

Most veterans returning from a combat zone undergo a period of adjustment. A recent study of young veterans (Pedersen, Marshall, & Kurz, 2016) identified that 70 percent screened as positive for behavioral health problems, less than a third of whom received adequate psychotherapy or psychotropic treatment. Many veterans have migraine headaches and experience cognitive difficulties, such as memory loss. Hypervigilance, insomnia, and jitteriness are common. The Substance Abuse and Mental Health Services Administration (SAMHSA) (Pemberton et al., 2016) reported that, particularly in the 18 to 25 age group of veterans, there was a higher incidence of nonmedical use of pain relievers, amphetamine use, and alcohol abuse or dependence than nonveterans and higher incidence of mental illness including major depressive episodes and severe mental illnesses. Plach and Sells (2013), identified in a study of veterans that over 50 percent screened positive for problem drinking, and over 90 percent had engaged in hazardous drinking (Cogan, 2014).

Traumatic Brain Injury

The incidence of **traumatic brain injury** (TBI) is a significant sequela of the Iraq and Afghanistan conflicts. Mild TBI is so frequent that it has been referred to as the "signature injury" of the wars in these countries (Cogan, 2014). The Defense and Veterans Brain Injury Center (DVBIC) reports a total of 339,462 TBIs since 2000, and in 2015 there were over 18,000 (DoD, 2018).

The Department of Veterans Affairs and Department of Defense offer the following definition of TBI:

> A traumatically induced structural injury and/or physiological disruption of brain function as a result of an external force that is indicated by new onset or worsening of at least one of the following clinical signs, immediately following the event:
>
> - Any period of loss of or a decreased level of consciousness
> - Any loss of memory for events immediately before or after the injury (post-traumatic amnesia)

- Any alteration in mental state at the time of the injury (confusion, disorientation, slowed thinking, etc.) (Alteration of consciousness/mental state)
- Neurological deficits (weakness, loss of balance, change in vision, praxis, paresis/plegia, sensory loss, aphasia, etc.) that may or may not be transient
- Intracranial lesion (DoD, 2018)

Symptoms may be classified as mild, moderate, or severe, according to their severity.

In the civilian population, the most common causes of TBI include child abuse in infants and toddlers, motor vehicle accidents in adolescents and young adults, and falls and associated subdural hematomas in older adults (Strong & Donders, 2012). Blasts from explosive devices are the leading cause of TBI for active-duty military personnel in combat (Birk, 2010; Cogan, 2014). Although the mechanism of damage from explosive blasts is not completely understood, researchers believe that it is "the pressure wave passing through the brain that significantly disrupts brain function" (Mayo Clinic, 2018). TBI also results from penetrating wounds, severe blows to the head with shrapnel or debris, and falls or bodily collisions with objects following a blast. Symptoms of TBI according to level of severity are presented in Table 28–1.

TABLE 28–1 Criteria and Symptomatology of Traumatic Brain Injury (TBI) According to Level of Severity

MILD	MODERATE	SEVERE
CRITERIA		
Structural imaging = normal	Structural imaging = normal or abnormal	Structural imaging = normal or abnormal
Loss of consciousness 0–30 min	Loss of consciousness >30 min and <24 hr	Loss of consciousness >24 hr
Alteration of consciousness/mental state = a moment up to 24 hr	Alteration of consciousness/mental state >24 hr; severity based on other criteria	Alteration of consciousness/mental state >24 hr; severity based on other criteria
Post-traumatic amnesia = 0–1 day	Post-traumatic amnesia = >1 and <7 days	Post-traumatic amnesia >7 days
Glasgow Coma Scale = 13–15 (best available score within first 24 hours)*	Glasgow Coma Scale = 9–12	Glasgow Coma Scale <9
SYMPTOMS		
Headache	Any of the symptoms of mild TBI	Any of the symptoms of mild TBI
Dizziness, ringing in the ears	Headache that gets worse or does not go away	Headache that gets worse or does not go away
Nausea	Repeated nausea and vomiting	Repeated nausea and vomiting
Trouble concentrating, confusion	Seizures	Seizures
Blurred vision	Difficulty awakening from sleep	Inability to awaken from sleep
Changes in sleep patterns	Dilation of one or both pupils of the eyes	Dilation of one or both pupils of the eyes
Mood changes	Slurred speech	Slurred speech
Sensitivity to light or sound	Weakness or numbness in the extremities Loss of coordination Increased confusion Restlessness Agitation	Weakness or numbness in the extremities Loss of coordination Profound confusion Restlessness Agitation

Source: Department of Veterans Affairs & Department of Defense (VA/DoD). (2016). *Clinical practice guideline for management of concussion /mild traumatic brain injury*. Retrieved from https://www.healthquality.va.gov/guidelines/Rehab/mtbi/mTBICPGFullCPG50821816.pdf

*In 2015, the DoD recommended against using the Glasgow Coma Scale to diagnose TBI.

Most soldiers who have sustained a mild TBI improve with no lasting clinical sequelae (VA/DoD, 2016). Many recover within hours to days, or at most, weeks. In a small minority, symptoms persist from 6 months to a year. The location and severity of the injury are factors that determine the long-term outcome for individuals with TBI. Severity is determined by the nature, speed, and location of the impact and by complications such as hypoxemia, hypotension, intracranial hemorrhage, and increased intracranial pressure (Ribbers, 2013).

The most common long-term sequelae related to TBI include problems with cognition (e.g., thinking, memory, and reasoning) and behavior or mental health (e.g., depression, anxiety, personality changes, aggression, acting out, and social inappropriateness) (Ribbers, 2013). Seizures occur in about 15 to 20 percent of individuals with TBI and commonly develop within the first 24 hours following the injury. With mild TBI, seizures usually subside within a week after the initial trauma. The potential for chronic epilepsy increases with severity of the injury. Language and communication problems, such as aphasia, dysarthria, and dysphasia, can be complications resulting from TBI (Byers & Jorge, 2017). Difficulties may also exist in the subtler aspects of communication, such as body language and nonverbal expression.

Studies show that TBI has long-term adverse effects on social functioning and productivity. Temkin and colleagues (2009) stated:

> Penetrating head injury sustained in wartime is clearly associated with increased unemployment. TBI also adversely affects leisure and recreation, social relationships, functional status, quality of life, and independent living. Although there is a dose-response relationship between severity of injury and social outcomes, there is insufficient evidence to determine at what level of severity the adverse effects are demonstrated. (p. 460)

Neurocognitive disorders, such as Alzheimer's disease (AD) and Parkinson's disease, are related to TBI (Ribbers, 2013). The risk for AD in individuals with moderate TBI is 2.3 times greater than it is in the general population. An association between Parkinson's disease and TBI has also been established. The disorder may develop years after TBI as a result of damage to the basal ganglia (Ribbers, 2013).

Several factors have also been identified that may worsen the condition for military personnel who sustain a TBI: being in a high-stress environment, being in extreme temperatures such as the 120-degree temperatures reported in Iraq, and having a TBI that is not recognized until the postdeployment period may all interfere with healing (Cogan, 2014). The prevalence as well as short- and long-term consequences suggest that screening for TBI should be conducted for all military personnel returning from active duty who present with physical, cognitive, or emotional symptoms.

Post-traumatic Stress Disorder

PTSD is the most common mental disorder among veterans returning from military combat. Gradus (2017) cites statistics that identify the lifetime prevalence for PTSD in the general population at 6.8 percent. In comparison, the following prevalence estimates for military veterans are identified:

- Veterans of OEF and OIF, 13.8 to 18.5 percent
- Gulf War veterans, 10 percent
- Vietnam veterans, 30 percent

The diagnostic criteria for PTSD from the *Diagnostic and Statistical Manual of Mental Disorders, Fifth Edition* (APA, 2013) are presented in Chapter 19, Trauma- and Stressor-Related Disorders. The disorder can occur when an individual is exposed to an accident or violence in which there is actual or threatened death or serious injury to the self or others. Symptoms of PTSD include the following:

- Reexperiencing the trauma through flashbacks, nightmares, and intrusive thoughts
- Intensive efforts to avoid activities, people, places, situations, or objects that arouse recollections of the trauma
- Chronic negative emotional state and diminished interest or participation in significant activities
- Aggressive, reckless, or self-destructive behavior
- Hypervigilance and exaggerated startle response
- Angry outbursts, problems with concentration, and sleep disturbances

Symptoms of PTSD may be delayed, in some instances for years. When emotions regarding the trauma are constricted, they may suddenly appear at some time in the future following a major life event, stressor, or an accumulation of stressors with time that challenge the person's defenses. Symptoms also may be masked by other physical or mental health problems that the veteran may be experiencing. In some instances, the symptoms do not appear to be problematic until the individual begins a readjustment to routine occupational or social functioning.

Reports indicate that some World War II veterans are only now, decades after returning from combat, being diagnosed with PTSD. At the time of their return, rarely did these veterans speak of their war experiences. But in many, the visions of horror have seeped to the surface in nightmares, flashbacks, anxiety, and emotional numbness. In a study at the University of Michigan, Dr. Helen Kales found that, in a group of World War II veterans being treated for depression, 38 percent of them met the criteria for PTSD (Albrecht, 2009). Langer (2011) reported that the PTSD symptoms for these veterans seemed to become more prominent in midlife and that the most significant precipitant was retirement. For many, their work gave meaning to their lives, and without it the symptoms of depression, anxiety, substance abuse, and PTSD began to emerge. Langer stated:

> Besides retirement, other precipitants [to PTSD in midlife] include the deaths of friends, one's own deteriorating health, children becoming autonomous, divorce, and other losses associated with aging. Other precipitants include current events that trigger memories of one's own combat experience, e.g., 9/11 and other wars.

Veterans with PTSD experience marital and relationship difficulties, including higher rates of physical and verbal aggression against their partners and children and higher rates of divorce (Monson, Fredman, & Adair, 2008). The IOM (2013), in its report on the readjustment needs of veterans, identified a significant rise in domestic violence among veterans of the Iraq and Afghanistan wars, and they recommended this issue be a high priority for assessment and intervention. The burden of caregiving to a partner with PTSD has been noted as an etiological factor in relationship difficulties. The caregiver's perception of how caring for the impaired partner affects their social life, health, and/or financial status is directly associated with the degree of difficulty experienced in the relationship (Lavender & Lyons, 2012). Some caregivers may experience what has been termed as *secondary trauma* or *vicarious traumatization,* a condition in which somatic symptoms and emotional distress occur as a response to caring for an individual who exhibits the symptoms of PTSD. Secondary symptoms are also common in children with a parent suffering from PTSD. Family members sometimes report having nightmares that mimic feelings and experiences of the veteran, difficulty sleeping, depression, and even visual hallucinations that are similar to the veteran's flashbacks.

Co-occurring disorders are common in individuals with PTSD, including major depressive disorder, substance use disorders, and anxiety disorders.

Individuals with TBI also may develop PTSD, depending on the degree of amnesia experienced immediately following the cerebral trauma.

Depression and Suicide

Depressive disorders have been identified as a growing problem among Americans in general, with an estimated 16 million adults having at least one depressive episode within the prior year (National Alliance on Mental Illness [NAMI], 2018). Depressive disorder has been identified as a significant problem among veterans as well. SAMHSA (2017) reports that 18.5 percent of veterans returning from Iraq or Afghanistan are being diagnosed with depression or PTSD; the two are often comorbidities. Impairments are observed in the domains of home management, interpersonal relationships, and occupational and social functioning.

Reports by the DoD and VA indicate that the number of suicides among veterans and active-duty military has risen dramatically since 2001, the year that detailed record-keeping began. This number reached an all-time high in 2012 with a rate of 22.7 suicides per 100,000 population (319) of active-duty military personnel, and although that number declined somewhat in 2013 to 18.7 per 100,000 (259), the number of suicides among reservists and national guardsmen remained alarmingly high at 23.4 to 28.9 per 100,000, respectively (Kime, 2015). When suicides among veterans are added to the numbers, the incidence is even higher. In 2017, the U.S. Department of Veterans Affairs released a report that examined suicide rates among veterans from 1979 to 2014. One significant finding was that the incidence of suicide among veterans is 22 percent higher than the general population and 65 percent of all military personnel who die by suicide are veterans aged 50 or older. For female veterans, the highest suicide rate is among those aged 18 to 29. Whereas the use of firearms as a method for suicide has declined in the civilian population, it remains high among veterans and has increased among female veterans. The U.S. Department of Veterans Affairs (2017) concludes "these results strongly suggest that firearms safety initiatives are likely an important component of an effective suicide prevention strategy for male and female veterans" (p. 47). The IOM report (2013) identified that compounding the risks for suicide is the fact that the VA has had a policy against restricting access to privately owned weapons. In 2014, VA policies were expanded to allow commanders to discuss access to firearms with at-risk populations and to provide for voluntary surrender of their firearms if they request it (Kime, 2015).

Suicide among military personnel is closely associated with the diagnoses of substance use disorder, major depressive disorder, PTSD, and TBI. A common theme among investigations of suicide attempts and completed suicides by military service members includes marital/relationship distress. Devries and associates (2012) stated:

> From 2005 to 2009, relationship problems were a factor in over 50 percent of the suicides in the Army. The health of our military fighting force is directly related to the health of our military marriages. What we see in the military is a common drama of relationship problems played out in an environment of uncommon stressors. (p. 7)

A study by Jakupcak and associates (2010) concluded that veterans who are unmarried or who report lower satisfaction with their social support networks are at increased risk for suicide.

The multiplicity of factors influencing these dramatic suicide rates makes it hard to pinpoint a specific cause, but it has captured the attention of the government and the general public. In 2015, President Obama signed into law the Clay Hunt SAV (suicide prevention for American veterans) Act, which, among other things, intends to expand peer support for troubled veterans, streamline transitions for exiting service people, and mandate annual surveying of VA mental health and suicide prevention programs (NAMI, 2015). Clayton Hunt was a decorated Marine who struggled with PTSD and depression after returning home from active duty and took his own life in 2011.

Substance Use Disorder

In addition to rising suicide rates, substance use disorder has also been on the rise in the military. The Army Suicide Prevention Task Force reported that 29 percent of active-duty military suicides between 2005 and 2009 involved alcohol or drugs, and in 2009, about one-third of these involved prescription drugs (National Institute on Drug Abuse [NIDA], 2013). Substance use disorder is a common co-occurring condition with PTSD. One study reports that almost 22 percent of veterans with PTSD also receive a diagnosis of substance use disorder (Brancu, Straits-Troster, & Kudler, 2011). Other studies have found that around 22 percent of all service members report heavy alcohol use (Herberman Mash et al., 2016). The combination of substance use, PTSD, depression, and TBI contributes to a significant risk for mental illness, relationship problems, difficult readjustment to home life, and, in many cases, suicide.

Among veterans who sought treatment for substance use disorder, 65 percent (almost double that of the nonveteran population) identified alcohol as their primary substance of abuse, 10 percent identified heroin as their primary drug, and 6.2 percent primarily used cocaine (SAMHSA, 2015). Herberman Mash and associates (2016), noting the high risk for suicide among heavy alcohol users, sought to identify reasons for heavy drinking and found that drinking to avoid rejection and the desire to "fit in" are associated with suicidality above overall alcohol consumption. This lack of a sense of connectedness with others has been identified as a risk factor for suicide in other populations as well, but these findings suggest that screening for alcohol use, the reasons for use, and one's sense of belonging or "fitting in" may be important in suicide prediction and prevention among service members.

Much like a trend that has been seen in U.S. civilians, opioid pain medication use and abuse among military personnel has been on the rise. NIDA (2013) reported that from 2005 to 2009, prescriptions for pain medications prescribed by military physicians quadrupled. Crosby (2015) reports that smoking tobacco is 24 percent higher among military personnel than in the general population. The IOM report (2013) on readjustment needs of veterans identified that as many as 39 percent of veterans are struggling with substance use issues, and their recommendations included supporting research to identify evidence-based treatments for substance use disorders as well as reevaluating policies about access to substances of abuse within the military. A firsthand account of what it was like for Josh, a soldier who served in Iraq, and his experience afterward, is presented in "Real People Real Stories: The Military Experience."

Diagnosis and Outcome Identification

Nursing diagnoses are formulated from the data gathered during the assessment phase and with background knowledge regarding predisposing factors to the disorder. Table 28–2 presents a list of selected client behaviors and the NANDA-International nursing diagnoses that correspond to those behaviors, which may be used in planning assistance for families as they confront the unique challenges associated with military life. Outcome criteria are presented for each.

Real People, Real Stories: The Military Experience

(The individual requested that his real name not be used.)

Karyn: What was it like for you when you returned from your tour of duty?

Sean: I was in Iraq for 360 days, and when we landed in the U.S., there was a little welcome home ceremony, and then we went to hang out at the NCO club. The next day, there was a lot of paper to process for benefits and release forms. There was an assessment by a doctor that was about 5 minutes. Basically, they ask if you're okay and they take your word for it. If you say you're not okay, then you can't leave with everyone else. The third day, they encouraged us to join the American Legion and VFW clubs and then bussed us home.

Karyn: You've mentioned before that you had postconcussion headaches and some nightmares. Were you still having these symptoms when you got home?

Sean: Yeah, I had been in an area, during my tour of duty, where a roadside bomb detonated. At the time, I was having extreme headaches, and I got pain medications, but no one talked about what had happened or how I was handling that. The role of the military was to make the soldier mission-capable, so that meant just treating the symptoms. When I got home, I was still having some nightmares and headaches, but I couldn't talk about it. My wife was in the military too, so we had both learned not to talk about emotions. Within a year, I was drinking heavily and separated from my wife. I sought out treatment at the VA, but I only went three times. I felt like they were primarily trying to validate my story as if they wanted to defend themselves against a potential claim. They never asked about alcohol use. I felt angry, and I had some aggression. I felt abandoned. Then I found out my mom had stolen my military checks and had spent them. At that point, I lost faith in everything. All of my core beliefs were gone. The only thing I had faith in was my fellow soldiers, and now that we were back home, they weren't there.

Karyn: Do you get together with any fellow vets?

Sean: Mostly people connect over Facebook, so they don't really get together. The military clubs are all about drinking, so there aren't any healthy options. I do know, though, that sometimes when vets have gotten wind through Facebook that one of us is suicidal, they've traveled across the country to track them down and try to get them help.

Karyn: The suicide rates have been tragically high among vets. Have you ever had thoughts yourself about suicide?

Sean: I have. I was in a very dark place. I thought I was such an awful person that the best option was to kill myself. I was drinking, I was making bad moral decisions, and I was nasty to friends. I didn't care about anything or any consequences. I just wanted momentary relief so I drank more, but, of course, that increased the depression. And it seems like every time we go to military exercises, we hear of another loss of someone to suicide. Last week, it was a fellow soldier who was a decorated hero for saving the lives of many of our guys. [Tearful.] So how do you rectify that someone saved all those lives and then comes home and takes their own life?

Karyn: It does seem like senseless, tragic loss. What has helped you get out of that dark place?

Sean: I have a brother who, even though he couldn't understand what I was going through, he kept checking in on me and repeatedly told me he was praying for me. He just kept showing up and telling me I had to get God back in my life. I knew he cared. I had a DUI and an accident, but I kept thinking "I just have to suck it up and be stronger than this." Instead, the drinking just increases exponentially faster than you can respond or try to control it. One night, I went home and trashed my house. I was ripping sinks out of walls. I remember a neighbor came over and told me I just needed to sober up, but I called the police and told them to take me in. I knew I was out of control.

When I got to the psych unit, I knew I wanted to be "fixed," but that mainly meant I wanted to be under control. I don't remember being asked if I wanted pills, but they gave me pills, and I didn't want to take them because it just made me feel less in control. There was an LPN there who told me that her husband was a vet and that she knew he was a good person. She said she never let his behavior define who he was. That gave me a lot of hope, like maybe I wasn't such an awful person. I reached out to God, and things started to change. I acknowledged that drinking was a primary issue, I cut ties with several unhealthy relationships, and there were supportive friends who came to visit me in the hospital, so I started to see that there were people who genuinely cared about me.

Karyn: What do you want healthcare providers and fellow soldiers to learn from your experience?

Sean: First, a soldier is not who you are; it's a job you do. I wish I had spent more time before my deployment literally writing down all those things that define who I am, like, I'm a loving father and a good friend and what is most important to me; what am I willing to die for. I think it would have helped me, when I came back home, to concretely remind myself of who I am. It's easy to lose all sense of that in the military.

Second, no mood-altering chemicals. There are a lot of things within the military that promote the use of chemicals such as alcohol and pain medication, and while it may keep people mission-ready or temporarily numb you, it becomes disastrous.

Third, reach out for support or, if you are a healthcare provider, help someone identify those people who will provide ongoing support. Supportive people and reaching out to God have been my lifelines.

TABLE 28–2 Nursing Diagnoses: Planning Care for Military Families

RISK FACTORS/DEFINING CHARACTERISTICS	NURSING DIAGNOSES	OUTCOME CRITERIA
POST-TRAUMATIC STRESS DISORDER		
Rage reactions, aggression, irritability, substance use, flashbacks, startle reaction	Risk for other-directed violence	Patient will demonstrate appropriate coping behaviors. Patient will not harm others.
Depression, perception of lack of social support, physical disabilities from combat injuries, feelings of hopelessness	Risk for suicide	Patient will not harm self.
Anger, aggression, depression, difficulty concentrating, flashbacks, guilt, headaches, hypervigilance, intrusive thoughts and dreams, nightmares, emotional numbness, panic attacks, substance abuse	Post-trauma syndrome related to having experienced the trauma of military combat	Patient will begin a healthy grief resolution, initiating the process of psychological healing. Patient will demonstrate ability to deal with emotional reactions in an individually appropriate manner.
Substance abuse	Ineffective coping; ineffective denial	Patient will verbalize understanding of the destructiveness of substance abuse and demonstrate a more adaptive method of coping.
Confusion, fear, and anxiety among family members and their inability to deal with the affected member's unpredictable behavior; ineffective family decision-making process	Interrupted family processes related to crisis associated with veteran member's illness	Family will verbalize understanding of trauma-related illness, demonstrate ability to maintain anxiety at manageable level, and make appropriate decisions to stabilize family functioning.
TRAUMATIC BRAIN INJURY		
Impaired physical mobility, limited range of motion, decreased muscle strength and control, perceptual or cognitive impairment, seizures	Risk for injury	Patient will remain free of physical injury.
Memory deficits; distractibility; altered attention span or concentration; impaired ability to make decisions, problem solve, reason, or conceptualize; personality changes	Disturbed thought processes*	Patient will regain cognitive ability to execute mental functions realistic with the extent of the injury.
Inability to perform desired or appropriate activities of daily living	Self-care deficit (specify)	Patient performs self-care activities within level of own ability.
Confusion, fear, and anxiety among family members and the inability to adapt to changes associated with veteran member's injury; difficulty accepting/receiving help; inability to express or to accept each other's feelings	Interrupted family processes related to situational transition and crisis; uncertainty about expectations and ultimate outcome	Family will verbalize understanding of trauma-related illness, demonstrate ability to maintain anxiety at manageable level, and make appropriate decisions to stabilize family functioning.
FAMILY MEMBERS' ISSUES		
Regressive behaviors, loss of appetite, temper tantrums, clinging behaviors, guilt and self-blame, sleep problems, irritability, aggression (children)	Risk for delayed development related to feelings of abandonment associated with parent's deployment	Parent/caregiver will identify behaviors at risk and initiate interventions to promote appropriate development. Child will develop healthy coping strategies and resume normal developmental progression.

Continued

TABLE 28–2 **Nursing Diagnoses: Planning Care for Military Families—cont'd**		
RISK FACTORS/DEFINING CHARACTERISTICS	**NURSING DIAGNOSES**	**OUTCOME CRITERIA**
Rebelliousness, irritability, acting-out behaviors, promiscuity, substance use (adolescents)	Ineffective coping related to feelings of abandonment associated with parent's deployment	Patient will work through stages of grief associated with the perceived loss and demonstrate healthy, age-appropriate coping strategies.
Depression, anxiety, loneliness, fear, feeling overwhelmed and powerless, anger (spouse/partner)	Risk for complicated grieving related to military deployment of spouse/partner	Patient will work through stages of grief, achieve a healthy acceptance, and express a sense of control over the present situation and future outcome.
Anger, anxiety, frustration, ineffective coping, sleep deprivation, somatic symptoms, fatigue (spouse/partner/caregiver)	Caregiver role strain related to complexity of caregiving responsibilities; lack of respite	Caregiver will demonstrate effective problem-solving skills and develop adaptive coping mechanisms to regain equilibrium.

*This diagnosis has been resigned from the NANDA-I list of approved diagnoses. It is used in this instance because it is most compatible with the identified behaviors.

Planning, Implementation, and Evaluation

Nurses provide care for service members, veterans, and their families in a variety of settings, including general hospitals, VA hospitals, community health centers, doctors' offices, long-term care centers, and community-based clinics. The care required by the veterans returning from combat in the war on terrorism is complex and multifaceted. War-related physical injuries are often striking and conspicuous in their visibility. However, it is the veteran's *invisible* injuries with which psychiatric mental health nurses are most often called upon for treatment. The need for nurses to provide care for the increasing number of veterans with these invisible injuries is intensifying, and the VA continues to search for more effective ways to ensure that military veterans and families receive the care that they desperately need and deserve. Clever and Segal (2013) caution that even though military families have some unique challenges, including compounding issues when both spouses are in the military, they are a diverse group and their needs are dynamic as they move through the transitions in their military career and family life.

Interventions for a selected number of nursing diagnoses relevant to veterans and military families are presented in Table 28–3. A sample teaching guide on PTSD, which may be used to instruct clients and families, is available online at Davis*Plus*. Evaluation is conducted by reassessing to determine if the nursing actions have been successful in meeting the outcome criteria.

Treatment Modalities

Treatment for PTSD and TBI includes psychosocial, rehabilitative, and medical approaches, which often can be combined for optimal response. Selection of appropriate therapy depends on accurate diagnosis and symptom assessment.

Post-Traumatic Stress Disorder

Psychosocial Therapies

Cognitive therapy, prolonged exposure therapy, group and family therapy, and eye movement desensitization and reprocessing have all been used successfully in the treatment of PTSD.

Psychopharmacology

Selective serotonin reuptake inhibitors (SSRIs) are now considered first-line treatment of choice for PTSD because of their efficacy, tolerability, and safety ratings. Other antidepressants that have also been effective include trazodone, the tricyclics amitriptyline and imipramine, and the monoamine oxidase inhibitor (MAOI) phenelzine. Benzodiazepines are sometimes prescribed for their antipanic effects, although their addictive properties make them less desirable. Antihypertensives, such as propranolol and clonidine, have been successful in alleviating symptoms such as nightmares, intrusive recollections, hypervigilance, insomnia, startle responses, and angry outbursts. More recently, intravenous ketamine infusions (in combination with psychotherapy) have demonstrated efficacy in treating PTSD (Chaverneff, 2016).

TABLE 28–3 Nursing Interventions for Veteran Patients and Military Families

Post-traumatic stress syndrome (PTSD)	Stay with the patient during periods of flashbacks and nightmares and offer reassurance of personal safety. Encourage the patient to talk about the traumatic experience at his or her own pace. Discuss maladaptive coping mechanisms being employed. Assist the patient in his or her effort to use more adaptive strategies. Include available support systems and make referrals for additional assistance where required. Help patient understand that use of substances merely numbs feelings and delays healing. Refer for treatment of substance use disorder. Discuss use of stress-management techniques, such as deep breathing, meditation, relaxation, and exercise. Administer medications as prescribed and provide medication education.
Risk for suicide (PTSD, TBI)	Assess degree of risk according to seriousness of threat, existence of a plan, and availability and lethality of the means. Ask directly if person is thinking of acting on thoughts or feelings. Ascertain presence of significant others for support. Determine whether substance use is a factor. Encourage expression of feelings, including appropriate expression of anger. Ensure that environment is safe. Help patient identify more appropriate solutions and offer hope for the future. Collaborate with the patient to develop an ongoing plan for safety.
Disturbed thought processes (TBI)	Evaluate mental status, including extent of impairment in thinking ability; remote and recent memory; orientation to person, place, and time; insight and judgment; changes in personality; attention span, distractibility, and ability to make decisions or problem solve; ability to communicate appropriately; anxiety level; evidence of psychotic behavior. Report to physician any cognitive changes that become obvious. Note behavior indicative of potential for violence and take appropriate action to prevent harm to client and others. Provide safety measures as required. Institute seizure precautions if indicated. Assist with limited mobility issues. Monitor medication regimen. Refer to appropriate rehabilitation providers.
Interrupted family processes (PTSD; TBI)	Emphasize the importance of and encourage continuous, open communication between family members to facilitate ongoing problem-solving. Assist the family to identify and use previously successful coping strategies. Encourage family participation in multidisciplinary team conference or group therapy. Involve family in social support and community activities of their interest and choice. Encourage use of stress-management techniques. Make necessary referrals (e.g., parent effectiveness, specific disease or disability support groups, self-help groups, clergy, psychological counseling, family therapy). Assist family to identify situations that may lead to fear or anxiety. Involve family in mutual goal-setting to plan for the future. Identify community agencies from which family may seek assistance (e.g., Meals on Wheels, visiting nurse, trauma support group, American Cancer Society, Veterans Administration).
Risk for complicated grieving (family of deployed service member)	Help family members to realize that all the feelings they are having are a normal part of the grieving process. Validate their feelings of anger, loneliness, fear, powerlessness, dysphoria, and distress at separation from their loved one.

Continued

TABLE 28–3	**Nursing Interventions for Veteran Patients and Military Families—cont'd**
	Help parent to understand that children's and adolescents' problematic behaviors are symptoms of grieving and that they should not be deemed unacceptable and result in punishment but rather be recognized as having their basis in grief.
	Children should be allowed an appropriate amount of time to grieve. Some experts believe that children need at least 4 weeks to adjust to a parent's deployment (Gabany & Shellenbarger, 2010). Refer for professional help if improvement is not observed in a reasonable period.
	Assess if maladaptive coping strategies, such as substance abuse, are being used.
	Identify and encourage patients to employ previously used successful coping strategies.
	Encourage resuming involvement in usual activities.
	Caution against spending too much time alone.
	Suggest keeping a journal of experiences and feelings.
	Refer to other resources, as needed, such as psychotherapy, family counseling, religious references or pastor, or grief support group.
Caregiver role strain (spouse/caregiver of injured service member)	Assess the spouse/caregiver's ability to anticipate and fulfill the injured service member's unmet needs. Provide information to assist the caregiver with this responsibility.
	Ensure that the caregiver encourages the injured service member to be as independent as possible.
	Encourage the caregiver to express feelings and to participate in a support group.
	Provide information or demonstrate techniques for dealing with acting-out, violent, or disoriented behavior by the injured service member.
	Identify additional needs, and ensure that resources are provided (e.g., physical therapy, occupational therapy, nutritionist, financial and legal help, and respite care).
	Assess for abuse of substances as a coping strategy.
	Refer to counseling or psychotherapy as needed.

Although these findings are still under further investigation, the researcher identifies that ketamine binds at N-methyl-D-aspartate receptors, which impacts fear learning and extinction. Keizer (2016; the researcher cited by Chaverneff) indicates that these treatments allow veterans to remember what happened to them but with less fear. He further notes that 50 percent of military veterans with PTSD also have chronic pain. The use of ketamine demonstrated efficacy in treating both issues.

Complementary Therapies

Acupuncture has been used successfully as an adjunctive therapy for individuals with PTSD. Relaxation techniques have been shown to alleviate symptoms associated with physiological hyperreactivity, and hypnosis may be helpful for symptoms such as pain, anxiety, dissociation, and nightmares (Brancu et al., 2011).

Traumatic Brain Injury

Type of care for the client with TBI depends on severity of the injury and area of the brain involved. Brancu and associates (2011) state, "Since 90 percent of patients have mild cases and experience full recovery, early intervention involving education and a focus on recovery is strongly recommended" (p. 59).

Psychosocial Therapies

Cognitive behavioral therapy (CBT) has been shown to be helpful to individuals with TBI. Scorer (2013) states, "An advantage of [CBT] interventions is that, given their highly structured content, they are amenable to specialized adaptation for memory, attention, and problem-solving impairments, reflecting the difficulties people with TBI often experience." Chard and associates (2011), as cited by Cogan (2014), found that cognitive processing therapy, which is a modification of CBT, was effective in reducing psychological symptoms for individuals with comorbid PTSD and mild TBI. Other therapies, such as prolonged exposure therapy, may also work well for veterans with mild TBI and emotional trauma (Brancu et al., 2011).

Rehabilitation Therapies

Rehabilitation therapy is multifaceted and determined by severity and location of the brain damage. Specialists in the care of the individual with TBI may include any or all of the following (Mayo Clinic, 2018):

■ **Physiatrist:** A physician trained in the medical specialty of physical medicine and rehabilitation. This physician oversees other professionals involved in the rehabilitation process.

- **Occupational therapist:** Helps the individual learn, relearn, or improve skills for everyday living.
- **Physical therapist:** Assists the veteran with mobility and relearning movement patterns, balance, and walking.
- **Recreational therapist:** Assists with leisure activities.
- **Speech and language pathologist:** Helps the person improve communication skills and use assistive communication devices, if necessary.
- **Neuropsychologist or psychiatrist:** Helps the veteran manage behaviors or learn coping strategies, provides talk therapy as needed for emotional and psychological well-being, and prescribes medication as needed.
- **Social worker or case manager:** Coordinates access to services, assists with care decisions and planning, and facilitates communication among various professionals, care providers, and family members.

Psychopharmacology

Medications for the individual with TBI are given to ameliorate specific symptoms. Antidepressants are prescribed for depression, which is very prevalent in individuals with TBI. SSRIs are commonly the antidepressants of choice, although tricyclics and others, such as venlafaxine, trazodone, bupropion, and duloxetine, are also used. Benzodiazepines or SSRIs may be administered for treatment of anxiety symptoms, and antipsychotics are prescribed if aggression, agitation, or psychotic behaviors occur. Anticonvulsants are given if seizures are a problem, and the physician may prescribe skeletal muscle relaxants for muscle spasms or spasticity. Methylphenidate or modafinil has been used to treat attention deficits and hyperactivity, and donepezil has been shown to be effective in enhancing cognitive performance of individuals with TBI (Foster & Spiegel, 2008).

Summary and Key Points

- About 3 million individuals currently are serving in the U.S. Armed Forces in more than 150 countries around the world.
- Veterans currently number more than 20 million.
- Since the beginning of the wars in Afghanistan and Iraq in 2001, more than 2.2 million U.S. military personnel have been deployed in 3 million tours of duty.
- The military lifestyle offers both positive and negative aspects to those who choose this way of life.

- To compensate for the extreme mobility, the focus of the military lifestyle turns inward to the military world rather than outward to the local community.
- In the OEF and OIF campaigns, there has been heavy dependence on the National Guard and Reserves and an escalation in the pace, duration, and number of deployments and redeployments experienced by these individuals.
- Military families face unique challenges, including frequent moves and many separations.
- Children and adolescents exhibit a number of problematic behaviors in response to the separation from a deployed parent.
- The cycle of deployment is described in five distinct stages: predeployment, deployment, sustainment, redeployment, and postdeployment.
- Special concerns of women in the military include sexual harassment, sexual assault, differential treatment and conditions, and issues related to being a parent.
- Evidence supports that a majority of young veterans screen positive for behavioral health problems and a third or less of those have had adequate treatment. Returning form a combat zone causes feelings and reactions that may contribute to difficulties with reintegration into civilian life.
- TBI is a traumatically induced structural injury and/or physiological disruption of brain function as a result of an external force to the head.
- Symptoms of TBI are related to the severity of the injury and the area of the brain that has been injured.
- The most common long-term sequelae related to TBI include problems with cognition and behavior or mental health.
- PTSD is the most common mental disorder among veterans returning from military combat.
- Symptoms of PTSD may occur shortly after the trauma, or they may be delayed, in some instances for years.
- Depression among military veterans is common, and suicide rates among veterans and service members have continued to be higher than in the general population.
- Substance use disorder is a common co-occurring condition with PTSD.
- Nursing care of military families and veterans is presented in the context of the six steps of the nursing process.
- Treatment modalities for PTSD and TBI include psychosocial therapies, psychopharmacology, complementary therapies, and rehabilitation therapies.

Review Questions
Self-Examination/Learning Exercise

Select the answer that is most appropriate for each of the following questions:

1. Dana's husband, who was deployed to Afghanistan a year ago, is returning home this week. Which of the following postdeployment situations may be likely to occur during the first few months of his return? (Select all that apply.)
   a. A honeymoon period of physical reconnection
   b. Resistance from the spouse regarding possible loss of autonomy
   c. Rejection by the children for perceived abandonment
   d. A period of adjustment to reconnect emotionally

2. Which of the following is the leading cause of traumatic brain injury (TBI) in active-duty military personnel in combat?
   a. Military vehicle accidents
   b. Blasts from explosive devices
   c. Falls
   d. Blows to the head from falling debris

3. Shane, a veteran of the war in Iraq, has been diagnosed with post-traumatic stress disorder (PTSD). He is a client of a VA outpatient clinic. He tells the nurse that he experiences panic attacks. Which of the following medications may be prescribed for Shane to treat his panic attacks?
   a. Alprazolam
   b. Lithium
   c. Carbamazepine
   d. Haldol

4. Shane, a veteran of the war in Iraq, has been diagnosed with post-traumatic stress disorder (PTSD). He has been hospitalized after swallowing a handful of his antipanic medication. His physical condition has been stabilized in the emergency department, and he has been admitted to the psychiatric unit. In developing his initial plan of care, which is the priority nursing diagnosis for Shane?
   a. Post-trauma syndrome
   b. Risk for suicide
   c. Complicated grieving
   d. Disturbed thought processes

5. Mike was injured during combat in Afghanistan. He has a diagnosis of traumatic brain injury (TBI). Which of the following medications might the physician prescribe to improve Mike's memory and thinking capability?
   a. Carbamazepine
   b. Duloxetine
   c. Donepezil
   d. Bupropion

6. Juan, a veteran of the war in Iraq, has been diagnosed with post-traumatic stress disorder (PTSD). He has been hospitalized on the psychiatric unit following an attempted suicide. In the middle of the night, he wakes up yelling and tells the nurse he was having a flashback to when his unit transport drove over an improvised explosive device (IED) and most of his fellow soldiers were killed. He is breathing heavily, perspiring, and his heart is pounding. The nurse's most appropriate *initial* intervention is which of the following?
   a. Contact the doctor on call to report the incident.
   b. Administer the prn order for chlorpromazine.
   c. Stay with Juan and reassure him of his safety.
   d. Have Juan sit outside the nurses' station until he is calm.

Review Questions—cont'd
Self-Examination/Learning Exercise

7. Mike, a veteran of combat in Afghanistan, has a diagnosis of mild traumatic brain injury (TBI). The psychiatric home health nurse from the VA medical center is assigned to make home visits to Mike and his wife, Marissa, who is his caregiver. Which of the following would be an appropriate nursing intervention by the home health nurse? (Select all that apply.)
   a. Assess for use of substances by Mike or Marissa.
   b. Encourage Marissa to do everything for Mike to prevent further deterioration in his condition.
   c. Assess Marissa's level of stress and potential for burnout.
   d. Encourage Marissa to allow Mike to be as independent as possible.
   e. Suggest that Marissa ask the physician for a nursing home placement for Mike.

8. Which of the following psychosocial therapies has been shown to be helpful for clients with traumatic brain injury (TBI)?
   a. Eye movement desensitization
   b. Psychoanalysis
   c. Reality therapy
   d. Cognitive behavioral therapy

9. Amy's husband of 1 year left 2 weeks ago for a year-long deployment in Afghanistan. Amy makes an appointment with the psychiatric nurse practitioner at the community mental health clinic. She tells the nurse that she can't sleep, has no appetite, is chronically fatigued, thinks about her husband constantly, and fears for his life. Which of the following might the nurse suggest/prescribe for Amy? (Select all that apply.)
   a. A prescription for sertraline, 50 mg/day
   b. Participation in a support group
   c. Resume involvement in usual activities
   d. Perform regular relaxation exercises

10. Sheila, a nurse, served as a captain in the military and returned from active duty 3 months ago. She reports experiencing nightmares and headaches since her return but denies being engaged in active combat during her tour of duty. Which of the following should the nurse include in the psychosocial assessment? (Select all that apply.)
    a. Folstein's mini-mental status exam
    b. History of sexual trauma
    c. History of military promotions
    d. Risks for substance use disorders

🏃 MOVIE CONNECTIONS

The Best Years of Our Lives (1946) • *The Deer Hunter* (1978) • *Jarhead* (2005) • *In the Valley of Elah* (2007) • *The Lucky Ones* (2008) • *A Walk in My Shoes* (2010)

References

Albrecht, B. (2009, July 16). Post-traumatic stress disorder hitting World War II veterans. *Cleveland Plain Dealer*, p. A1. Retrieved from http://www.cleveland.com/news/plaindealer/index.ssf?/base/cuyahoga/1247733140222090.xml&coll=2

American Academy of Child & Adolescent Psychiatry. (2017). *Military Families.* Retrieved from https://www.aacap.org/AACAP/Families_and_Youth/Facts_for_Families/FFF-Guide/Families-In-The-Military-088.aspx

American Psychiatric Association. (2013). Diagnostic and statistical manual of mental disorders (5th ed.) Washington, DC: American Psychiatric Publishing.

Birk, M. (2010). Traumatic brain injury. *Army Medicine.* Retrieved from http://www.armymedicine.army.mil/hc/healthtips/08/201003mtbi.cfm

Brancu, M., Straits-Troster, K., & Kudler, H. (2011). Behavioral health conditions among military personnel and veterans: Prevalence and best practices for treatment. *North Carolina Medical Journal, 72*(1), 54–60.

Burgess, A. W., Slattery, D. M., & Herlihy, P. A. (2013). Military sexual trauma: A silent syndrome. *Journal of Psychosocial Nursing, 51*(2), 20–26.

Byers, J. A., & Jorge, R. E. (2017). Neuropsychiatric consequences of traumatic brain injury. In B. J. Sadock, V. A. Sadock, &

P. Ruiz (Eds.), *Comprehensive textbook of psychiatry* (pp. 522–540). Philadelphia, PA: Wolters Kluwer.

Chard, K. M., Schumm, J. A., McIlvain, S. M., Bailey, G. W., & Parkinson, R. B. (2011). Exploring the efficacy of a residential treatment program incorporating cognitive processing therapy-cognitive for veterans with PTSD and traumatic brain injury. *Journal of Traumatic Stress, 24,* 347–351. doi:10.1002/jts.20644

Chaverneff, F. (2016). *Ketamine shows signs of efficacy in treating PTSD.* Retrieved from http://www.clinicalpainadvisor.com/aapmanagement-2016/ketamine-to-treat-both-complex-regional-pain-syndrome-and-post-traumatic-stress-disorder/article/524792

Clever, M., & Segal, D. R. (2013). The demographics of military children and families. *The Future of Children, 23*(2), 13–39. doi:10.1353/foc.2013.0018

Cogan, A. M. (2014). Occupational needs and intervention strategies for military personnel with mild traumatic brain injury and persistent post-concussion symptoms: A review. *OTJR: Occupation, Participation, and Health, 34*(3), 150–159.

Crosby, K. (2015). FDA and the Department of Defense: A joint force to reduce tobacco use in the military (FDA blog, September 2015). Retrieved from http://blogs.fda.gov/fdavoice/index.php/2015/09/fda-and-the-departmentof-defense-a-joint-force-to-reduce-tobacco-use-in-themilitary-2/?utm_source=CTPtwitter&utm_medium=socialmedia&utm_campaign=HealthyBase

Department of Defense (DoD). (2017a). *About the Department of Defense.* Retrieved from http://www.defense.gov/About-DoD

Department of Defense (DoD). (2017b). *2016 demographics: Profile of the military community.* Retrieved from http://download.militaryonesource.mil/12038/MOS/Reports/2016-Demographics-Report.pdf

Department of Defense (DoD). (2017c). *Department of Defense annual report on sexual assault in the military, Fiscal year 2016.* Washington, DC: Author.

Department of Defense. (2018). *DoD worldwide numbers for TBI.* Retrieved from http://dvbic.dcoe.mil/files/tbi-numbers/worldwide-totals-2017-Q1-Q4_feb-14-2018_v1.0_2018-03-08_0.pdf

Department of Veterans Affairs & Department of Defense (VA/DoD). (2016). *Clinical practice guideline for management of concussion/mild traumatic brain injury.* Retrieved from http://www.healthquality.va.gov/guidelines/Rehab/mtbi/mTBICPGClinicianSummary50821816.pdf

Devries, M. R., Hughes, H. K., Watson, H., & Moore, B. A. (2012). Understanding the military culture. In B. A. Moore (Ed.), *Handbook of counseling military couples* (pp. 7–18). New York, NY: Routledge.

Foster, M., & Spiegel, D. R. (2008). Use of donepezil in the treatment of cognitive impairments of moderate traumatic brain injury. *Journal of Neuropsychiatry and Clinical Neurosciences, 20*(1), 106.

Gabany, E., & Shellenbarger, T. (2010). Caring for families with deployment stress: How nurses can make a difference in the lives of military families. *American Journal of Nursing, 110*(11), 36–41.

Gradus, J. L. (2017). Epidemiology of PTSD. *National Center for PTSD.* Retrieved from http://www.ptsd.va.gov/professional/PTSD-overview/epidemiological-facts-ptsd.asp

Hall, L. K. (2008). *Counseling military families.* New York, NY: Taylor & Francis.

Hall, L. K. (2011). The military culture, language, and lifestyle. In R. B. Everson & C. R. Figley (Eds.), *Families under fire* (pp. 31–52). New York, NY: Routledge.

Hall, L. K. (2012). The military lifestyle and the relationship. In B. A. Moore (Ed.), *Handbook of counseling military couples* (pp. 137–156). New York, NY: Routledge.

Herberman Mash, H. B., Fullerton, C. S., Ng, T. H. H., Nock, M. K., Wynn, G. H., & Ursano, R. J. (2016). Alcohol use and reasons for drinking as risk factors for suicidal behavior in the U.S. army. *Military Medicine, 181*(8), 811.

Institute of Medicine (IOM). (2013). *Returning home from Iraq and Afghanistan: Readjustment needs of veterans, service members, and their families.* Washington, DC: National Academies Press.

Jakupcak, M., Vannoy, S., Imel, Z., Cook, J. W., Fontana, A., Rosenheck, R., & McFall, M. (2010). Does PTSD moderate the relationship between social support and suicide risk in Iraq and Afghanistan war veterans seeking mental health treatment? *Depression and Anxiety, 27*(11), 1001–1005.

Keizer, B. (2016). Interdisciplinary treatment for the war on co-morbid CRPS and PTSD. Presented at AAPM 2016, September 21-25, San Antonio, TX.

Kelly Temps in Uniform. (2012). *This ain't Hell, but you can see it from here.* Retrieved from http://thisain thell.us/blog/?p=30410

Kime, P. (2015). DoD military suicide rate declining. *Military Times.* Retrieved from http://www.militarytimes.com/story/military/pentagon/2015/01/16/defense-department-suicides-2013-report/21865977

Langer, R. (2011). Combat trauma, memory, and the World War II veteran. *War, Literature & the Arts, 23*(1). Retrieved from http://wlajournal.com/23_1/images/langer.pdf

Lavender, J. M., & Lyons, J. A. (2012). Posttraumatic stress disorder. In B. A. Moore (Ed.), *Handbook of counseling military couples* (pp. 183–200). New York, NY: Routledge.

Mathewson, J. (2011). In support of military women and families. In R. B. Everson & C. R. Figley (Eds.), *Families under fire* (pp. 215–235). New York, NY: Routledge.

Mayo Clinic. (2018). *Traumatic brain injury.* Retrieved from http://www.mayoclinic.com/health/traumatic-brain-injury/DS00552

Monson, C. M., Fredman, S. J., & Adair, K. C. (2008). Cognitive-behavioral conjoint therapy for posttraumatic stress disorder: Application to Operation Enduring and Iraqi Freedom veterans. *Journal of Clinical Psychology, 64,* 958–971.

National Alliance on Mental Illness (NAMI). (2015). President Obama signs Veterans Suicide Prevention Act [blog]. Retrieved from https://www.nami.org/Search?searchtext=Clayton+Hunt+Act&searchmode=anyword

National Alliance on Mental Illness (NAMI). (2018). *Tell me about depression.* Retrieved from http://www.nami.org/Videos/ Tell-Me-About-Depression

National Institute on Drug Abuse (NIDA). (2013). *Drug facts: Substance abuse among the military.* Retrieved from http://www.drugabuse.gov/publications/drugfacts/substance-abuse-in-military

Pedersen, E. R., Marshall, G. N., & Kurz, J. (2016). Behavioral health treatment receipt among a community sample of young adult veterans. *Journal of Behavioral Health Services & Research.* doi:10.1007/s11414-016-9534-7

Pemberton, M. R., Forman-Hoffman, V. L., Lipari, R. N., Ashley, O. S., Heller, D. C., & Williams, M. R. (2016). *Prevalence of past year substance use and mental illness by veteran status in a nationally representative sample.* Retrieved from https://www.samhsa.gov/data/sites/default/files/NSDUH-DR-VeteranTrends-2016/NSDUH-DR-VeteranTrends-2016.htm

Pincus, S. H., House, R., Christenson, J., & Alder, L. E. (2013). The emotional cycle of deployment: A military family perspective. *Operation: Military kids.* Retrieved from http://4h.missouri .edu/programs/military/resources/manual/deployment-cycles.pdf

Plach, H. L., & Sells, C. H. (2013). Occupational performance needs of young veterans. *American Journal of Occupational Therapy, 67,* 73–81. doi:10.5014/ajot.2013.003871

Ribbers, G. M. (2013). Brain injury: Long-term outcome after traumatic brain injury. In J. H. Stone & M. Blouin (Eds.), *International encyclopedia of rehabilitation.* Retrieved from http://cirrie .buffalo.edu/encyclopedia/en/article/338

Scorer, R. (2013). *Psychological therapies for victims of traumatic brain injury.* Retrieved from http://www.pannone.com/media /articles/clinical-negligence/medical-negligence/psychological-therapies-for-victims-of-traumatic-brain-injury-and-how-medical-evidence-plays-a-crucial-role

Smith, R. (2012). Military children and families. *Helping Hands for Freedom.* Retrieved from http://helpinghandsforfreedom. org/remaining-programs-2012-arizona-military-children-families/#more-567

Strong, C. H., & Donders, J. (2012). Traumatic brain injury. In B. A. Moore (Ed.), *Handbook of counseling military couples* (p. 279–294). New York, NY: Routledge.

Substance Abuse and Mental Health Services Administration (SAMHSA). (2015). Veterans' primary substance of abuse is alcohol in treatment admissions. *The CBHSQ Report.* Retrieved from http://www.samhsa.gov/data/sites/default/files/report_2111/Spotlight-2111.pdf

Substance Abuse and Mental Health Services Administration (SAMHSA). (2017). *Veterans and military families.* Retrieved from http://www.samhsa.gov/veterans-military-families

Temkin, N. R., Corrigan, J. D., Dikmen, S. S., & Machamer, J. (2009). Social functioning after traumatic brain injury. *Journal of Head Trauma Rehabilitation, 24*(6), 460–467.

U.S. Census Bureau. (2016). *Quick facts United States.* Retrieved from http://www.census.gov/quickfacts/table/PST045215/00

U.S. Department of Veteran Affairs. (2017). *VA releases veteran suicide statistics by state.* Retrieved from https://www.va.gov/opa/pressrel/pressrelease.cfm?id=2951

U.S. Equal Employment Opportunity Commission (EEOC). (n.d.). *Sexual harassment.* Retrieved from https://www.eeoc.gov/laws/types/sexual_harassment.cfm

Vlahos, K. B. (2012). The rape of our military women. *Anti-War.Com.* Retrieved from http://original.antiwar.com/vlahos/2012/05/14/the-rape-of-our-military-women

Wakefield, M. (2007). Guarding the military home front. *Counseling Today.* Retrieved from http://ct.counseling.org/2007/01/from-the-president-guarding-the-military-home-front

Wolf, N. (2012). A culture of cover-up: Rape in the ranks of the U.S. military. *The Guardian.* Retrieved from http://www.guardian.co.uk/commentisfree/2012/jun/14/culture-coverup-rape-ranks-us-military

Wolfe, J., Sharkansky, E. J., Read, J. P., Dawson, R., Martin, J. A., & Oimette, P. C. (1998). Sexual harassment and assault as predictors of PTSD symptomatology among U.S. female Persian Gulf military personnel. *Journal of Interpersonal Violence, 13*(1), 40–57.

Classic References

Wertsch, M. E. (1996). *Military brats: Legacies of childhood inside the fortress.* St. Louis, MO: Brightwell.

Appendix A

Mental Status Assessment

Gathering the correct information about the patient's mental status is essential to the development of an appropriate plan of care. The mental status examination is a description of all the areas of the patient's mental functioning. The following are the components that are considered critical in the assessment of a patient's mental status. Examples of interview questions and criteria for assessment are included.

Identifying Data

1. Name
2. Gender
3. Age
   a. How old are you?
   b. When were you born?
4. Race/culture
   a. What country did you (your ancestors) come from?
5. Occupational/financial status
   a. How do you make your living?
   b. How do you obtain money for your needs?
6. Educational level
   a. What was the highest grade level you completed in school?
7. Significant other
   a. Are you married?
   b. Do you have a significant relationship with another person?
8. Living arrangements
   a. Do you live alone?
   b. With whom do you share your home?
9. Religious preference
   a. Do you have a religious preference?
10. Allergies
    a. Are you allergic to anything?
    b. Foods? Medications?
11. Special diet considerations
    a. Do you have any special diet requirements?
    b. Diabetic? Low sodium?
12. Chief complaint
    a. For what reason did you come for help today?
    b. What seems to be the problem?
13. Medical diagnosis

General Description

Appearance

1. Grooming and dress
   a. Note unusual modes of dress.
   b. Evidence of soiled clothing?
   c. Use of makeup?
   d. Neat; unkempt?
2. Hygiene
   a. Note evidence of body or breath odor.
   b. Note condition of skin, fingernails.
3. Posture
   a. Note if standing upright, rigid, slumped over.
4. Height and weight
   a. Perform accurate measurements.
5. Level of eye contact
   a. Intermittent?
   b. Occasional and fleeting?
   c. Sustained and intense?
   d. No eye contact?
6. Hair color and texture
   a. Is hair clean and healthy looking?
   b. Greasy, matted, tangled?
7. Evidence of scars, tattoos, or other distinguishing skin marks
   a. Note any evidence of swelling or bruises.
   b. Birthmarks?
   c. Rashes?
8. Evaluation of patient's appearance compared with chronological age

Motor Activity

1. Tremors
   a. Do hands or legs tremble?
   b. Continuously?
   c. At specific times?

2. Tics or other stereotypical movements
   a. Any evidence of facial tics?
   b. Jerking or spastic movements?
3. Mannerisms and gestures
   a. Specific facial or body movements during conversation?
   b. Nail biting?
   c. Covering face with hands?
   d. Grimacing?
4. Hyperactivity
   a. Gets up and down out of chair.
   b. Paces.
   c. Unable to sit still.
5. Restlessness or agitation
   a. Lots of fidgeting.
   b. Clenching hands.
6. Aggressiveness
   a. Overtly angry and hostile.
   b. Threatening.
   c. Uses sarcasm.
7. Rigidity
   a. Sits or stands in a rigid position.
   b. Arms and legs appear stiff and unyielding.
8. Gait patterns
   a. Any evidence of limping?
   b. Limitation of range of motion?
   c. Ataxia?
   d. Shuffling?
9. Echopraxia
   a. Evidence of mimicking the actions of others?
10. Psychomotor retardation
    a. Movements are very slow.
    b. Thinking and speech are very slow.
    c. Posture is slumped.
11. Freedom of movement (range of motion)
    a. Note any limitation in ability to move.

Speech Patterns

1. Slowness or rapidity of speech
   a. Note whether speech seems very rapid or slower than normal.
2. Pressure of speech
   a. Note whether speech seems frenzied.
   b. Unable to be interrupted?
3. Intonation
   a. Are words spoken with appropriate emphasis?
   b. Are words spoken in monotone, without emphasis?
4. Volume
   a. Is speech very loud? Soft?
   b. Is speech low-pitched? High-pitched?

5. Stuttering or other speech impairments
   a. Hoarseness?
   b. Slurred speech?
6. Aphasia
   a. Difficulty forming words.
   b. Use of incorrect words.
   c. Difficulty thinking of specific words.
   d. Making up words (neologisms).

General Attitude

1. Cooperative/uncooperative
   a. Answers questions willingly.
   b. Refuses to answer questions.
2. Friendly/hostile/defensive
   a. Is sociable and responsive.
   b. Is sarcastic and irritable.
3. Uninterested/apathetic
   a. Refuses to participate in interview process.
4. Attentive/interested
   a. Actively participates in interview process.
5. Guarded/suspicious
   a. Continuously scans the environment.
   b. Questions motives of interviewer.
   c. Refuses to answer questions.

Emotions

Mood

1. Depressed; despairing
   a. Reports overwhelming feeling of sadness.
   b. Reports loss of interest in regular activities.
2. Irritable
   a. Easily annoyed and provoked to anger.
3. Anxious
   a. Demonstrates or verbalizes feeling of apprehension.
4. Elated
   a. Expresses feelings of joy and intense pleasure.
   b. Is intensely optimistic.
5. Euphoric
   a. Demonstrates a heightened sense of elation.
   b. Expresses feelings of grandeur ("Everything is wonderful!").
6. Fearful
   a. Demonstrates or verbalizes feeling of apprehension associated with real or perceived danger.
7. Guilty
   a. Expresses a feeling of discomfort associated with real or perceived wrongdoing.
   b. Expresses associated feelings of sadness and despair.

8. Labile
   a. Exhibits mood swings that range from eupho-ria to depression or anxiety.

Affect

1. Congruence with mood
   a. Outward emotional expression is consistent with mood (e.g., if depressed, emotional ex-pression is sadness, eyes downcast, may be crying).
2. Constricted or blunted
   a. Minimal outward emotional expression is observed.
3. Flat
   a. There is an absence of outward emotional expression.
4. Appropriate
   a. The outward emotional expression is what would be expected in a certain situation (e.g., crying upon hearing of a death).
5. Inappropriate
   a. The outward emotional expression is in-compatible with the situation (e.g., laughing upon hearing of a death).

Thought Processes

Form of Thought

1. Flight of ideas
   a. Verbalizations are continuous and rapid and flow from one to another.
2. Loose association
   a. Verbalizations shift from one unrelated topic to another.
3. Circumstantiality
   a. Verbalizations are lengthy and tedious and, because of numerous details, are delayed in reaching the intended point.
4. Tangentiality
   a. Verbalizations that are lengthy and tedious and never reach an intended point.
5. Neologisms
   a. The individual is making up nonsensical-sounding words, which have meaning only to him or her.
6. Concrete thinking
   a. Thinking is literal; elemental.
   b. Absence of ability to think abstractly.
   c. Unable to translate simple proverbs.
7. Clang associations
   a. Speaking in puns or rhymes; using words that sound alike but have different meanings.

8. Word salad
   a. Using a mixture of words that have no mean-ing together; sounding incoherent.
9. Perseveration
10. Repetition of words or phrases in the absence or cessation of socially appropriate context. Echolalia
   a. Persistently repeating what another person says.
11. Mutism
   a. Does not speak (either cannot or will not).
12. Poverty of speech
   a. Speaks very little; may respond in monosyl-lables.
13. Ability to concentrate and disturbance of atten-tion
   a. Does the person hold attention to the topic at hand?
   b. Is the person easily distractible?
   c. Is there selective attention (e.g., blocks out topics that create anxiety)?

Content of Thought

1. Delusions (Does the person have unrealistic ideas or beliefs?)
   a. Persecutory: A belief that someone is out to get him or her is some way (e.g., "The FBI will be here at any time to take me away").
   b. Grandiose: An idea that he or she is all-powerful or of great importance (e.g., "I am the king, and this is my kingdom! I can do anything!").
   c. Reference: An idea that whatever is happen-ing in the environment is about him or her (e.g., "Just watch the movie on TV tonight. It is about my life").
   d. Control or influence: A belief that his or her behavior and thoughts are being controlled by external forces (e.g., "I get my orders from Channel 27. I do only what the forces dictate").
   e. Somatic: A belief that he or she has a dysfunc-tional body part (e.g., "My heart is at a stand-still. It is no longer beating").
   f. Nihilistic: A belief that he or she, a part of the body, or even the world does not exist or has been destroyed (e.g., "I am no longer alive").
2. Suicidal or homicidal ideas
   a. Is the individual expressing ideas of harming self or others?
3. Obsessions
   a. Is the person verbalizing about a persistent thought or feeling that the person is unable to eliminate from his or her consciousness?

4. Paranoia/suspiciousness
   a. Continuously scans the environment.
   b. Questions motives of interviewer.
   c. Refuses to answer questions.
5. Magical thinking
   a. Is the person speaking in a way that indicates belief that his or her words or actions have the ability to cause and effect that is, in fact, irrational? (e.g., "If you step on a crack, you break your mother's back!" or "If I raise my hand the rain pours down.")
6. Impaired religiosity
   a. Is the individual demonstrating obsession with religious ideas and behavior that is causing marked distress and impairing ability to function?
7. Phobias
   a. Is there evidence of irrational fears (of a specific object or a social situation)?
8. Poverty of thought
   a. Is the individual vague, stereotypical, or limited in ability to share information? Does the patient express feeling of emptiness or being devoid of thought?

Perceptual Disturbances

1. Hallucinations (Is the person experiencing unrealistic sensory perceptions?)
   a. Auditory (Is the individual hearing voices or other sounds that do not exist?)
   b. Visual (Is the individual seeing images that do not exist?)
   c. Tactile (Does the individual feel unrealistic sensations on the skin?)
   d. Olfactory (Does the individual smell odors that do not exist?)
   e. Gustatory (Does the individual have a false perception of an unpleasant taste?)
2. Illusions
   a. Does the individual misperceive or misinterpret real stimuli within the environment (e.g., sees something and thinks it is something else)?
3. Depersonalization (altered perception of the self)
   a. The individual verbalizes feeling "outside the body"; visualizing himself or herself from afar.
4. Derealization (altered perception of the environment)
   a. The individual verbalizes that the environment feels "strange or unreal." A feeling that the surroundings have changed.

Sensorium and Cognitive Ability

1. Level of alertness/consciousness
   a. Is the individual clear-minded and attentive to the environment?
   b. Or is there disturbance in perception and awareness of the surroundings?
2. Orientation. Is the person oriented to the following?
   a. Time
   b. Place
   c. Person
   d. Circumstances
3. Memory
   a. Recent (Is the individual able to remember occurrences of the past few days?)
   b. Remote (Is the individual able to remember occurrences of the distant past?)
   c. Confabulation (Does the individual fill in memory gaps with experiences that have no basis in fact?)
4. Capacity for abstract thought
   a. Can the individual interpret proverbs correctly? For example, "What does 'no use crying over spilled milk' mean?"

Impulse Control

1. Ability to control impulses (Does psychosocial history reveal problems with any of the following?)
   a. Aggression
   b. Hostility
   c. Fear
   d. Guilt
   e. Affection
   f. Sexual feelings

Judgment

1. Ability to solve problems and make decisions
   a. What are your plans for the future?
   b. What do you plan to do to reach your goals?
2. Adaptive versus maladaptive use of coping strategies.

Insight

1. Knowledge about self
   a. Awareness of limitations.
   b. Awareness of consequences of actions.
   c. Awareness of illness.
      i. "Do you think you have a problem?"
      ii. "Do you think you need treatment?"
   d. Awareness of use of ego defense mechanisms (e.g., rationalization, projection, displacement, denial).

Appendix B

Glossary

A

abandonment. A unilateral severance of the professional relationship between a healthcare provider and a client without reasonable notice at a time when there is still a need for continuing healthcare.

abreaction. "Remembering with feeling"; bringing into conscious awareness painful events that have been repressed and reexperiencing the emotions that were associated with the events.

abuse. To use wrongfully or in a harmful way. Improper treatment or conduct that may result in injury.

acculturation. To change one's cultural beliefs, behaviors, and/or values as a result of engagement with people of a different culture.

acquaintance rape. Rape perpetrated by someone with whom the victim has met or priorly been acquainted.

acupoints. In Chinese medicine, areas along the body that link pathways of healing energy.

acupressure. A technique in which the fingers, thumbs, palms, or elbows are used to apply pressure to certain points along the body. This pressure is thought to dissolve any obstructions in the flow of healing energy and to restore the body to a healthier functioning.

acupuncture. A technique in which hair-thin, sterile, disposable, stainless-steel needles are inserted into points along the body to dissolve obstructions in the flow of healing energy and restore the body to a healthier functioning.

acute stress disorder. The *DSM-5* diagnostic category describing a trauma- and stressor-related disorder that is short term (from 3 days to 1-month duration) and results in significant distress or impairment in function. (For a complete list of diagnostic criteria, refer to Chapter 19, Trauma- and Stressor-Related Disorders.

adaptation. Restoration of the body to homeostasis following a physiological and/or psychological response to stress.

addiction. A compulsive or chronic requirement. The need is so strong as to generate distress (either physical or psychological) if left unfulfilled.

adjustment. The process of modifying one's behavior in changed circumstances or an altered environment in order to fulfill psychological, physiological, and social needs.

adjustment disorder. A maladaptive reaction to an identifiable psychosocial stressor that occurs within 3 months after onset of the stressor. The individual shows impairment in social and occupational functioning or exhibits symptoms that are in excess of a normal and expectable reaction to the stressor.

advance directive. A legal document that a competent individual may sign to convey wishes regarding future healthcare decisions intended for a time when the individual is no longer capable of informed consent. It may include one or both of the following: (1) a living will, in which the individual identifies the type of care that he or she does or does not wish to have performed and (2) a durable power of attorney for healthcare, in which the individual names another person who is given the right to make healthcare decisions for the individual who is incapable of doing so.

advocacy. The act of pleading for, supporting, or representing a cause or individual. Advocacy in nursing applies to any act in which the nurse is serving in the best interests of the patient, from simple procedures such as hand washing to protect the patient from infection to complex ethically and morally charged issues in which certain clients are unable to advocate for themselves. Nurses also advocate for their patients indirectly by serving in organizations that support and serve to improve healthcare for all individuals and by participating in policy-making legislation that affects healthcare of the public.

affect. The behavioral expression of emotion; may be appropriate (congruent with the situation), inappropriate (incongruent with the situation), constricted or blunted (diminished range and intensity), or flat (absence of emotional expression).

affective domain. A category of learning that includes attitudes, feelings, and values.

aggression. Harsh physical or verbal actions intended (either consciously or unconsciously) to harm or injure another.

aggressive. Behavior that defends an individual's own basic rights by violating the basic rights of others (as contrasted with **assertiveness**).

agoraphobia. The fear of being in places or situations from which escape might be difficult (or embarrassing) or in which help might not be available in the event of a panic attack.

agranulocytosis. Extremely low levels of white blood cells. Symptoms include sore throat, fever, and malaise. This may be a side effect of long-term therapy with some antipsychotic medications.

akathisia. Restlessness; an urgent need for movement; a type of extrapyramidal side effect associated with some antipsychotic medications.

akinesia. Muscular weakness or a loss or partial loss of muscle movement; a type of extrapyramidal side effect associated with some antipsychotic medications.

Alcoholics Anonymous (AA). A major self-help organization for the treatment of alcoholism. It is based on a 12-step program to help members attain and maintain sobriety. Once individuals have achieved sobriety, they in turn are expected to help other alcoholic persons.

allopathic medicine. Traditional medicine; the type of medicine traditionally and currently practiced in the United States and taught in U.S. medical schools.

alternative medicine. Practices that differ from usual traditional (allopathic) medicine.

altruism. One therapeutic factor of group therapy (identified by Irvin Yalom) in which individuals gain self-esteem through mutual sharing and concern. Providing assistance and support to others creates a positive self-image and promotes self-growth.

altruistic suicide. Suicide based on behavior of a group in which an individual is excessively integrated.

amenorrhea. Cessation of the menses; may be a side effect of some antipsychotic medications and may be a symptom in anorexia nervosa.

amnesia. An inability to recall important personal information that is too extensive to be explained by ordinary forgetfulness.

amnesia, generalized. The inability to recall anything that has happened during the individual's entire lifetime.

amnesia, localized. The inability to recall all incidents associated with a traumatic event for a specific time period following the event.

amnesia, selective. The inability to recall only certain incidents associated with a traumatic event for a specific time period following the event.

amphetamine. A racemic sympathomimetic amine that acts as a central nervous system stimulant. It (and its derivatives such as methamphetamine and dextroamphetamine) is a commonly abused substance but has therapeutic use in the treatment of narcolepsy and attention deficit-hyperactivity disorder.

andropause. Also called *male menopause.* A syndrome of symptoms related to the decline of testosterone levels in men. Some symptoms include depression, weight gain, insomnia, hot flashes, decreased libido, mood swings, decreased strength, and erectile dysfunction.

anger. An emotional response to one's perception of a situation. Anger has both positive and negative functions.

anger management. The use of various techniques and strategies to control responses to anger-provoking situations. The goal of anger management is to reduce both the emotional feelings and the physiological arousal that anger engenders.

anhedonia. The inability to experience or even imagine any pleasant emotion.

anomic suicide. Suicide that occurs in response to changes that occur in an individual's life that disrupt cohesiveness from a group and cause that person to feel without support from the formerly cohesive group.

anorexia nervosa. An illness characterized by morbid fear of obesity, distorted body image, preoccupation with food, and refusal to eat.

anorexiants. Drugs that suppress appetite.

anorgasmia. Inability to achieve orgasm.

anosmia. Inability to smell.

anosognosia. A symptom of some mental illnesses, such as schizophrenia, in which the individual is manifesting overt symptoms of illness but is unaware of the presence of symptoms/unaware that there is anything wrong.

anticipatory grief. A subjective state of emotional, physical, and social responses to an anticipated loss of a valued entity. The grief response is repeated once the loss actually occurs, but it may not be as intense as it might have been if anticipatory grieving has not occurred.

antisocial personality disorder. A pattern of socially irresponsible, exploitative, and guiltless behavior, evident in the tendency to fail to conform to the law, develop stable relationships, or sustain consistent employment; exploitation and manipulation of others for personal gain is common.

anxiety. Vague, diffuse apprehension that is associated with feelings of uncertainty and helplessness.

aphasia. Inability to communicate through speech, writing, or signs, caused by dysfunction of brain centers.

aphonia. Inability to speak.

apraxia. Inability to carry out motor activities despite intact motor function or inability to use objects properly.

arbitrary inference. In cognitive therapy this is a type of thinking error in which the individual automatically comes to a conclusion about an incident without the facts to support it or even sometimes despite contradictory evidence to support it.

ascites. Excessive accumulation of serous fluid in the abdominal cavity, occurring in response to portal hypertension caused by cirrhosis of the liver.

assault. An act that results in a person's genuine fear and apprehension that he or she will be touched without consent. Nurses may be guilty of assault for threatening to place an individual in restraints against his or her will.

assertive. Behavior that enables individuals to act in their own best interests, to stand up for themselves without undue anxiety, to express their honest feelings comfortably, or to exercise their own rights without denying those of others.

assessment. A systematic, dynamic process by which the registered nurse, through interaction with the patient, family, groups, communities, populations, and healthcare providers, collects and analyzes data. Assessment may include the following dimensions: physical, functional, psychosocial, emotional, cognitive, sexual, cultural, age-related, environmental, spiritual/transpersonal, and economic.[1]

assimilation. Adopting the behaviors, beliefs, and values of the majority culture.

associative looseness. Sometimes called *loose associations,* a thinking process characterized by speech in which ideas shift from one unrelated subject to another. The individual is unaware that the topics are unconnected.

ataxia. Muscular incoordination.

attachment. Connectedness with others in interpersonal relationship.

attachment theory. The hypothesis that individuals who maintain close relationships with others into old age are more likely to remain independent and less likely to be institutionalized than those who do not.

attitude. A frame of reference around which an individual organizes knowledge about his or her world. It includes an emotional element and can have a positive or negative connotation.

autism. A focus inward on a fantasy world while distorting or excluding the external environment; common in schizophrenia.

autism spectrum disorder. A disorder that is characterized by impairment in social interaction skills and interpersonal communication and a restricted repertoire of activities and interests.

autocratic. A leadership style in which the leader makes all decisions for the group. Productivity is very high with this type of leadership, but morale is often low because of the lack of member input and creativity.

autoimmunity. A condition in which the body produces a disordered immunological response against itself. In this situation, the body fails to differentiate between what is normal and what is a foreign substance. When this occurs, the body produces antibodies against normal parts of the body to such an extent as to cause tissue injury.

automatic thoughts. Thoughts that occur rapidly in response to a situation and without rational analysis. They are often negative and based on erroneous logic.

autonomy. Independence; self-governance. An ethical principle that emphasizes the status of persons as autonomous moral agents whose right to determine their destinies should always be respected.

aversive stimulus. A stimulus that follows a behavioral response and decreases the probability that the behavior will recur; also called punishment.

avoidant personality disorder. A personality disorder characterized by social withdrawal rooted in extreme fear of rejection and feelings of inadequacy.

axon. The cellular process of a neuron that carries impulses away from the cell body.

B

battering. A pattern of repeated physical assault, usually of a woman by her spouse or intimate partner. Men are also battered, although this occurs much less frequently.

---

[1] American Nurses Association. (2010). *Nursing: Scope and standards of practice.* Silver Spring, MD: Author.

battery. The unconsented touching of another person. Nurses may be charged with battery should they participate in the treatment of a client without his or her consent and outside of an emergency situation.

behavior modification. A treatment modality aimed at changing undesirable behaviors using a system of reinforcement to bring about the modifications desired.

behavior therapy. A form of psychotherapy, the goal of which is to modify maladaptive behavior patterns by reinforcing more adaptive behaviors.

behavioral objectives. Statements that indicate to an individual what is expected of him or her. Behavioral objectives are a way of measuring learning outcomes and are based on the affective, cognitive, and psychomotor domains of learning.

belief. A belief is an idea that one holds to be true. It can be rational, irrational, taken on faith, or a stereotypical idea.

beneficence. An ethical principle that refers to one's duty to benefit or promote the good of others.

bereavement. The period of grief and sadness that is the normal process of reacting to a loss and may include mental, physical, social, and emotional reactions.

bereavement overload. An accumulation of grief that occurs when an individual experiences many losses over a short period and is unable to resolve one before another is experienced. This phenomenon is common among the elderly.

binging. A symptom of some eating disorders, notably binge eating disorder and bulimia nervosa in which an individual consumes thousands of calories at one sitting.

binge eating disorder. An illness characterized by recurrent episodes of binging on food.

bioethics. The term used with ethical principles that refer to concepts within the scope of medicine, nursing, and allied health.

biofeedback. The use of instrumentation to become aware of processes in the body that usually go unnoticed and to bring them under voluntary control (e.g., the blood pressure or pulse); used as a method of stress reduction.

bipolar disorder. Characterized by mood swings from profound depression to extreme euphoria (mania) with intervening periods of normalcy. Psychotic symptoms may or may not be present.

body dysmorphic disorder. An exaggerated belief that the body is deformed or defective in some specific way.

body image. One's perception of his or her own body. It may also be how one believes others perceive his or her body. (See also **physical self.**)

borderline personality disorder. A disorder characterized by a pattern of intense and chaotic relationships with affective instability; fluctuating and extreme attitudes regarding other people; impulsivity; direct and indirect self-destructive behavior; and lack of a clear or certain sense of identity, life plan, or values.

boundaries. The level of participation and interaction between individuals and between subsystems. Boundaries denote physical and psychological space that individuals identify as their own. They are sometimes referred to as *limits.* Boundaries are appropriate when they permit appropriate contact with others while preventing excessive interference. Boundaries may be clearly defined (healthy) or rigid or diffuse (unhealthy).

bulimia nervosa. An illness characterized by recurrent binge eating followed by compensatory purging behaviors, such as vomiting, laxative use, excessive exercise, medication use, and others, to prevent weight gain.

C

cachexia. A state of ill health, malnutrition, and wasting; extreme emaciation.

cannabis. The dried flowering tops of the hemp plant. It produces euphoric effects when ingested or smoked and is commonly used in the form of marijuana or hashish.

carcinogen. Any substance or agent that produces or increases the risk of developing cancer in humans or lower animals.

case management. A healthcare delivery process, the goals of which are to provide quality healthcare, decrease fragmentation, enhance the client's quality of life, and contain costs. A case manager coordinates the client's care from admission to discharge and sometimes following discharge. Critical pathways of care are the tools used for the provision of care in a case management system.

case manager. The individual responsible for negotiating with multiple healthcare providers to obtain a variety of services for a client.

catastrophic thinking. Always thinking that the worst will occur without considering the possibility of more likely, positive outcomes.

catatonia. A type of psychological disturbance that is typified by stupor or excitement. Stupor is characterized by extreme psychomotor retardation, mutism, negativism, and posturing; excitement, by psychomotor agitation, in which the movements are frenzied and purposeless. Catatonic symptoms may be associated with other mental or physical disorders.

catharsis. One curative factor of group therapy (identified by Irvin Yalom), in which members in a group can express both positive and negative feelings in a nonthreatening atmosphere.

cell body. The part of the neuron that contains the nucleus and is essential for the continued life of the neuron.

child sexual abuse. Any sexual act, such as indecent exposure or improper touching to penetration (sexual intercourse), that is carried out with a child.

chiropractic medicine. A system of alternative medicine based on the premise that the relationship between structure and function in the human body is a significant health factor and that such relationships between the spinal column and the nervous system are important because the normal transmission and expression of nerve energy are essential to the restoration and maintenance of health.

Christian ethics. The ethical philosophy, based on Christian doctrine stating that we should treat others as moral equals and treat others as we would want to be treated were we in similar situations; sometimes referred to as *the ethic of the golden rule.*

circadian rhythm. A 24-hour biological rhythm controlled by a "pacemaker" in the brain that sends messages to other systems in the body. Circadian rhythm influences various regulatory functions, including the sleep–wake cycle, body temperature regulation, patterns of activity such as eating and drinking, and hormonal and neurotransmitter secretion.

circumstantiality. In speaking, the delay of an individual to reach the point of a communication, owing to unnecessary and tedious details.

cisgender. Describes individuals whose gender identity matches their assigned sex at birth.

civil law. Law that protects the private and property rights of individuals and businesses.

clang association. A pattern of speech in which the choice of words is governed by sounds. Clang associations often take the form of rhyming.

classical conditioning. A type of learning that occurs when an unconditioned stimulus (UCS) that produces an unconditioned response (UCR) is paired with a conditioned stimulus (CS), until the CS alone produces the same response, which is then called a conditioned response (CR). Pavlov's example: food (i.e., UCS) causes salivation (i.e., UCR); ringing bell (i.e., CS) with food (i.e., UCS) causes salivation (i.e., UCR), ringing bell alone (i.e., CS) causes salivation (i.e., CR).

clinging. A common symptom of separation anxiety disorders in which the child excessively clings to the mother or other individual from whom the child fears being separated.

codependency. An exaggerated dependent pattern of learned behaviors, beliefs, and feelings that make life painful. It is a dependence on people and things outside the self, along with neglect of the self to the point of having little self-identity.

cognition. Mental operations that relate to logic, awareness, intellect, memory, language, and reasoning powers.

cognitive. Relating to the mental processes of thinking and reasoning.

cognitive development. A series of stages described by Piaget through which individuals progress, demonstrating at each successive stage a higher level of logical organization than at each previous stage.

cognitive domain. A category of learning that involves knowledge and thought processes within the individual's intellectual ability. The individual must be able to synthesize information at an intellectual level before the actual behaviors are performed.

cognitive maturity. The capability to perform all mental operations needed for adulthood.

cognitive therapy. A type of therapy in which the individual is taught to control thought distortions that are considered to be a factor in the development and maintenance of emotional disorders.

collaborative safety plan. A plan that is developed in collaboration with a suicidal patient to identify strategies for maintaining ongoing safety and prevention of suicide.

collectivist culture. A type of culture that highly values interdependence among its members.

colposcope. An instrument that contains a magnifying lens and to which a 35-mm camera can be attached. A colposcope is used to examine for tears and abrasions inside the vaginal area of a sexual assault victim.

common law. Laws that are derived from decisions made in previous cases.

communication. An interactive process of transmitting information between two or more entities.

community. A group of people living close to and depending to some extent on each other.

compensation. An ego defense mechanism in which an individual covers up a real or perceived weakness by emphasizing a trait that one considers more desirable.

complementary medicine. Practices that differ from usual traditional (allopathic) medicine but may in fact supplement it in a positive way.

compounded rape reaction. Symptoms that are in addition to the typical rape response of physical complaints, rage, humiliation, fear, and sleep disturbances. They include depression and suicide, substance abuse, and even psychotic behaviors.

compulsions. Unwanted repetitive behavior patterns or mental acts (e.g., praying, counting, repeating words silently) that are intended to reduce anxiety, not to provide pleasure or gratification.[2] They may be performed in response to an obsession or in a stereotyped fashion.

concept mapping. A diagrammatic teaching and learning strategy that allows students and faculty to visualize interrelationships between medical diagnoses, nursing diagnoses, assessment data, and treatments. A diagram of client problems and interventions.

concrete thinking. Thought processes that are focused on specifics rather than on generalities and immediate issues rather than eventual outcomes. Individuals who are experiencing concrete thinking are unable to comprehend abstract terminology.

conditioned response. In classical conditioning, a response that is a *learned* response (not reflexive) following repeated exposure to a target stimulus.

conditioned stimulus. In classical conditioning, an unrelated stimulus that is presented to a subject with a target stimulus and that, with repeated exposure, comes to elicit the same response as the original target stimulus.

confabulation. Creating imaginary events to fill in memory gaps.

confidentiality. The right of an individual to the assurance that his or her case will not be discussed outside the boundaries of the healthcare team.

contextual stimuli. Conditions present in the environment that support a focal stimulus and influence a threat to self-esteem.

contingency contracting. A written contract between individuals used to modify behavior. Benefits and consequences for fulfilling the terms of the contract are delineated.

controlled response pattern. The response to rape in which feelings are masked or hidden, and a calm, composed, or subdued affect is seen.

counselor. One who listens as the client reviews feelings related to difficulties he or she is experiencing in any aspect of life; one of the nursing roles identified by H. Peplau.

countertransference. In psychoanalytic theory, countertransference refers to the counselor's behavioral and emotional response to the client. These responses may be related to unresolved feelings toward significant others from the counselor's past or they may be generated in response to the client's behavior toward the counselor.

covert sensitization. An aversion technique used to modify behavior that relies on the individual's imagination to produce unpleasant symptoms. When the individual is about to succumb to undesirable behavior, he or she visualizes something that is offensive or even nauseating in an effort to block the behavior.

criminal law. Law that provides protection from conduct deemed injurious to the public welfare. It provides for punishment of those found to have engaged in such conduct.

crisis. Psychological disequilibrium in a person who confronts a hazardous circumstance that constitutes an important problem that he or she can neither escape nor solve with usual problem-solving resources.

crisis intervention. An emergency type of assistance in which the intervener becomes a part of the individual's life situation. The focus is to provide guidance and support to help mobilize the resources needed to resolve the crisis and restore or generate an improvement in previous level of functioning. Usually lasts no longer than 6 to 8 weeks.

critical pathways of care (CPCs). An abbreviated plan of care that provides outcome-based guidelines for goal achievement within a designated length of time.

cultural syndromes. Syndromes that are specific to a cultural group.

culture. A particular society's entire way of living, encompassing shared patterns of belief, feeling, and knowledge that guide people's conduct and are passed down from generation to generation.

cycle of battering. Three phases of predictable behaviors that are repeated over time in a relationship between a batterer and a victim: tension-building phase; the acute battering incident; and the calm, loving, respite (honeymoon) phase.

cyclothymic disorder. A chronic mood disturbance involving numerous episodes of hypomania and depressed mood of insufficient severity or duration to meet the criteria for bipolar disorder.

---

[2]American Psychiatric Association. (2013). *Diagnostic and statistical manual of mental disorders* (5th ed.). Washington, DC: Author.

D

date rape. A situation in which the rapist is known to the victim. This may occur during dating or with acquaintances or schoolmates. (Also called *acquaintance rape*.)

decatastrophizing. In cognitive therapy, with this technique the therapist assists the client to examine the validity of a negative automatic thought. Even if some validity exists, the client is then encouraged to review ways to cope adaptively, moving beyond the current crisis situation.

defamation of character. An individual may be liable for defamation of character by sharing with others information about a person that is detrimental to that person's reputation.

deinstitutionalization. The removal of mentally ill individuals from institutions and the subsequent plan to provide care for these individuals in the community setting.

delayed grief. The absence of evidence of grief when it ordinarily would be expected.

delayed ejaculation. Delayed or absent ejaculation, even though the man has a firm erection and has had more than adequate stimulation.

delirious mania. A grave form of mania characterized by severe clouding of consciousness and representing an intensification of the symptoms associated with mania. The symptoms of delirious mania have become relatively rare since the availability of antipsychotic medications.

delirium. A state of mental confusion and excitement characterized by disorientation for time and place, often with hallucinations, incoherent speech, and a continual state of aimless physical activity.

delusions. False personal beliefs not consistent with a person's intelligence or cultural background. The individual continues to have the belief in spite of obvious proof that it is false and/or irrational.

dementia. See **neurocognitive disorder.**

democratic leadership. A leadership style employed in group interventions that focuses on full participation of the members in decision making and problem-solving.

dendrites. The cellular processes of a neuron that carry impulses toward the cell body.

denial. Refusal to acknowledge the existence of a real situation and/or the feelings associated with it.

density. The number of people in a given environmental space, influencing interpersonal interaction.

dependent personality disorder. A personality disorder characterized by pervasive, excessive dependency needs, submissiveness, and exaggerated fears of inability to care for oneself.

depersonalization. An alteration in the perception or experience of the self so that the feeling of one's own reality is temporarily lost.

deployment. A term used in the military to describe movement of troops into an active-duty environment.

depression. An alteration in mood that is expressed by feelings of sadness, despair, and pessimism. There is a loss of interest in usual activities, and somatic symptoms may be evident. Changes in appetite and sleep patterns are common.

derealization. An alteration in the perception or experience of the external world so that it seems strange or unreal.

detoxification. The process of managed withdrawal from a substance to which one has become addicted.

diagnosis related groups (DRGs). A system used to determine prospective payment rates for reimbursement of hospital care based on the client's diagnosis.

Diagnostic and Statistical Manual of Mental Disorders, Fifth Edition (DSM-5). Standard nomenclature of emotional illness published by the American Psychiatric Association (APA) and used by all healthcare practitioners. It classifies mental illness and presents guidelines and diagnostic criteria for various mental disorders.

diagnostic overshadowing. A phenomenon in which a person's physical symptoms are assumed to be attributed to his or her mental illness.

dichotomous thinking. In this type of thinking, situations are viewed in all-or-nothing, black-or-white, good-or-bad terms.

directed association. A technique used to help clients bring into consciousness events that have been repressed. Specific thoughts are guided and directed by the psychoanalyst.

disaster. A natural or man-made occurrence that overwhelms the resources of an individual or community and increases the need for emergency evacuation and medical services.

discriminative stimulus. A stimulus that precedes a behavioral response and predicts that a particular reinforcement will occur. Individuals learn to discriminate between various stimuli that will produce the responses they desire.

disengagement. In family theory, disengagement refers to extreme separateness among family members. It is promoted by rigid boundaries or lack of communication among family members.

disengagement theory. This theory suggests there is a process of mutual withdrawal of aging persons and society from each other that is correlated with successful aging. This theory has been challenged by many investigators.

displacement. Feelings that are transferred from one target to another that is considered less threatening or neutral.

dissociation. The splitting off of clusters of mental contents from conscious awareness, a mechanism central to hysterical conversion and dissociative disorder.

distance. A cultural characteristic that defines the means by which various cultures use interpersonal space to communicate.

distraction. In cognitive therapy, when dysfunctional cognitions have been recognized, activities are identified that can be used to distract the client and divert him or her from the intrusive thoughts or depressive ruminations that are contributing to the client's maladaptive responses.

disulfiram. A drug that is administered to individuals who abuse alcohol as a deterrent to drinking. Ingestion of alcohol while disulfiram is in the body results in a syndrome of symptoms that can produce a great deal of discomfort and can even result in death if the blood alcohol level is high.

domains of learning. Categories in which individuals learn or gain knowledge and demonstrate behavior. There are three domains of learning: affective, cognitive, and psychomotor.

double-bind communication. An emotionally distressing situation in which an individual receives conflicting messages in the communication process, whereby one message is negated by another. This creates a condition in which a successful response to one message results in a failed response to the other.

dual diagnosis. A client has a dual diagnosis when it is determined that he or she has a co-existing substance disorder and mental illness. Treatment is designed to target both problems.

dysthymia. A depressive neurosis. The symptoms are similar to, if somewhat milder than, those ascribed to major depressive disorder. There is no loss of contact with reality.

dystonia. Involuntary muscular movements (spasms) of the face, arms, legs, and neck; may occur as an extrapyramidal side effect of some antipsychotic medications.

E

echolalia. The parrot-like repetition, by an individual with loose ego boundaries, of the words spoken by another.

echopraxia. An individual with loose ego boundaries attempting to identify with another person by imitating movements that the other person makes.

ego. One of the three elements of the personality identified by Freud as the rational self or "reality principle." The ego seeks to maintain harmony between the external world, the id, and the superego.

ego defense mechanisms. Strategies employed by the ego for protection in the face of threat to biological or psychological integrity. (See individual defense mechanisms.)

egoistic suicide. The response of an individual who feels separate and apart from the mainstream of society.

electroconvulsive therapy (ECT). A type of somatic treatment in which electric current is applied to the brain through electrodes placed on the temples. A grand mal seizure produces the desired effect. This is used with severely depressed patients refractory to antidepressant medications.

emaciated. The state of being excessively thin or physically wasted.

emotional abuse. A pattern of behavior on the part of the parent or caretaker that results in serious impairment of the child's social, emotional, or intellectual functioning.

emotional neglect. A chronic failure by the parent or caretaker to provide the child with the hope, love, and support necessary for the development of a sound, healthy personality.

empathy. The ability to see beyond outward behavior and sense accurately another's inner experiencing. With empathy, one can accurately perceive and understand the meaning and relevance in the thoughts and feelings of another.

enculturation. The process of learning the norms within a culture.

enmeshment. Exaggerated connectedness among family members. It occurs in response to diffuse boundaries in which there is overinvestment, overinvolvement, and lack of differentiation between individuals or subsystems.

esophageal varices. Veins in the esophagus that become distended because of excessive pressure from defective blood flow through a cirrhotic liver.

essential hypertension. Persistent elevation of blood pressure for which there is no apparent cause or associated underlying disease.

ethical dilemma. A situation that arises when, based on moral considerations, an appeal can be made for taking each of two opposing courses of action.

ethical egoism. An ethical theory espousing that what is "right" and "good" is what is best for the individual making the decision.

ethics. A branch of philosophy dealing with values related to human conduct, to the rightness and wrongness of certain actions, and to the goodness and badness of the motives and ends of such actions.

ethnicity. The concept of people identifying with each other because of a shared heritage.

evaluation. The process of determining the progress toward attainment of expected outcomes, including the effectiveness of care.[3]

exhibitionistic disorder. A paraphilic disorder characterized by a recurrent urge to expose one's genitals to a stranger.

expressed response pattern. Pattern of behavior in which the victim of rape expresses feelings of fear, anger, and anxiety through such behavior as crying, sobbing, restlessness, and tenseness; in contrast to the rape victim who withholds feelings in the controlled response pattern.

extinction. In behavior therapy, the gradual decrease in frequency or disappearance of a response when the positive reinforcement is withheld.

extrapyramidal symptoms (EPS). A variety of responses that originate outside the pyramidal tracts and in the basal ganglion of the brain. Symptoms may include tremors, chorea, dystonia, akinesia, akathisia, and others. May occur as a side effect of some antipsychotic medications.

F

factitious disorder. Disorders that involve conscious, intentional feigning of physical or psychological symptoms. Individuals with factitious disorder pretend to be ill in order to receive emotional care and support commonly associated with the role of "patient."

false imprisonment. The deliberate and unauthorized confinement of a person within fixed limits by the use of threat or force. A nurse may be charged with false imprisonment by placing a patient in restraints against his or her will in a nonemergency situation.

family. Two or more individuals who depend on one another for emotional, physical, and economical support. The members of the family are self-defined.

family structure. A set of invisible principles that influence the interaction among family members.

These principles are established over time and become the "laws" that govern the conduct of various family members.

family system. A system in which the parts of the whole may be the marital dyad, parent-child dyad, or sibling groups. Each of these subsystems are is further divided into subsystems of individuals.

family therapy. A type of therapy in which the focus is on relationships within the family. The family is viewed as a system in which the members are interdependent, and a change in one creates change in all.

fetishistic disorder. A paraphilic disorder characterized by recurrent sexual urges and sexually arousing fantasies involving the use of nonliving objects.

"fight-or-flight" syndrome. A syndrome of physical symptoms that results from an individual's real or perceived notion that harm or danger is imminent.

flexible boundary. A personal boundary is flexible when, because of unusual circumstances, individuals can alter limits that they have set for themselves. Flexible boundaries are healthy boundaries.

flight of ideas. A symptom common in bipolar manic episodes in which the individual's thoughts are racing and they rapidly switch topics when communicating.

flooding. Sometimes called *implosion therapy,* this technique is used to desensitize individuals to phobic stimuli. The individual is "flooded" with a continuous presentation (usually through mental imagery) of the phobic stimulus until it no longer elicits anxiety.

focal stimulus. A situation of immediate concern that results in a threat to self-esteem.

Focus Charting. A type of documentation that follows a data, action, and response (DAR) format. The main perspective is a client "focus," which can be a nursing diagnosis, a client's concern, a change in status, or a significant event in the client's therapy. The focus cannot be a medical diagnosis.

forensic. Pertaining to the law; legal.

forensic nursing. The application of forensic science combined with the biopsychological education of the registered nurse in the scientific investigation, evidence collection and preservation, analysis, prevention, and treatment of trauma- and/or death-related medical-legal issues.

free association. A technique used to help individuals bring to consciousness material that has been repressed. The individual is encouraged to verbalize whatever comes into his or her mind, drifting naturally from one thought to another.

frotteuristic disorder. A paraphilic disorder characterized by the recurrent preoccupation with in-

---

[3]American Nurses Association. (2010). *Nursing: Scope and standards of practice.* Silver Spring, MD: Author.

tense sexual urges or fantasies involving touching or rubbing against a nonconsenting person.

fugue. A sudden, unexpected travel away from home or customary work locale with the assumption of a new identity and an inability to recall one's previous identity; usually occurring in response to severe psychosocial stress.

G

gains. The reinforcements an individual receives for somaticizing.

Gamblers Anonymous (GA). An organization of inspirational group therapy, modeled after Alcoholics Anonymous (AA), for individuals who desire to, but cannot, stop gambling.

gay. An accepted term to describe men who prefer partnership with other men.

gender. The condition of being either male or female.

gender dysphoria. A sense of marked distress and mood disturbances associated with an incongruence between biologically assigned gender and subjectively experienced gender.

general adaptation syndrome. The general biological reaction of the body to a stressful situation, as described by Hans Selye. It occurs in three stages: the alarm reaction stage, the stage of resistance, and the stage of exhaustion.

generalized anxiety disorder. A disorder characterized by chronic (at least 6 months), unrealistic, and excessive anxiety and worry.

genetics. Study of the biological transmission of certain characteristics (physical and/or behavioral) from parent to offspring.

genogram. A graphic representation of a family system. It may cover several generations. Emphasis is on family roles and emotional relatedness among members. Genograms facilitate recognition of areas requiring change.

genotype. The total set of genes present in an individual at the time of conception and coded in the DNA.

genuineness. The ability to be open, honest, and "real" in interactions with others; the awareness of what one is experiencing internally and the ability to project the quality of this inner experiencing in a relationship.

geriatrics. The branch of clinical medicine specializing in the care of the elderly and concerned with the problems of aging.

gerontology. The study of normal aging.

geropsychiatry. The branch of clinical medicine specializing in psychopathology of the elderly.

"granny-dumping." Media-generated term for abandoning elderly individuals at emergency departments, nursing homes, or other facilities—literally, leaving them in the hands of others when the strain of caregiving becomes intolerable.

grief. A subjective state of emotional, physical, and social responses to the real or perceived loss of a valued entity. Change and failure can also be perceived as losses. The grief response consists of a set of relatively predictable behaviors that describe the subjective state that accompanies mourning.

grief, exaggerated. A reaction in which all of the symptoms associated with normal grieving are exaggerated out of proportion. Pathological depression is a type of exaggerated grief.

grief, inhibited. The absence of evidence of grief when it ordinarily would be expected.

group. A collection of individuals whose association is founded on shared commonalities of interest, values, norms, or purpose. Membership in a group is generally by chance (born into the group), by choice (voluntary affiliation), or by circumstance (the result of life-cycle events over which an individual may or may not have control).

group therapy. A therapy group, founded in a specific theoretical framework, led by a person with an advanced degree in psychology, social work, nursing, or medicine. The goal is to encourage improvement in interpersonal functioning.

gynecomastia. Enlargement of the breasts in men; may be a side effect of some antipsychotic medications.

H

habit-reversal therapy. A type of behavior therapy in which the individual develops awareness of unhealthy habits and learns to substitute more adaptive coping strategies in an effort to extinguish unwanted behaviors.

hallucinations. False sensory perceptions not associated with real external stimuli. Hallucinations may involve any of the five senses.

hepatic encephalopathy. A brain disorder resulting from the inability of the cirrhotic liver to convert ammonia to urea for excretion. The continued rise in serum ammonia results in progressively impaired mental functioning, apathy, euphoria or depression, sleep disturbances, increasing confusion, and progression to coma and eventual death.

histrionic personality disorder. A type of personality disorder characterized by excessively emotional and attention-seeking behavior, often presented in a very colorful and dramatic fashion.

HIV-associated neurocognitive disorder. A neuropathological syndrome, possibly caused by chronic HIV encephalitis and myelitis and manifested by cognitive, behavioral, and motor symptoms that become more severe with progression of the disease.

hoarding disorder. A disorder in which the individual has extreme difficulty parting with possessions, regardless of their value, and may also be accompanied by excessive acquisition of material possessions.

home care. A wide range of health and social services that are delivered at home to recovering, disabled, and chronically or terminally ill persons in need of medical, nursing, social, or therapeutic treatment and/or assistance with essential activities of daily living.

homocysteine. An amino acid produced by the catabolism of methionine. Elevated levels may be linked to increased risk of cardiovascular disease.

homosexuality. A sexual preference for persons of the same gender.

hope. A guiding principle of The Recovery Model that stresses potential for improved quality of life and recovery from illness.

hospice. A program that provides palliative and supportive care to meet the special needs arising out of the physical, psychosocial, spiritual, social, and economic stresses that are experienced during the final stages of illness and during bereavement.

hyperactivity. Excessive psychomotor activity that may be purposeful or aimless, accompanied by physical movements and verbal utterances that are usually more rapid than normal. Inattention and distractibility are common with hyperactive behavior.

hypersomnia. Excessive sleepiness or seeking excessive amounts of sleep.

hypertensive crisis. A potentially life-threatening syndrome that results when an individual taking monoamine oxidase inhibitors (MAOIs) eats a product high in tyramine. Symptoms include severe occipital headache, palpitations, nausea and vomiting, nuchal rigidity, fever, sweating, marked increase in blood pressure, chest pain, and coma. Foods with tyramine include aged cheeses or other aged, overripe, and fermented foods; broad beans; pickled herring; beef or chicken liver; preserved meats; beer and wine; yeast products; chocolate; caffeinated drinks; canned figs; sour cream; yogurt; soy sauce; and some over-the-counter cold medications and diet pills.

hypnosis. A treatment for disorders brought on by repressed anxiety. The individual is directed into a state of subconsciousness and assisted, through suggestions, to recall certain events that he or she cannot recall while conscious.

hypomania. A mild form of mania. Symptoms are excessive hyperactivity but not severe enough to cause marked impairment in social or occupational functioning or to require hospitalization.

I

id. One of the three components of the personality identified by Freud as the "pleasure principle." The id is the locus of instinctual drives; is present at birth; and compels the infant to satisfy needs and seek immediate gratification.

identification. An attempt to increase self-worth by acquiring certain attributes and characteristics of an individual one admires.

illusion. A misperception of a real external stimulus.

implosion therapy. See **flooding**.

impulsivity. The urge or inclination to act without consideration of the possible consequences of one's behavior.

incest. Sexual exploitation of a child under 18 years of age by a relative or nonrelative who holds a position of trust in the family.

informed consent. Permission granted to a physician by a client to perform a therapeutic procedure, prior to which information about the procedure has been presented to the client with adequate time given for consideration about the pros and cons.

insomnia. Difficulty initiating or maintaining sleep.

insulin coma therapy. The induction of a hypoglycemic coma aimed at alleviating psychotic symptoms; a dangerous procedure, questionably effective, no longer used in psychiatry.

integration. The process used with individuals with dissociative identity disorder in an effort to bring all the subpersonalities together into one; usually achieved through hypnosis.

intellectualization. An attempt to avoid expressing actual emotions associated with a stressful situation by using the intellectual processes of logic, reasoning, and analysis.

interdisciplinary care. A concept of providing care for a client in which members of various disciplines work together with common goals and shared responsibilities for meeting those goals.

intimate distance. The closest distance that individuals will allow between themselves and others. In the United States, this distance is 0 to 18 inches.

intimate partner violence. A pattern of abusive behavior that is used by an intimate partner to gain or maintain power andcontrol over the other intimate partner.

intoxication. A physical and mental state of exhilaration and emotional frenzy or lethargy and stupor.

introjection. The beliefs and values of another individual are internalized and symbolically become a part of the self to the extent that the feeling of separateness or distinctness is lost.

isolation. The separation of a thought or a memory from the feeling tone or emotions associated with it (sometimes called *emotional isolation*).

J

justice. An ethical principle reflecting that all individuals should be treated equally and fairly.

K

Kantianism. The ethical principle espousing that decisions should be made and actions taken out of a sense of duty.

kleptomania. A recurrent failure to resist impulses to steal objects not needed for personal use or monetary value.

Korsakoff's psychosis. A syndrome of confusion, loss of recent memory, and confabulation in alcoholics caused by a deficiency of thiamine. It often occurs together with Wernicke's encephalopathy and may be termed *Wernicke-Korsakoff syndrome*.

L

laissez-faire leadership. A leadership type in which the leader lets group members do as they please. There is no direction from the leader. Member productivity and morale may be low owing to frustration from lack of direction.

lanugo. Fine, neonatal-like hair growth on the body and a symptom sometimes seen in indviduals with anorexia nervosa.

lesbian. A female homosexual.

libel. An action with which an individual may be charged for sharing with another individual, in writing, information that is detrimental to someone's reputation.

libido. Freud's term for the psychic energy used to fulfill basic physiological needs or instinctual drives, such as hunger, thirst, and sexuality.

limbic system. Parts of the brain that collectively make up what is often called the *emotional brain*. The limbic system is associated wtih feelings such as fear, anger, love, joy , hope, and with sexuality, and social behavior. As research has progressed it has become more difficult to define the boundaries of the limbic system.

long-term memory. Memory for remote events or those that occurred many years ago. The type of memory that is preserved in the elderly individual.

loose association. A thinking process characterized by speech in which ideas shift from one unrelated topic to another. The individual is unaware that topics are unconnected. (See also *associative looseness*.)

loss. The experience of separation from something of personal importance.

M

magical thinking. A primitive form of thinking in which an individual believes that thinking about a possible occurrence can make it happen.

magnification. A type of thinking in which the negative significance of an event is exaggerated.

maladaptation. A failure of the body to return to homeostasis following a physiological and/or psychological response to stress, disrupting the individual's integrity.

malpractice. The failure of one rendering professional services to exercise that degree of skill and learning commonly applied under all the circumstances in the community by the average prudent reputable member of the profession, with the result of injury, loss, or damage to the recipient of those services or to those entitled to rely upon them.

managed care. A concept purposefully designed to control the balance between cost and quality of care. Examples of managed care are health maintenance organizations (HMOs) and preferred provider organizations (PPOs). The amount and type of healthcare that the individual receives is determined by the organization providing the managed care.

mania. A manifestation of bipolar disorder in which the predominant mood is elevated, expansive, or irritable. Motor activity is frenzied and excessive. Psychotic features may or may not be present.

marital rape. Sexual violence directed at a marital partner against that person's will.

marital schism. A state of severe chronic disequilibrium and discord within the marital dyad with recurrent threats of separation.

marital skew. A marital relationship in which there is lack of equal partnership. One partner dominates the relationship and the other partner.

Medicaid. A system established by the federal government to provide medical care benefits for indigent Americans. The Medicaid program is jointly funded by state and federal governments, and coverage varies significantly from state to state.

Medicare. A system established by the federal government to provide medical care benefits for elderly Americans.

medication-assisted treatment. The use of various medications to decrease the intensity of symptoms in an individual who is withdrawing from, or who is experiencing the effects of excessive use of, alcohol and other drugs and to decrease cravings by administering a controlled dose of another medication.

meditation. A method of relaxation in which an individual sits in a quiet place and focuses total concentration on an object, a word, or a thought.

melancholia. A severe form of major depressive episode. Symptoms are exaggerated, and interest or pleasure in virtually all activities is lost.

menopause. The period marking the permanent cessation of menstrual activity; usually occurs at approximately 48 to 51 years of age.

mental health. The successful adaptation to stressors from the internal or external environment, evidenced by thoughts, feelings, and behaviors that are age-appropriate and congruent with local and cultural norms.

mental illness. Maladaptive responses to stressors from the internal or external environment, evidenced by thoughts, feelings, and behaviors that are incongruent with the local and cultural norms and interfere with the individual's social, occupational, and/or physical functioning.

mental imagery. A method of stress reduction that employs the imagination. The individual focuses imagination on a scenario that is particularly relaxing to him or her (e.g., a scene on a quiet seashore, a mountain atmosphere, or floating through the air on a fluffy white cloud).

meridians. In Chinese medicine, pathways along the body in which the healing energy (qi) flows and which are links between acupoints.

milieu. French for "middle"; the English translation connotes "surroundings or environment."

milieu therapy. Also called therapeutic community or therapeutic environment, this type of therapy consists of a scientific structuring of the environment in order to effect behavioral changes and to improve the individual's psychological health and functioning.

minimization. A type of thinking in which the positive significance of an event is minimized or undervalued.

mobile outreach units. Programs in which volunteers and paid professionals drive or walk around and seek out homeless individuals who need assistance with physical or psychological care.

modeling. Learning new behaviors by imitating the behaviors of others.

mood. An individual's sustained emotional tone, which significantly influences behavior, personality, and perception.

moral behavior. Conduct that results from serious critical thinking about how individuals ought to treat others; reflects respect for human life, freedom, justice, or confidentiality.

moral-ethical self. That aspect of the personal identity that functions as observer, standard setter, dreamer, comparer, and most of all evaluator of who the individual says he or she is. This component of the personal identity makes judgments that influence an individual's self-evaluation.

mourning. The psychological process (or stages) through which the individual passes on the way to successful adaptation to the loss of a valued entity.

multidisciplinary care. A concept of providing care for a client in which individual disciplines provide specific services for the client without formal arrangement for interaction between the disciplines.

Munchausen syndrome. See **factitious disorder.**

N

narcissism. Self-love or self-admiration.

narcissistic personality disorder. A disorder characterized by an exaggerated sense of self-worth. These individuals lack empathy and are hypersensitive to the evaluation of others.

narcolepsy. A disorder in which the characteristic manifestation is sleep attacks. The individual cannot prevent falling asleep even in the middle of a sentence or performing a task.

National Standards for Culturally and Linguistically Appropriate Services (NCLAS). A set of standards established by the U.S. Department of Health and Human Services Office of Minority Health for health care organizations and providers focusing on culturally competent care.

natural law theory. The ethical theory that has as its moral precept to "do good and avoid evil" at all costs. Natural law ethics are grounded in a concern for the human good that is based on people's ability to live according to the dictates of reason.

negative reinforcement. Increasing the probability that a behavior will recur by removal of an undesirable reinforcing stimulus.

negativism. Strong resistance to suggestions or directions; exhibiting behaviors contrary to what is expected.

neglect of a child. *Physical neglect* of a child includes refusal of or delay in seeking healthcare, abandonment, expulsion from the home or refusal to allow a runaway to return home, and inadequate supervision. *Emotional neglect* refers to a chronic failure by the parent or caretaker to provide the child with the hope, love, and support necessary for the development of a sound, healthy personality.

negligence. The failure to do something that a reasonable person, guided by those considerations that ordinarily regulate human affairs, would do or doing something that a prudent and reasonable person would not do.

neologism. New words that an individual invents that are meaningless to others but have symbolic meaning to the psychotic person.

neurocognitive disorder (NCD). The *DSM-5* diagnostic label for disorders of global impairment of cognitive functioning that is progressive and interferes with social and occupational abilities. These disorders include Alzheimer's disease and lewy body dementia among others.

neuroendocrinology. The study of hormones functioning within the neurological system.

neuroleptic. Antipsychotic medication used to prevent or control psychotic symptoms.

neuroleptic malignant syndrome (NMS). A rare but potentially fatal complication of treatment with neuroleptic drugs. Symptoms include severe muscle rigidity, high fever, tachycardia, fluctuations in blood pressure, diaphoresis, and rapid deterioration of mental status to stupor and coma.

neuron. A nerve cell; consists of a cell body, an axon, and dendrites.

neurosis. An unconscious conflict that produces anxiety and other symptoms and leads to maladaptive use of defense mechanisms.

neurotransmitter. A chemical that is stored in the axon terminals of the presynaptic neuron. An electrical impulse through the neuron stimulates the release of the neurotransmitter into the synaptic cleft, which in turn determines whether or not another electrical impulse is generated.

nonassertive. Individuals who are nonassertive (sometimes called *passive*) seek to please others at the expense of denying their own basic human rights.

nonmaleficence. The ethical principle that espouses abstaining from negative acts toward another, including acting carefully to avoid harm.

nursing diagnosis. A clinical judgment about individual, family, or community responses to actual and potential health problems/life processes. Nursing diagnoses provide the basis for selection of nursing interventions to achieve outcomes for which the nurse is accountable.

Nursing Interventions Classification (NIC). A comprehensive, research-based, standardized classification of interventions that nurses perform.

Nursing Outcomes Classification (NOC). A comprehensive, standardized classification of patient/client outcomes developed to evaluate the effects of nursing interventions.[4]

nursing process. A dynamic, systematic process by which nurses assess, diagnose, identify outcomes, plan, implement, and evaluate nursing care. It has been called "nursing's scientific methodology." Nursing process gives order and consistency to nursing intervention.

O

obesity. The state of having a body mass index of 30 or above.

object constancy. The phase in the separation/individuation process when the child learns to relate to objects in an effective, constant manner. A sense of separateness is established, and the child is able to internalize a sustained image of the loved object or person when out of sight.

obsessions. Unwanted, intrusive, persistent ideas, thoughts, impulses, or images that cause marked anxiety or distress. Common ones include repeated thoughts about contamination, repeated doubts, a need to have things in a particular order, aggressive or sexual impulses, and fears of harm to oneself or others.[5]

obsessive-compulsive disorder. Recurrent thoughts or ideas (obsessions) that an individual is unable to put out of his or her mind and actions that an individual is unable to refrain from performing (compulsions). The obsessions and compulsions are severe enough to interfere with social and occupational functioning.

obsessive-compulsive personality disorder. A type of personality disorder in which the individual has an intense fear of making mistakes, which manifests in inflexible and perfectionistic behavior. It is differentiated from obsessive-compulsive disorder in that there is no evidence of the obsessive-compulsive rituals in the individual with this personality disorder.

---

[4] Moorhead, S., Johnson, M., Maas, M., & Swanson, E. (2013). *Nursing outcomes classification (NOC)* (5th ed.). St. Louis, MO: Mosby.

[5] American Psychiatric Association. (2013). *Diagnostic and statistical manual of mental disorders* (5th ed.). Washington, DC: Author.

oculogyric crisis. An attack of involuntary deviation and fixation of the eyeballs, usually in the upward position. It may last for several minutes or hours and may occur as an extrapyramidal side effect of some antipsychotic medications.

operant conditioning. The learning of a particular action or type of behavior that is followed by a reinforcement.

opioids. A synthetic or naturally occurring substance that acts on opiate receptors to produce opiate-like effects.

orgasm. A peaking of sexual pleasure with release of sexual tension and rhythmic contraction of the perineal muscles and pelvic reproductive organs.

osteoporosis. A reduction in the mass of bone per unit of volume that interferes with the mechanical support function of bone. This process occurs because of demineralization of the bones and is escalated in women about the time of menopause.

outcomes. End results that are measurable, desirable, and observable and translate into observable behaviors.

overgeneralization. Also called *absolutistic thinking*. In cognitive therapy, this refers to a distorted thinking pattern in which sweeping conclusions are made based on one incident—an "all-or-nothing" type of thinking.

overt sensitization. A type of aversion therapy that produces unpleasant consequences for undesirable behavior. An example is the use of disulfiram therapy with alcoholics, which induces an undesirable physical response if the individual has consumed any alcohol.

P

palilalia. Repeating one's own sounds or words (a type of vocal tic associated with Tourette's disorder).

panic. A sudden overwhelming feeling of terror or impending doom. This most severe form of emotional anxiety is usually accompanied by behavioral, cognitive, and physiological signs and symptoms considered to be outside the expected range of normalcy.

panic disorder. A disorder characterized by recurrent panic attacks, the onset of which are unpredictable and manifested by intense apprehension, fear, or terror, often associated with feelings of impending doom and accompanied by intense physical discomfort.

paradoxical intervention. In family therapy, "prescribing the symptom." The therapist requests that the family continue to engage in the behavior that they are trying to change. Tension is relieved, and the family is able to view more clearly the possible solutions to their problem.

paralanguage. The gestural component of the spoken word. It consists of pitch, tone, loudness of spoken messages, the rate of speaking, expressively placed pauses, and emphasis assigned to certain words.

paranoia. A term that implies extreme suspiciousness. In schizophrenia, paranoia is characterized by persecutory delusions and hallucinations of a threatening nature.

paranoid personality disorder. A type of personality disorder in which the individual intensely mistrusts others and assumes that they have malevolent intentions toward them.

paraphilic disorder. Repetitive behaviors or fantasies that involve nonhuman objects, real or simulated suffering or humiliation, or nonconsenting partners.

parasomnia. Unusual or undesirable behaviors that occur during sleep (e.g., nightmares, sleep terrors, and sleepwalking).

passive-aggressive. Behavior that defends an individual's own basic rights by expressing resistance to social and occupational demands. Sometimes called *indirect aggression,* this behavior takes the form of sly, devious, and undermining actions that express the opposite of what the person is really feeling.

pathological gambling. A failure to resist impulses to gamble and gambling behavior that compromises; disrupts; or damages personal, family, or vocational pursuits.

patient-centered care. An approach to patient care that focuses on listening to the patient, empowering them as central to decision-making about their care, developing a collaborative partnership, and only make decisions for the patient (such as involuntary hospitalization) when he or she is clearly unable to and when it is necessary to protect the patient's safety.

pedophilic disorder. Recurrent urges and sexually arousing fantasies involving sexual activity with a prepubescent child.

peer assistance programs. Programs established by the American Nurses Association to assist impaired nurses. The individuals who administer these efforts are nurse members of the state associations as well as nurses who are in recovery themselves.

perseveration. Persistent repetition of the same word or idea in response to different questions.

personal distance. The distance between individuals who are having interactions of a personal nature, such as a close conversation. In the U.S. culture, personal distance is approximately 18 to 40 inches.

personal identity. An individual's self-perception that defines his or her functions as observer, standard setter, and self-evaluator. It strives to maintain a stable self-image and relates to what the individual strives to become.

personal self. See **personal identity**.

personality. Deeply ingrained patterns of behavior, which include the way one relates to, perceives, and thinks about the environment and oneself.

personalization. Taking complete responsibility for situations without considering that other circumstances may have contributed to the outcome.

phencyclidine. An anesthetic used in veterinary medicine; used illegally as a hallucinogen, referred to as *PCP* or *angel dust*.

phenotype. Characteristics of physical manifestations that identify a particular genotype. Examples of phenotypes include eye color, height, blood type, language, and hairstyle. Phenotypes may be genetic or acquired.

phobia. An irrational fear.

physical neglect of a child. The failure on the part of the parent or caregiver to provide for a child's basic needs, such as food, clothing, shelter, medical and dental care, and supervision.

physical self. A personal appraisal by an individual of his or her physical being; includes physical attributes, functioning, sexuality, wellness-illness state, and appearance.

PIE charting. More specifically called *APIE*, this method of documentation has an assessment, problem, intervention, and evaluation (APIE) format and is a problem-oriented system used to document nursing process.

positive reinforcement. A reinforcement stimulus that increases the probability that the behavior will recur.

postpartum depression. Depression that occurs during the postpartum period. It may be related to hormonal changes, tryptophan metabolism, or alterations in membrane transport during the early postpartum period. Other predisposing factors may also be influential.

post-traumatic stress disorder (PTSD). A syndrome of symptoms that develops following a psychologically distressing event that is outside the range of usual human experience (e.g., rape, war). The individual is unable to cope with the associated anxiety and has nightmares, flashbacks, and panic attacks.

posturing. The voluntary assumption of inappropriate or bizarre postures.

preassaultive tension state. Behaviors predictive of potential violence. They include excessive motor activity; tense posture; defiant affect; clenched teeth and fists; and other arguing, demanding, and threatening behaviors.

precipitating event. A stimulus arising from the internal or external environment that is perceived by an individual as taxing or exceeding his or her resources and endangering his or her well-being.

predisposing factors. A variety of elements that influence how an individual perceives and responds to a stressful event. Types of predisposing factors include genetic influences, past experiences, and existing conditions.

Premack principle. This principle states that a frequently occurring response (R1) can serve as a positive reinforcement for a response (R2) that occurs less frequently. For example, a girl may talk to friends on the phone (R2) only if she does her homework (R1).

premature ejaculation. Ejaculation that occurs with minimal sexual stimulation or before, upon, or shortly after penetration and before the person wishes it.

premenstrual dysphoric disorder. A disorder that is characterized by depressed mood, anxiety, mood swings, and decreased interest in activities during the week prior to menses and subsiding shortly after the onset of menstruation.

priapism. Prolonged painful penile erection, may occur as an adverse effect of some antidepressant medications, particularly trazodone.

primary gain. The receipt of positive reinforcement for somaticizing by being able to avoid difficult situations because of physical complaint.

primary neurocognitive disorder (NCD). NCD, such as Alzheimer's disease, in which the NCD itself is the major sign of some organic brain disease not directly related to any other organic illness.

primary prevention. Reduction of the incidence of mental disorders within the population by helping individuals to cope more effectively with stress and by trying to diminish stressors within the environment.

privileged communication. A doctrine common to most states that grants certain privileges under which healthcare professionals may refuse to reveal information about and communications with clients.

problem-oriented recording (POR). A system of documentation that follows a subjective data, objective data, assessment, plan, implementation, and evaluation (SOAPIE) format. It is based on a list of identified patient problems to which each entry is directed.

prodromal syndrome. A syndrome of symptoms that often precede the onset of aggressive or violent behavior. These symptoms include anxiety and tension, verbal abuse and profanity, and increasing hyperactivity.

progressive relaxation. A method of deep muscle relaxation in which each muscle group is alternately tensed and relaxed in a systematic order with the person concentrating on the contrast of sensations experienced from tensing and relaxing.

projection. Attributing to another person feelings or impulses unacceptable to oneself.

prospective payment. The program of cost containment within the healthcare profession directed at setting forth pre-established amounts that would be reimbursed for specific diagnoses.

pseudocyesis. A condition in which an individual has nearly all the signs and symptoms of pregnancy but is not pregnant; a conversion reaction.

pseudodementia. Symptoms of depression that mimic those of neurocognitive disorder.

pseudohostility. A family interaction pattern characterized by a state of chronic conflict and alienation among family members. This relationship pattern allows family members to deny underlying fears of tenderness and intimacy.

pseudomutuality. A family interaction pattern characterized by a façade of mutual regard with the purpose of denying underlying fears of separation and hostility.

pseudoparkinsonism. A side effect of some antipsychotic medications. Symptoms mimic those of Parkinson's disease, such as tremor, shuffling gait, drooling, and rigidity.

psychiatric home care. Care provided by psychiatric nurses in the client's home. Psychiatric home-care nurses must have physical and psychosocial nursing skills to meet the demands of the client population they serve.

psychoanalysis. An approach to treatment of mental and emotional distress, originated by Sigmund Freud, that focuses on bringing unconscious thoughts and drives into conscious awareness.

psychobiology. The study of the biological foundations of cognitive, emotional, and behavioral processes.

psychodrama. A specialized type of group therapy that employs a dramatic approach in which patients become "actors" in life situation scenarios. The goal is to resolve interpersonal conflicts in a less-threatening atmosphere than the real-life situation would present.

psychodynamic nursing. Being able to understand one's own behavior, to help others identify felt difficulties, and to apply principles of human relations to the problems that arise at all levels of experience.

psychoimmunology. The study of the implications of the immune system in psychiatry.

Psychological Recovery Model. A model of treatment that focuses on the importance of hopefulness, self-determination, and positive self-concept in recovery from mental illnesses or emotional stress.

psychomotor domain. A category of learning in which the behaviors are processed and demonstrated. The information has been intellectually processed, and the individual is displaying motor behaviors.

psychomotor retardation. Extreme slowdown of physical movements. Posture slumps; speech is slowed; digestion becomes sluggish. Common in severe depression.

psychophysiological. Referring to psychological factors contributing to the initiation or exacerbation of a physical condition. Either a demonstrable organic pathology or a known pathophysiological process is involved.

psychosis. A mental state in which there is a severe loss of contact with reality. Symptoms may include delusions, hallucinations, disorganized speech patterns, and bizarre or catatonic behaviors.

psychosomatic. See **psychophysiological**.

psychotic disorder. A serious psychiatric disorder in which there is a gross disorganization of the personality, a marked disturbance in reality testing, and the impairment of interpersonal functioning and relationship to the external world.

psychotropic medication. Medication that affects psychic function, behavior, or experience.

public distance. Appropriate interactional distance for speaking in public or yelling to someone some distance away. U.S. culture defines this distance as 12 feet or more.

purging. The act of attempting to rid the body of calories by self-induced vomiting or excessive use of laxatives or diuretics.

purpose. A guiding principle in The Recovery Model that stresses the importance of finding purpose in life for the process of recovery from mental illness.

pyromania. An inability to resist the impulse to set fires.

Q

qi. In Chinese medicine, the healing energy that flows through pathways in the body called *meridians*. (Also called *chi*.)

R

rape. The expression of power and dominance by means of sexual violence, most commonly by men over women, although men may also be rape victims. Rape is considered an act of aggression, not of passion.

rape trauma syndrome. A variable group of symptoms that are indicative of the trauma associated with rape. Symptoms may include expressed response patterns, controlled responses, or silent reactions.

rapport. The development between two people in a relationship of special feelings based on mutual acceptance, warmth, friendliness, common interest, a sense of trust, and a nonjudgmental attitude.

rationalization. Attempting to make excuses or formulate logical reasons to justify unacceptable feelings or behaviors.

reaction formation. Preventing unacceptable or undesirable thoughts or behaviors from being expressed by exaggerating opposite thoughts or types of behaviors.

reality therapy. A type of therapy developed by William Glasser, rooted in control theory, which stresses individual responsibility for choosing how to respond to present situations.

receptor sites. Molecules that are situated on the cell membrane of the postsynaptic neuron that will accept only molecules with a complementary shape. These complementary molecules are specific to certain neurotransmitters that determine whether an electrical impulse will be excited or inhibited.

reciprocal inhibition. Also called *counterconditioning*, this technique serves to decrease or eliminate a behavior by introducing a more adaptive behavior but one that is incompatible with the unacceptable behavior (e.g., introducing relaxation techniques to an anxious person; relaxation and anxiety are incompatible behaviors).

reframing. Changing the conceptual or emotional setting or viewpoint in relation to which a situation is experienced and placing it in another frame that fits the "facts" of the same concrete situation equally well or even better and thereby changing its entire meaning. The behavior may not actually change, but the consequences of the behavior may change because of a change in the meaning attached to the behavior.

regression. A retreat to an earlier level of development and the comfort measures associated with that level of functioning.

relaxation. A decrease in tension or intensity, resulting in refreshment of body and mind. A state of refreshing tranquility.

religion. A set of beliefs, values, rites, and rituals adopted by a group of people. The practices are usually grounded in the teachings of a spiritual leader.

religiosity. When identified as a symptom of illness, refers to excessive demonstration of or obsession with religious ideas and behavior that causes marked distress and impairs ability to function; common in schizophrenia.

reminiscence therapy. A process of life review by elderly individuals that promotes self-esteem and provides assistance in working through unresolved conflicts from the past.

repression. The involuntary blocking of unpleasant feelings and experiences from one's awareness.

residual stimuli. Certain beliefs, attitudes, experiences, or traits that may contribute to an individual's low self-esteem.

retrograde ejaculation. Ejaculation of the seminal fluid backward into the bladder; may occur as a side effect of antipsychotic medications.

right. That which an individual is entitled (by ethical, legal, or moral standards) to have, or to do, or to receive from others within the limits of the law.

rigid boundaries. A person with rigid boundaries is "closed" and difficult to bond with. Such a person has a narrow perspective on life, sees things one way, and cannot discuss matters that lie outside his or her perspective.

ritualistic behavior. Purposeless activities that an individual performs repeatedly in an effort to decrease anxiety (e.g., hand washing); common in obsessive-compulsive disorder.

S

safe house or shelter. An establishment set up by many cities to provide protection for battered women and their children.

SBIRT. An acronym for Screening, Brief Intervention, and Referral for Treatment, SBIRT is an evidence-based approach that can be used in emergency departments, trauma centers, primary care, and other community settings to quickly identify the severity of substance use disorders and refer for treatment as necessary.

scapegoating. Occurs when hostility exists in a marriage dyad and an innocent third person (usually a child) becomes the target of blame for the problem.

schemas. Also called *core beliefs*, cognitive structures that consist of the individual's fundamental beliefs and assumptions, which develop early in life from personal experiences and identification with significant others. These concepts are reinforced by further learning experiences and, in turn, influence the formation of other beliefs, values, and attitudes.

schizoid personality disorder. A type of personality disorder characterized by extreme detachment from personal relationships and restricted expression of emotions.

schizotypal personality disorder. A disorder characterized by odd and eccentric behavior, not decompensating to the level of schizophrenia.

screening. An aspect of the assessment process in which broad questions are used to identify issues requiring further evaluation.

secondary gain. The receipt of positive reinforcement for somaticizing through added attention, sympathy, and nurturing.

secondary neurocognitive disorder (NCD). Neurocognitive disorder that is caused by or related to another disease or condition, such as HIV disease or a cerebral trauma.

secondary prevention. Healthcare that is directed at reduction of the prevalence of psychiatric illness by shortening the course (duration) of the illness. This is accomplished through early identification of problems and prompt initiation of treatment.

selective abstraction. Sometimes called *mental filter*, a type of thinking in which a conclusion is drawn based on only a selected portion of the evidence.

self-concept. The composite of beliefs and feelings that one holds about oneself at a given time, formed from perceptions of others' reactions. The self-concept consists of the physical self or body image, the personal self or identity, and the self-esteem.

self-consistency. The component of the personal identity that strives to maintain a stable self-image.

self-esteem. The degree of regard or respect that individuals have for themselves. It is a measure of worth that they place on their abilities and judgments.

self-expectancy. The component of the personal identity that is the individual's perception of what he or she wants to be, to do, or to become.

self-ideal. See **self-expectancy**.

sensate focus. A therapeutic technique used to treat individuals and couples with sexual dysfunction. The technique involves touching and being touched by another and focusing attention on the physical sensations encountered thereby. Clients gradually move through various levels of sensate focus that progress from nongenital touching to touching that includes the breasts and genitals; touching done in a simultaneous, mutual format rather than by one person at a time; and touching that extends to and allows eventually for the possibility of intercourse.

serotonin syndrome. A syndrome that is an adverse reaction to serotonergic medications. It may range from mild to severe and is potentially fatal. Symptoms may include significantly elevated temperature, agitation, muscle rigidity or twitching, sweating, irregular heartbeat, and seizures.

sexual assault nurse examiner (SANE). A clinical forensic registered nurse who has received specialized training to provide care to the sexual assault victim.

sexual exploitation of a child. The inducement or coercion of a child into engaging in sexually explicit conduct for the purpose of promoting any performance (e.g., child pornography).

sexual masochism disorder. Sexual stimulation derived from being humiliated, beaten, bound, or otherwise made to suffer.

sexual sadism disorder. Recurrent urges and sexually arousing fantasies involving acts (real, not simulated) in which the psychological or physical suffering (including humiliation) of the victim is sexually exciting.

sexuality. Sexuality is the constitution and life of an individual relative to characteristics regarding intimacy. It reflects the totality of the person and does not relate exclusively to the sex organs or sexual behavior.

shaping. In learning, one shapes the behavior of another by giving reinforcements for increasingly closer approximations to the desired behavior.

shelters. A variety of places designed to help the homeless, ranging from converted warehouses that provide cots or floor space on which to sleep overnight to significant operations that provide a multitude of social and healthcare services.

"ship of fools." The term given during the Middle Ages to sailing boats filled with severely mentally ill people who were sent out to sea with little guidance and in search of their lost rationality.

short-term memory. The ability to remember events that occurred very recently. This ability deteriorates with age.

silent rape reaction. The response of a rape victim in which he or she tells no one about the assault.

slander. An action with which an individual may be charged for orally sharing information that is detrimental to a person's reputation.

social anxiety disorder. A disorder in which the individual experiences extreme fear of doing something embarrassing or being negatively evaluated by others in a social situation.

social distance. The distance considered acceptable in interactions with strangers or acquaintances, such as at a cocktail party or in a public building. U.S. culture defines this distance as 4 to 12 feet.

social distancing. An aspect of stigma that refers to the tendency of healthcare workers and others to avoid people with mental illness or addiction.

social phobia. The fear of being humiliated in social situations.

social skills training. Educational opportunities through role play for the person with schizophrenia to learn appropriate social interaction skills and functional skills that are relevant to daily living.

Socratic questioning. When the therapist questions the client with Socratic questioning (also called *guided discovery*), the client is asked to describe feelings associated with specific situations. Questions are stated in a way that may stimulate in the client a recognition of possible dysfunctional thinking and may produce a dissonance about the validity of the thoughts.

somatization. A method of coping with psychosocial stress by developing physical symptoms.

specific phobia. A persistent fear of a specific object or situation, other than the fear of being unable to escape from a situation (agoraphobia) or the fear of being humiliated in social situations (social phobia).

spirituality. The human quality that gives meaning and sense of purpose to an individual's existence. Spirituality exists within each individual regardless of belief system and serves as a force for interconnectedness between the self and others, the environment, and a higher power.

splitting. A primitive ego defense mechanism in which the person is unable to integrate and accept both positive and negative feelings. In the view of these individuals, people—including themselves—

and life situations are either all good or all bad. This trait is common in borderline personality disorder.

statutory law. A law that has been enacted by legislative bodies, such as a county or city council, state legislature, or the U.S. Congress.

statutory rape. Unlawful intercourse between a person who is over the age of consent and a person who is under the age of consent. Legal age of consent varies from state to state. An individual can be arrested for statutory rape even when the interaction has occurred between consenting individuals.

stereotyping. The process of classifying all individuals from the same culture or ethnic group as identical.

stigmatization. The devaluing, marginalizing, and disenfranchising of certain patients because of symptoms or conditions.

stimulus. In classical conditioning, that which elicits a response.

stimulus generalization. The process by which a conditioned response is elicited from all stimuli *similar* to the one from which the response was learned.

store-front clinics. Establishments that have been converted into clinics that serve the homeless population.

stress. A state of disequilibrium that occurs when there is a disharmony between demands occurring within an individual's internal or external environment and his or her ability to cope with those demands.

stress management. Various methods used by individuals to reduce tension and other maladaptive responses to stress in their lives; includes relaxation exercises, physical exercise, music, mental imagery, or any other technique that is successful for a person.

stressor. A demand from within an individual's internal or external environment that elicits a physiological and/or psychological response.

sublimation. The rechanneling of personally and/or socially unacceptable drives or impulses into activities that are more tolerable and constructive.

subluxation. The term used in chiropractic medicine to describe vertebrae in the spinal column that have become displaced, possibly pressing on nerves and interfering with normal nerve transmission.

substance abuse. Use of psychoactive drugs that poses significant hazards to health and interferes with social, occupational, psychological, or physical functioning.

substance addiction. Physical addiction is identified by the inability to stop using a substance despite attempts to do so; a continual use of the substance despite adverse consequences; a developing tolerance; and the development of withdrawal symptoms upon cessation or decreased intake. Psychological addiction is said to exist when a substance is perceived by the user to be necessary to maintain an optimal state of personal well-being, interpersonal relations, or skill performance.

substitution therapy. The use of various medications to decrease the intensity of symptoms in an individual who is withdrawing from, or experiencing the effects of excessive use of, substances.

subsystems. The smaller units of which a system is composed. In family systems theory, the subsystems are composed of husband–wife, parent–child(ren), or sibling–sibling.

suicide prevention. The collective efforts including screening, assessment, referral for treatment, and collaborative partnership with the patient to prevent suicide as an outcome.

suicide risk factors. Situations, stressors, or demographics that have been statistically related to increased vulnerability toward suicide.

suicide warning signs. Behaviors and communication that are associated with more imminent risk for suicide and requiring immediate intervention. These include threats of suicide, a plan with access to means, hopelessness, and others.

sundowning. A phenomenon in neurocognitive disorder in which the symptoms seem to worsen in the late afternoon and evening.

superego. One of the three elements of the personality identified by Freud that represents the conscience and the culturally determined restrictions that are placed on an individual.

suppression. The voluntary blocking from one's awareness of unpleasant feelings and experiences.

surrogate. One who serves as a substitute figure for another.

symbiosis. One of the stages of development in Object Relations Theory in which the child views himself or herself as an extension of his or her mother rather than a separate entity.

symbiotic relationship. A type of "psychic fusion" that occurs between two people; it is unhealthy in that severe anxiety is generated in either or both if separation is indicated. A symbiotic relationship is normal between infant and mother.

sympathy. The actual sharing of another's thoughts and behaviors. Differs from **empathy** in that with empathy one experiences an objective understanding of what another is feeling rather than actually sharing those feelings.

synapse. The junction between two neurons. The small space between the axon terminals of one neuron and the cell body or dendrites of another is called the synaptic cleft.

systematic desensitization. A treatment for phobias in which the individual is taught to relax and then asked to imagine various components of the phobic stimulus on a graded hierarchy, moving from that which produces the least fear to that which produces the most.

T

tangentiality. The inability to get to the point of a story. The speaker introduces many unrelated topics until the original topic of discussion is lost. Tangentiality can be symptomatic of cognitive disruptions common in schizophrenia.

tardive dyskinesia. Syndrome of symptoms characterized by bizarre facial and tongue movements, a stiff neck, and difficulty swallowing. It may occur as an adverse effect of long-term therapy with some antipsychotic medications.

technical expert. Peplau's term for one who understands various professional devices and possesses the clinical skills necessary to perform the interventions that are in the best interest of the client.

temperament. A set of inborn personality characteristics that influence an individual's manner of reacting to the environment and ultimately influences his or her developmental progression.

territoriality. The innate tendency of individuals to own space. Individuals lay claim to areas around them as their own. This phenomenon can have an influence on interpersonal communication.

tertiary gain. The receipt of positive reinforcement for somaticizing by causing the focus of the family to switch to the individual and away from conflict that may be occurring within the family.

tertiary prevention. Healthcare that is directed toward reduction of the residual effects associated with severe or chronic physical or mental illness.

therapeutic communication. Caregiver verbal and nonverbal techniques that focus on the care receiver's needs and advance the promotion of healing and change. Therapeutic communication encourages exploration of feelings and fosters understanding of behavioral motivation. It is nonjudgmental, discourages defensiveness, and promotes trust.

therapeutic community. Also called *milieu therapy*, this approach strives to manipulate the environment so that all aspects of the client's hospital experience are considered therapeutic.

therapeutic group. Differs from group therapy in that there is a lesser degree of theoretical foundation. Focus is on group relations, interactions between group members, and the consideration of a selected issue. Leaders of therapeutic groups do not require the degree of educational preparation required of group therapy leaders.

therapeutic relationship. An interaction between two people (usually a caregiver and a care receiver) in which input from both participants contributes to a climate of healing, growth promotion, and/or illness prevention.

thought-stopping technique. A self-taught technique that an individual uses each time he or she wishes to eliminate intrusive or negative, unwanted thoughts from awareness.

Tidal Model. A nursing-developed, person-centered approach to the recovery model, which stresses the individual's personal story as significant to working on recovery.

time out. An aversive stimulus or punishment during which the individual is removed from the environment where the unacceptable behavior is being exhibited.

token economy. In behavior modification, a type of contracting in which the reinforcers for desired behaviors are presented in the form of tokens, which may then be exchanged for designated privileges.

tolerance. The need for increasingly larger or more frequent doses of a substance in order to obtain the desired effects originally produced by a lower dose.

tort. The violation of a civil law in which an individual has been wronged. In a tort action, one party asserts that wrongful conduct on the part of the other has caused harm, and compensation for harm suffered is sought.

transcendence. A developmental task more recently identified by Eric Erikson and associate in which the older adult must learn to move from materialistic, rational thinking to a broader worldview that includes increased sense of meaning in life, well-being, and a sense of satisfaction.[6]

transference. Transference occurs when a client unconsciously displaces (or "transfers") to the nurse or therapist feelings formed toward a person from his or her past.

transgender. An individual, despite having the anatomical characteristics of a given gender, has the self-perception of being of the opposite gender and may seek to have gender changed through surgical intervention.

transvestic disorder. A *DSM-5* diagnostic category identified as one of a group of paraphilic disorders in which recurrent sexual urges, sexually arousing fantasies or behaviors arise from dressing in the clothes of the opposite gender *and* the outcome is clinically significant distress or impairment in social, occupational, or other important areas of functioning.

trauma-informed care. An approach to care that assesses for history of physical, sexual, or psychosocial trauma and provides care with consideration for how trauma history may influence an individual's response to interventions and treatments.

traumatic brain injury. Injury to the brain that is the result of head trauma.

triangles. A three-person emotional configuration that is considered the basic building block of the family system. When anxiety becomes too great between two family members, a third person is brought in to form a triangle. Triangles are dysfunctional in that they offer relief from anxiety through diversion rather than through resolution of the issue.

trichotillomania (hair-pulling disorder). The recurrent failure to resist impulses to pull out one's own hair.

type A personality. The personality characteristics attributed to individuals prone to coronary heart disease, including excessive competitive drive, chronic sense of time urgency, easy anger, aggressiveness, excessive ambition, and inability to enjoy leisure time.

type B personality. The personality characteristics attributed to individuals who are not prone to coronary heart disease; includes characteristics such as ability to perform even under pressure but without the competitive drive and constant sense of time urgency experienced by the type A personality. Type Bs can enjoy their leisure time without feeling guilty, and they are much less impulsive than type A individuals; that is, they think things through before making decisions.

type C personality. The personality characteristics attributed to the cancer-prone individual. Includes characteristics such as suppression of anger, calm, passive, puts the needs of others before his or her own but holds resentment toward others for perceived "wrongs."

type D personality. Personality characteristics attributed to individuals who are at increased risk of

---

[6]Erikson, E. H., & Erikson, J. M. (1997). *The life cycle completed: Extended version with new chapters on the ninth stage of development.* New York, NY: W W Norton.

cardiovascular morbidity and mortality. The characteristics include a combination of negative emotions and social inhibition.

tyramine. An amino acid found in aged cheeses or other aged, overripe, and fermented foods; broad beans; pickled herring; beef or chicken liver; preserved meats; beer and wine; yeast products; chocolate; caffeinated drinks; canned figs; sour cream; yogurt; soy sauce; and some over-the-counter cold medications and diet pills. If foods high in tyramine content are consumed while an individual is taking monoamine oxidase inhibitors, a potentially life-threatening syndrome called *hypertensive crisis* can result.

U

unconditional positive regard. Carl Rogers's term for the respect and dignity of an individual regardless of his or her unacceptable behavior.

unconditioned response. In classical conditioning, an unconditioned response refers to a reflexive response to a specific target stimulus.

unconditioned stimulus. In classical conditioning, a specific stimulus that elicits an unconditioned, reflexive response.

undoing. A mechanism used to symbolically negate or cancel out a previous action or experience that one finds intolerable.

universality. One curative factor of groups (identified by Irvin Yalom) in which individuals realize that they are not alone in a problem and in the thoughts and feelings they are experiencing. Anxiety is relieved by the support and understanding of others in the group who share similar experiences.

utilitarianism. The ethical theory that espouses the greatest happiness for the greatest number. Under this theory, action would be taken based on the end results that will produce the most good (happiness) for the most people.

V

values. Personal beliefs about the truth; beauty; or worth of a thought, object, or behavior that influences an individual's actions.

values clarification. A process of self-discovery by which people identify their personal values and their value rankings. This process increases awareness about why individuals behave in certain ways.

veracity. An ethical principle that refers to one's duty to always be truthful.

veterans. Individuals who have served in the military.

voyeuristic disorder. Recurrent urges and sexually arousing fantasies involving the act of observing unsuspecting people, usually strangers, who are either naked, in the process of disrobing, or engaging in sexual activity.

W

waxy flexibility. A condition by which the individual with schizophrenia passively yields all movable parts of the body to any efforts made at placing them in certain positions.

Wernicke's encephalopathy. A brain disorder caused by thiamine deficiency and characterized by visual disturbances, ataxia, somnolence, stupor, and, without thiamine replacement, death.

withdrawal. The physiological and mental readjustment that accompanies the discontinuation of an addictive substance.

word salad. A group of words that are put together in a random fashion without any logical connection.

WRAP Model. An approach to the recovery model (Wellness Recovery Action Plan) that stresses learning a distinct set of skills necessary for managing symptoms of mental illness or emotional distress in everyday life.

Y

yin and yang. The fundamental concept of Asian health practices. Yin and yang are opposite forces of energy, such as negative/positive, dark/light, cold/hot, hard/soft, and feminine/masculine. Food, medicines, and herbs are classified according to their yin and yang properties and are used to restore a balance, thereby restoring health.

yoga. A system of beliefs and practices, the ultimate goal of which is to unite the human soul with the universal spirit. In Western countries, yoga uses body postures, along with meditation and breathing exercises, to achieve a balanced, disciplined workout that releases muscle tension; tones the internal organs; and energizes the mind, body, and spirit so that natural healing can occur.

Appendix C

Answers to Review Questions

CHAPTER 1. Mental Health and Mental Illness
1. c **2.** d **3.** b **4.** a **5.** b **6.** d **7.** c
8. a, b, c, d **9.** c **10.** b

CHAPTER 2. Biological Implications
1. d **2.** d **3.** a **4.** b **5.** c **6.** a **7.** d **8.** c
9. b **10.** a **11.** a, b, c **12.** b, c, d

CHAPTER 3. Ethical and Legal Issues
1. b **2.** a **3.** c **4.** b **5.** c **6.** d **7.** a, b, d **8.** b, d
9. a, b **10.** c

CHAPTER 4. Psychopharmacology
1. a **2.** c **3.** d **4.** b **5.** c **6.** b **7.** a **8.** b
9. a **10.** b **11.** a, b, c

CHAPTER 5. Relationship Development and Therapeutic Communication
1. c **2.** a **3.** a, b, c **4.** b **5.** a **6.** d **7.** c **8.** a
9. b **10.** b, e **11.** d **12.** d

CHAPTER 6. The Nursing Process in Psychiatric Mental Health Nursing
1. b **2.** a **3.** d **4.** a **5.** c **6.** b **7.** a, b, c, d
8. d **9.** c **10.** a, c, d

CHAPTER 7. Milieu Therapy—The Therapeutic Community
1. a, b, c **2.** b **3.** c **4.** b **5.** a **6.** d **7.** c **8.** b
9. a, b, d, e **10.** a, b

CHAPTER 8. Intervention in Groups
1. b **2.** d **3.** a **4.** c **5.** c **6.** d **7.** c **8.** b
9. d **10.** a

CHAPTER 9. Crisis Intervention
1. c **2.** d **3.** a **4.** b **5.** c **6.** a **7.** d **8.** b
9. b **10.** d **11.** c **12.** c **13.** e

CHAPTER 10. The Recovery Model
1. b, d **2.** c **3.** d **4.** a **5.** c

CHAPTER 11. Suicide Prevention
1. a **2.** a, c, d, e **3.** c **4.** a **5.** d **6.** c **7.** b
8. b, e **9.** a, b, c **10.** b

CHAPTER 12. Caring for Patients With Mental Illness and Substance Use Disorders in General Practice Settings
1. a, b, c **2.** c **3.** a, d **4.** b **5.** d

CHAPTER 13. Neurocognitive Disorders
1. c, e **2.** d **3.** b **4.** a, b, e **5.** b **6.** a, c, e **7.** d
8. c **9.** a **10.** b **11.** c, e

CHAPTER 14. Substance Use and Addiction Disorders
1. a **2.** c **3.** b **4.** b **5.** a **6.** c **7.** a **8.** b
9. d **10.** a **11.** a, b, c, d, e

CHAPTER 15. Schizophrenia Spectrum and Other Psychotic Disorders
1. b **2.** b **3.** c **4.** d **5.** d **6.** a **7.** c **8.** b
9. c **10.** d **11.** c **12.** a, b, e

CHAPTER 16. Depressive Disorders
1. c **2.** b **3.** a **4.** d **5.** a, b, d **6.** a, b, c, e
7. a **8.** c **9.** b **10.** a, b, d **11.** a, d

CHAPTER 17. Bipolar and Related Disorders
1. b **2.** c **3.** a **4.** a, c, d **5.** b **6.** d **7.** b **8.** c
9. 1 = b, 2 = d, 3 = a, 4 = c **10.** c

CHAPTER 18. Anxiety, Obsessive-Compulsive, and Related Disorders
1. d **2.** c **3.** d **4.** a **5.** b **6.** c **7.** a, b, c
8. c **9.** a **10.** b

CHAPTER 19. Trauma- and Stressor-Related Disorders
1. b **2.** c **3.** a **4.** d **5.** b **6.** b **7.** c **8.** a
9. a **10.** d **11.** a, c

CHAPTER 20. Somatic Symptom and Dissociative Disorders
1. a **2.** b **3.** d **4.** b **5.** c **6.** d **7.** b **8.** a
9. b **10.** d

CHAPTER 21. Eating Disorders
1. c **2.** a **3.** b **4.** b **5.** c **6.** b **7.** c **8.** b
9. c **10.** a, b, c, d

CHAPTER 22. **Personality Disorders**
1. d **2.** a **3.** b **4.** d **5.** a **6.** b **7.** c **8.** a
9. d **10.** b

CHAPTER 23. **Children and Adolescents**
1. b **2.** c **3.** a **4.** b **5.** b **6.** b, c, d **7.** c
8. d **9.** a **10.** b

CHAPTER 24. **The Aging Individual**
1. c **2.** d **3.** b **4.** a **5.** c **6.** d **7.** a **8.** a
9. c **10.** a

CHAPTER 25. **Survivors of Abuse or Neglect**
1. b **2.** c **3.** a **4.** d **5.** b **6.** d **7.** a **8.** b
9. b **10.** d

CHAPTER 26. **Community Mental Health Nursing**
1. a **2.** b **3.** a **4.** c **5.** d **6.** b **7.** c **8.** d
9. a **10.** a, b, c, d

CHAPTER 27. **The Bereaved Individual**
1. a, b, c, d **2.** c **3.** c **4.** d **5.** a **6.** a **7.** b
8. c **9.** a **10.** c

CHAPTER 28. **Military Families**
1. a, b, d **2.** b **3.** a **4.** b **5.** c **6.** c **7.** a, c, d
8. d **9.** a, b, c, d **10.** b, d

CHAPTER 29. **Concepts of Personality Development**
1. b **2.** c **3.** d **4.** b **5.** b **6.** b **7.** a **8.** c
9. a **10.** b

CHAPTER 30. **Complementary and Psychosocial Therapies**
1. a, c, e, f **2.** a, b, d **3.** c, d **4.** a, d, e **5.** c **6.** d
7. a **8.** b **9.** a **10.** b **11.** a

CHAPTER 31. **Cultural and Spiritual Concepts Relevant to Psychiatric Mental Health Nursing**
1. c **2.** d **3.** a **4.** d **5.** b **6.** c **7.** b **8.** b
9. a **10.** d

CHAPTER 32. **Issues Related to Human Sexuality and Gender Dysphoria**
1. b **2.** c **3.** a, b, c, d **4.** a **5.** b **6.** d **7.** b
8. c **9.** a, b, d, e

Appendix D

Examples of Answers to Communication Exercises

CHAPTER 9 Crisis Intervention

1. "I'll try to help you to the best of my ability. Please tell me what is upsetting you." Establish rapport, convey respect, and assess precipitating events.
2. "Hi Shelley, my name is Mrs. Smith, and I am a registered nurse here to help you. I'm so glad you came in to seek help. I'd like to ask you some questions about the events you've experienced. Alright?" Convey respect, reassurance of help, and empower the client to be involved in decision making.
3. "Thomas, last evening you became very upset, stating you thought the FBI was trying to kill you, and you struck another patient." (Giving information) "Do you remember any of those events?" (Assessing the patient's perception and memory) "Restraint is an intervention that we only use when other efforts have failed to protect your safety and the safety of others." (Giving information) "Let's talk about what you think would be helpful in preventing that from happening again." (Formulating a plan, empowering the client to be involved in problem-solving)

CHAPTER 10 The Recovery Model

1. Because inability to sit still may be a side effect of many antipsychotic medications, one response is to assess the client's medications, assess the client's symptoms, and educate him about akathisia as appropriate. This response supports the principle that recovery should empower the client to make informed decisions through providing information and resources. Asking the client how he wishes to proceed supports the principle that recovery is person-driven.

   For example:

   "Joshua, I see that you are taking Thorazine, and the inability to sit still may be a side effect of this medication. There are other medications that will treat your symptoms and that don't have the same risk for this side effect. Would you like to explore these options further?"

2. Using the recovery model principles of respect and the importance of support through peers and allies, one possible response may be, "Kelly, I haven't been in an active combat situation, but I hope to earn your trust as a mental health professional and try to understand, to the best of my ability, the issues you've been struggling with. Many veterans identify, as you have, that fellow veterans are better able to provide on-going support with an appreciation for the shared experiences you've endured. Are you interested in exploring some of those options, too?"

CHAPTER 11 Suicide Prevention

1. "Mr. J, it sounds like you have been feeling hopeless; this is a common symptom of depression." (Giving information) "Have you been having any thoughts of taking your own life?" (Closed-ended, directive questioning to assess for the presence of suicide ideation)
2. Communication at this point should be focused on thorough assessment of Mr. J's expressed suicide ideas. Assessment questions include (but are not comprehensive):
   "When you have these ideas do you have a plan in mind?"
   "How strong is your intention to die?"
   "Do you have access to the means for implementing this plan?"
3. "It sounds like you are grieving, that must be very painful, tell me more about your experience and feelings related to losing your wife." (Empathy, exploring/encouraging description)

CHAPTER 13 Neurocognitive Disorders

1. "Mrs. B, you are not in a restaurant. This is the General Hospital. I am your nurse, Mary. How may I help you?" (Reality orientation)
2. "Mrs. B, you have already eaten your breakfast. Would you like a snack?"
   "Please tell me what it was like when you lived on the farm." (Reminiscing)

CHAPTER 14 Substance Use and Addiction Disorders

1. "Tom, you are here because it has been determined that drinking alcohol is causing problems for you at home and at your work." (Confronting reality)
2. "Tom, you are experiencing symptoms related to your body's withdrawal from alcohol. When did you have your last drink? I will bring you a cup of coffee." (Confrontation with caring)
3. "You are feeling angry toward your boss and your wife, but your drinking is apparently interfering with your job and your marriage. Unless you abstain from alcohol, you are at risk of losing both." (Confronting reality)

CHAPTER 15 Schizophrenia Spectrum and Other Psychotic Disorders

1. "I know that you believe what you are saying is true, but I find it very hard to accept." (Voicing doubt) "Please understand that you are safe here." (Reassurance of safety)
2. The nurse should slowly and carefully approach Hal so that he is not startled by his or her presence. "Hal, are you hearing the voices again? What do you hear the voices saying to you?" (Encouraging description of perceptions. This type of information may help to protect the client and others from potential violence associated with command hallucinations.) "I know the voices seem real to you, but I do not hear any voices speaking." (Presenting reality)
3. "I don't understand what you are saying, Hal. What message do you want to give me? Might you be telling me that you are lonely?" (Seeking clarification; attempting to translate words into feelings)

CHAPTER 16 Depressive Disorders

1. "You have had a lot of losses. You are feeling very much alone right now." (Verbalizing the implied)
2. "You feel sad because you can no longer do the things that you used to do . . . the things that made you feel good about yourself." (Statement that focuses on feelings)
3. Direct questions assessing suicide potential: "Are you or have you been thinking about harming yourself? Do you have a plan for doing so? Have you ever acted on that plan?"

Demonstrations of genuine concern and caring: "I care about you. I will stay here with you." Expressions of empathy: "It must be frightening to feel so all alone. But you are not alone. There are many people who care about you, and I am one of those people."

CHAPTER 17 Bipolar and Related Disorders

1. "Bob, I'm not sure I understand what you are saying. Are your thoughts racing?" (Clarifying, assessing)
2. "John, I have an activity in the next room that I could use your help with. Would you please come with me?" (Offering an alternative activity, redirecting, reducing stimulation)

CHAPTER 18 Anxiety, Obsessive-Compulsive, and Related Disorders

1. "John, I'd like to check your vital signs and then discuss how I can best help you feel more comfortable."
2. "Often, when people become very anxious they develop irrational thinking patterns that contribute to worsening their mood and impacting their behavior in negative ways. By becoming aware of thought patterns that increase your anxiety you can learn how to replace those automatic thoughts with more rational patterns in a way that improves your mood, symptoms, and behavior."

CHAPTER 21 Eating Disorders

1. "Helena, we've established a treatment plan that limits going to the restroom immediately after a meal because we are trying to help you avoid the urge to purge the food you just ate. Let's talk about how you are feeling right now and see if we can identify some other options for your behaviors before and after meals."
2. "John, many people with this kind of eating disorder report feeling a loss of control, and I understand how that can alter your self-esteem. These are symptoms of an illness with many contributing factors. I want to support you in your efforts to manage this illness, and there is good evidence that recovery is achievable."

CHAPTER 22 Personality Disorders

1. "My name is Nancy. I am your nurse on this shift, and you will be in my care until 11 p.m. You may

ask for me by my name if you have any requests."
(Giving information)

2. "You were arrested because you broke the law."
(Confronting reality)

3. "I do not give out personal information to patients, and I do not go out with patients. I hope that you will be able to get your life straightened out in a positive way." (Confrontation with caring)

CHAPTER 25 Survivors of Abuse or Neglect

1. "You are not to blame, Sarah. You do not deserve to be abused in this way. He is responsible for his behavior."

2. "There are places you can go where you and your children will be safe. I will give you that information."
"You need to consider whether you want to press charges against him."

3. "You must consider the safety of yourself and your children. You have the phone number of the safe house. It is your decision what to do now."

CHAPTER 27 The Bereaved Individual

1. "I believe we did everything we could to provide care for your husband, and it's so hard to lose someone you love even when they are terminally ill. I'll stay with you and try to answer any questions you have."

2. "Yes, John, it's probable that you are in the end stage of life. Let's talk about how to prepare for this."

3. "Nancy, these are difficult spiritual questions. Would you like to talk more with the chaplain?"

CHAPTER 32 Issues Related to Human Sexuality and Gender Dysphoria

1. "Are you having thoughts of taking your own life?" (Assessment for suicide ideation and intentions are the priority because Jamie has expressed feeling that he wants to die)

2. "I'd be glad to discuss with you the benefits and disadvantages of this option. What do you already know about hormone treatments?" (Conveys respect, collaboration, assessment)

Appendix E

DSM-5 Classification: Categories and Codes*

International Classification of Diseases, 10th revision, Clinical Modification (ICD-10-CM) codes are provided.

Neurodevelopmental Disorders

Intellectual Disabilities

	Intellectual Disability (Intellectual Developmental Disorder)
	Specify current severity:
70	Mild
71	Moderate
72	Severe
73	Profound
F88	Global Developmental Delay
F79	Unspecified Intellectual Disability (Intellectual Developmental Disorder)

Communication Disorders

F80.9	Language Disorder
F80.0	Speech Sound Disorder
F80.81	Childhood-Onset Fluency Disorder (Stuttering)
	Note: Later-onset cases are diagnosed as 307.0 (F98.5) adult-onset fluency disorder.
F80.89	Social (Pragmatic) Communication Disorder
(F80.9)	Unspecified Communication Disorder

*Reprinted with permission from the *Diagnostic and Statistical Manual of Mental Disorders, Fifth Edition.* (Copyright 2013). American Psychiatric Association.

Autism Spectrum Disorder

F84.0	Autism Spectrum Disorder *Specify* if: Associated with a known medical or genetic condition or environmental factor; Associated with another neurodevelopmental, mental, or behavioral disorder *Specify* current severity for Criterion A and Criterion B: Requiring very substantial support, Requiring substantial support, Requiring support *Specify* if: With or without accompanying intellectual impairment, With or without accompanying language impairment, With catatonia (use additional code 293.89 [F06.1])

Attention-Deficit/Hyperactivity Disorder

	Attention-Deficit/Hyperactivity Disorder *Specify* whether:
F90.2	Combined presentation
F90.0	Predominantly inattentive presentation
F90.1	Predominantly hyperactive/impulsive presentation *Specify* if: In partial remission *Specify* current severity: Mild, Moderate, Severe
F90.8	Other Specified Attention Deficit-Hyperactivity Disorder
F90.9	Unspecified Attention Deficit-Hyperactivity Disorder

Specific Learning Disorder

	Specific Learning Disorder *Specify* if:
F81.0	With impairment in reading (*specify* if with word reading accuracy, reading rate or fluency, reading comprehension)
F81.81	With impairment in written expression (*specify* if with spelling accuracy, grammar and punctuation accuracy, clarity or organization of written expression)
F81.2	With impairment in mathematics (*specify* if with number sense, memorization of arithmetic facts, accurate or fluent calculation, accurate math reasoning) *Specify* current severity: Mild, Moderate, Severe

Motor Disorders

F82	Developmental Coordination Disorder
F98.4	Stereotypic Movement Disorder *Specify* if: With self-injurious behavior, Without self-injurious behavior *Specify* if: Associated with a known medical or genetic condition, neurodevelopmental disorder, or environmental factor *Specify* current severity: Mild, Moderate, Severe

Tic Disorders

F95.2	Tourette's Disorder
F95.1	Persistent (Chronic) Motor or Vocal Tic Disorder *Specify* if: With motor tics only, With vocal tics only
F95.0	Provisional Tic Disorder
F95.8	Other Specified Tic Disorder
F95.9	Unspecified Tic Disorder

Other Neurodevelopmental Disorders

F88	Other Specified Neurodevelopmental Disorder
F89	Unspecified Neurodevelopmental Disorder

Schizophrenia Spectrum and Other Psychotic Disorders

The following specifiers apply to Schizophrenia Spectrum and Other Psychotic Disorders where indicated:

[a] *Specify* if: The following course specifiers are only to be used after a 1-year duration of the disorder: First episode, currently in acute episode; First episode, currently in partial remission; First episode, currently in full remission; Multiple episodes, currently in acute episode; Multiple episodes, currently in partial remission; Multiple episodes, currently in full remission; Continuous; Unspecified

[b] *Specify* if: With catatonia (use additional code 293.89 [F06.1])

[c] *Specify* current severity of delusions, hallucinations, disorganized speech, abnormal psychomotor behavior, negative symptoms, impaired cognition, depression, and mania symptoms

F21	Schizotypal (Personality) Disorder
F22	Delusional Disorder[a, c] *Specify* whether: Erotomanic type, Grandiose type, Jealous type, Persecutory type, Somatic type, Mixed type, Unspecified type *Specify* if: With bizarre content
F23	Brief Psychotic Disorder[b, c] *Specify* if: With marked stressor(s), Without marked stressor(s), With postpartum onset
F20.81	Schizophreniform Disorder[b, c] *Specify* if: With good prognostic features, Without good prognostic features
F20.9	Schizophrenia[a, b, c]
	Schizoaffective Disorder[a, b, c] *Specify* whether:
F25.0	Bipolar type
F25.1	Depressive type
	Substance/Medication-Induced Psychotic Disorder[c] **Note:** See the criteria set and corresponding recording procedures for substance-specific codes and ICD-10-CM coding. *Specify* if: With onset during intoxication, With onset during withdrawal
	Psychotic Disorder Due to Another Medical Condition[c] *Specify* whether:
F06.2	With delusions
F06.0	With hallucinations
F06.1	Catatonia Associated With Another Mental Disorder (Catatonia Specifier)
F06.1	Catatonic Disorder Due to Another Medical Condition

F06.1	Unspecified Catatonia **Note:** Code first 781.99 (R29.818) other symptoms involving nervous and musculo-skeletal systems.
F28	Other Specified Schizophrenia Spectrum and Other Psychotic Disorder
F29	Unspecified Schizophrenia Spectrum and Other Psychotic Disorder

Bipolar and Related Disorders

The following specifiers apply to Bipolar and Related Disorders where indicated:

[a]*Specify*: With anxious distress (*specify* current severity: mild, moderate, moderate-severe, severe); With mixed features; With rapid cycling; With melancholic features; With atypical features; With mood-congruent psychotic features; With mood-incongruent psychotic features; With catatonia (use additional code 293.89 [F06.1]); With peripartum onset; With seasonal pattern

	Bipolar I Disorder[a]
	Current or most recent episode manic
F31.11	Mild
F31.12	Moderate
F31.13	Severe
F31.2	With psychotic features
F31.73	In partial remission
F31.74	In full remission
F31.9	Unspecified
F31.0	Current or most recent episode hypomanic
F31.73	In partial remission
F31.74	In full remission
F31.9	Unspecified
	Current or most recent episode depressed
F31.31	Mild
F31.32	Moderate
F31.4	Severe
F31.5	With psychotic features

F31.75	In partial remission
F31.76	In full remission
F31.9	Unspecified
F31.9	Current or most recent episode unspecified
F31.81	Bipolar II Disorder[a] *Specify* current or most recent episode: Hypomanic, Depressed *Specify* course if full criteria for a mood episode are not currently met: In partial remission, In full remission *Specify* severity if full criteria for a mood episode are not currently met: Mild, Moderate, Severe
F34.0	Cyclothymic Disorder *Specify* if: With anxious distress
	Substance/Medication-Induced Bipolar and Related Disorder **Note:** See the criteria set and corresponding recording procedures for substance-specific codes and ICD-10-CM coding. *Specify* if: With onset during intoxication, With onset during withdrawal
	Bipolar and Related Disorder Due to Another Medical Condition *Specify* if:
F06.33	With manic features
F06.33	With manic- or hypomanic-like episode
F06.34	With mixed features
F31.89	Other Specified Bipolar and Related Disorder
F31.9	Unspecified Bipolar and Related Disorder

Depressive Disorders

The following specifiers apply to Depressive Disorders where indicated:

[a]*Specify*: With anxious distress (*specify* current severity: mild, moderate, moderate-severe, severe); With mixed features; With melancholic features; With atypical features; With mood-congruent psychotic features; With mood-incongruent psychotic features; With catatonia (use additional code 293.89 [F06.1]); With peripartum onset; With seasonal pattern

F34.8	Disruptive Mood Dysregulation Disorder
	Major Depressive Disorder[a]
	Single episode
F32.0	Mild
F32.1	Moderate
F32.2	Severe
F32.3	With psychotic features
F32.4	In partial remission
F32.5	In full remission
F32.9	Unspecified
	Recurrent episode
F33.0	Mild
F33.1	Moderate
F33.2	Severe
F33.3	With psychotic features
F33.41	In partial remission
F33.42	In full remission
F33.9	Unspecified
F34.1	Persistent Depressive Disorder (Dysthymia)[a] *Specify* if: In partial remission, In full remission *Specify* if: Early onset, Late onset *Specify* if: With pure dysthymic syndrome; With persistent major depressive episode; With intermittent major depressive episodes, with current episode; With intermittent major depressive episodes, without current episode *Specify* current severity: Mild, Moderate, Severe
N94.3	Premenstrual Dysphoric Disorder
	Substance/Medication-Induced Depressive Disorder **Note:** See the criteria set and corresponding recording procedures for substance-specific codes and ICD-10-CM coding. *Specify* if: With onset during intoxication, With onset during withdrawal
	Depressive Disorder Due to Another Medical Condition
	Specify if:
F06.31	With depressive features

F06.32	With major depressive-like episode
F06.34	With mixed features
F32.8	Other Specified Depressive Disorder
F32.9	Unspecified Depressive Disorder

Anxiety Disorders

F93.0	Separation Anxiety Disorder
F94.0	Selective Mutism
	Specific Phobia
	Specify if:
F40.218	Animal
F40.228	Natural environment
	Blood-injection injury
F40.230	Fear of blood
F40.231	Fear of injections and transfusions
F40.232	Fear of other medical care
F40.233	Fear of injury
F40.248	Situational
F40.298	Other
F40.10	Social Anxiety Disorder (Social Phobia) *Specify* if: Performance only
F41.0	Panic Disorder
	Panic Attack Specifier
F40.00	Agoraphobia
F41.1	Generalized Anxiety Disorder
	Substance/Medication-Induced Anxiety Disorder **Note:** See the criteria set and corresponding recording procedures for substance-specific codes and ICD-10-CM coding. *Specify* if: With onset during intoxication, With onset during withdrawal, With onset after medication use
F06.4	Anxiety Disorder Due to Another Medical Condition
F41.9	Unspecified Anxiety Disorder

Obsessive-Compulsive and Related Disorders

The following specifier applies to Obsessive-Compulsive and Related Disorders where indicated:

[a] *Specify* if: With good or fair insight, With poor insight, With absent insight/delusional beliefs

F42	Obsessive-Compulsive Disorder[a] *Specify* if: Tic-related
F45.22	Body Dysmorphic Disorder[a] *Specify* if: With muscle dysmorphia
F42	Hoarding Disorder[a] *Specify* if: With excessive acquisition
F63.3	Trichotillomania (Hair-Pulling Disorder)
L98.1	Excoriation (Skin-Picking) Disorder
	Substance/Medication-Induced Obsessive-Compulsive and Related Disorder **Note:** See the criteria set and corresponding recording procedures for substance-specific codes and ICD-9-CM and ICD-10-CM coding. *Specify* if: With onset during intoxication, With onset during withdrawal, With onset after medication use
F06.8	Obsessive-Compulsive and Related Disorder Due to Another Medical Condition *Specify* if: With obsessive-compulsive disorder-like symptoms, With appearance preoccupations, With hoarding symptoms, With hair-pulling symptoms, With skin-picking symptoms
F42	Other Specified Obsessive-Compulsive and Related Disorder
F42	Unspecified Obsessive-Compulsive and Related Disorder

Trauma- and Stressor-Related Disorders

F94.1	Reactive Attachment Disorder *Specify* if: Persistent *Specify* current severity: Severe
F94.2	Disinhibited Social Engagement Disorder *Specify* if: Persistent *Specify* current severity: Severe
F43.10	Post-traumatic Stress Disorder (includes Post-traumatic Stress Disorder for Children 6 Years and Younger) *Specify* whether: With dissociative symptoms *Specify* if: With delayed expression
F43.0	Acute Stress Disorder
	Adjustment Disorders *Specify* whether:
F43.21	With depressed mood
F43.22	With anxiety
F43.23	With mixed anxiety and depressed mood
F43.24	With disturbance of conduct
F43.25	With mixed disturbance of emotions and conduct
F43.20	Unspecified
F43.8	Other Specified Trauma- and Stressor-Related Disorder
F43.9	Unspecified Trauma- and Stressor-Related Disorder

Dissociative Disorders

F44.81	Dissociative Identity Disorder
F44.0	Dissociative Amnesia *Specify* if:
F44.1	With dissociative fugue
F48.1	Depersonalization/Derealization Disorder
F44.89	Other Specified Dissociative Disorder
F44.9	Unspecified Dissociative Disorder

Somatic Symptom and Related Disorders

F45.1	Somatic Symptom Disorder *Specify* if: With predominant pain *Specify* if: Persistent *Specify* current severity: Mild, Moderate, Severe
F45.21	Illness Anxiety Disorder *Specify* whether: Care seeking type, Care avoidant type
	Conversion Disorder (Functional Neurological Symptom Disorder) *Specify* symptom type:
F44.4	With weakness or paralysis
F44.4	With abnormal movement
F44.4	With swallowing symptoms
F44.4	With speech symptom
F44.5	With attacks or seizures

F44.6	With anesthesia or sensory loss
F44.6	With special sensory symptom
F44.7	With mixed symptoms *Specify* if: Acute episode, Persistent *Specify* if: With psychological stressor (specify stressor), Without psychological stressor
F54	Psychological Factors Affecting Other Medical Conditions *Specify* current severity: Mild, Moderate, Severe, Extreme
F68.10	Factitious Disorder (includes Factitious Disorder Imposed on Self, Factitious Disorder Imposed on Another) *Specify* Single episode, Recurrent episodes
F45.8	Other Specified Somatic Symptom and Related Disorder
F45.9	Unspecified Somatic Symptom and Related Disorder

Feeding and Eating Disorders

The following specifiers apply to Feeding and Eating Disorders where indicated:

[a]*Specify* if: In remission
[b]*Specify* if: In partial remission, In full remission
[c]*Specify* current severity: Mild, Moderate, Severe, Extreme

	Pica[a]
F98.3	In children
F50.8	In adults
F98.21	Rumination Disorder[a]
F50.8	Avoidant/Restrictive Food Intake Disorder[a]
	Anorexia Nervosa[b, c] *Specify* whether:
F50.01	Restricting type
F50.02	Binge-eating/purging type
F50.2	Bulimia Nervosa[b, c]
F50.8	Binge-Eating Disorder[b, c]
F50.8	Other Specified Feeding or Eating Disorder
F50.9	Unspecified Feeding or Eating Disorder

Elimination Disorders

F98.0	Enuresis *Specify* whether: Nocturnal only, Diurnal only, Nocturnal and diurnal
F98.1	Encopresis *Specify* whether: With constipation and overflow incontinence, Without constipation and overflow incontinence
	Other Specified Elimination Disorder
N39.498	With urinary symptoms
R15.9	With fecal symptoms
	Unspecified Elimination Disorder
R32	With urinary symptoms
R15.9	With fecal symptoms

Sleep-Wake Disorders

The following specifiers apply to Sleep-Wake Disorders where indicated:

[a]*Specify* if: Episodic, Persistent, Recurrent
[b]*Specify* if: Acute, Subacute, Persistent
[c]*Specify* current severity: Mild, Moderate, Severe

G47.00	Insomnia Disorder[a] *Specify* if: With non-sleep disorder mental comorbidity, With other medical comorbidity, With other sleep disorder
G47.10	Hypersomnolence Disorder[b, c] *Specify* if: With mental disorder, With medical condition, With another sleep disorder
	Narcolepsy[c] *Specify* whether:
G47.419	Narcolepsy without cataplexy but with hypocretin deficiency
G47.411	Narcolepsy with cataplexy but without hypocretin deficiency
G47.419	Autosomal dominant cerebellar ataxia, deafness, and narcolepsy
G47.419	Autosomal dominant narcolepsy, obesity, and type 2 diabetes
G47.429	Narcolepsy secondary to another medical condition

Breathing-Related Sleep Disorders

G47.33	Obstructive Sleep Apnea Hypopnea[c]
	Central Sleep Apnea *Specify* whether:
G47.31	Idiopathic central sleep apnea
R06.3	Cheyne-Stokes breathing
G47.37	Central sleep apnea comorbid with opioid use **Note:** First code opioid use disorder, if present. *Specify* current severity
	Sleep-Related Hypoventilation *Specify* whether
G47.34	Idiopathic hypoventilation
G47.35	Congenital central alveolar hypoventilation
G47.36	Comorbid sleep-related hypoventilation *Specify* current severity Circadian Rhythm Sleep-Wake Disorders[a] *Specify* whether:
G47.21	Delayed sleep phase type *Specify* if: Familial, Overlapping with non-24-hour sleep-wake type
G47.22	Advanced sleep phase type *Specify* if: Familial
G47.23	Irregular sleep-wake type
G47.24	Non-24-hour sleep-wake type
G47.26	Shift work type
G47.20	Unspecified type

Parasomnias

	Non-Rapid Eye Movement Sleep Arousal Disorders *Specify* whether:
F51.3	Sleepwalking type *Specify* if: With sleep-related eating, With sleep-related sexual behavior (sexsomnia)
F51.4	Sleep terror type
F51.5	Nightmare Disorder[b, c] *Specify* if: During sleep onset *Specify* if: With associated non-sleep disorder, With associated other medical condition, With associated other sleep disorder
G47.52	Rapid Eye Movement Sleep Behavior Disorder
G25.81	Restless Legs Syndrome

	Substance/Medication-Induced Sleep Disorder **Note:** See the criteria set and corresponding recording procedures for substance-specific codes and ICD-10-CM coding. *Specify* whether: Insomnia type, Daytime sleepiness type, Parasomnia type, Mixed type *Specify* if: With onset during intoxication, With onset during discontinuation/withdrawal
G47.09	Other Specified Insomnia Disorder
G47.00	Unspecified Insomnia Disorder
G47.19	Other Specified Hypersomnolence Disorder
G47.10	Unspecified Hypersomnolence Disorder
G47.8	Other Specified Sleep-Wake Disorder
G47.9	Unspecified Sleep-Wake Disorder

Sexual Dysfunctions

The following specifiers apply to Sexual Dysfunctions where indicated:

[a]*Specify* whether: Lifelong, Acquired
[b]*Specify* whether: Generalized, Situational
[c]*Specify* current severity: Mild, Moderate, Severe

F52.32	Delayed Ejaculation[a, b, c]
F52.21	Erectile Disorder[a, b, c]
F52.31	Female Orgasmic Disorder[a, b, c] *Specify* if: Never experienced an orgasm under any situation
F52.22	Female Sexual Interest/Arousal Disorder[a, b, c]
F52.6	Genito-Pelvic Pain/Penetration Disorder[a, c]
F52.0	Male Hypoactive Sexual Desire Disorder[a, b, c]
F52.4	Premature (Early) Ejaculation[a, b, c]
	Substance/Medication-Induced Sexual Dysfunction[c] **Note:** See the criteria set and corresponding recording procedures for substance-specific codes and ICD-10-CM coding. *Specify* if: With onset during intoxication, With onset during withdrawal, With onset after medication use
F52.8	Other Specified Sexual Dysfunction
F52.9	Unspecified Sexual Dysfunction

Gender Dysphoria

	Gender Dysphoria
F64.2	Gender Dysphoria in Children *Specify* if: With a disorder of sex development
F64.1	Gender Dysphoria in Adolescents and Adults *Specify* if: With a disorder of sex development *Specify* if: Post-transition **Note:** Code the disorder of sex development if present, in addition to gender dysphoria.
F64.8	Other Specified Gender Dysphoria
64.9	Unspecified Gender Dysphoria

Disruptive, Impulse-Control, and Conduct Disorders

F91.3	Oppositional Defiant Disorder
	Specify current severity: Mild, Moderate, Severe
F63.81	Intermittent Explosive Disorder
	Conduct Disorder *Specify* whether:
F91.1	Childhood-onset type
F91.2	Adolescent-onset type
F91.9	Unspecified onset *Specify* if: With limited prosocial emotions *Specify* current severity: Mild, Moderate, Severe
F60.2	Antisocial Personality Disorder
F63.1	Pyromania
F63.2	Kleptomania
F91.8	Other Specified Disruptive, Impulse-Control, and Conduct Disorder
F91.9	Unspecified Disruptive, Impulse-Control, and Conduct Disorder

Substance-Related and Addictive Disorders

The following specifiers and note apply to Substance-Related and Addictive Disorders where indicated:

[a] *Specify* if: In early remission, In sustained remission
[b] *Specify* if: In a controlled environment
[c] *Specify* if: With perceptual disturbances

[d] The ICD-10-CM code indicates the comorbid presence of a moderate or severe substance use disorder, which must be present in order to apply the code for substance withdrawal.

Substance-Related Disorders

Alcohol-Related Disorders

	Alcohol Use Disorder[a, b]
	Specify current severity:
F10.10	Mild
F10.20	Moderate
F10.20	Severe
	Alcohol Intoxication
F10.129	With use disorder, mild
F10.229	With use disorder, moderate or severe
F10.929	Without use disorder
	Alcohol Withdrawal[c, d]
F10.239	Without perceptual disturbances
F10.232	With perceptual disturbances
	Other Alcohol-Induced Disorders
F10.99	Unspecified Alcohol-Related Disorder

Caffeine-Related Disorders

F15.929	Caffeine Intoxication
F15.93	Caffeine Withdrawal
	Other Caffeine-Induced Disorders
F15.99	Unspecified Caffeine-Related Disorder

Cannabis-Related Disorders

	Cannabis Use Disorder[a, b] *Specify* current severity
F12.10	Mild
F12.20	Moderate
F12.20	Severe
	Cannabis Intoxication[c]
	Without perceptual disturbances
F12.129	With use disorder, mild

F12.229	With use disorder, moderate or severe
F12.929	Without use disorder
	With perceptual disturbances
F12.122	With use disorder, mild
F12.222	With use disorder, moderate or severe
F12.922	Without use disorder
F12.288	Cannabis Withdrawal[d]
	Other Cannabis-Induced Disorders
F12.99	Unspecified Cannabis-Related Disorder

Hallucinogen-Related Disorders

	Phencyclidine Use Disorder[a, b]
	Specify current severity:
F16.10	Mild
F16.20	Moderate
F16.20	Severe
	Other Hallucinogen Use Disorder[a, b] *Specify* the particular hallucinogen *Specify* current severity:
F16.10	Mild
F16.20	Moderate
F16.20	Severe
	Phencyclidine Intoxication
F16.129	With use disorder, mild
F16.229	With use disorder, moderate or severe
F16.929	Without use disorder
	Other Hallucinogen Intoxication
F16.129	With use disorder, mild
F16.229	With use disorder, moderate or severe
F16.929	Without use disorder
F16.983	Hallucinogen Persisting Perception Disorder
	Other Phencyclidine-Induced Disorders
	Other Hallucinogen-Induced Disorders
F16.99	Unspecified Phencyclidine-Related Disorder
F16.99	Unspecified Hallucinogen-Related Disorder

Inhalant-Related Disorders

	Inhalant Use Disorder[a, b] *Specify* the particular inhalant *Specify* current severity:
F18.10	Mild
F18.20	Moderate
F18.20	Severe
	Inhalant Intoxication
F18.129	With use disorder, mild
F18.229	With use disorder, moderate or severe
F18.929	Without use disorder
	Other Inhalant-Induced Disorders
F18.99	Unspecified Inhalant-Related Disorder

Opioid-Related Disorders

	Opioid Use Disorder[a] *Specify* if: On maintenance therapy, In a controlled environment *Specify* current severity:
F11.10	Mild
F11.20	Moderate
F11.20	Severe
	Opioid Intoxication[c]
	Without perceptual disturbances
F11.129	With use disorder, mild
F11.229	With use disorder, moderate or severe
F11.922	Without use disorder
F11.23	Opioid Withdrawal[d]
	Other Opioid-Induced Disorders
F11.99	Unspecified Opioid-Related Disorder

Sedative-, Hypnotic-, or Anxiolytic-Related Disorders

	Sedative, Hypnotic, or Anxiolytic Use Disorder[a, b] *Specify* current severity:
F13.10	Mild
F13.20	Moderate
F13.20	Severe
	Sedative, Hypnotic, or Anxiolytic Intoxication

F13.129	With use disorder, mild
F13.229	With use disorder, moderate or severe
F13.929	Without use disorder
	Sedative, Hypnotic, or Anxiolytic Withdrawal[c, d]
F13.239	Without perceptual disturbances
F13.232	With perceptual disturbances
	Other Sedative-, Hypnotic-, or Anxiolytic-Induced Disorders
F13.99	Unspecified Sedative-, Hypnotic-, or Anxiolytic-Related Disorder

Stimulant-Related Disorders

	Stimulant Use Disorder[a, b] *Specify* current severity:
	Mild
F15.10	Amphetamine-type substance
F14.10	Cocaine
F15.10	Other or unspecified stimulant
	Moderate
F15.20	Amphetamine-type substance
F14.20	Cocaine
F15.20	Other or unspecified stimulant
	Severe
F15.20	Amphetamine-type substance
F14.20	Cocaine
F15.20	Other or unspecified stimulant
	Stimulant Intoxication[c] *Specify* the specific intoxicant
	Amphetamine or other stimulant, Without perceptual disturbances
F15.129	With use disorder, mild
F15.229	With use disorder, moderate or severe
F15.929	Without use disorder
	Cocaine, Without perceptual disturbances
F14.129	With use disorder, mild
F14.229	With use disorder, moderate or severe
F14.929	Without use disorder

	Amphetamine or other stimulant, With perceptual disturbances
F15.122	With use disorder, mild
F15.222	With use disorder, moderate or severe
F15.922	Without use disorder
	Cocaine, With perceptual disturbances
F14.122	With use disorder, mild
F14.222	With use disorder, moderate or severe
F14.922	Without use disorder
	Stimulant Withdrawal[d] *Specify* the specific substance causing the withdrawal syndrome
F15.23	Amphetamine or other stimulant
F14.23	Cocaine
	Other Stimulant-Induced Disorders
	Unspecified Stimulant-Related Disorder
F15.99	Amphetamine or other stimulant
F14.99	Cocaine

Tobacco-Related Disorders

	Tobacco Use Disorder[a] *Specify* if: On maintenance therapy, In a controlled environment *Specify* current severity:
Z72.0	Mild
F17.200	Moderate
F17.200	Severe
F17.203	Tobacco Withdrawal[d]
	Other Tobacco-Induced Disorders
F17.209	Unspecified Tobacco-Related Disorder

Other (or Unknown) Substance-Related Disorders

	Other (or Unknown) Substance Use Disorder[a, b] *Specify* current severity:
F19.10	Mild
F19.20	Moderate
F19.20	Severe
	Other (or Unknown) Substance Intoxication

F19.129	With use disorder, mild
F19.229	With use disorder, moderate or severe
F19.929	Without use disorder
F19.239	Other (or Unknown) Substance Withdrawal[d]
	Other (or Unknown) Substance-Induced Disorders
F19.99	Unspecified Other (or Unknown) Substance-Related Disorder

Non-Substance-Related Disorders

F63.0	Gambling Disorder[a] *Specify* if: Episodic, Persistent *Specify* current severity: Mild, Moderate, Severe

Neurocognitive Disorders

	Delirium[a] **Note:** See the criteria set and corresponding recording procedures for substance-specific codes and ICD-10-CM coding. *Specify* whether:
	Substance intoxication delirium[a]
	Substance withdrawal delirium[a]
	Medication-induced delirium[a]
F05	Delirium due to another medical condition
F05	Delirium due to multiple etiologies *Specify* if: Acute, Persistent *Specify* if: Hyperactive, Hypoactive, Mixed level of activity
R41.0	Other Specified Delirium
R41.0	Unspecified Delirium

Major and Mild Neurocognitive Disorders

Specify whether due to: Alzheimer's disease, Frontotemporal lobar degeneration, Lewy body disease, Vascular disease, Traumatic brain injury, Substance/medication use, HIV infection, Prion disease, Parkinson's disease, Huntington's disease, Another medical condition, Multiple etiologies, Unspecified

[a] *Specify* Without behavioral disturbance, With behavioral disturbance. *For possible major neurocognitive disorder and for mild neurocognitive disorder, behavioral disturbance cannot be coded but should still be indicated in writing.*

[b] *Specify* current severity: Mild, Moderate, Severe. *This specifier applies only to major neurocognitive disorders (including probable and possible).*

NOTE: As indicated for each subtype, an additional medical code is needed for probable major neurocognitive disorder or major neurocognitive disorder. An additional medical code should *not* be used for possible major neurocognitive disorder or mild neurocognitive disorder.

Major or Mild Neurocognitive Disorder Due to Alzheimer's Disease

	Probable Major Neurocognitive Disorder Due to Alzheimer's Disease[b] **Note:** Code first G30.9 Alzheimer's disease.
F02.81	With behavioral disturbance
F02.80	Without behavioral disturbance
G31.9	Possible Major Neurocognitive Disorder Due to Alzheimer's Disease[a, b]
G31.84	Mild Neurocognitive Disorder Due to Alzheimer's Disease[a]

Major or Mild Frontotemporal Neurocognitive Disorder

	Probable Major Neurocognitive Disorder Due to Frontotemporal Lobar Degeneration[b] **Note:** Code first G31.09 frontotemporal disease.
F02.81	With behavioral disturbance
F02.80	Without behavioral disturbance
G31.9	Possible Major Neurocognitive Disorder Due to Frontotemporal Lobar Degeneration[a, b]
G31.84	Mild Neurocognitive Disorder Due to Frontotemporal Lobar Degeneration[a]

Major or Mild Neurocognitive Disorder With Lewy Bodies

	Probable Major Neurocognitive Disorder With Lewy Bodies[b] **Note:** Code first G31.83 Lewy body disease.
F02.81	With behavioral disturbance
F02.80	Without behavioral disturbance
G31.9	Possible Major Neurocognitive Disorder With Lewy Bodies[a, b]
G31.84	Mild Neurocognitive Disorder With Lewy Bodies[a]

Major or Mild Vascular Neurocognitive Disorder

	Probable Major Vascular Neurocognitive Disorder[b] **Note:** No additional medical code for vascular disease.
F01.51	With behavioral disturbance
F01.50	Without behavioral disturbance
G31.9	Possible Major Vascular Neurocognitive Disorder[a, b]
G31.84	Mild Vascular Neurocognitive Disorder[a]

Major or Mild Neurocognitive Disorder Due to Traumatic Brain Injury

	Major Neurocognitive Disorder Due to Traumatic Brain Injury[b] **Note:** For ICD-9-CM, code first 907.0 late effect of intracranial injury without skull fracture. For ICD-10-CM, code first S06.2X9S diffuse traumatic brain injury with loss of consciousness of unspecified duration, sequela.
F02.81	With behavioral disturbance
F02.80	Without behavioral disturbance
G31.84	Mild Neurocognitive Disorder Due to Traumatic Brain Injury[a]

Substance/Medication-Induced Major or Mild Neurocognitive Disorder[a]

NOTE: No additional medical code. See the criteria set and corresponding recording procedures for substance-specific codes and ICD-10-CM coding.

Specify if: Persistent

Major or Mild Neurocognitive Disorder Due to HIV Infection

	Major Neurocognitive Disorder Due to HIV Infection[b] **Note:** Code first B20 HIV infection.
F02.81	With behavioral disturbance
F02.80	Without behavioral disturbance
G31.84	Mild Neurocognitive Disorder Due to HIV Infection[a]

Major or Mild Neurocognitive Disorder Due to Prion Disease

	Major Neurocognitive Disorder Due to Prion Disease[b] **Note:** Code first A81.9 prion disease.
F02.81	With behavioral disturbance
F02.80	Without behavioral disturbance
G31.84	Mild Neurocognitive Disorder Due to Prion Disease[a]

Major or Mild Neurocognitive Disorder Due to Parkinson's Disease

	Major Neurocognitive Disorder Probably Due to Parkinson's Disease[b] **Note:** Code first 332.0 (G20) Parkinson's disease.
F02.81	With behavioral disturbance
F02.80	Without behavioral disturbance
G31.9	Major Neurocognitive Disorder Possibly Due to Parkinson's Disease[a, b]
G31.84	Mild Neurocognitive Disorder Due to Parkinson's Disease[a]

Major or Mild Neurocognitive Disorder Due to Huntington's Disease

	Major Neurocognitive Disorder Due to Huntington's Disease[b] **Note:** Code first G10 Huntington's disease.
F02.81	With behavioral disturbance
F02.80	Without behavioral disturbance
G31.84	Mild Neurocognitive Disorder Due to Huntington's Disease[a]

Major or Mild Neurocognitive Disorder Due to Another Medical Condition

	Major Neurocognitive Disorder Due to Another Medical Condition[b] **Note:** Code first the other medical condition.
F02.81	With behavioral disturbance
F02.80	Without behavioral disturbance
G31.84	Mild Neurocognitive Disorder Due to Another Medical Condition[a]

Major or Mild Neurocognitive Disorder Due to Multiple Etiologies

	Major Neurocognitive Disorder Due to Multiple Etiologies[b] **Note:** Code first all the etiological medical conditions (with the exception of vascular disease).
F02.81	With behavioral disturbance
F02.80	Without behavioral disturbance
G31.84	Mild Neurocognitive Disorder Due to Multiple Etiologies[a]

Unspecified Neurocognitive Disorder

R41.9	Unspecified Neurocognitive Disorder[a]

Personality Disorders

Cluster A Personality Disorders

F60.0	Paranoid Personality Disorder
F60.1	Schizoid Personality Disorder
F21	Schizotypal Personality Disorder

Cluster B Personality Disorders

F60.2	Antisocial Personality Disorder
F60.3	Borderline Personality Disorder
F60.4	Histrionic Personality Disorder
F60.81	Narcissistic Personality Disorder

Cluster C Personality Disorders

F60.6	Avoidant Personality Disorder
F60.7	Dependent Personality Disorder
F60.5	Obsessive-Compulsive Personality Disorder

Other Personality Disorders

F07.0	Personality Change Due to Another Medical Condition *Specify* whether: Labile type, Disinhibited type, Aggressive type, Apathetic type, Paranoid type, Other type, Combined type, Unspecified type
F60.89	Other Specified Personality Disorder
F60.9	Unspecified Personality Disorder

Paraphilic Disorders

The following specifier applies to Paraphilic Disorders where indicated:

[a]*Specify* if: In a controlled environment, In full remission

F65.3	Voyeuristic Disorder[a]
F65.2	Exhibitionistic Disorder[a] *Specify* whether: Sexually aroused by exposing genitals to prepubertal children, Sexually aroused by exposing genitals to physically mature individuals, Sexually aroused by exposing genitals to prepubertal children and to physically mature individuals
F65.81	Frotteuristic Disorder[a]
F65.51	Sexual Masochism Disorder[a] *Specify* if: With asphyxiophilia
F65.52	Sexual Sadism Disorder[a]
F65.4	Pedophilic Disorder *Specify* whether: Exclusive type, Nonexclusive type *Specify* if: Sexually attracted to males, Sexually attracted to females, Sexually attracted to both *Specify* if: Limited to incest
F65.0	Fetishistic Disorder[a] *Specify*: Body part(s), Nonliving object(s), Other
F65.1	Transvestic Disorder[a] *Specify* if: With fetishism, With autogynephilia
F65.89	Other Specified Paraphilic Disorder
F65.9	Unspecified Paraphilic Disorder

Other Mental Disorders

F06.8	Other Specified Mental Disorder Due to Another Medical Condition
F09	Unspecified Mental Disorder Due to Another Medical Condition
F99	Other Specified Mental Disorder
F99	Unspecified Mental Disorder

Medication-Induced Movement Disorders and Other Adverse Effects of Medication

G21.11	Neuroleptic-Induced Parkinsonism
G21.19	Other Medication-Induced Parkinsonism
G21.0	Neuroleptic Malignant Syndrome
G24.02	Medication-Induced Acute Dystonia
G25.71	Medication-Induced Acute Akathisia
G24.01	Tardive Dyskinesia
G24.09	Tardive Dystonia
G25.71	Tardive Akathisia
G25.1	Medication-Induced Postural Tremor
G25.79	Other Medication-Induced Movement Disorder
	Antidepressant Discontinuation Syndrome
T43.205A	Initial encounter
T43.205D	Subsequent encounter
T43.205S	Sequelae
	Other Adverse Effect of Medication
T50.905A	Initial encounter
T50.905D	Subsequent encounter
T50.905S	Sequelae

Other Conditions That May Be a Focus of Clinical Attention

Relational Problems
Problems Related to Family Upbringing

Z62.820	Parent-Child Relational Problem
Z62.891	Sibling Relational Problem
Z62.29	Upbringing Away From Parents
Z62.898	Child Affected by Parental Relationship Distress

Other Problems Related to Primary Support Group

Z63.0	Relationship Distress With Spouse or Intimate Partner
Z63.5	Disruption of Family by Separation or Divorce
Z63.8	High Expressed Emotion Level Within Family
Z63.4	Uncomplicated Bereavement

Abuse and Neglect
Child Maltreatment and Neglect Problems
Child Physical Abuse, Confirmed

T74.12XA	Initial encounter
T74.12XD	Subsequent encounter

Child Physical Abuse, Suspected

T76.12XA	Initial encounter
T76.12XD	Subsequent encounter

Other Circumstances Related to Child Physical Abuse

Z69.010	Encounter for mental health services for victim of child abuse by parent
Z69.020	Encounter for mental health services for victim of nonparental child abuse
Z62.810	Personal history (past history) of physical abuse in childhood
Z69.011	Encounter for mental health services for perpetrator of parental child abuse
Z69.021	Encounter for mental health services for perpetrator of nonparental child abuse

Child Sexual Abuse, Confirmed

T74.22XA	Initial encounter
T74.22XD	Subsequent encounter

Child Sexual Abuse, Suspected

T76.22XA	Initial encounter
T76.22XD	Subsequent encounter

Other Circumstances Related to Child Sexual Abuse

Z69.010	Encounter for mental health services for victim of child sexual abuse by parent
Z69.020	Encounter for mental health services for victim of nonparental child sexual abuse
Z62.810	Personal history (past history) of sexual abuse in childhood
Z69.011	Encounter for mental health services for perpetrator of parental child sexual abuse
Z69.021	Encounter for mental health services for perpetrator of nonparental child sexual abuse

Child Neglect, Confirmed

T74.02XA	Initial encounter
T74.02XD	Subsequent encounter

Child Neglect, Suspected

T76.02XA	Initial encounter
T76.02XD	Subsequent encounter

Other Circumstances Related to Child Neglect

Z69.010	Encounter for mental health services for victim of child neglect by parent
Z69.020	Encounter for mental health services for victim of nonparental child neglect
Z62.812	Personal history (past history) of neglect in childhood
Z69.011	Encounter for mental health services for perpetrator of parental child neglect
Z69.021	Encounter for mental health services for perpetrator of nonparental child neglect

Child Psychological Abuse, Confirmed

T74.32XA	Initial encounter
T74.32XD	Subsequent encounter

Child Psychological Abuse, Suspected

T76.32XA	Initial encounter
T76.32XD	Subsequent encounter

Other Circumstances Related to Child Psychological Abuse

Z69.010	Encounter for mental health services for victim of child psychological abuse by parent
Z69.020	Encounter for mental health services for victim of nonparental child psychological abuse
Z62.811	Personal history (past history) of psychological abuse in childhood
Z69.011	Encounter for mental health services for perpetrator of parental child psychological abuse
Z69.021	Encounter for mental health services for perpetrator of nonparental child psychological abuse

Adult Maltreatment and Neglect Problems

Spouse or Partner Violence, Physical, Confirmed

T74.11XA	Initial encounter
T74.11XD	Subsequent encounter

Spouse or Partner Violence, Physical, Suspected

T76.11XA	Initial encounter
T76.11XD	Subsequent encounter

Other Circumstances Related to Spouse or Partner Violence, Physical

Z69.11	Encounter for mental health services for victim of spouse or partner violence, physical
Z91.410	Personal history (past history) of spouse or partner violence, physical
Z69.12	Encounter for mental health services for perpetrator of spouse or partner violence, physical

Spouse or Partner Violence, Sexual, Confirmed

T74.21XA	Initial encounter
T74.21XD	Subsequent encounter

Spouse or Partner Violence, Sexual, Suspected

T76.21XA	Initial encounter
T76.21XD	Subsequent encounter

Other Circumstances Related to Spouse or Partner Violence, Sexual

Z69.81	Encounter for mental health services for victim of spouse or partner violence, sexual
Z91.410	Personal history (past history) of spouse or partner violence, sexual
Z69.12	Encounter for mental health services for perpetrator of spouse or partner violence, sexual

Spouse or Partner Neglect, Confirmed

T74.01XA	Initial encounter
T74.01XD	Subsequent encounter

Spouse or Partner Neglect, Suspected

T76.01XA	Initial encounter
T76.01XD	Subsequent encounter

Other Circumstances Related to Spouse or Partner Neglect

Z69.11	Encounter for mental health services for victim of spouse or partner neglect
Z91.412	Personal history (past history) of spouse or partner neglect
Z69.12	Encounter for mental health services for perpetrator of spouse or partner neglect

Spouse or Partner Abuse, Psychological, Confirmed

T74.31XA	Initial encounter
T74.31XD	Subsequent encounter

Spouse or Partner Abuse, Psychological, Suspected

T76.31XA	Initial encounter
T76.31XD	Subsequent encounter

Other Circumstances Related to Spouse or Partner Abuse, Psychological

Z69.11	Encounter for mental health services for victim of spouse or partner psychological abuse
Z91.411	Personal history (past history) of spouse or partner psychological abuse
Z69.12	Encounter for mental health services for perpetrator of spouse or partner psychological abuse

Adult Physical Abuse by Nonspouse or Nonpartner, Confirmed

T74.11XA	Initial encounter
T74.11XD	Subsequent encounter

Adult Physical Abuse by Nonspouse or Nonpartner, Suspected

T76.11XA	Initial encounter
T76.11XD	Subsequent encounter

Adult Sexual Abuse by Nonspouse or Nonpartner, Confirmed

T74.21XA	Initial encounter
T74.21XD	Subsequent encounter

Adult Sexual Abuse by Nonspouse or Nonpartner, Suspected

T76.21XA	Initial encounter
T76.21XD	Subsequent encounter

Adult Psychological Abuse by Nonspouse or Nonpartner, Confirmed

T74.31XA	Initial encounter
T74.31XD	Subsequent encounter

Adult Psychological Abuse by Nonspouse or Nonpartner, Suspected

T76.31XA	Initial encounter
T76.31XD	Subsequent encounter

Other Circumstances Related to Adult Abuse by Nonspouse or Nonpartner

Z69.81	Encounter for mental health services for victim of nonspousal adult abuse
Z69.82	Encounter for mental health services for perpetrator of nonspousal adult abuse

Educational and Occupational Problems
Educational Problems

Z55.9	Academic or Educational Problem

Occupational Problems

Z56.82	Problem Related to Current Military Deployment Status
Z56.9	Other Problem Related to Employment

Housing and Economic Problems
Housing Problems

Z59.0	Homelessness
Z59.1	Inadequate Housing
Z59.2	Discord With Neighbor, Lodger, or Landlord
Z59.3	Problem Related to Living in a Residential Institution

Economic Problems

Z59.4	Lack of Adequate Food or Safe Drinking Water
Z59.5	Extreme Poverty
Z59.6	Low Income
Z59.7	Insufficient Social Insurance or Welfare Support
Z59.9	Unspecified Housing or Economic Problem

Other Problems Related to the Social Environment

Z60.0	Phase of Life Problem
Z60.2	Problem Related to Living Alone
Z60.3	Acculturation Difficulty
Z60.4	Social Exclusion or Rejection
Z60.5	Target of (Perceived) Adverse Discrimination or Persecution
Z60.9	Unspecified Problem Related to Social Environment

Problems Related to Crime or Interaction With the Legal System

Z65.4	Victim of Crime
Z65.0	Conviction in Civil or Criminal Proceedings Without Imprisonment

Z65.1	Imprisonment or Other Incarceration
Z65.2	Problems Related to Release From Prison
Z65.3	Problems Related to Other Legal Circumstances

Other Health Service Encounters for Counseling and Medical Advice

Z70.9	Sex Counseling
Z71.9	Other Counseling or Consultation

Problems Related to Other Psychosocial, Personal, and Environmental Circumstances

Z65.8	Religious or Spiritual Problem
Z64.0	Problems Related to Unwanted Pregnancy
Z64.1	Problems Related to Multiparity
Z64.4	Discord With Social Service Provider, Including Probation Officer, Case Manager, or Social Services Worker
Z65.4	Victim of Terrorism or Torture
Z65.5	Exposure to Disaster, War, or Other Hostilities
Z65.8	Other Problem Related to Psychosocial Circumstances
Z65.9	Unspecified Problem Related to Unspecified Psychosocial Circumstances

Other Circumstances of Personal History

Z91.49	Other Personal History of Psychological Trauma
Z91.5	Personal History of Self-Harm
Z91.82	Personal History of Military Deployment
Z91.89	Other Personal Risk Factors
Z72.9	Problem Related to Lifestyle
Z72.811	Adult Antisocial Behavior
Z72.810	Child or Adolescent Antisocial Behavior

Problems Related to Access to Medical and Other Healthcare

Z75.3	Unavailability or Inaccessibility of Health-care Facilities
Z75.4	Unavailability or Inaccessibility of Other Helping Agencies

Nonadherence to Medical Treatment

Z91.19	Nonadherence to Medical Treatment
E66.9	Overweight or Obesity
Z76.5	Malingering
Z91.83	Wandering Associated With a Mental Disorder
R41.83	Borderline Intellectual Functioning

Index

References followed by the letter "f" are for figures, "t" are tables, and "b" are boxes.

A

Q